# Nursing Diagnosis Index

# Nursing Diagnosis

## Application to Clinical Practice

# Nursing Diagnosis

## Application to Clinical Practice

**LYNDA JUALL CARPENITO-MOYET,** RN, MSN, CRNP

**Family Nurse Practitioner**
ChesPenn Health Services
Chester, Pennsylvania

**Nursing Consultant**
Mullica Hill, New Jersey

Wolters Kluwer | Lippincott Williams & Wilkins
Health

Philadelphia · Baltimore · New York · London
Buenos Aires · Hong Kong · Sydney · Tokyo

*Acquisitions Editor:* Jean Rodenberger
*Product Manager:* Michelle Clarke
*Director of Nursing Production:* Helen Ewan
*Vendor Manager:* Cynthia Rudy
*Art Director, Design:* Joan Wendt
*Art Director, Illustration:* Brett MacNaughton
*Manufacturing Coordinator:* Karin Duffield
*Compositor:* Cadmus

Printed in China

13th Edition

ISBN 13: 978-0-7817-7792-6
Library of Congress Cataloging-in-Publication Data Available on Request

Care has been taken to confirm the accuracy of the information presented and to describe generally accepted practices. However, the authors, editors, and publisher are not responsible for errors or omissions or for any consequences from application of the information in this book and make no warranty, expressed or implied, with respect to the currency, completeness, or accuracy of the contents of the publication. Application of this information in a particular situation remains the professional responsibility of the practitioner; the clinical treatments described and recommended may not be considered absolute and universal recommendations.

The authors, editors, and publisher have exerted every effort to ensure that drug selection and dosage set forth in this text are in accordance with the current recommendations and practice at the time of publication. However, in view of ongoing research, changes in government regulations, and the constant flow of information relating to drug therapy and drug reactions, the reader is urged to check the package insert for each drug for any change in indications and dosage and for added warnings and precautions. This is particularly important when the recommended agent is a new or infrequently employed drug.

Some drugs and medical devices presented in this publication have Food and Drug Administration (FDA) clearance for limited use in restricted research settings. It is the responsibility of the health care provider to ascertain the FDA status of each drug or device planned for use in his or her clinical practice.

LWW.COM

Nursing Diagnosis - Definitions and Classifications 2009–2011 @ 2009, 2007, 2005, 2003, 2001, 1998, 1996, 1994 NANDA International. Used by arrangement with Wiley-Blackwell Publishing, a company of John Wiley & Sons, Inc. In order to make safe and effective judgments using NANDA-I nursing diagnoses it is essential that nurses refer to the definitions and defining characteristics of the diagnoses listed in this work.

# To My Earth Angels

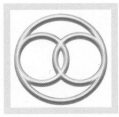

In the eighth edition of this book, I introduced the reader to Earth angels. The dictionary defines "angel" as a "spiritual being . . . an attendant spirit or guardian . . . one who aids or supports." Earth angels can be friends, strangers, adults, or children. Most often, the Earth angel does not even know the profound effects of the angelic encounter.

These Earth angels were always there, giving me permission to be imperfect, to grieve, and to heal. These Earth angels—Ginny, Donna, Heather, Tere, and Tracey—continue to not be afraid of my grief, my anger, or riding the emotional roller-coaster with me, their wings flapping in the wind. Thank you Earth angels, friends and strangers.

> *Para mi Jorge*
> Man meets woman
> Woman wants to run like a rabbit
> She has had her share of sorrow
> But she waits
> She realizes the man has had his share of sorrow too.
> So they both wait,
> And learn to trust and love again.
>
> *Gracias, mi esposo*
> Jorge Luis Moyet-Gonzalez

On July 7, 2006, my husband Jorge died suddenly. I will pass on the gifts he gave to me, protecting the vulnerable, forgiving wrongs, and that love is patient. Te amo Jorge.

# Current Contributors

**Virginia Arcangelo, RN, MSN, PhD**
Family Nurse Practitioner
Private Practice
Berlin, New Jersey
(Risk for Complications of Medication Adverse Events)

**Susan Bohnenkaup, RN, MSN, CNS, BC, CCM**
Clinical Nurse Specialist
University Medical Center
Tucson, Arizona
(Impaired Oral Mucous Membrane)

**Tere Bryant, PT, MBA**
Physical Therapist
Private Practice
Tucson, Arizona
(Impaired Physical Mobility, Self-Care Deficit)

**Jeanne Fenn, RN, BC, MEd, CDE**
Clinical nurse educator
University Medical Center
Tucson, Arizona
(Pediatric Pain)

**Gloria J. Gdovin, RN, MSN, CCRN**
Clinical Nurse Educator, Critical Care
Carondelet Health Network
St. Joseph's Hospital
Tucson, Arizona
(All Collaborative Problems except Reproductive and Medication Adverse Events)

**Pauline Green, PhD, RN**
Professor
Howard University
Washington, D.C.
(Contamination)

**Donna Jarzya, MS, APRN-BC**
Acute Pain Clinical Specialist
University Medical Center
Tucson, Arizona
(Altered Comfort, Acute Pain, Chronic Pain)

**Gabrielle Anne Jurecky, RN, MSN**
Staff Nurse III
University Medical Center
Tucson, Arizona
(Pediatric Pain)

**Debra L. Luisi, RN, MSN**
Cardiac Surgical Nurse
St. Luke's Hospital

Bethlehem, Pennsylvania
(Risk for Imbalanced Body [section], Imbalanced Nutrition [section], Ineffective Protection [section], Impaired Urinary Elimination)

**Laura V. Polk, DNSc, RN**
Associate Professor
College of Southern Maryland
La Plata, Maryland
(Contamination)

**Linda Rankin, RN,BS, MJ**
NICU Clinical Specialist
Carondelet Saint Joseph's Hospital
Tucson, Arizona
(Ineffective Thermoregulation, Ineffective Infant Feeding Pattern, Disorganized Infant Behavior)

**Michael Ryan, RN, MS, MAHCT**
Administrator
Heartland Hospice
Tucson, Arizona
(Grieving, Spiritual Distress, Impaired Religiosity)

**Tracy A. Schreiner, RN, MSN, MBA**
President, Schreiner Consulting
Adjunct Faculty
Grand Canyon University
Phoenix, Arizona
Chamberlain College of Nursing
Addison, Illinois
Phoenix, Arizona
(Risk for Imbalanced Body [section], Imbalanced Nutrition [section], Ineffective Protection [section], Impaired Urinary Elimination)

**Ann Sprengel, RN, EdD**
Professor
Southeast Missouri University
Cape Girardeau, Missouri
(Hopelessness, Powerlessness)

**Janet Weber, RN, EdD**
Professor
Southeast Missouri University
Cape Girardeau, Missouri
(Hopelessness, Powerlessness)

**Teresa Wilson**
OB Clinical Nurse Educator
Carondelet Health Network
Tucson, Arizona
(Reproductive Collaborative Problems, Hyperbilirubinemia, Ineffective Breastfeeding)

## Past Contributors

**Rosalinda Alfaro-LeFevre, RN, MSN,** President, Teaching Smart/Learning Easy, Stuart, Florida
(Risk for Ineffective Respiratory Function; Ineffective Airway Clearance; Ineffective Breathing Patterns; Deficient Diversional Activity; Impaired Verbal Communication; Deficient Fluid Volume; Excess Fluid Volume; Risk for Imbalanced Body Temperature; Hyperthermia and Hypothermia)

**Ann H. Barnhouse, RN, MSN,** Nurse Educator, Hudson, Ohio
(Relocation Stress)

**Christine J. Brugler, RN, MSN,** Private Practice, Warren, Ohio
(Relocation Stress)

**Margaret Edwards, RN, MSN, CAN BC,** Director, Behavioral Health, Carondelet Health Network, Tucson, Arizona
(Co-authored with Lori Minus: Anxiety, Ineffective Coping, Post-Trauma Syndrome, Disturbed Self-Concept, Risk for Self-Harm, Disturbed Sensory Perception, Disturbed Thought Processes, Risk for Violence [12th ed.])

**Joan T. Harkulich, RN, MSN,** Director of Research and Professional Services, Care Services, Beachwood, Ohio
(Relocation Stress)

**Lori Minus, BSN, RN-C,** Manager, Behavior Health Services, Carondelet Health Network, St. Mary's Hospital, Tucson, Arizona
(Co-authored with Margaret Edwards: Anxiety, Ineffective Coping, Post-Trauma Syndrome, Disturbed Self-Concept, Risk for Self-Harm, Disturbed Sensory Perception, Disturbed Thought Processes, Risk for Violence [12th ed.])

**John M. Dugan, RN, BSN,** Manager, Intensive Care, Carondelet Health Network, St. Joseph's Hospital, Tucson, Arizona
(Collaborative Problems except Reproductive [12th ed.])

## Reviewers

**Anita G. Kinser, EdD, RN-BC**
Associate Professor, Nursing/Nursing Education Resource Specialist
School of Nursing
Riverside Community College
Riverside, CA

**Brenda Morris, EdD, MS, BSN, RN**
Baccalaureate Program Director and Clinical Associate Professor of Nursing
College of Nursing & Healthcare Innovation
Arizona State University
Phoenix, AZ

**Laura B. Patton, BSN, MN, RN**
Professor
School of Nursing
Gordon College
Barnesville,GA

**Hazel L. Ruff, MS, APRN-BC, FNP**
Instructor
School of Nursing
Norfolk State University
Norfolk, VA

**Marcia Stevens, RN, MEd, DNSc**
Professor
School of Nursing
Minnesota State University, Mankato
Mankato, MN

# Preface

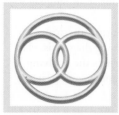

Rapid change continues to occur in health care and in the nursing profession. Hospitals continue to try to increase their nursing staffs, while the acuity of clients continues to rise. Many nurses, and even some faculty, question the usefulness of nursing diagnosis. Unfortunately, nursing diagnosis is still joined at the hip with traditional care planning. It is time to separate these Siamese twins so that both can function separately. Nursing diagnosis defines the science and art of nursing. It is as imperative to nursing as medical diagnoses are to physicians. It serves to organize nursing's knowledge in the literature, in research, and in the clinician's mind. Do not underestimate the importance of this classification. A clinician with expertise with nursing diagnoses can hypothesize several explanations for a client's anger, such as fear, anxiety, powerlessness, or spiritual distress. Without this knowledge, the client is simply angry.

Care planning as it is taught in schools of nursing is an academic exercise. This is not wrong, but as the student progresses into the senior year, this academic care plan must be transformed into a clinically useful product. Nursing diagnosis must be presented as clinically useful. Nurses who are expert in certain nursing diagnoses should be consulted, just as our medical colleagues consult other physicians for their expertise. Health care facilities should publish a list of nursing experts in their facility for consultation. Faculty, nurse managers, administrators, and clinicians need to do their part. Change is imperative. The documentation requirements are unrealistic. There is little time to think and analyze with these documentation mandates. Nursing must defend its right to determine its documentation requirements just as medicine has.

If nursing continues to do business as usual, nursing as we want it—nursing as clients need it—will cease to exist. Nursing will continue to be defined by what we do and write and not by what we know. From assessment criteria to specific interventions, the book focuses on nursing. It provides a condensed, organized outline of clinical nursing practice designed to communicate creative clinical nursing. It is not meant to replace textbooks of nursing, but rather to provide nurses in a variety of settings with the information they need without requiring a time-consuming review of the literature. It will assist students in transferring their theoretical knowledge to clinical practice; it can also be used by experienced nurses to recall past learning and to intervene in those clinical situations that previously went ignored or unrecognized.

The author agrees that nursing needs a classification system to organize its functions and define its scope. Use of such a classification system would expedite research activities and facilitate communication between nurses, consumers, and other health care providers. After all, medicine took over 100 years to develop its taxonomy. Our work, at the national level, only began in 1973. It is hoped that the reader will be stimulated to participate at the local, regional, or national level in the utilization and development of these diagnoses.

Since the first edition was published, the use of nursing diagnosis has increased markedly throughout the United States, Canada, and internationally. Practicing nurses vary in experience with nursing diagnosis from just beginning to full practice integration for over 30 years. With such a variance in use, questions posed by the neophyte, such as:

- What does the label really mean?
- What kinds of assessment questions will yield nursing diagnoses?
- How do I differentiate one diagnosis from another?
- How do I tailor a diagnosis for a specific individual?
- How should I intervene after I formulate the diagnostic statement?
- How do I care-plan with nursing diagnoses?

These questions differ dramatically from such questions from experts as:

- Should nursing diagnoses represent the only diagnoses on the nursing care plan?
- Can medical diagnoses be included in a nursing diagnosis statement?
- What are the ethical issues in using nursing diagnoses?
- What kind of problem statement should I write to describe a person at risk for hemorrhage?
- How can I efficiently use nursing diagnosis?

- What kind of nursing diagnosis should I use to describe a healthy person?
- Do I need nursing diagnoses with critical pathways?

This 13th edition of *Nursing Diagnosis: Application to Clinical Practice* seeks to continue to answer these questions.

In Section One, Chapter 1 addresses issues and controversies. It explores arguments regarding the ethics and cultural implications of nursing diagnoses. It discusses the implications of a consistent language for nurses as members of a multidisciplinary team.

Chapter 2 focuses on the development of nursing diagnosis and the work of the North American Nursing Diagnosis Association (NANDA). The chapter explores the concepts of nursing diagnosis, classification, and taxonomic issues. It discusses the review process of NANDA and describes the evolving taxonomy of NANDA. Chapter 2 also covers the use of non–NANDA-approved diagnoses and practice dilemmas associated with nursing diagnoses.

Chapter 3 differentiates among actual, risk, and possible nursing diagnoses. It also presents a discussion of wellness and syndrome diagnoses. It outlines guidelines for writing diagnostic statements and avoiding errors.

Chapter 4 describes the Bifocal Clinical Practice Model. This chapter includes a more detailed discussion of nursing diagnoses and collaborative problems, covering their relationship to assessment, goals, interventions, and evaluation.

Chapter 5 describes the process of care planning and discusses various care planning systems. Topics covered include priority identification, nursing goals versus client goals, case management and nursing accountability. The chapter differentiates interventions for nursing diagnoses and collaborative problems. It also clarifies evaluation, distinguishing evaluation of nursing care from evaluation of the client's condition. It presents a discussion of multidisciplinary care, along with a three-tiered care planning system aimed at increasing the clinical use of care plans without increasing writing. Samples of nursing records appear throughout the chapter.

Section Two is organized into four parts:

Part One: Individual Nursing Diagnoses
Part Two: Family/Home Nursing Diagnoses
Part Three: Community Nursing Diagnoses
Part Four: Health Promotion and Wellness Nursing Diagnoses

Each part includes an introduction, assessment for specific population, key concepts, author's notes, and specific diagnoses for the population. Diagnoses are discussed under the following subheads:

- Definition
- Defining Characteristics or Risk Factors
- Related Factors
- Author's Notes
- Errors in Diagnostic Statements
- Maternal Considerations
- Pediatric Considerations
- Geriatric Considerations
- Transcultural Considerations

Author's Notes and Errors in Diagnostic Statements are designed to help the nurse understand the concept behind the diagnosis, differentiate one diagnosis from another, and avoid diagnostic errors. Maternal, Pediatric, and Geriatric Considerations for all relevant diagnoses provide additional pertinent information. Transcultural Considerations strive to increase the reader's sensitivity to cultural diversity without stereotyping.

Each nursing diagnosis is addressed with generic interventions and rationale. If applicable, Maternal, Pediatric, and Geriatric focus interventions and rationale are included. Each nursing diagnosis is then followed by one or more specific nursing diagnoses that relate to familiar clinical situations. Goals for the diagnosis are provided with the related interventions, which represent activities in the independent domain of nursing derived from the physical and applied sciences, pharmacology, nutrition, mental health, and nursing research.

Each nursing diagnosis has NIC major intervention categories and NOC outcome categories. This inclusion was to assist those in the development of electronic care planning. The goals, indicators, and interventions are the work of this author, not NIC or NOC.

Every attempt has been made to provide the reader with the most recent literature and research findings on the subject. Frequently, students are instructed not to use references over 5 years old. This can be problematic. however, as at times an original paper or research on a topic remains, even 10 years later, the state of science on that topic. If a subsequent author or researcher uses the original work, often his or her citation is substituted for the older one. I disagree with this practice; both citations should be listed. Therefore, throughout this book, the reader will find citations of various ages and many older than 5 years. Web site addresses for diagnoses have been added for the nurse and consumer.

Section Three consists of a Manual of Collaborative Problems. In this section, each of the nine generic collaborative problems is explained under the following subheads:

- Physiologic Overview
- Definition
- Diagnostic Considerations
- Focus Assessment Criteria
- Significant Laboratory Assessment Criteria

Discussed under their appropriate problems are 52 specific collaborative problems, covering:

- Definition
- High-Risk Populations
- Nursing Goals
- Interventions

The author invites comments or suggestions from readers. Correspondence can be directed to the publisher or to the author: e-mail Juall46@msn.com

*Lynda Juall Carpenito-Moyet,* RN, MSN, CRNP

# Acknowledgments

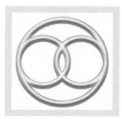

This 13th edition was made possible with the intensive help of Michelle Clarke and Jean Rodenberger, my editors at Lippincott Williams & Wilkins. A special thank you to my daughter-in-law Heather, for all her assistance with manuscript preparation. God did not give me a daughter, but gave me a very special daughter-in-law. Thank you, Heather.

This edition would not have been possible without the patience, kindness, and expertise of Michelle Clarke. The winds behind my sails were Donna Zazworsky, Ginny Arcangelo, Heather Carpenito, Tracey Shriner, Tere Bryant, and my brother Gene—I love you all.

The support for this book continues nationally and internationally. It has been translated into 11 languages.

Finally, I would like to thank the group in Detroit (Jo Ann Maklebust, Mary Sieggreen, and Linda Mondoux) for their moral support while I wrote the first edition. Rosalinda Alfaro-LeFevre recognized the need for this book in 1983 and sought me out to make it a reality.

On a personal level, my son Olen Juall Carpenito and his wife Heather have given me two special gifts—my grandsons Olen, Jr. and Aiden. They light up my world.

# Contents

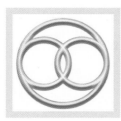

# SECTION 3

## Manual of Collaborative Problems   843

### Introduction   843

# The Focus of Nursing Care

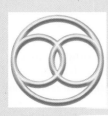

## Introduction

*Nursing is primarily assisting individuals (sick or well) with those activities contributing to health or its recovery (or to a peaceful death) that they perform unaided when they have the necessary strength, will, or knowledge; nursing also helps individuals carry out prescribed therapy and to be independent of assistance as soon as possible\* (Henderson & Nite, 1960).*

All of us are constantly responding and interacting with outside events, things, and other persons. We are also responding to what is occurring in our mind, spirit, and body. We are in a constant state interactions and reactions.

Our *health* is a dynamic, ever-changing state influenced by past and present interaction patterns. It is the state of wellness as the individual defines it; it is no longer defined as the presence of a biologic disease.

- When we seek advice or care about our health, we can choose to accept it or not accept it.
- We define our own health.
- We are responsible for our health.
- We make choices—some healthy, some not.

Societal health needs have changed in the last few decades; so must the nurse's view of the consumers of health care as individuals, families, or communities. An *individual* becomes a client not only when an actual or potential problem compromises health but also when he or she desires assistance to achieve a higher level of health. The use of *client* in place of *patient* to identify the health care consumer suggests an autonomous person who has freedom of choice in seeking and selecting assistance. *Family* is used to describe any persons who serve as support systems to the client. *Community* is used to describe support systems, geographical locations (e.g., sections of a city as well as groups, such as senior citizen centers).

The definition of nursing cited earlier, now almost 50 years old, is as relevant today as it was then. The services of the art and science of nursing are needed when an individual's strength, will or, knowledge are insufficient for them to participate in activities contributing to their health, recovery, or peaceful death. Nurses enable clients, families, and communities to carry out their chosen therapies and to be independent of our assistance as soon as possible.

---

\*We as clients are active participants who assume responsibility for our choices.

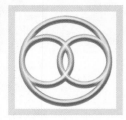

# 1

# NURSING DIAGNOSES: ISSUES AND CONTROVERSIES

**Learning Objectives**

After reading the chapter, the student should be able to answer the following questions:

- Why can't we just use the words we have always used?
- Are care plans a waste of time?
- Will other disciplines understand our language?
- Will clients understand our language?
- Are nursing diagnoses culturally sensitive?
- Is it unethical to not label client behaviors?
- Does the use of nursing diagnoses violate client confidentiality?

Nursing diagnosis arouses some emotion in almost every nurse. Responses range from apathy to excitement, from rejection to enthusiasm for scientific investigation. Although nursing diagnoses have been an accepted part of professional nursing practice for more than 25 years, some nurses continue to resist using them. This chapter explores some of the most commonly cited reasons.

## Why Can't We Just Use the Words We've Always Used?

What words have nurses always used? Diabetes mellitus? Prematurity? Pneumonia? Difficult? Cystic fibrosis? For many years, nurses used only medical diagnoses to describe the client problems that they addressed. Gradually, however, nurses have learned that medical diagnoses do not describe many client problems in sufficient detail to enable other nurses to provide continuing care for clients with special needs.

The fact is that nurses always have shared with other disciplines, such as medicine, respiratory therapy, and physical therapy, a common language for certain client problems. Examples of terms from this language include *hypokalemia*, *hypovolemic shock*, *hyperglycemia*, and *increased intracranial pressure*. Any attempt to rename labels such as these should be viewed as foolhardy and unnecessary. For instance, *dysrhythmias* should not be renamed *decreased cardiac output*, nor should *hyperglycemia* be relabeled as *altered carbohydrate metabolism*.

This author takes the position that nurses should use pre-established terminology when appropriate, whether as a collaborative problem (e.g., *Risk for Complications of Hyperglycemia*) or as a nursing diagnosis (e.g., *Risk for Pressure Ulcer*). Nursing should continue to use the terminology that clearly communicates a client situation or problem to other nurses and other disciplines.

Having said this, let us now examine the discipline-specific language of nurses. Have nurses had a common language or set of labels for client problems that they diagnose and treat in addition to the shared language previously discussed? Before the advent of nursing diagnoses, how did nurses describe client problems such as:

- Inability to dress self
- Difficulty selecting among treatment options
- Risk for infection
- Breastfeeding problems
- Ineffective cough
- Spiritual dilemmas

Sometimes a nurse would use the terms listed above, but sometimes not. Often the nurse had many options available to describe a problem. For example, a nurse could use any of the following terms to describe a client at risk for pressure ulcers:

- Immobility
- Comatose
- Decubitus ulcers

- Reddened skin
- Incontinence
- Inability to turn in bed
- Bed sores
- Paralysis

An examination of this list reveals the inconsistency of the terms. Some are signs and symptoms. Some are causative factors. Some are risk factors. Some are problems.

Some nurses, particularly those with much experience, want to be able to describe client problems in any way they wish. Although an experienced nurse may be able to decipher inconsistent terminology, how can the nursing profession teach its science to its students if each instructor, textbook, and staff nurse uses different words to describe the same situation? Consider medicine: How could medical students learn the difference between cirrhosis and cancer of the liver if "impaired liver function" was used to describe both situations? Medicine relies on a standardized classification system to teach its science and to communicate client problems to other disciplines. Nursing needs to do likewise.

So, although nurses traditionally have had a common language for certain problems, this language has been incomplete to describe all the client responses that nurses diagnose and treat. It also is important to emphasize that some responses labeled as nursing diagnoses (e.g., *Decisional Conflict*, *Powerlessness*) were nonexistent in the nursing literature as recently as 15 years ago. The official classification of these responses as nursing diagnoses has advanced their investigation and increased their presence in the nursing literature. For example, in 1982 there were two citations in the literature on powerlessness; the number increased to 113 by 1994 and there were over 500 by 2008.

## Care Plans Are a Waste of Time

Students are often told by practicing nurses that the care plans they write or type are not useful in clinical nursing. It is important to distinguish between care plans of students and care plans in practice.

Students create care plans to assist them in problem solving and to prioritize and individualize their care for a client. Student care plans are directions for a student with a particular client. The majority of these care plans are standard or expected care for a particular problem or situation. After caring for a client, the student can then revise the plan with additions or deletions. As the student progresses in the program, these plans should be more concise with less basic, standard care.

This type of care plan is not necessary in clinical practice. Predictive standard care should be known by experienced nurses on a unit. For example, if a surgical nurse is unfamiliar with the care needed for a person post-hip replacement, he or she should have access to the care plan for the specific postoperative situation in a reference or online.

#### ◀◀ Carp's Cues
The only time a nurse should create a care plan for another nurse to follow is when it is necessary to alert that nurse to additional care that is needed beyond the standard. The system should be easy to use to encourage these additions.

## Other Disciplines Will Not Understand Our Diagnoses

According to Seahill (1991), the use of nursing diagnosis in a multidisciplinary inpatient child psychiatry setting proved problematic because this setting emphasized the "whole patient" and the importance of effective information sharing among disciplines. Let us examine the validity of this assertion. For the purposes of this discussion, health care disciplines are separated into three groups: medicine, licensed health care disciplines, and nonlicensed health care personnel.

### Medicine

Because it is important for nurses to understand certain aspects of medical diagnoses, nurses have committed to learning them and to be knowledgeable about current changes in conditions and treatments. But as physicians originally defined these conditions, how often did they say, "Do you think that nurses will understand (for example) disseminated intravascular coagulation?" Most likely never.

If it is important for a physician to understand such nursing diagnoses as *Spiritual Distress* or *Decisional Conflict*, then the physician can seek the pertinent knowledge as a nurse does. The nurse also should share information with the physician concerning nursing diagnoses that the client and nurse have identified as priorities. Multidisciplinary conferences provide an opportunity for this sharing. Some nursing diagnoses may prove useful to some physicians, such as those in primary care.

## Licensed Health Care Disciplines

In addition to nursing, licensed health care disciplines include physical, occupational, speech, nutritional, respiratory, and recreational therapies and social service. Each of these disciplines is involved in care planning for clients—some in their individual departments and some as part of multidisciplinary teams. These disciplines should be introduced to the language of nursing diagnosis and encouraged to use any applicable diagnoses. Box 1.1 lists examples of nursing diagnoses that are often useful to other disciplines. Sharing nursing diagnosis terminology with other disciplines can only strengthen the role of nursing and emphasize a multidisciplinary approach. Keep in mind, however, that other disciplines should not use nursing diagnoses to determine interventions that nurses should perform. For example, a physical therapist using the nursing diagnosis *Impaired Physical Mobility* will write interventions only for physical therapy, not for nursing. Refer to Chapter 5 for a discussion of multidisciplinary care planning.

## Nonlicensed Health Care Personnel

In most acute, long-term, and community health care settings in the United States and Canada, registered nurses, licensed practical nurses, and registered nurse assistants, nursing aides, or technicians provide nursing care. It is not important that all nursing team members understand nursing diagnoses, but it is important for each team member to understand the interventions for which he or she is responsible. For example, an aide may be expected to explain why a client needs to be repositioned every 2 h and given assistance to the bathroom after eating, but may not be expected to explain the difference between functional and total incontinence.

## Clients Will Not Understand Our Diagnoses

It is important for the client and family to understand and agree with nursing diagnoses and the associated goals and interventions. The nurse should emphasize to the client and family that nursing diagnosis terminology is designed primarily to give nurses consistent language for communicating this information. The nurse also can explain why a medical diagnosis does not describe the client's problems or concerns

---

**BOX 1.1 EXAMPLES OF NURSING DIAGNOSES USEFUL FOR OTHER DISCIPLINES**

**Physical Therapy**
*Self-Care Deficit*
*High Risk for Injury*
*Impaired Physical Mobility*
*Noncompliance*
*Unilateral Neglect*
*Fatigue*

**Occupational Therapy**
*Deficient Diversional Activity*
*Fatigue*
*Impaired Home Maintenance*
*Instrumental Self-Care Deficit*

**Social Service**
*Caregiver Role Strain*
*Ineffective Family Coping*
*Decisional Conflict*
*Interrupted Family Processes*
*Impaired Home Maintenance*
*Instrumental Self-Care Deficit*
*Social Isolation*

**Speech Therapy**
*Impaired Communication*
*Impaired Swallowing*
*Confusion*

**Nutritional Therapy**
*Imbalanced Nutrition: More Than Body Requirements*
*Imbalanced Nutrition: Less Than Body Requirements*
*Impaired Swallowing*
*Feeding Self-Care Deficit*

**Respiratory Therapy**
*High Risk for Aspiration*
*High Risk for Impaired Respiratory Function*
*Ineffective Airway Clearance*
*Dysfunctional Weaning Response*

from a nurse–client perspective. Keep in mind that, regardless of the specific terminology used, the nurse must tailor all explanations to the client's and family's ability and readiness to learn, cultural background, educational level, and so forth. This will help promote understanding and decision making.

## Nurse Practitioners, Nurse Anesthetists, and Nurse Midwives Do Not Need Nursing Diagnoses*

Advanced nursing practice has been a hot topic of discussion in legislative forums. Many state boards of nursing have defined or are in the process of defining advanced practice.

### ◂◂ Carp's Cues

This author disagrees with the notion that nurse practitioners, nurse midwives or nurse anesthetists are advanced practice nurses but rather they practice in an expanded role. The term advanced practice is sometimes confused with expert nursing. Expertise in nursing should not be defined by a role but rather the depth of knowledge the nurse has regardless of the role. Expert nurses have complex assessment skills and engage in rapid decision-making to provide appropriate and timely care to complex client and family health situations. Expert nurses can be staff nurses in traditional roles. Some nurses in expanded roles focus too heavily on becoming experts in medicine not nursing.

Nurse practitioners diagnose and treat acute and chronic medical conditions. In addition, the nurse practitioner assesses the person's overall health habits and functional status. Therefore, a problem list for a client of a nurse practitioner should include medical and nursing diagnoses.

For example, during an appointment with a 52-year-old man, the man complains of back pain, has high blood pressure, and also reports that he has blackouts from alcohol abuse. After discussing his alcohol use, it is determined that the man drinks excessively every day after work. He, however, denies that he has a problem. His problem list would include:

1. Low back pain unknown etiology
2. Hypertension
3. Chronic alcoholism

Ineffective denial
Advanced nurses demonstrate expert nursing practice by diagnosing client responses to varied situations (e.g., medical diagnoses, personal or maturational crises, which are nursing diagnoses). An advanced nurse would explore such questions as:

• How has the client's ability to function changed since his cerebrovascular accident?
• How has a family system changed, or how is it vulnerable because of an ill newborn who required several months of hospitalization?

Compared with nursing, medicine has little to offer clients and families experiencing chronic disease such as multiple sclerosis or diabetes. Clients' most common complaints do not involve the medical care they receive, but rather focus on dissatisfaction with how their other problems are addressed. Nurses are in the optimum position to address such problems and increase client satisfaction with health care.

Nurse practitioners, nurse anesthetists, or nurse midwives who do not formulate or treat nursing diagnoses may be too focused on medicine. To evaluate this practice, a nurse in advanced practice should ask: Do I consult with physician colleagues for complex medical problems? Do physicians consult with me for complex nursing diagnoses? If the answer is no, the nurse should explore why. Does the problem lie with the physician's attitude, or is the nurse not overtly demonstrating diagnosis and treatment of nursing diagnoses? Or is the nurse not practicing nursing?

If nurse practitioners, nurse anesthetists, and nurse midwives do not practice as expert nurses, who diagnose and treat selected medical diagnoses using protocols, and formulate and treat nursing diagnoses, 5 years from now these nurses may still be struggling to define their roles. Carpenito (1995) uses nursing diagnoses to differentiate the discipline-specific expertise of nurse practitioners and physicians in primary care. Figure 1.1 illustrates this relationship.

*Carpenito, L. J. (1992, February). *Are nurse practitioners expert nurses?* Paper presented at the 11th Annual National Nursing Symposium, Advanced Practice Within a Restructured Health Care Environment, Los Angeles.

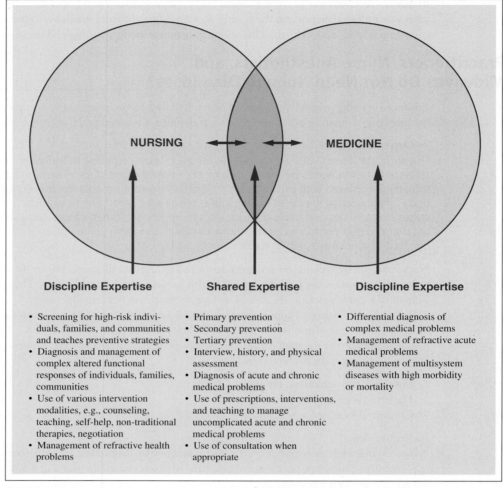

**Discipline Expertise**

- Screening for high-risk individuals, families, and communities
  and teaches preventive strategies
- Diagnosis and management of
  complex altered functional
  responses of individuals, families,
  communities
- Use of various intervention
  modalities, e.g., counseling,
  teaching, self-help, non-traditional
  therapies, negotiation
- Management of refractive health
  problems

**Shared Expertise**

- Primary prevention
- Secondary prevention
- Tertiary prevention
- Interview, history, and physical
  assessment
- Diagnosis of acute and chronic
  medical problems
- Use of prescriptions, interventions,
  and teaching to manage
  uncomplicated acute and chronic
  medical problems
- Use of consultation when
  appropriate

**Discipline Expertise**

- Differential diagnosis of
  complex medical problems
- Management of refractive acute
  medical problems
- Management of multisystem
  diseases with high morbidity
  or mortality

**FIGURE 1.1** Domains of expertise of primary care nurse practitioners and primary care physicians. (© 1995 by Lynda Juall Carpenito; written permission needed to duplicate.)

## Nursing Diagnoses Are Not Culturally Sensitive

Nursing diagnoses, specifically the North American Nursing Diagnosis Association (NANDA) classifications, have been accused of being insensitive to cultural considerations. According to Leininger (1990),
major concerns with the NANDA classifications are the "problems of using, promoting, and implementing the taxonomy with such limited international or transcultural data, including theoretical cultural
ideas, conditions, and practices in diverse cultures." Leininger (1990) also states that there are "a host of
culture-specific illnesses and culture-bound syndromes that need to be documented and understood by
nurses," because expressions of health care, wellness, and illness are different in different cultures.

NANDA is the clearinghouse for nursing diagnosis work from nurses in the United States, and
throughout the world. Nursing diagnoses accepted by NANDA are based primarily on the dominant
Anglo-American cultural values, norms, and standards. Never has this work been portrayed or disseminated as relevant to other cultures. Clearly, North America is home to hundreds of distinctly diverse
ethnic groups, but the NANDA classifications do not address this cultural diversity.

How can nursing diagnosis represent the wide cultural diversity in North America? Only those nurses
who deeply understand a particular culture can develop the culture-specific defining characteristics and
risk factors to make a nursing diagnosis relevant. For example, Native American nurses and non–Native
American nurses who care for Native American clients can examine NANDA's work and determine its relevance to Native American culture. They can promote necessary additions and revisions to the NANDA

classifications and also can develop and submit culturally specific responses currently not on the NANDA list.

Many texts on nursing diagnosis have been translated for use outside North America. Although nurses from different cultures do these translations, all too often they do not address important cultural differences. If nursing diagnosis is determined to be useful as a concept, then nurses in other countries will need to develop diagnoses relevant to their particular cultures. The following two books specifically address nursing diagnoses from different cultural perspectives: *Planification des Soins Infirmiers* (Grondin, Lussier, Phaneuf, & Riopelle, 2005) from a French-Canadian perspective, and *Diagnostico de Enfermeria* (Luis, 2008) from a Spanish perspective.

Keep in mind that a nursing diagnosis is not a judgment that nurses make about a client's or family's responses, values, or health based on *their own* cultural perspectives. Rather, it represents a response that the client or family finds problematic according to their cultural perspective. For example, some cultures believe in fatalism (i.e., outside forces control one's fate and health). The nurse unfamiliar with this belief may incorrectly diagnose the problem as *Powerlessness*.

*Transcultural Considerations* are incorporated into Section Two to increase the nurse's appreciation of cultural diversity.

## Nursing Diagnosis Is Unethical

Some have criticized nursing diagnosis as emphasizing problem-based practice, encouraging professional arrogance, and requiring "value judgments by nurses about another's way of living, viewing self, being or relating with others" (Mitchell, 1991, p. 102). Case studies cited in the literature (Mitchell, 1991) of nursing diagnosis that caused poor or unethical nursing care are interesting. Close examination of these cases reveals that the origin of the unacceptable nursing care rested in the nurse, not in the nursing diagnosis. Obviously, unsatisfactory, irresponsible, and unethical nursing care existed before the advent of nursing diagnosis.

According to Mitchell (1991), "when an individual's definition of health is not consistent with the nurse's, the person's health value is judged as ineffective, maladaptive, or dysfunctional" (p. 100). The nurse's determination of a client's response as ineffective, maladaptive, or dysfunctional should be based on the client's perspective of the problem and on the nurse's knowledge and expertise. A client's ineffective response is not ineffective for the nurse, but rather is ineffective for the client.

To illustrate, let us examine the diagnosis *Grieving*, with the defining characteristics of unsuccessful adaptation to loss, prolonged denial, depression, and delayed emotional reaction. How can a nurse diagnose complicated grieving? What may be a sign or symptom of complicated grieving in one person may not be such in another. The question is: For whom is the grieving dysfunctional? The client? The family? Or the nurse? For grieving to be dysfunctional, it must be dysfunctional for the person experiencing the grief. For example, if a mother visits the gravesite of her deceased child every day for 1 year after the child's death, is this dysfunctional? To determine if it is, the nurse should explore with this client whether these visits interfere with other necessary or enjoyable activities. What does she do when she is not visiting the gravesite? What would happen if she decreased the visits? Only through such a dialogue could the nurse and client be able to identify whether the client's grieving is dysfunctional or whether, perhaps, the client finds the visits comforting and an effective coping mechanism.

## Nursing Diagnoses Can Violate Confidentiality

Nurses and other health professionals commonly are privy to significant personal concerns of clients under their care. According to the American Nurses Association Code of Ethics, "the nurse safeguards the client's right to privacy by judiciously protecting information of a confidential nature." The professional mandate to apply the nursing process for all clients, however, sometimes places the nurse in a position of conflict. Certain information recorded in assessments and diagnostic statements may compromise a client's right to privacy, choice, or confidentiality. Nurses should never use nursing diagnostic statements to influence others to view or treat an individual, family, or group negatively. They must take great caution to ensure that a nursing diagnosis does no harm!

Nurses have a responsibility to make nursing diagnoses and to prescribe nursing treatments. Inherent in the diagnostic process and planning of care is the responsibility to ascertain that there is permission to write, treat, or refer the diagnosis as appropriate.

When a client shares personal information or emotions with the nurse, does this information automatically become part of the client's record or care plan? The nurse has two basic obligations to a client: (1) to address applicable nursing diagnoses and (2) to protect the client's confidentiality. The nurse is *not* obligated to pass on all of a client's nursing diagnoses to other nurses, as long as the nurse can ensure that all diagnoses are addressed.

Consider the following example: Ms. Jackson, 45 years old, is hospitalized for treatment of ovarian cancer. At one point, she states to the nurse, "The God I worship did this to me, and I hate Him for it." Further discussion validates that Ms. Jackson is disturbed about her feelings and changes in her previous beliefs. From these assessment data, the nurse develops the nursing diagnosis *Spiritual Distress related to conflict between disease occurrence and religious faith*. But what should the nurse do with the information, which Ms. Jackson makes clear she considers confidential? The nurse can assist Ms. Jackson with this nursing diagnosis through several different avenues:

1. Apprising her of available community resources for follow-up assistance in dealing with her spiritual distress
2. Continuing to assist her to explore her feelings and using the nurse's notes to reflect discussions (without using quotation marks to denote her actual words)
3. Recording the nursing diagnosis *Spiritual Distress* on the care plan and developing appropriate interventions

Referring her to an appropriate spiritual advisor

Option 1 returns the problem to the client for management after discharge. Sometimes the nature of a problem and its priority among the client's other problems make providing the client or family with information on available resources for use after discharge the most appropriate option. The nurse should, however, be cautioned against using this option merely to "wash one's hands" of a problem.

Option 2 allows the nurse to continue a dialogue with the client about the issue, but without divulging it specifically. The problem with this option is that the client's care plan will not reflect this problem as a nursing diagnosis on the active list. As a result, should the client's nurse become unable to care for the client, this diagnosis likely would not be addressed.

Option 3 incorporates the problem, as a nursing diagnosis, into the client's care plan, where the entire nursing staff can address it. To help protect the confidentiality of very sensitive disclosed information, the nurse should make a few modifications, such as not quoting the client's statements exactly.

Documentation of the nursing diagnosis on the care plan raises another possible dilemma. What if the primary nurse in whom the client or family has confided cannot follow the diagnosis full-time? How can the primary nurse involve others in addressing this diagnosis without violating the client's confidentiality? The primary nurse should encourage the client to allow another nurse to intervene in his or her absence. If the client refuses referral or another nurse, the nurse should document this in the progress notes, continuing to protect the client's confidentiality. For example:

> *Discussed with Ms. Jackson the feasibility of another nurse intervening with her regarding her spiritual concerns in my absence. Ms. Jackson declined involvement of another nurse. Instructed her on whom to contact if she changes her mind.*

This note documents the nurse's responsibility to the client as well as the nurse's accountability.

It is also important to note that, in most cases, the nurse should not share confidential information with family members without the client's permission. Exceptions to preserving confidentiality, however, "may be necessary if the information the client shares with the nurse contains indications of a threat to the lives of the patient or others" (Curtin & Flaherty, 1982).

Option 4 is a commonly chosen action for clients with spiritual conflicts. Before referring a client, however, the nurse should ascertain the client's receptivity to such a referral. To assume receptivity without first consulting the client can be problematic. The client chose to share very personal information with a particular nurse, who then is obligated to assist the client with the problem. If the nurse believes that a religious leader or another professional would be beneficial to the client, the nurse should approach the client with the option. An example of such a dialogue follows:

> *Ms. Jackson, we've been discussing your concerns about your illness and how it has changed your spiritual beliefs. I know someone who has been very helpful for people with concerns similar to yours. I'd like to ask her to visit you. What do you think about this?*

Such a dialogue clearly designates the choice as Ms. Jackson's. Just as nurses have an obligation to inform clients and families of available resources, clients have the right to accept or reject these resources.

# Summary

Nursing diagnosis has sparked much debate. Too often, those opposed to nursing diagnosis practice in isolation as primary providers and see no need for diagnoses in their nurse–client relationships. If they engage in therapeutic interventions, they are engaged in treating phenomena. They see no need for diagnoses, yet they must analyze responses, which directs them to future interventions. If intervening is not part of a nurse–client relationship, then perhaps there is no nurse–client relationship. Nursing actively assists clients, families, or communities to reduce or eliminate problems, reduce risk factors, prevent problems, and promote healthier lifestyles.

Nursing diagnosis provides nursing with a framework within which to organize its science. It is, however, each individual nurse's responsibility to apply nursing diagnoses with caution and care.*

---

*Carpenito, L. J., & Duespohl, T. A. (1985). *A guide to effective clinical instruction* (2nd ed.). Rockville, MD: Aspen Systems.

# 2 DEVELOPMENT OF NURSING DIAGNOSIS

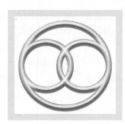

**Learning Objectives**

After reading the chapter, the student should be able to answer the following questions:

- What are the benefits of a uniform language in nursing?
- What is NANDA-I?
- How are nursing diagnoses approved for clinical use?

## What Are the Benefits of a Uniform Language in Nursing?

Before the development of a classification or list of nursing diagnoses, nurses used whatever word they wanted to describe client problems. For example, nurses might have described a client recovering from surgery as "the appendectomy," another client as "the diabetic," and another client as "difficult." Clearly, knowing that a person has diabetes brings to mind blood sugar problems and risk for infection, so the focus was on common problems or risk factors derived from medical diagnoses. If the client with diabetes or surgery had another problem that needed nursing attention, this problem would have gone undiagnosed. Before 1972, not only did nurses lack the terms to describe problems (except medical diagnoses), but also they did not have assessment questions to uncover such problems.

The need for a common, consistent language for medicine was identified more than 200 years ago. If physicians chose to use random words to describe their clinical situations, then:

- How could they communicate with one another? With nurses?
- How could they organize research?
- How could they educate new physicians?
- How could they improve quality if they could not retrieve data systematically to determine which interventions improved the client's condition?

For example, before the formal labeling of acquired immunodeficiency syndrome (AIDS), defining or studying the disease was difficult, if not impossible. Often, medical records of affected clients would show various diagnoses or causes of death, such as sepsis, cerebral hemorrhage, or pneumonia, because the AIDS diagnosis did not exist. Every physician in the world uses the same terminology for medical diagnoses. As new diagnoses are discovered, all medical clinicians can access the research using the same words.

### ◀◀ Carp's Cues

By definition, *diagnosis* is the careful, critical study of something to determine its nature. The question is not *whether* nurses can diagnose, but *what* nurses can diagnose.

## What Is NANDA-I?

In 1953, V. Fry introduced the term *nursing diagnosis* to describe a step necessary in developing a nursing care plan. Over the next 20 years, references to nursing diagnosis appeared sporadically in the literature.

In 1973, the American Nurses Association (ANA) published its *Standards of Practice*; in 1980, it followed with its *Social Policy Statement*, which defined nursing as "the diagnosis and treatment of human response to actual or potential health problems." Most state nurse practice acts describe nursing in accordance with the ANA definition.

In March 1990, at the Ninth Conference of the North American Nursing Diagnosis Association (NANDA), the General Assembly approved an official definition of nursing diagnosis (NANDA, 1990):

> *Nursing diagnosis is a clinical judgment about individual, family, or community responses to actual or potential health problems/life processes. Nursing diagnosis provides the basis for selection of nursing interventions to achieve outcomes for which the nurse is accountable.*

This definition was revised from "the nurse is accountable" to "the nurse has accountability" at the National Conference of NANDA-I in Miami (November 2008).

It is important also to emphasize that the responses called nursing diagnoses can be to illness and life events. Previously, nurses focused more on responses to medical conditions or treatments. Nurses now diagnose and treat responses to life events such as parenting, aging parents, and school failure.

## The North American Nursing Diagnosis Association International

In 1973, the first conference on nursing diagnosis was held to identify nursing knowledge and to establish a classification system suitable for computerization. From this conference developed the National Group for the Classification of Nursing Diagnosis, composed of nurses from different regions of the United States and Canada, representing all elements of the profession: practice, education, and research.

In 2003, the organization was renamed the North American Nursing Diagnosis Association International (NANDA). In addition to reviewing and accepting nursing diagnoses for addition to the list, NANDA also reviews previously accepted nursing diagnoses. Since the first conference, NANDA has grown with membership of nurses from every continent.

In March 1990, the first issue of *Nursing Diagnosis*, NANDA's official journal, was published. This journal aims to promote the development, refinement, and application of nursing diagnoses and to serve as a forum for issues pertaining to the development and classification of nursing knowledge. The journal is now named *International Journal of Nursing Terminologies and Classification*.

## NANDA Taxonomy

A *taxonomy* is a type of classification, the theoretical study of systematic classifications including their bases, principles, procedures, and rules. The work of the initial theorist group at the third national conference and subsequently of the NANDA taxonomic committee produced the beginnings of a conceptual framework for the diagnostic classification system. This framework was named NANDA Nursing Diagnosis Taxonomy I, which comprised nine patterns of human response. In 2000, NANDA approved a new Taxonomy II, which has 13 domains, 106 classes, and 155 diagnoses (NANDA, 2001).

Table 2.1 illustrates the 13 domains and associated definitions. The second level, classes, may be useful as assessment criteria. The third level (diagnostic concepts), most useful for clinicians, is the nursing

### TABLE 2.1 TAXONOMY II DOMAINS AND DEFINITIONS

| | | |
|---|---|---|
| Domain 1 | Health Promotion | Awareness of well-being or normality of function and the strategies used to maintain control of and enhance that well-being or normality of function |
| Domain 2 | Nutrition | Activities of taking in, assimilating, and using nutrients for the purposes of tissue maintenance, tissue repair, and production of energy |
| Domain 3 | Elimination | Secretion and excretion of waste products from the body |
| Domain 4 | Activity/Rest | Production, conservation, expenditure, or balance of energy resources |
| Domain 5 | Perception/Cognition | Human information-processing system including attention, orientation, sensation, perception, cognition, and communication |
| Domain 6 | Self-perception | Awareness about the self |
| Domain 7 | Role Relationships | Positive and negative connections or associations between persons or groups of persons and the means by which those connections are demonstrated |
| Domain 8 | Sexuality | Sexual identity, sexual function, and reproduction |
| Domain 9 | Coping/Stress Tolerance | Contending with life events/life processes |
| Domain 10 | Life Principles | Principles underlying conduct, thought, and behavior about acts, customs, or institutions viewed as being true or having intrinsic worth |
| Domain 11 | Safety/Protection | Freedom from danger, physical injury, or immune system damage, preservation from loss, and protection of safety and security |
| Domain 12 | Comfort | Sense of mental, physical, or social well-being or ease |
| Domain 13 | Growth/Development | Age-appropriate increases in physical dimensions, organ systems, and/or attainment of developmental milestones |

North American Nursing Diagnosis Association. (2001). *Nursing diagnosis: Definitions and classification 2001–2002.* Philadelphia: NANDA.

diagnosis labels. Changes in terminology were made for consistency; for example, *Altered Nutrition* was changed to *Imbalanced Nutrition*. An example of one domain is:

| | | | |
|---|---|---|---|
| Domain 4 | Activity/Rest | | |
| Class 1 | Sleep/Rest | | |
| Diagnostic Concepts | 00095 | Insomnia | |
| | 00096 | Sleep Deprivation | |

## How Are Nursing Diagnoses Approved for Clinical Use?

Some believe that nursing diagnoses are created by NANDA-I. Often it is asked why NANDA does not have more nursing diagnoses for persons with mental illnesses? Nursing diagnoses are not developed by NANDA.

◂◂ **Carp's Cues**
NANDA-approved Nursing Diagnoses can only be clinically relevant if clinical nurses are involved in their development. Missing nursing diagnoses are the responsibility of clinical nurses to submit.

The Diagnosis Development Committee (DDC) of NANDA –I is responsible for reviewing and assisting others to develop and refine their proposed diagnoses. The committee responds to submissions from nurses worldwide. After the committee determines that a submitted diagnosis meets the definition criteria for a nursing diagnosis and contains all of the required elements, the diagnosis is released for membership review and approval. Submission can be for new nursing diagnoses or for recommendations for revisions. In addition, the DDC regularly critiques previously accepted Nursing Diagnosis for revision and sometimes for deletion. The process is ongoing and with the product nursing diagnosis always in refinement.

## Summary

A classification system for nursing diagnoses has been in continual development for the past 30 years. During this period, the initial question, "Does nursing really need a classification system?" has been replaced by, "How can such a system be developed in a scientifically sound manner?" The ANA has designated NANDA as the official organization to develop this classification system. Despite problems, through the concerted effort of many fine clinical nurses, nurse researchers, and other nursing professionals and organizations, this evolving classification system increasingly reflects both the art and science of nursing.

# 3

# TYPES AND COMPONENTS OF NURSING DIAGNOSES

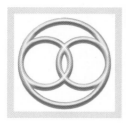

## Learning Objectives

After reading the chapter, the student should be able to answer the following questions:

- What are the differences between actual, risk, and possible nursing diagnoses?
- What is a wellness diagnosis?
- What are syndrome nursing diagnoses?
- When can a non-NANDA nursing diagnosis be used?
- When should unknown etiology be used?
- How can errors be avoided in diagnostic statements?

This chapter will focus on types of nursing diagnoses and writing diagnostic statements. There are four types of nursing diagnoses: actual, risk, possible, wellness, and syndrome.

## Actual Nursing Diagnoses

An *actual nursing diagnosis* represents a problem that has been validated by the presence of major defining characteristics. This type of nursing diagnosis has four components: label, definition, defining characteristics, and related factors.

### Label

The label should be in clear, concise terms that convey the meaning of the diagnosis.

### Definition

The definition should add clarity to the diagnostic label. It also should help to differentiate a particular diagnosis from similar diagnoses.

### Defining Characteristics

For actual nursing diagnoses, defining characteristics are signs and symptoms that, when seen together, represent the nursing diagnosis. Defining characteristics are separated into major and minor designations.

- *Major.* For nonresearched diagnoses, at least one must be present for validation of the diagnosis. For researched diagnoses, at least one must be present under the 80%–100% grouping.
- *Minor.* These characteristics provide supporting evidence but may not be present.

The nursing diagnoses in Section 2 will have researched and nonresearched defining characteristics. Table 3.1 represents major and minor defining characteristics for the researched diagnosis *Defensive Coping* (Norris & Kunes-Connell, 1987).

### Related Factors

In actual nursing diagnoses, related factors are contributing factors that have influenced the change in health status. Such factors can be grouped into four categories:

- *Pathophysiologic, Biologic, or Psychological.* Examples include compromised oxygen transport, and compromised circulation. Inadequate circulation can cause Impaired Skin Integrity.
- *Treatment-Related.* Examples include medications, therapies, surgery, and diagnostic study. Specifically, medications can cause nausea. Radiation can cause fatigue. Scheduled surgery can cause Anxiety.
- *Situational.* Examples include environmental, home, community, institution, personal, life experiences, and roles. Specifically a flood in a community can contribute to Risk for Infection; Divorce can cause Grieving; Obesity can contribute to Activity Intolerance.

| TABLE 3.1 FREQUENCY SCORES FOR DEFINING CHARACTERISTICS OF DEFENSIVE COPING | |
|---|---|
| **Defining Characteristics** | **Frequency Scores** |
| **Major (80%–100%)** | |
| Denial of obvious problems/weaknesses | 88% |
| Projection of blame/responsibility | 87% |
| Rationalizes failures | 86% |
| Hypersensitive to slight criticism | 84% |
| **Minor (50%–79%)** | |
| Grandiosity | 79% |
| Superior attitude toward others | 76% |
| Difficulty in establishing/maintaining relationships | 74% |
| Hostile laughter or ridicule of others | 71% |
| Difficulty in testing perceptions against reality | 62% |
| Lack of follow-through or participation in treatment or therapy | 56% |

Norris, J. & Kunes-Connell, M. (1987). Self-esteem disturbance: A clinical validation study. In A. McLane (Ed.), *Classification of nursing diagnoses: Proceedings of the seventh NANDA national conference.* St. Louis: CV Mosby.

- *Maturational.* Examples include age-related influences, such as in children and the elderly. Specifically the elderly are a risk for Social Isolation; Infants are at Risk for Injury; adolescents are at Risk for Infection Transmission.

**INTERACTIVE EXERCISE 3.1**

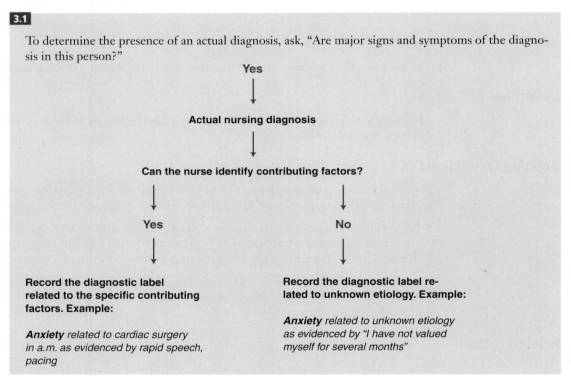

To determine the presence of an actual diagnosis, ask, "Are major signs and symptoms of the diagnosis in this person?"

Yes

↓

**Actual nursing diagnosis**

↓

**Can the nurse identify contributing factors?**

Yes → **Record the diagnostic label related to the specific contributing factors. Example:**

*Anxiety* related to cardiac surgery in a.m. as evidenced by rapid speech, pacing

No → **Record the diagnostic label related to unknown etiology. Example:**

*Anxiety* related to unknown etiology as evidenced by "I have not valued myself for several months"

## Risk and High-Risk Nursing Diagnoses

NANDA defines a *risk nursing diagnosis* as "a clinical judgment that an individual, family, or community is more vulnerable to develop the problem than others in the same or similar situation." The concept of "at risk" is useful clinically. Nurses routinely prevent problems in people experiencing similar situations such as surgery or childbirth who are not at high risk. For example, all postoperative clients are at risk for infection. All women postdelivery are at risk for hemorrhage. Thus there are expected or predictive diagnoses for all clients who have undergone surgery while on chemotherapy or with a fractured hip.

◀◀ **Carp's Cues**

Nurses do not need to include it on the client's care plan in the hospital. In fact it is a waste of time for nurses (not students) to write text of the same predicted care repeatedly. Students are expected to write the predicted care until they are experienced with that care. Instead, this diagnosis is part of the unit's standard of care (see Chapter 5 for a discussion of standards; refer also to THE POINT. Log in to http://thepoint.lww.com/CarpenitoApp13e for a Medical Care Plan for the Hospitalized Adult Client.

All persons admitted to the hospital are at Risk for Infection related to increased microorganisms in the environment, risk of person-to-person transmission, and invasive tests and therapies. Refer to Box 3.1 for an illustration of this standard diagnosis and how it is individualized to become a High Risk diagnosis. The high-risk concept is very useful for persons who have additional risk factors that make them more vulnerable for the problem to occur. Pregnant women are at risk for injury, but they are at high risk during their third trimester. A pregnant woman with multiple sclerosis can be at higher risk, (e.g., Risk for Falls related to unstable gait secondary to multiple sclerosis).

## Label

In a risk nursing diagnosis, the term *Risk for* precedes the nursing diagnosis label or High Risk if this concept is used.

## Definition

As in an actual nursing diagnosis, the definition in a risk nursing diagnosis expresses a clear, precise meaning of the diagnosis.

## Risk Factors

Risk factors for risk and high-risk nursing diagnoses represent those situations that increase the vulnerability of the client or group. These factors differentiate high-risk clients and groups from all others in the same population who are at some risk. The validation to support an actual diagnosis is signs and symptoms (e.g., *Impaired Skin Integrity related to immobility secondary to pain as evidenced by 2-cm erythematous sacral lesion*). In contrast, the validation to support a high-risk diagnosis is risk factors (e.g., *High Risk for Impaired Skin Integrity related to immobility secondary to pain*).

## Related Factors

The related factors for risk nursing diagnoses are the same risk factors previously explained for actual nursing diagnoses. The components of a risk nursing diagnostic statement are discussed later in this chapter.

---

### BOX 3.1  REVISING A STANDARD SURGICAL CARE PLAN NURSING DIAGNOSIS

**Standard Nursing Diagnosis**
Risk for Infection related to incision and loss of protective skin barrier

**Client Nursing Diagnosis**
High Risk for Infection related to incision, loss of protective skin barrier and high blood glucose levels secondary to diabetes mellitus

INTERACTIVE
EXERCISE   3.2

To determine the presence of a risk diagnosis, ask, "Are major signs and symptoms of the diagnosis found in this person?"

```
                                   No
                                   ↓
                          Validation of risk factors
                        ↙                            ↘
                  Yes                                    No
                   ↓                                      ↓
          Risk nursing diagnosis              Do you suspect a problem
                   ↓                                 may be present?
    Record "Risk for" before the              ↙                ↘
    diagnostic label related to            Yes                    No
    the risk factors. Example:              ↓                      ↓
                                       Possible              No problem
    Risk for Impaired Skin In-        nursing diagnosis        at
    tegrity related to immobility          ↓                 this time
    and fatigue                       Collect more data         ↓
                                      to confirm            Monitor
                                      or rule out.
                                           ↓
                                 Record "Possible" before the
                                 diagnostic label. Example:

                                 Possible Feeding Self-Care Deficit
                                 related to fatigue and IV in right hand
```

## Possible Nursing Diagnoses

*Possible nursing diagnoses* are statements that describe a suspected problem requiring additional data. It is unfortunate that many nurses have been socialized to avoid appearing tentative. In scientific decision making, a tentative approach is not a sign of weakness or indecision, but an essential part of the process. The nurse should delay a final diagnosis until he or she has gathered and analyzed all necessary information to arrive at a sound scientific conclusion. Physicians demonstrate tentativeness with the statement *rule out (R/O)*. Nurses also should adopt a tentative position until they have completed data collection and evaluation and can confirm or rule out.

### ◀◀ Carp's Cues
NANDA does not address possible nursing diagnoses because they are not a classification issue; they are an option for clinical nurses. With a possible nursing diagnosis, the nurse has some, but insufficient, data to support a confirmed diagnosis.

Possible nursing diagnoses are two-part statements consisting of:

• The possible nursing diagnosis
• The "related to" data that lead the nurse to suspect the diagnosis

An example is *Possible Disturbed Self-Concept related to recent loss of role responsibilities secondary to worsening of multiple sclerosis*.

When a nurse records a possible nursing diagnosis, he or she alerts other nurses to assess for more data to support or rule out the tentative diagnosis. After additional data collection, the nurse may take one of three actions:

• Confirm the presence of major signs and symptoms, thus labeling an actual diagnosis.
• Confirm the presence of potential risk factors, thus labeling a risk diagnosis.
• Rule out the presence of a diagnosis (actual or risk) at this time.

# Wellness Nursing Diagnoses

According to NANDA, a wellness nursing diagnosis is "a clinical judgment about an individual, group, or community in transition from a specific level of wellness to a higher level of wellness" (1992, p. 84). For an individual or group to have a wellness nursing diagnosis, two cues should be present: (1) a desire for increased wellness, and (2) effective present status or function.

Diagnostic statements for wellness nursing diagnoses are one part, containing the label only. The label begins with "Readiness for Enhanced," followed by the higher-level wellness that the individual or group desires (e.g., *Readiness for Enhanced Family Processes*).

Wellness nursing diagnoses do not contain related factors. Inherent in these diagnoses is a client or group who understands that higher-level functioning is available. The related goals would give direction for interventions:

**Nursing Diagnosis:** Readiness for Enhanced Family Processes
**Goals:**
The family will:

* Eat dinner together 5 days/week.
* Include children in discussions of family decisions.
* Report respect for privacy of each member.

Stolte describes wellness nursing diagnoses as "a conclusion from assessment data which focuses on patterns of wellness, healthy responses, or client strengths" (1996, p. 9). Interventions focus on attainment of health behaviors or achievement of developmental tasks.

Since 1973, many nurses have expressed concern that the NANDA list primarily represents alteration or dysfunction with too little emphasis on wellness (Popkess-Vawter, 1984). Many nurses interact with healthy clients, such as new parents, school-aged children, and clients of college health services and well-baby clinics. Nurses also help ill clients to pursue optimal health through interventions such as stress management, exercise programs, and nutritional counseling.

"Strengths are qualities or factors that will help the person to recover, cope with stressors, and progress to his or her original health or as close as possible before hospitalization, illness, or surgery" (Carpenito-Moyet, 2007, p. 84). Examples of strength are as follows:

* Positive support system
* High motivation
* Financial stability
* Alert, good memory

◄◄ **Carp's Cues**
Strengths are different from wellness diagnoses. Table 3.2 lists statements that describe strengths for each of the 11 functional health patterns. When the nurse and client conclude that there is positive functioning in a functional health pattern, this conclusion is an assessment conclusion, but by itself is not a nursing diagnosis. The nurse uses these data to help the client reach a higher level of functioning or to plan interventions for altered or at risk for altered functioning.

| TABLE 3.2 FUNCTIONAL HEALTH PATTERNS AND ASSOCIATED POSITIVE FUNCTIONING ASSESSMENT STATEMENTS | |
| --- | --- |
| **Functional Health Pattern** | **Positive Functioning Assessment Statements** |
| 1. Health perception–health management pattern | 1. Positive health perception / Effective health management |
| 2. Nutritional–metabolic pattern | 2. Effective nutritional–metabolic pattern |
| 3. Elimination pattern | 3. Effective elimination pattern |
| 4. Activity–exercise pattern | 4. Effective activity–exercise pattern |
| 5. Sleep–rest pattern | 5. Effective sleep–rest pattern |
| 6. Cognitive–perceptual pattern | 6. Positive cognitive–perceptual pattern |
| 7. Self-perception pattern | 7. Positive self-perception pattern |
| 8. Role–relationship pattern | 8. Positive role–relationship pattern |
| 9. Sexuality–reproductive pattern | 9. Positive sexuality–reproductive pattern |
| 10. Coping–stress intolerance pattern | 10. Effective coping–stress tolerance pattern |
| 11. Value–belief pattern | 11. Positive value–belief pattern |

One could incorporate positive functioning assessment statements under each functional health pattern on the admission assessment tool, as illustrated by sleep-rest pattern. Wellness/ Promotion Nursing Diagnoses can all be found in Part 4.

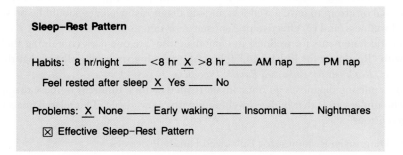

**Sleep–Rest Pattern**

Habits:  8 hr/night _____  <8 hr _X_  >8 hr _____  AM nap _____  PM nap _____

   Feel rested after sleep _X_ Yes _____ No

Problems: _X_ None _____ Early waking _____ Insomnia _____ Nightmares

   ☒ Effective Sleep–Rest Pattern

INTERACTIVE
EXERCISE   **3.3**

If you assess a client and find no problems of functioning, ask, "Is the person or group at high risk for a problem?"

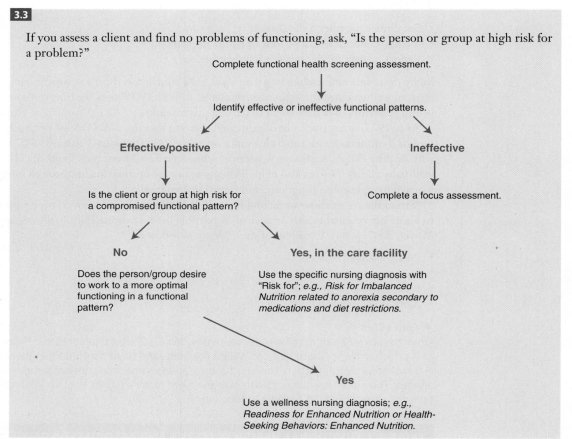

Complete functional health screening assessment.

Identify effective or ineffective functional patterns.

**Effective/positive**        **Ineffective**

Is the client or group at high risk for a compromised functional pattern?        Complete a focus assessment.

**No**        **Yes, in the care facility**

Does the person/group desire to work to a more optimal functioning in a functional pattern?        Use the specific nursing diagnosis with "Risk for"; *e.g., Risk for Imbalanced Nutrition related to anorexia secondary to medications and diet restrictions.*

**Yes**

Use a wellness nursing diagnosis; *e.g., Readiness for Enhanced Nutrition or Health-Seeking Behaviors: Enhanced Nutrition.*

# Syndrome Nursing Diagnoses

*Syndrome nursing diagnoses* are an interesting development in nursing diagnosis. They comprise a cluster of predicted actual or high-risk nursing diagnoses related to a certain event or situation. For example, Carlson-Catalino (1998) used an exploratory qualitative study of post–acute-phase battered women to identify 24 nursing diagnoses in all the subjects. This research supports a diagnosis of *Battered Woman Syndrome*. In medicine, syndromes cluster signs and symptoms, not diagnoses. In nursing, a cluster of signs and symptoms represents a single nursing diagnosis, not a syndrome nursing diagnosis.

   Nurses should approach the development of syndrome diagnosis carefully. They also must dialogue with clients to determine other nursing diagnoses indicating the need for client–nurse interventions. The clinical advantage of a syndrome diagnosis is that it alerts the nurse to a "complex clinical condition requiring expert nursing assessments and interventions" (McCourt, 1991).

| TABLE 3.3  REVISION OF RAPE TRAUMA SYNDROME | |
|---|---|
| **Signs/Symptom Cluster (abridged)** | **Nursing Diagnosis Cluster** |
| *Aggression* | *Anxiety* |
| *Agitation* | *Disturbed Sleep Pattern* |
| *Anger* | *Fear* |
| *Anxiety* | *High Risk for Ineffective Sexuality Patterns* |
| *Confusion* | *Grieving* |
| *Fear* | *Pain* |
| *Shock* | *Risks for Chronic Sorrow* |
| *Shame* | *Risk for Infection Transmission* |
| *Nightmares* | *Interrupted Family Processes* |
| *Phobias* | *Social Isolation* |

◀◀ **Carp's Cues**

There continues to be differing opinions on syndrome nursing diagnoses.

Syndrome nursing diagnoses are diagnostic statements with the etiologic or contributing factors contained in the diagnostic label (e.g., *Rape Trauma Syndrome*). NANDA has five syndrome diagnoses: *Rape Trauma Syndrome*, *Disuse Syndrome*, *Post-Trauma Syndrome*, *Relocation Stress Syndrome*, and *Impaired Environmental Interpretation Syndrome*. Some of these syndrome diagnoses do not adhere to a cluster of nursing diagnoses but have a cluster of signs and symptoms. NANDA continues to explore how syndrome diagnoses differ from other types of nursing diagnoses.

Two diagnoses—Rape Trauma Syndrome and Disuse Syndrome—were accepted with signs and symptoms (defining characteristics) instead of a cluster of actual / risk nursing diagnoses with nursing diagnoses. Table 3.3 illustrates how this diagnosis can be revised to represent a syndrome diagnosis.

## Non–NANDA-Approved Diagnoses

The issue of whether nurses should use only NANDA-approved diagnoses continues to spark debate. Some agencies and schools of nursing mandate use of NANDA-approved diagnoses only. Others do not support these restrictions.

Several authors, including Alfaro (1990), Gordon (1990), and Carpenito (1990), have made recommendations about using non-NANDA nursing diagnoses. Every agency and school of nursing should have an approved list containing all NANDA-approved nursing diagnoses as well as any other that the agency or school has approved for use. This list would help nurses avoid using unknown and possibly confusing labels.

Nurses, faculty members, or students could submit a non–NANDA-approved diagnosis to be considered for inclusion within the agency or school list for further clinical development. (Of course, any proposed diagnosis should contain all of its appropriate components—definition, defining characteristics, risk factors.) Refer to Appendix A for NANDA Diagnosis Submission Guidelines. Including non–NANDA-approved diagnoses on agency or school lists can help encourage orderly, scientific development of nursing diagnoses while avoiding terminologic chaos.

## Diagnostic Statements

Nursing diagnostic statements can have one, two, or three parts. One-part statements contain only the diagnostic label, as in wellness and syndrome nursing diagnoses. Two-part statements contain the label and the factors that have contributed or could contribute to a change in health status, as in risk and possible diagnoses. Three-part statements contain the label, contributing factors, and signs and symptoms of the diagnosis, as in actual diagnoses. Box 3.2 lists diagnostic statements with examples.

## Writing Diagnostic Statements

Three-part diagnostic statements contain the following elements:

| Problem | *related to* | Etiology | *as evidenced by* | Symptom |
|---|---|---|---|---|
| Diagnostic label | | Contributing factors | | Signs and symptoms |

**BOX 3.2 TYPES OF DIAGNOSTIC STATEMENTS**

**One-Part Statement**
- Wellness nursing diagnoses (e.g., *Readiness for Enhanced Parenting, Readiness for Enhanced Nutrition*)
- Syndrome nursing diagnoses (e.g., *Disuse Syndrome, Rape Trauma Syndrome*)

**Two-Part Statement**
- Risk nursing diagnoses (e.g., *Risk for Injury related to lack of awareness of hazards*)
- Possible nursing diagnoses (e.g., *Possible Disturbed Body Image related to isolating behaviors postsurgery*)

**Three-Part Statement**
- Actual nursing diagnoses (e.g., *Impaired Skin Integrity related to prolonged immobility secondary to fractured pelvis, as evidenced by a 2-cm lesion on back*)

In two-part and three-part diagnostic statements, *related to* reflects a relationship between the first and second parts of the statement. The more specific that the second part of the statement is, the more specialized the interventions can be. For example, the diagnosis *Noncompliance* stated alone usually conveys the negative implication that the client is not cooperating. When the nurse relates the noncompliance to be a factor, however, this diagnosis can transmit a very different message:

- *Noncompliance related to negative side effects of a drug (reduced libido, fatigue), as evidenced by "I stopped my blood pressure medicine."*
- *Noncompliance related to inability to understand the need for weekly blood pressure measurements, as evidenced by "I don't keep my appointments if I'm busy."*

## Using "Unknown Etiology" in Diagnostic Statements

If the defining characteristics of a nursing diagnosis are present but the etiologic and contributing factors are unknown, the statement can include the phrase *unknown etiology* (e.g., *Fear related to unknown etiology, as evidenced by rapid speech, pacing, and "I'm worried."*). The use of *unknown etiology* alerts the nurse and other members of the nursing staff to assess for contributing factors as they intervene for the current problem.

If the nurse suspects certain factors or a relationship between certain factors and the nursing diagnosis, he or she can use the term *possible* (e.g., *Anxiety related to possible marital discord*).

Syndrome diagnoses that may represent exceptions to the need to use the phrase *related to* are *Rape Trauma Syndrome* and *Disuse Syndrome*. As more specific diagnoses evolve, it may become unnecessary for the nurse to write *related to* statements. Instead, many future nursing diagnoses may be one-part statements, such as *Functional Incontinence* or *Death Anxiety*.

## Avoiding Errors in Diagnostic Statements

As with any other skill, writing diagnostic statements takes knowledge and practice. To increase the accuracy and usefulness of diagnostic statements (and to reduce frustration), nurses should avoid several common errors. See Table 3.4 for examples of errors to avoid.

Nursing diagnostic statements should not be written in terms of:

- Cues (e.g., crying, hemoglobin level)
- Inferences (e.g., dyspnea)
- Goals (e.g., should perform own colostomy care)
- Client needs (e.g., needs to walk every shift; needs to express fears)
- Nursing needs (e.g., change dressing, check blood pressure)

Nurses should avoid legally inadvisable or judgmental statements, such as:

- *Fear related to frequent beatings by husband*
- *Ineffective Family Coping related to mother-in-law's continual harassment of daughter-in-law*
- *Risk for Impaired Parenting related to low IQ of mother*

| TABLE 3.4 | EXAMPLES OF ERRORS TO AVOID WHEN WRITING DIAGNOSTIC STATEMENTS | |
|---|---|
| **Incorrect** | **Correct** |
| **Medical diagnoses** | |
| Risk for Infection related to diabetes mellitus | Risk for Infection related to increased microorganism activity with hyperglycemia |
| **Treatments or equipment** | |
| Imbalanced Nutrition related to feeding tube | Impaired Comfort related to irritation of feeding tube |
| **Medication side effects** | |
| Risk for Infection related to chemotherapy | Risk for Infection related to decreased white blood cells secondary to chemotherapy |
| **Diagnostic studies** | |
| Cardiac catheterization | Anxiety related to scheduled cardiac cauterization |
| **Situations** | |
| Dying | Powerlessness related to his course of terminal illness |

#### ◀◀ Carp's Cues

A nursing diagnosis should not be related to a medical diagnosis, such as *Disturbed Self-Concept related to multiple sclerosis* or *Anxiety related to myocardial infarction*. If the use of a medical diagnosis adds clarity to the diagnosis, the nurse can link it to the statement with the phrase *secondary to* (e.g., *Disturbed Self-Concept related to recent losses of role responsibilities secondary to multiple sclerosis, as evidenced by, "My mother comes every day to run my house,"* or *"I can no longer be the woman in charge of my house.")*.

**INTERACTIVE EXERCISE** `3.4`

Examine the following diagnostic statements and determine whether they are written correctly or incorrectly.

1. *Anxiety related to AIDS*
2. *Chronic Sorrow related to crying and episodes of inability to sleep*
3. *Risk for Injury related to dizziness secondary to high blood pressure*
4. *Impaired Parenting related to frequent screaming at child*
5. *Risk for Constipation related to reports of bowel movements once a week*

## Summary

On the surface, nursing diagnosis appears to be a convenient, simple solution to some of professional nursing's problems. This impression has led many nurses to use nursing diagnoses; however, many still do not integrate diagnosis into their nursing practice. Integrating nursing diagnosis into practice is a collective and personal process. Collectively, the nursing profession has developed the structure of nursing diagnosis and continues to identify and refine specific diagnoses. Individually, each nurse struggles with diagnostic reasoning and confirmation as well as with related ethical implications. Collectively and individually, these struggles will continue.

## ANSWERS TO INTERACTIVE EXERCISES

`3.4`

1. *Incorrect.* The related factor AIDS does not communicate what interventions are needed. Is this diagnosis of AIDS new? Has the disease worsened?
2. *Incorrect.* Crying and inability to sleep are signs and symptoms, not related factors, of a problem. Correct presentation would be *Chronic Sorrow related to ongoing losses as a result of multiple sclerosis as evidenced by crying and inability to sleep*.
3. *Correct.*
4. *Incorrect.* Frequent screaming at a child is a sign of a problem, not a "related to." Correct presentation would be *Impaired Parenting related to unknown etiology as evidenced by frequent screaming at child*.
5. *Incorrect.* Weekly bowel movements are a symptom of constipation, not related to a risk diagnosis. Correct presentation would be *Constipation related to unknown etiology as manifested by weekly bowel movements*.

# 4 NURSING DIAGNOSIS: WHAT IT IS, WHAT IT IS NOT

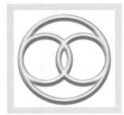

**Learning Objectives**

After reading the chapter, the student should be able to answer the following questions:

- What is the bifocal clinical practice model?
- How do nursing diagnoses differ from collaborative problems?
- How are collaborative problems written?
- Is monitoring an intervention?

As discussed in Chapter 2, the official NANDA definition of nursing diagnosis reads: "Nursing diagnosis is a clinical judgment about an individual, family, or community response to actual or potential health problems or life processes. Nursing diagnosis provides the basis for selection of nursing interventions to achieve outcomes for which the nurse has accountability" (NANDA, 2008). But what about other clinical situations—those that nursing diagnosis does not cover, those that necessitate nursing intervention and medical interventions? Where do they fit within the scope of nursing practice? What about clinical situations in which the nurses and physicians must both prescribe interventions to achieve outcomes?

## Collaboration with Other Disciplines

The practice of nursing requires three different types of nursing responsibilities:

1. Validating nursing diagnoses, providing interventions to treat, and evaluating progress
2. Monitoring for physiologic instability and collaborating with physicians and nurse practitioners, who determine medical treatment

Consulting with other disciplines (physical therapists, occupational therapists, social service, respiratory therapy, pharmacists) to increase the nurse's expertise in providing care to a particular client
When nurses collaborate with other disciplines such as physical therapy, nutritionists, respiratory therapy, and social service, they may offer recommendations for management of a problem. These recommendations can either be made informally to the nurse and added to the care plan at the discretion of the nurse or ordered by the discipline on the order record according to the institutional policies.

### ◀◀ Carp's Cues

Other disciplines should not add interventions to the care plan unless it is a multidiscipline care plan. These interventions on a multidiscipline care plan would indicate what care that discipline is providing.

When the care plan is not multidisciplinary and a physical therapist has recommendations for nursing interventions for a client, the nurse will determine if these interventions are to be added to the care plan.

This is the same as when a physician requests a specialist to see a client. The specialist does not write orders for the client but instead communicates recommendations in a consultation report.

This is a very important distinction. Prior to adding interventions for nursing staff to implement, the nurse must evaluate available resources and appropriateness for this client situation. When nurses collaborate with physicians to co-treat problems, the physician prescribes treatments, diagnostic studies, and therapies. These prescriptions are not optional. They are legal. If the nurse disagrees with the orders for the client, the nurse must discuss this with the physician and/or nurse manager. As with any collaborative relationships, functions and activities sometimes overlap.

## Bifocal Clinical Practice Model

In 1983, Carpenito introduced a model for practice that describes the clinical focus of professional nurses in addition to NANDA nursing diagnoses. This *bifocal clinical practice model* identifies the two clinical situations in which nurses intervene: one as primary prescriber and the other in collaboration with medicine. This model not only organizes the focus of nursing practice, but also helps distinguish nursing from other health care disciplines.

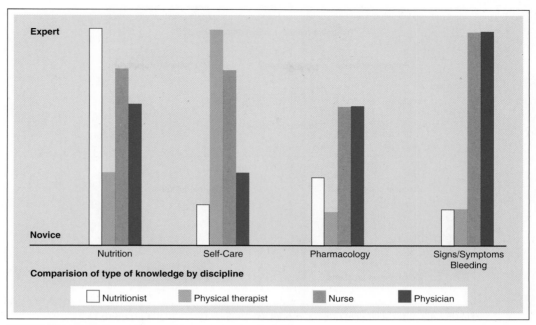

**FIGURE 4.1** Comparison of type of knowledge by discipline.

◀◀ **Carp's Cues**

Collaborative problems are specifically defined as problems that require both medicine and nursing interventions to treat. Collaboration with other disciplines (e.g., physical therapy, nutritionists, respiratory therapists, and the use nursing diagnosis) is discussed in Chapter 1.

Nursing derives its knowledge from various disciplines, including biology, medicine, pharmacology, psychology, nutrition, and physical therapy. Nursing differs from other disciplines in its wide range of knowledge. Figure 4.1 illustrates the varied types of such knowledge as compared with other disciplines. Certainly, the nutritionist has more expertise in the field of nutrition, and the pharmacist in the field of therapeutic pharmacology, than any nurse has. But every nurse brings knowledge of nutrition and pharmacology to client interactions that is sufficient for most clinical situations. (And when a nurse's knowledge is insufficient, nursing practice calls for consultation with appropriate disciplines.)

No other discipline has this wide knowledge base, possibly explaining why past attempts to substitute other disciplines for nursing have proved costly and ultimately unsuccessful. For this reason, any workable model for nursing practice must encompass all the varied situations in which nurses intervene, while also identifying situations in nursing that non-nursing personnel must address.

Nursing prescribes for and treats client and group *responses* to situations. These situations can be organized into five categories:

1. Pathophysiologic (e.g., myocardial infarction, borderline personality, burns)
2. Treatment-related (e.g., anticoagulant therapy, dialysis, arteriography)
3. Personal (e.g., dying, divorce, relocation)
4. Environmental (e.g., overcrowded school, no handrails on steps, rodents)

Maturational (e.g., peer pressure, parenthood, aging)
The bifocal clinical practice model, diagrammed in Figure 4.2, identifies these responses as either *nursing diagnoses* or *collaborative problems*. Together, nursing diagnoses and collaborative problems represent the range of conditions that necessitate nursing care. The major assumptions in the bifocal clinical practice model:

1. **Client***
   • Has the power for self-healing
   • Continually interrelates with the environment
   • Makes decisions according to individual priorities

---

*The term client can be an individual, a family, significant others, a group, or a community.

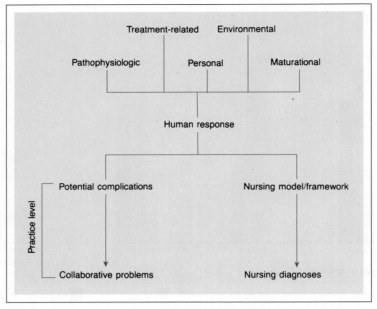

FIGURE 4.2 Bifocal clinical nursing model. (© 1985 by Lynda Juall Carpenito.)

- Is a unified whole, seeking balance
- Has individual worth and dignity
- Is an expert on own health

2. **Health**
   - Is a dynamic, ever-changing state
   - Is defined by the client
   - Is an expression of optimum well-being
   - Is the responsibility of the client

3. **Environment**
   - Represents external factors, situations, and people who influence or are influenced by the client
   - Includes physical and ecologic environments, life events, and treatment modalities

4. **Nursing**
   - Is accessed by the client when he or she needs assistance to improve, restore, or maintain health or to achieve a peaceful death (Henderson & Nite, 1960)
   - Ensures the client has the needed information for an informed consent
   - Supports the right of the client to refuse recommendations
   - Engages the client to assume responsibility in self-healing decisions and practices
   - Reduces or eliminates environmental factors that can or do cause compromised functioning

# Understanding Collaborative Problems

Carpenito (1999) defines collaborative problems as:

> Certain physiologic complications that nurses monitor to detect onset or changes in status. Nurses manage collaborative problems using physician-prescribed and nursing-prescribed interventions to minimize the complications of the events.

The designation *certain* clarifies that all physiologic complications are not collaborative problems. If the nurse can prevent the onset of the complication or provide the primary treatment for it, then the diagnosis is a nursing diagnosis. For example:

| Nurses can prevent: | Nursing diagnosis: |
| --- | --- |
| Pressure ulcers | *Risk for Impaired Skin Integrity* |
| Thrombophlebitis | *Ineffective Peripheral Tissue Perfusion* |
| Complications of immobility | *Disuse Syndrome* |
| Aspiration | *Risk for Aspiration* |

| Nurses can treat: | Nursing diagnosis: |
| --- | --- |
| Stage I or II pressure ulcers | *Impaired Skin Integrity* |

| Swallowing problems | *Impaired Swallowing* |
|---|---|
| Ineffective cough | *Ineffective Airway Clearing* |
| **Nurses cannot prevent:** | **Collaborative problems:** |
| Seizures | Seizures |
| Bleeding | Bleeding |

## Prevention Versus Detection

Nurses can prevent some physiologic complications, such as pressure ulcers and infection from invasive lines. Prevention differs from detection. Nurses do not prevent hemorrhage or seizure; instead, they monitor to detect its presence early to prevent greater severity of complication or even death. Physicians cannot treat collaborative problems without nursing's knowledge, vigilance, and judgment. For collaborative problems, nurses institute orders, such as position changes, client teaching, or specific protocols, in addition to monitoring.

Unlike medical diagnoses, however, nursing diagnoses represent situations that are the primary responsibility of nurses, who diagnose onset and manage changes in status. When a situation no longer requires nursing management, the client is discharged from nursing care.

For a collaborative problem, nursing focuses on monitoring for onset or change in status of physiologic complications and on responding to any such changes with physician-prescribed and nurse-prescribed nursing interventions. The nurse makes independent decisions for both collaborative problems and nursing diagnoses. The difference is that for nursing diagnoses, nursing prescribes the definitive treatment to achieve the desired outcome; in contrast, for collaborative problems, prescription for definitive treatment comes from both nursing and medicine.

Even though a nurse cannot prevent bleeding, early detection will prevent hemorrhage. Thus, for collaborative problems, nurses can detect onset of a physiologic problem such as urinary bleeding or decreased urine output. The nurse can also monitor for changes in an existing problem such as high blood pressure or pneumonia.

## Collaborative Problem Diagnostic Statements

This edition has changed the label for all collaborative problems to *Risk for Complications of* (RC of). For example:

- *Risk for Complications of Renal Failure*
- *Risk for Complications of Peptic Ulcer*
- *Risk for Complications of Asthma*

This label indicates that the nursing focus is to reduce the severity of certain physiologic factors or events. For example, *Risk for Complications of Hypertension* alerts the nurse that this client is either experiencing or at high risk for hypertension. In either event, the nurse will receive a report on the status of the collaborative problem or will proceed to evaluate the client's blood pressure. Changing the terminology to distinguish whether the client is actually hypertensive or simply at risk is not necessary or realistic, given the fluctuating condition of most clients. The following illustrates this difference.

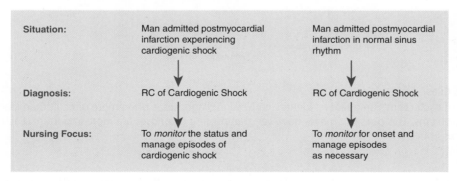

| Situation: | Man admitted postmyocardial infarction experiencing cardiogenic shock | Man admitted postmyocardial infarction in normal sinus rhythm |
|---|---|---|
| Diagnosis: | RC of Cardiogenic Shock | RC of Cardiogenic Shock |
| Nursing Focus: | To *monitor* the status and manage episodes of cardiogenic shock | To *monitor* for onset and manage episodes as necessary |

If the nurse is managing a cluster or group of complications, he or she may record the collaborative problems together:

- *Risk for Complications of Cardiac Dysfunction*
- *Risk for Complications of Pacemaker Insertion*

The nurse also can word the collaborative problem to reflect a specific cause, as in *Risk for Complications of Hyperglycemia related to long-term corticosteroid therapy.* In most cases, however, such a link is unnecessary.

#### ◄◄ Carp's Cues

When writing collaborative problem statements, the nurse must make sure not to omit the stem *Risk for Complications of.* This stem designates that nurse-prescribed interventions are required for treatment. Without the stem, the collaborative problem could be misread as a medical diagnosis, in which case nursing involvement becomes subordinate to medicine, the discipline primarily responsible for the diagnosis and treatment of medical conditions.

## Differentiating Nursing Diagnoses from Collaborative Problems _____

Both nursing diagnoses and collaborative problems involve all steps of the nursing process: assessment, diagnosis, planning, implementation, and evaluation. Each, however, requires a different approach from the nurse.

### Assessment and Diagnosis

For nursing diagnoses, assessment involves data collection to identify signs and symptoms of actual nursing diagnoses or risk factors for high-risk nursing diagnoses. For collaborative problems, assessment focuses on determining physiologic stability or risk for instability. The nurse identifies a collaborative problem when certain situations increase the client's vulnerability for a complication or the client has experienced one.

Collaborative problems usually are associated with a specific pathology or treatment. For example, all clients who have undergone abdominal surgery are at some risk for such problems as hemorrhage and urinary retention. Expert nursing knowledge is required to assess a particular client's specific risk for these problems and to identify them early to prevent complications and death. Table 4.1 illustrates the difference.

Medical diagnoses are not useful problem statements for nurses. For example, diabetes mellitus is not the problem focus. Instead, hypoglycemia or hyperglycemia is used. Sometimes the medical diagnosis and the collaborative problem use the same terminology, such as seizures or hyperkalcemia. The key is: Can the nurse monitor the condition? The nurse monitors for hyperglycemia or hypoglycemia, not diabetes mellitus.

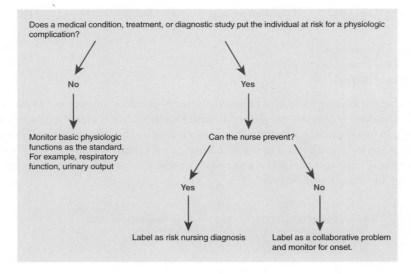

#### ◄◄ Carp's Cues

Because of each client's uniqueness, identifying nursing diagnoses is often more difficult than identifying collaborative problems. This does not mean, however, that nursing diagnoses are more important. Each client's situation determines importance.

### Goals

Nursing diagnoses and collaborative problems have different implications for goals. Bulechek and McCloskey (1985) define *goals* as "guideposts to the selection of nursing interventions and criteria in the evaluation of nursing interventions." These authors continue by saying that "readily identifiable and logical links should exist between the diagnoses and the plan of care, and the activities prescribed should assist or enable the client to meet the identified expected outcome." Thus, goals and interventions can be critical to differentiating nursing diagnoses from collaborative problems that nurses treat.

**TABLE 4.1  NURSING DIAGNOSES AND COLLABORATIVE PROBLEMS**

|  | Nursing Diagnoses | Collaborative Problems |
|---|---|---|
| Assessment | Requires data collection of risk factors (risk dx) or sign/symptoms of actual nursing diagnoses | No specific assessment is needed because certain collaborative problems will be addressed when specific medical conditions, treatments of diagnostic studies make the client high risk for a physiologic complication to occur |
| **Focus of interventions** |  | **Monitoring for physiological instability** |
|  | To prevent risk nsg dx | Institute nursing interventions to minimize the severity of the complication |
|  | To reduce or eliminate an actual dsg dx | Consult with medicine for medical orders for the client |

INTERACTIVE EXERCISE

**4.1**

You read on a care plan the following:

*Risk for Deficient Fluid Volume related to loss of fluids during surgery and possible hemorrhage postoperatively*
**Goal:** The client will demonstrate BP and pulse within normal limits and no bleeding.
**Interventions:**

1. Monitor intake of IV fluids.
2. Monitor vital signs every hour.
3. Inspect dressing for s/s of bleeding.
4. Monitor urine output hourly.

Notify physician with changes as needed.
During your care of this client, his urine output decreases and his pulse increases. What would you do? (Answer at the end of this chapter.)

Client goals are inappropriate for collaborative problems. They represent criteria that nurses cannot use to evaluate the effectiveness or appropriateness of nursing interventions. Collaborative problems have nursing goals such as RC of Hypoglycemia.

## Nursing Goal

The nurse will monitor for early signs and symptoms of hypoglycemia and collaboratively intervene to stabilize the client.

## Indicators

Fasting blood sugar        70–110 mg/dL
Clear, oriented

The indicators are used as monitoring criteria.

## Interventions

Nursing interventions can be classified as two types: nurse-prescribed and physician-prescribed (*delegated*). Regardless of type, all nursing interventions require astute nursing judgment because the nurse is legally accountable for intervening appropriately.

For both nursing diagnoses and collaborative problems, the nurse makes independent decisions concerning nursing interventions. The nature of these decisions differs, however. For nursing diagnoses, the nurse independently prescribes the primary treatment for goal achievement. In contrast, for collaborative problems, the nurse confers with a physician and implements physician-prescribed as well as nurse-prescribed nursing interventions.

*Primary treatment* describes those interventions that are most responsible for successful outcome achievement. Nevertheless, these are not the only interventions used to treat the diagnosed condition. For example, interventions for a client with the nursing diagnosis *Impaired Physical Mobility related to incisional pain* might include the following:

- Explain the need for moving and ambulation.
- Teach client how to splint the incision before coughing, deep breathing, sitting up, or turning in bed.
- If pain relief medication is scheduled PRN, instruct the client to request medication as soon as the pain returns.
- Evaluate if pain relief is satisfactory; if not, contact the physician for increased dosages or decreased interval between doses.
- Schedule activities, bathing, and ambulation to correspond with times when the client's comfort level is highest.
- Discuss and negotiate ambulation goals with the client.

All of these are nurse-prescribed interventions. A physician-prescribed intervention for this client might be Demerol 75 mg IM q4h. This medication is important to manage the client's postoperative pain; however, it alone cannot be considered a primary treatment.

The difference between a nursing diagnosis and a collaborative problem is illustrated on p. 28.

**INTERACTIVE EXERCISE** 4.2

Refer to Section 3 under collaborative problem RC of GI Bleeding, p. 911. Review the interventions and label each one as nurse-prescribed or physician-prescribed. (Refer to answers at the end of the chapter.)

## Monitoring Versus Prevention

Is monitoring an intervention? Interventions are directed at improving a person's condition or preventing a problem. *Monitoring* involves continually collecting selected data to evaluate whether the client's condition has changed (improved, deteriorated, not improved, or remained within a normal range). Monitoring does not improve a client's health status or prevent a problem; rather, it provides information necessary to determine *if* or *what type* of interventions are needed. Monitoring detects problems. It is associated with every type of nursing diagnosis and collaborative problem:

- For actual nursing diagnosis, monitor the client's condition for improvement.
- For risk nursing diagnosis, monitor the client for signs of the problem.
- For wellness nursing diagnosis, monitor the client's participation in lifestyle changes.
- For collaborative problems, monitor for onset or change in status of a problem.

Although monitoring does not qualify as an intervention, it is an activity. For convenience, monitoring is included with the interventions for the diagnoses presented in Sections 2 and 3.

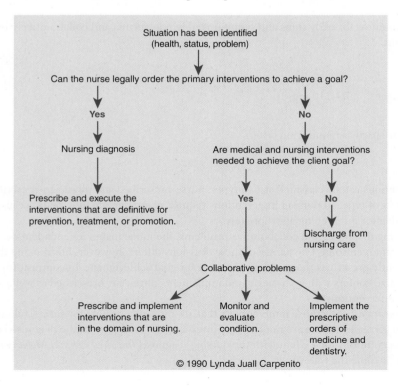

© 1990 Lynda Juall Carpenito

# Evaluation

The nurse evaluates a client's status and progress differently for nursing diagnoses and collaborative problems. When evaluating nursing diagnoses, the nurse:

* Assesses the client's status
* Compares this response to the goals
* Concludes whether the client is progressing toward outcome achievement

For example, a client has the following goal:

* Will walk 25 feet with assistance by June 18.

Today (June 16) the client walked 20 feet with assistance.

The nurse concludes that he is progressing to goal achievement by June 18. The nurse can record this evaluation on a flow record or on a progress note.

In contrast, to evaluate collaborative problems, the nurse:

* Collects selected data
* Compares data with established norms
* Judges whether the data are within an acceptable range

For example, a client has a nursing goal:

* The nurse will detect early signs/symptoms of pneumonia and collaboratively intervene to stabilize the client.

**INTERACTIVE**
**EXERCISE**  4.3

## Case Study 1

Mr. Smith, 35 years old, is admitted for a possible concussion after a motor vehicle collision, with a physician's order for a clear liquid diet and a neurologic assessment every hour. On admission, the nurse records the following on a flow record:

* Oriented and alert
* Pupils 6 mm, equal, and reactive to light
* BP 120/72, pulse 84, resp 20, temp 99°F

Two hours later, the nurse records the following on the nurse's or progress note:

* Vomiting
* Restlessness
* Pupils 6 mm, equal, with a sluggish response to light
* BP 140/60, pulse 65, resp 12, temp 99°F

*Problem:* Possible increased intracranial pressure (ICP)
Now, apply the following criteria questions:
Q: Can the nurse legally order the primary interventions to achieve the client goal (which would be a reversal of the increasing ICP)?
Q: Are medical and nursing interventions needed for goal achievement? (Answers at the end of chapter.)

## Case Study 2

Mr. Green, 45 years old, has a cholecystectomy incision (10 days postop) that is not healing and has continual purulent drainage. The nursing care consists of:

* Inspecting and cleansing the incision and the surrounding area q8h
* Applying a drainage pouch
* Promoting optimal nutrition and hydration to enhance healing

*Problem:* Adjacent skin at risk for erosion
Now apply the criteria questions:
Q: Can the nurse legally order the definitive interventions to achieve the goals (which would be continued intact surrounding tissue)? (Answer at end of chapter.)

## *Indicators*

Respiration 16 to 20 per minute, breath sounds equal, no adventitious sounds.
Oxygen saturation (pulse oximetry) greater than 95

Today the clinical data were respirations 18, breath sounds equal, no adventitious sounds and a pulse ox of 98. The nurse concludes that the client is stable.

The nurse records the assessment data for collaborative problems on flow records or on progress notes if findings are significant. Nurses evaluate whether the collaborative problem has improved, has worsened, is stable, or is unchanged. They also notify physicians if changes in treatment are indicated.

Thus, evaluation of nursing diagnoses focuses on progress toward achieving client goals, whereas evaluation for collaborative problems focuses on the client's status compared with established norms. Evaluation is discussed further in Chapter 5.

## Summary

According to Wallace and Ivey (1989), "Understanding which nursing diagnoses are most effective and the situations in which the term collaborative problem is best applied helps group the mass of data the nurse must consider." The bifocal clinical practice model provides a structure for forming this understanding. In doing so, it uniquely distinguishes nursing from other health care professions, while providing nurses with a logical description of the focus of clinical nursing.

## ANSWERS TO INTERACTIVE EXERCISES

### 4.1

Call the physician because the interventions needed are medical treatments. This situation is not a nursing diagnosis, because the nurse does not order the treatment needed. As a collaborative problem, it would be better described as *Risk for Complications of Bleeding*. A goal would be "The nurse will monitor for and manage changes in status."

### 4.2

Of the 11 interventions, the first five are nurse-prescribed, and the remaining six are physician-prescribed. Nursing is responsible for all 11 interventions, although medicine prescribes some.

### 4.3

#### Case Study 1

1. No, nurses do not definitively treat or prevent increased ICP. They collaborate with the physician for definitive treatment.
2. Yes, medical and nursing interventions are needed.

Yes
↓
Collaborative problem
RC of Increased Intracranial Pressure

| ↓ | | ↓ |
| --- | --- | --- |
| Prescribes and implements interventions within the domain of nursing | Monitors and evaluates the client's condition | Implements the prescriptive orders of medicine |

In this situation, the nurse would monitor to detect increasing ICP. The nurse also prescribes interventions that reduce ICP, but these interventions are not considered primary and must be accompanied by physician-prescribed treatments. This problem is the joint responsibility of medicine and nursing.

#### Case Study 2

Yes, nurses do prescribe interventions that will prevent skin erosion as a result of wound drainage.

↓
Nursing diagnosis
↓

*Risk for Impaired Skin Integrity related to draining purulent wound*

In this situation, the nurse would prescribe the interventions to preserve adjacent skin. No collaboration with medicine is warranted.

Because each client is unique, developing exclusive criteria that will always differentiate nursing diagnoses from other client problems is difficult. Ultimately, the decision to use or not to use a nursing diagnosis label rests with the individual nurse until more refined defining characteristics for each diagnosis are developed and tested.

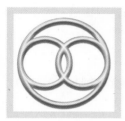

# 5

# PLANNING CARE WITH NURSING DIAGNOSIS

### Learning Objectives

After reading the chapter, the student should be able to answer the following questions:

- What are functional health patterns?
- How are priority nursing diagnoses identified?
- What is the difference between nursing and client goals?
- How is evaluation different for nursing diagnoses and collaborative problems?
- What are standardized care plans?

Because clients require nursing care 7 days a week and 24 hours a day, nurses must rely on one another and nonlicensed nursing personnel to help clients achieve outcomes of care. Obviously, some system of communication is necessary. For more than 30 years, this system consisted of handwritten care plans or verbal reports, neither of which was very useful. This chapter addresses the varied methods that nurses use today to communicate a client's care to other caregivers.

## Data Collection Formats

Data collection usually consists of two formats: the nursing baseline or screening assessment and the focus or ongoing assessment. The nurse can use each alone or together. As discussed in Chapter 3, nurses encounter, diagnose, and treat two types of response: nursing diagnoses and collaborative problems. Each type requires a different assessment focus.

### Initial, Baseline, or Screening Assessment

An initial, baseline, or screening assessment involves collecting a predetermined set of data during initial contact with the client (e.g., on admission, first home visit). This assessment serves as a tool for "narrowing the universe of possibilities" (Gordon, 1994). During this assessment, the nurse interprets data as significant or insignificant. This process is explored later in this chapter.

The nurse should organize the initial assessment to permit systematic, efficient data collection. Appendix B illustrates an assessment form with checking or circling options, which can help save time during documentation. The nurse always can elaborate with additional questions and comments. Open-ended questions are better for assessment of certain functional areas, such as fear or anxiety. Nurses should view printed assessment forms as guides, not mandates. Before requesting information from a client, nurses should ask themselves, "What am I going to do with the data?" If certain information is useless or irrelevant for a particular client, then its collection is unnecessary and potentially distressing. For example, asking a terminally ill client how much he or she smokes is unnecessary unless the nurse has a specific goal. If a client will be NPO, collecting data about eating habits is probably unnecessary. Such assessment will be indicated if the client resumes eating.

If a client is extremely stressed, the nurse should collect only necessary data and defer the assessment of functional patterns to another time. A stressed client is not the best source of data, because stress may cloud the memory.

### *Functional Health Patterns*

As discussed earlier, nursing assessment focuses on collecting data that validate nursing diagnoses. Gordon's system of functional health patterns provides an excellent, relevant format for nursing data collection to determine an individual's or group's health status and functioning (1994). After data collection is complete, the nurse and client can determine positive functioning, altered functioning, or at-risk for altered functioning. Altered functioning is defined as functioning that the client (individual or group) perceives as negative or undesirable. Refer to Box 5.1 for functional health patterns.

Refer to Appendix B for a sample initial assessment organized according to functional health patterns. It is designed to assist the nurse in gathering subjective and objective data. Should questions arise

## BOX 5.1 FUNCTIONAL HEALTH PATTERNS

1. **Health Perception–Health Management Pattern**
   - Perceived pattern of health, well-being
   - Knowledge of lifestyle and relationship to health
   - Knowledge of preventive health practices
   - Adherence to medical, nursing prescriptions

2. **Nutritional–Metabolic Pattern**
   - Usual pattern of food and fluid intake
   - Types of food and fluid intake
   - Actual weight, weight loss or gain
   - Appetite, preferences

3. **Elimination Pattern**
   - Bowel elimination pattern, changes
   - Bladder elimination pattern, changes
   - Control problems
   - Use of assistive devices
   - Use of medications

4. **Activity–Exercise Pattern**
   - Pattern of exercise, activity, leisure, recreation
   - Ability to perform activities of daily living (self-care, home maintenance, work, eating, shopping, cooking)

5. **Sleep–Rest Pattern**
   - Patterns of sleep, rest
   - Perception of quality, quantity

6. **Cognitive–Perceptual Pattern**
   - Vision, learning, taste, touch, smell
   - Language adequacy
   - Memory
   - Decision-making ability, patterns
   - Complaints of discomforts

7. **Self-Perception–Self-Concept Pattern**
   - Attitudes about self, sense of worth
   - Perception of abilities
   - Emotional patterns
   - Body image, identity

8. **Role–Relationship Patterns**
   - Patterns of relationships
   - Role responsibilities
   - Satisfaction with relationships and responsibilities

9. **Sexuality–Reproductive Pattern**
   - Menstrual, reproductive history
   - Satisfaction with sexual relationships, sexual identity
   - Premenopausal or postmenopausal problems
   - Accuracy of sex education

10. **Coping–Stress Tolerance Patterns**
    - Ability to manage stress
    - Knowledge of stress tolerance
    - Sources of support
    - Number of stressful life events in last year

11. **Value–Belief Pattern**
    - Values, goals, beliefs
    - Spiritual practices
    - Perceived conflicts in values

concerning a pattern, the nurse would gather more data about the diagnosis by using the focus assessment under the diagnosis.

When collecting data according to the functional health patterns, the nurse questions, observes, and evaluates the client or family. For example, under the Cognitive–Perceptual Pattern, the nurse asks the client if he or she has difficulty hearing, observes if the client is wearing a hearing aid, and evaluates if the client understands English.

## Physical Assessment

In addition to functional health pattern assessment, the nurse also collects data related to body system functioning. Physical assessment, the collection of objective data concerning the client's physical status, incorporates head-to-toe examination, with a focus on the body systems. The techniques used include inspection, palpation, percussion, and auscultation.

Appendix B lists those areas of physical assessment in which nurse generalists should be proficient. Physical assessment by nurses should be clearly "nursing" in focus. By examining their philosophy and definition of nursing, nurses should seek to develop expertise in those areas that will enhance nursing practice.

Keep in mind that separation of functional health patterns from physical assessment is done for organizational purposes only. No useful nursing assessment framework can restrict actual data collection in such a manner. Because humans are open systems, a problem in one functional health pattern invariably influences body system functioning or functioning in another functional health pattern. Anxiety can effect appetite; Sleep problems can increase coping difficulties

INTERACTIVE **5.1**
EXERCISE

Mr. Gene, 61 years old, is admitted for neurologic surgery. He has a history of peripheral vascular disease and Parkinson's disease. The nurse's initial assessment reveals the following under the functional health pattern Activity–Exercise and physical assessment of musculoskeletal function:

**ACTIVITY-EXERCISE PATTERN**
SELF-CARE ABILITY:

0 = Independent     1 = Assistive device     2 = Assistance from others
3 = Assistance from person and equipment     4 = Dependent/Unable

| | 0 | 1 | 2 | 3 | 4 |
|---|---|---|---|---|---|
| Eating/Drinking | ✓ | | | | |
| Bathing | | | ✓ | | |
| Dressing/Grooming | | | ✓ | | |
| Toileting | | | ✓ | | |
| Bed Mobility | | | ✓ | | |
| Transferring | | | ✓ | | |
| Ambulating | | ✓ | | | |
| Stair Climbing | ✓ | | | | |
| Shopping | | | | | ✓ |
| Cooking | | | | | ✓ |
| Home Maintenance | | | | | ✓ |

ASSISTIVE DEVICES: ____ None ____ Crutches ____ Bedside commode _✓_ Walker
____ Cane ____ Splint/Brace ____ Wheelchair ____ Other ____

**PHYSICAL ASSESSMENT**
MUSCULAR–SKELETAL
Range of Motion: _✓_ Full ____ Other _____
Balance and Gait: ____ Steady _✓_ Unsteady
Hand Grasps: _✓_ Equal _✓_ Strong ____ Weakness/Paralysis (____ Right ____ Left)
Leg Muscles: ____ Equal ____ Strong _✓_ Weakness/Paralysis (_✓_ Right ____ Left)

Examine the above assessment data. What data are significant? (Answers at end of chapter)

## Focus Assessment

Focus assessment is the acquisition of selected or specific data as determined by the nurse and the client or family, or by the client's condition. The nurse who assesses the condition of a new postoperative client (vital signs, incision, hydration, comfort) is performing a focus assessment. These are ongoing assessments.

The nurse also can perform a focus assessment during the initial interview if collected data suggest a possible problem that the nurse must validate or rule out. For example, during the baseline interview, the nurse suspects that certain data $(S_1, S_2)$ may represent a nursing diagnosis. The nurse considers a possible or tentative diagnosis. The nurse then collects additional data (focus assessment) to confirm or rule out the tentative diagnosis.

## The Care Planning Process

Today, the methods used to communicate client care between nurses and other caregivers vary. Critical pathways, automated care planning systems, and preprinted standardized care plans have replaced handwritten care plans. Later in this chapter, types of care planning systems will be discussed.

Critical pathways and standardized care plans reflect the expected diagnoses and associated goals and interventions commonly related to a client's medical or surgical problem. This type of system frees nurses from the repetitive writing of routine care. The care outlined on the standardized plan or critical pathway should represent the responsible care to which the client is entitled.

Before discussing the care planning process, the nurse must identify the type, as well as the duration, of needed care. People receiving nursing care for less than 8 h, as in the emergency department, short-stay surgery, or recovery room, have a specific medical diagnosis or need a specific procedure. The nursing care must be specific for the condition and length of stay, which can be organized on a standardized care plan or pathway. Additions to this predicted care must be made according to client needs and length of stay. This is also true for hospital admissions for acute illness or surgical procedures.

In nonacute settings such as long-term care, community or home care, or assisted-living and rehabilitation units, nurses usually must supplement critical pathways and standardized plans with personalized care plans. The longer the nurse–client relationship is, the more data are available to individualize the plan.

People with an acute episode of a chronic illness (multiple sclerosis), rehabilitation needs (stroke), or a terminal illness require a different approach. They need care plans and problem lists.

## Planning

Care plans represent the planning, not the delivery, of care. This planning phase of the nursing process has three components:

1.  Establishing a priority set of diagnoses
2.  Designating client goals and nursing goals
3.  Prescribing nursing interventions

### Establishing a Priority Set of Diagnoses

Realistically, a nurse cannot hope to address all, or even most, of the nursing diagnoses and collaborative problems that can apply to an individual, family, or community. By identifying a priority set—a group of nursing diagnoses and collaborative problems that take precedence over others—the nurse can best direct resources toward goal achievement. Differentiating priority diagnoses from non-priority diagnoses is crucial:

- *Priority diagnoses* are those nursing diagnoses or collaborative problems that, if not managed now, will deter progress to achieve outcomes or will negatively affect functional status.
- *Non-priority diagnoses* are those nursing diagnoses or collaborative problems for which treatment can be delayed without compromising present functional status.

#### ◀◀ Carp's Cues

Numbering the diagnoses on a problem list does not indicate priority; rather, it shows the order in which the nurse entered them on the list. Assigning absolute priority to nursing diagnoses or collaborative problems can create the false assumption that number one is automatically the first priority. In the clinical setting, priorities can shift rapidly as the client's condition changes. For this reason, the nurse must view the entire problem list as the priority set, with priorities shifting within the list periodically.

### Priority Diagnoses

In an acute care setting, the client enters the hospital for a specific purpose, such as surgery or other treatments for acute illness. In such a situation, certain nursing diagnoses or collaborative problems requiring specific nursing interventions often apply. Carpenito (1995) uses the term *diagnostic cluster* to describe such a group; this cluster can appear in a critical pathway or standardized plan of care.

For example, the following is a diagnostic cluster for a person having abdominal surgery.

## ▪▪▪▪▪■ DIAGNOSTIC CLUSTER

### Preoperative

*Nursing Diagnosis*
- Anxiety/Fear related to surgical experience, loss of control, unpredictable outcome, and insufficient knowledge of preoperative routines, postoperative exercises and activities, and postoperative changes and sensations

## ▪▪▪▪▪▪ DIAGNOSTIC CLUSTER *Continued*

### Preoperative

*Collaborative Problems*

RC of Hemorrhage
RC of Hypovolemia/Shock
RC of Evisceration/Dehiscence
RC of Paralytic Ileus
RC of Infection (Peritonitis)
RC of Urinary Retention
RC of Thrombophlebitis

*Nursing Diagnosis*

- Risk for Ineffective Respiratory Function related to immobility secondary to postanesthesia state and pain
- Risk for Infection related to a site for organism invasion secondary to surgery
- Acute Pain related to surgical interruption of body structures, flatus, and immobility
- Risk for Imbalanced Nutrition: Less Than Body Requirements related to increased protein and vitamin requirements for wound healing and decreased intake secondary to pain, nausea, vomiting, and diet restrictions
- Risk for Constipation related to decreased peristalsis secondary to immobility and the effects of anesthesia and opioids
- Activity Intolerance related to pain and weakness secondary to anesthesia, tissue hypoxia, and insufficient fluid and nutrient intake
- Risk for Ineffective Therapeutic Regimen Management related to insufficient knowledge of care of operative site, restrictions (diet, activity), medications, signs and symptoms of complications, and follow-up care.

All of these diagnoses are priority diagnoses.

When should additional diagnoses (other than in the diagnostic cluster) be added to the problem list or care plan:

- What nursing diagnoses or collaborative problems are associated with the primary condition (e.g., surgery)?
- Are there additional collaborative problems associated with coexisting medical conditions that require monitoring (e.g., hypoglycemia)?
- Are there additional nursing diagnoses that, if not managed or prevented now, will deter recovery or affect the client's functional status (e.g., *High Risk for Constipation*)?
- What problems does the client perceive as priority?

## INTERACTIVE EXERCISE    **5.2**

Mr. Stanley, 76 years old, is admitted for emergency gastric surgery for repair of a bleeding ulcer. He also has diabetes mellitus and peripheral vascular disease. After completing a functional assessment, the nurse identifies the following:

- Compromised gait
- Occasional incontinence when walking to the bathroom
- Wife complaining of many caregiver responsibilities and an unmotivated husband

Examine the data above and begin to formulate nursing diagnoses and collaborative problems that need nursing interventions. Refer to the four questions above to assist with this analysis and to determine whether Mr. Stanley and his family have other diagnoses that require nursing interventions. Mr. Stanley's priority list (diagnostic cluster) follows.

*RC of Urinary retention*
*RC of Hemorrhage*
*RC of Hypovolemia/shock*
*RC of Pneumonia (stasis)*
*RC of Peritonitis*
*RC of Thrombophlebitis*
*RC of Paralytic ileus*
*RC of Evisceration*
*RC of Dehiscence*

Risk for Infection related to destruction of first line of defense
    against bacterial invasion
Risk for Impaired Respiratory Function related to postanesthesia
    state, postoperative immobility, and pain
Impaired Physical Mobility related to pain and weakness secondary
    to anesthesia, tissue hypoxia, and insufficient fluids/nutrients
Risk for Imbalanced Nutrition: Less Than Body Requirements
    related to increased protein/vitamin requirements for wound
    healing and decreased intake secondary to pain, nausea, vomiting,
    and diet restrictions
Risk for Compromised Human Dignity related to multiple factors
    associated with hospitalization
Risk for Ineffective Therapeutic Regimen Management related to
    insufficient knowledge of home care, incisional care, signs and
    symptoms of complications, activity restriction, and follow-up care

> From postoperative standard of care (diagnostic cluster)

*RC of Hypo/Hyperglycemia*

> From medical history of diabetes mellitus

Possible Functional Incontinence related to reports of occasional
    incontinence when walking to bathroom

> From nursing admission assessment

High Risk for Caregiver Role Strain (wife) related to multiple
    caregiver responsibilities and progressive deterioration of husband

> From nursing admission assessment

High Risk for Injury related to altered gait and deconditioning
    secondary to peripheral vascular disease and decreased motivation

> From medical history of peripheral vascular disease and reports of prolonged immobility

## Non-Priority Nursing Diagnoses

Non-priority diagnoses that are identified are referred for management after discharge. For example, for a client who is 50 lb overweight and hospitalized after myocardial infarction, the nurse eventually would want to explain the effects of obesity on cardiac function and refer the client to a weight-reduction program after discharge. The discharge summary record would reflect the teaching and referral; a nursing diagnosis related to weight reduction would not need to appear on the problem list.

Mr. and Mrs. Stanley probably have many other important but non-priority nursing diagnoses; however, because of the limited length of stay, nursing resources must be directed toward those problems that will deter progress at this time. The nurse can discuss important diagnoses with the client and family, with recommendations for future attention (e.g., referral to a community agency).

## Designating Client Goals and Nursing Goals

Client goals (outcome criteria) and nursing goals are standards or measures used to evaluate the client's progress (outcome) or the nurse's performance (process). According to Alfaro (2009), *client goals* are statements describing a measurable behavior of the client, family, or group that denotes a favorable status (changed or maintained) after the delivery of nursing care. *Nursing goals* are statements describing measurable actions that denote the nurse's accountability for the situation or diagnosis. As discussed in Chapter 4, nursing diagnoses have client goals, whereas collaborative problems have nursing goals.

Certain situations may call for involvement from several disciplines. For example, for a client experiencing extreme anxiety, the physician may prescribe an antianxiety medication, an occupational therapist may provide diversional activities, and a nurse may institute nonpharmacologic anxiety-reducing measures, such as relaxation exercises. According to Gordon (1994), "Saying a nursing diagnosis is a health problem a nurse can treat does not mean that non-nursing consultants cannot be used. The critical element is whether the nurse-prescribed interventions can achieve the outcome established with the client."

INTERACTIVE
EXERCISE

**5.3**

Examine the following goals:

*The client will*

- Demonstrate stable vital signs
- Have electrolytes within normal range
- Have cardiac rhythm and rate within normal limits
- Have blood loss within acceptable limits after surgery

While you are caring for this client, his cardiac rhythm becomes abnormal and his surgical wound begins to bleed. What would you do?

- Change the nursing interventions.
- Revise the goal.
- Change the diagnosis.
- Call the doctor for physician-prescribed interventions.

(Answer at end of chapter)

## Revaluating the Goal

If a client goal is not achieved or progress toward achievement is not evident, the nurse must reevaluate the attainability of the goal or review the nursing care plan, asking the following questions (Carpenito, 1999):

- Is the diagnosis correct?
- Has the goal been set mutually? Is the client participating?
- Is more time needed for the plan to work?
- Does the goal need to be revised?
- Does the plan need to be revised?
- Are physician-prescribed interventions needed?

## Goals for Collaborative Problems

As discussed earlier, identifying client goals for collaborative problems is inappropriate and can imply erroneous accountability for nurses. Rather, collaborative problems involve nursing goals that reflect nursing accountability in situations requiring physician-prescribed and nurse-prescribed interventions. This accountability includes (1) monitoring for physiologic instability, (2) consulting standing orders and protocols or a physician to obtain orders for appropriate interventions, (3) performing specific actions to manage and to reduce the severity of an event or situation, and (4) evaluating client responses.

Nursing goals for collaborative problems can be written as "The nurse will manage and minimize the problem." The following are examples of goals for collaborative problems:

| Collaborative Problem | Nursing Goal |
|---|---|
| *Risk for Complications of Bleeding* | The nurse will monitor to detect early signs/symptoms of bleeding and collaboratively intervene to stabilize the client. |
| | Indicators |
| | Calm, alert, oriented |
| | Urine output 5 ml/kg/hr |
| | Pulse 60–100 breaths/min |

## Goals for Nursing Diagnoses

Client goals can represent predicted resolution of a problem, evidence of progress toward resolution of a problem, progress toward improved health status, or continued maintenance of good health or function. Nurses and clients use these goals to direct interventions to achieve desired changes or maintenance and to measure the effectiveness and validity of interventions. Nurses can formulate goals (outcome criteria) to direct and measure positive results or to prevent complications. Goals (outcome criteria) seek to direct interventions to provide the client with:

- Improved health status by increasing comfort (physiologic, psychological, social, spiritual) and coping abilities (e.g., The client will discuss relationship between activity and carbohydrate requirements and walk unassisted to end of hall four times a day.)
- Maintenance of present optimal level of health (e.g., The client will continue to share fears.)
- Optimal levels of coping with significant others (e.g., The client will relate an intent to discuss with her husband her concern about returning to work.)
- Optimal adaptation to deterioration of health status (e.g., The client will visually scan the environment to prevent injury while walking.)
- Optimal adaptation to terminal illness (e.g., The client will compensate for periods of anorexia and nausea.)
- Collaboration and satisfaction with health care providers (e.g., The client will ask questions concerning the care of his colostomy.)

Alternatively, goals (outcome criteria) seek to direct interventions to prevent negative alterations in the client, such as:

- Complications (e.g., The client will not experience the complications of imposed bed rest as evidenced by continued intact skin; full range of motion, no calf tenderness, and clear lung fields.)
- Disabilities (e.g., The client will elevate left arm on pillow and exercise fingers on sponge ball to reduce edema.)
- Unwarranted death (e.g., The infant will be attached to an apnea monitor at night.)

## Components of Goals

The essential characteristics of goals are as follows:

- Long-term or short-term
- Measurable behavior
- Specific in content and time
- Attainable

### Long and Short Term Goals

A *long-term goal* is an objective that the client is expected to achieve over weeks or months. A *short-term goal* is an objective that the client is expected to achieve in a few days or as a stepping stone toward a long-term goal. Long-term goals are appropriate for all clients in long-term care facilities and for some clients in rehabilitation units, mental health units, community nursing settings, and ambulatory services. For a client with a nursing diagnosis of *Risk for Suicide* (Varcarolis, 2007):

| | |
|---|---|
| Long-term Goal | Client will state that she wants to live. |
| Short-term Goals | Client will discuss painful feelings. |
| | Client will make no-suicide contract with nurse by end of first session. |

Measurable behavior is expressed by use of *measurable verbs*, or verbs that describe the exact action that the nurse expects the client to display when he or she has met the goal. The action or behavior must be such that the nurse can validate it through seeing or hearing. (The nurse may occasionally use touch, taste, and smell to measure goal achievement.) If the verb does not describe a result that can be seen or heard (e.g., The client *will experience* less anxiety), the nurse can change it to a behaviorally measurable one (e.g., The client *will report* less anxiety).

**INTERACTIVE EXERCISE** 5.4

Examine the following goals:

*The client will*

- Accept the death of his wife
- State the signs and symptoms of high blood glucose
- Know the signs and symptoms of low blood glucose
- Administer insulin correctly
- Understand the importance of a low-fat diet

Which goals can you evaluate by seeing or hearing? (Answer at end of chapter)

Nurses can make the measurement of goal achievement easier by:

- Using the phrase *as evidenced by* to introduce measurable evidence of reduced signs and symptoms, (e.g., The client will experience less anxiety, as evidenced by reduced pacing;

The client will demonstrate tolerance to activity, as evidenced by a return to resting pulse (76) 3 min after activity)

- Adding the phrase *within normal limits* (WNL) (e.g., The client will demonstrate healing WNL.)

A student may be asked to define what WNL is. For example, the client will demonstrate healing WNL as evidenced by intact, approximate wound edges and no or little abnormal drainage. The process of writing measurable goals is diagrammed below.

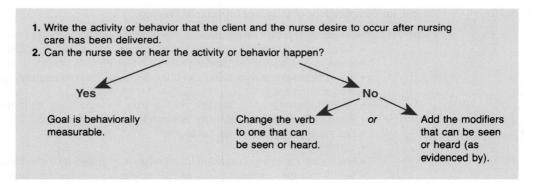

Goals should be *specific in content and time*. Three elements add to the specificity of a goal: (1) content, (2) modifiers, and (3) achievement time. The *content* indicates what the client is to do, experience, or learn (e.g., drink, walk, cough, verbalize). *Modifiers* add individual preferences to the goal and are usually adjectives or adverbs explaining what, where, when, and how. Nurses can add the *time for achievement* to a goal using one of three options:

1. By discharge (e.g., The client will relate intent to discuss fears regarding diagnosis with wife at home.)
2. Continued (e.g., The client will demonstrate continued intact skin.)

By date (e.g., The client will walk half the length of the hallway with assistance by Friday morning.) Finally, a goal must be *attainable*, meaning that the client must be able to achieve the goal based on his or her age, condition, mental status, and motivation.

## Goals for Possible Nursing Diagnoses

It is inappropriate for nurses to formulate client goals for collaborative problems and possible nursing diagnoses because they have not been confirmed. Consider the following possible nursing diagnosis and associated goal:

- **Nursing diagnosis:** *Possible Feeding Self-Care Deficit related to IV in right hand*
- **Goal:** the client will feed himself

Possible nursing diagnoses do not have goals until they are confirmed. How can the nurse write a client goal for a diagnosis that has not been confirmed or ruled out yet?

## Prescribing Nursing Interventions

As previously discussed (see Chapter 4), the two types of nursing interventions are nurse prescribed and physician prescribed (delegated). *Nurse-prescribed interventions* are those that nurses formulate for themselves or other nursing staff to implement. *Physician-prescribed (delegated) interventions* are prescriptions for clients that physicians formulate for nursing staff to implement. Physicians' orders are not orders for nurses; rather, they are orders for clients that nurses implement if indicated.

Both types of interventions require independent nursing judgment, because legally the nurse must determine whether it is appropriate to initiate the action, regardless of whether it is independent or delegated. Box 5.2 shows a sample nursing care plan with both types of interventions.

Note that nurses can and should consult with other disciplines, such as social workers, nutritionists, and physical therapists, as appropriate. Nevertheless, doing so is consultative only; if interventions for nursing diagnoses result from such consultation, the nurse writes these orders on the nursing care plan for other nursing staff to implement. (A discussion of other disciplines and their role in nursing care plans is included later in this chapter.)

---

### BOX 5.2 NURSE-PRESCRIBED AND DELEGATED INTERVENTIONS

*Standard of Care*

**Risk for Complications of Increased Intracranial Pressure**

NP 1. Monitor for signs and symptoms of increased intracranial pressure.
- Pulse changes: slowing rate to 60 or below; increasing rate to 100 or above
- Respiratory irregularities: slowing rate with lengthening periods of apnea
- Rising blood pressure or widening pulse pressure with moderately elevated temperature
- Temperature rising
- Level of responsiveness: variable change from baseline (alert, lethargic, comatose)
- Pupillary changes (size, equality, reaction to light, movements)
- Eye movements (doll's eyes, nystagmus)
- Vomiting
- Headache: constant, increasing in intensity; aggravated by movement/standing
- Subtle changes: restlessness, forced breathing, purposeless movements, and mental cloudiness
- Paresthesia, paralysis

NP 2. Avoid:
- Carotid massage
- Prone position
- Neck flexion
- Extreme neck rotation
- Valsalva maneuver
- Isometric exercises
- Digital stimulation (anal)

NP 3. Maintain a position with slight head elevation.
NP 4. Avoid rapidly changing positions.
NP 5. Maintain a quiet, calm environment (soft lighting).
NP 6. Plan activities to reduce interruptions.
NP 7. Intake and output; use infusion pump to ensure accuracy.
NP 8. Consult for stool softeners.
Del 9. Maintain fluid restrictions as ordered (may be restricted to 1000 mL/day for a few days).
Del 10. Administer fluids at an even rate as prescribed.
Del 11. Administer medications (osmotic diuretics [e.g., mannitol] and corticosteroids [e.g., dexamethasone, methylprednisolone if administered]).

(Del = Delegated; NP = Nurse-prescribed)

## Evaluating Nursing Diagnoses

Nurses need client goals (outcome criteria) to evaluate a nursing diagnosis. After the nurse and client mutually set client goals, the nurse will (1) assess the client's status, (2) compare this response to the outcome criteria, and (3) conclude whether the client is progressing toward outcome achievement. The example below illustrates this evaluation process:

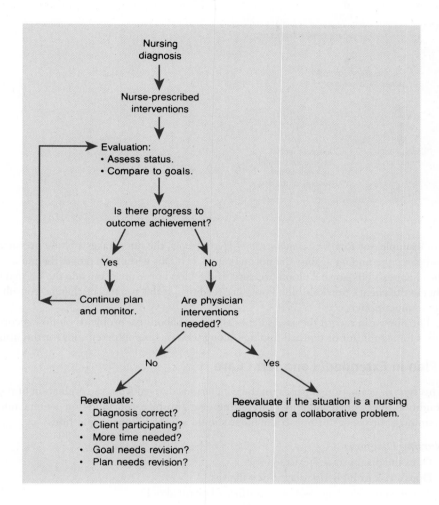

If a goal is "The client will walk unassisted half the length of the hall by 6/5," the nurse would observe the client's response to interventions, asking, "How far did the client walk?" and "Did he or she need assistance?" The nurse then would compare the client's response after interventions with the established goals.

The nurse can record the client's response on flow charts or progress notes. Flow charts record clinical data, such as vital signs, skin condition, any side effects, and wound assessments. Progress notes record specific responses that are not appropriate for flow charts, such as response to counseling, response of family members to the client, and any unusual responses.

## Evaluating Collaborative Problems

Because collaborative problems do not have client goals, the nurse evaluates them differently than nursing diagnoses. For collaborative problems, the nurse will (1) assess the client's status, (2) compare the data to established norms, (3) judge whether the data fall within acceptable ranges, and (4) conclude if the client's condition is stable, improved, unimproved, or worse.

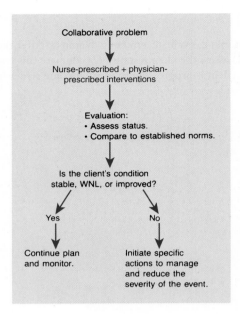

For example, for *Risk for Complications of Hypertension*, the nurse takes a blood pressure reading and compares the finding against the normal range. If it falls within the range, the nurse concludes that the client exhibits normal blood pressure. If the blood pressure is outside the normal range, the nurse checks the client's previous blood pressure readings. If this is a recent change, consult with a physician or nurse-practitioner.

The nurse can record the assessment data for collaborative problems on flow records and use progress notes for significant or unusual findings, along with nursing interventions for the situation.

## Evaluating the Care Plan in Extended/ Long Term Care

This type of evaluation depends on the conclusions derived from the evaluation of the client's progress or condition in extended and long term settings, e.g., hospice, rehabilitation centers, nursing homes. After examining the client's response, the nurse should ask the following questions:

*Nursing Diagnosis*
- Does the diagnosis still exist?
- Does a risk or high-risk diagnosis still exist?
- Has the possible diagnosis been confirmed or ruled out?
- Does a new diagnosis need to be added?

*Goals*
- Have they been achieved?
- Do they reflect the present focus of care?
- Can more specific modifiers be added?
- Are they acceptable to the client?

*Interventions*
- Are they acceptable to the client?
- Are they specific to the client?
- Do they provide clear instructions to the nursing staff?

*Collaborative Problems*
- Is continuing monitoring indicated?

In reviewing the problems and interventions, the nurse records one of the following decisions in the evaluation column or in the progress notes at the time prescribed for evaluation:

- *Continue.* The diagnosis is still present, and the goals and interventions are appropriate.

- *Revised.* The diagnosis is still present, but the goals or nursing orders require revision. The revisions are then recorded.
- *Ruled Out/Confirmed.* Additional data collection has confirmed or ruled out a possible diagnosis. Goals and nursing orders are written.
- *Achieved.* The goals have been achieved, and that portion of the care plan is discontinued.
- *Reinstate.* A diagnosis that had been resolved returns.

The nurse caring for or directing the client's care can make minor revisions on a care plan daily. He or she can use a yellow felt-tip marker (highlighter) to mark those areas no longer in use. Because it is still possible to read through the yellow marking, the nurse can refer to previous planning. In addition, the marking will not interfere with photocopying. Examples of evaluation documentation are presented later in this chapter.

## Multidisciplinary Care Planning

Commonly, multiple disciplines provide the care of individuals, families, or groups. Good coordination of this care is critical for optimal use of resources and to prevent duplication. Given overall knowledge level and time spent with clients, nurses typically are in the best position to coordinate this care. The case management model subscribes to this philosophy.

Agencies take various steps to promote coordinated multidisciplinary planning:

- Conducting regular multidisciplinary planning conferences
- Creating multidisciplinary problem lists
- Creating multidisciplinary care plans

Some of these strategies, however, can be problematic for nurses. As discussed in this chapter, care plans serve as directions for nursing staff in providing client care. Should staff from other disciplines—physical therapy, social services, nutrition—write on nursing care plans? If so, should they write interventions for nurses to follow or specific to their discipline?

When a client requires services other than nursing, the physician orders a consultation of the services. Staff members from the needed discipline then create a plan of care with goals and interventions relating specifically to their discipline, not to nursing. Should this plan be part of a multidisciplinary care plan? Yes, but only if the plan clearly designates which sections apply only to specific disciplines.

Physician-prescribed interventions are transferred from the chart to appropriate documents, such as medication administration records, treatment records, and Kardexes. It is not necessary to enter physician-prescribed interventions on nursing care plans.

A nurse is accountable for following the interventions that other professional nurses prescribe. If a nurse disagrees with another nurse's care plan, the two nurses should consult and discuss the problem. If doing so is impossible, then the disagreeing nurse can delete or revise the existing nursing orders. Professional courtesy dictates that the nurse should leave a note to the previous nurse explaining the change, if it could be problematic.

Should other disciplines add interventions for nursing staff to the nursing care plan? When a discipline other than nursing or medicine has suggestions for nursing management of a nursing diagnosis, the nurse should view these suggestions as expert advice. The nurse may or may not incorporate such advice into the nursing care plan. This situation is similar to that of a consulting physician, who may make recommendations but does not write medical orders for another physician's client.

When a nurse enters an intervention on the care plan based on a suggestion from another discipline, that the nurse credit the order to that discipline.

For example:

*Gently perform passive ROM to arms after meals and at 8–9 pm, per consult with C. Levy, RPT.*

Historically, nurses exclusively have used nursing diagnoses and collaborative problems to describe the focus of nursing care. But nursing diagnoses and collaborative problems also can describe the focus of care for other non-physician disciplines, such as physical therapy, respiratory therapy, social service, occupational therapy, nutritional therapy, and speech therapy. Other disciplines could add their discipline-specific interventions to standardized care plans with the designation that the interventions are prescribed and provided by that discipline (not nursing). These disciplines also would be encouraged to revise or add to care plans for their interventions. Box 5.3 illustrates a multidisciplinary care plan. Note that all nursing diagnoses or collaborative problems do not have non–nurse-prescribed interventions.

### BOX 5.3 SAMPLE MULTIDISCIPLINARY CARE PLAN FOR A CLIENT AFTER TOTAL HIP REPLACEMENT

**Nursing Diagnosis:**
*Impaired Physical Mobility related to pain, stiffness, fatigue, restrictive equipment, and prescribed activity restrictions*

**Goal:**
The client will increase activity to walking with walker for 15 mins tid and demonstrate proper positioning and transfer techniques.

**Interventions:**

| | | |
|---|---|---|
| PT | 1. | Establish an exercise program tailored to the client's ability. |
| | 2. | Implement exercises at regular intervals. |
| PT/Nsg | 3. | Teach body mechanics and transfer techniques. |
| | 4. | Encourage independence. |
| PT/Nsg | 5. | Teach and supervise use of ambulatory aids. |

Multidisciplinary conferencing provides an excellent way to review and evaluate a client's, families, or group status and progress. In some facilities, such conferencing is required for all applicable clients.

# Care Planning Systems

Standards of care are detailed guidelines that represent the predicted care for specific situations. They do not direct nurses to provide medical interventions; rather, they provide an efficient method for retrieving predicted generic nursing interventions. Standards of care identify a set of problems (actual or at risk) that typically occur in a particular situation—a diagnostic cluster. An efficient, professional, and useful care planning system encompasses standards of care, client problem lists, and standardized and addendum care plans.

## Standardization

Like any concept or system, standardized care planning forms have both advantages and disadvantages. Advantages include the following:

- Eliminate the need to write routine nursing interventions
- Illustrate to new or part-time employees the unit standard of care
- Direct nursing staff to selected documentation requirements
- Provide the criteria for a quality improvement program and resource management
- Allow the nurse to spend more time delivering than documenting care

Disadvantages are as follows:

- May replace a needed individualized intervention
- May encourage nurses to focus on predictable instead of additional problems

Some nurses experienced these disadvantages when standardized care plans were introduced into their clinical setting. In such cases, the solution was to eliminate standardized care plans. Follow-up care plan audits revealed that the nurses were writing what previously was contained on the standard of care (e.g., *turn q2h, administer pain relief medication*).

Keep in mind that standards of care should represent the care that nurses are responsible for providing, not an ideal level of care. Unrealistic, ideal standards merely frustrate nurses and hold them legally accountable for care that they cannot provide

#### ◀◀ Carp's Cues

Nurses also have been socialized to view standardization as mediocre and unprofessional care. Standards of care or standardized care plans should represent responsible nursing care predicted for certain situations. Nurses should view these predictions as scientific. When problems arise with the use of standardized forms, the solution is not to change the forms but to address their misuse.

# Levels of Care

As discussed earlier, the nurse cannot hope to address all—or, usually, even most—of a client's problems. Rather, the nurse must focus on the client's most serious, or priority, problems. The nurse should refer problems that will not be addressed in the health care facility to both the client and family for interventions after discharge. Referrals to community agencies, such as weight loss or smoking cessation programs and psychological counseling, may be indicated after discharge. Nurses must create realistic standards based on client acuity, length of stay, and available resources.

A care planning system can be structured with three tiers or levels of care:

1. Level I—generic unit standard of care
2. Level II—diagnostic cluster or single-diagnosis standardized care plan
3. Level III—addendum care plans

## Level I—Unit Standards of Care

Level I standards of care represent the predicted generic care required for all or most clients on a unit. These standards contain nursing diagnoses or collaborative problems (the diagnostic cluster) applicable to the specific situation. Box 5.4 presents a sample diagnostic cluster for standards of care in a general medical unit. Each unit—orthopedics, oncology, pediatrics, surgical, postanesthesia, neonatal, emergency, mental health, postpartum and so on—should have a generic unit standard of care.

Level I standards can be laminated and placed in each client care area as a reference for nurses. Because these standards apply to all clients, the nurse does not have to write these nursing diagnoses or collaborative problems on an individual client's care plan. Instead, institutional policy can specify that the generic standard will be implemented for all clients if indicated.

The concept of high risk is not useful at the unit standard level. At this level, all or most clients are at risk, but not at *high* risk. For example, after surgery all individuals are at risk for infection, but not all are at high risk.

---

**BOX 5.4 GENERIC DIAGNOSTIC CLUSTER FOR HOSPITALIZED ADULTS WITH MEDICAL CONDITIONS**

**Collaborative Problems**
- *Risk for Complications of Cardiovascular*
- *Risk for Complications of Respiratory*

**Nursing Diagnosis**
- *Anxiety* related to unfamiliar environment, routines, diagnostic tests and treatments, and loss of control
- *Risk for Injury* related to unfamiliar environment and physical/mental limitations secondary to condition, medications, therapies, and diagnostic tests
- *Risk for Infection* related to increased microorganisms in environment, the risk of person-to-person transmission, and invasive tests and therapies
- *Self-Care Deficit* related to sensory, cognitive, mobility, endurance, or motivation problems
- *Risk for Imbalanced Nutrition: Less Than Body Requirements* related to decreased appetite secondary to treatments, fatigue, environment, and changes in usual diet, and increased protein/vitamin requirements for healing
- *Risk for Constipation* related to change in fluid/food intake, routine and activity level, effects of medications, and emotional stress
- *Disturbed Sleep Patterns* related to unfamiliar, noisy environment, change in bedtime ritual, emotional stress, and change in circadian rhythm
- *Risk for Spiritual Distress* related to separation from religious support system, lack of privacy, or inability to practice spiritual rituals
- *Interrupted Family Process* related to disruption of routines, change in role responsibilities, and fatigue associated with increased workload and visiting hour requirements
- *Risk for Compromised Human Dignity* related to multiple factors associated with hospitalization

To document Level I standards of care, the nurse should use flow chart notations unless he or she finds unusual data or significant incidents occur. Although standards of care do not have to be part of the client's record, the record should specify what standards have been selected for the client. The problem list, representing the priority nursing diagnoses and collaborative problems for an individual client, can serve this purpose.

## Level II—Standardized Care Plans

Preprinted care plans that represent care to provide for a client, family, or group in addition to the Level I unit standards of care, Level II standardized care plans are supplements to the generic unit standard. Thus, a client admitted to a medical unit will receive nursing care based on both Level I unit standards and the Level II standardized care plan for the specific condition that led to admission.

A Level II standardized care plan contains either a diagnostic cluster or a single nursing diagnosis or collaborative problem, such as *High Risk for Impaired Skin Integrity* or *RC of Fluid/Electrolyte Imbalances*. Box 5.5 presents a Level II standardized care plan for the collaborative problem *RC of Hypo/Hyperglycemia*.

A diagnostic cluster Level II standard would contain additional nursing diagnoses and collaborative problems that are predicted to be present and prior because of a medical condition, surgical intervention, or therapy. For example, the following presents a problem list of the client who is 1 day after total hip replacement surgery, and the source of the care.

RC of Dislocation of Joint
RC of Neurovascular Compromise
RC of Emboli (fat, blood)
Impaired Physical Mobility
High Risk for Impaired Skin Integrity
High Risk for Injury
High Risk for Ineffective Therapeutic Regimen Management

Client's problem list
from Level II
Standard—Post
Total Hip
Replacement

---

### BOX 5.5 LEVEL II STANDARDIZED CARE PLAN FOR RISK FOR COMPLICATIONS OF HYPO/HYPERGLYCEMIA

**Risk for Complications of Hypo/Hyperglycemia**
Nursing Goal: The nurse will manage and minimize hypo- or hyperglycemia episodes.
1. Monitor for signs and symptoms of hypoglycemia:
   - Blood glucose less than 70 mg/dL
   - Pale, moist, cool skin
   - Tachycardia, diaphoresis
   - Jitteriness, irritability
   - Headache, slurred speech
   - Incoordination
   - Drowsiness
   - Visual changes
   - Hunger, nausea, abdominal pain
2. Follow protocols when indicated, e.g., concentrated glucose (oral, IV).
3. Monitor for signs and symptoms of ketoacidosis:
   - Blood glucose greater than 300 mg/dL
   - Positive plasma ketone, acetone breath
   - Headache, tachycardia
- Kussmaul's respirations, decreased BP
- Anorexia, nausea, vomiting
- Polyuria, polydipsia
   - If ketoacidosis occurs, follow protocols, e.g., initiation of IV fluids, insulin IV.
   - If episode is severe, monitor vital signs, urine output, specific gravity, ketones, blood glucose electrolytes q 30 mins or PRN.
   - Document blood glucose findings and other assessment data on flow record. Document unusual events or responses on progress notes.

If this client also had diabetes mellitus, the nurse would add the following single diagnosis standard to the problem list: *RC of Hypo/Hyperglycemia*.

After the nursing staff are well oriented to the details of the unit standard, the diagnoses on the Level I unit standard can be omitted from individual client problem lists or care plans. Policy would indicate that this standard would apply to all the clients on the unit.

## Level III—Addendum Care Plans

An addendum care plan lists additional interventions beyond the Level I and II standards that an individual client requires. These specific interventions may be added to a standardized care plan or may be associated with additional priority nursing diagnoses or collaborative problems not included on the Level II standardized care plan or Level I unit standards.

For many hospitalized clients, the nurse can direct initial care responsibility using standards of care. Assessment information obtained during subsequent nurse–client interactions may warrant specific additions to the client's care plan to ensure outcome achievement. The nurse can add or delete from standardized plans or handwrite or free-text (by computer) an addendum diagnosis with its applicable goals and interventions.

The documentation of implementation does not take place on a care plan but on flow charts, graphic charts, or nursing progress notes, depending on the types of data being recorded.

### ◀◀ Carp's Cues

The uniqueness of all persons predicts that the nurse can always add additional nursing diagnoses to every client problem list. However, given the shortened length of stay of hospitalized persons, the nurse must determine if the additional diagnoses are priority. The standardized care plan should address most of the priority nursing diagnoses. It is important to note that the nurse will always individualize interventions for standardized nursing diagnoses for each client.

## Problem List/Care Plan

As discussed earlier, a problem list represents the priority set of nursing diagnoses and collaborative problems that the nursing staff will manage for a particular client. When appropriate, the term *diagnostic* can be used in place of *problem* (i.e., diagnosis list/care plan) to accommodate wellness diagnoses.

The problem list is a permanent chart record that identifies both the nursing diagnoses and collaborative problems receiving nursing management and also the source for interventions: standard of care, standardized care plan, or addendum care plan. Figure 5.2 illustrates a sample nursing problem list/care plan for a client with a history of type 1 diabetes mellitus who is admitted to a medical unit for treatment of pneumonia. This sample includes the client's priority set of diagnoses as well as the addendum interventions that the nurse has added to the standardized care plan under the diagnosis *Acute Pain*.

### ◀◀ Carp's Cues

*Problem lists are an excellent method to communicate the specific nursing focus for an individual client. They can easily cross reference to a standardized plan or addendum individualized plan.*

## Summary

The repetitive writing or selecting of routine care items in an electronic record of the same care predicted to be present because of a particular medical condition or surgical procedure continues today.

It is a waste of nurses' time.

It consumes time better spent with clients and families.

It deters nurses from writing individualized plans when needed.

All nursing units can provide care using standardized care plans and can be more motivated to individualize this care when the needless writing is eliminated.

**NURSING PROBLEM LIST/CARE PLAN**

| NURSING DIAGNOSIS/ COLLABORATIVE PROBLEM | STATUS | STANDARD | ADDENDUM | EVALUATION OF PROGRESS | | | | |
|---|---|---|---|---|---|---|---|---|
| *Med Unit Standard* | 9/20 A | ✔ | | 9/21 P/LJC | 9/22 P/Pw | 9/23 P-GA | | |
| *RC of Hyperthermia* | 9/20 | | | S/LJC | S/Pw | S-GA | | |
| *RC of Hyper/Hypoglycemia* | 9/20 A | ✔ | | | | | | |
| *Acute Pain* | 9/20 A | ✔ | ✔ | | | | | |
| | | | | | | | | |
| | | | | | | | | |
| | | | | | | | | |

STATUS CODE: A = Active  R = Resolved  RO = Ruled-out
EVALUATION CODE: S = Stable, I = Improved, *W = Worsened, U = Unchanged, *P = Not Progressing, P = Progressing

Reviewed With Client/Family ___9/21 LJC___ , _____ , _____ , (Date)

**ADDENDUM CARE PLAN**

| Nsg Dx/ Coll Prob | Client/ Nursing Goals | Date/ Initials | Interventions |
|---|---|---|---|
| *Acute Pain* | — | 9/23 LJC | 1. *Provide a gentle back rub in evening.* |
| | | | 2. *Leave blanket at foot of bed for easy access.* |
| | | | |
| | | | |
| | | | |
| | | | |
| | | | |
| | | | |
| | | | |

| Initials/Signature | | | |
|---|---|---|---|
| 1. *LJC Lynda J. Carpenito* | 3. | 5. | 7. |
| 2. *Pw Poti Wychoff* | 4. *G. Arcangelo* | 6. | 8. |

**FIGURE 5.2** Sample problem list/care plan.

# ANSWERS TO INTERACTIVE EXERCISES

**5.1**

Significant data:
  Needs assistance for five activities
  Could not perform three activities
  Walks with walker
  Shows unsteady gait
  Has right leg weakness

**5.2**

Possible nursing diagnoses:
  Self-care Deficit
  Risk for Injury
  Disuse Syndrome

**5.3**

The only appropriate choice is the fourth. If physician-prescribed interventions are needed when goals are not achieved, then the problem is a collaborative problem. The goals would be nursing goals, not client goals. The goals listed on p. 37 should be replaced with "The nurse should monitor for changes in physiologic states and minimize complications."

**5.4**

You can see or hear goals 2 and 4. You cannot see or hear "accept," "know," or "understand." To measure knowledge or understanding, the person has to tell (hear) you what he or she knows or demonstrate (see) how to do something.

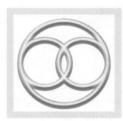

# 6 ELEVEN STEPS TO PUTTING IT ALL TOGETHER WITH CONCEPT MAPPING

### Learning Objectives

After reading the chapter, the student should be able to answer the following questions:

- What is concept mapping?
- How to focus your assessment for a particular client?
- How do you write a care plan if you have not met the client?
- What additional information should you add to the care plan?
- After providing care, how do you evaluate the client's progress?

## Concept Mapping

"Concept mapping is a technique that can help you organize data for analysis. It uses diagrams to demonstrate the relationship of one concept or piece of information to other concepts or pieces of information." (Carpenito-Moyet, 2007)

Concept mapping can help you:

- Explain relationships of data
- Identify both strengths and risk factors in clients
- Determine if there is sufficient data to support your diagnosis

The concept map is composed of a center circle with a ring of outer circles that are connected to the center. This is the diagram that you can use to map clinical data on your client.

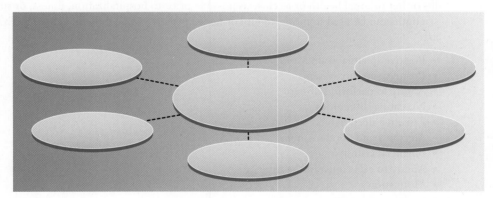

For example, below and on the next page are concept maps for a client.

His strengths are mapped below:

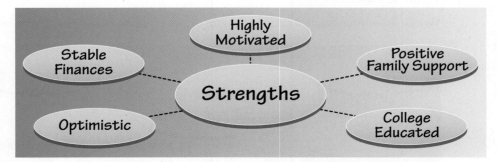

His risk factors are mapped below:

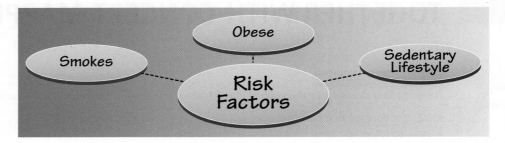

Throughout the 11 steps you can use concept mapping to help organize the data. Refer to http://thepoint.lww.com/CarpenitoApp13e for a sample concept map diagram that you can use clinically for your client's data.

Now you have learned the five steps in the nursing process. You will have the tools to create a plan of care (or care plan) for your assigned client

# Step 1: Assessment

If you need to write a care plan before you can interview the client, go to Step 2 now. If you interview your assigned client before you write your care plan, complete your assessment using the form recommended by your faculty. After you complete your assessment, you will now need to identify:

- Strengths
- Risk factors
- Problems in functioning

Strengths are qualities or factors that will help the person to recover, cope with stressors, and progress to his or her original health or as close as possible prior to hospitalization, illness, or surgery. The client's strengths can be used to motivate him or her to perform some difficult activities. Examples of strengths are:

- Positive spiritual framework
- Positive support system
- Ability to perform self-care
- No eating difficulties
- Effective sleep habits
- Alertness and good memory
- Financial stability
- Ability to relax most of the time
- Motivation
- Positive self-esteem
- Internal locus of control
- Self responsibility
- Positive self-efficacy

Write a list of your assigned client's strengths or use a concept map with strengths as the center.

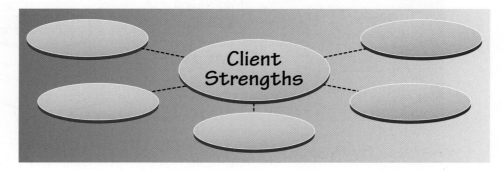

Risk factors are situations, personal characteristics, disabilities, or medical conditions that can hinder the person's ability to heal, cope with stressors, and progress to his or her original health prior to hospitalization, illness, or surgery. Examples of risk factors are as follows:

- No or ineffective support system
- No or little regular exercise
- Inadequate or poor nutritional habits
- Learning difficulties
- Denial
- Poor coping skills
- Communication problems
- Obesity
- Fatigue
- Limited ability to speak or understand English
- Memory problems
- Hearing problems
- Self-care problems before hospitalization
- Difficulty walking
- Financial problems
- Negative self-efficacy

Write a list of risk factors for your assigned client or create a concept map of risk factors

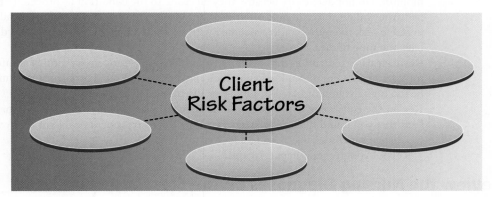

**◄◄ Carp's Cues**

When someone is ill there is an obvious focus on the illness, problems and risk factors. Unfortunately, strengths are often overlooked. Everyone has strengths. Some have more than others do. Our strengths help us through hard times. With sudden illness, trauma, or with deteriorating conditions, the strengths of the client and family can be mobilized to cope effectively. Sometimes the strength of clients and families are not obvious. Search for them!

## Step 2: Same-Day Assessment

If you have not completed a screening assessment of your assigned client, determine the following as soon as you can by asking the client, family, or nurse assigned to your client the following questions.

- Before hospitalization:
  — Could the client perform self-care?
  — Did the client need assistance?
  — Could the client walk unassisted?
  — Did the client have memory problems?
  — Did the client have hearing problems?
  — Did the client smoke cigarettes?
- What conditions or diseases does the client have that make him or her more vulnerable to:
  — Falling
  — Infection
  — Nutrition/fluid imbalance

— Pressure ulcers
— Severe or panic anxiety
— Physiological instability (e.g., electrolytes, blood glucose, blood pressure, respiratory function, healing problems)
- When you meet the assigned client, determine if any of the risk factors are present:
  — Obesity
  — Communication problems
  — Movement difficulties
  — Inadequate nutritional status

Write significant data on an index card. Go to Step 3.

## Step 3: Create Your Initial Care Plan

If your client is in the hospital for a medical problem, refer to the generic medical care plan online (http://thePoint.lww.com/CarpenitoApp13e). If your client is in the hospital for a surgical condition, refer to the generic surgical care plan B online. These generic care plans reflect the usual predicted care a client needs. Ask your instructor if you can use them and revise them electronically for your specific client.

## Step 4: Review the Collaborative Problems on the Generic Plan

- Review the collaborative problems listed. These are the physiological complications that you need to monitor. Do not delete any because they all relate to the condition or procedure that your client has had. You will need to add how often you should take vital signs, record intake and output, change dressings, etc. Ask the nurse you are assigned with for these times and review the Kardex, which also may have the time frames.
- Review each intervention for collaborative problems. Are any interventions unsafe or contraindicated for your client? For example, if your client has edema and renal problems, the fluid requirements may be too high for him or her. Ask a nurse or instructor for help here.
- Review the collaborative problems on the standard plan. Also review all additional collaborative problems that you found that are related to any medical or treatment problems. For example, if your client has diabetes mellitus, you need to add:
  RC of hypoglycemia/hyperglycemia

## Step 5: Review the Nursing Diagnoses on the Standard Plan

Review each nursing diagnosis on the plan.

- Does it apply to your assigned client?
- Does your client have any risk factors (see your index card) that could make this diagnosis worse?

An example on the Generic Medical Care Plan is *Risk for Injury related to unfamiliar environment and physical or mental limitations secondary to condition, medication, therapies, or diagnostic tests*.

Now look at your list of risk factors for your assigned client.

Can any factors listed contribute to the client's sustaining an injury? For example, is he or she having problems walking or seeing? Is he or she experiencing dizziness?

If your client has an unstable gait related to peripheral vascular disease (PVD), you would add the following diagnosis: *Risk for Injury related to unfamiliar environment and unstable gait secondary to peripheral vascular disease*. Review the goals listed for the nursing diagnosis:

- Are they pertinent to your client?
- Can the client demonstrate achievement of the goal on the day you provide care?
- Do you need more time?
- Do you need to make the goal more specific for your client?

Delete goals that are inappropriate for your client. If your client will need more time to meet the goal, add "by discharge." If the client can accomplish the goal this day, write, "by (insert date)" after the goal.

Using the same diagnosis *Risk for injury related to unfamiliar environment and physical and mental limitations secondary to the condition, therapies, and diagnostic tests*, consider this goal:

The client will request assistance with activities of daily living (ADLs).

## Indicators

- Identify factors that increase risk of injury.
- Describe appropriate safety measures.

If it is realistic for your client to achieve all the goals on the day of your care, you should add the date to all of them.

If your client is confused, you can add the date to the main goal, but you would delete all the indicators because the person is confused

Or you could modify the goal by writing:

Family member will identify factors that increase the client's risk of injury.

Review the goals listed for the nursing diagnosis:

- Are they pertinent to your client?
- Can the client demonstrate achievement of the goal on the day you provide care?
- Do you need more time?
- Do you need to make the goal more specific for your client?

Delete goals that are inappropriate for your client. If your client will need more time to meet the goal, add "by discharge." If the client can accomplish the goal this day, write, "by (insert date)" after the goal.

Using the same diagnosis *Risk for injury related to unfamiliar environment and physical and mental limitations secondary to the condition, therapies, and diagnostic tests*, consider this goal:

The client will request assistance with ADLs.

## Indicators

- Identify factors that increase risk of injury.
- Describe appropriate safety measures.

If it is realistic for your client to achieve all the goals on the day of your care, you should add the date to all of them.

If your client is confused, you can add the date to the main goal, but you would delete all the indicators because the person is confused.

Or you could modify the goal by writing:

Family member will identify factors that increase the client's risk of injury.

Review each intervention for each nursing diagnosis:

- Are they relevant for your client?
- Will you have time to provide them?
- Are any interventions not appropriate or contraindicated for your assigned client?
- Can you add any specific interventions?
- Do you need to modify any interventions because of risk factors (see index card)?

#### ◀◀ Carp's Cues

Remember that you cannot individualize a care plan for a client until you spend time with him or her, but you can add or delete interventions based on your preclinical knowledge of this client (e.g., medical diagnosis, coexisting medical conditions).

## Step 6: Prepare the Care Plan (Written or Printed)

You can prepare the care plan by:

- Typing the online generic care plan into your word processor, then deleting or adding specifics for your client (use another color for additions/deletions or a different type font)
- Photocopying a section from this book, then adding or deleting specifics for your client
- Writing the care plan

#### ◀◀ Carp's Cues

Ask your faculty person what options are acceptable. Using different colors or fonts allows him or her to clearly see your analysis. Be prepared to provide rationales for why you added or deleted items.

## Step 7: Initial Care Plan Completed

Now that you have a care plan of the collaborative problems and nursing diagnoses, are there any risk factors or other medical problems that present? Confused? Diabetes Mellitus?

## Step 8: Additional Risk Factors

If your client has risk factors (on the index card) that you identified in Steps 1 and 2, evaluate if these risk factors make your assigned client more vulnerable to develop a problem.

The following questions can help to determine if the client or family has additional diagnoses that need nursing interventions:

- Are additional collaborative problems associated with coexisting medical conditions that require monitoring (e.g., hypoglycemia)?
- Are there additional nursing diagnoses that, if not managed or prevented now, will deter recovery or affect the client's functional status (e.g., *High Risk for Constipation*)?
- What problems does the client perceive as priority?
- What nursing diagnoses are important but treatment for them can be delayed without compromising functional status?

### ◄◄ Carp's Cues

You can address nursing diagnoses not on the priority list by referring the client for assistance after discharge (e.g., counseling, weight loss program). Limited time and resources mandate that these problems be referred back to the client for management after discharge. Do not create a care plan that is impossible for you to provide to the client and family.

Priority identification is a very important but difficult concept. Because of shortened hospital stays and because many clients have several chronic diseases at once, nurses cannot address all nursing diagnoses for every client. Nurses must focus on those for which the client would be harmed or not make progress if they were not addressed. Ask your clinical faculty to review your list. Be prepared to provide rationales for your selections.

## Step 9: Evaluate the Status of Your Client (After You Provide Care)

### Collaborative Problems

Review the nursing goals for the collaborative problems:

- Assess the client's status.
- Compare the data to established norms (indicators).
- Judge if the data fall within acceptable ranges.
- Conclude if the client is stable, improved, unimproved, or worse.

Is your client stable or improved?

- If yes, continue to monitor the client and to provide interventions indicated.
- If not, has there been a dramatic change (e.g., elevated blood pressure and decreased urinary output)? Have you notified the physician or advanced practice nurse? Have you increased your monitoring of the client? Communicate your evaluations of the status of collaborative problems to your clinical faculty and to the nurse assigned to your client.

### Nursing Diagnosis

Review the goals or outcome criteria for each nursing diagnosis.
Did the client demonstrate or state the activity defined in the goal?
If yes, then communicate (document) the achievement on your plan.
If not and the client needs more time, change the target date.
If time is not the issue, evaluate why the client did not achieve the goal.
Was the goal:

- Not realistic because of other priorities?
- Not acceptable to the client?

Review the interventions for each nursing diagnosis.
> Are they acceptable to the client?
> Can you make them more specific?
> Are there any interventions that should be revised or deleted?

## Step 10: Document the Care on the Agency's Forms, Flow Records, and Progress Notes

## Step 11: Evaluation of the Care Plan

After each day of caring for the client, go back to Step 9 and repeat the evaluation and make revisions to the plan if needed

## Summary

More than one nurse has told you that care planning is a useless, waste of time. Probably this nurse has experienced care-planning systems that require mindless writing or repetitive data selection on an electronic charting system.

As a student of nursing, it is important for you to learn the standard of care that is expected in to be needed in many clinical situations.

Some clinical examples are:

- Post-abdominal surgery
- Newborn care
- Postpartum care
- Client with pneumonia
- Client after a stroke (CVA)
- Client post-myocardial infarction

After you have experienced giving care to several persons after abdominal surgery, you will know the care that is indicated. This will allow you to focus on other possible nursing diagnoses. You need to become expert in the standard of care. Care planning that does not require you to write the same care repeatedly will allow you more opportunities to individualize the care. Learning the nursing process by writing can help you to understand this type of scientific problem solving. As a practicing nurse, you will then be able to **think** critically and specifically about each client without **writing** it.

# Manual of Nursing Diagnoses

## Part One

# INDIVIDUAL NURSING DIAGNOSES

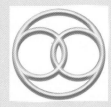

## Introduction

The *Manual of Nursing Diagnoses* consists of nursing diagnoses. This section has been divided into four parts with the diagnoses placed in the appropriate categories:

- Part One—Individual Nursing Diagnoses
- Part Two—Family/Home Nursing Diagnoses
- Part Three—Community Nursing Diagnoses
- Part Four—Health Promotion/Wellness Nursing Diagnoses

They are described with the three NANDA-required elements first:

- Definition
- Defining characteristics, signs and symptoms, or risk factors of the diagnosis
- Related factors, organized according to pathophysiologic, treatment-related, situational, and maturational, that may contribute to or cause the actual diagnosis

Additional components include the following:

- *Author's Note*, which clarifies the concept and clinical use of the diagnosis
- *Errors in Diagnostic Statements*, which explain common mistakes in formulating diagnoses and ways to correct them
- *Key Concepts*, which list scientific explanations about the diagnosis and interventions, categorized as *Generic, Pediatric, Maternal, Geriatric*, and *Transcultural Considerations*

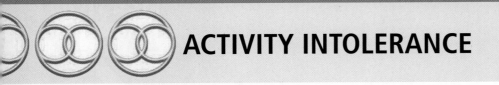

# ACTIVITY INTOLERANCE

**Activity Intolerance**

Related to Insufficient Knowledge of Adaptive Techniques Needed Secondary to COPD
Related to Insufficient Knowledge of Adaptive Techniques Needed Secondary to Impaired
    Cardiac Function

## DEFINITION

The state in which a person experiences a reduction in one's physiologic capacity to endure activities to the degree desired or required (Magnan, 1987)

## DEFINING CHARACTERISTICS

### Major (Must Be Present)

An altered physiologic response to activity

**Respiratory**

| | |
|---|---|
| Dyspnea | Excessively increased rate |
| Shortness of breath | Decreased rate |

**Pulse**

| | |
|---|---|
| Weak | Decreased |
| Excessively increased | Failure to return to pre-activity level after 3 min |
| Rhythm change | |

**Blood Pressure**

| | |
|---|---|
| Failure to increase with activity | Increased diastolic pressure greater than 15 mm Hg |

### Minor (May Be Present)

| | |
|---|---|
| Weakness | Fatigue |
| Pallor or cyanosis | Confusion |
| Vertigo | |

## RELATED FACTORS

Any factors that compromise oxygen transport, physical conditioning, or create excessive energy demands that outstrip the client's physical and psychological abilities can cause activity intolerance. Some common factors follow.

### Pathophysiologic

*Related to compromised oxygen transport system secondary to:*

*Cardiac*

| | |
|---|---|
| Cardiomyopathies | Congestive heart failure |
| Dysrhythmias | Angina |
| Myocardial infarction (MI) | Valvular disease |
| Congenital heart disease | |

*Respiratory*

| | |
|---|---|
| Chronic obstructive pulmonary disease (COPD) | Bronchopulmonary dysplasia |
| | Atelectasis |

*Circulatory*

Anemia                          Peripheral arterial disease

Hypovolemia

***Related to increased metabolic demands secondary to:***

***Acute or Chronic Infections***

Viral infection                 Mononucleosis

Endocrine or metabolic disorders   Hepatitis

***Chronic Diseases***

Renal                           Hepatic

Inflammatory                    Musculoskeletal

Neurologic

***Related to inadequate energy sources secondary to:***

Obesity                         Inadequate diet

Malnourishment

## Treatment-Related

***Related to increased metabolic demands secondary to:***

Malignancies                    Surgery

Diagnostic studies              Treatment schedule/frequency

***Related to compromised oxygen transport secondary to:***

Hypovolemia                     Prolonged bed rest

## Situational (Personal, Environmental)

***Related to inactivity secondary to:***

Depression                      Sedentary lifestyle

Inadequate social support       Insufficient knowledge

***Related to increased metabolic demands secondary to:***

Assistive equipment (walkers, crutches, braces)

Extreme stress

Pain

Environmental barriers (e.g., stairs)

Climate extremes (especially hot, humid climates)

Air pollution (e.g., smog)

Atmospheric pressure (e.g., recent relocation to high-altitude living)

***Related to inadequate motivation secondary to:***

Fear of falling                 Pain

Depression                      Dyspnea

Obesity

## Maturational

Older adults may have decreased muscle strength and flexibility, as well as sensory deficits. These factors can undermine body confidence and may contribute directly or indirectly to activity intolerance.

■■■■■■ **AUTHOR'S NOTE**

*Activity Intolerance* is a diagnostic judgment that describes a client with compromised physical conditioning. This client can engage in therapies to increase strength and endurance. Activity Intolerance is different than Fatigue; fatigue is a pervasive, subjective draining feeling. Rest does treat fatigue but it can also cause tiredness. Moreover, in *Activity Intolerance*, the goal is to increase tolerance to activity; in *Fatigue*, the goal is to assist the client to adapt to the fatigue, not to increase endurance.

# ERRORS IN DIAGNOSTIC STATEMENTS

1. *Activity Intolerance related to dysrhythmic episodes in response to increased activity secondary to recent MI*

    The current goals would be to monitor cardiac response to activity and to prevent decreased cardiac output, not to increase tolerance to activity. This situation would be labeled more appropriately as a collaborative problem: *RC of Decreased Cardiac Output.*

2. *Activity Intolerance related to fatigue secondary to chemotherapy*

    Rest does not relieve fatigue associated with chemotherapy, nor is such fatigue amenable to interventions to increase endurance. The correction would be: *Fatigue related to anemia and chemical changes secondary to toxic effects of chemotherapy.*

# KEY CONCEPTS

## Generic Considerations

* *Endurance* is the ability to continue a specified task; *fatigue* is the inability to continue a specified task. Conceptually, endurance and fatigue are opposites. Nursing interventions, such as work simplification, aim to delay task-related fatigue by maximizing efficient use of the muscles that control motion, movement, and locomotion.
* The ability to maintain a given level of performance depends on *personal factors:* strength, coordination, reaction time, alertness, and motivation; and on *activity-related factors:* frequency, duration, and intensity.
* In healthy people, the work of breathing is very limited. In those with COPD, however, it may increase five to 10 times above normal. Under such conditions, the oxygen required *just for breathing* may be a large fraction of total oxygen consumption.
* The effects of bed rest deconditioning develop rapidly and may take weeks or months to reverse. All people confined to bed are at risk for activity intolerance as a result of bed-rest–induced deconditioning.

## Pediatric Considerations

* Children at special risk for activity intolerance include those with respiratory conditions, cardiovascular conditions, anemia, and chronic illnesses (Hockenberry & Wilson, 2007).
* Research shows that supervised exercise training at moderate intensity is safe and produces significant beneficial changes in hemodynamics and exercise time in children with cardiac disease (Balfour, 1991).

## Geriatric Considerations

* Decreased cardiac output in older adults has been attributed to disease-related, not age-related, processes (Miller, 2009). Fleg (1986) found no age-related changes in resting cardiac output in a study of healthy people between 30 and 80 years of age.
* Studies have demonstrated an average decline of 5% to 10% per decade in maximum oxygen consumption ($\dot{V}o_2$max) from 25 to 75 years of age. Very athletic people have declines in $\dot{V}o_2$max; however, it is only half of the 10% per decade decline that less athletic people exhibit. There seems to be either decreased efficiency in mobilizing blood to exercising muscles or increased difficulty for muscles to extract and use oxygen because of decreased muscle mass.
* By 75 years of age, only 10% of the pacemaker cells in the SA node remain, which could account for slowed conduction during exercise.
* Prolonged immobility and inactivity through self-imposed restrictions, mental status changes, or pathophysiologic changes can contribute to decreased activity tolerance (Cohen et al., 2000).
* Decreased muscle mass leads to decreased strength, which, in turn, leads to decreased endurance. Muscle strength, which is maximal between 20 to 30 years of age, drops to 80% of that value by 65 years of age (Cohen, Gorenberg, & Schader, 2000).
* Increased chest wall rigidity with aging leads to decreased lung expansion, resulting in decreased tissue oxygenation. This immediately affects activity tolerance.

# Focus Assessment Criteria

Assessing for Activity Intolerance:

1. Starting with preactivity assessment, the nurse establishes baseline "at rest" measurements of blood pressure, pulse, and respiration.

     If pathology is known in a particular organ system (e.g., exertional dyspnea in pulmonary disease, angina in cardiac disease, increased spasticity in neuromuscular disease), then during activity focus on signs and symptoms indicating intolerance in that system.
2. During postactivity evaluation, the nurse assesses recovery time, the time required for blood pressure, pulse, and respiration to return to preactivity levels, which reflects physiologic tolerance for activity.

## Subjective Data

### Assess for Defining Characteristics

| | |
|---|---|
| Weakness | Fatigue |
| Dyspnea | |

### Assess for Related Factors

Lack of incentive
Lack of confidence in ability to perform activity
Pain that interferes with performance of activities
Fear of injury or aggravating disease as a result of participation in activity

## Objective Data

### Assess for Defining Characteristics

Assess strength and balance; evaluate client's ability to:

| | |
|---|---|
| Reposition self in bed | Maintain erect posture |
| Rise to standing position | Perform activities of daily living (ADLs) |
| Ambulate | |
| Assume and maintain sitting position | |

Assess response to activity:

1. Take resting vital signs (Table II.1): pulse (rate, rhythm, quality); respirations (rate, depth, effort); and blood pressure.
2. Have the client perform the activity.
3. Take vital signs immediately after the activity.
4. Have the client rest for 3 min; take vital signs again. Compare finding with resting vital signs (Table II.1).
5. Assess for pallor, cyanosis, chest pain, confusion, vertigo, and use of accessory muscles.

### TABLE II.1  PHYSIOLOGY RESPONSE TO ACTIVITY (EXPECTED AND ABNORMAL)

| | Pulse | Blood Pressure | Respiration |
|---|---|---|---|
| **Resting** | | | |
| Normal | 60–90 | <140/90 | <20 |
| Abnormal | >100 | >140/90 | >20 |
| **Immediately After Activity** | | | |
| Normal | ↑Rate ↑Strength | ↑Systolic | ↑Rate ↑Depth |
| Abnormal | ↑Rate ↑Strength Irregular rhythm | Decrease or no change in systolic | Excessive ↓Rate or ↑Rate |
| **3 Minutes After Activity** | | | |
| Normal | Within 6 beats of resting pulse | | |
| Abnormal | >7 beats of resting pulse | | |

## Assess for Related Factors

Refer to Related Factors

For more information on Focus Assessment Criteria, visit http://thepoint.lww.com.

**NOC**
Activity Intolerance

> ## Goal

The client will progress activity to (specify level of activity desired).

### Indicators

- Identify factors that aggravate activity intolerance.
- Identify methods to reduce activity intolerance.
- Maintain blood pressure within normal limits 3 min after activity.

**NIC**
Activity,
Therapy Energy
Management,
Exercise Promotion,
Sleep Enhancement,
Mutual Goal Setting

> ## General Interventions

### Monitor the Client's Response to Activity and Record Response

Take resting pulse, blood pressure, and respirations.
Consider rate, rhythm, and quality (if signs are abnormal—e.g., pulse above 100—consult with physician about advisability of increasing activity).
Have client perform the activity.
Take vital signs immediately after activity.
Have client rest for 3 min; take vital signs again

**R:** Response to activity can be evaluated by comparing preactivity blood pressure, pulse, and respiration with postactivity results. These, in turn, are compared with recovery time.
**R:** Strenuous activity may increase the pulse by 50 beats. This rate is still satisfactory as long as it returns to resting pulse within 3 min.

Discontinue the activity if the client responds with:

- Complaints of chest pain, vertigo, or confusion
- Decreased pulse rate
- Failure of systolic blood pressure to increase
- Decreased systolic blood pressure
- Increased diastolic blood pressure by 15 mm Hg
- Decreased respiratory response

Reduce the intensity or duration of the activity if:

- The pulse takes longer than 3 to 4 min to return to within 6 beats of the resting pulse.
- The respiratory rate increase is excessive after the activity.

**R:** Clinical responses that require discontinuation or reduction in the activity level are evidence of compromised cardiac or respiratory ability.

## Increase the Activity Gradually

Increase tolerance for activity by having the client perform the activity more slowly, for a shorter time with more rest pauses, or with more assistance.
Minimize the deconditioning effects of prolonged bed rest and imposed immobility:

- Begin active range of motion (ROM) at least twice a day. For the client who is unable, the nurse should perform passive ROM.
- Encourage isometric exercise.
- Encourage the client to turn and lift self actively unless contraindicated.
- Promote optimal sitting balance and tolerance by increasing muscle strength.
- Gradually increase tolerance by starting with 15 min the first time out of bed.
- Have the client get out of bed three times a day, increasing the time out of bed by 15 min each day.
- Practice transfers. Have the client do as much active movement as possible during transfers.

- Promote ambulation with or without assistive devices.
- Provide support when the client begins to stand.
- If the client cannot stand without buckling the knees, he or she is not ready for ambulation; help the client to practice standing in place with assistance.
- Choose a safe gait. (If the gait appears awkward but stable, continue; stay close by and give clear coaching messages, e.g., "Look straight ahead, not down.")
- Allow the client to gauge the rate of ambulation.
- Provide sufficient support to ensure safety and prevent falling.
- Encourage the client to wear comfortable walking shoes (slippers do not support the feet properly).

**R:** Activity tolerance develops cyclically through adjusting frequency, duration, and intensity of activity until the desired level is achieved. Increasing activity frequency precedes increasing duration and intensity (work demand). Increased intensity is offset by reduced duration and frequency. As tolerance for more intensive activity of short duration develops, frequency is once again increased.

## Discuss Effects of Condition on Role Responsibilities, Occupation, and Finances

**R:** Knowledge, values, beliefs, and perceived capability for action influence a client's decision to engage in a particular activity (Magnan, 1987).

## Determine Adequacy of Sleep (See Disturbed Sleep Pattern for More Information)

Plan rest periods according to the client's daily schedule. (They should occur throughout the day and between activities.)

Encourage client to rest during the first hour after meals. (Rest can take many forms: napping, watching TV, or sitting with legs elevated.)

**R:** Rest relieves the symptoms of activity intolerance. The daily schedule is planned to allow for alternating periods of activity and rest and coordinated to reduce excess energy expenditure.

## Promote a Sincere "Can-Do" Attitude

Identify factors that undermine client's confidence, such as fear of falling, perceived weakness, and visual impairment.

Explore possible incentives with the client and the family; consider what the client values:

| | |
|---|---|
| Playing with grandchildren | Going fishing |
| Returning to work | Performing a task, such as a craft |

Allow the client to set the activity schedule and functional activity goals. If the goal is too low, negotiate (e.g., "Walking 25 ft seems low. Let's increase it to 50 ft. I'll walk with you.").

Plan a purpose for the activity, such as sitting up in a chair to eat lunch, walking to a window to see the view, or walking to the kitchen to get some juice.

Help client to identify progress. Do not underestimate the value of praise and encouragement as effective motivational techniques. In selected cases, assisting the client to keep a written record of activities may help to demonstrate progress.

**R:** Nursing interventions for activity intolerance promote participation in activities to achieve a level of activity desired by the client for the therapeutic regimen. Strategies that are individualized can increase motivation.

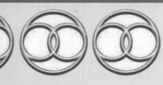

# ACTIVITY INTOLERANCE

## ▶ Related to Insufficient Knowledge of Adaptive Techniques Needed Secondary to COPD

**NOC**
Activity Tolerance

### ➤ Goal

The client will progress activity to (specify level of activity desired).

### *Indicators*

- Demonstrate methods of controlled breathing to conserve energy.
- Demonstrate ability to perform controlled coughing.

**NIC**
Same as for Generic, Smoking Cessation Assistance, Nutrition Management, Respiratory Monitoring, Teaching: Prescribed Activity/Exercise

### ➤ General Interventions

The following interventions apply to people experiencing *Activity Intolerance* resulting from a known cause: COPD. Nurses use these interventions in conjunction with the interventions identified for general cases of *Activity Intolerance* (see pp. 62–63).

### Eliminate or Reduce Contributing Factors

#### *Lack of Knowledge*

Assess understanding of prescribed therapeutic regimen; proceed with health teaching using simple, clear instructions; include family members.
Specifically assess knowledge of pulmonary hygiene and adaptive breathing techniques.

**R:** Pulmonary rehabilitation can decrease anxiety and depression associated with severe COPD.

#### *Inadequate Pulmonary Hygiene Routine*

Explain the importance of adhering to daily coughing schedule for clearing the lungs and that doing so is a lifetime commitment.
Teach the proper method of controlled coughing:

1. Breathe deeply and slowly while sitting up as upright as possible.
2. Use diaphragmatic breathing.
3. Hold the breath for 3 to 5 s; then slowly exhale as much of this breath as possible through the mouth. (Lower rib cage and abdomen should sink down with exhaling.)
4. Take a second deep breath, hold, and cough forcefully from deep in the chest (not from the back of the mouth or throat); use two short, forceful coughs.

Rest after coughing sessions.
Instruct the client to practice controlled coughing four times a day: 30 min before meals and at bedtime. Allow 15 to 30 min of rest after coughing session and before meals.
Consider use of inhaled humidity, postural drainage, and chest clapping before coughing session. Assess for use of prescribed aerosol bronchodilators to dilate airways and thin secretions.

**R:** Clearing and defense of the airways are of utmost importance in meeting tissue demands for increased oxygen during periods of rest and periods of increased activity.

#### *Suboptimal Breathing Techniques*

Beginning instruction in physical and mental relaxation techniques is helpful before teaching controlled breathing.

**R:** Techniques of physical relaxation minimize muscle tension. Relaxation is an essential preliminary step in teaching controlled breathing to eliminate wasteful and unproductive motions of the upper chest, shoulders, and neck.

Instruct the client by demonstrating the desired breathing technique; then direct him or her to mimic your breathing pattern.

For pursed-lip breathing, the client should breathe in through the nose, then breathe out slowly through partially closed lips while counting to 7 and making a "pu" sound. (Often, people with progressive lung disease learn this naturally.)

For diaphragmatic breathing:

1. Place your hands on the client's abdomen below the base of the ribs and keep them there while he or she inhales.
2. To inhale, the client relaxes the shoulders, breathes in through the nose, and pushes the stomach outward against your hands. The client holds the breath for 1 to 2 s to keep the alveoli open, then exhales.
3. To exhale, the client breathes out slowly through the mouth while you apply slight pressure at the base of the ribs.
4. Have the client practice this breathing technique several times with you; then, the client should place his or her own hands at the base of the ribs to practice alone.
5. Once the client has learned the technique have him or her practice it a few times each hour.

**R:** People with COPD can benefit from specific breathing exercises, which involve retraining of breathing patterns, and from general exercise programs that support normal daily activities (Bauldoff et al., 1996).

**R:** Therapeutic efforts to improve respiratory muscle function need to be tailored to each client, according to the muscle group most likely to benefit. In the early stages of COPD, treatment should focus on the diaphragm, whereas for more advanced disease, the focus must shift to the inspiratory muscles of the rib cage and of exhalation.

## Insufficient Activity Level

Assess current activity level. Consider:

- Current pattern of activity/rest
- Distribution of energy demand over the course of the day
- Perceptions of the most demanding required activities
- Perceptions of the areas for which the client desires or requires increased participation
- Efficacy of current adaptive techniques

Identify physical barriers at home and work (e.g., number of stairs) that seem insurmountable or limit participation in activities.

Identify ways to reduce the work demand of frequently performed tasks (e.g., sitting, rather than standing, to prepare vegetables; keeping frequently used utensils on a countertop to avoid unnecessary overhead reaching or bending).

Identify ways of alternating periods of exertion with periods of rest to overcome barriers (e.g., place a chair in the bathroom near the sink so the client can rest during daily hygiene).

Keep in mind that a plan including frequent short rest periods during an activity is less demanding and more conducive to completing the activity than a plan that calls for a burst of energy followed by a long period of rest.

**R:** Symptom-limited endurance training has been shown effective for improving performance and reducing perceived breathlessness (Punzal, Ries, Kaplan, & Prewitt, 1991). The minimal duration and frequency of exercise required to improve performance appears to be 20 to 30 min three to five times per week. Not all people, however, are candidates for exercise reconditioning. A pulmonologist should be consulted.

## Poor Health-Related Behaviors

Teach the client to avoid factors that aggravate symptoms and advance disease (e.g., excessive allergens, pollution).

Discourage smoking. Smoking cessation should be considered of highest priority in any program of comprehensive care of clients with COPD.

If the client chooses to smoke, discourage smoking before meals and activity.

If the client wishes to reduce or stop smoking, see further interventions under Risk-Prone Health Behavior in Section 2, Part 4.

**R:** An integrated program incorporates the principles of physical relaxation, pulmonary hygiene, controlled breathing, and adequate nutrition and hydration; energy conservation through work simplification and smoking cessation maximizes activity tolerance.

## Monitor the Client's Response to Activity

Refer to Focus Assessment Criteria under Objective Data.

### *Increase Activity Gradually*

Reassure the client that some increase in daily activity is possible.
Instruct the client in controlled breathing techniques.
Encourage the client to use controlled breathing techniques to decrease work of breathing during activities.
After the client masters controlled breathing in relaxed positions, begin to increase activity.
Teach the client to maintain a controlled breathing pattern while sitting or standing.
Progress the client to maintaining controlled breathing during bed-to-chair transfers and walking.
Many clients can learn to maintain rhythmic breathing during walking by using a simple 2:4 ratio: two steps during inspiration and four steps during expiration.
Do not progress the client to more demanding activity until breathing is well controlled during less demanding activities.

**R:** People with COPD can benefit from specific breathing exercises, which involve retraining of breathing patterns, and from general exercise programs that support normal daily activities (Bauldoff et al., 1996).

## Encourage Discussion of Sexuality

Encourage the client to discuss the effects of the condition on sexuality.
Refer to *Ineffective Sexuality Patterns*.

## Initiate Health Teaching

Teach the client to observe sputum; note changes in color, amount, and odor; and seek professional advice if sputum changes. Discuss the need for annual influenza immunizations. (The usefulness of one-time-only pneumococcal vaccinations has recently been questioned; therefore, administration should be on an individual basis.)
Instruct the client to wear warm, dry clothing; avoid crowds, heavy smoke, fumes, and irritants; avoid exertion in cold, hot, or humid weather; and balance work, rest, and recreation to regulate energy expenditure.
Emphasize the importance of maintaining a nutritious diet (high calorie, high vitamin C, high protein, and 2 to 3 quarts of liquid a day, unless on fluid restriction).

**R:** Clients with COPD are susceptible to infection and must detect symptoms early and consult with physician for treatment (frequently, early antibiotic therapy is necessary). Strategies to increase resistance to infection include immunizations, avoiding environmental irritants and crowds, and maintaining optimal nutrition and hydration.

Teach the importance of supporting arm weight to reduce the need for respiratory muscles to stabilize the chest wall (Bauldoff et al., 1996; Breslin, 1992).
Teach how to increase unsupported arm endurance with lower extremity exercises performed during the exhalation phase of respiration (Bauldoff et al., 1996; Breslin, 1992).

**R:** The physiologic demands of unsupported arm tasks lead to both exercise-induced increases in respiratory muscle work and nonventilatory recruitment of respiratory muscles to maintain chest wall position (Breslin, 1992). Research has shown that arm support during performance of arm tasks reduces diaphragmatic recruitment, increases respiratory endurance (Bauldoff et al., 1996), and increases arm exercise endurance. Providing arm support (e.g., resting elbows on a tabletop while shaving or eating) may enhance independence and improve functional capacity (Bauldoff et al., 1996).

Evaluate the client's knowledge of the care, cleansing, and use of inhalator equipment.

**R:** Inhalator equipment can harbor microorganisms and must be disinfected properly.

## Make Referrals as Indicated

Refer to a community nurse for follow-up.
Consult a physical therapist for a comprehensive exercise program especially for people with COPD.

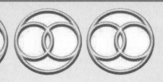

# ACTIVITY INTOLERANCE

## ▌ Related to Insufficient Knowledge of Adaptive Techniques Needed Secondary to Impaired Cardiac Function

**NOC**
Activity Intolerance

### ➤ Goal

The client will demonstrate tolerance for increased activity by maintaining pulse, respirations, and blood pressure within predetermined ranges.

### *Indicators*

- Identify factors that increase cardiac workload.
- Describe adaptive techniques needed to perform ADLs.
- Identify cues for stopping activity: fatigue, shortness of breath, chest pain.

**NIC**
Same as for Generic, Smoking Cessation Assistance, Weight Reduction Assistance, Knowledge: Illness Care, Teaching: Prescribed Activity/ Exercise, Nutrition Management

### ➤ General Interventions

### Assess for Causative/Contributing Factors

Refer to Related Factors.

### Eliminate or Reduce Contributing Factors

### *Assess Knowledge and Behavior Related to the Four "E's": Eating, Exertion, Exposure, and Emotional Stress (Adapted from Day, 1984)*

Eating
Assess knowledge of restricted diet.
Explain importance of adhering to prescribed salt-restricted diet.
Explore alternatives for seasoning foods to taste using natural herbs and spices.
Encourage a light meal in the evening to promote a more comfortable night's rest.
Initially provide easily digestible and chewable foods.
Schedule meals to avoid interfering with other activities.
Offer food preferences, avoiding dislikes.
Consider sociocultural influences.

Exertion
Teach the client to modify approaches to activities to regulate energy expenditure and reduce cardiac workload (e.g., take rest periods during activities, at intervals during the day, and for 1 h after meals; sit rather than stand when performing activities; when performing a task, rest every 3 min for 5 min to allow

the heart to recover; stop an activity if exertional fatigue or signs of cardiac hypoxia, such as markedly increased pulse rate, dyspnea, or chest pain, occur).

Instruct the client to avoid certain types of exertion: isometric exercises (e.g., using arms to lift self, carry objects) and Valsalva maneuver (e.g., bending at the waist in a sit-up fashion to rise from bed, straining during a bowel movement).

### Exposure

Instruct the client to avoid unnecessary exposure to environmental extremes and exertion during hot, humid weather or extreme cold weather, which places additional demands on the heart.

Instruct the client to dress warmly during cold weather (e.g., create a barrier to cold weather by wearing layers of clothing).

### Emotional Stress

Assist the client to identify emotional stressors (e.g., at home, at work, socially).

Discuss usual responses to emotional stress (e.g., anger, depression, avoidance, discussion).

Explain the effects of emotional stress on the cardiovascular system (increased heart rate, blood pressure, respirations).

Discuss various methods for stress management/reduction (e.g., deliberate problem solving, relaxation techniques, yoga or meditation, biofeedback, regular exercise).

**R:** An integrated program of medically supervised exercise, dietary restriction, stress management, and limited exposure to environmental extremes maximizes activity tolerance.

People with impaired cardiac function can achieve some immediate gains in activity tolerance by modifying their approach (e.g., pacing activities, avoiding isometric work, limiting the duration of dynamic work by taking frequent rests).

## Discuss the Effects of Smoking

Discuss the effects of smoking on the cardiovascular, respiratory, circulatory, and muscular-skeletal systems.

Teach the client when not to smoke: before and immediately after an activity.

Discuss methods that can help the client to quit smoking (refer to Risk-Prone Health Behavior).

Advise the client that at least several attempts may be needed to be successful.

**R:** Tobacco is a potent vasoconstrictor that increases the workload of the heart, damages lung tissue, damages blood vessels, and decreases circulation to muscles and bones.

## Address Overweight/Obesity

Assess whether client is overweight or obese by measuring height and weight and comparing findings with a standardized height–weight chart, or use anthropometric measurements (see Risk-Prone Health Behavior for charts of weight for height and anthropometric norms and strategies for weight loss).

**R:** People with impaired cardiac function can increase both activity level and tolerance through weight loss, modifications in approach to activities, and careful monitoring of responses.

## Monitor Response to Activity (See General Interventions, pp. 62–63) and Teach Self-Monitoring Techniques

Take resting pulse.

Take pulse during or immediately after activity.

Take pulse 3 min after cessation of activity.

Instruct the client to stop activity and report:

- Decreased pulse rate during activity
- Pulse rate greater than 112 beats/min
- Irregular pulse
- Pulse rate that does not return to within 6 beats of resting pulse after 3 min
- Dyspnea
- Chest pain
- Palpitations

• Perceptions of exertional fatigue

**R:** Response to activity can be evaluated by comparing preactivity blood pressure, pulse, and respiration with postactivity blood pressure, pulse, and respiration. These, in turn, are compared with recovery time.

## Increase the Activity Gradually

Allow for periods of rest before and after planned periods of exertion, such as treatments, ambulation, meals.
Encourage gradual increases in activity and ambulation to prevent a sudden increase in cardiac workload.
Assess the client's perceived capability for increased activity.
Assist the client in setting short-term activity goals that are realistic and achievable.
Reassure the client that even small increases in activity will lift spirits and restore self-confidence.

**R:** An exercise program that is monitored can improve both exercise capacity and quality of life in clients with moderate heart failure (Rees et al., 2004).

## Initiate Health Teaching and Referrals as Indicated

Instruct the client to consult his or her physician or nurse practitioner for a long-term exercise program.
Explain dietary restrictions to both client and family. Give them written instructions or refer them to pertinent literature or web sites for information on diets.
Explain dosage, side effects, administration, and storage of prescribed drug therapy (e.g., diuretics, vasodilators).

**R:** Specific instructions will be needed for management of condition and treatments.

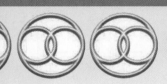

# INEFFECTIVE ACTIVITY PLANNING

## DEFINITION

The state in which an individual has an inability to prepare for a set of actions fixed in time and under certain circumstances.

## DEFINING CHARACTERISTICS

Verbalization of fear toward a task to be undertaken
Verbalization of worries toward a task to be undertaken
Excessive anxieties toward a task to be undertaken
Failure pattern of behavior
Lack of plan
Lack of resources
Lack of sequential organization
Procrastination
Unmet goals for chosen activity

## RELATED FACTORS

Compromised ability to process information
Defensive flight behavior when faced with proposed solution
Hedonism

Lack of family support
Lack of friend support
Unrealistic perception of events
Unrealistic perception of personal competence

■■■■■■ **AUTHOR'S NOTE**

This newly accepted NANDA-I nursing diagnosis can represent a problematic response that related to many existing nursing diagnoses as Chronic Confusion, Self-Care Deficit, Anxiety, Ineffective Denial, Ineffective Coping and Ineffective Self-Health Management. This author recommends that ineffective activity planning should be seen as a sign or symptom. The questions are:

• What activities are not being planned effectively? Self-care? Self-Health management?
• What is preventing effective activity planning? Confusion? Anxiety? Fear? Denial? Stress Overload?
• Examples are:
• Stress Overload related to unrealistic perception of events as evidence by impaired ability to plan ….(specify activity}
• Ineffective Self-Health Management related to lack of plan, lack of resources, lack of social support as evidence by impaired ability to plan…(specify activity)
• Anxiety related to compromised ability to process information and unrealistic perception of personal competence as evident by impaired ability to plan{specify activity}

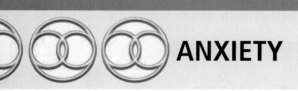

# ANXIETY

**Anxiety**

**Death Anxiety**

## DEFINITION

The state in which an individual experiences a vague feeling of dread or apprehension; it is a response to external or internal stimuli that can have behavioral, emotional, cognitive, and physical symptoms.

## DEFINING CHARACTERISTICS

### Major (Must Be Present)

Manifested by symptoms from each category—physiologic, emotional, and cognitive; symptoms vary according to level of anxiety (Whitley, 1994).

**Physiologic**

| | |
|---|---|
| Increased heart and respiratory rates | Elevated blood pressure |
| | Dilated pupils |
| Diaphoresis | Trembling, twitching |
| Voice tremors/pitch changes | Nausea or vomiting |
| Palpitations | Diarrhea |
| Frequent urination | Fatigue and weakness |
| Insomnia | Dry mouth |
| Flushing or pallor | Restlessness |
| Body aches and pains | Faintness/dizziness |

(especially chest, back, neck)    Hot and cold flashes
Paresthesias    Anorexia

### Emotional
*Client states feelings of:*

| | |
|---|---|
| Apprehension | Helplessness |
| Nervousness | Lack of self-confidence |
| Loss of control | Tension or being "keyed up" |
| Inability to relax | Anticipation of misfortune |

*Client exhibits:*

| | |
|---|---|
| Irritability/impatience | Angry outbursts |
| Crying | Tendency to blame others |
| Startle reaction | Criticism of self and others |
| Withdrawal | Lack of initiative |
| Self-deprecation | Poor eye contact |

### Cognitive

| | |
|---|---|
| Inability to concentrate | Lack of awareness of surroundings |
| Forgetfulness | Rumination |
| Orientation to past | Blocking of thoughts (inability to remember) |
| Hyperattentiveness | Preoccupation |
| Diminished learning ability | Confusion |

## RELATED FACTORS

### Pathophysiologic

Any factor that interferes with the basic human needs for food, air, comfort, and security.

### Situational (Personal, Environmental)

*Related threat to self-concept secondary to:*

| | |
|---|---|
| Change in status and prestige | Lack of recognition from others |
| Failure (or success) | Loss of valued possessions |
| Ethical dilemma | |

*Related to loss of significant others secondary to:*

| | |
|---|---|
| Death | Divorce |
| Cultural pressures | Moving |
| Temporary or permanent separation | |

*Related to threat to biologic integrity secondary to:*

| | |
|---|---|
| Dying | Assault |
| Invasive procedures | Disease (specify) |

*Related to change in environment secondary to:*

| | | |
|---|---|---|
| Hospitalization | Moving | Natural disasters |
| Retirement | Safety hazards | Refugee issues |
| Environmental pollutants | Incarceration | Military or political deployment |

*Related to change in socioeconomic status secondary to:*

| | |
|---|---|
| Unemployment | New job |
| Promotion | Displacement |

*Related to idealistic expectations of self and unrealistic goals (specify)*

### Maturational

#### Infant/Child
*Related to separation*
*Related to unfamiliar environment, people*
*Related to changes in peer relationships*
*Related to death of (specify) with unfamiliar rituals and grieving adults*

**Adolescent**
*Related to death of (specify)*
*Related to threat to self-concept secondary to:*
Sexual development     Peer relationships changes

**Adult**
*Related to threat to self-concept secondary to:*
Pregnancy             Parenting
Career changes        Effects of aging
*Related to previous pregnancy complications, miscarriage, or fetal death*
*Related to lack of knowledge of changes associated with pregnancy*
*Related to lack of knowledge about labor experience*

**Older Adult**
*Related to threat to self-concept secondary to:*
Sensory losses        Motor losses
Financial problems    Retirement changes

## AUTHOR'S NOTE

Several researchers have examined the nursing diagnoses of *Anxiety* and *Fear* (Jones & Jacob, 1984; Taylor-Loughran, O'Brien, LaChapelle, & Rangel, 1989; Whitley, 1994; Yokom, 1984). Differentiation of these diagnoses focuses on whether the threat can be identified. If so, the diagnosis is *Fear*; if not, it is *Anxiety* (NANDA, 2001). This differentiation, however, has not proved useful for clinicians (Taylor-Loughran et al., 1989).

Anxiety is a vague feeling of apprehension and uneasiness in response to a threat to one's value system or security pattern (May, 1977). The client may be able to identify the situation (e.g., surgery, cancer), but actually the threat to self relates to the enmeshed uneasiness and apprehension. In other words, the situation is the source of, but is not itself, the threat. In contrast, fear is feelings of apprehension related to a specific threat or danger to which one's security patterns respond (e.g., flying, heights, snakes). When the threat is removed, fear dissipates (May, 1977). Anxiety is distinguished from fear, which is feeling afraid or threatened by a clearly identifiable external stimulus that represents danger to the person. Anxiety is unavoidable in life and can serve many positive functions by motivating the person to take action to solve a problem or to resolve a crisis (Varcarolis et al., 2006).

Anxiety and fear produce a similar sympathetic response: cardiovascular excitation, pupillary dilation, sweating, tremors, and dry mouth. Anxiety also involves a parasympathetic response of increased gastrointestinal (GI) activity; in contrast, fear is associated with decreased GI activity. Behaviorally, the fearful person exhibits increased alertness and concentration, with avoidance, attack, or decreasing the risk of threat. Conversely, the anxious person experiences increased tension, general restlessness, insomnia, worry, and helplessness and vagueness concerning a situation that cannot be easily avoided or attacked.

Clinically, both anxiety and fear may coexist in a response to a situation. For example, a client facing surgery may be fearful of pain and anxious about possible cancer. According to Yokom (1984), "Fear can be allayed by withdrawal from the situation, removal of the offending object, or by reassurance. Anxiety is reduced by admitting its presence and by being convinced that the values to be gained by moving ahead are greater than those to be gained by escape."

## ERRORS IN DIAGNOSTIC STATEMENTS

### Fear related to upcoming surgery

Anticipated surgery can be a source of many threats, including threats to security patterns, health, values, self-concept, role functioning, goal achievement, and relationships. These threats can produce vague feelings ranging from mild uneasiness to panic. Identifying a threat as merely surgery is too simplistic; personal threats also are involved. Moreover, although some uneasiness may be attributed to fear (which teaching can eliminate), the remaining feelings relate to anxiety. Because this situation is inescapable, the nurse must assist the client with coping mechanisms for managing anxiety and fear.

## ■■■■■■ KEY CONCEPTS

### Generic Considerations

- Anxiety refers to feelings aroused by a nonspecific threat to a client's self-concept that impinges on health, assets, values, environment, role functioning, needs fulfillment, goal achievement, personal relationships, and sense of security (Miller, 2009). It varies in intensity depending on the severity of the perceived threat and the success or failure of efforts to cope with the feelings.
- Anxiety attacks at a deeper level than fear (Varcarolis, 2006). Anxiety affects the central core of personality. It erodes feelings of self-esteem and personal worth.
- A client uses both interpersonal and intrapsychic mechanisms to reduce or relieve anxiety. The effectiveness of coping strategies depends on the client and situation, not on the behavior itself.
- *Interpersonal patterns* of coping include the following:
  - Acting out: converting anxiety into anger (either overtly or covertly expressed)
  - Paralysis or retreating behaviors: withdrawing or being immobilized by anxiety
  - Somatizing: converting anxiety into physical symptoms
  - Constructive action: using anxiety to learn and to solve problems (includes goal setting, learning new skills, and seeking information)
- Defense mechanisms lower anxiety and protect self-esteem. Some are maladaptive if they interfere with overall adjustment. Examples include repression, sublimation, regression, displacement, projection, denial, conversion, rationalization, suppression, and identification.
- People develop a range of coping behaviors, both maladaptive and adaptive. Maladaptive coping mechanisms are characterized by the inability to make choices, conflict, repetition, rigidity, alienation, and secondary gains.
- Anxiety can be classified as normal, acute (state), and chronic (trait) (Varcarolis, 2006).

  1. Normal anxiety also known as state is necessary for survival. It prompts constructive behaviors, such as being on time or studying for a test. State anxiety is the response to an imminent loss or change that disrupts one's sense of security. Examples include apprehension before a speech or the death of a close relative or friend.
  2. Chronic, or trait, anxiety is anxiety that one lives with daily. In children, chronic anxiety may manifest as permanent apprehension or overreaction to unexpected stimuli. In adults, chronic anxiety may manifest as poor concentration, insomnia, relationship problems, and chronic fatigue.

The effects of anxiety on a client's abilities vary with degree:

- *Mild*
  - Heightened perception and attention; alertness
  - Ability to deal with problems
  - Ability to integrate past, present, and future experiences
  - Use of learning and consensual validation
  - Mild tension-relieving behaviors (nail biting, hair twisting)
  - Sleeplessness
- *Moderate*
  - Slightly narrowed perception; selective inattention, which can be directed
  - Slight difficulty concentrating; learning requires more effort
  - View of present experiences in terms of past
  - Possible failure to notice what is happening in a peripheral situation; some difficulty adapting and analyzing
  - Voice/pitch changes
  - Increased respiratory and heart rates
  - Tremors, shakiness
- *Severe*
  - Distorted perception; focus on scattered details; inability to attend to more even when instructed
  - Severely impaired learning; high distractibility and inability to concentrate
  - View of present experiences in terms of past; almost cannot understand current situation
  - Poor function; communication difficult to understand
  - Hyperventilation, tachycardia, headache, dizziness, nausea
  - Complete self-absorption

*(continued)*

■■■■■■ **KEY CONCEPTS** *Continued*

- *Panic*
  - Irrational reasoning; focuses on blown-up detail
  - Inability to learn
  - Inability to integrate experiences; focus only on present; inability to see or understand situation; lapses in recall of thoughts
  - Inability to function; usually increased motor activity or unpredictable responses to minor stimuli; communication not understandable
  - Feelings of impending doom (dyspnea, dizziness/faintness, palpitations, trembling, choking, paresthesia, hot/cold flashes, sweating)
  - Thoughts related to loss of control, death, illness
- Lyons (2002) has identified five factors that contribute to stressful lifestyles as idealistic expectations of self, unrealistic goals, toxic thoughts, negative self-talk, and procrastination.

## Pediatric Considerations

### Anxiety

- Signs of anxiety in children vary greatly depending on developmental stage, temperament, past experience, and parental involvement (Hockenberry & Wilson, 2009). The most common sign in children and adolescents is increased motor activity. Signs of anxiety can be viewed developmentally and may be reflected in the following ways:
  - *Birth to 9 months:* Disruption in physiologic functioning (e.g., sleep disorders, colic)
  - *9 months to 4 years:* Major source is loss of significant others and loss of love. Therefore, anxiety may be seen as anger when parents leave; somatic illnesses; motor restlessness; regressive behaviors (thumb sucking, rocking); regression in toilet training.
  - *4 to 6 years:* Major source is fear of body damage; belief that bad behavior causes bad things (e.g., illness); somatic complaints of headache, stomachache
  - *6 to 12 years:* Excessive verbalization, compulsive behavior (e.g., repeating tasks)
  - *Adolescence:* Similar to 6 to 12 years plus negativistic behavior
  - Separation from parents, change in usual routines, strange environments, painful procedures, and parental anxiety may heighten anxiety (Hockenberry & Wilson, 2009). Assess for alterations in the functional health patterns to detect anxiety.
- Sources of anxiety for children and adolescents are related to school (e.g., performance, peer pressure), separation, social situations, and family.
- Refer children who manifest disorders of avoidance, overanxiousness, severe separation anxiety, and school phobia to mental health experts.

### Responses to Death

- A child's concept of death has three stages:
  1. Less than 5 years old: Death is reversible, seen as asleep or unable to move.
  2. 5 to 9 years old: Death is perceived as a person (angel or monster) carrying away people. Believes own death can be avoided.
  3. After 9 or 10 years old: Death is final and inevitable.
- A child's involvement in funeral rituals should be encouraged if age-appropriate. Shielding children from these rituals does not promote a healthy adaptation to the reality of death.
- An adolescent inexperienced with death and wanting to appear in control may not openly grieve. He or she may continue in usual actions such as online activities and meeting friends as if nothing has happened (Hockenberry & Wilson, 2009).

## Maternal Considerations

- Multiple sources of anxiety are fear for personal or fetal well-being, previous miscarriages or complications, anticipated labor, responsibilities of parenthood, and relationship with partner (Pillitteri, 2009).

## Geriatric Considerations

Older adults may manifest anxiety with complaints of nervousness, "nerve trouble," or feelings of uneasiness (Mohr, 2007).
- Additional signs and symptoms of anxiety are pacing, fidgeting, changes in sleeping or eating patterns, and complaints of fatigue, pain, insomnia, or GI upsets (Miller, 2009).
- Anxiety that starts for the first time in late life is frequently associated with another condition such as depression, dementia, physical illness, or medication toxicity or withdrawal. Phobias, particularly agoraphobia, and generalized anxiety disorder are the most common late-life disorders. Initial treatment involves doses lower than the usual starting doses for adults to ensure the elderly client can tolerate the medication (Varcarolis et al., 2006).

## Transcultural Considerations

- Clients and families from different cultures face many challenges when they seek health care in the dominant culture's health care delivery systems. In addition to usual sources of anxiety (e.g., unfamiliar people, unknown prognosis), they may be anxious about language difficulties, privacy, separation from support systems, and cost (Andrews & Boyle, 2008).
- Members of cultures that depend on kin for caring will expect more humanistic kinds of nursing care and less scientific–technologic care (Andrews & Boyle, 2008).
- Each culture has rules governing the appropriate ways to express and deal with anxiety. Culturally competent nurses should be aware of them while being careful not to stereotype clients (Varcarolis et al., 2006).

# Focus Assessment Criteria

## Subjective Data

### Assess for Defining Characteristics

**Palpitations, Dyspnea, Dry Mouth, Nausea, Diaphoresis**
Precipitating factors
Frequency
Duration

**Feelings**
Extreme Sadness and Worthlessness, Guilt, Apprehension, Rejection or Isolation, Inability to Cope, Falling Apart, Racing Thoughts

**Usual Coping Behavior**
"How do you usually handle a particular situation (i.e., anger, disappointment, loss, rejection)?"
"What did you usually do when you faced similar situations in the past?"
"What happens when you do that?" (relevant coping mechanism)

## Subjective and Objective Data

### Assess for Defining Characteristics

**General Appearance**
Facial expression (e.g., sad, hostile, expressionless)
Dress (e.g., meticulous, disheveled, seductive, eccentric)

**Behavior During Interview**
*Communication Pattern*

| | |
|---|---|
| Appropriate | Rambling |
| Denial of problem | Suspicious |
| Hallucinations | Delusions |

*Flow of Thought (e.g., appropriate, difficulty concentrating)*

*Nonverbal Behavior (appropriate or inappropriate)*
Affect to verbal content
Gestures, mannerisms, facial grimaces, postures

## Interaction Skills
### With Nurse
*Appropriate*
Shows dependency          Relates well
Demanding/pleading        Withdrawn/preoccupied with self
Hostile

### With Significant Others
Relates appropriately with all family members
Problematic behavior toward one-member/all members

## Present Coping Behavior
*Appropriate*                *"Acting-out" Behaviors*
Derogatory                  Manipulating others to do tasks for him or her
Arguing, Threatening        Restlessness
Intimidating                Pacing
Ritualistic behavior
Smoking, using/abusing alcohol/drugs

### Problematic Behaviors
Withdrawing                 Avoiding talking about self
Showing signs of depression Minimizing signs and symptoms
Engaging in denial          Developing dissociation
Diverting attention         Engaging in ritualistic behavior
Sleeping                    Blocking

### Somatizing
Headache                    Anorexia
Dyspnea                     Colitis
Multiple complaints         Syncope
Hives, eczema               Menstrual disturbance

For more information on Focus Assessment Criteria, visit http://thepoint.lww.com.

**NOC**
Anxiety Level, Coping, Impulse Self-Control

## ➤ Goal

The client will relate increased psychological and physiologic comfort.

### Indicators:

- Describe own anxiety and coping patterns.
- Identifies two strategies to reduce anxiety.

**NIC**
Anxiety Reduction, Impulse Control Training, Anticipatory Guidance

## ➤ General Interventions

Nursing interventions for *Anxiety* can apply to any client with anxiety regardless of etiologic and contributing factors.

### Assist the Client to Reduce Present Level of Anxiety

### Assess Level of Anxiety (See Key Concepts): Mild, Moderate, Severe, or Panic

Provide reassurance and comfort.
Stay with the client.
Do not make demands or ask the client to make decisions.

Support present coping mechanisms (e.g., allow the client to talk, cry); do not confront or argue with defenses or rationalizations.

Speak slowly and calmly.

Be aware of your own concern and avoid reciprocal anxiety.

Convey empathic understanding (e.g., quiet presence, touch, allowing crying, talking).

Provide reassurance that a solution can be found.

Remind the client that feelings are not harmful.

Respect personal space.

**R:** Nursing strategies differ depending on the level of anxiety (Tarsitano, 1992).

### If Anxiety Is at Severe or Panic Level:

Provide a quiet, nonstimulating environment with soft lighting.

Remain calm in your approach.

Use short, simple sentences; speak slowly.

Give concise directions.

Focus on the present.

Remove excess stimulation (e.g., take the client to a quieter room); limit contact with others (e.g., other clients, family) who are also anxious.

Provide physical measures that will aid in relaxation such as warm baths, back massage, aromatherapy, and music.

Consult a physician for possible pharmacologic therapy, if indicated.

Provide an opportunity to exercise (e.g., walk fast).

**R:** Some fears are based on inaccurate information, which accurate data can relieve. A client with severe anxiety or panic does not retain learning.

**R:** The anxious client tends to overgeneralize, assume, and anticipate catastrophe. Resulting cognitive problems include difficulty with attention and concentration, loss of objectivity, and vigilance. Providing emotional support and relaxation techniques and encouraging sharing may help a client clarify and verbalize fears, allowing the nurse to give realistic feedback and reassurance. Exercise helps to dispel some anxiety.

### If the Client Is Hyperventilating or Experiencing Dyspnea

Demonstrate breathing techniques; ask the client to practice the technique with you.

Acknowledge the client's fear and give positive reinforcement for efforts.

Acknowledge feelings of helplessness.

Avoid suggesting that the client "relax." Do not leave the client alone.

Provide assistance with all tasks during acute episodes of dyspnea.

During an acute episode, do not discuss preventive measures.

During nonacute episodes, teach relaxation techniques (e.g., tapes, guided imagery).

**R:** An anxious client has a narrowed perceptual field with a diminished ability to function.

**R:** Anxiety tends to feed on itself, trapping the client in a spiral of increasing anxiety, hyperventilation, and physical pain.

**R:** Research has shown that involving family members in care increases client cooperation and positive adjustment to the experience (Leske, 1993).

## When Anxiety Diminishes, Assist the Client in Recognizing Anxiety and Causes.

Help the client to see that mild anxiety can be a positive catalyst for change does not need to be avoided.

Request validation of your assessment of anxiety (e.g., "Are you uncomfortable now?").

If the client says yes, continue with the learning process; if the client cannot acknowledge anxiety, continue supportive measures until he or she can.

When the client can learn, determine usual coping mechanisms: "What do you usually do when you get upset?" (e.g., read, discuss problems, distance, use substances, and seek social support).

Assess for unmet needs or expectations; encourage recall and description of what client experienced immediately before feeling anxious.

Assist in reevaluation of perceived threat by discussing the following:

- Were expectations realistic? Too idealistic?
- Was it possible to meet expectations?
- Where in the sequence of events was change possible?

**R:** Verbalization allows sharing and provides an opportunity to correct misconceptions.
Teach anxiety interrupters to use when client cannot avoid stressful situations:

- Look up. Lower shoulders.
- Control breathing.
- Slow thoughts. Alter voice.
- Give self-directions (out loud, if possible).
- Exercise.
- "Scruff your face"—changes facial expression.
- Change perspective: imagine watching situation from a distance (Grainger, 1990).

**R:** Relaxation techniques help the person switch the autonomous system from the fight-or-flight response to a more relaxed response (Varcarolis 2006).

## Reduce or Eliminate Problematic Coping Mechanisms

Depression, withdrawal (see *Ineffective Coping*)
Violent behavior (see *Risk for Other-Directed Violence*)
Denial

- Develop an atmosphere of empathic understanding.
- Assist in lowering the level of anxiety.
- Focus on the present situation.
- Give feedback about current reality; identify positive achievements.
- Have the client describe events in detail; focus on specifics of who, what, when, and where.

**R:** Denial can be an effective defense mechanism when the situation is too stressful to cope.

Numerous physical complaints with no known organic base (Maynard, 2004)
- Encourage expression of feelings.
- Give positive feedback when the client is symptom free.
- Acknowledge that symptoms must be burdensome.
- Encourage interest in the external environment (e.g., volunteering, helping others).
- Listen to complaints.
- Evaluate secondary gains the client receives and attempt to interrupt the cycle; see the client regularly, not simply in response to somatic complaints.
- Engage in discussions not related to symptoms.
- Avoid "doing something" to each complaint; set limits consistently.

**R:** The conversion of emotional distress into physical symptoms is called somatization. Psychological concepts that may underlie somatization are amplification of body sensations, the need to be sick, the need for one family member to be the identified client, and avoidance of the emotional stressors (Maynard, 2004).

Anger (e.g., demanding behavior, manipulation; with adults, see *Ineffective Coping*)
Unrealistic expectations of self (Lyon, 2002)

- Help to set realistic goals with short-term daily or weekly goals.
- Allow for setbacks.
- Use positive self-talk.
- Practice "thought stopping" with toxic thinking.

**R:** Unrealistic expectations will heighten expectations of self and increase anxiety. Participating in decision-making can give a client a sense of control, which enhances coping ability. Perception of loss of control can result in a sense of powerlessness, then hopelessness (Courts, Barba, & Tesh, 2001).

Toxic thoughts (Lyon, 2002)

- Avoid assigning negative meaning to an event.
- Avoid "reading someone else's mind."
- Avoid all-or-nothing, black-or-white thinking.
- Avoid making the worst of a situation.
- Attempt to fix the problem; avoid assigning blame.

**R:** Toxic thoughts can confuse the situation, increase anxiety, and reduce effective coping (Varcarolis, 2006).

Promote resiliency

- Avoid minimizing positive experiences.
- Gently encourage humor.
- Encourage optimism.
- Encourage discussion with significant others.
- Encourage the client to seek spiritual comfort through religion, nature, prayer, meditation, or other methods.

**R:** Resilience is a combination of abilities and characteristics that interact to allow an individual to bounce back, cope successfully, and function above the norm in spite of significant stress or adversity (Tusaie & Dyer, 2004). Environmental factors that favor resilience are perceived social support or a sense of connectiveness (Tusaie & Dyer, 2004).

## Initiate Health Teaching and Referrals as Indicated

Refer people identified as having chronic anxiety and maladaptive coping mechanisms for ongoing mental health counseling and treatment.
Instruct in nontechnical, understandable terms regarding illness and associated treatments.

**R:** Simple and repeating explanations are needed because anxiety may interfere with learning.

Instruct (or refer) the client for assertiveness training.

**R:** Assertiveness training helps one ask for what he or she wants, learn how to say no, and reduce the stress of unrealistic expectations of others.

Instruct the client to increase exercise and reduce TV watching (refer to Risk-Prone Health Behavior for specific interventions).

**R:** Exercise can effectively reduce anxiety (Blanchard, Courneya, & Laing, 2001). Exercise is an effective method for reducing state anxiety in breast cancer survivors (Blanchard, Courneya, & Laing, 2001).

Instruct in use of relaxation techniques (e.g., aromatherapy, hydrotherapy, music therapy, massage).
Explain the benefits of foot massage and reflexology (Grealish et al., 2000; Stephenson et al., 2000).
**R:** Complementary therapies such as massage, aromatherapy, and hydrotherapy are useful in managing stress and anxiety (Wong, Lopez-Wahas, & Molassiotis, 2001).
**R:** Music therapy is an effective nursing intervention in decreasing anxiety (Wong, Lopez-Nahas, & Molassiotis, 2001).

Provide telephone numbers for emergency intervention: hotlines, psychiatric emergency room, and on-call staff if available.

**R:** Providing access to help in the community can reduce feelings of aloneness and powerlessness.

## Pediatric Considerations

### Actions

Explain events that are sources of anxiety using simple, age-appropriate terms and illustrations, such as puppets, dolls, and sample equipment.

**R:** Explanations that are age-appropriate can reduce anxiety.

Allow child to wear underwear and have familiar toys or objects.

**R:** Any strategy that increases comfort and familiarity can reduce anxiety.

Assist the child to cope with anxiety (Hockenberry & Wilson, 2009):

- Establish a trusting relationship.
- Minimize separation from parents.
- Encourage expression of feelings.
- Involve the child in play.
- Prepare the child for new experiences (e.g., procedures, surgery).
- Provide comfort measures.
- Allow for regression.
- Encourage parental involvement in care.
- Allay parental apprehension and provide them information.

**R:** The presence of parents provides a familiar, stabilizing support. Parental anxiety influences the child's anxiety.

Assist a child with anger.

- Encourage the child to share anger (e.g., "How did you feel when you had your injection?").
- Tell the child that being angry is okay (e.g., "I sometimes get angry when I can't have what I want.").
- Encourage and allow the child to express anger in acceptable ways (e.g., loud talking, running outside around the house).

**R:** Children need opportunities and encouragement to express anger in a controlled, acceptable way (e.g., choosing not to play a particular game or with a particular person, slamming a door, voicing anger). Unacceptable expressions of anger include throwing or breaking objects and hitting others. Children who are not permitted to express anger may develop hostility and perceive the world as unfriendly.

## Maternal Considerations

### Actions

Discuss expectations and concerns regarding pregnancy and parenthood with the woman alone, her partner alone, and then together as indicated.

**R:** Some fears are based on inaccurate information, which accurate data can relieve.

Acknowledge anxieties and their normality (Lugina et al., 2001):

- 1 week postpartum: worried about feeling tired and nervous about breasts, perineum, and infection
- 1 week postpartum: worried about baby's eyes, respirations, temperature, safety, and crying
- 6 weeks' postpartum: worried about partner's reaction to her and baby

**R:** Providing emotional support and encouraging sharing may help a client clarify and verbalize fears, allowing the nurse to give realistic feedback and reassurance. If there was a previous fetal or neonatal death, provide opportunities for both mother and father to share their feelings and fears.

**R:** Partners of women with a previous pregnancy loss or neonatal death are often expected to appear strong to support their partner. Research reported that men who experience this very personal tragedy need as much emotional support and opportunities to share their grief as the mother (McCreight, 2004).

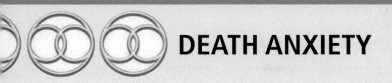

# DEATH ANXIETY

## DEFINITION

The state in which an individual experiences a vague uneasy feeling of discomfort or dread generated by perceptions of a real or imagined threat to one's existence

## DEFINING CHARACTERISTICS

Worrying about the effects of one's own death on significant others

Feeling powerless over issues related to dying

Fear of loss of mental abilities when dying

Fear of anticipated pain related to dying

Fear of suffering related to dying

Deep sadness

Fear of the process of dying

Concerns of overworking the caregiver as terminal illness incapacitates self

Total loss of control over any aspect of one's own death

Negative thoughts related to death or dying

Fear of prolonged dying

Fear of premature death

## RELATED FACTORS

A diagnosis of a potentially terminal condition or impending death can cause this diagnosis. Additional factors can contribute to death anxiety.

### Situational (Personal, Environmental)

*Related to personal conflict with palliative versus curative care*

*Related to conflict with family regarding palliative versus. curative care*

*Related to fear of being a burden*

*Related to fear of unmanageable pain*

*Related to fear of abandonment*

*Related to unresolved conflict (family, friends)*

*Related to fear that one's life lacked meaning*

*Related to social disengagement*

*Related to powerlessness and vulnerability*

*Related to nonacceptance of own mortality*

*Related to uncertainty about life after death*

*Related to uncertainty about an encounter with a higher power*

*Related to uncertainty about the existence of a higher power*

*Related to experiencing the dying process*

*Related to anticipated impact of death on others*

### ■■■■■ AUTHOR'S NOTE

The inclusion of *Death Anxiety* in the NANDA classification creates a diagnostic category with the etiology in the label. This opens the NANDA list to thousands of diagnostic labels with etiology (e.g., separation anxiety, failure anxiety, and travel anxiety). Many diagnostic labels can take this same path: fear as claustrophobic fear, diarrhea as traveler's diarrhea, decisional conflict as end-of-life decisional conflict.

Specifically end-of life situations create multiple responses in clients and significant others. Some of these are shared and expected of those involved. These responses could be described with a syndrome diagnosis as End-of-Life Syndrome. This author recommends its development by nurses engaged in palliative and hospice care.

## ■■■■■■ ERRORS IN DIAGNOSTIC STATEMENTS

### Death anxiety related to terminal illness

This diagnosis reflects multiple issues and responses to terminal illness as fear, pain, powerlessness, grieving, interrupted family processes, etc. Without a syndrome diagnosis, the nurse must assess for problematic responses and use specific nursing diagnoses as pain, grieving.

Reserve death anxiety for those related factors that will inhibit the client to a peaceful death psychologically and spiritually (e.g., an unresolved conflict with a friend).

## ■■■■■■ KEY CONCEPTS

In a research study of the reactions of 153 rehabilitation counselors to possible client death, 22% reported they preferred not to work with clients with life-threatening illnesses. Death anxiety scores were higher in younger respondents (younger than 44 years of age). Educational programs and support groups help reduce death anxiety in health care workers (Hunt & Rosenthal, 2000).

In response to the difficult situation of attempting to help a client understand the seriousness of metastatic cancer, Campbell reports he says, "When cancer has spread from where it has started to somewhere else in the body, it means it is metastatic and cannot be cured. That means that while we can treat your cancer, hopefully lengthening your life and controlling symptoms, we can never make it go away. And because you are otherwise healthy, it means it's likely you will one day die from this cancer" (2008, p. 5). When the prognosis is very poor, Campbell reports he says, "I am afraid you are dying" (2008, p. 5).

### Transcultural Considerations

Truth-telling is critical to the dominant culture of Americans and Canadians to preserve individual autonomy. Other cultures may not value truth-telling if it disrupts family solidarity. Refer to Spiritual Distress for a review of religious beliefs and rituals regarding death.

## Focus Assessment Criteria

See *Anxiety* and *Grieving*.

**NOC**
Dignified Life Closure, Fear Self-Control, Client Satisfaction, Decision-Making, Family Coping

### ➤ Goal

The client will report diminished anxiety or fear.

### *Indicators:*

• Share feelings regarding dying.
• Identify specific requests that will increase psychological comfort.

**NIC**
Limit Setting, Patient Rights Protection, Family Support, Dying Care, Coping Enhancement, Active Listening, Emotional Support, Spiritual Support

### ➤ General Interventions

For a client with a new or early diagnosis of a potentially terminal condition:

• Allow the client and family separate opportunities to discuss their understanding of the condition. Correct misinformation.
• Access valid information regarding condition, treatment options, and stage of condition from primary provider (physician, nurse practitioner).
• Ensure a discussion of the prognosis if known.

**R:** With a diagnosis of a potential terminal illness, clients and families should be given opportunities to talk about treatments, cures, and goals regarding quality of life (e.g., curative vs. symptomatic comfort care.

For the client experiencing a progression of a terminal illness:
Explore with the client his or her understanding of the situation and feelings.

**R:** It is important to determine the client's understanding of the situation and personal preferences or requests.

Ensure that the primary physician or nurse practitioner initiate a discussion regarding the situation and options desired by the client.

**R:** These discussions provide insight into the client's understanding and directs treatment decisions. Research reports that only 31% of persons with terminal conditions reported end-of-life discussions with a physician (Wright, 2008b).

Encourage the client to reconstruct his or her world view:

• Allow the client to verbalize feelings about the meaning of death.
• Advise the client that there are no right or wrong feelings.
• Advise the client that responses are his or her choice.
• Acknowledge struggles.
• Encourage dialogue with a spiritual mentor or soul friend.

**R:** When a client is facing death, reconstructing a world view involves balancing thoughts about the painful subject with avoiding painful thoughts.

Allow significant others opportunities to share their perceptions and concerns. Advise them that sadness is expected and normal.
Clarify the difference between healthy grieving with pathological depression.

**R:** Clarification is needed to determine if their concerns regarding end-of-life care is consistent with the client. "It is normal and healthy to feel sad at the end of life, to grieve the impending loss of everything a person holds dear" (Coombs-Lee, 2008, p.12).

Discuss the value of truthful conversations, e.g., sorrow, mistakes, disagreements,

**R:** "Avoiding truthful conversations does not bring hope and comfort: it brings isolation and loneliness" (Coombs-Lee, 2008, p12).

To foster psychospiritual growth, dialogue with the client specifically (Yokimo, 2009, p. 700):

• If your time is indeed shortened, what do you need to get done?
• Are there people whom you need to contact in order to resolve feeling or unfinished business?
• What do you want to do with whatever time you have left?

If appropriate, offer to help the client contact others to resolve conflicts (old or new) verbally or in writing. Validate that forbygiveness is not a seeking reconciliation, "but a letting go of a hurt" (Yakimo, 2009, p. 707).

**R:** "Asking for or providing forgiveness is a powerful healing tool" (Yakimo, 2009, p.706).

The nurse through listening can help the client with personal growth.
Explain preparatory depression and associate behaviors to significant others (Yakimo, 2009).

• Realization of impending death
• Reviewing what their life has meant
• Reflections on life review and sorrow of impeding losses

**R:** Preparatory depression is when the person realizes his or her approaching death and desires to be released from suffering (Yakimo, 2009).

Encourage significant others to allow for life review and sorrow and not to try and "cheer him or her up."

**R:** Acceptance of the final separation in life is not reached until the dying client's life review and sorrow is listened to (Yakimo, 2009).

Respect the dying client's wishes (e.g., few or no visitors, modifications in care, no heroic measures, or food or liquid preferences).

**R:** If the person is ready to release life and die and others expect him or her to want to continue to live, or the person's own depression, grief, and turmoil are increased (Yakimo, 2009, p. 700).

Encourage the client to:

• Tell life stories and reminisce.
• Discuss leaving a legacy: donation, personal articles, or taped messages.

**R:** Strategies that help the client find meaning in failures and successes can reduce anxiety and depression.

Encourage reflective activities, such as personal prayer, meditation, and journal writing.
Return to a previously pleasurable activity. Examples include painting, music, woodworking, and quilting.
Return of the gift of love to others by listening, praying for others, sharing personal wisdom gained from illness, and creating legacy gifts.

**R:** Promoting and restoring interests, imagination, and creativity enhance quality of life (Brant, 1998).

Aggressively manage unrelieved symptoms:
Nausea   Vomiting
Pruritus   Fatigue
Pain

Explain palliative care and advance directives and assist in the process if desired.

**R:** Serious unrelieved symptoms can cause a distressing death and needless added suffering for families (Nelson et al., 2000).

## Initiate Referrals and Health Teaching as Indicated

### Explain Palliative Care (Miller, 2009)

• Has the primary focus of ensuring comfort and psychosocial and spiritual well-being rather than improving physical function
• Management of distressing symptoms (e.g., pain, thirst, nausea, dyspnea, constipation, dry mouth)
• Education and support of family and significant others
• Consultation, education, and support of professional caregivers.

**R:** Palliative care is a holistic approach to caring for persons with advanced progressive illness. Palliative care can be provided at any point during the course of an illness. Palliative care will always be a part of hospice care, but it can be provided to persons not in a hospice program (Miller, 2009).

Explain hospice care:

• Hospice has designated caregivers, nurses, social service, physicians, and nurse practitioners in the program
• Hospice provides palliative care in homes and health care settings
• Refer to educational resources (e.g., National Hospice and Palliative Organization: www.nhpco.org)

 **Pediatric Considerations**

**Educate Parents about the Need to Explain Honestly and Age-Appropriately the Child's Impending Death; Consult with Experts as Needed**

**R:** Chronically ill children with poor prognoses or termini illnesses often know more about death than is thought by adults. "Children are harmed by what they do not know, by what they are not told, and by their misconceptions" (Yakimo, 2009).

**When Someone Else or a Pet Is Dying or Has Died (Yakimo, 2009):**
• Explain what is happening or what happened
• Ask the child how he or she feels.
• Have a funeral for the pet.

- Be specific that the child is not responsible for the death.
- Explain the funeral service and discuss if the child will attend.
- Explain that adults will be sad and crying. Limit exposure.

**Do Not:**

Associate death with sleep.

Force a young child to attend the funeral.

Tell the child not to cry.

Give a long, detailed explanation beyond the child's level of understanding.

**R:** Explanations regarding death need to be age-appropriate and factual to avoid misconceptions and escalation of fears (Hockenberry & Wilson, 2009). Shielding older children from death and funerals does not prepare them from the reality of death.

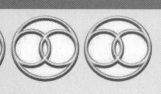

# RISK FOR BLEEDING

## ▶ Risk for Complications of Bleeding

## DEFINITION (NANDA)

At risk for a decrease in blood volume that may compromise health

## RISK FACTORS (NANDA)

Aneurysm

Circumcision

Deficient knowledge

Disseminated intravascular coagulation

History of falls

Gastrointestinal disorders (e.g., gastric ulcer disease, polyps, varices)

Impaired liver function (e.g., cirrhosis, hepatitis)

Inherent coagulopathies (e.g., thrombocytopenia)

Postpartum complications (e.g., uterine atony, retained placenta)

Pregnancy-related complications (e.g., placenta previa, molar pregnancy, abruption placenta)

Trauma

Treatment-related side effects (e.g., surgery, medications, administration of platelets deficient blood products, chemotherapy)

### ▪▪▪▪▪ AUTHOR'S NOTES

This new NANDA-I diagnosis represents several collaborative problems.

## Interventions/Goals

Refer to Section 3 for the specific collaborative problem such as Risk for Complications of Hypovolemia, Risk for Complications of Bleeding, Risk for Complications of GI Bleeding, Risk for Complications of Prenatal Bleeding, Risk for Complications of Postpartum Hemorrhage, or Risk for Complications of Anticoagulant Therapy

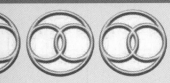

# RISK FOR UNSTABLE BLOOD GLUCOSE

▶ **Risk for Complications of Hypoglycemia/Hyperglycemia**

## DEFINITION (NANDA)

Risk for Variation of Blood Glucose/Sugar Levels from the Normal Range

## RISK FACTORS (NANDA)

Deficient knowledge of diabetes management (e.g., action plan)
Developmental level
Dietary intake
Inadequate blood glucose monitoring
Lack of acceptance of diagnosis
Lack of adherence to diabetes management (e.g., action plan)
Lack of diabetes management (e.g., action plan)

Medication management
Physical activity level
Physical health status
Pregnancy
Rapid growth periods
Stress
Weight gain
Weight loss

### ■■■■■■ AUTHOR'S NOTE

This new nursing diagnosis represents a situation that requires collaborative intervention with medicine. This author recommends that the Collaborative Problem Hyper/Hyperglycemia be used instead. Students should consult with their faculty for advice to use Risk for Unstable Blood Glucose or Risk for Complications of Hypoglycemia/Hyperglycemia.

Refer to Section 3 for interventions for these diagnoses.

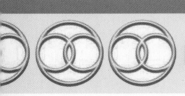

# RISK FOR IMBALANCED BODY TEMPERATURE

Hyperthermia
Hypothermia
Ineffective Thermoregulation
Related to Newborn Transition to Extrauterine Environment

## DEFINITION

The state in which the individual is at risk for failing to maintain body temperature within normal range (36° to 37.5° C or 98° to 99.5° F) (Smeltzer & Bare, 2008)

## RISK FACTORS

Presence of risk factors (see Related Factors).

# RELATED FACTORS

## Treatment Related

### *Related to cooling effects of:*

| | |
|---|---|
| Parenteral fluid infusion/blood transfusion | Dialysis |
| Cooling blanket | Operating suite |

## Situational (Personal, Environmental)

### *Related to:*

| | |
|---|---|
| Exposure to cold, rain, snow, wind/exposure to heat, sun, and humidity extremes | Inability to pay for shelter, heat, or air conditioning |
| | Extremes of weight |
| | Consumption of alcohol |
| Inappropriate clothing for climate | Dehydration/malnutrition |
| Newborn birth environment exposure | Insufficient drying |

## Maturational

### *Related to ineffective temperature regulation secondary to extremes of age (e.g., newborn, older adult)*

■■■■■■ **AUTHOR'S NOTE**

*Risk for Imbalanced Body Temperature* includes those at risk for *Hyperthermia, Hypothermia, Ineffective Thermoregulation,* or all of these. If the client is at risk for only one (e.g., *Hypothermia* but not *Hyperthermia*), then it is more useful to label the problem with the specific diagnosis (*Risk for Hypothermia*). If the client is at risk for two or more, then *Risk for Imbalanced Body Temperature* is more appropriate. The focus of nursing care is preventing abnormal body temperatures by identifying and treating those with normal temperature who demonstrate risk factors that nurse-prescribed interventions (e.g., removing blankets, adjusting environmental temperature) can control. If the imbalance is related to a pathophysiologic complication that requires nursing and medical interventions, then the problem should be labeled as a collaborative problem (e.g., *RC of Severe Hypothermia related to hypothalamus injury*). The focus of concern then becomes monitoring to detect and report significant temperature fluctuations and implementing collaborative interventions (e.g., a warming or cooling blanket) as ordered. See also Author's Notes for *Hyperthermia* and *Hypothermia.*

■■■■■ **KEY CONCEPTS**

## Generic Considerations

- The body has two major compartments: the *shell* (skin and subcutaneous tissue) and the *core* (vital internal organs, intestinal tract, and large muscle groups). Heat transfer involves shell and core; it is possible for the shell to be warm while the core is cold, and vice versa.
- Regulation of body temperature is a dynamic process involving four mechanisms (Porth, 2006):
  - *Conduction:* Direct transfer of heat from the body to cooler objects without motion (e.g., from cells and capillaries to skin and onto clothing)
  - *Convection:* Transfer of heat by circulation (e.g., from warmer core areas to peripheral areas and from air movement next to the skin)
  - *Radiation:* Transfer of heat between the skin and the environment
  - *Evaporation:* Transfer of heat when skin or clothing is wet and heat is lost through moisture into the environment
- Heat production occurs in the core, which is innervated by thermoreceptor stimulation from the hypothalamus.
- Normothermia is defined as a core temperature of 36.6° to 37.5° C or 98° to 99.5° F (Smeltzer & Bare, 2008).
- Heat loss and gain vary in individuals and are influenced by body surface area, peripheral vasomotor tone, and quantity of subcutaneous tissue.

*(continued)*

■ ■ ■ ■ ■ ■ **KEY CONCEPTS** *Continued*

- Shivering, the body's physiologic attempt to create more heat, produces profound physiologic responses:
  - Increased oxygen consumption to two to five times the normal rate
  - Increased metabolic demand to as much as 400% to 500%
  - Increased myocardial work, carbon dioxide production, cutaneous vasoconstriction, and eventual lactic acid production

The reliability of temperature depends on accurate temperature-taking technique, minimization of variables affecting the temperature measurement device, and the site chosen for measurement.

- Oral temperature readings may be unreliable (from such variables as poor contact between the thermometer and mucosa, air movement, and smoking or drinking before temperature taking); oral temperatures measure 0.5° below core temperature (Giuliano et al., 2000).
- Rectal temperature readings, which have fewer affecting variables and are more reliable than oral readings, measure 0.5° C above core temperature at normothermia, and at temperatures less than 36.5° C measure *peripheral* temperature rather than *core* temperature. Rectal temperatures measure 1° *higher* than oral temperature readings.
- Axillary temperature readings are reliable only for skin temperature; they measure 1° *lower* than oral temperature readings.

## Hyperthermia

- The body responds to hot environments by increasing heat dissipation through increased sweat production and dilation of peripheral blood vessels.
- Increased metabolic rate increases body temperature and vice versa (increased body temperature increases metabolic rate).
- Fever is a major sign of onset of infection, inflammation, and disease: treatment with aspirin or acetaminophen without medical consultation may mask important symptoms that should receive medical attention.
- Blood is the body's cooling fluid: low blood volume from dehydration predisposes one to fever.

## Hypothermia

- The body responds to cold environments with mechanisms aimed at preventing heat loss and increasing heat production:

  | | |
  |---|---|
  | Muscle contraction | Peripheral vasoconstriction |
  | Increased heart rate | Dilation of blood vessels in muscles |
  | Shivering and vasodilatation | Release of thyroxine and corticosteroids |

- Severe hypothermia can cause life-threatening dysrhythmias and must be referred to a physician.
- Without safe and effective re-warming, hypothermia (a core temperature <35° C [95° F]) in the postoperative period has many profound negative effects (decreased myocardial and cerebral functions, respiratory acidosis, impaired hematologic and immunologic functions, and cold diuresis). Hypothermia also reduces blood pressure and contributes to shock.
- Vasodilatation promotes heat loss and predisposes to hypothermia.

## Pediatric Considerations

Almost every child experiences a fever of 100° to 104° F at some time. It usually does not harm normal children; only approximately 4% of febrile children are susceptible to convulsions. Children younger than 18 years with fever accompanied by symptoms of influenza should never be medicated with aspirin or products containing aspirin because of the risk of development of potentially fatal Reye's syndrome.

- Newborns are vulnerable to heat loss because of the following (Varda & Behnke, 2000). The following sequence illustrates this mechanism:

Large body surface area relative to body mass
Less adipose tissue for insulation
Environment (delivery room, nursery)

Increased basal metabolism rate
Prematurity
Malfunction of surroundings providing
   warmth (Isolette, radiant warmer)

- Hyperthermia may result from malfunction of warming equipment (Isolette, radiant warmer).
- Nonshivering thermogenesis is a heat production mechanism located in brown fat (highly vascular adipose tissue) found only in infants. When skin temperature begins to drop, thermal receptors transmit impulses to the central nervous system. The following sequence illustrates this mechanism:
  Central nervous system (CNS) → Stimulates sympathetic nervous system → Release of norepinephrine from adrenal gland and at nerve endings in brown fat → Heat production. Thermoregulation is controlled by hypothalamus. Untreated hypothermia can result in newborn weigh loss, glucose utilization, metabolic hypoxemia, hypoxia, and death.
- Treating all fevers in children is unnecessary. Fevers related to heat stroke can be treated with tepid or cold sponging. Fevers (less than 104° F or 40° C) in previously well children with no history of febrile convulsions and without a threatening illness can be left untreated or, if desired, treated with acetaminophen. Sponging increases the child's discomfort.
- Tepid sponging instead of antipyretic drugs is indicated for very young infants and children with severe liver disease or a history of hypersensitivity to antipyretic drugs.

## Geriatric Considerations

Older adults can become hypothermic or hyperthermic in moderately cold or hot environments, compared with younger adults, who require exposure to severe cold or hot temperatures (Miller, 2009).
- Age-related changes that interfere with the body's ability to adapt to cold temperature include inefficient vasoconstriction, decreased cardiac output, decreased subcutaneous tissue, and delayed and diminished sweating (Miller, 2009).
- Older adults have a higher threshold for onset and decreased efficiency of sweating.
- Older adults have a dulled perception of cold and warmth and thus may lack the stimulus to initiate protective actions.
- The thirst mechanism becomes less efficient with aging, as does the kidney's ability to concentrate urine, increasing the risk of heat-related dehydration.
- Inactivity and immobility increase susceptibility to hypothermia by suppressing shivering and reducing heat-generating muscle activity.
- Seventy percent of all victims of heat stroke are older than 60 years.

# Focus Assessment Criteria

## Subjective Data

### Assess for Defining Characteristics

History of symptoms (abnormal skin temperature, altered mentation, headaches, nausea, lethargy, vertigo)
Onset

### Assess for Related Factors

Hyperthermia
Dehydration
Recent exposure to communicable disease without known immunity
   (e.g., measles without vaccine or previous illness)
Recent overexposure to sun, heat, humidity
Recent overactivity
Radiation/chemotherapy/immunosuppression
Alcohol use
Impaired judgment
Home environment
Adequate ventilation?          Air conditioning?
Automobile environment?      Room temperature?

Medications

| | | |
|---|---|---|
| Diuretics | Anticholinergics | CNS depressants |
| Antidepressants | Vasoconstrictors | |

How often taken? Last dose taken when?

### Hypothermia

Recent exposure to cold/dampness

Inactivity

Impaired judgment

Medications

| | |
|---|---|
| Vasodilators | CNS depressants |

Home environment

| | | |
|---|---|---|
| Heating, blankets | Clothing (e.g., socks, hat, gloves) | Shelter |

### Problems That May Contribute to Hyperthermia or Hypothermia

| | | |
|---|---|---|
| Smoking | Circulatory problems (specify) | History of frostbite |
| Diabetes | Mobility problems | Cardiovascular disorders |
| Repeated infections | Neurologic disorders | Peripheral vascular disease |

## Objective Data

### Assess for Defining Characteristics

#### Vital Signs

| | | |
|---|---|---|
| Normal baseline temperature | Present temperature | Abnormal respiratory rate |
| Abnormal heart rate, rhythm | Abnormal blood pressure | |

#### Mental Status

#### Skin and Circulation

#### Signs of Dehydration

| | |
|---|---|
| Parched mouth/furrowed tongue/dry lips | Increased urine specific gravity |

For more information on Focus Assessment Criteria, visit http://thepoint.lww.com.

---

**NOC**
Thermoregulation

## ➤ Goal

The client will demonstrate a temperature within normal limits for age.

### Indicators:

Report measures to prevent temperature fluctuations.
Report episodes of chills, diaphoresis, shivering, cool skin

---

**NIC**
Temperature Regulation, Temperature Regulation: Intraoperative, Environmental Management

## ➤ Interventions

Monitor temperature as needed (1 to 4 hours). Use continuous temperature monitoring for vulnerable individuals as critically ill adults, neonates, and infants.

**R:** Continuous temperature monitoring will provide early detection of temperature changes to prevent cardiovascular complications (Smith, 2004).

Use oral thermometers if possible.

**R:** The oral route is more reliable than tympanic or axillary (Giuliano et al., 2000).

Maintain consistent room temperature of 22.2° C (72° F). Avoid drafts.

**R:** This temperature will prevent heat loss through radiation.

During bathing, expose only small sections of the body. After washing, cover the area with absorbent blanket.

**R:** These interventions will reduce heat loss from evaporation.

Ensure that optimal nutrition and hydration is achieved.

**R:** Dehydration can decrease body temperature by reducing fluid volume. Increased calories are needed to maintain metabolic functioning during fever (Edwards, 1999).

Refer to Ineffective Thermoregulation for interventions for newborns.
Refer to Hypothermia or Hyperthermia for interventions to prevent body temperature disruptions.

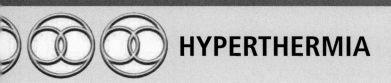

# HYPERTHERMIA

## DEFINITION

The state in which an individual has or is at risk of having a sustained elevation of body temperature greater than 37.8° C (100° F) orally or 38.8° C (101° F) rectally due to external factors

## DEFINING CHARACTERISTICS

### Major (Must Be Present)

Temperature higher than 37.8° C (100° F) orally or 38.8° C (101° F) rectally

### Minor (May Be Present)

Flushed skin                    Dehydration
Warm to touch                   Specific or generalized aches and pains (e.g., headache)
Increased respiratory rate      Malaise/fatigue/weakness
Tachycardia                     Loss of appetite
Shivering/goose pimples

## RELATED FACTORS

### Treatment-Related

Decreased ability to sweat secondary to (specify medication)

### Situational (Personal, Environmental)

*Related to:*
Exposure to heat, sun
Inappropriate clothing for climate
No access to air conditioning
Newborn hospital environment warming equipment
*Related to decreased circulation secondary to:*
Extremes of weight
Dehydration
*Related to insufficient hydration for vigorous activity*

### Maturational

*Related to ineffective temperature regulation secondary to age (refer to* Ineffective Thermoregulation)

## ■■■■■■ AUTHOR'S NOTE

The nursing diagnoses *Hypothermia* and *Hyperthermia* represent people with temperature below and above normal, respectively. Some of these states are treatable by nursing interventions, such as correcting external causes (e.g., inappropriate clothing, exposure to elements [heat or cold], and dehydration). Nursing care centers on preventing or treating mild hypothermia and hyperthermia. As life-threatening situations that require medical and nursing interventions, severe hypothermia and hyperthermia represent collaborative problems and should be labeled *RC of Hypothermia* or *RC of Hyperthermia*.

Temperature elevation from infections, other disorders (e.g., hypothalamic), or treatments (e.g., hypothermia units) require collaborative treatment. If desired, the nurse could use the nursing diagnosis *Impaired Comfort* and the collaborative problem *RC of Hypothermia* or *RC of Hyperthermia*.

## ■■■■■■ ERRORS IN DIAGNOSTIC STATEMENTS

1. *Hyperthermia related to intraoperative pharmacogenic hypermetabolism*
   This situation describes malignant hyperthermia, a life-threatening, inherited disorder resulting in a hypermetabolic state related to use of anesthetic agents and depolarizing muscle relaxants. *RC of Malignant Hypertension* would more appropriately describe this situation, which necessitates rapid detection and treatment by both nursing and medicine.
2. *Hyperthermia related to effect of circulating endotoxins on hypothalamus secondary to sepsis*
   Nursing for people with elevated temperature in acute care focuses on monitoring and managing the fever with nursing and physician orders or promoting comfort through nursing orders. *Impaired Comfort* would more appropriately describe a situation that nurses treat, with *RC of Sepsis* representing the physiologic complication that nurses monitor for and manage with nurse-prescribed and physician-prescribed interventions.

## Focus Assessment Criteria

See *Risk for Imbalanced Body Temperature*.
For more information on Focus Assessment Criteria, visit http://thepoint.lww.com.

| **NOC** |
| --- |
| Thermoregulation |

## ➤ Goal

The client will maintain body temperature.

### Indicators:

- Identify risk factors for hyperthermia.
- Reduce risk factors for hyperthermia.

| **NIC** |
| --- |
| Fever Treatment, Temperature Regulation, Environmental Management, Fluid Management |

## ➤ General Interventions

### Remove or Reduce Contributing Risk Factors

#### Dehydration

Monitor intake and output and provide favorite Teach importance of maintaining adequate fluid intake (at least 2,000 mL a day of cool liquids unless contraindicated by heart or kidney disease. Explain the importance of not relying on thirst sensation as an indication of the need for fluid.

**R:** Increased calories and fluids are required to maintain metabolic functions during fever.

Recommended fluid replacement for moderate activities in hot weather (DeFabio, 2000) is as follows:

- 78° F to 84.9° F       16 oz/h
- 85° F to 89.9° F       24 oz/h
- Greater than 90° F    32 oz/h

See also *Deficient Fluid Volume*.

**R:** Strategies are used to maintain balance between intake and output.

Avoid caffeine and alcohol.

**R:** Caffeine and alcohol are diuretics and therefore further dehydrate.

## *Environmental Warmth/Exercise*

Assess whether clothing or bedcovers are too warm for the environment or planned activity.

Remove excess clothing or blankets (remove hat, gloves, or socks, as appropriate) to promote heat loss. Encourage wearing loose cotton clothing.

**R:** Adding clothes or blankets inhibits the body's natural ability to reduce body temperature; removing clothes or blankets enhances the body's natural ability to reduce body temperature.

**R:** Exposure of the head, face, hands, and feet can affect body temperature greatly. Heat is conducted from the blood vessels of these vascular areas to the skin and from the skin to the air, and where cold is conducted from the air to the skin and from the skin to the blood vessels.

Provide air conditioning, dehumidifiers, fans, or cool baths or compresses as appropriate.

Teach the importance of increasing fluid intake during warm weather and exercise. Advise against exercising in hot weather.

**R:** Activity level and environmental temperature greatly affect body temperature; high humidity increases the effect of cold or heat on the body.

**Initiate Health Teaching as Indicated**

Explain that children and older adults are more at risk for hyperthermia.

Teach the early signs of hyperthermia or heat stroke:

Flushed skin       Headache/confusion

Fatigue             Loss of appetite

Teach the client to take cool baths several times a day in hot temperatures, avoiding soap to prevent skin drying.

Teach the client to apply ice packs or cool, wet towels to the body, especially on the axillae and groin.

Explain the need to avoid alcohol, caffeine, and large, heavy meals during hot weather.

Stress the need to report persistent elevated temperature.

Teach the need to wear a hat or use an umbrella during sun exposure.

**R:** Explanations are given for appropriate dressing of children and infants related to warm weather and prevention of hyperthermia in adults.

# HYPOTHERMIA*

## DEFINITION

The state in which an individual has or is at risk of having a sustained reduction of body temperature of below 35.5° C (96° F) rectally because of increased vulnerability to external factors*

## DEFINING CHARACTERISTICS†

### Major (80% to 100%)

Reduction in body temperature below 35.5° C (96° F) rectally†
Cool skin
Pallor (moderate)
Shivering (mild)

### Minor (50% to 79%)

Mental confusion/drowsiness/restlessness
Decreased pulse and respiration
Cachexia/malnutrition

## RELATED FACTORS

### Situational (Personal, Environmental)

*Related to:*
Exposure to cold, rain, snow, wind
Inappropriate clothing for climate
Inability to pay for shelter or heat
*Related to decreased circulation secondary to:*

| | |
|---|---|
| Extremes of weight | Dehydration |
| Consumption of alcohol | Inactivity |

### Maturational

*Related to ineffective temperature regulation secondary to age (e.g., neonate, older adult).*

■■■■■■ **AUTHOR'S NOTE**

Because more serious hypothermia (temperatures below 35° C or 95° F rectally) can cause severe pathophysiologic consequences, such as decreased myocardial and respiratory function, the nurse must report these low readings to the physician. This is a Collaborative Problem: *RC of Hypothermia*. Nurses most often initiate nurse-prescribed interventions for mild hypothermia (temperatures between 35° C [95° F] and 36° C [97° F] rectally) to prevent more serious hypothermia. Nurses are commonly responsible for identifying and preventing *Risk for Hypothermia*. See also *Risk for Imbalanced Body Temperature*.

---

*Temperatures below 35° C (95° F) rectally should be reported to the physician for collaborative management of re-warming.

†Adapted from Carroll, S. M. (1989). Nursing diagnosis: Hypothermia. In R. M. Carroll-Johnson (Ed.). *Classification of nursing diagnosis: Proceedings of the eighth conference.* Philadelphia: J. B. Lippincott.

■ ■ ■ ■ ■ ■ **ERRORS IN DIAGNOSTIC STATEMENTS**
See *Risk for Imbalanced Body Temperature* and *Hyperthermia*.

## Focus Assessment Criteria

See *Risk for Imbalanced Body Temperature*.
For more information on Focus Assessment Criteria, visit http://thepoint.lww.com.

**NOC**
Thermoregulation

## ➤ Goal

The client will maintain body temperature within normal limits.

### Indicators:

- Identify risk factors for hypothermia.
- Reduce risk factors for hypothermia.

**NIC**
Hypothermia
Treatment,
Temperature
Regulation,
Temperature
Regulation:
Intraoperative,
Environmental
Management

## ➤ General Interventions

### Assess for Risk Factors

Refer to Related Factors.

### Monitor Body and Environmental Temperatures

### Reduce or Eliminate Causative or Contributing Factors, If Possible

#### Prolonged Exposure to Cold Environment

Assess room temperatures at home.
Teach the client to keep room temperatures at 70° F to 75° F or to layer clothing with sweaters.
Explain the importance of wearing a hat, gloves, and warm socks and shoes to prevent heat loss.
Discourage going outside when temperatures are very cold.
Acquire an electric blanket, warm blankets, or down comforter and flannel sheets for the bed.
Provide a hot bath before the client is cold.
Teach the client to wear close-knit undergarments to prevent heat loss.
Explain that more clothes may be needed in the morning, when body metabolism is lowest.
Consult with social service to identify sources of financial assistance/warm clothing/blankets, shelter.
Teach the importance of preventing heat loss before body temperature is actually lowered.
Acquire warm socks, sweaters, gloves, and hats.

**R:** Minimizing evaporation, convections, conduction, and radiation can prevent significant heat losses.

### Neurovascular/Peripheral Vascular Disease

Keep room temperature at 70° F to 74° F.
Assess for adequate circulation to the extremities (i.e., satisfactory peripheral pulses).
Instruct the client to wear warm gloves and socks to reduce heat loss.
Teach the client to take a warm bath if he or she cannot get warm.

**R:** Decreased circulation cause cold extremities.

## Initiate Health Teaching If Indicated

Explain the relationship of age as a risk for hypothermia.
Teach the early signs of hypothermia: cool skin, pallor, blanching, and redness.

Explain the need to drink 8 to 10 glasses of water daily and to consume frequent, small meals with warm liquids.

Explain the need to avoid alcohol during periods of very cold weather.

**R:** Early detection of hypothermia can prevent tissue damage.

## Reduce Heat Loss During Surgery

Warmed blankets
Limit exposed areas
Warmed fluids (intravenous, irrigating)
Heating and humidifying inhaled gases

**R:** People whose temperatures are maintained at normal levels during the intraoperative period experience fewer adverse outcomes; hospital costs also are lower.

The greatest reduction in temperature is during the first hour of surgery.

**Pediatric and Geriatric Interventions**

### For Extremes of Age (Newborns, Older Adults)

Maintain room temperature at 70° F to 74° F.

Instruct the adult client to wear hat, gloves, and socks if necessary to prevent heat loss.

Explain to family members that newborns, infants, and older adults are more susceptible to heat loss (see also *Ineffective Thermoregulation*).

**R:** Older adults can become hypothermic or hyperthermic in moderately cold or hot environments, compared with younger adults, who require exposure to severe cold or hot temperatures (Miller, 2009).

**R:** Infants are vulnerable to heat loss because of large body surface area relative to body mass, increased basal metabolism rate, and less adipose tissue for insulation (Varda & Behnke, 2000).

### During Intraoperative Experience

For children and older adults, unless hypothermia is desired to reduce blood loss, consider the following interventions (Puterbough, 1991):

- Increase ambient temperature of operating room (OR) before the case.
- Use a portable radiant heating lamp to provide additional heat during surgery.
- Cover with warm blankets when arriving in the OR.
- When possible, use a warming mattress.
- During prepping and surgery, keep as much of body surface covered as possible.
- Warm prep set, blood, fluids, anesthesia, and irrigants.
- Replace wet gowns and drapes with dry ones.
- Keep head well covered.
- Continue heat-conserving interventions postoperatively.

**R:** Children and older adults can become hypothermic in moderately cold OR environments (Miller, 2009; Hockenberry et al., 2009).

During the immediate postoperative period, clients are prone to hypothermia related to prolonged exposure to cold in the OR and the infusion of large quantities of cool intravenous fluids.

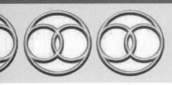

# INEFFECTIVE THERMOREGULATION

## DEFINITION

The state in which an individual experiences or is at risk of experiencing an inability to maintain a stable core normal body temperature in the presence of adverse or changing external factors

## DEFINING CHARACTERISTICS

Temperature fluctuations related to limited metabolic compensatory regulation in response to environmental factors

## RELATED FACTORS

### Situational (Personal, Environmental)

*Related to:*

Fluctuating environmental temperatures
Cold or wet articles (clothes, cribs, equipment)
Inadequate housing

Wet body surface
Inadequate clothing for weather (excessive, insufficient)

### Maturational

***Related to limited metabolic compensatory regulation secondary to age (e.g., neonate, older adult)***

## ■■■■■■ AUTHOR'S NOTE

*Ineffective Thermoregulation* is a useful diagnosis for people with difficulty maintaining a stable core body temperature over a wide range of environmental temperatures. This diagnosis most commonly applies to older adults and newborns. Thermoregulation involves balancing heat production and heat loss. Nursing care focuses on manipulating external factors (e.g., clothing and environmental conditions) to maintain body temperature within normal limits, and on teaching prevention strategies.

## ■■■■■■ ERRORS IN DIAGNOSTIC STATEMENTS

1. *Ineffective Thermoregulation related to effects of a hypothalamic tumor*
   Hypothalamic tumors can affect the temperature-regulating centers, resulting in body temperature shifts. This situation requires constant surveillance and rapid response to changes with appropriate nursing and medical treatments. Thus, this situation would be better described as a collaborative problem: *RC of Hypo/Hyperthermia.*
2. *Ineffective Thermoregulation related to temperature fluctuations*
   Temperature fluctuations represent a manifestation of the diagnosis, not a related factor. If the fluctuations result from age-related limited compensatory regulation, the diagnosis would be written: *Ineffective Thermoregulation related to decreased ability to acclimatize to heat or cold secondary to age*, as evidenced by temperature fluctuations.

## Focus Assessment Criteria

### Objective Data

#### *Assess for Defining Characteristics*

**Skin**
Color
Temperature

Nailbeds
Rashes

**Temperature**

Environment (home, infant [ambient, radiant warmer; Isolette])

Body (adult, child [rectal, oral], newborn [axillary])

**Respiration**

Rate            Rhythm

Any retractions     Breath sounds

**Heart Rate**

For more information on Focus Assessment Criteria, visit http://thepoint.lww.com.

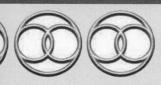

# INEFFECTIVE THERMOREGULATION

## ▌ Related to Newborn Transition to Extrauterine Environment

**NOC**
Thermoregulation

## ➤ Goals

The infant will have a temperature between 36.4° and 37° C.

The parent will explain techniques to avoid heat loss at home.

### Indicators:

- List situations that increase heat loss.
- Demonstrate how to conserve heat during bathing.
- Demonstrate how to take an infant's temperature.
- State appropriate newborn attire for various outdoor and indoor climates.

**NIC**
Temperature
Regulation,
Environmental
Management,
Newborn
Monitoring, Vital
Sign Monitoring

## ➤ General Interventions

### Assess for Contributing Factors

Environmental sources of heat loss

Lack of knowledge (caregivers, parents)

### Reduce or Eliminate Sources of Heat Loss

#### Evaporation

In the delivery room, quickly dry skin and hair with a heated towel and place infant in a pre-warmed heated environment.

When bathing, provide a warm environment or bath under heat source.

Wash and dry the infant in sections to reduce evaporation.

Limit time in contact with wet diapers or blankets.

#### Convection

Reduce drafts in the delivery room.

Place the sides of the radiant warmer bed up at all times.

Use only portholes for infant access in the Isolette whenever possible

Avoid drafts on the infant (air conditioning, fans, windows, open portholes on Isolette).

## Conduction

Warm all articles for care (stethoscopes, scales, hands of caregivers, clothes, bed linens, cribs).
Place the infant very close to the mother to conserve heat (and foster bonding).
Warm or cover any equipment that may come in contact with the infant's skin.

## Radiation

Place the infant next to the mother in the delivery room.
Reduce objects in the room that absorb heat (metal).
Place the crib or Isolette as far away from walls (outside) or windows as possible.
Preheat incubator.

**R:** The newborn loses heat through (Hockenberry & Wilson 2009):

- Evaporation (loss of heat when water on skin changes to vapor)
- Convection (loss of heat when cool air flows over skin)
- Conduction (transfer of heat when skin surface is in direct contact with a cool surface)

## Monitor Temperature of Newborn

### Assess Axillary Temperature Initially Every 30 Min Until Stable, Then Every 4 to 8 h

**If Temperature Is Less Than 36.3° C**
**R:** Axillary temperatures should be measured for 5 minutes. The most accurate temperature measurement is the oral route (Fallis, 2000).

1. Wrap infant in two blankets.
2. Put stockinette cap on.
3. Assess for environmental sources of heat loss.
4. If hypothermia persists over 1 h, notify a physician.

Assess for complications of cold stress: hypoxia, respiratory acidosis, hypoglycemia, fluid and electrolyte imbalances, and weight loss.
**R:** Significant heat losses the first few moments after birth can drop the newborn's temperature 1° to 3° C. Drying, heated blankets, and swaddling can reduce these losses (Varda & Behnke, 2000).
**R:** Premature or low–birth-weight infants are more susceptible to heat loss because of the reduced metabolic reserves available (e.g., glycogen), increased brown adipose tissue, increased total body water, and thin skin.

**If Temperature Is Greater Than 37° C**

1. Loosen blanket.
2. Remove cap, if on.
3. Assess environment for thermal gain.
4. If hyperthermia persists over 1 h, notify a physician.

**R:** Exposure of the head, face, hands, and feet can affect body temperature greatly. Heat is conducted from blood vessels of these vascular areas to the skin and from the skin to the air, and where cold is conducted from the air to the skin and from the skin to the blood vessels.

## Initiate Health Teaching

Teach caregiver why infant is vulnerable to temperature fluctuations (cold and heat).
Explain sources of environmental heat loss.
Demonstrate how to conserve heat during bathing.
Instruct that it is not necessary routinely to check temperature at home.
Teach to check temperature if infant is hot, sick, or irritable, as follows:

1. Shake down the thermometer.
2. Place the thermometer in the femoral fold.
3. Hold the thermometer in place for 11 min.

4. Read at eye level.
5. Report temperature greater than 37.5° C to a health care professional.

**R:** Parents are taught how to prevent heat loss via evaporation, convection, and radiation during infant care and in the home environment (Hockenberry &Wilson, 2009).

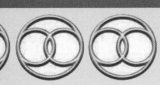

# BOWEL INCONTINENCE

## DEFINITION

A state in which an individual experiences a change in normal bowel habits characterized by involuntary passage of stool

## DEFINING CHARACTERISTICS

Involuntary passage of stool

## RELATED FACTORS

### Pathophysiologic

*Related to impaired rectal sphincter secondary to:*

| | |
|---|---|
| Anal or rectal surgery | Obstetric injuries |
| Anal or rectal injury | Peripheral neuropathy |

*Related to overdistention of rectum secondary to chronic constipation*

*Related to lack of voluntary sphincter control secondary to:*

| | |
|---|---|
| Progressive neuromuscular disorder | Spinal cord injury |
| Spinal cord compression | Multiple sclerosis |
| Cerebral vascular accident | |

*Related to impaired reservoir capacity secondary to:*

| | |
|---|---|
| Inflammatory bowel disease | Chronic rectal ischemia |

### Treatment-Related

*Related to impaired reservoir capacity secondary to:*

| | |
|---|---|
| Colectomy | Radiation proctitis |

### Situational (Personal, Environmental)

*Related to inability to recognize, interpret, or respond to rectal cues secondary to:*

| | |
|---|---|
| Depression | Cognitive impairment |

### ERRORS IN DIAGNOSTIC STATEMENTS

#### Bowel Incontinence Related to Oozing of Stool

Oozing of stool does not cause bowel incontinence; rather, it is evidence. If the etiology is unknown, the diagnosis should be written: *Bowel Incontinence related to unknown etiology*, as evidenced by oozing of stool. When the etiology is known, the diagnosis should reflect this (e.g., *Bowel Incontinence related to relaxed anal sphincter secondary to S4 lesion*).

## ■■■■■ KEY CONCEPTS

### Generic Considerations

- Bowel incontinence has three major causes: underlying disease of the colon, rectum, or anus; long-standing constipation or fecal impaction; and neurogenic rectal changes.
- Complete spinal cord injury, spinal cord lesions, neurologic disease, or congenital defects that interrupt the sacral reflex arc (at the sacral segments S2, S3, S4) result in an areflexic (autonomous) or flaccid bowel. Flaccid paralysis at this level, known as an LMN lesion, results in loss of the defecation reflex, loss of sphincter control (flaccid anal sphincter), and no bulbocavernosus reflex.
- Because of an interrupted sacral reflex arc and a flaccid anal sphincter, bowel incontinence can occur without rectal stimulation whenever stool is in the rectal vault. The stool may leak out if too soft or remain (if not extracted), predisposing the client to fecal impaction or constipation. Some intrinsic contractile abilities of the colon remain, but peristalsis is sluggish, leading to stool retention with contents in the rectal vault.
- Complete central nervous system (CNS) lesions or trauma above sacral cord segments S2, S3, S4 (T12–L1–L2 vertebral level) result in an areflexic neurogenic bowel. They interrupt the ascending sensory signals between the sacral reflex center and the brain, resulting in the inability to feel the urge to defecate. They also interrupt descending motor signals from the brain, causing loss of voluntary control over the anal sphincter. Because the sacral reflex center is preserved, it is possible to develop a stimulation–response bowel evacuation program using digital stimulation or digital stimulation devices.

 **Geriatric Considerations**

Age-related changes in the large intestines include reduced mucus production, decreased elasticity of the rectal wall, and diminished perception of rectal wall distention (Miller, 2009).

These age-related changes require a larger rectal volume in order to perceive the urge to defecate and may predispose the client to constipation (Miller, 2009).

## Focus Assessment Criteria

See *Constipation*.

For more information on Focus Assessment Criteria, visit http://thepoint.lww.com.

**NOC**
Bowel Continence,
Tissue Integrity

## ➤ Goal

The client will evacuate a soft, formed stool every other day or every third day.

### Indicators

- Relate bowel elimination techniques.
- Describe fluid and dietary requirements.

**NIC**
Bowel Incontinence
Care, Bowel Training,
Bowel Management,
and Skin Surveillance

## ➤ General Interventions

### Assess Contributing Factors

Refer to Related Factors.

## Assess the Client's Ability to Participate in Bowel Continence

| | |
|---|---|
| Orientation, Motivation | Ability to reach toilet |
| Control of Rectal Sphincter | Intact anorectal sensation |

**R:** To maintain bowel continence, a client must be motivated, have intact anorectal sensation, be able to store feces consciously, be able to contract puborectalis and external anal sphincter muscles, and have access to a toileting facility.

**R:** Cognitive impairments can impede recognition of bowel cues. Another cause of bowel incontinence is rectal sphincter abnormalities.

## Plan a Consistent, Appropriate Time for Elimination

Institute a daily bowel program for 5 days or until a pattern develops, then move to an alternate-day program (morning or evening).
Provide privacy and a nonstressful environment.
Give reassurance and protect from embarrassment while establishing the bowel program.

**R:** Long-standing constipation or fecal impaction causes overdistention of the rectum by feces. This causes continuous reflex stimulation which reduces sphincter tone. Incontinence will be either diarrhea leaking around the impaction or leaking of feces from a full rectum.

## Teach Effective Bowel Elimination Techniques

Position a functionally able client upright or sitting. If he or she is not functionally able (e.g., quadriplegic), place the client in left side-lying position.

**R:** Techniques that facilitate gravity and increase intra-abdominal pressure to pass stool enhance bowel elimination.

For a functionally able client, use assistive devices (e.g., dil stick, digital stimulator, raised commode seat, lubricant, and gloves) as appropriate.

**R:** Digital stimulation results in reflex peristalsis and evacuation.

For a client with impaired upper extremity mobility and decreased abdominal muscle function, teach bowel elimination facilitation techniques as appropriate:

Valsalva maneuver          Forward bends
Sitting push-ups          Abdominal massage
Pelvic floor exercises

**R:** These techniques increase intra-abdominal pressure to aid in stool evacuation. Pelvic floor exercises can increase the strength of the puborectalis and external anal sphincter muscles.

Maintain an elimination record or a flow sheet of the bowel schedule that includes time, stool characteristics, assistive methods used, and number of involuntary stools, if any.

**R:** This record will assist in planning an individualized bowel schedule.

## Explain Fluid and Dietary Requirements for Good Bowel Movements

Ensure client drinks 8 to 10 glasses of water daily.
Design a diet high in bulk and fiber.
Refer to *Constipation* for specific dietary instructions.

**R:** Stool consistency and volume are important for continence. Large volumes of loose stool overwhelm the continence mechanism. Small, hard stools that do not distend or stimulate the rectum do not alert the client to the need to defecate.

## Explain Effects of Activity on Peristalsis

Assist in determining the appropriate exercises for the client's functional ability.

**R:** Exercise increases gastrointestinal motility and hastens bowel function.

## Initiate Health Teaching, as Indicated

Explain the hazards of using stool softeners, laxatives, suppositories, and enemas.
Explain the signs and symptoms of fecal impaction and constipation. (Refer to *Dysreflexia* for additional information.)

Initiate teaching of a bowel program before discharge. If the client is functionally able, encourage independence with the bowel program; if not, incorporate assistive devices or attendant care, as needed. Explain the effects of stool on the skin and ways to protect the skin (refer to *Diarrhea* for interventions).

**R:** Laxatives cause unscheduled bowel movements, loss of colon tone, and inconsistent stool consistency. Enemas can overstretch the bowel and decrease tone. Stool softeners are not needed with adequate food or fluid intake.

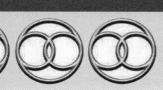

# INEFFECTIVE BREASTFEEDING

## DEFINITION

The state in which a mother, infant, or child experiences or is at risk of experiencing dissatisfaction or difficulty with the breastfeeding process

## DEFINING CHARACTERISTICS

Unsatisfactory breastfeeding process:

- Actual or perceived inadequate milk supply
- Inability of infant to attach onto maternal breast correctly (poor latch)
- Observable signs of inadequate infant intake
- Nonsustained suckling at the breast
- Persistence of sore nipples beyond the first week of breastfeeding
- Fussiness and crying of infant within the first hour after breastfeeding; lack of response to other comfort measures
- Infant arching and crying at the breast, resisting latching on
- Unsustained sucking

## RELATED FACTORS

### Physiologic

*Related to difficulty of neonate to attach or suck secondary to:*
Cleft lip/palate                Prematurity
Previous breast surgery         Inverted nipples, inadequate let-down reflex stress

### Situational (Personal, Environmental)

*Related to maternal fatigue*
*Related to maternal anxiety*
*Related to maternal ambivalence*
*Related to multiple birth*
*Related to inadequate nutrition intake*
*Related to inadequate fluid intake*
*Related to history of unsuccessful breastfeeding*
*Related to nonsupportive partner/family*
*Related to lack of knowledge*
*Related to interruption in breastfeeding secondary to ill mother, ill infant*
*Related to work schedule and/or barriers in the work environment*

## ■■■■■ AUTHOR'S NOTE

In managing breastfeeding, nurses strive to reduce or eliminate factors that contribute to *Ineffective Breastfeeding* or factors that can increase vulnerability for a problem using the diagnosis *Risk for Ineffective Breastfeeding*.

In the acute setting after delivery, too little time will have elapsed for the nurse to conclude that there is no problem in breastfeeding, unless the mother is experienced. For many mother–infant dyads, *Risk for Ineffective Breastfeeding related to inexperience with the breastfeeding process* would represent a nursing focus on preventing problems in breastfeeding. *Risk* would not be indicated for all mothers.

## ■■■■■ ERRORS IN DIAGNOSTIC STATEMENTS

### Ineffective Breastfeeding related to reports of no symptoms of let-down reflex

When a mother reports or the nurse observes no signs of let-down reflex, *Ineffective Breastfeeding* is validated. If contributing factors are unknown, the diagnosis could be written as *Ineffective Breastfeeding related to unknown etiology*, as evidenced by reports of no signs of let-down reflex and mother's anxiety regarding feeding.

If the nurse has validated contributing factors, he or she can add them. The nurse should assess for various possible contributing factors, rather than prematurely focusing on a common etiology that may be incorrect for the specific situation.

## ■■■■■ KEY CONCEPTS

### Generic Considerations

- Lactation results from complex interactions among the mother's health and nutrition status, the infant's health status, and breast tissue development under the influence of estrogen and progesterone.
- Prolactin and oxytocin are pituitary hormones that control milk production and are stimulated by infant sucking and maternal emotions.
- Many medications are excreted in breast milk. Some are harmful to the infant. Advise the mother to consult with a health care professional (nurse, physician, pharmacist) before taking a medication (prescribed or over-the-counter).
- The advantages of breast milk for the infant are as follows:
  - Is easier to digest
  - Meets nutritional needs
  - Reduces allergies and asthma
  - Provides antibodies and macrophages for early immunization
  - Causes fewer gastrointestinal infections and almost no constipation
  - Improves tooth alignment
  - Reduces childhood infections throughout childhood if nursing continues for 1 year (respiratory, ear)
  - In juvenile diabetes, can significantly stall the onset of diabetes, perhaps even into adulthood
  - Results in fewer incidents of sudden infant death syndrome
  - Gives bowel movements a pleasant odor
  - Does not smell sour or stain clothing in vomitus
  - The advantages of breastfeeding for the mother are as follows:
  - Hastens uterine involution and postpartum resolution
  - Reduces risks for breast cancer
  - Allows more time to rest during feedings
  - Requires less preparation and decreased costs
  - Promotes faster bonding
- The disadvantages of breastfeeding are:
  - Alternate person cannot substitute.
  - Breastfeeding is a learned process for mother and baby. It requires about 2 to 3 weeks of commitment to adjust to and learn the skills of breastfeeding.
  - Breast milk is nearly completely digested—intestinal emptying is faster and newborn may need to feed more often than with formula.

## Pediatric Considerations

Physical and psychosocial pressure influence an adolescent's eating habits, which may put the teenage mother and her infant at risk during the breastfeeding period.

## Focus Assessment Criteria

### Subjective Data

*Assess for Related Factors*

History of breastfeeding (self, sibling, friend)
Supportive people (partner, friend, sibling, parent)
Daily intake

| | |
|---|---|
| Calories | Basic food groups |
| Calcium | Fluids |
| Vitamin supplements | Medications |

History of breast surgery

### Objective Data

*Assess for Defining Characteristics*

Breast condition (soft, firm, engorged)
Nipples (cracked, sore, inverted)
For more information on Focus Assessment Criteria, visit http://thepoint.lww.com.

**NOC**
Breastfeeding Establishment: Infant, Breastfeeding Establishment: Maternal, Breastfeeding Management, Knowledge: Breastfeeding

## Goals

The mother will report confidence in establishing satisfying, effective breastfeeding.
The mother will demonstrate effective breastfeeding independently.

### Indicators:

- Identify factors that deter breastfeeding.
- Identify factors that promote breastfeeding.
- Demonstrate effective positioning.

### Infant Shows Signs of Adequate Intake

#### Indicators:

Wet diapers, weight gain, relaxed, and feeding

**NIC**
Breastfeeding Assistance, Lactation Counseling

## General Interventions

### Assess for Causative or Contributing Factors

Lack of knowledge
Lack of role model
Lack of support (partner, physician, family)
Discomfort

| | |
|---|---|
| Leaking | Engorgement |
| Loss of control of bodily fluid | Nipple soreness |

Embarrassment
Attitudes and misconceptions of mother
Social pressure against breastfeeding
Change in body image
Change in sexuality

Feelings of being tied down
Stress
Lack of conviction regarding decision to breastfeed
Sleepy, unresponsive infant
Infant with hyperbilirubinemia
Fatigue
Separation from infant (premature or sick infant, sick mother)
Barriers in workplace

## Promote Open Dialogue

### Assess Knowledge

Has the woman taken a class in breastfeeding?
Has she read anything on the subject?
Does she have friends who are breastfeeding their babies?
Did her mother breastfeed?

### Explain Myths and Misconceptions

Ask her to list anticipated difficulties. Common myths include the following:

- My breasts are too small.
- My breasts are too large.
- My mother couldn't breastfeed.
- How do I know my milk is good?
- How do I know the baby is getting enough?
- The baby will know that I'm nervous.
- I have to go back to work, so what's the point of breastfeeding for a short time?
- I'll never have any freedom.
- Breastfeeding will cause my breasts to sag.
- My nipples are inverted, so I can't breastfeed.
- My husband won't like my breasts anymore.
- I'll have to stay fat if I breastfeed.
- I can't breastfeed if I have a cesarean section.
- You cannot get pregnant when breastfeeding

**R:** Listening to mother's and partner's concerns can help prioritize concerns.

### Build on Mother's Knowledge

Clarify misconceptions.
Explain process of breastfeeding.
Offer literature.
Show video.
Discuss advantages and disadvantages.
Bring breastfeeding mothers together to talk about breastfeeding and their concerns.
Discuss contraindications to breast feeding

### Support Mother's Decision to Breast- or Bottle-Feed

**R:** Constant positive feedback is essential for an inexperienced mother. The decision to breastfeed is very personal and should not be made without adequate information (Hockenberry et al., 2009).

## Assist Mother During First Feedings

### Promote Relaxation

Position comfortably, using pillows (especially cesarean-section mothers).
Use a footstool or phone book to bring knees up while sitting.

Use relaxation breathing techniques.

**R:** Inadequate let-down reflex can result from a tense or nervous mother, pain, insufficient milk, engorgement, or inadequate sucking position or motions.

### Demonstrate Different Positions and Rooting Reflex

| | |
|---|---|
| Sitting | Football hold |
| Lying | Skin to skin |

Cradle hold: instruct the woman to place a supporting hand on the baby's bottom and turn the body toward the mother's (promotes security in infant). Cradle hold stabilizes the head and reduces force.

Show the mother how she can use it to help the infant latch on.

Show how to grasp breast with fingers under the breast and thumbs on top; this way she can point the nipple directly at the baby's mouth (avoid scissors hold, which constricts milk flow).

Make sure the baby grasps a good portion of the areola, not just the nipple.

Observe gliding action of the jaw, which indicates proper latch-on and suck.

The infant should not be chewing or simply sucking with the lips.

Observe for bruising after feeding.

**R:** Successful breastfeeding is dependent on the ability of the infant to latch on.

## Promote Successful Breastfeeding

### Advise the Mother to Increase Feeding Times Gradually

Start at 10 min per side.
Build up over the next 3 to 5 days.

### Instruct the Mother to Offer Both Breasts at Each Feeding

Alternate the beginning side each time.

**Demonstrate:**
- How to use a finger to keep breast tissue from obstructing the infant's nose
- Use of finger in the infant's mouth to break the seal before removing from the breast
- Ways to awaken infant (may be necessary before offering the second breast)

### Discuss Burping

Inform the mother that burping may be unnecessary with breastfed infants.
If the infant grunts and seems full between breasts, the mother should attempt to burp the infant, then continue feeding.

**R:** Successful breastfeeding depends on both physical and emotional support. Physical support includes promotion of comfort and proper technique (Pillitteri, 2009).

## Provide Follow-Up Support During Hospital Stay

Develop a care plan so other health team members are aware of any problems or needs. Try to establish a consistent plan so the breastfeeding mother does not receive mixed and opposing opinions from her health care providers.

Allow for flexibility of feeding schedule; avoid scheduling feedings. Strive for 10 to 12 feedings/24 h according to the infant's size and need. (Frequent feedings help prevent or reduce breast engorgement.)

Promote rooming in.

Allow for privacy during feedings.

Be available for questions.

Be positive even if the experience is difficult.

Reassure the mother that this is a learning time for her and the infant. They will develop together as the days pass.

**R:** Mothers need continuous support to enhance the breastfeeding experience.

## Teach Ways to Control Specific Nursing Problems (May Need Assistance of Lactation Consultant).

### Engorgement

Wear correctly fitting support brassiere day and night.

Apply warm compresses for 15 to 20 min before breastfeeding.

Nurse frequently (on demand).

Use hand expression, hand pump, or electric pump to tap off some of the tension before putting the infant to the breast.

Massage breasts and apply warm washcloth before expression.

Encourage rooming-in and feeding on demand.

**R:** Providing enough time for adequate sucking position or motions.

### Sore Nipples

Apply warm, moist compress for 5 to 10 min after breastfeeding.

Keep nipples warm and dry.

Decrease breastfeeding time to 5 to 10 min per side. Start the baby on nontender side first. Allow for more frequent, short feedings. Suggest alternate positions to rotate the infant's grasps. Allow the breasts to dry after each feeding.

Keep nursing pads dry.

Coat the nipples with breast milk (which has healing properties) and allow to air-dry.

Use breast shield as the last measure and remove after milk has let down.

Explain that nipple soreness usually resolves within 7 to 10 days.

**R:** Nipple shields diminish milk supply and should not be recommended routinely. The newborn may develop a nipple shield preference.

### Stasis, Mastitis

If one area of the breast is sore or tender, apply moist heat before each breastfeeding session.

Gently massage from the base of the breast toward the nipple before beginning to breastfeed and during feeding.

Breastfeed frequently and change position during feeding.

Rest frequently.

If stasis lasts more than 48 h, consult with nurse practitioner, midwife, or physician for antibiotic therapy.

Monitor for signs and symptoms of mastitis: chills, body aches, fatigue, and fever above 100.4° F.

**R:** Early self-management may prevent complications.

### Difficulty with Baby Grasping Nipple

Cup the breast with fingers underneath.

Position the baby for mother's and infant's comfort (turn the baby's abdomen toward mother's body).

Stroke the infant's cheek for rooting reflex.

Hand-express some milk into the infant's mouth.

Roll nipples to bring them out before feeding.

Use a nipple shell between feedings to help extend inverted nipples. Remove shield after let-down.

Assess the infant's suck—the baby may need assistance in development of suck. Use a lactation consultant if indicated.

**R:** The infant at the breast must be in relaxed, correct alignment, have correct tongue and areolar placement, have sufficient motion for areolar compression, and demonstrate audible swallowing.

## Encourage Verbal Expression of Feelings Regarding Changes in Body.

Many women dislike leaking and lack of control. Explain that this is temporary.

Demonstrate use of a nursing pad. With a disposable pad, the client should not use waterproof backing, to prevent irritation; cotton (washable) seems to reduce irritation.

Breasts change from "sexual objects" to implements of nutrition, which can affect the sexual relationship. Sexual partners will get milk if they suck on the woman's nipples. Orgasm releases milk. Infant suckling is "sensual"—this may cause guilt or confusion in the woman. Encourage discussion with other mothers. Include the partner in at least one discussion to assess his or her feelings and how they most affect the breastfeeding experience.

Explore the woman's feelings about self-consciousness during feedings.

Where?

Around whom?

What is partner's reaction to when and where she breastfeeds?

Demonstrate the use of a shawl for modesty, allowing breastfeeding in public.

Remind the woman that what she is doing is normal and natural.

**R:** Dialogue can alienate fears which can deter breastfeeding.

## Assist the Family with the Following:

### Sibling Reaction

Explore feelings and anticipation of problems. An older child may be jealous of contact with the baby. Mother can use this time to read to the older child.

The older child may want to breastfeed. Allow him or her to try; usually, the child will not like it.

Stress the older child's attributes: freedom, movement, and choices.

### Fatigue and Stress

Explore the situation.

Encourage the mother to make herself and infant a priority.

Encourage her to limit visits from relatives for the first 4 weeks.

Emphasize that the mother will need support and assistance during first 4 weeks. Encourage the support person to help as much as possible.

Encourage the mother not to try to be "superwoman," but to ask directly for help from friends or relations, or to hire someone.

### Feelings of Being Enslaved

Allow the mother to express feelings.

Encourage her to seek assistance and to pump milk to allow others to feed the baby.

Advise her that she can store harvested breast milk for 8 h at room temperature, 3 days in the refrigerator, and 6 months in the freezer. (*Note:* Tell the woman never to microwave frozen breast milk, as doing so destroys its immune properties.)

Remember that time between feedings will get longer (every 2 h for 4 weeks, then every 3 to 4 h for 3 months).

**R:** Mothers who are prepared for possible problems at home will have more confidence and be more likely to continue breastfeeding (Ertem et al., 2001).

## Initiate Referrals, as Indicated

Refer to lactation consultant if indicated by:

- Lack of confidence
- Ambivalence
- Problems with infant suck and latch-on
- Infant weight drop or lack of urination
- Barriers in workplace
- Prolonged soreness
- Hot, tender spots on breast

Refer to La Leche League.

Refer to childbirth educator and childbirth class members.

Refer to other breastfeeding mothers.

**R:** Referrals to community resources can provide continued support and information.

**R:** Company-sponsored lactation programs enable employed mothers to continue breastfeeding as long as they desire (Ortiz, McGilligan, & Kelly, 2004).

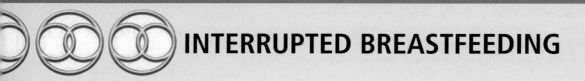# INTERRUPTED BREASTFEEDING

## DEFINITION (NANDA)

A break in the continuity of the breastfeeding process as a result of inability or inadvisability to put baby to breast for feeding

## DEFINING CHARACTERISTICS (NANDA)

Infant receives no nourishment at the breast for some or all feedings
Maternal desire to eventually provide breast milk for child's nutritional needs
Maternal desire to maintain breastfeeding for child's nutritional needs

## RELATED FACTORS (NANDA)

Maternal or infant illness          Prematurity
Maternal employment                 Contraindications (e.g., drugs, true breast milk jaundice)
Need to wean infant abruptly

### ■■■■■■ AUTHOR'S NOTE

This diagnosis represents a situation, not a response. Nursing interventions do not treat the interruption but, instead, its effects. The situation is interrupted breastfeeding; the responses can vary. For example, if continued breastfeeding or use of a breast pump is contraindicated, the nurse focuses on the loss of this breastfeeding experience using the nursing diagnosis *Grieving*.

If breastfeeding continues with expression and storage of breast milk, teaching, and support, the diagnosis will be *Risk for Ineffective Breastfeeding related to continuity problems secondary to (e.g., maternal employment)*. If difficulty is experienced, the diagnosis would be *Ineffective Breastfeeding related to interruption secondary to (specify) and lack of knowledge*.

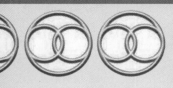

# DECREASED CARDIAC OUTPUT

## ▶ Risk for Complications of Decreased Cardiac Output

## DEFINITION (NANDA)

Inadequate blood pumped by the heart to meet metabolic demands of the body

## DEFINING CHARACTERISTICS

Altered heart rate/rhythm
Altered preload
Altered contractibililty
Altered afterload

## RELATED FACTORS (NANDA)

Altered heart rate          Altered afterload
Altered rhythm              Altered contractibility
Altered stroke volume       Altered preload

## ▪▪▪▪▪▪ AUTHOR'S NOTE

This nursing diagnosis represents a situation in which nurses have multiple responsibilities. People experiencing decreased cardiac output may display various responses that disrupt functioning (e.g., activity intolerance, disturbed sleep–rest, anxiety, fear). Or they may be at risk for developing such physiologic complications as dysrhythmias, cardiogenic shock, and congestive heart failure.

When *Decreased Cardiac Output* is used clinically, associated goals usually are written:

Systolic blood pressure is greater than 100     Cardiac output is greater than 5
Urine output is greater than 30 mL/h            Cardiac rate and rhythm are within normal limits

These goals do not represent parameters for evaluating nursing care, but for evaluating the client's status. Because they are monitoring criteria that the nurse uses to guide implementation of nurse-prescribed and physician-prescribed interventions, students consult with faculty to determine which diagnosis to use: Decreased Cardiac Output or Risk for Complications of Decreased Cardiac Output. Refer to *Activity Intolerance related to insufficient knowledge of adaptive techniques needed secondary to impaired cardiac function* and to *RC of Cardiac/Vascular Dysfunction* (Section 3) for specific interventions.

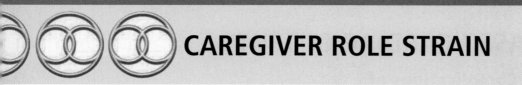

# CAREGIVER ROLE STRAIN

Caregiver Role Strain

Risk for Caregiver Role Strain

## DEFINITION

A state in which a client is experiencing physical, emotional, social, and/or financial burden(s) in the process of giving care to another

## DEFINING CHARACTERISTICS—EXPRESSED OR OBSERVED

Insufficient time or physical energy
Difficulty performing required caregiving activities
Conflicts between caregiving responsibilities and other important roles (e.g., work, relationships)
Apprehension about the future for the care receiver's health and ability to provide care
Apprehension about care receiver's care when caregiver is ill or deceased
Feelings of depression or anger
Feelings of exhaustion and resentment

## RELATED FACTORS

### Pathophysiologic

*Related to unrelenting or complex care requirements secondary to:*

Debilitating conditions (acute, progressive)  Progressive dementia
Addiction  Chronic mental illness
Unpredictable illness course  Disability

### Treatment-Related

*Related to 24-hour care responsibilities*
*Related to time-consuming activities (e.g., dialysis, transportation)*

### Situational (Personal, Environmental)

*Related to unrealistic expectations of caregiver by care receiver, self, or others*
*Related to pattern of ineffective coping*
*Related to compromised physical health*
*Related to history of poor relationship or family dysfunction*
*Related to duration of caregiving required*
*Related to isolation*
*Related to insufficient respite or recreation or finances*
*Related to no or unavailable support*
*Related to insufficient resources and/or finances*

### Maturational

Infant, child, and adolescent related to unrelenting care requirements secondary to:

Mental disabilities (specify)  Physical disabilities (specify)

## AUTHOR'S NOTE

"Health care policies that rely on caregiver sacrifice can be made to appear cost-effective only if the emotional, social, physical, and financial costs incurred by the caregiver are ignored" (Winslow & Carter, 1999, p. 285). Family caregivers provide care for people of all ages. The care receivers have physical and/or mental disabilities, which can be temporary or permanent. Some disabilities are permanent but stable (e.g., blindness); others signal progressive deterioration (e.g., Alzheimer's disease).

Caring and caregiving are intrinsic to all close relationships. They are "found in the context of established roles such as wife–husband, child–parent" (Pearlin, Mullan, Semple, & Skaff, 1990, p. 583). Under some circumstances, caregiving is "transformed from the ordinary exchange of assistance among people standing in close relationship to one another to an extraordinary and unequally distributed burden" (ibid.). It becomes a dominant, overriding component occupying the entire situation (ibid.).

Chronic sorrow has been associated with caregivers of people with mental illness and children with chronic illness. See *Chronic Sorrow* for more information.

*Caregiver Role Strain* represents the burden of caregiving on the physical and emotional health of the caregiver and its effects on the family and social system of the caregiver and care receiver. *Risk for Caregiver Role Strain* can be a very significant nursing diagnosis because nurses can identify those at high risk and assist them to prevent this grave situation.

## ERRORS IN DIAGNOSTIC STATEMENTS

1. *Caregiver Role Strain related to depression and anger at family, as evidenced by unrealistic expectations of caregiver for self and by others*

Too often, caregivers with multiple, unrelenting responsibilities are reluctant to admit they need help. Others may interpret this reluctance as not needing help. The caregiver is further isolated, feeling no one really cares or appreciates the work involved, which can contribute to depression and anger. Thus, this diagnosis must be rewritten to reflect the unrealistic expectations as the related factors and the resulting symptoms as evidence. It is helpful to quote the data if relevant: *Caregiver Role Strain related to unrealistic expectations of caregiver for self and by others, as evidenced by depressed feelings and anger at family who "don't understand my burden."*

## KEY CONCEPTS

### Generic Considerations

- According to the National Women's Health Information Center (2006), about one in four American families, or 22.4 million households, care for someone over the age of 50.
- A 2006 study from MetLife Mature Market Institute and the National Alliance for Caregiving reports the cost to U.S. business due to lost productivity of working caregivers is $17.1 billion to $33.6 billion per year. Nearly 40% of the caregivers are men, and approximately 15% provide care at a distance of greater than one hour away.
- Nearly one third of young adults age 18-44 suffer from a chronic illness, and there has been an increase in the survival of low birth weight and premature infants (National Center for Health Statistics, 2003).
- With the growing aging population and advances in medicine increasing the longevity of chronically ill people, the need for health care escalates. Of 4 million Americans with Alzheimer's disease, more than 70% live at home (Winslow & Carter, 1999). One family member largely provides such home health care. Women (e.g., wife, daughter, daughter-in-law) represent 70% of these caregivers.
- Family caregivers in particular play significant roles in the care of elders with advanced chronic disease and in the context of palliative and end-of-life care.
- Burden is related to the caregiver's gender, age, social support, income, and resources and the care receiver's cognitive and functional limitations (Winslow & Carter, 1999).
- Caregiving responsibilities often create conflict with obligations to work and family (Lund, 2005).

*(continued)*

▪▪▪▪▪▪ **KEY CONCEPTS** *Continued*

- Smith, Smith, and Toseland (1991) reported the following problems (by priority) identified by family caregivers:
  - Improving coping skills (e.g., time management, stress management)
  - Family issues (sibling conflict, other role conflicts)
  - Responding to care receiver's needs (emotional, physical, financial)
  - Eliciting formal and informal support
  - Guilt and feelings of inadequacy
  - Long-term planning
  - Quality of relationship with care receiver

## Pediatric Considerations

Children considered candidates for home care services are those:
- Dependent on mechanical ventilation
- Needing prolonged intravenous nutritional or drug therapy
- With terminal illness
- Requiring nutritional (e.g., tube feedings) or respiratory support (e.g., tracheostomy, suctioning)
- Needing daily or near-daily nursing care for apnea monitoring, dialysis, urinary catheters, or colostomy pouches

The child and family provide the basis for home care and collaborate with the nurse to provide its direction.

Caregivers of preterm infants on apnea monitors experienced more fatigue than caregivers of preterm infants not on apnea monitors. This fatigue increased in the caregivers of monitored infants over 1 month and decreased in caregivers of non-monitored infants. This fatigue interfered with activities of daily living (ADLs), socialization, and leisure.

## Transcultural Considerations

Dilworth-Anderson, Williams, & Gibson (2002) reported that ethnic minority families used fewer formal services but more informal family member support for family caregiving activities.

# Focus Assessment Criteria

## Subjective Data

### *Assess for Defining Characteristics*

How well do you manage your:

| Caregiving responsibilities? | Household responsibilities? | Life outside caregiving |
| Work responsibilities? | Family responsibilities? | Social Life |

On a scale from 0 to 10 (0 = not tired, peppy, to 10 = total exhaustion), rate the fatigue you usually feel. Does it change during the day or week? If so, why?

Do you feel stressed between caring for your _____ and trying to meet other responsibilities?

How would you describe your usual emotional state? (Calm, stressed, angry, anxious, depressed, exhausted, or guilty)

What do you do when you are very stressed?

What are you most concerned about?

For present        For future

When was the last time you went out to eat?

What have you done for fun lately? When was your last vacation?

## *Assess for Related Factors*

### Caregiver History
*Lifestyle*

| | |
|---|---|
| Typical day | Work history |
| Weekly hobbies | Leisure activities |

*Health*

| | |
|---|---|
| Ability to perform ADLs | Chronic conditions |

*Family Members*

| | |
|---|---|
| Parents, spouse | Children, siblings |
| Extended family | In-laws |
| Grandparents | |

*Economic Resources*

| | |
|---|---|
| Sources | Adequacy (present, future) |

Factors increasing caregiver strain

| | |
|---|---|
| Poor insight into situation | Unrealistic expectations (caregiver, family) |
| Reluctance or inability to access help | Unsatisfactory relationship |
| Insufficient resources (e.g., help, financial) | Social isolation |
| Insufficient leisure | Competing roles (spouse, parenting, work) |

### Care Receiver Characteristics
*Cognitive Status (e.g., Memory, Speech)*
*History of relationship with caregiver*
*Problematic Behaviors (Pearlin et al., 1990)*

| | |
|---|---|
| Wanders | Cries easily |
| Threatens | Repeats questions and requests |
| Uses foul language | Clings |
| Incontinence | Depressed |
| Suspicious | Up at night |
| Sexually inappropriate | |

*Activities with Which the Care Receiver Needs Assistance*

| | |
|---|---|
| Bathing | Medicines |
| Dressing, grooming | Transportation |
| Eating | Laundry |
| Toileting, Incontinence | Shopping |
| Mobility | |

### Caregiver–Care Receiver Relationship
*Support System*
Who? (Family, friends, clergy, agency, group)
What? (Visits, respite, chores, empathy)
How often?
What have you lost because of your caregiver responsibilities?

### Care Issues Related to Chronically Ill Child
*Parenting Issues*

| | |
|---|---|
| Discipline of ill child | Discipline of well siblings |

*Family Adaptations*

| | |
|---|---|
| Living arrangements | Day-to-day management |
| Vacations | Work arrangements |

*Support Systems*

| | |
|---|---|
| School issues | Church, synagogue, mosque, or faith community |

# ➤ Goals

The caregiver will report a plan to decrease caregiver's burden.

## *Indicators*

- Share frustrations regarding caregiving responsibilities.
- Identify one source of support.
- Identify two changes that, if made, would improve daily life.

The family will establish a plan for weekly support or help.

## *Indicators:*

- Relate two strategies to increase support.
- Convey empathy to caregiver regarding daily responsibilities.

# ➤ General Interventions

## Assess for Causative or Contributing Factors

Refer to Related Factors

## Provide Empathy and Promote a Sense of Competency.

Allow caregiver to share feelings.
Emphasize the difficulties of the caregiving responsibilities.
Convey admiration of the caregiver's competency.
Evaluate effects of caregiving periodically (depression, burnout).

**R:** Lindgren (1990) reported that burnout in caregivers was related to emotional exhaustion and a low sense of accomplishment. Caregivers who were commended for their accomplishments reported lower levels of burnout.

**R:** Caregiving to a chronically ill family member or friend with many behavioral problems is the most stressful situation one can encounter.

## Promote Realistic Appraisal of the Situation.

Determine how long the caregiving has been occurring (Winslow & Carter, 1999).
Ask the caregiver to describe future life in 3 months, 6 months, and 1 year.
Discuss the effects of present schedule and responsibilities on physical health, emotional status, and relationships.
Discuss positive outcomes of caregiving responsibilities (for self, care receiver, family).
Evaluate if behavior is getting worse.

**R:** Coping with the burdens of caregiving requires "constantly changing cognitive and behavioral efforts to manage specific external and/or internal demands that are appraised as taxing or exceeding the resources of the person" (Lazarus & Folkman, 1984).

**R:** The most critical period for caregiver stress is the 2- to 4-year period (Gaynor, 1990).

## Promote Insight into the Situation.

Ask the caregiver to describe "a typical day":

| | |
|---|---|
| Caregiving tasks | Household tasks |
| Work outside the home | Role responsibilities |

Ask the caregiver to describe:

At-home leisure activities (daily, weekly)
Outside-the-home social activities (weekly)
Engage other family members in discussion, as appropriate

Discuss the danger of viewing helpers as less competent or less essential

Explain that dementia causes memory loss, which results in (Young, 2001):

| | |
|---|---|
| Repetitive questions | Denial of memory loss |
| Forgetting | Fluctuations in memory |

**R:** Caregiver stress is not an event but "a mix of circumstances, experiences, responses, and resources that vary considerably among caregivers and that consequently vary in their impact on caregivers' health and behavior" (Pearlin et al., 1990, p. 584).

**R:** Pruchno, Kleban, Michaels, and Dempsey (1990) reported that in female caregiving spouses, depression predicts a decline in physical health over 6 months. The amount of care provided had few effects on levels of depression, feelings of burden, or health.

## Assist Caregiver to Identify Activities for Which He or She Desires Assistance.

Care receiver's needs (hygiene, food, treatments, mobility; refer to Self-Care Deficits)

| | |
|---|---|
| Laundry | House cleaning |
| Meals | Shopping, errands |
| Transportation | Appointments (doctor, hairdresser) |
| Yard work | House repairs |
| Respite (hours per week) | Money management |

**R:** Shields (1992) reported a primary source of conflict among family members and the caregiver as unsatisfied needs. The caregiver wishes for others to affirm the burden, when, in fact, the family responds to the caregiver's complaints with problem-solving techniques. The caregiver appears to reject suggestions, which annoys the family. The results are a "caregiver feeling unappreciated, unsupported, and depressed, and family members feeling angry and rejecting toward the caregiver" (Shields, 1992).

## Engage Family (Apart from Caregiver) to Appraise Situation (Shields, 1992).

Allow the family to share frustrations.
Share the need for the caregiver to feel appreciated.
Discuss the importance of regularly acknowledging the burden of the situation for the caregiver.
Discuss the benefits of listening without giving advice.
Differentiate the types of social support (emotional, appraisal, informational, instrumental).
Emphasize the importance of emotional and appraisal support.

| | |
|---|---|
| Regular phone calls | Cards, letters |
| Visits | |

Stress "that in many situations, there are no problems to be solved, only pain to be shared" (Shields, 1992, p. 31).
Discuss the need to give the caregiver "permission" to enjoy self (e.g., vacations, day trips).
Allow caregiver opportunities to respond to "How can I help you?"

**R:** Numerous researchers have identified consistent social supports as the single most significant factor that reduces or prevents caregiver role strain (Clipp & George, 1990; Pearlin et al., 1990; Shields, 1992).

## Assist with Accessing Informational and Instrumental Support.

Role play how to ask for help with activities (e.g., "I have three appointments this week, could you drive me to one?" "I could watch your children once or twice a week in exchange for you watching my husband.").
Identify all possible sources of volunteer help: family (siblings, cousins), friends, neighbors, church, and community groups.

Discuss how most people feel good when they provide a "little help."

**R:** The number of people in a household influences how many secondary, informal caregivers assist the primary caregiver. Spouse primary caregivers are less likely to have secondary caregivers to help them with care activities. Older people cared for by spouses received "about 15% to 20% fewer person-days of help than those cared for by adult children."

## If Appropriate, Discuss If and When an Alternative Source of Care (e.g., Nursing Home) May Be Indicated.

Evaluate factors that reduce the stress of deciding on nursing home placement (Hagen, 2001):

- Low level of guilt
- Independence in the relationship
- Availability of support from others
- Low fear of loneliness
- Positive or neutral nursing home attitudes
- Positive sense of life without care burden

**R:** Institutionalization of a family member has many admission-related stressors (e.g., financial constraints, transferring belongings, emotional strain, feelings of failure [Hagen, 2001]).

**R:** Guilt, negative attitudes about nursing homes, sense of existential self, independence in the relationship, fear of loneliness, and perceived presence of support affect the decision-making process for nursing home placement (Hagen, 2001; Larrimore, 2003).

## Initiate Health Teaching and Referrals, If Indicated.

Explain the benefits of sharing with other caregivers.
Support group
Telephone buddy system with another caregiver
Identify community resources available.

Counseling     Social service
Day care

Arrange a home visit by a physical or occupational therapist to evaluate the environment (safety, assistive devices, home alterations).
Arrange a home visit by professional nurse or physical therapy to provide strategies to improve communication, time management, and caregiving.
Engage others to work actively to increase state, federal, and private agencies' financial support for resources to enhance caregiving in the home.

**R:** These strategies emphasize the need for caregiver to protect their health with a balance of work, sleep, leisure, and support and identify sources of help in the community

**Pediatric Interventions**

### Determine Parents' Understanding of and Concerns About Child's Illness, Course, Prognosis, and Related Care Needs

*Elicit the Effects of Caregiving Responsibility on*

Personal life (work, rest, leisure)
Marriage (time alone, communication, decisions, attention)

**R:** Strategies to promote family cohesiveness reduce isolation or aloneness.

*Assist Parents to Meet the Well Siblings' Needs for*

Knowledge of sibling's illness and relationship to own health
Sharing feelings of anger, unfairness, embarrassment
Discussions of future of ill sibling and self (e.g., family planning, care responsibilities)

*(continued)*

**Pediatric Interventions**
*Continued*

**R:** Addressing the developmental tasks of the ill child and the well siblings provides opportunities to grow, develop, gain independence, and master effective coping skills.

### Discuss Strategies to Help Siblings Adapt

Include in family decisions when appropriate.
Keep informed about ill child's condition.
Maintain routines (e.g., meals, vacations).
Prepare for changes in home life.
Promote activities with peers.
Avoid making the ill child the center of the family.
Determine what daily assistance in caregiving is realistic.
Plan for time alone.
Advise teachers of home situation.
Address developmental needs. See *Delayed Growth and Development.*

**R:** Strategies to promote family cohesiveness and individual family needs can enhance effective stress management (Williams, 2000).

### Advise that Caregiving Activities Produce Fatigue that Can Increase Over Time (Williams, 2000)

### Discuss Strategies to Reduce Caregiver Fatigue (Williams, 2000)

Partner support            Household help
Child care for siblings    Provisions to ensure adequacy of caregiver's sleep

**R:** Helping the family identify predictable stressors can assist them to plan coping strategies.
**R:** All family members are encouraged to learn specific skills to balance the responsibilities.

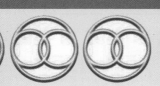

# RISK FOR CAREGIVER ROLE STRAIN

## DEFINITION

A state in which a client is at high risk to experience physical, emotional, social, and/or financial burden(s) in the process of giving care to another

## RELATED OR RISK FACTORS

Primary caregiver responsibilities for a recipient who requires regular assistance with self-care or supervision because of physical or mental disabilities in addition to one or more of the following:

*Related to unrelenting or complex care requirements secondary to:*
*Care receiver characteristics*
Inability to perform self-care            Lack of motivation to perform self-care
Cognitive problems                        Psychological problems
Unrealistic expectations
*Caregiver/spouse characteristics*
Pattern of ineffective coping             Compromised physical health
Unrealistic expectations of self

*Related to history of poor relationship or family dysfunction*
*Related to unrealistic expectations for caregiver by others (society, other family members)*
*Related to duration of caregiving required*
*Related to isolation*
*Related to insufficient respite or recreation or finances*

### ■■■■■■ AUTHOR'S NOTE

See *Caregiver Role Strain.*

### ■■■■■■ ERRORS IN DIAGNOSTIC STATEMENTS

See *Caregiver Role Strain.*

### ■■■■■■ KEY CONCEPTS

See *Caregiver Role Strain.*

## Focus Assessment Criteria

See *Caregiver Role Strain.*

**NOC**
Refer to *Caregiver Role Strain*

## ➤ Goal

The client will relate a plan on how to continue social activities despite caregiving responsibilities.

### Indicators:

- Identify activities that are important for self.
- Relate intent to enlist the help of at least two people weekly.

**NIC**
Refer to *Caregiver Role Strain*

## ➤ General Interventions

### Explain Causes of Caregiver Role Strain

See Related Factors.

## Teach Caregiver and Significant Others to Be Alert for Danger Signals (Murray, Zentner, & Yakimo, 2009, p. 567):

- No matter what you do it is never enough.
- You believe you are the only client in the world doing this.
- You have no time or place to be alone for a brief respite.
- Family relationships are breaking down because of the caregiving pressures.
- Your caregiving duties are interfering with your work and social life.
- You are in a "no-win situation" and will not admit difficulty.
- You are alone because you have shut out everyone who could help.
- You are overeating, or undereating, abusing drugs or alcohol, or being harsh and abusive with your relative.
- There are no more happy times; loving and caring have given way to exhaustion and resentment and you no longer feel good about yourself or take pride in what you are doing.

**R:** Danger signals must be addressed to preserve health and relationships and to prevent abuse.

## Explain the Four Types of Social Support to All Involved.

Emotional (concern, trust)
Appraisal (affirms self-worth)

Informational (useful advice, information for problem solving)

Instrumental (caregiving) or tangible assistance (money, help with chores)

**R:** Identifying the various sources of social support can help the caregiver seek out specific support.

## Discuss the Implications of Daily Responsibilities with the Primary Caregiver (Irvin & Acton, 1997).

Encourage caregiver to set realistic goals for self and care recipient.

Discuss the need for respite and short-term relief.

Encourage caregiver to accept offers of help.

Practice asking for help; avoid "they should know I need help" thinking and martyrdom behavior.

Caution on viewing others as not "competent enough."

Discuss that past conflicts will not disappear. Try to work on resolution and emphasize today.

**R:** The caregiver role may require a relabeled perspective of putting aside guilt and accepting that a good son or daughter can be concerned with the well-being of their parent without feeling great affection (Murray, Zentner, & Yakimo, 2009).

## Stress Importance of Daily Health Promotion Activities (see Health-Seeking Behaviors):

- Rest–exercise balance
- Effective stress management
- Low-fat, high–complex-carbohydrate diet
- Supportive social networks
- Appropriate screening practices for age

Maintain a good sense of humor; associate with others who laugh.

Advise caregivers to initiate phone contacts or visits with friends or relatives rather than waiting for others to do it.

**R:** Caregivers must maintain their own health in order to be successful with coping with caregiving responsibilities.

## Assist Those Involved to Appraise the Situation.

What is at stake? What are the choices?

Provide accurate information and answers to encourage a realistic perspective.

Initiate discussions concerning stressors of home care (physical, emotional, environmental, financial).

Emphasize the importance of respites to prevent isolating behaviors that foster depression.

Discuss with nonprimary caregivers their responsibilities in caring for the primary caregiver.

Where is there help? Direct the family to community agencies, home health care organizations, and sources of financial assistance as needed. (See *Impaired Home Maintenance Management*.)

**R:** These strategies can assist the family to reorganize roles at home and set priorities to maintain family integrity and reduce stress.

## Discuss with All Household Members the Implications of Caring for an Ill Family Member.

Available resources (finances, environmental)

24-hour responsibility

Effects on other household members

Likelihood of progressive deterioration

Sharing of responsibilities (with other household members, siblings, neighbors)

Likelihood of exacerbation of long-standing conflicts

Effects on lifestyle

Alternative or assistive options (e.g., community-based providers, group living, nursing home)

**R:** Shields (1992) reported a primary source of conflict among family members and the caregiver as unsatisfied needs. The caregiver wishes for others to affirm the burden, when, in fact, the family responds to the caregiver's complaints with problem-solving techniques. The caregiver appears to reject suggestions, which annoys the family. The results are a "caregiver feeling unappreciated and unsupported and depressed and family members feeling angry and rejecting toward the caregiver" (Shields, 1992).

## Assist Caregiver to Identify Activities for Which He or She Desires Assistance.

See *Caregiver Role Strain*.

## Assist with Accessing Informational and Instrumental Support.

See *Caregiver Role Strain*.

## Initiate Health Teaching and Referrals, If Indicated.

See *Caregiver Role Strain*.

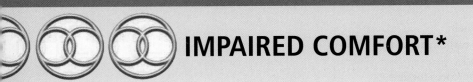

# IMPAIRED COMFORT*

**Impaired Comfort**

Acute Pain
Chronic Pain
Nausea

## DEFINITION

The state in which a person experiences an uncomfortable sensation in response to a noxious stimulus

## DEFINING CHARACTERISTICS

### Major (Must Be Present)

The person reports or demonstrates discomfort.

### Minor (May Be Present)

Autonomic response in acute pain
    Increased blood pressure    Diaphoresis
    Increased pulse    Dilated pupils
    Increased respirations
Guarded position
Facial mask of pain
Crying, moaning
Abdominal heaviness
Nausea
Vomiting
Malaise
Pruritus

*This diagnosis was developed by this author and was added by NANDA in 2002.

# RELATED FACTORS

Any factor can contribute to impaired comfort. The most common are listed below.

## Biopathophysiologic

*Related to uterine contractions during labor*
*Related to trauma to perineum during labor and delivery*
*Related to involution of uterus and engorged breasts*
*Related to tissue trauma and reflex muscle spasms secondary to:*

### Musculoskeletal Disorders

| | |
|---|---|
| Fractures | Arthritis |
| Contractures | Spinal cord disorders |
| Spasms | |

### Visceral Disorders

| | |
|---|---|
| Cardiac | Intestinal |
| Renal | Pulmonary |
| Hepatic | |

### Cancer

### Vascular Disorders

| | |
|---|---|
| Vasospasm | Phlebitis |
| Occlusion | Vasodilation (headache) |

*Related to inflammation of, or injury*

| | |
|---|---|
| Nerve | Joint |
| Tendon | Muscle |
| Bursa | Juxta-articular structures |

*Related to fatigue, malaise, or pruritus secondary to contagious diseases:*

| | |
|---|---|
| Rubella | Chicken pox |
| Hepatitis | Mononucleosis |
| Pancreatitis | |

*Related to effects of cancer on (specify)*
*Related to abdominal cramps, diarrhea, and vomiting secondary to:*

| | |
|---|---|
| Gastroenteritis | Influenza |
| Gastric ulcers | |

Related to inflammation and smooth muscle spasms secondary to:

| | |
|---|---|
| Renal calculi | Gastrointestinal infections |

## Treatment-Related

*Related to tissue trauma and reflex muscle spasms secondary to:*

| | |
|---|---|
| Surgery | Diagnostic tests (venipuncture, invasive scanning, biopsy) |
| Burns | |
| Accidents | |

*Related to nausea and vomiting secondary to:*

| | |
|---|---|
| Chemotherapy | Anesthesia |
| Side effects of (specify) | |

## Situational (Personal, Environmental)

*Related to fever*
*Related to immobility/improper positioning*
*Related to overactivity*
*Related to pressure points (tight cast, elastic bandages)*

*Related to allergic response*
*Related to chemical irritants*
*Related to unmet dependency needs*
*Related to severe repressed anxiety*

## Maturational

*Related to tissue trauma and reflex muscle spasms secondary to:*
Infancy: Colic
Infancy and early childhood: Teething, ear pain
Middle childhood: Recurrent abdominal pain, growing pains
Adolescence: Headaches, chest pain, dysmenorrhea

### ■■■■■■ AUTHOR'S NOTE

A diagnosis not on the current NANDA list, Impaired Comfort can represent various uncomfortable sensations (e.g., pruritus, immobility, NPO status). For a person experiencing nausea and vomiting, the nurse should assess whether Impaired Comfort, Risk for Impaired Comfort, or Risk for Imbalanced Nutrition: Less Than Body Requirements is appropriate. Short-lived episodes of nausea, vomiting, or both (e.g., postoperatively) is best described with Impaired Comfort related to effects of anesthesia or analgesics. When nausea/vomiting may compromise nutritional intake, the appropriate diagnosis may be Risk for Imbalanced Nutrition: Less Than Body Requirements related to nausea and vomiting secondary to (specify). Impaired Comfort also can be used to describe a cluster of discomforts related to a condition or treatment, such as radiation therapy.

### ■■■■■■ ERRORS IN DIAGNOSTIC STATEMENTS

1. Impaired Comfort related to immobility
   Although immobility can contribute to impaired comfort, the nursing diagnosis Disuse Syndrome describes a cluster of nursing diagnoses that apply or are at high risk to apply as a result of immobility. Impaired Comfort can be included in Disuse Syndrome; thus, the diagnosis should be written as Disuse Syndrome.
2. Impaired Comfort related to nausea and vomiting secondary to chemotherapy
   Nausea and vomiting represent signs and symptoms, not contributing factors, of impaired comfort. Impaired Comfort can be used to describe a cluster of discomforts associated with chemotherapy, such as Impaired Comfort related to the effects of chemotherapy on bone marrow production and irritation of emetic center, as evidenced by complaints of nausea, vomiting, anorexia, and fatigue.

### ■■■■■■ KEY CONCEPTS

#### Generic Considerations

* Pruritus (itching) is the most common skin alteration. It can be a response to an allergen or a sign or symptom of a systemic disease, such as cancer, renal dysfunction, or diabetes.
* Pruritus, described as a tickling or tormenting sensation, originates exclusively in the skin and provokes the urge to scratch.
* Although the same neurons are likely to transmit signals for itching as for pressure, pain, and touch, each sensation is perceived and mediated differently (Porth, 2007).
* Pruritus arises from subepidermal nerve stimulation by proteolytic enzymes, which the epidermis releases as a result of either primary irritation or secondary allergic responses (Porth, 2007).
* The same unmyelinated nerves that act for burning pain also serve for pruritus. As a pruritic sensation increases in intensity, it may become burning (Porth, 2007).
* Areas that immediately surround body openings are most susceptible to itching. This apparently is related to a concentration of sensory nerve endings and vulnerability to external contamination (Porth, 2007).

## Geriatric Considerations

Asteatosis (excessive skin dryness) is the most common cause of pruritus in older adults. Its incidence ranges from 40% to 80%, as a result of varying criteria and climate differences. With scratching, small breaks in the epidermis can increase the risk of infection owing to age-related changes in the immune system (Miller, 2009).

## Transcultural Considerations

- Pain is a universally recognized "private experience that is greatly influenced by cultural heritage" (Ludwig-Beymer, 1989, p. 283).
- U.S. nurses are preponderantly white, middle-class women socialized to believe "that in any situation self-control is better than open displays of strong feelings" (Ludwig-Beymer, 1989, p. 294). Nurses should not stereotype members of a particular culture, but instead accept a wide range of pain expressions (Ludwig-Beymer, 1989).
- The nurses' own cultural background influences interpretation of a patients' pain (Lovering, 2006).
- Families transmit to their children cultural norms related to pain (Ludwig-Beymer, 1989).
- Zborowski (1952), in his classic studies on the influence of culture on the pain experience, found that the pain event, its meaning, and responses are culturally learned and culturally specific. He reported the following cultural variations in interpretation and responses to pain:
  - *Third-generation Americans:* Unexpressive; concerned with implications; controlled emotional response
  - *Jewish:* Concerned about the implication of the pain; readily seek relief; frequently express pain to others
  - *Irish:* See pain as private; unexpressive; unemotional
  - *Italian:* Concerned with immediate pain relief; present oriented
  - *Japanese:* Value self-control; will not express pain or ask for relief
  - *Hispanic:* Present oriented; use folk medicine frequently; view suffering as a positive spiritual experience
  - *Chinese:* May ignore symptoms; use alternative health practices
  - *Black Americans:* May respond stoically because of dominant culture pressure or belief that pain is God's will
  - Chinese women believe they will dishonor themselves and their family if they are loud during labor (Weber, 1996).
  - Women from many South and Central American cultures believe the more intense the expression of pain during labor, the stronger the love toward the infant (Weber, 1996).

# Focus Assessment Criteria

This nursing assessment of pain is designed to acquire data for assessing a person's adaptation to pain, not for determining the cause or existence of pain.

## Subjective Data

### Assess for Defining Characteristics

**Pain**

"Where is your discomfort located; does it radiate?" (Ask child to point to place).

"When did it begin?"

"Can you relate the cause of this discomfort?" or "What do you think has caused your discomfort?"

"Describe the discomfort and its pattern."

Time of day

Frequency (constant, intermittent, transient)

Duration

Quality/intensity

Ask person to rate the pain: at its best, after pain-relief measures, and at its worst. Use consistent scale, language, or set of behaviors to assess pain.

For adults, use an oral or visual analogue scale of 0 to 10 (0 = no pain, 10 = worst pain ever).

For children, select a scale appropriate for developmental age: can use scale for assessed age or younger; include child in selection:

- 3 years and older: Use drawings or photographs of faces (Oucher scale) ranging from smiling to frowning to crying with numeric scale.
- 4 years and older: Use four white poker chips to ask child how many pieces of hurt he or she feels (no hurt = no chips).
- 6 years and older: Use a numeric scale, 0 to 5 or 0 to 10 (verbally or visually); use blank drawing of body, front and back, asking child to use three different crayons to color places with a little pain, medium pain, and a lot of pain (Eland Color Tool).

"How do you usually react to pain (crying, anger, silence)?"

"Are any other symptoms associated with your discomfort (nausea, vomiting, numbness)?"*

### Effects of Pain

"Do you talk to others about your discomfort (spouse, friends, nurse)?" "To whom do you talk?" Ask client to indicate if each of the following increases, decreases, or has no effect on discomfort.*

| | | |
|---|---|---|
| Liquor | Vibration | Defecation |
| Stimulants (e.g., caffeine) | Pressure | Tension |
| Eating | No movement | Bright lights |
| Heat | Movement/activity | Loud noises |
| Cold | Sleep, rest | Going to work |
| Damp | Lying down | Intercourse |
| Weather changes | Distraction (e.g., TV) | Mild exercise |
| Massage | Urination | Fatigue |

Ask person what effect pain has had or is anticipated to have on the following patterns:

Work/activity (work/home activities, leisure/play)

Relationships/relating (wanting to be alone, with people)

Sleep (difficulty falling asleep/staying asleep)

Eating (appetite, weight gain/loss)

Elimination (bowel, constipation/diarrhea, bladder)

Menses

Sex (libido, function)

### Cultural Effects on Pain (Weber, 1996)

| | |
|---|---|
| Country of origin | Religious practices (blood |
| Time in United States | transfusion, specific |
| Native language | clothing, male attendants) |
| Ability to understand/speak | Food, beverage preferences |
| Availability of interpreter | Hygiene practices |

### Pruritus

| | |
|---|---|
| Onset | Relieved by what |
| Precipitated by what | History of allergy (individual, family) |
| Site(s) | |

### Nausea/Vomiting

| | |
|---|---|
| Onset, duration | Frequency, severity |
| Vomitus (amount, appearance) | Relief measures |

## Objective Data (Acute/Chronic Pain)

## *Assess for Defining Characteristics*

### Behavioral Manifestations

| | |
|---|---|
| Mood | Eye Movements |
| Calmness | Fixed |

*Adapted from the McGill Pain Questionnaire.

Moaning                                Searching
Crying                                 Open
Grimacing                              Closed
Pacing                                 Perceptions
Restlessness                           Oriented to time and place
Withdrawn

### Musculoskeletal Manifestations

Mobility of Painful Part               Muscle Tone
Full                                   Spasm
Limited/guarded                        Tenderness
No movement                            Tremors (in effort to hide pain)

### Dermatologic Manifestations

Color (redness)                        Moisture/diaphoresis
Temperature                            Edema

### Cardiorespiratory Manifestations

*Cardiac*                              *Respiratory*
Rate                                   Rate
Blood pressure                         Rhythm
Palpitations present                   Depth

### Sensory Alterations

Paresthesia                            Dysesthesias

### Developmental Manifestations

*Infant*
Irritability                           Changes in eating or sleeping
Inconsolability                        Generalized body movements

*Toddler*
Irritability                           Changes in eating or sleeping
Aggression (kicking, biting)           Rocking
Sucking                                Clenched teeth

*Preschool*
Irritability                           Changes in eating or sleeping
Aggression                             Verbal expressions of pain

*School-Aged*
Changes in eating or sleeping          Change in play patterns
Verbal expressions of pain             Denial of pain

*Adolescent*
Mood changes                           Behavior extremes ("acting out")
Verbal expressions when asked          Changes in eating or sleeping

For more information on Focus Assessment Criteria, visit http://thepoint.lww.com.

**NOC**
Symptom Control;
Comfort Status

## Goal

The client will report acceptable control of symptoms.

### Indicators

- Describe factors that increase symptoms.
- Describe measures to improve comfort.

**NIC**
Pruritus
Management,
Fever Treatment,
Environmental
Management:
Comfort

# ➤ General Interventions

## Assess for Sources of Discomfort

Pruritus       Prolonged bed rest
Fever

## Reduce Pruritus and Promote Comfort.

### *Maintain Hygiene without Producing Dry Skin*

Encourage frequent baths:

- Use cool water when acceptable.
- Use mild soap (Castile, lanolin) or a soap substitute.
- Blot skin dry; do not rub.

Apply cornstarch lightly to skin folds by first sprinkling on hand (to avoid caking of powder); for fungal conditions, use antifungal or antiyeast powder preparations [Mycostatin (nystatin)] or miconazole cream.
Massage pruritic scar tissue with cocoa butter daily (Field et al., 2000).

**R:** Massaging pruritic scars decreases itching, pain, and anxiety (Field et al., 2000).
**R:** Coolness reduces vasodilatation.

### *Prevent Excessive Dryness*

Lubricate skin with a moisturizer unless contraindicated; pat on with hand or gauze.
Apply lubrication after bath, before skin is dry, to encourage moisture retention.
Apply wet dressings continuously or intermittently to relieve itching and remove crusts and exudate.
Provide 20- to 30-min tub soaks of 32°F to 38°F; water can contain oatmeal powder, Aveeno, cornstarch, or baking soda.

**R:** Excessive warmth or dryness, rough fabrics, fatigue, stress, and monotony (lack of distractions) aggravate pruritus (Thorns & Edmonds, 2000).

### *Promote Comfort and Prevent Further Injury*

Advise against scratching; explain the scratch–itch–scratch cycle.
Secure order for topical corticosteroid cream for local inflamed pruritic areas; apply sparingly and occlude area with plastic wrap at night to increase effectiveness of cream and prevent further scratching.
Secure an antihistamine order if itching is unrelieved.
Use mitts (or cotton socks), if necessary, on children and confused adults.
Maintain trimmed nails to prevent injury; file after trimming.
Remove particles from bed (food crumbs, caked powder).
Use old, soft sheets and avoid wrinkles in bed; if bed protector pads are used, place draw sheet over them to eliminate direct contact with skin.
Avoid using perfumes and scented lotions.
Avoid contact with chemical irritants/solutions.
Wash clothes in a mild detergent and put through a second rinse cycle to reduce residue; avoid use of fabric softeners.
Prevent excessive warmth by use of cool room temperatures and low humidity, light covers with bed cradle; avoid overdressing.
Apply ointments with gloved or bare hand, depending on type, to lightly cover skin; rub creams into skin.
Use frequent, thin applications of ointment, rather than one thick application.

**R:** Scratching stimulates histamine release, increasing pruritus.
**R:** Dryness increases skin sensitivity by stimulating nerve endings.

### *Proceed with Health Teaching, when Indicated*

Explain causes of pruritus and possible prevention methods.
Explain factors that increase symptoms (e.g., low humidity, heat).

Explain interventions that relieve symptoms (e.g., fluid intake of 3,000 mL/day unless contraindicated).

Advise about exposure to sun and heat and protective products.

Teach person to avoid fabrics that irritate skin (wool, coarse textures).

Teach person to wear protective clothing (rubber gloves, apron) when using chemical irritants.

Refer for allergy testing, if indicated.

Provide opportunity to discuss frustrations.

For further interventions, refer to Ineffective Coping if pruritus is stress related.

**R:** Refer to rationales listed above.

### For a Person on Bed Rest:

Vary position at least every 2 h unless other variables necessitate more frequent changes.

Use small pillows or folded towels to support limbs.

Vary positions with flexion and extension, abduction, or adduction.

Use prone position if tolerable.

**R:** Frequent position changes maintain musculoskeletal function and prevent contractures.

## Pediatric Interventions

Explain to children why they should not scratch.

Dress child in long sleeves, long pants, or a one-piece outfit to prevent scratching.

Avoid overdressing child, which will increase warmth.

Give child a tepid bath before bedtime; add two cups of cornstarch to bath water.

Apply Caladryl lotion to weeping pruritic lesions; apply with small paintbrush.

Use cotton blankets or sheets next to skin.

Remove furry toys that may increase lint and pruritus.

Teach child to press or (if permitted) put a cool cloth on the area that itches, but not to scratch.

**R:** See Rationales for General Interventions.

## Maternal Interventions

Teach the following to prevent strain on back muscles:

- Avoid heavy lifting; use leg muscles, not back muscles.
- Place one foot higher than the other when standing for prolonged periods.
- Wear heels lower than 1 inch.
- Wear maternity girdle and exercise daily (e.g., walk, stretch).
- Apply heat or cold to back two or three times daily.

If leg cramps occur and are not caused by thrombophlebitis, teach client to flex or bend foot and not massage. Instruct client to stretch calf muscles before going to bed.

**R:** Approximately 50% of all pregnant women report backache; causes include postural changes, relaxation of pelvic ligaments, and movement of symphysis pubis (Davis, 1996).

**R:** Lowered serum calcium and increased phosphate levels are thought to increase neuromuscular irritability.

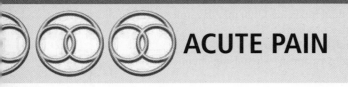

# ACUTE PAIN

## DEFINITION

The state in which a person experiences and reports the presence of severe discomfort or an uncomfortable sensation, lasting from 1 s to less than 6 months

## DEFINING CHARACTERISTICS

### Self Report of Pain Quality and Intensity

(Attempt to use with all patients)

### For Patients Unable to Provide Self-Report (in order of preference):

- Presence of pathological condition or procedure known to cause pain
- Physical responses such as diaphoresis, changes in blood pressure or pulse, pupil dilation, change in respiratory rate, guarding, grimacing, moaning, crying, or restlessness
- Surrogate reporting (family members, caregivers)
- Response to an analgesic trial (Herr et al., 2006)

## RELATED FACTORS

See Impaired Comfort.

### ◼◼◼◼◼◼ AUTHOR'S NOTE

Nursing management of pain presents specific challenges. Is acute pain a response that nurses treat as a nursing diagnosis or collaborative problem? Is acute pain the etiology of another response that better describes the condition that nurses treat? Does some cluster of nursing diagnoses represent a pain syndrome or chronic pain syndrome (e.g., Fear, Risk for Ineffective Family Coping, Impaired Physical Mobility, Social Isolation, Ineffective Sexuality Patterns, Risk for Colonic Constipation, Fatigue)? McCafferty and Beebe (1989) cite 18 nursing diagnoses that can apply to people experiencing pain. Viewing pain as a syndrome diagnosis can provide nurses with a comprehensive nursing diagnosis for people in pain to whom many related nursing diagnoses could apply.

### ◼◼◼◼◼◼ ERRORS IN DIAGNOSTIC STATEMENTS

1. Pain related to surgical incision
   Viewing incisional pain as an etiology rather than a response may better relate to nursing's focus. For a client who has undergone surgery, the nurse focuses on reducing pain to permit increased participation in activities and to reduce anxiety, as described by the nursing diagnosis Impaired Physical Mobility related to fear of pain and weakness secondary to anesthesia and insufficient fluids and nutrients.
2. Pain related to cardiac tissue ischemia
   The nurse has several responsibilities for a person experiencing chest pain: evaluating cardiac status, reducing activity, administering PRN medication, and reducing anxiety. Before discharge, the nurse teaches self- monitoring, self-medication, signs and symptoms of complications, follow-up care, and necessary lifestyle modifications. Management of chest pain involves nurse-prescribed and physician-prescribed interventions, so this situation should be described as the collaborative problem *RC of Cardiac Dysfunction*. This collaborative problem encompasses various cardiac complications (e.g., dysrhythmias, decreased cardiac output, angina). In addition, two nursing diagnoses would apply: Anxiety related to present situation, unknown future, and perceived effects on self and significant others, and Ineffective Health Maintenance related to insufficient knowledge of condition, signs and symptoms of complications, risk factors, activity restrictions, and follow-up care.

■■■■■■ **KEY CONCEPTS**

### Generic Considerations

- "Pain has been described as an experience that overwhelms the individual and consumes every aspect of life" (Ferrell, 1995, p. 609).
- All pain is real, regardless of its cause. Pure psychogenic pain is probably rare, as is pure organic pain. Most bodily pain is a combination of mental events (psychogenic) and physical stimuli (organic).
- Pain has two components: sensory, which is neurophysiologic, and perceptual or experiential, which has cognitive and emotional origins. The interaction of these two components determines the amount of suffering.
- Pain tolerance means the duration and intensity of pain that a person is willing to endure. It differs among people and may vary in one person in different situations.
- Personal factors that influence pain tolerance are as follows:

| | |
|---|---|
| Knowledge of pain and its cause | Energy level (fatigue) |
| | Stress level |
| Meaning of pain | Genetic factors |
| Ability to control pain | |

- Social and environmental factors that influence pain tolerance are as follows:

| | |
|---|---|
| Interactions with others | Secondary gains |
| Response of others (family, friends) | Sensory overload or deprivation |
| | Stressors |

- Pain threshold is the point at which a person reports that a stimulus is painful (Pasero & McCaffery, 2004)
- Studies have shown that diagnosed physiologic pain does respond to placebos, so a positive response to placebo cannot be used to diagnose pain as psychogenic.
- Pain can be classified as acute or chronic, according to cause and duration, not intensity.
  - *Acute pain* has a duration of 1 month to less than 6 months. The cause is usually organic disease or injury. With healing, the pain subsides and eventually disappears.
  - *Chronic pain* lasts for 6 months or longer. It can be described as limited, intermittent, or persistent.
  - *Limited pain* results from a known physical lesion, and an end of the pain will come (e.g., burns).
  - *Intermittent pain* provides the person with pain-free periods. The cause may or may not be known (e.g., headaches).
  - *Persistent pain* usually occurs daily. The cause may or may not be known and is usually not a threat to life (e.g., low back pain).
- The person may respond to acute pain physiologically by diaphoresis and increased blood pressure and heart and respiratory rates and behaviorally by crying, moaning, or showing anger.
- The person with chronic pain usually has adapted to it, both physiologically and behaviorally. Thus, he or she may not show visible signs of the pain.
  - *Addiction* is "a primary chronic neurobiologic disease with genetic, psychosocial and environmental factor influencing its development and manifestations. It is characterized by impaired control over drug use, compulsive use, continued use despite harm and craving" (Savage et al., 2001).
  - *Addiction Risk:* Available data suggest the risk of iatrogenic addiction is low in the treatment of acute pain and cancer pain
  - *Pseudoaddiction* is an iatrogenic syndrome created by the under treatment of pain which may present with behaviors similar to that of addiction such as drug craving and clockwatching (APS, 2003).
  - *Drug tolerance* is "a state of adaptation in which exposure to a drug induces changes that result in a diminution of one or more of its effects over time" (Savage et al., 2001).
  - *Drug dependence* is "a state of adaptation manifested by a drug class specific abstinence syndrome following abrupt cessation of that drug." (Savage et al., 2001)
  - *Multimodal Therapy (Balanced Analgesia)* "includes drugs from each of the three analgesia groups (nonsteroidal anti-inflammatory agents, opioids, and local anesthetics). Lower doses of several analgesics reduces the likelihood of significant side effects from a single agent or method" (McCaffery & Pasero, 1999).

# Pediatric Considerations

- Studies have shown that, when adults and children undergo the same surgery, children are under medicated (Hockenberry & Wilson, 2009). In one study, 52% of the children received no analgesic postoperatively, whereas the remaining 48% received preponderantly aspirin or acetaminophen.
- Maturational and chronologic age, cause of pain, coping style, parental response, culture, past pain experiences, and whether pain is acute or chronic influence the child's response to pain.

### Infant
- Associates environment with painful experience
- Cries loudly and makes verbal protests long after the stimulus is withdrawn

### Toddler
- Fears body intrusion
- Does not understand rationale for pain or have ability to conceptualize the duration of the experience, even if told
- Seeks out parental figures as a source of comfort

### Pre-schooler
- Engages in magical thinking or fantasies (e.g., believes something they thought or did caused the pain)
- Uses increased verbal skills to communicate pain
- Has limited understanding of time
- After pain passes, talks to toys or other children about the pain experience
- Denies pain, especially if he or she associates it with adverse consequences (e.g., injection, ridicule if not brave)

### School-Aged
- Fears body injury
- Can describe the cause, type, quality, and severity of pain
- Can rate the severity of pain
- Attempts to relate the pain experience to previous events and gain control over actions
- Denies pain, especially if he or she associates it with adverse consequences
- May be influenced by presence of parents in expressing pain

### Adolescent
- Considers body image as very important
- May use overconfidence to compensate for fear
- May use more "socially acceptable" behavioral responses to pain than do younger children, but fear and anxiety are not decreased
- May be influenced by presence of parents in expressing pain

# Maternal Considerations

- The discomforts of labor vary: backaches, leg cramps, imposed immobility, and contractions.
- Chapman (1991) reported that expectant fathers assumed that their roles during labor are to act as coach, teammate, or witness.
- Prolonged latent phase of labor (>20 h for primigravida or 14 h for multipara) usually results from an unripe cervix. Other causes are abnormal fetal position, dysfunctional labor, cephalopelvic disproportion, or sedation or analgesia used too early.

# Geriatric Considerations

- Pain is omnipresent in older adults and may be accepted by them and professionals as a normal and unavoidable accompaniment to aging. Unfortunately, many chronic diseases that are common in older adults, such as osteoarthritis and rheumatoid arthritis, may not receive adequate pain management.
- Older adults may not demonstrate objective signs and symptoms of pain because of years of adaptation and increased pain tolerance. They may eventually accept the pain, thereby lowering expectations for comfort and mobility. Pain-coping mechanisms cultivated throughout life are important to identify

and reinforce in pain management. Effective pain management can greatly improve overall physical functioning and emotional well-being.

- Pain is omnipresent in older adults and may be accepted by them and professionals as a normal and unavoidable accompaniment to aging. Unfortunately, many chronic diseases that are common in older adults, such as osteoarthritis and rheumatoid arthritis, may not receive adequate pain management.
- Older adults may not demonstrate objective signs and symptoms of pain because of years of adaptation and increased pain tolerance. They may eventually accept the pain, thereby lowering expectations for comfort and mobility. Pain-coping mechanisms cultivated throughout life are important to identify and reinforce in pain management. Effective pain management can greatly improve overall physical functioning and emotional well-being.
- The effects of narcotic opioid analgesics are prolonged in older adults because of decreased metabolism and clearance of the drug. Also, side effects seem to be more frequent and pronounced, especially anticholinergic effects, extrapyramidal effects, and sedation. For older adults, it is advised that drugs be started at a lower dosage. Because older adults often take multiple drugs, drug interactions should be monitored.

## Transcultural Considerations

See Impaired Comfort.

## Focus Assessment Criteria

See Impaired Comfort.

**NOC**
Comfort Level, Pain Control

## Goal

The person will experience a satisfactory relief measure as evidenced by (specify).

### Indicators

- Increased participation in activities of recovery
- Reduction in pain behaviors (specify)
- Improvement in mood, coping

**NIC**
Pain Management, Medication Management, Emotional Support, Teaching: Individual, Hot/Cold Application, Simple Massage

## General Interventions

### Assess for Factors that Decrease Pain Tolerance.

Disbelief from others  Uncertainty of prognosis
Fear (e.g., of addiction or loss of control)          Fatigue
Monotony   Financial and social stressors
Lack of knowledge

### Reduce or Eliminate Factors that Increase Pain.

### Disbelief from Others

Establish a supportive accepting relationship:

- Acknowledge the pain.
- Listen attentively to client's discussion of pain.
- Convey that you are assessing pain because you want to understand it better (not determine if it really exists).

Assess the family for any misconceptions about pain or its treatment:

- Explain the concept of pain as an individual experience.
- Discuss factors related to increased pain and options to manage.

- Encourage family members to share their concerns privately (e.g., fear that the person will use pain for secondary gains if he or she receives too much attention).

## Lack of Knowledge/Uncertainty

Explain the cause of the pain, if known.

Relate the severity of the pain and how long it will last, if known.

Explain diagnostic tests and procedures in detail by relating the discomforts and sensations that the client will feel; approximate the duration

Support individual in addressing specific questions regarding diagnosis, risks, benefits of treatment, and prognosis. Consult with the specialist or primary care provider.

**R:** Trying to convince health care providers that he or she is experiencing pain will cause the client anxiety, which compounds the pain. Both are energy depleting.

**R:** People who are prepared for painful procedures by explanations of the actual sensations experience less stress than those who receive vague explanations.

## Fear

Provide accurate information to reduce fear of addiction.

- Explore reasons for the fear.
- Explain the difference between drug tolerance and drug addiction (see Key Concepts).

Assist in reducing fear of losing control.

- Include client in setting a realistic pain goal and in adopting strategies for pain control which are congruent with his/her beliefs and experiences.
- Provide privacy for the client's pain experience.
- Attempt to limit the number of health care providers who provide care.
- Allow client to share intensity of pain; express to client how well he or she tolerated it.
- Involve the social worker or case manager if social or financial concerns exist.

Provide information to reduce fear that the medication will gradually lose its effectiveness.

- Discuss drug tolerance.
- Discuss interventions for drug tolerance with the physician (e.g., changing the medication, increasing the dose, decreasing the interval, adding adjunct therapy).
- Discuss the effect of relaxation techniques on medication effects.

**R:** Addiction is a psychological syndrome characterized by compulsive drug-seeking behavior generally associated with a desire for drug administration to produce euphoria or other effects, not pain relief. Addiction is believed to be rare, and there is no evidence that adequate administration of opioids for pain produces addiction.

**R:** The use of noninvasive pain-relief measures (e.g., relaxation, massage, distraction) can enhance the therapeutic effects of pain-relief medications.

**R:** People who are prepared for painful procedures by explanations of the actual sensations experience less stress than those who receive vague explanations.

**R:** Studies have shown that the human brain secretes endorphins, which have opiatelike properties that relieve pain. The release of endorphins may be responsible for the positive effects of placebos and noninvasive pain-relief measures.

## Fatigue

Determine the cause of fatigue (sedatives, analgesics, sleep deprivation).

Explain that pain contributes to stress, which increases fatigue.

Assess present sleep pattern and the influence of pain on sleep.

Provide opportunities to rest during the day and with periods of uninterrupted sleep at night (must rest when pain is decreased).

Consult with physician for an increased dose of pain medication at bedtime.

Refer to *Insomnia* for specific interventions to enhance sleep.

**R:** Relaxation and guided imagery effectively manage pain by increasing sense of control, reducing feelings of helplessness and hopelessness, providing a calming diversion, and disrupting the pain–anxiety–tension cycle (Sloman, 1995).

### Monotony

Discuss with client and family the therapeutic uses of distraction, along with other methods of pain relief.

Emphasize that the degree to which a person can be distracted from the pain is not at all related to the existence or intensity of the pain.

Explain that distraction usually increases pain tolerance and decreases pain intensity; however, after the distraction ceases, the person may have an increased awareness of pain and fatigue.

Vary the environment if possible.

*If the client is on bed rest:*
- Encourage family to personalize the room with flowers, plants, and pictures.
- Provide music, videos, and video games.
- Consult with a recreational therapist for appropriate tasks.

*If the client is at home:*
- Encourage person to plan an activity for each day, preferably outside the home.
- Discuss the possibility of learning a new skill (e.g., a craft, a musical instrument).
- Teach a method of distraction during acute pain that is not a burden (e.g., count items in a picture, count silently to self, play cards); breathe rhythmically; listen to music and increase the volume as pain increases.

**R:** Include the patient's home opioid dose and schedule in the nursing history. This is critical in patients who are tolerant to opioids as the dose required to manage acute pain in tolerant patients may be 2 to 3 times greater than opioid naive patients (Mitra & Sinatra, 2004). Collaborate with the physician in the use of an appropriate dose and in the use of a multi-modal approach.

**R:** Establish a realistic pain goal with the patient.

**R:** Studies have shown that the human brain secretes endorphins, which have opiatelike properties that relieve pain. The release of endorphins may be responsible for the positive effects of placebos and noninvasive pain-relief measures.

**R:** The use of noninvasive pain-relief measures (e.g., relaxation, massage, distraction) can enhance the therapeutic effects of pain-relief medications.

**R:** Nonpharmacologic interventions provide a major treatment approach for pain, specifically chronic pain (McGuire, Sheidler, & Polomano, 2000). They provide clients with an increased sense of control, promote active involvement, reduce stress and anxiety, elevate mood, and raise the pain threshold (McGuire, Sheidler, & Polomano, 2000).

## Collaborate with Client about Possible Methods to Reduce Pain Intensity.

*Consider the Following Before Selecting a Specific Pain-relief Method:*

Client's willingness (motivation) and ability to participate

Preference

Support of significant others for method

Contraindications (allergy, health problem)

Method's cost, complexity, precautions, and convenience

## Explain the Various Noninvasive Pain-relief Methods to the Client and Family and Why They Are Effective.

**Discuss the Use of Heat Applications,\* Their Therapeutic Effects, Indications, and Related Precautions**

Hot water bottle                    Moist heat pack

_____

\*May require a primary care provider's order.

Warm tub

Hot summer sun

Electric heating pad

Thin plastic wrap over

painful area to retain body

heat (e.g., knee, elbow)

**Discuss the Use of Cold Applications,\* Their Therapeutic Effects, Indications, and Related Precautions.**

Cold towels (wrung out)

Ice bag

Ice massage

Cold water immersion for

small body parts

Cold gel pack

**Explain the Therapeutic Uses of Menthol Preparations, Massage, and Vibration.**

**Teach Client to Avoid Negative Thoughts about Ability to Cope with Pain.**

**Practice Distraction (e.g., Guided Imagery, Music).**

**Practice Relaxation Techniques.**

**R:** Studies have shown that the human brain secretes endorphins, which have opiatelike properties that relieve pain. The release of endorphins may be responsible for the positive effects of placebos and noninvasive pain-relief measures.

**R:** The use of noninvasive pain-relief measures (e.g., relaxation, massage, distraction) can enhance the therapeutic effects of pain-relief medications.

**R:** Nonpharmacologic interventions provide a major treatment approach for pain, specifically chronic pain (McGuire, Sheidler, & Polomano, 2000). They provide clients with an increased sense of control, promote active involvement, reduce stress and anxiety, elevate mood, and raise the pain threshold (McGuire, Sheidler, & Polomano, 2000).

## Provide Optimal Pain Relief with Prescribed Analgesics.

Use oral route when feasible, intravenous or rectal routes if needed with permission.

Avoid intermuscular routes due to erratic absorption and unnecessary pain.

Assess vital signs, especially respiratory rate, before administration.

Consult with pharmacist for possible adverse interactions with other medications (e.g., muscle relaxants, tranquilizers).

Understand pain therapies, including the peak and duration of selected routes of administration of opioid therapy. (Dunwoody, Krenzischek, Pasero, Rathmell, Polomano, 2008).

Use a preventive approach:

- Medicate before an activity (e.g., ambulation) to increase participation, but evaluate the hazard of sedation.
- Instruct client to request PRN pain medication before the pain is severe.
- Collaborate with physician to order medications on a 24-h schedule basis rather than PRN unless the person is sedated.

**R:** Pain management should be aggressive and individualized to eliminate any unnecessary pain, with drugs administered on a regular schedule rather than PRN in the early postoperative period (AHCPR, 1992).

**R:** The preventive approach may reduce the total 24-h dose compared with the PRN approach; it provides a constant blood level of the drug, it reduces craving for the drug, and it reduces the anxiety of having to ask and wait for PRN relief (AHCPR, 1992).

**R:** Oral administration is preferred when possible. Liquid medications can be given to those who have difficulty swallowing (AHCPR, 1992).

**R:** If frequent injections are necessary, the IV route is preferred because it is not painful and absorption is guaranteed. Side effects (decreased respirations and blood pressure), however, may be more profound.

## Assess Client's Response to the Pain-Relief Medication.

After administration, return in 30 min to assess effectiveness.

Ask client to rate severity of pain before the medication and amount of relief received.

---

\*May require a primary care provider's order.

Ask person to indicate when the pain began to increase.

Consult with physician if a dosage or interval change is needed; the dose may be increased by 50% until effective (Agency for Health Care Policy and Research [AHCPR], 1992).

Collaborate with the physician to use opioid sparing adjuvants when appropriate (Lussier, Huskey, Portenoy, 2004; Elia, Lysakowski, & Tramer, 2005).

Communicate the patient's pain descriptors to the physician as they may suggest pain which might better respond to adjuvants or opioid/adjuvant combinations.

Visceral or soft tissue pain is typically described as aching and generally not localized. It is responsive to opioids and nonsteroidal anti-inflammatory drugs (NSAIDs).

Bone or connective tissue pain is described as a dull, steady ache which worsens with movement. It is somewhat responsive to opioids and very responsive to NSAIDs.

Neuropathic pain is described as burning, stabbing, stinging, electric, shooting or numbness. It is responsive to anticonvulsants (gabapentin), selective serotonin reuptake inhibitors (SSRIs), tricyclic antidepressants (TCAs), clonidine, Lidoderm patches®, and N-methyl-D-aspartate receptor antagonists (NMDAs) such as ketamine or methadone.

Muscle spasm is described as cramping, spasm or tightening and responds to muscle relaxants.

## Reduce or Eliminate Common Side Effects of Opioids.

### Sedation

Assess whether the cause is the opioid, fatigue, sleep deprivation, or other drugs (sedatives, antiemetics).

Assess for signs of respiratory depression (decreased level of consciousness, respiratory rate below 8, decreased oxygen saturation) and report to physician or nurse practitioner.

Inform person that drowsiness usually occurs the first 2 to 3 days, then subsides.

If drowsiness is excessive, consult with physician to slightly reduce the dose and/or add non-sedating adjuvant pain medication.

### Constipation

Explain the effects of opioids on peristalsis.

For long-term drug use, consult with physician on the use of a stool softener with a mild pro-motility agent, e.g., Senna.

Refer to Constipation for additional interventions.

### Nausea and Vomiting (see also Nausea/Vomiting)

Instruct person that nausea usually subsides after a few doses.

Refrain from withholding opioid doses because of nausea; rather, secure an order for an antiemetic.

If nausea persists, consult with physician for the appropriate antiemetic or for a change of narcotic opioid that produces less nausea (e.g., morphine) or decrease the opiod dose by 25%.

### Dry Mouth

Explain that opioid decrease saliva production.

Instruct person to rinse mouth often, suck on sugarless sour candies, eat pineapple chunks or watermelon (if permissible), and drink liquids often.

Explain the necessity of good oral hygiene and dental care.

**R:** Management of side effects can increase comfort level and use of medications.

## Assist Family to Respond Optimally to Client's Pain Experience

Assess family's knowledge of pain and response to it.

Give accurate information to correct misconceptions (e.g., addiction, doubt about pain).

Provide each family member with opportunities to discuss fears, anger, and frustrations privately; acknowledge the difficulty of the situation.

Incorporate family members in the pain-relief modality, if possible (e.g., stroking, massage).

Praise their participation and concern.

Minimize procedural and diagnostic pain:

- Anticipate pain and pre-medicate the patient prior to painful procedures.
- Consider the use of either intradermal 0.9% sodium chloride next to the vein or a topical anesthetic (per protocol or physician order) prior to intravenous starts.

- Encourage the use of relaxation or guided imagery during procedures.

**R:** Helping the family to understand the pain experience can enhance positive coping (Pasero & McCaffery, 2004).

## Reduce the Potential for Chronic Pain Syndromes

Acute pain that is poorly controlled can lead to debilitating chronic pain syndromes (Pasero & McCaffery, 2004).

Chronic pain syndromes may occur after mastectomy, thoracotomy, and amputation (phantom pain) (Perkins et al., 2000).

Prolonged pain after surgery may create sensitization of the nervous system. Such pain is more responsive to adjuvant therapy appropriate for neuropathic pain. (See "Client's response to pain medication:" type of pain, descriptor and medication to which each pain is most responsive.)

Risk factors include prolonged severe pain prior to and after surgery.

Nerve damage is an intraoperative factor which contributes to chronic post operative pain (Perkins & Kehlet, 2000).

Collaborate with the physician to minimize postoperative pain.

Request a pain service consultation or (if unavailable) an outpatient referral to a pain service for patients with severe ongoing postoperative pain.

## Initiate Health Teaching, as Indicated

Discuss with client and family noninvasive pain-relief measures (relaxation, distraction, massage).

Teach the techniques of choice to the person and family.

Explain the expected course of the pain (resolution) if known (e.g., fractured arm, surgical incision).

Provide the patient with written guidelines for weaning from pain medications when the acute event is relieved.

**Pediatric Interventions**

### Assess for Pain

#### Assess the Child's Pain Experience

Determine the child's concept of the cause of pain, if feasible.

Ask child to point to the area that hurts. See Focus Assessment under Impaired Comfort.

Determine the intensity of the pain at its worst and best. Use a pain assessment scale appropriate for the child's developmental age. Use the same scale the same way each time, and encourage its use by parents and other health care professionals. Indicate on the care plan which scale to use and how (introduction of scale, language specific for child); attach copy if visual scale. (See p. 128 for a description of pain scales.)

Ask the child what makes the pain better and what makes it worse.

Include the parents' rating of their child's pain in assessment. Parents and nurses can rate a child's pain differently. The parents' observation is often more accurate.

Assess whether fear, loneliness, or anxiety is contributing to pain.

Assess effect of pain on sleep and play. Note: A child who sleeps, plays, or both can still be in pain (sleep and play can serve as distractions) or adequately medicated for pain.

With infants, assess crying, facial expressions, body postures, and movements. Infants exhibit distress from environmental stimuli (light, sound) as well as from touch and treatments. Use tactile and vocal stimuli to comfort infants, but assess the effect of comfort measures (does it increase or decrease distress?) and individualized intervention.

Explain the pain source to the child using verbal and sensory (visual, tactile) explanations (e.g., allow child to handle equipment, perform treatment on doll). Explicitly explain and reinforce to the child that he or she is not being punished.

*(continued)*

**Pediatric
Interventions**
*Continued*

### Assess the Child and Family for Misconceptions About Pain or Its Treatment

Explain to the parents the necessity of good explanations to promote trust.

Explain to the parents that the child may cry more openly when they are present, but that their presence is important for promoting trust.

Parents and older children may have misconceptions about analgesia and may fear narcotic use/abuse. Emphasize that narcotic use for moderate or severe pain does not lead to addiction. Discuss with parents and older children that "say no to drugs" does not apply to analgesia for pain prescribed by physicians and monitored by physicians and nurses.

**R:** Assessment of pain in children consists of three parts: the nature of the pain-producing pathology, the autonomic responses of acute pain, and the child's behaviors. It never should be based only on behavior.

**R:** Nurses, physicians, and parents should identify and use consistent pain assessment criteria (e.g., assessment scale, specific behaviors) to assess pain in a child.

## Promote Security with Honest Explanations and Opportunities for Choice

### Promote Open, Honest Communication.

Tell the truth; explain:

- How much it will hurt
- How long it will last
- What will help the pain

Do not threaten (e.g., do not tell the child, "If you don't hold still, you won't go home").

Explain to the child that the procedure is necessary so he or she can get better and that holding still is important so it can be done quickly.

Discuss with parents the importance of truth-telling. Instruct them to:

- Tell child when they are leaving and when they will return.
- Relate to the child that they cannot take away pain, but that they will be with him or her (except in circumstances when parents are not permitted to remain).

Allow parents opportunities to share their feelings about witnessing their child's pain and their helplessness.

**R:** Anxiety, fear, and separation can increase pain.

### Prepare the Child for a Painful Procedure

Discuss the procedure with the parents; determine what they have told the child.

Explain the procedure in words suited to the child's age and developmental level (see Delayed Growth and Development for age-related needs).

Relate the likely discomforts (e.g., what the child will feel, taste, see, or smell).

- "You will get an injection that will hurt for a little while and then it will stop."
- Be sure to explain when an injection will cause two discomforts: the prick of the needle and the absorption of the drug.

Encourage the child to ask questions before and during the procedure; ask the child to share what he or she thinks will happen and why.

Share with the child older than 12 years that:

- You expect the child to hold still and that it will please you if he or she can.
- It is all right to cry or squeeze your hand if it hurts.

Find something to praise after the procedure, even if child could not hold still.

Arrange to have parents present for procedures (especially for children younger than 10 years); describe what to expect to parents before procedure, and give them a role during procedure (e.g., hold the child's hand, talk to the child).

**R:** Verbal communication usually is not sufficient or reliable to explain pain or painful procedures with children younger than 7 years. The nurse can explain by demonstrating with pictures or dolls. The more senses that are stimulated in explanations to children, the greater the communication. When possible, parents should be included in preparation.

## Reduce the Pain During Treatments When Possible

If restraints must be used, have sufficient personnel available so the procedure is not delayed.

If injections are ordered, try to obtain an order for oral or IV analgesics instead. If injections must be used:

1. Expect the child (older than 2 or 3 years) to hold still.
2. Have the child participate by holding the Band-Aid for you.
3. Tell the child how pleased you are that he or she helped.
4. Pull the skin surface as taut as possible (for IM).
5. Comfort the child after the procedure.

Tell child step-by-step what is going to happen right before it is done.

Offer the child the option of learning distraction techniques for use during the procedure. (The use of distraction without the child's knowledge of the impending discomfort is not advocated because the child will learn to mistrust.):

- Tell a story with a puppet.
- Blow a party noisemaker.
- Ask the child to name or count objects in a picture.
- Ask the child to look at the picture and to locate certain objects ("Where is the dog?").
- Ask child to tell you about his or her pet.
- Ask child to count your blinks.

Avoid rectal thermometers in preschoolers; if possible, use electronic oral or ear probes.

Provide the child with privacy during the painful procedure; use a treatment room rather than the child's bed.

The child's bed should be a "safe" place.

No procedures should be done in the playroom or schoolroom.

**R:** School-aged children can understand why a procedure needs to be done. Assessment tools can be used.

### Provide the Child Optimal Pain Relief with Prescribed Analgesics

Medicate child before painful procedure or activity (e.g., ambulation).

Consult with physician for a change of the IM route to the IV route.

Assess appropriateness of medication, dose, and schedule for cause of pain, child's weight, and child's response, not age.

Along with using pain assessment scales, observe for behavioral signs of pain (because the child may deny pain); if possible, identify specific behaviors that indicate pain in an individual child.

Assess the potential for use of patient-controlled analgesia (PCA), which provides intermittent controlled doses of IV analgesia (with/without continuous infusion) as determined by the child's need. Children as young as 5 years of age can use PCA. Parents of children physically unable can administer it to them. PCA has been found safe and to provide superior pain relief compared with conventional-demand analgesia.

Consult with physician about the use of epidural infusion of morphine for treatment of postoperative pain. Epidural morphine infusion has been used safely in both adults and children in nonintensive care settings.

**R:** Assessment of pain in children consists of three parts: the nature of the pain-producing pathology, the autonomic responses of acute pain, and the child's behaviors. It never should be based only on behavior.

**R:** Nurses, physicians, and parents should identify and use consistent pain assessment criteria (e.g., assessment scale, specific behaviors) to assess pain in a child.

**R:** Children and adolescents often deny pain to avoid injections. Although oral administration of analgesia is the route of choice for children, followed by IV administration, O'Brien and Konsler (1988) found that 40% of medications for postoperative pain were administered IM.

## Reduce or Eliminate the Common Side Effects of Opioids

### Sedation

Assess whether the cause is the opioid, fatigue, sleep deprivation, or other drugs (sedatives, antiemetics).
If drowsiness is excessive, consult with physician to slightly reduce the dose.

### Constipation

Explain to older children why pain medications cause constipation.
Increase roughage in diet (e.g., fruits; 1 teaspoon of bran on cereal).
Encourage child to drink 8 to 10 glasses of liquid each day.
Teach child how to do abdominal isometric exercises if activity is restricted (e.g., "Pull in your tummy; now relax your tummy; do this ten times each hour during the day").
Instruct child to keep a record of exercises (e.g., make a chart with a star sticker placed on it whenever the exercises are done).
Refer to Constipation for additional interventions.

### Dry Mouth

Explain to older children that narcotics decrease saliva production.
Instruct child to rinse mouth often, suck on sugarless sour candies, eat pineapple chunks and watermelon, and drink liquids often.
Explain the necessity of brushing teeth after every meal.

**R:** Management of side effects will increase comfort and use of medications.

## Assist Child with the Aftermath of Pain

Tell the child when the painful procedure is over. Pick up the small child to indicate it is over.
Encourage child to discuss pain experience (draw or act out with dolls).
Encourage child to perform the painful procedure using the same equipment on a doll under supervision.
Praise the child for his or her endurance and convey that he or she handled the pain well regardless of actual behavior (unless the child was violent to others).
Give the child a souvenir of the pain (Band-Aid, badge for bravery).
Teach child to keep a record of painful experiences and to plan a reward each time he or she achieves a behavioral goal, such as a gold star (reward) for each time the child holds still (goal) during an injection. Encourage achievable goals; holding still during an injection may not be possible for every child, but counting or blowing may be.

**R:** Provides an opportunity to discuss experience.

## Collaborate with Child to Initiate Appropriate Noninvasive Pain-relief Modalities

Encourage mobility as much as indicated, especially when pain is lowest.
Discuss with child and parents activities that they like, and incorporate them in daily schedule (e.g., clay modeling, painting).
Discuss with the child older than 7 years that thinking about something else can decrease the pain, and demonstrate the effects.

1. Ask child to count to 100 (or count your eye blinks).
2. As child is counting, apply gentle pressure to Achilles tendon (pinch back of heel).
3. Gradually increase the pressure.
4. Ask child to stop counting but keep pressure on heel.

Ask if the child can feel the discomfort in his or her heel now and if the child felt it during counting.

Consider the use of transcutaneous electrical nerve stimulation (TENS) for procedural, acute, and chronic pain. TENS has been studied and used effectively in children with postoperative pain, headache, and procedural pain, without adverse effects.

Refer to guidelines for noninvasive pain-relief measures.

**R:** Pharmacologic measures combined with noninvasive techniques provide the most effective means of treating pain in children.

### Assist Family to Respond Optimally to Child's Pain Experience

Assess family's knowledge of and response to pain (e.g., do parents support the child who has pain?).

Assure parents that they can touch or hold their child, if feasible (e.g., demonstrate that touching is possible even with tubes and equipment).

Give accurate information to correct misconceptions (e.g., the necessity of the treatment even though it causes pain).

Provide parents opportunities to discuss privately their fears, anger, and frustrations.

Acknowledge the difficulty of the situation.

Incorporate parents in the pain-relief modality if possible (e.g., stroking, massage, distraction).

Praise their participation and concern.

Negotiate goals of pain management plan; reevaluate regularly (e.g., pain-free, decreased pain).

## Initiate Health Teaching and Referrals, If Indicated.

Provide child and family with ongoing explanations.

Use the care plan to promote continuity of care for hospitalized child.

Use available mental health professionals, if needed, for assistance with guided imagery, progressive relaxation, and hypnosis.

Use available pain service (pain team) at pediatric health care centers for an interdisciplinary and comprehensive approach to pain management in children.

Refer parents to pertinent literature for themselves and children (see Bibliography).

**Maternal Interventions**

Advise the woman that she will be assisted in managing her labor. Explore her wishes.

Determine the role the expectant father chooses for the labor and birth experience: coach, teammate, or witness, or support the doula or coach.

Explain all procedures before initiation.

Provide comfort techniques as desired (e.g., walking, music, massage, acupressure, shower, baths, hot or cold applications, hypnosis, imagery) (Pillitteri, 2009).

Instruct woman not to use breathing techniques too early.

Engage the woman in pleasant dialogue and thoughts about specific subjects (e.g., other children, favorite friends, new baby, memorable vacation).

As labor progresses to active stage:

1. Evaluate effectiveness of breathing techniques.
2. If pain or anxiety is not reduced, consult with midwife or physician for a new plan.
3. Evaluate fatigue level.
4. Assess how well labor partner is anticipating the woman's needs.
5. Encourage ambulation and position changes every 20 to 30 min.
6. Approach the woman in an unhurried, gentle manner.
7. Experiment with rhythmic chanting or moaning with contractions.

**R:** Labor pain belongs to the woman experiencing it (Lowe, 1996).

**R:** Lowe (1996) found that women who engage in positive dialogue and thinking experience less pain.

*(continued)*

**Maternal**
**Interventions**
*Continued*

**R:** Depending on the choice of roles by the expectant father, the nurse supplements, supervises, or provides the supportive care.
**R:** Calm explanations can reduce fear and anxiety.
**R:** Sensory overload can contribute to anxiety and fear.
**R:** Walking promotes less frequent, more efficient contractions.
**R:** Position changes can prevent or correct malposition of the fetus, promote rotation and labor progress, and reduce lower back pain.
**R:** If prolonged latent labor is expected, a new plan of care is needed to prevent sleep deprivation, maternal exhaustion, and increased anxiety.
**R:** Maternal exhaustion can occur if breathing techniques are used too early.

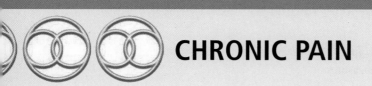

# CHRONIC PAIN

## DEFINITION

The state in which a person experiences pain that is persistent or intermittent and lasts for more than 6 months

## DEFINING CHARACTERISTICS

### Major (Must Be Present)

The person reports that pain has existed for more than 6 months (may be the only assessment data present).

### Minor (May Be Present)

| | |
|---|---|
| Discomfort | Guarded movement |
| Anger, frustration, depression because of situation | Muscle spasms |
| Facial mask of pain | Redness, swelling, heat |
| Anorexia, weight loss | Color changes in affected area |
| Insomnia | Reflex abnormalities |

## RELATED FACTORS

See *Impaired Comfort*.

■■■■■■ **AUTHOR'S NOTE**

It is well known that chronic pain affects coping, sleep, sexual activity, socialization, family processes, nutrition, spirituality, and activity tolerance. Cruz and Pimenta reported possible components of *Chronic Pain Syndrome* as *Risk for Constipation*, *Disturbed Sleep Pattern*, *Deficient Knowledge*, *Impaired Physical Mobility*, *Anxiety/Fear*, *Activity Intolerance*, and *Imbalanced Nutrition*. This author proposes that *Chronic Pain Syndrome* could represent only the effects of chronic pain on the psychosocial domain. When chronic pain affects sleep, self-care, nutrition, elimination, activity tolerance, or sexual activity, individual diagnoses may be more useful clinically.

■■■■■ **ERRORS IN DIAGNOSTIC STATEMENTS**

See *Impaired Comfort*.


■■■■■ **KEY CONCEPTS**

Refer to *Acute Pain*.


## Focus Assessment Criteria

See *Impaired Comfort*.

**NOC**
Comfort Level,
Pain: Disruptive
Effects, Pain Control,
Depression Control

> ## Goals

The person will relate improvement of pain and increased daily activities as evidenced by (specify).

### Indicators

• Relate that others validate that their pain exists.
• Practice selected noninvasive pain-relief measures.

The child will demonstrate coping mechanism for pain, methods to control pain, and the pain cause/disease, as evidenced by increased play and usual activities of childhood, and (specify).

### Indicators

• Communicate improvement in pain verbally, by pain assessment scale, or by behavior (specify).
• Maintain usual family role and relationships throughout pain experience, as evidenced by (specify).

**NIC**
Pain Management,
Medication
Management,
Exercise Promotion,
Mood Management,
Coping
Enhancement

> ## General Interventions

### Assess the Person's Pain Experience.

### Assess for Factors that Decrease Pain Tolerance.

See Acute Pain.

### Reduce or Eliminate Factors that Increase Pain.

See Acute Pain.

### Determine with Client and Family the Effects of Chronic Pain on the Person's Life (Ferrell, 1995).

Physical well-being (fatigue, strength, appetite, sleep, function, constipation, nausea)
Psychological well-being (anxiety, depression, coping, control, concentration, sense of usefulness, fear, enjoyment)
Spiritual well-being (religiosity, uncertainty, positive changes, sense of purpose, hopefulness, suffering, meaning of pain, transcendence)
Social well-being (family support, family distress, sexuality, affection, employment, isolation, financial burden, appearance, roles, relationships)

**R:** Pain is an intense experience for the client and family members. Interventions focus on helping families understand pain's effects on roles and relationships.
**R:** Ferrell (1995) validated that pain affects quality of life. Assessment of the specific effects is essential.

## Assist Client and Family to Reduce the Effects of Depression on Lifestyle.

Explain the relationship between chronic pain and depression.

Encourage verbalization concerning difficult situations.

Listen carefully.

See *Ineffective Coping for additional interventions.*

**R:** The person with chronic pain may respond with withdrawal, depression, anger, frustration, and dependency, all of which can affect the family in the same way.

## Collaborate with Client about Possible Methods to Reduce Pain Intensity.

See *Acute Pain.*

## Collaborate with Client to Initiate Appropriate Nonpharmaceutical Pain-Relief Measures.*

See *Acute Pain.*

## Provide Pain Relief with Prescribed Analgesics.*

Determine preferred route of administration: oral, IM, IV, rectal (refer to Key Concepts).

Assess client's response to the medication. For those admitted to acute care settings:

After administration, return in 30 min to assess effectiveness.

Ask person to rate severity of pain before the medication and amount of relief received.

Ask client to indicate when the pain began to increase.

Consult with the physician if a dosage or interval change is needed.

For outpatients:

Ask person to keep a record of when he or she takes medication and kind of relief received.

Instruct person to consult physician with questions concerning medication dosage.

Encourage the use of oral medications as soon as possible

- Consult with physician for a schedule to change from IM to IV or oral.
- Explain to client and family that oral medications can be as effective as IM.

Explain how the transition will occur:

1. Begin oral medication at a larger dose than necessary (loading dose).
2. Continue PRN IV medication but use as a backup for pai unrelieved by oral medication.
3. Gradually reduce IM IV medication dose.

Use the person's account of pain to regulate oral doses.

Consult with physician about possibly adding aspirin or acetaminophen to medication regimen.

**R:** The oral route is preferred because it is convenient and cost effective. Intramuscular routes are painful and have unreliable absorption rates (McCaffery, 2003).

## Discuss Fears (Individual, Family) of Addiction and Under Treatment of Pain.

Explain tolerance versus addiction.

**R:** Control of pain effectively requires clarifying misconception about addiction and overdose. Opioid tolerance and physical dependence are expected with long-term opioid treatment. Addiction is different and not usual in persons who use opioids for pain management. (APS, 2004; McCaffery, Pasero, & Portenoy, 2004).

## Reduce or Eliminate Common Side Effects of Opioids.

See *Acute Pain.*

---

*May require a primary care provider's order.

## Assist Family to Respond Optimally to the Client's Pain Experience.

See *Acute Pain*.

Encourage family to seek assistance if needed for specific problems, such as coping with chronic pain: family counselor; financial and service agencies (e.g., American Cancer Society).

## Promote Optimal Mobility.

Discuss the value of exercise, e.g., walking, yoga, or stretching.

**R:** Exercise or stretching exercises.

Plan daily activities when pain is at its lowest level.

## Initiate Health Teaching and Referrals as Indicated.

Discuss with client and family the various treatment modalities available:

| | |
|---|---|
| Family therapy | Group therapy |
| Behavior modification | Biofeedback |
| Hypnosis | Acupuncture |
| Exercise program | |

**Pediatric
Interventions
Interventions**

Assess pain experiences by using developmentally appropriate assessment scales and by assessing behavior. Incorporate child and family in ongoing assessment. Identify potential for secondary gain for reporting pain (e.g., companionship, attention, concern, caring, distraction); include strategies for meeting identified needs in plan of care.

Set short-term and long-term goals for pain management with child and family and evaluate regularly (e.g., totally or partially relieve pain, control behavior or anxiety associated with pain).

Promote normal growth and development; involve family and available resources, such as occupational, physical, and child life therapists.

Promote the "normal" aspects of the child's life: play, school, family relationships, physical activity.

Promote a trusting environment for child and family.

Believe the child's pain.

Encourage child's perception that interventions are attempts to help.

Provide continuity of care and pain management by health care providers (nurse, physician, pain team) and in different settings (inpatient, outpatient, emergency department, home).

Use interdisciplinary team for pain management as necessary (e.g., nurse, physician, child life therapist, mental health therapist, occupational therapist, physical therapist, nutritionist).

Identify myths and misconceptions about pediatric pain management (e.g., IM analgesia, narcotic use and dosing, assessment) in attitudes of health care professionals, child, and family; provide accurate information and opportunities for effective communication.

Provide parents and siblings with opportunities to share their experiences and fears.

**R:** See Rationales for Acute Pain.

**R:** Parents of a child with pain report unendurable pain, helplessness, total commitment, feeling the pain physically, being unprepared, agony, terror, and wishing for death in cases of terminal illness (Ferrell, 1995). Interventions attempt to elicit these feelings and experiences.

**R:** Assessing the child's cognitive level and age is important to provide appropriate explanations.

**R:** Preschoolers assume their pain has resulted from bad deeds. Nurses must attempt to reduce their sense of personal blame.

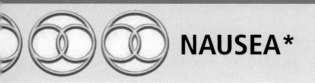

# NAUSEA*

## DEFINITION

The state in which a person experiences an unpleasant, wavelike sensation in the back of the throat, epigastrium, or throughout the abdomen that may or may not lead to vomiting

## DEFINING CHARACTERISTICS

### Major

A vague, unpleasant, subjective sensation of being "sick to stomach"
Can be accompanied by watery salivation, pallor, sweating, tachycardia
May precede vomiting

## RELATED FACTORS

### Biopathophysiologic

*Related to tissue trauma and reflex muscle spasms secondary to:*
Acute gastroenteritis
Peptic ulcer disease
Irritable bowel syndrome
Pancreatitis
Infections (e.g., food poisoning)
Drug overdose
Renal calculi
Uterine cramps associated with menses
Motion sickness

### Treatment-Related

*Related to effects of chemotherapy, theophylline, digitalis, antibiotics*
*Related to effects of anesthesia*

## ERRORS IN DIAGNOSTIC STATEMENTS

Refer to *Impaired Comfort*.

## KEY CONCEPTS

### Generic Considerations

Nausea results from stimulation of the medullary vomiting center in the brain (Porth, 2007).

Nausea and vomiting, when determined to have emotional origins, may result from developmental adjustment and adaptation. A child learns that vomiting is unacceptable and thus learns to control it. He or she receives approval for not vomiting. Should childhood situations or conflicts resurface, the adult may experience nausea and vomiting.

Nausea is the third most common side effect of chemotherapy after alopecia and fatigue.

Inadequate management of previous nausea causes anticipatory nausea before chemotherapy (Eckert, 2001).

*This diagnosis was developed by this author prior to being accepted by NANDA.

**Maternal Considerations**

The etiology of nausea during pregnancy is unknown. Contributing factors include fatigue and hormonal, neurologic, and psychological changes (Davis, 1996).

## Focus Assessment Criteria

### Subjective Data

Onset/duration
　Time of day, pattern
Frequency
Vomitus (amount, time of day)
Associated with
　Medications　　Activity
　Specific foods　Pain
　Position
　Relief measures
For more information on Focus Assessment Criteria, visit http://thepoint.lww.com.

**NOC**
Comfort Level, Nutrition Status, Hydration

➤ ## Goal

The client will report decreased nausea.

### Indicators

• Name foods or beverages that do not increase nausea.
• Describe factors that increase nausea.

**NIC**
Medication Management, Nausea Management, Fluid/Electrolyte Management, Nutrition Management

➤ ## General Interventions

### Teach How to Use Antiemetic Medications Before and After Chemotherapy

**R:** Aggressive management before, during, and after chemotherapy can prevent nausea (Eckert, 2002).

### Promote Comfort During Nausea and Vomiting

Protect people at risk for aspiration (immobile clients, children).
Address the cleanliness of the person and environment.
Provide an opportunity for oral care after each episode.
Apply a cool, damp cloth to the person's forehead, neck, and wrists.

**R:** Comfort measures also reduce the stimuli for vomiting.

## Reduce or Eliminate Noxious Stimuli

### Pain

Plan care to avoid unpleasant or painful procedures before meals.
Medicate clients for pain 30 min before meals according to physician's orders.
Provide a pleasant, relaxed atmosphere for eating (no bedpans in sight; do not rush); try a "surprise" (e.g., flowers with meal).
Arrange the plan of care to decrease or eliminate nauseating odors or procedures near mealtimes.

### Fatigue

Teach or assist client to rest before meals.
Teach client to spend minimal energy preparing food (cook large quantities and freeze several meals at a time; request assistance from others).

## Odor of Food

Teach client to avoid cooking odors—frying food, brewing coffee—if possible (take a walk; select foods that can be eaten cold).

Suggest using foods that require little cooking during periods of nausea.

Suggest trying sour foods.

**R:** Unpleasant sights or odors can stimulate the vomiting center.

## Decrease Stimulation of the Vomiting Center

Reduce unpleasant sights and odors. Restrict activity.

Provide good mouth care after vomiting.

Teach client to practice deep breathing and voluntary swallowing to suppress the vomiting reflex.

Instruct the person to sit down after eating, but not to lie down.

Encourage the person to eat smaller meals and to eat slowly.

Restrict liquids with meals to avoid overdistending the stomach; also, avoid fluids 1 h before and after meals.

Loosen clothing.

Encourage client to sit in fresh air or use a fan to circulate air.

Advise client to avoid lying flat for at least 2 h after eating. (A person who must rest should sit or recline so the head is at least 4 inches higher than the feet.)

Advise client to listen to music.

Offer small amounts of clear fluids and foods and beverages with ginger.

**R:** Music can serve as a diversional adjunct to antiemetic therapy (Ezzone et al., 1998).

**R:** Ginger has been found effective for treatment of nausea.

Maternal Interventions

### Teach that Various Interventions Have Been Reported to Help Control Nausea during Pregnancy

Avoid fatigue; greasy, high-fat foods; and strong odors.

Eat high-protein meals and a snack before retiring.

Chew gum or suck hard candies.

Eat carbohydrates (crackers) on arising; eat immediately when hungry.

Consume carbonated beverages, Coke syrup, orange juice, ginger ale, and herbal teas, e.g., ginger.

Lie down to relieve symptoms.

**R:** From 50% to 80% of all pregnant women experience "morning sickness" (Davis, 1996). Fatigue has been reported to precipitate such nausea/vomiting (Voda & Randall, 1982).

**R:** Voda and Randall (1982) reported that eating a high-protein snack before going to bed at night decreases morning nausea in some pregnant women.

### Instruct the Pregnant Woman to Try One Food or Beverage Type at a Time (e.g., High-Protein Meals/Bedtime Snack); If Nausea Is Not Relieved, Try Another Measure

Explain use of acupressure and acupuncture. Refer to resources.

**R:** Acupressure and acupuncture have proven effective for nausea and vomiting in pregnancy.

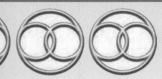

# IMPAIRED COMMUNICATION*

**Impaired Communication**

Related to Effects of Hearing Loss
Related to Effects of Aphasia on Expression or Interpretation
Related to Foreign Language Barrier
Impaired Verbal Communication

## DEFINITION

The state in which a person experiences, or is at risk to experience, difficulty exchanging thoughts, ideas, wants, or needs with others

## DEFINING CHARACTERISTICS

### Major (Must Be Present)

Inappropriate or absent speech or response
Impaired ability to speak or hear

### Minor (May Be Present)

Incongruence between verbal and nonverbal messages
Stuttering
Slurring
Word-finding problems
Weak or absent voice
Statements of being misunderstood or not understanding
Dysarthria
Aphasia
Language barrier

## RELATED FACTORS

### Pathophysiologic

***Related to disordered, unrealistic thinking secondary to:***

| | |
|---|---|
| Schizophrenic disorder | Psychotic disorder |
| Delusional disorder | Paranoid disorder |

***Related to impaired motor function of muscles of speech secondary to:***

Cerebrovascular accident
Oral or facial trauma
Brain damage (e.g., birth/head trauma)
Central nervous system (CNS) depression/increased intracranial pressure
Tumor (of the head, neck, or spinal cord)
Chronic hypoxia/decreased cerebral blood flow
Nervous system diseases (e.g., myasthenia gravis, multiple sclerosis, muscular dystrophy, Alzheimer's disease)
Vocal cord paralysis/quadriplegia

***Related to impaired ability to produce speech secondary to:***

Respiratory impairment (e.g., shortness of breath)

---

*Note: This diagnosis was developed by Rosalinda Alfaro-LeFevre and is not currently on the NANDA list, but is included here for clarity and usefulness

Laryngeal edema/infection
Oral deformities
　　Cleft lip or palate　　　　　　　Missing teeth
　　Malocclusion or fractured jaw　　Dysarthria
***Related to auditory impairment***

## Treatment-Related

***Related to impaired ability to produce speech secondary to:***
Endotracheal intubation　　　　　　　Tracheostomy/tracheotomy/laryngectomy
Surgery of the head, face, neck, or mouth　　Pain (especially of the mouth or throat)
CNS depressants

## Situational (Personal, Environmental)

***Related to decreased attention secondary to fatigue, anger, anxiety, or pain***
***Related to no access to or malfunction of hearing aid***
***Related to psychological barrier (e.g., fear, shyness)***
***Related to lack of privacy***
***Related to unavailable interpreter***

## Maturational

**Infant/Child**
***Related to inadequate sensory stimulation***

**Older Adult (Auditory Losses)**
***Related to hearing impairment***
***Related to cognitive impairments secondary to (specify)***

### ■ AUTHOR'S NOTE

*Impaired Communication* may not be useful to describe communication problems that are a manifestation of psychiatric illness or coping problems. If nursing interventions focus on reducing hallucinations, fear, or anxiety, *Confusion, Fear,* or *Anxiety* would be more appropriate.

### ■ ERRORS IN DIAGNOSTIC STATEMENTS

#### Impaired Communication related to failure of staff to use effective communication techniques

The diagnostic statement should not be used as a vehicle to reveal a problem resulting from incorrect or insufficient nursing intervention. Instead, the diagnosis should be *Impaired Verbal Communication related to effects of tracheotomy on ability to talk.* The care plan should specify the communication techniques to use.

### ■ KEY CONCEPTS

#### Generic Considerations

- Messages are sent more by body language and tone of voice than by words.
- Speech represents the fundamental way for humans to express needs, desires, and feelings. If only one person expresses information without any feedback from a listener, effective communication cannot be said to have happened.
- Any of the following can cause problems with *sending* information:
- Inability or failure to send messages that the listener can clearly understand (e.g., language or word-meaning problems, failure to speak when listener is ready)

*(continued)*

■■■■■■ **KEY CONCEPTS** *Continued*

- Fear of being overheard, judged, or misunderstood (e.g., lack of privacy, confidentiality, trust, or nonjudgmental attitude)
- Concern over response (e.g., "I don't want to hurt or anger anyone.")
- Use of words that "talk down" to the receiver (e.g., talking to an elderly or handicapped person as if he or she were a child)
- Failure to allow sufficient time for listening or providing feedback
- Physical problems that interfere with the ability to see, talk, or move
- Any of the following can cause problems with *receiving* information:
- Language or vocabulary problems
- Fatigue, pain, fear, anxiety, distractions, attention span problems
- Not realizing the importance of the information
- Problems that interfere with the ability to see or hear
- Therapeutic communication begins with:
- Offering *unconditional positive regard*, or genuine warmth for the person being helped
- Caring about the other person and being free of judgment of what he or she thinks or feels
- Ongoing therapeutic communication requires:
- A capacity for empathic understanding of the client's *internal frame of reference*
- This means working to understand how the person really feels and remaining unbiased
- The ability to be genuine, human, and *authentic*
- Dysarthria is a disturbance in the voluntary muscular control of speech. It is caused by conditions such as Parkinson's disease, multiple sclerosis, myasthenia gravis, cerebral palsy, and CNS damage. The same muscles are used in eating and swallowing.
- *Expressive aphasia* is a disturbance in the ability to speak, write, or gesture understandably.
- *Receptive aphasia* is a disturbance in the ability to comprehend written and spoken language. Those with receptive aphasia may have intact hearing, but cannot process or are unaware of their own sounds.
- Understanding of and respect for differences in personality and thinking styles are essential for communicating in ways that enhance interpersonal relations.

## Pediatric Considerations

- Although most verbal communication occurs between the nurse and parents, the adults should not ignore the child's input. Nurses should assess writing, drawing, play, and body language (facial expressions, gestures).
- Play therapy can be invaluable in establishing rapport and communicating true feelings.
- The child with hearing loss may exhibit alterations in the following responses:
- Orientation (e.g., lack of startle reflex to a loud sound)
- Vocalizations and sound production (e.g., lack of babbling by 7 months of age)
- Visual attention (e.g., responding more to facial expression than verbal explanation)
- Social/emotional behavior (e.g., becomes irritable at inability to make self understood)
- For deaf infants, visual and tactile modalities are particularly important for communicating, interacting, and gaining information about the environment (Koester et al., 1998).

## Geriatric Considerations

- Hearing loss is the third most prevalent condition affecting institutionalized older adults, exceeded only by arthritis and hypertension (Lindblade & McDonald, 1995). Only 18% of older adults with hearing loss own hearing aids. Many deny hearing loss because of fear of pressure to buy a hearing aid.
- About 40% of people older than 65 years have a significant hearing impairment that interferes with communication (Miller, 2009).
- Reduced auditory acuity correlates positively with social isolation. Understanding speech in group conversation has been identified as a prime area of difficulty for older adults. Some withdraw from social gatherings because they feel frustrated asking people to repeat things. Friends and family may refrain from entertaining hearing-impaired people because they misperceive their turning their heads away

during conversation or failure to participate as disinterest. They may also misperceive hearing impairments as mental impairments because of inappropriate comments during conversation, irritability, and inattention.
- Older adults have a high prevalence of chronic conditions that can interfere with speech or understanding of speech.

## Transcultural Considerations

- The dominant U.S. culture tends to conceal feelings and is considered low touch (Giger & Davidhizar, 2007). Difficulties can occur if the person or family does not communicate in a way that the nurse expects.
- In some cultures, a nod is a polite response meaning "I heard you, but I do not necessarily understand or agree" (Giger & Davidhizar, 2007).
- Touch is a strong form of communication with many meanings and interpretations.
- Cultural uses of touch vary, with touch between same-sex people as taboo in some cultures but expected in others (Giger & Davidhizar, 2009).
- English and German cultures do not encourage touching.
- Some highly tactile cultures are Spanish, Italian, French, Jewish, and South American.
- All cultures have rules about who touches whom, when, and where.
- The dominant U.S. culture views eye contact as an indication of a positive self-concept, openness, and honesty. It views lack of eye contact as low self-esteem, guilt, or lack of interest. Some cultures are not accustomed to eye contact, including Filipino, Native American, and Vietnamese (Giger & Davidhizar, 2007).
- The client and family should be encouraged to communicate their interpretations of health, illness, and health care (Giger & Davidhizar, 2007) within the context of their specific culture.
- African Americans speak English with varied geographic dialects. Some African Americans pronounce certain syllables or consonants differently (e.g., they may pronounce *th* as *d*, as in "*des*" for "these"). These different pronunciations should not be viewed as substandard or ungrammatical. In addition, some slang words may have different meanings—for example, "the birth of my daughter was a real bad experience." The person may mean it was unique and positive (Giger & Davidhizar, 2007).
- Mexican Americans speak Spanish, which has more than 50 dialects; thus, a nurse who speaks Spanish may have difficulty understanding a different dialect. Both men and women are very modest and restrict self-disclosure to those whom they know well. They consider direct confrontation and arguments rude; thus, agreeing may be a courtesy, not a commitment. A folk illness called *mal ojo* (evil eye) is thought to harm a child when the child is admired, but not touched, by a person thought to have special powers. When interacting with children, touch them lightly to avoid *mal ojo*. These clients may view kidding as rude and deprecating.
- Chinese Americans value silence and avoid disagreeing or criticizing. Whereas many Americans of other cultural backgrounds naturally raise the voice to make a point, Chinese Americans associate raising the voice with anger and loss of control. They rarely use "no," and "yes" can mean "perhaps" or "no." Touching the head is a serious breach of etiquette. Hesitation, ambiguity, and subtlety dominate Chinese speech (Giger & Davidhizar, 2007).

# Focus Assessment Criteria

## Subjective Data

### *Assess for Defining Characteristics*

Note the usual pattern of communication as described by the person or family.

| | |
|---|---|
| Very verbal | Responds inappropriately |
| Sometimes verbal | Does not speak/respond |
| Uses sign language | Speaks only when spoken to |
| Writes only | Gestures only |

Does the person feel he or she is communicating normally today?

If not, what does the client feel may help him or her to communicate better?

Would the client like to talk with or have present a specific person to help express ideas?

Does the client have trouble hearing?

Hearing problem                      Use of a hearing aid
Both ears or one                     Family history of hearing loss
How long? Gradual? Sudden?           History of exposure to loud noises
Ask person/caregiver to:
   Rate the ability to communicate on a scale of 0 to 10, with 0 signifying "completely unable to communicate" and 10 signifying "communicates well."
Describe factors that aid communication.

## Assess for Related Factors

Does the person feel that barriers hinder his or her ability to communicate?
Lack of privacy
Fear of uncertain origin
Fear of being inappropriate or "stupid"
Not enough time to gather thoughts and ask questions
Need for significant other or familiar face
Language, dialect, or cultural barrier (specify)
Lack of knowledge of subject being discussed
Pain, stress, or fatigue

# Objective Data

## Assess for Defining Characteristics

### Describe Ability to Form Words
Not able          Fair          Good

### Speech Pattern
Slurred speech        Voice weakness (whisper)
Lisping               Language barrier
Stuttering

### Ability to Comprehend
Follows simple commands or ideas
Can follow complex instructions or ideas
Sometimes can follow instructions or ideas
Can follow simple instructions or ideas
Follows commands and ideas only if the hearing aid is working
Follows commands and ideas only if he or she can see the speaker's mouth (lip-reads)

### What Is the Developmental Age?

### Describe Ability to Form Sentences
Good              Nonsensical or confused
Slow              Can make short, simple sentences
Not able
Unclear ideas     Language barrier

### Is Eye Contact Maintained?
Yes               Rarely
No                Blind/impaired vision
Occasionally

### Hearing Loss (Check Each Ear Separately)
*External Ear*
Deformities       Lesions
Lumps or tenderness

*Middle and Inner Ear*
Cerumen           Discharge
Redness           Swelling

*Auditory Acuity*
Can hear ticking watch or whispered words

*With Decreased Hearing*
Weber and Rinne test results

*Hearing Aid?*
Left ear                Right ear

## Assess for Related Factors

**Barriers**
Tracheostomy
Endotracheal tube

**Affect or Manner**

| | | |
|---|---|---|
| Nervous | Flat | Anxious |
| Angry | Attentive | Uncomfortable |
| Fearful | Comfortable | Withdrawn |

**Contributing Factors**
Do contributing factors inhibit the ability to communicate? (see Related Factors)
For more information on Focus Assessment Criteria, visit http://thepoint.lww.com.

---

**NOC**
Communication

# ➤ Goal

The person will report improved satisfaction with ability to communicate.

## Indicators:

- Demonstrates increased ability to understand.
- Demonstrates improved ability to express self.
- Uses alternative methods of communication, as indicated.

---

**NIC**
Communication
Enhancement:
Speech,
Communication
Enhancement:
Hearing Active
Listening,
Socialization
Enhancement

# ➤ General Interventions

## Identify a Method to Communicate Basic Needs

### Assess Ability to Comprehend, Speak, Read, and Write

### Provide Alternative Methods of Communication

Use a computer, pad and pencil, hand signals, eye blinks, head nods, and bell signals.
Make flash cards with pictures or words depicting frequently used phrases (e.g., "Wet my lips," "Move my foot," "I need a glass of water" or "I need a bedpan").
Encourage the person to point, use gestures, and pantomime.

**R:** Effective communication is an interactive process involving the *mutual exchange* of information (thoughts, ideas, feelings, and perceptions) between two or more people. Problems with *sending* or *receiving* messages (or both) can hamper this process.
Using alternative forms of communication can help decrease anxiety, isolation, and alienation; promote a sense of control; and enhance safety (Iezzoni et al., 2004).

## Identify Factors that Promote Communication

## Create Atmosphere of Acceptance and Privacy

## Provide a Nonrushed Environment

## Use Techniques to Increase Understanding

Face the client and establish eye contact if possible.
Use uncomplicated one-step commands and directives.

Have only one person talk (following a conversation with multiple parties can be difficult).

Encourage the use of gestures and pantomime.

Match words with actions; use pictures.

Terminate the conversation on a note of success (e.g., move back to an easier item).

Validate that the client understands the message.

Give information in writing to reinforce.

**R:** The nurse should make every attempt to understand the client. Each success, regardless of how minor, decreases frustration and increases motivation.

**R:** Communication is the core of all human relations. Impaired ability to communicate spontaneously is frustrating and embarrassing. Nursing actions should focus on decreasing tension and conveying understanding of how difficult the situation must be for the client (Underwood, 2004).

## Initiate Health Teaching and Referrals, If Needed

Seek consultation with a speech or audiology specialist.

**R:** Specialists may be needed after discharge.

**Pediatric Interventions**

Use age-appropriate words and gestures (see *Growth and Development Delayed*, Table II.8).

Initially talk to parent and allow the child to observe. Gradually include the child.

1. Approach the child slowly and speak in a quiet, unhurried, confident voice.
2. Assume an eye-level position.
3. Use simple words and short sentences.
4. Talk about something not related to the present situation (e.g., school, toy, hair, clothes).

Offer choices as much as possible.

Encourage the child to share concerns and fears.

Allow the child an opportunity to touch and use articles (e.g., stethoscope, tongue blade).

**R:** Communication with children must be based on developmental stage, language abilities, and cognitive level.

**R:** In children, receptive language is always more advanced than expressive language; children understand more than they can articulate. (See Table II.8 in the diagnostic category *Growth and Development, Delayed*, under Language/Cognition.)

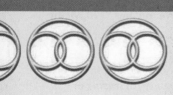

# IMPAIRED COMMUNICATION

## ▶ Related to Effects of Hearing Loss

**NOC**
Communication,
Communication:
Receptive,
Communication
Expressive

## ➤ Goal

The person will relate/demonstrate an improved ability to communicate.

### Indicators

- Wear functioning hearing aid if appropriate.
- Communicate through alternative methods.

| NIC |
|---|
| Active Listening, Communication Enhancement: Hearing Deficit |

## ➤ Interventions

### Ask the Person What Mode of Communication He or She Desires

#### *Record on Care Plan the Method to Use (May Be Combination of the Following):*

Writing          Speech-reading (or lip-reading)
Speaking
Gesturing      Sign language

**R:** Successful interaction with deaf or hearing-impaired clients requires knowing background issues, including age of onset, choice of language, cultural background, education level, and type of hearing loss.

## Assess Ability to Receive Verbal Messages

### *If Client Can Hear With a Hearing Aid, Make Sure that It Is On and Functioning*

Check batteries by turning volume all the way up until it whistles. (If it does not whistle, insert new batteries.)
Make sure volume is at a level that enhances hearing. (Many people with hearing aids turn the volume down occasionally for peace and quiet.)
Make a special effort to ensure client wears the hearing aid during off-the-unit visits (e.g., special studies, the operating room [OR]).

### *If Client Can Hear With Only One Ear, Speak Slowly and Clearly Directly into the Good Ear. It Is More Important to Speak Distinctly than Loudly*

Place bed in a position so the person's good ear faces the door.
Stand or sit on the side on which client hears best (e.g., if left ear is better, sit on the left).

**R:** Many older adults with hearing impairments don't wear hearing aids. Those who wear them must be encouraged to use them consistently, clean and maintain them, and replace batteries. They should be assertive in letting significant others know about situations and environmental areas in which they experience difficulty because of background noise.

### *If the Person Can Speech-Read*

Look directly at the person and talk slowly and clearly.
Avoid standing in front of light—have the light on your face so the person can see your lips.
Minimize distractions that may inhibit the person's concentration.
Minimize conversations if the person is fatigued or use written communication.
Reinforce important communications by writing them down.

**R:** Ten percent of deaf people have the skill and language level to read lips. Only 40% of the English language is visible. Lip or speech reading is difficult and fatiguing in the hospital. Unfamiliar terminology, anxiety, and poor lighting all can contribute to errors.

### *If Client Can Read and Write, Provide Pad and Pencil at All Times. If Client Can Understand Only Sign Language, Have an Interpreter with Him or Her as Much as Possible*

Address all communication to the person, not to the interpreter (e.g., do not say, "ask Mrs. Jones . . ."). Record name and phone number of interpreter(s) on the care plan.
If in a group setting (e.g., diabetes class), place client at front of the room near the instructor or send interpreter with him or her.
Carefully evaluate the person's understanding of required knowledge.
Give information in writing.

**R:** When using an interpreter, some things may be omitted or misunderstood. Whenever possible, give information in writing as well as through the interpreter.

### Use Factors that Promote Hearing and Understanding

Talk distinctly and clearly, facing the person.
Minimize unnecessary sounds in the room:
Have only one person talk.
Be aware of background noises (e.g., close the door, turn off the television or radio).
Repeat, then rephrase a thought, if the person does not seem to understand the whole meaning.
Use gestures to enhance communication.
Encourage the person to maintain contact with other deaf people to minimize feelings of social isolation.
Write as well as speak all important messages.
Validate the person's understanding by asking questions that require more than "yes" or "no" answers. Avoid asking, "Do you understand?"
**R:** Hearing aids magnify all sounds. Therefore, extraneous sounds (e.g., rusting of papers, minor squeaks) can inhibit understanding of voiced messages.
**R:** The following are available to assist clients with hearing impairment:
- DEAFNET, a computer system that allows clients to type messages to a computer at the phone company, which a voice synthesizer translates verbally.

## Initiate Referrals as Needed

Seek consultation with a speech or audiology specialist for assistance with communication.
- Telecommunication devices for the deaf (known as TDD) that operate by communicating electronically, messages that are typed, infrared systems, computers, voice amplifiers, amplified telephones, low-frequency doorbells and telephone ringers, closed-caption TV decoders, flashing alarm clocks, flashing smoke detectors, hearing aids, and lip reading and signing instruction.
- Deaf service centers available in most communities to help with housing, job seeking, travel arrangements, recreation, and adult education opportunities.

**R:** Under the Rehabilitation Act of 1973 and the Americans with Disabilities Act (ADA) of 1990, hospitals must offer reasonable accommodations for hearing-impaired clients. For example, they must provide qualified interpreters and auxiliary tools such as teletype machines, unless doing so imposes an undue financial or other burden.*

---

*Accessed from: http://www.mweb.com/legal/legal1a.html#2.

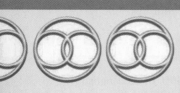

# IMPAIRED COMMUNICATION

## ▶ Related to Effects of Aphasia on Expression or Interpretation

Aphasia is a communication impairment—a difficulty in expressing, a difficulty in understanding, or a combination of both—resulting from cerebral impairments.

**NOC**
Communication:
Expressive

## ▶ Goal

The person will report decreased frustration with communication.

### Indicators

- Demonstrate increased ability to understand.
- Demonstrate improved ability to express ideas, thoughts, needs.

**NIC**
Communication
Enhancement:
Speech Deficit,
Active Listening,
Anxiety Reduction

# ➤ Interventions

## Use Techniques that Enhance Verbal Expression

### *Make a Concerted Effort to Understand the Person*

Allow enough time to listen.

Rephrase messages aloud to validate what was said.

Acknowledge when you understand, and do not be concerned with imperfect pronunciation at first.

Ignore mistakes and profanity.

Do not pretend you understand if you do not.

Observe nonverbal cues for validation (e.g., answers yes and shakes head no).

Allow person time to respond; do not interrupt; supply words only occasionally.

**R:** Deliberate actions can improve speech. As speech improves, confidence increases and the client will make more attempts at speaking.

## *Teach Techniques to Improve Speech*

Ask to slow speech down and say each word clearly, while providing the example.

Encourage client to speak in short phrases.

Explain that client's words are not clearly understood (e.g., "I can't understand what you're saying.").

Suggest a slower rate of talking, or taking a breath before beginning to speak.

Ask client to write down message, or to draw a picture, if verbal communication is difficult.

Focus on the present; avoid controversial, emotional, abstract, or lengthy topics.

**R:** Poor communication can cause frustration, anger, hostility, depression, fear, confusion, and isolation.

## *Explain the Benefits of Daily Speech Practice. Consult with Speech Therapist for Specific Exercises*

**R:** Daily exercises help improve the efficiency of speech musculature and increase rate, volume, and articulation.

## Acknowledge Client's Frustration and Improvements

Verbally address frustration over inability to communicate, and explain that both nurse and client need to use patience.

Maintain a calm, positive attitude (e.g., "I can understand you if we work at it.").

Use reassurance (e.g., "I know it's difficult, but you'll get it."); use touch if acceptable.

Maintain a sense of humor.

Allow tears (e.g., "It's OK. I know it's frustrating. Crying can let it all out.").

Give the person opportunities to make care-related decisions (e.g., "Would you rather have orange juice or prune juice?").

Provide alternative methods of self-expression:

Humming/singing

Dancing/exercising/walking

Writing/drawing/painting/coloring

Helping (tasks such as opening mail, choosing meals)

**R:** Good communicators are also good listeners, who listen for both facts and feelings.

"Presencing," or just being present and available, even if one says or does little, can effectively communicate caring to another.

## Identify Factors that Promote Comprehension

### *Provide Sufficient Light and Remove Distractions*

### *Speak When the Person Is Ready to Listen*

Achieve eye contact, if possible.

Gain the person's attention by a gentle touch on the arm and a verbal message of "Listen to me" or "I want to talk to you."

**R:** Deliberate actions can improve speech. As speech improves, confidence increases and the client will make more attempts at speaking.

## *Modify Your Speech*

Speak slowly; enunciate distinctly.

Use common adult words.

Do not change subjects or ask multiple questions in succession.

Repeat or rephrase requests.

Do not increase volume of voice unless person has a hearing deficit.

Match your nonverbal behavior with your verbal actions to avoid misinterpretation (e.g., do not laugh with a coworker while performing a task).

Try to use the same words with the same task (e.g., bathroom vs. toilet, pill vs. medication).

Keep a record at bedside of the words to maintain continuity.

As the person improves, allow him or her to complete your sentences (e.g., "This is a . . . [pill]").

**R:** Improving the client's comprehension can help decrease frustration and increase trust. Clients with aphasia can correctly interpret tone of voice.

## *Use Multiple Methods of Communication*

Use pantomime.

Point.

Use flash cards.

Show what you mean (e.g., pick up a glass).

Write key words on a card, so client can practice them while you show the object (e.g., paper).

**R:** Using alternative forms of communication can help to decrease anxiety, isolation, and alienation (Iezzoni et al., 2004).

## Show Respect When Providing Care

Avoid discussing the person's condition in his or her presence; assume client can understand despite deficits.

Monitor other health care providers for adherence to plan of care.

Talk to the person whenever you are with him or her.

**R:** Nursing care should focus on increasing comfort.

**R:** After survival, perhaps the most basic human need is to communicate with others. Communication provides security by reinforcing that clients are not alone and that others will listen. Poor communication can cause frustration, anger, hostility, depression, fear, confusion, and isolation.

## Initiate Health Teaching and Referrals, If Indicated

Explain the reasons for labile emotions and profanity

**R:** Emotional lability (swings between crying and laughing) is common in people with aphasia. This behavior is not intentional and declines with recovery.

Teach communication techniques and repetitive approaches to significant others.

Encourage family to share feelings concerning communication problems.

Explain the need to include the person in family decision making.

Seek consultation with a speech pathologist early in treatment regimen.

**R:** Speech represents the fundamental way for humans to express needs, desires, and feelings. If only one person expresses information without any feedback from a listener, effective communication cannot be said to have happened.

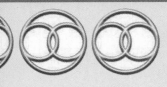

# IMPAIRED COMMUNICATION

## ▶ Related to Foreign Language Barrier

➤ **Goal**

The person will communicate needs and concerns (through interpreter if needed).

### *Indicators*

* Demonstrate ability to understand information.
* Relate feelings of reduced frustration and isolation.

➤ **Interventions**

### Assess Ability to Communicate in English*

Assess language the client speaks best.
Assess client's ability to read, write, speak, and comprehend English.

**R:** Knowledge of a foreign language depends on four elements: how to speak, understand, read, and write the language.

Do not evaluate understanding based on "yes" or "no" responses

**R:** An answer of "yes" may be an effort to please, rather than a sign of understanding.

## Identify Factors that Promote Communication Without a Translator

Face the person and give a pleasant greeting, in a normal tone of voice.
Talk clearly and somewhat slower than normal (do not overdo it).

**R:** An attempt on the nurse's part to communicate over a language barrier encourages the client to do the same.
**R:** People should overcome the human tendency either to ignore or to shout at people who do not speak the dominant language.

If the person does not understand or speak (respond), use an alternative communication method:

* Write message.
* Use gestures or actions.
* Use pictures or drawings.
* Make flash cards that translate words or phrases.

Encourage client to teach others some words or greetings of his or her own language (helps to promote acceptance and willingness to learn).
Do not correct a client or family's pronunciation.
Clarify the exact meaning of an unclear word.
Use medical terms and the slang word when indicated (e.g., vomiting/throwing up).

**R:** Be aware that, when one learns a language, one usually learns only one meaning for a word. Some words in English have more than one meaning, such as "discharge" and "pupil."
**R:** During the initial assessment, start with general questions. Allow time for the person to talk even if it is not related. Use non-direct, open-ended questions when possible. Delay asking very personal questions, if possible.

---

*English is used as an example of the dominant language.

## Be Cognizant of Possible Cultural Barriers

Be careful when touching the person; some cultures may consider touch inappropriate.

Be aware of different ways the culture expects men and women to be treated (cultural attitudes may influence whether a man speaks to a woman about certain matters, or vice versa).

**R:** Communicating through touch or holding varies among cultures. Some cultures view touch as an extremely familiar gesture, some shy away from touching a given part of the body (a pat on the head may be offensive), and some consider it appropriate for men to kiss one another and for women to hold hands.

Make a conscious effort to be nonjudgmental about cultural differences.

**R:** Nurses must have transcultural sensitivity, understand how to impart knowledge, and know how to advocate to represent the client's needs. Interpreting with cultural sensitivity is much more complex than simply putting words in another language (Giger & Davidhizar, 2009).

Make note of what seems to be a comfortable distance from which to speak.

**R:** Appropriate distance between communicators varies across cultures. Some normally stand face to face, whereas others stand several feet apart to be comfortable.

## Initiate Referrals, When Needed

Use a *fluent* translator when discussing important matters (e.g., taking a health history, signing an operation permit). Reinforce communications through the translator with written information.

If possible, allow the translator to spend as much time as the person wishes (be flexible with visitors' rules and regulations).

If a translator is unavailable, plan a daily visit from someone who has some knowledge of the person's language. (Many hospitals and social welfare offices keep a "language" bank with names and phone numbers of people who are willing to translate.)

Use AT&T telephone translating system when necessary.

**R:** Effective communication is critical and must be ensured with persons who do not speak or understand English.

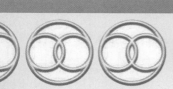

# IMPAIRED VERBAL COMMUNICATION

## DEFINITION

The state in which a person experiences, or is at high risk to experience, a decreased ability to speak but can understand others

## DEFINING CHARACTERISTICS

### Major (One Must Be Present)

Inability to speak words but can understand others
Articulation or motor planning deficits

### Minor (May Be Present)

Shortness of breath

## RELATED FACTORS

See *Impaired Communication*.

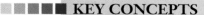

## KEY CONCEPTS

See *Impaired Communication*.

## Focus Assessment Criteria

See *Impaired Communication*.

**NOC**
Communication:
Expressive Ability

## ➤ Goal

The person will demonstrate improved ability to express self.

### Indicators:

- Relate decreased frustration with communication.
- Use alternative methods as indicated.

**NIC**
Active Listening,
Communication
Enhancement:
Speech Deficit

## ➤ General Interventions

### Identify a Method for Communicating Basic Needs

See *Impaired Communication for general interventions*.

### Identify Factors that Promote Communication

#### For Clients with Dysarthria

Reduce environmental noise (e.g., radio, TV) to increase the caregiver's ability to listen to words.

Do not alter your speech or messages, because the client's comprehension is not affected; speak on an adult level.

Encourage the client to make a conscious effort to slow down speech and to speak louder (e.g., "Take a deep breath between sentences.").

Ask the client to repeat unclear words; observe for nonverbal cues to help understanding.

If the client is tired, ask questions that require only short answers.

If speech is unintelligible, teach use of gestures, written messages, and communication cards.

**R:** Dysarthria is a disturbance in the voluntary muscular control of speech. People with dysarthria usually do not have problems with comprehension.

#### For Those Who Cannot Speak (e.g., Endotracheal Intubation, Tracheostomy)

Reassure that speech will return, if it will. If not, explain available alternatives (e.g., esophageal speech, sign language).

Do not alter your speech, tone, or type of message; speak on an adult level.

Read lips for cues.

**R:** The person's ability to understand is not affected.

### Promote Continuity of Care to Reduce Frustration

#### Observe for Signs of Frustration or Withdrawal

Verbally address frustration over inability to communicate, and explain that both nurse and client must use patience.

Maintain a calm, positive attitude (e.g., "I can understand you if we work at it.").

Use reassurance (e.g., "I know it's difficult, but you'll get it").

Maintain a sense of humor.

Allow tears (e.g., "It's OK. I know it's frustrating. Crying can let it all out.").

For the client with limited speaking ability (e.g., can make simple requests, but not lengthy statements), encourage letter writing or keeping a diary to express feelings and share concerns.

Anticipate needs and ask questions that need a simple yes or no answer.

**R:** After survival, perhaps the most basic human need is to communicate with others. Communication provides security by reinforcing that clients are not alone and that others will listen. Poor communication can cause frustration, anger, hostility, depression, fear, confusion, and isolation.

## *Maintain a Specific Care Plan*

Write the method of communication that is used (e.g., "Uses word cards," "Points for bedpan").

Record directions for specific measures (e.g., allow him to keep a urinal in bed).

**R:** Written directions will help to reduce communication problems and frustration.

## Initiate Health Teaching and Referrals, as Indicated

Teach communication techniques and repetitive approaches to significant others.

Encourage the family to share feelings concerning communication problems.

**R:** After survival, perhaps the most basic human need is to communicate with others. Communication provides security by reinforcing that clients are not alone and that others will listen. Poor communication can cause frustration, anger, hostility, depression, fear, confusion, and isolation.

Seek consultation with a speech pathologist early in the treatment regimen.

**R:** Expert consultation may be needed after discharge.

**Pediatric Interventions**

Establish a method of communication appropriate for age.

**R:** The ability to communicate with people in the environment increases the child's independence, self-esteem, and self-actualization and decreases fear.

If a young child is deprived of vocalization, teach basic language gestures (time, food, family relationships, emotions, animals, numbers, frequent requests).

**R:** Children who cannot vocalize are at risk for delays in receptive and expressive language development (i.e., vocal speech, voice production).

Consult with a speech pathologist for ongoing assistance.

Discuss with parents or caregivers the importance of providing the child with a method of communication.

**R:** Communication promotes bonding and attachment with the child's caregiver as the primary social reinforcer.

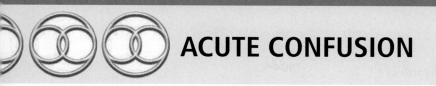

# ACUTE CONFUSION

## DEFINITION

The state in which there is an abrupt onset of a cluster of global, fluctuating disturbances in consciousness, attention, perception, memory, orientation, thinking, sleep–wake cycle, and psychomotor behavior (American Psychiatric Association [APA], 2004)

## DEFINING CHARACTERISTICS

### Major (Some Must Be Present)

*Abrupt Onset of:*

| | |
|---|---|
| Reduced ability to focus | Disorientation |
| Restlessness | Hypervigilance |
| Incoherence | Fear |
| Anxiety | Excitement |

*Symptoms worse at nights or when fatigued or in new situations.*

### Minor (May Be Present)

| | |
|---|---|
| Illusions | Hallucinations |
| Delusions | Misperception of stimuli |

## RISK FACTORS

Presence of risk factors (see Related Factors).

## RELATED FACTORS

*Related to abrupt onset of cerebral hypoxia or disturbance in cerebral metabolism secondary to (Miller, 2009):*
*Sample Nursing Diagnosis: Acute Confusion related to abrupt onset of cerebral hypoxia secondary to dehydration and*

### Fluid and Electrolyte Disturbances

| | |
|---|---|
| Dehydration | Hypokalemia |
| Volume depletion | Hyponatremia/hypernatremia |
| Acidosis/alkalosis | Hypoglycemia/hyperglycemia |
| Hypercalcemia/hypocalcemia | |

### Nutritional Deficiencies

| | |
|---|---|
| Folate or vitamin $B_{12}$ deficiency | Niacin deficiency |
| Anemia | Magnesium deficiency |

### Cardiovascular Disturbances

| | |
|---|---|
| Myocardial infarction | Heart block |
| Congestive heart failure | Temporal arteritis |
| Dysrhythmias | Subdural hematoma |

### Respiratory Disorders

| | |
|---|---|
| Chronic obstructive pulmonary disease | Tuberculosis |
| Pulmonary embolism | Pneumonia |

### Infections

Sepsis

Meningitis, encephalitis

Urinary tract infection (especially elderly)

### Metabolic and Endocrine Disorders

Hypothyroidism/
hyperthyroidism

Hypopituitarism/
hyperpituitarism

Parathyroid disorders

Hypoadrenocorticism/
hyperadrenocorticism

Postural hypotension

Hypothermia/hyperthermia

Hepatic or renal failure

### Central Nervous System (CNS) Disorders

Cerebral vascular accident

Multiple infarctions

Tumors

Normal-pressure hydrocephalus

Head trauma

Seizures and postconvulsive states

## Treatment-Related

*Related to a disturbance in cerebral metabolism secondary to:*

### Surgery

Therapeutic drug intoxication

    Neuroleptics

    General anesthesia

Side effects of medication

    Narcotics

| | | |
|---|---|---|
| Diuretics | Barbiturates | Sulfa drugs |
| Digitalis | Methyldopa | Ciprofloxacin |
| Propranolol | Disulfiram | Metronidazole |
| Atropine | Lithium | Acyclovir |
| Oral hypoglycemics | Phenytoin | H2 receptor antagonists |
| Antiinflammatories | Over-the-counter cold, cough, | Anticholinergics |
| Antianxiety agents |   and sleeping preparations | |

Phenothiazines

Benzodiazepines

## Situational (Personal, Environmental)

*Related to disturbance in cerebral metabolism secondary to:*

Withdrawal from alcohol, sedatives, hypnotics

Heavy metal or carbon monoxide intoxication

*Related to:*

| | | |
|---|---|---|
| Pain | Immobility | Unfamiliar situations |
| Bowel impaction | Depression | |

*Related to chemical intoxications or medications (specify):*

| | |
|---|---|
| Alcohol | Methamphetamines |
| Cocaine | PCP |
| Methadone | Heroin |

■ ■ ■ ■ ■ ■ **AUTHOR'S NOTE**

The addition of *Acute Confusion* and *Chronic Confusion* to the NANDA list provides the nurse with more diagnostic clarity than *Disturbed Thought Processes*. *Acute Confusion* has an abrupt onset with fluctuating symptoms; *Chronic Confusion* describes long-standing or progressive degeneration. *Disturbed Thought Processes* is also a disruption of cognitive processes; however, the causes are coping problems or personality disorders.

## ■■■■■ ERRORS IN DIAGNOSTIC STATEMENTS

1. *Acute Confusion related to advanced age*

This diagnosis does not represent an understanding of confusion, aging, and its effects on cognition. An aged person who is confused could have various reasons for confusion (e.g., electrolytic imbalance, fever, cerebral infarctions, Alzheimer's disease). He or she needs a medical and nursing assessment. Before the causes are known, this diagnosis can be stated as *Chronic Confusion related to unknown etiology.*

## ■■■■■ KEY CONCEPTS

### Generic Considerations

- "Confusion" is a term nurses use frequently to describe an array of cognitive impairments. "Identifying a person as confused is just an initial step" (Rasin, 1990; Roberts, 2001). Confusion is a behavior that indicates a disturbance in cerebral metabolism. Reduced cerebral metabolism decreases neurotransmitter levels in the brain, especially acetylcholine and epinephrine. Acetylcholine is necessary for attention, learning, memory, and information processing (Rasin, 1990; Roberts, 2001).
- *Acute confusion* or delirium results from transient biochemical disruptions caused by medications, infections, dehydration, electrolyte imbalances, and metabolic disturbances (Foreman et al., 1999). It usually lasts less than 5 days when the underlying causes are treated. Early detection and treatment can prevent unnecessarily long hospital stays (Foreman et al., 1999).
- Behavior patterns of acutely confused patients include hyperactivity, hypoactivity, and mixed (Cacchione, Culp, Laing, & Tripp, 2003).
- Chronic confusion results from progressive degeneration of the cerebral cortex. Diseases that cause such degeneration vary but manifest similar behavioral disturbances. Alzheimer's disease causes about 60% of cases of chronic confusion, whereas multiple infarctions or strokes cause about 10% of the pathology labeled multi-infarct disease (MID). A combination of senile dementia of Alzheimer's type (SDAT) and MID cause another 17%. Rare and occasionally reversible conditions such as Pick's disease, Creutzfeldt-Jakob disease, and chronic chemical intoxication (e.g., alcohol, lead, opioids, cocaine) cause the remaining 13% (Hall, 1991). People with chronic confusion can experience delirium, also.

### Geriatric Considerations

- Moderate to severe cognitive impairment in older adults can result from dementia, delirium, or depression. Nurses must approach their assessment carefully and cautiously; they should not base the diagnosis on a single symptom or physical finding.
- Infection is one of the most common causes of changes of mental status in seniors (Bishop, 2006).
- Falls and confusion are frequently encountered in the very old who have pneumonia (Janssens & Krause, 2004).
- Thinking and arithmetic abilities, memory, judgment, and problem solving are measured in older adults to give a general index of overall cognitive ability. Short-term memory may decline somewhat, but long-term memory often remains intact (Miller, 2009).
- With age, intelligence does not alter (perhaps until the very later years), but the person needs more time to process information. Reaction time increases as well. There may be some difficulty in learning new information because of increased distractibility, decreased concrete thinking, and difficulty solving new problems. Older adults usually compensate for these deficiencies by taking more time to process the information, screening out distractions, and using extreme care in making decisions. Marked cognitive decline usually is attributed to disease processes such as atherosclerosis, loss of neurons, and other pathologic changes (Miller, 2009).
- Most older adults exhibit no cognitive impairment. Severe cognitive impairment, a consequence of disease process, occurs in only 1% of people older than 65 years and 20% of people older than 85 years (Miller, 2009).
- Age-related changes can influence medication actions and produce negative consequences. See Table II.2.

| TABLE II.2 AGE-RELATED CHANGES THAT MAY INFLUENCE MEDICATION CONCENTRATIONS | |
|---|---|
| **Age-Related Change** | **Effect on Some Medications** |
| Decreased body water, decreased lean tissue, increased body fat | Increased or decreased serum concentration |
| Decreased serum albumin | Increased amount of the active portion of protein-bound medications |
| Decreased renal and liver functioning | Increased serum concentration |
| Decreased gastric acid, increased gastric pH | Altered absorption of medications that are sensitive to stomach pH |
| Altered homeostatic mechanisms | Increased potential for adverse effects |
| Altered receptor sensitivity | Increased or decreased therapeutic effect |

Miller, C. (2009). Nursing care for wellness in older adults (5th ed.). Philadelphia: Lippincott Williams & Wilkins.

- Dementia describes impairments of intellectual, not behavioral, functioning. It refers to a group of symptoms, not a disease (Miller, 2009). Alzheimer's disease, the fourth leading case of death in adults, is one type of dementia.
- Blazer (1986) reported depressive symptoms in 27% of community-living older adults. According to Parmelee, Katz, and Lawton (1989), 12% of older adults living in nursing homes met the criteria for major depression, whereas 30% were identified with minor depressive symptoms.
- Suicide is always a possibility, especially in the early stage of dementia, for numerous reasons: depression, loss of self-worth, and impaired judgment.

## Focus Assessment Criteria

From client and significant others.

### Subjective Data

### *History of the Individual*

**Lifestyle**

| | | |
|---|---|---|
| Interests | Strengths and limitations | Work history |
| Past and present coping | Education | Use of alcohol/drugs |
| Previous functioning | Previous handling of stress | |

**Support System (Availability)**
**History of Medical Problems and Treatments (Medications)**
**Activities of Daily Living (ADLs; Ability and Desire to Perform)**

### *History of Symptoms (Onset and Duration):*

| | | |
|---|---|---|
| Acute or chronic | Time of day | Sudden or gradual |
| Downward progression | Continuous or intermittent | |

### *Assess for Feelings of:*

| | | |
|---|---|---|
| Extreme sadness | Worthlessness | Mistrust or suspicion |
| Guilt for past actions | Excessive self-importance | Apprehension |
| Being rejected or isolated | Depersonalization | Living in an unreal world |
| Others controlling client | | |

### *Assess for Fears*

| | | |
|---|---|---|
| Harm from others | Thoughts racing | External agents control mind |
| Being held prisoner | Being unable to cope | Falling apart |

### *Assess for Hallucinations*

| | | |
|---|---|---|
| Visual | Tactile (includes objective component) | Gustatory |
| Olfactory | | |
| Auditory | | |

## Assess for Behaviors Associated with Depression, Dementia, and Delirium (Dellasega, 1998)

| Depression | Dementia | Delirium |
|---|---|---|
| Sudden or gradual onset | Gradual, insidious onset | Sudden, acute onset |
| Sleep difficulties | May sleep less; restlessness | Behavior worsens at night |
| Slowed motor behavior | Wandering behavior | Hypo/hyperarousal |
| Sadness, loss of interest and pleasure | Defensiveness | Hallucinations and illusions in attention |
| Memory intact | Gradual loss of ability to remember | Fluctuating performance |

# Objective Data (Includes a Subjective Component)

## General Appearance

Facial expression (alert, sad, hostile, expressionless)
Dress (meticulous, disheveled, seductive, eccentric)

## Behavior During Interview

| Withdrawn | Level of anxiety | Hostile |
|---|---|---|
| Cooperative | Apathetic | Quiet |
| Attention/concentration | Negativism | |

## Communication Pattern

| Appropriate | Obsessions | Rambling |
|---|---|---|
| Sexual preoccupations | Suspicious | Homicidal plans |
| Denying problem | Suicidal ideas | Worthlessness |
| Delusions | | |

## Speech Pattern

| Appropriate | Loose connections | Blocking (cannot finish idea) |
|---|---|---|
| Topic jumping | Circumstantial | Cannot reach a conclusion |

## Rate of Speech

| Appropriate | Reduced | Excessive |
|---|---|---|
| Pressured | | |

## Affect

| Blunted | Congruent with content | Bright |
|---|---|---|
| Appropriate to content | Flat | Inappropriate to content |
| Sad | | |

## Interaction Skills

**With Nurse**

| Inappropriate | Demanding/pleading | Relates well |
|---|---|---|
| Hostile | Withdrawn/preoccupied | |

**With Significant Others**

| Relates with all (some) family members | Hostile toward all (some) family members | Does not seek interaction |
|---|---|---|
| | | Does not have visitors |

## Activities of Daily Living

Capable of self-care (observed, reported)

## Nutrition–Hydration Status

| Appetite | Weight | Eating patterns |
|---|---|---|

## Sleep–Rest Pattern

| | | |
|---|---|---|
| Sleeps too much or too little | Early wakefulness | Cycle reversed |
| Insomnia | Fragmented sleep | |

## Personal Hygiene

| | | |
|---|---|---|
| Cleanliness | Clothes | Grooming |

## Motor Activity

| | | |
|---|---|---|
| Within normal limits | Agitated | Decreased/stuporous |

For more information on Focus Assessment Criteria, visit http://thepoint.lww.com.

**NOC**
Cognition, Cognitive Orientation, Distorted Thought Self-Control

### ➤ Goal

The person will have diminished episodes of delirium.

### Indicators:

- Be less agitated.
- Participate in ADLs.
- Be less combative.

**NIC**
Cognitive Stimulation, Calming Technique, Reality Orientation, Environmental Management: Safety

### ➤ General Interventions

#### Assess for Causative and Contributing Factors

Ensure that a thorough diagnostic workup has been completed.

**Laboratory**

| | |
|---|---|
| CBC and electrolytes | TSH, $T_4$ |
| Vitamin $B_{12}$ and folate, thiamine | Serum thyroxine and serum-free thyroxine |
| Rapid plasma reagin (RPR) | Calcium and phosphate |
| Na and K | Creatinine, BUN |
| AST, ALT, and bilirubin | Serum glucose and fasting blood sugar |
| Urinalysis | |

**Diagnostic**

| | |
|---|---|
| EEG | CT scan |
| Chest x-ray | ECG |

**Psychiatric Evaluation**
Evaluate for depression. (See Focus Assessment Criteria in *Ineffective Coping*.)

**R:** *Acute confusion* or delirium results from transient biochemical disruptions caused by medications, infections, dehydration, electrolyte imbalances, and metabolic disturbances (Foreman et al., 1999). It usually lasts less than 5 days when the underlying causes are treated. Early detection and treatment can prevent unnecessarily long hospital stays (Foreman et al., 1999).

## Promote Client's Sense of Integrity

### Examine Knowledge and Attitudes About Confusion Especially in the Aged

Educate family, significant others, and caregivers about the situation and coping methods (Young, 2001):
Explain the cause of the confusion.
Explain that the client does not realize the situation.
Explain the need to remain patient, flexible, and calm.
Stress the need to respond to the client as an adult.
Explain that the behavior is part of a disorder and is not voluntary.

**R:** Differentiating between acute (reversible) and chronic (irreversible) confusion is important for family and caregivers (Miller, 2009).

## *Maintain Standards of Empathic, Respectful Care*

Be an advocate when other caregivers are insensitive to the client's needs.

Function as a role model with coworkers.

Provide other caregivers with up-to-date information on confusion.

Expect empathic, respectful care and monitor its administration.

Attempt to obtain information for conversation (likes, dislikes; interests, hobbies; work history). Interview early in the day.

Encourage significant others and caregivers to speak slowly with a low voice pitch and at an average volume (unless hearing deficits are present), with eye contact, and as if expecting the client to understand.

**R:** Communication can be enhanced with useful and meaningful topics as one adult to another.

## *Provide Respect and Promote Sharing*

Pay attention to what the client says.

Pick out meaningful comments and continue talking.

Call the client by name and introduce yourself each time you make contact; use touch if welcomed.

Use the name the client prefers; avoid "Pops" or "Mom," which can increase confusion and is unacceptable.

Convey to the client that you are concerned and friendly (through smiles, an unhurried pace, humor, and praise; do not argue).

Focus on the feeling behind the spoken word or action.

**R:** This demonstrates unconditional positive regard and communicates acceptance and affection to a person who has difficulty interpreting the environment (Hall 1994).

## Provide Sufficient and Meaningful Sensory Input

## *Reduce Abrupt Changes in Schedule or Relocation*

Keep the client oriented to time and place.

Refer to time of day and place each morning.

Provide the client with a clock and calendar large enough to see.

If confusion is severe, remove all visible mirrors.

Use nightlights or dim lights at night.

Use indirect lighting and turn on lights before dark.

Provide the client with the opportunity to see daylight and dark through a window, or take the client outdoors.

Single out holidays with cards or pins (e.g., wear a red heart for Valentine's Day).

**R:** Sensory input is carefully planned to reduce excess stimuli that increases confusion. Reduce or eliminate:

- Fatigue
- Change in routine, environment, or caregiver
- High-stimulus activity (e.g., crowds) or images (e.g., frightening pictures or movies)
- Frustration from trying to function beyond capabilities or from being restrained
- Pain, discomforts, illness, or side effects from medications
- Competing or misleading stimuli (e.g., mirrors, television, costumes)

**R:** These factors can interfere with achieving maximum cognitive function.

## *Use Adaptive Devices to Diminish Sensory Impediments (e.g., Lighting, Glasses, Hearing Aids)*

## *Encourage the Family to Bring in Familiar Objects from Home (e.g., Photographs with Nonglare Glass, Afghan)*

Ask the client to tell you about the picture.

Focus on familiar topics.

**R:** "Functional or baseline behavior is likely to occur when the external demands (stressors) on the individual are adjusted to the level to which the person has adapted" (Hall, 1991).

### *In Teaching a Task or Activity—Such as Eating—Break It into Small, Brief Steps by Giving Only One Instruction at a Time*

Remove covers from food plate and cups.

Locate the napkin and utensils.

Add sugar and milk to coffee.

Add condiments to food (sugar, salt, pepper).

Cut foods.

Offer simple explanations of tasks.

Allow the client to handle equipment related to each task.

Allow the client to participate in the task, such as washing his face.

Acknowledge that you are leaving and say when you will return.

**R:** Memory loss and diminished intellectual functioning create a need for consistency.

**R:** Sensory input is carefully planned to reduce excess stimuli, which increase confusion (Miller, 2004).

## Promote a Well Role

Allow former habits (e.g., reading in the bathroom).

Encourage the wearing of dentures.

Ask client/significant others his usual grooming routine and encourage him to follow it.

Provide privacy at all times; when it is necessary to expose a body surface, take precautions to cover all other areas (e.g., if washing a back, use towels or blankets to cover legs and front torso).

Provide for personal hygiene according to the client's preferences (hair grooming, showers or bath, nail care, cosmetics, deodorants and fragrances).

Discourage the use of nightclothes during the day; have the client wear shoes, not slippers.

Promote mobility as much as possible.

Have the client eat meals out of bed, unless contraindicated.

Promote socialization during meals (e.g., set up lunch for four individuals in the lounge).

Plan an activity each day to look forward to (e.g., bingo, ice cream sundae gathering).

Encourage participation in decision-making (e.g., selecting what he wishes to wear).

## Discuss Current Events, Seasonal Events (Snow, Water Activities); Share Your Interests (Travel, Crafts)

**R:** Strategies that emphasize normalcy can contribute to positive self-esteem and reduce confusion.

## Do Not Endorse Confusion

Do not argue with the client.

Determine the best response to confused statements.

Sometimes the confused client may be comforted by a response that reduces his or her fear; for example, "I want to see my mother," when his or her mother has been dead for 20 years. The nurse may respond with, "I know that your mother loved you."

Direct the client back to reality; do not allow him or her to ramble.

Adhere to the schedule; if changes are necessary, advise the client of them.

Avoid talking to coworkers about other topics in the client's presence.

Provide simple explanations that cannot be misinterpreted.

Remember to acknowledge your entrance with a greeting and your exit with a closure ("I will be back in 10 minutes").

Avoid open-ended questions.

Replace five- or six-step tasks with two- or three-step tasks.

**R:** Unconditional positive regard communicates acceptance and affection to a person who has difficulty interpreting the environment.

**R:** Careful listening is critical to evaluate responses to prevent escalation of anxiety and to detect physiologic discomforts (Miller, 2009).

### Prevent Injury to the Individual

Follow institutional procedures for protecting confused persons, for example, sitters

Explore other alternatives instead of restraints (Rateau, 2000). Put the client in a room with others who can help watch him.

Enlist the aid of family or friends to watch the client during confused periods.

If the client is pulling out tubes, use mitts instead of wrist restraints.

Refer to *Risk for Injury* for strategies for assessing and manipulating the environment for hazards.

Register with an emergency medical system, including the "wanderers' list" with the local police department.

**R:** Restraints are a violation of a client's rights and increase anxiety. All attempts to protect the client should be used instead.

### Initiate Referrals, as Needed

Refer caregivers to appropriate community resources.

**R:** Additional community services may be needed for management at home.

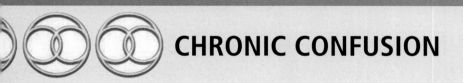

# CHRONIC CONFUSION

## DEFINITION

A state in which a person experiences an irreversible, long-standing, and/or progressive deterioration of intellect and personality

## DEFINING CHARACTERISTICS

### Major (Must Be Present)

*Progressive or long-standing:*

Cognitive or intellectual losses
  Loss of memory                                   Inability to make choices, decisions
Loss of time sense
Inability to solve problems, reason
  Altered perceptions                               Poor judgment
Loss of language abilities
Affective or personality losses
  Loss of affect                                    Increasing self-preoccupation
  Diminished inhibition                             Psychotic features
  Loss of tact, control of temper                   Antisocial behavior
  Loss of recognition (others, environment, self)   Loss of energy reserve
Cognitive or planning losses
Loss of general ability to plan                     Impaired ability to set goals, plan
Progressively lowered stress threshold
  Purposeful wandering                              Purposeless behavior
  Violent, agitated, or anxious behavior            Withdrawal or avoidance behavior
  Compulsive repetitive behavior

# RELATED FACTORS

## Pathophysiologic (Hall, 1991)

Related to progressive degeneration of the cerebral cortex secondary to:

| | |
|---|---|
| Alzheimer's disease | Multi-infarct disease (MID) |
| Combination | |

Related to disturbance in cerebral metabolism, structure, or integrity secondary to:

| | |
|---|---|
| Pick's disease | Creutzfeldt-Jakob disease |
| Toxic substance injection | Degenerative neurologic disease |
| Brain tumors | Huntington's chorea |
| End-stage diseases | Psychiatric disorders |

(AIDS, cirrhosis, cancer, renal failure, cardiac failure, chronic obstructive pulmonary disease)

## ▪▪▪▪▪ AUTHOR'S NOTE

Refer to *Acute Confusion*.

## ▪▪▪▪▪ ERRORS IN DIAGNOSTIC STATEMENTS

Refer to *Acute Confusion*.

## ▪▪▪▪▪ KEY CONCEPTS

- See *Acute Confusion*.
- Progressive dementing illnesses have four clusters of symptoms (Hall, 1991).

### Intellectual Losses

| | |
|---|---|
| Loss of memory (recent initially) | Inability to make choices |
| Loss of sense of time | Altered ability to identify visual or auditory stimuli |
| Inability to solve problems and reason | Loss of expressive and receptive language |

### Affective Personality Losses

| | |
|---|---|
| Loss of affect | Emotional lability |
| Decreased attention span | Loss of tact |
| Decreased inhibitions | Increased self-preoccupation |

### Cognitive or Planning Losses

| | |
|---|---|
| Loss of ability to plan | Loss of energy reserves |
| Loss of instrumental functions (e.g., money management, mail, shopping) | Motor apraxia |
| | Frustration, refusal to participate |
| Functional losses (e.g., bathing, choosing clothes) | |

### Progressively Lowered Stress Threshold

| | |
|---|---|
| Confused or agitated night awakening | Violent, agitated, anxious behavior |
| Purposeful wandering | Compulsive repetitive behavior |

Both depression and dementia cause cognitive impairments. Differentiating the underlying cause is critical, because depression is treatable (Miller, 2009).

# Focus Assessment Criteria

Refer to *Acute Confusion*.

**NOC**

Cognitive Ability, Cognitive Orientation, Distorted Thought Self-Control, Surveillance: Safety, Emotional Support, Environmental Management, Fall Prevention, Calming Technique

## ➤ Goal

The person will participate to the maximum level of independence in a therapeutic milieu.

### *Indicators:*

- Decreased frustration
- Diminished episodes of combativeness
- Increased hours of sleep at night
- Stabilized or increased weight

**NIC**

Cognitive Stimulation, Calming Technique, Reality Orientation, Environmental Management: Safety

## ➤ General Interventions

### Refer to Interventions Under Acute Confusion

### Assess Who the Person Was Before the Onset of Confusion

Educational level, career        Hobbies, lifestyle
Coping styles

**R:** Assessing the client's personal history can provide insight into current behavior patterns and communicates the nurse's interest (Hall, 1994).

**R:** Specific personal data can improve individualization of care (Hall, 1994).

## Observe the Client to Determine Baseline Behaviors

Best time of day        Response time to a simple question
Amount of distraction tolerated        Judgment
Insight into disability        Signs/symptoms of depression
Routine

**R:** Baseline behavior can be used to develop a plan for activities and daily care routines (Hall, 1994).

## Promote the Client's Sense of Integrity (Miller, 2009)

Adapt communication to client's level:

- Avoid "baby talk" and a condescending tone of voice.
- Use simple sentences and present one idea at a time.
- If the client does not understand, repeat the sentence using the same words.

Use positive statements; avoid "don'ts."
Unless a safety issue is involved, do not argue.
Avoid general questions, such as, "What would you like to do?" Instead, ask, "Do you want to go for a walk or work on your rug?"
Be sensitive to the feelings the client is trying to express.
Avoid questions you know the client cannot answer.
If possible, demonstrate to reinforce verbal communication.
Use touch to gain attention or show concern unless a negative response is elicited.
Maintain good eye contact and pleasant facial expressions.
Determine which sense dominates the client's perception of the world (auditory, kinesthetic, olfactory, or gustatory). Communicate through the preferred sense.

**R:** Alzheimer's disease-related dementia affects communication abilities (i.e., receptive and expressive; Hall, 1994).

## Promote the Client's Safety

Ensure that the client carries identification.
Adapt the environment so the client can pace or walk if desired.

Keep the environment uncluttered.

**R:** Confused persons are at high risk for injury.

Reevaluate whether treatment is needed. If needed, provide the following to promote safety:

### Intravenous Therapy

Camouflage tubing with loose gauze.

Consider an intermittent access device instead of continuous IV therapy.

If dehydration is a problem, institute a regular schedule for offering oral fluids.

Use the least restrictive sites.

### Urinary Catheters

Evaluate causes of incontinence.

Institute a specific treatment depending on type. Refer to *Impaired Urinary Elimination*.

Place urinary collection bag at the end of the bed with catheter between rather than draped over legs. Velcro bands can hold the catheter against the leg.

### Gastrointestinal Tubes

Check frequently for pressure against nares.

Camouflage gastrostomy tube with a loosely applied abdominal binder.

If the client is pulling out tubes, use mitts instead of wrist restraints.

Evaluate if restlessness is associated with pain. If analgesics are used, adjust dosage to reduce side effects.

Put the client in a room with others who can help watch him or her.

Enlist the aid of family or friends to watch the client during confused periods.

Give the client something to hold (e.g., stuffed animal).

**R:** Treatments and equipment can increase confusion and agitation.

## If Combative, Determine the Source of the Fear and Frustration

| | |
|---|---|
| Fatigue | Misleading or inappropriate stimuli |
| Change in routine, environment, caregiver | Pressure to exceed functional capacity |
| Physical stress, pain, infection, acute illness, discomfort | |

**R:** Fatigue is the most frequent cause of dysfunctional episodes. Physical stressors can precipitate a dysfunctional episode (e.g., urinary tract infections, caffeine, constipation).

## If a Dysfunctional Episode or Sudden Functional Loss Has Occurred:

Address the client by surname.

Assume a dependent position to the client.

Distract the client with cues that require automatic social behavior (e.g., "Mrs. Smith, would you like some juice now?").

After the episode has passed, discuss the episode with the client.

Document antecedents, behavior observed, and consequences.

**R:** These strategies can reduce aggression and may prevent future episodes with careful recording of the episode.

## Ensure Physical Comfort and Maintenance of Basic Health Needs

Refer to *Self-Care Deficits*.

## Select Modalities that Provide Favorable Stimuli for the Client

### Music Therapy

Determine the client's preferences. Play this music before the usual level of agitation for at least 30 min; assess response.

Provide soft, familiar music during meals.
Arrange group songfests with consideration to cultural/ethical orientation.
Play music during other therapies (physical, occupational, and speech).
Have the client exercise to music.
Organize guest entertainment.
Use client-developed songbooks (large print and decorative covers).

### Recreation Therapy

Encourage arts and crafts          Suggest creative writing
Provide puzzles                    Organize group games

### Remotivation Therapy

Organize group sessions into five steps (Dennis, 1984):

*Step 1:* Create a climate of acceptance (approx. 5 min).

- Maintain a relaxed atmosphere; introduce leaders and participants.
- Provide large-letter name tags and names on chairs.
- Maintain assigned places for every session.

*Step 2:* Creating a bridge to reality (approx. 15 min).

- Use a prop (visual, audio, song, picture, object, poem) to introduce the theme of the session.

*Step 3:* Share the world we live in (approx. 15 min).

- Discuss the topic as a group.
- Promote stimulation of senses.

*Step 4:* Appreciate the work of the world (approx. 20 min).

- Discuss how the topic relates to their past experiences (work, leisure).

*Step 5:* Create a climate of appreciation (approx. 5 min).

- Thank each member individually.
- Announce the next session's topic and meeting date.
- Use associations and analogies (e.g., "If ice is cold, then fire is . . . ?"
  "If day is light, then night is . . . ?").

Choose topics for remotivation sessions based on suggestions from group leaders and group interests. Examples are pets, bodies of water, canning fruits and vegetables, transportation, and holidays.

### Sensory Training

Stimulate vision (with brightly colored items of different shape, pictures, colored decorations, kaleidoscopes).
Stimulate smell (with flowers, coffee, cologne).
Stimulate hearing (ring a bell, play music).
Stimulate touch (sandpaper, velvet, steel-wool pads, silk, stuffed animals).
Stimulate taste (spices, salt, sugar, sour substances).

### Reminiscence Therapy

Consider instituting reminiscence therapy on a one-to-one or group basis. Discuss the purpose and goals with the client care team. Prepare well before initiating.

**R:** These therapies can focus the person and can reduce confusion.
**R:** Music therapy at least 30 min before the person's usual peak level of agitation can reduce agitation (Gerdner, 1999).

## Implement Techniques to Lower the Stress Threshold (Hall & Buckwalter, 1987; Miller, 2009)

### Reduce Competing or Excessive Stimuli

Keep the environment simple and uncluttered.

Use simple written cues to clarify directions for use of radio and television.

Eliminate or minimize unnecessary noise.

**R:** Overstimulation, understimulation, or misleading stimuli can cause dysfunctional episodes because of impaired sensory interpretation (Hall, 1994).

### Plan and Maintain a Consistent Routine

Attempt to assign the same caregivers.

Elicit from family members specific methods that help or hinder care.

Arrange personal care items in order of use (clothes, toothbrush, mouthwash, and so forth).

Determine a daily routine with the client and family.

Write down the sequence for all caregivers.

Reduce the stress when change is anticipated:

- Keep the change as simple as possible (e.g., minimal holiday decorations).
- Ensure the client is well rested.
- Institute change during the client's best time of day if possible.

**R:** Consistency can reduce confusion and increase comfort.

### Focus on the Client's Ability Level

Do not request performance of function beyond ability.

Express unconditional positive regard for the client.

Modify environment to compensate for ability (e.g., use of Velcro fasteners, loose clothing, elastic waistbands).

Use simple sentences; demonstrate activity.

Do not ask questions that the client cannot answer.

Avoid open-ended questions (e.g., "What do you want to eat?" "When do you want to take a bath?").

Avoid using pronouns; name objects.

Offer simple choices (e.g., "Do you want a cookie or crackers?").

Use finger foods (e.g., sandwiches) to encourage self-feeding.

**R:** Attempting to perform functions that exceed cognitive capacity will result in fear, anger, and frustration (Hall, 1994).

### Minimize Fatigue (Hall, 1994)

Provide rest periods twice daily.

Choose a rest activity with the client, such as reading or listening to music.

Encourage napping in recliner chairs, not bed.

Plan high-stress or fatiguing activities during the best time for the client.

Allow the person to cease an activity at any time.

Incorporate regular exercise in the daily plan.

Be alert to expressions of fatigue and increased anxiety; immediately reduce stimuli.

**R:** Fatigue can increase confusion.

### Initiate Health Teaching and Referrals, as Needed

Support groups

Community-based programs (e.g., day care, respite care)

Alzheimer's association (www.alz.org)

Long-term–care facilities

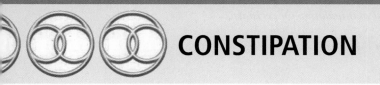

# CONSTIPATION

Constipation

Related to Effects of Immobility on Peristalsis
Perceived Constipation

## DEFINITION

The state in which a client experiences or is at high risk of experiencing stasis of the large intestine resulting in infrequent (two or less weekly) elimination and/or hard, dry feces

## DEFINING CHARACTERISTICS

### Major (Must Be Present)

Hard, formed stool   Defecation fewer than two times a week
Prolonged and difficult evacuation

### Minor (May Be Present)

Decreased bowel sounds                    Straining on defecation
Reported feeling of rectal fullness       Palpable impaction
Reported feeling of pressure in rectum    Feeling of inadequate emptying

## RELATED FACTORS

### Pathophysiologic

*Related to defective nerve stimulation, weak pelvic floor muscles, and immobility secondary to:*
Spinal cord lesions          Cerebrovascular accident (CVA, stroke)
Spinal cord injury           Neurologic diseases (multiple sclerosis, Parkinson's)
Spina bifida                 Dementia
*Related to decreased metabolic rate secondary to:*
Obesity            Hyperparathyroidism      Hypopituitarism
Pheochromocytoma   Uremia                   Diabetic neuropathy
Hypothyroidism
*Related to decreased response to urge to defecate secondary to:*
Affective disorders
*Related to pain (on defecation):*
Hemorrhoids                  Back injury
*Related to decreased peristalsis secondary to hypoxia (cardiac, pulmonary)*
*Related to motility disturbances secondary to irritable bowel syndrome*
*Related to failure to relax anal sphincter or high resting pressure in the anal canal secondary to:*
Multiple vaginal deliveries   Chronic straining

### Treatment-Related

*Related to side effects of (specify):*
Antidepressants              Calcium channel blockers
Antacids (calcium, aluminum) Calcium
Iron                         Anticholinergics
Barium                       Anesthetics
Aluminum                     Narcotics (codeine, morphine)
Aspirin                      Diuretics
Phenothiazines               Anti-Parkinson agents

*Related to effects of anesthesia and surgical manipulation on peristalsis*
*Related to habitual laxative use*
*Related to mucositis secondary to radiation*

## Situational (Personal, Environmental)

*Related to decreased peristalsis secondary to:*
    Immobility     Stress
    Pregnancy    Lack of exercise
*Related to irregular evacuation patterns*
*Related to cultural/health beliefs*
*Related to lack of privacy*
*Related to inadequate diet (lack of roughage, fiber, thiamine) or fluid intake*
*Related to fear of rectal or cardiac pain*
*Related to faulty appraisal*
*Related to inability to perceive bowel cues*

## ■■■■■■ AUTHOR'S NOTE

Constipation results from delayed passage of food residue in the bowel because of factors that the nurse can treat (e.g., dehydration, insufficient dietary roughage, immobility). Perceived constipation refers to a faulty perception of constipation with self-prescribed overuse of laxatives, enemas, and/or suppositories.

When constipation stems from factors amenable to nursing interventions other than those related to colonic or perceived constipation, the nursing diagnosis *Constipation* can apply.

## ■■■■■■ ERRORS IN DIAGNOSTIC STATEMENTS

1. *Constipation related to reports of infrequent hard, dry feces*
   A report of infrequent hard, dry feces validates constipation—it is not a contributing factor. If the nurse does not know the cause, he or she can write: *Constipation related to unknown etiology,* as evidenced by reports of infrequent hard, dry feces.

## ■■■■■■ KEY CONCEPTS

### Generic Considerations

- Irritable bowel syndrome affects 10% to 15% of the U.S. population to some degree and can include constipation, diarrhea, and pain (Hadley & Gaarder, 2006). Constipation is a predominant symptom in many clients with irritable bowel syndrome (Heisch, 2005).
- Bowel elimination is controlled primarily by muscular and neurologic activity. Undigested food or feces passes through the large intestine propelled by involuntary muscles within the intestinal walls. At the same time, water that was needed for digestion is reabsorbed. The feces pass through the sigmoid colon, which empties into the rectum. At some point, the amount of stool in the rectum stimulates a defecation reflex, which causes the anal sphincter to relax and defecation to occur (Shua-Haim, Sabo, & Ross, 1999). Table II.3 illustrates the components needed for normal bowel elimination and the conditions that impede them.
- Chronic constipation subtypes include slow transit constipation, pelvic floor dyssynergia, functional constipation, and irritable bowel syndrome with constipation (Prather, 2004).
- Bowel patterns are culturally or family determined. Range of normal is wide, from three times a day to once every 3 days (Shua-Haim et al., 1999).
- Undigested fiber absorbs water, which adds bulk and softness to the stool, speeding its passage through the intestines. Fiber without adequate fluid can aggravate, not facilitate, bowel function.
- Laxatives and enemas are not components of a bowel management program. They are for emergency use only.
- Chronic use of stool softeners can cause fecal incontinence and is not recommended for treatment of chronic constipation in nonambulatory individuals (Shua-Haim et al., 1999).

## TABLE II.3  COMPONENTS FOR NORMAL BOWEL ELIMINATION AND CORRESPONDING BARRIERS

| Components | Barriers |
|---|---|
| Daily diet of fiber (15–25 g) | Lack of access to fresh foods<br>Financial constraints<br>Insufficient knowledge* |
| 8–10 glasses of water a day | Mobility problems<br>Fear of incontinence<br>Impaired thought process*<br>Low motivation |
| Daily exercise | Minimal activity level<br>Pain, fatigue<br>Fear of falling |
| Cognitive appraisal | Impaired thought process<br>Faulty appraisal |
| Toileting routine | Low motivation<br>Change in routine<br>Stress |
| Response to rectal cues | Mobility problems<br>Decreased awareness<br>Environmental constraints<br>Self-care deficits |

*These barriers can impede all the components.

## Pediatric Considerations

- Unlike in adults, constipation in children is not defined by frequency, but by the character of stool. Passage of firm or hard stool with symptoms of difficulty in expulsion, blood-streaked bowel movements, and abdominal discomfort characterize constipation in children.
- As the infant ages, the stomach enlarges to hold more food, and the peristaltic activity of the gastrointestinal (GI) tract slows. Thus, stools change in color, consistency, and frequency (Hockenberry & Wilson, 2009).
- Voluntary withholding (functional constipation) is the most common cause of constipation beyond the neonatal period. Conflicts in toilet training or pain on defecation may lead to stool retention (Hockenberry & Wilson, 2009).
- Encopresis is fecal soiling or incontinence secondary to constipation. Previously toilet-trained children with encopresis should be evaluated psychologically.
- Children with functional constipation associate defecation with discomfort. When the sensation of relaxation of the internal anal sphincter occurs, the child contracts the external sphincter to prevent the expulsion of stools. Eventually the rectum dilates, resulting in more stool retention and diminished sensory response.

## Maternal Considerations

Constipation in pregnancy results from:
- Displacement of the intestines
- Increased water absorption from colon
- Hormonal influences
- Prolonged intestinal time
- Use of iron supplements

Postpartum causes of constipation are:
- Relaxed abdominal tone
- Decreased peristalsis
- Food and fluid restrictions during labor

### Geriatric Considerations

- Older adults experience reduced mucus secretion in the large intestines and decreased elasticity of the rectal wall (Miller, 2004).
- Sensory dysfunction in the anorectal area of older adults can reduce the ability to sense rectal distention (Shua-Haim et al., 1999).
- Some older adults are prone to constipation owing to such factors as decreased activity, insufficient dietary fiber and bulk, insufficient fluid intake, side effects of medications, laxative abuse, and inattention to defecation cues (Miller, 2009).
- Thirty percent of older adults complain of constipation compared to 2% of the general population (Shaefer & Cheskin, 1998).

### Transcultural Considerations

Some cultures have folk medicine for elimination problems. For example, Mexican Americans differentiate diarrhea as hot or cold. If the stool is green or yellow, it is hot and treated with cold tea. If white, the stool is cold and treated with hot tea (Giger & Davidhizar, 2003).

## Focus Assessment Criteria

### Subjective Data

#### Assess for Defining Characteristics

Elimination pattern
    Usual           Present
What frequency is considered normal?
Laxative/enema use
    Type           How often
Episodes of diarrhea
    How often?        Frequency?        Duration?
Precipitated by what?
Associated symptoms/complaints of:

| | | |
|---|---|---|
| Headache | Thirst | Weakness |
| Pain | Lethargy | Cramping |
| Anorexia | Weight loss/gain | Awareness of bowel cues |

### Assess for Related Factors

#### Lifestyle

*Activity level*
*Occupation*
*Exercise (what? how often?)*

*Nutrition*

| | |
|---|---|
| 24-h recall of foods and liquids taken | Protein |
| | Usual 24-h intake |
| Carbohydrates | Fiber |
| Fat | Liquids |

*Current drug therapy*

| | |
|---|---|
| Antibiotics | Antacids |
| Iron | Central nervous system (CNS) depressants |
| Steroids | |

*Medical–surgical history*

| | |
|---|---|
| Present conditions | Past conditions |
| Surgical history | Awareness of bowel cues |
|   (colostomy? ileostomy?) | |

## Objective Data

### *Assess for Defining Characteristics*

**Stool**

*Color*
*Odor*
*Consistency*

*Components*

| | |
|---|---|
| Blood | Undigested food |
| Parasites | Pus |
| Mucus | |

***Gastrointestinal Motility (Auscultation, Light Palpation)***

**Bowel Sounds**

| | |
|---|---|
| High-pitched, gurgling | High-pitched, frequent, loud, pushing (5/min) |
| Weak and infrequent | Absent |

### *Assess for Related Factors*

**Nutrition**

| *Food intake* | *Fluid intake* |
|---|---|
| Type | Type |
| Amounts | Amounts |

**Perianal Area/Rectal Examination**

| | |
|---|---|
| Hemorrhoids | Irritation |
| Fissures | Impaction |
| Control of rectal sphincter | Stool in rectum |
|   (presence of anal wink, | |
|   bulbocavernosus reflex) | |

For more information on Focus Assessment Criteria, visit http://thepoint.lww.com.

---

**NOC**
Bowel Elimination,
Hydration,
Knowledge: Diet

## ➤ Goal

The client will report bowel movements at least every 2 to 3 days.

### *Indicators:*

- Describe components for effective bowel movements.
- Explain rationale for lifestyle change(s).

---

**NIC**
Bowel Management,
Fluid Management,
Constipation/
Impaction
Management

## ➤ General Interventions

### Assess Contributing Factors

Refer to Related Factors.

### Promote Corrective Measures

### *Regular Time for Elimination*

Review daily routine.
Advise the client to include time for defecation as part of his or her daily routine.
Discuss a suitable time (based on responsibilities, availability of facilities, and so forth).

Provide a stimulus to defecation (e.g., coffee, prune juice).

Advise the client to attempt to defecate about 1 h or so after meals and that remaining in the bathroom for a suitable length of time may be necessary.

Use the bathroom instead of a bedpan if possible.

Provide privacy (close door, draw curtains around the bed, play the television or radio to mask sounds, have a room deodorizer available).

Provide comfort (reading material as diversion) and safety (call bell available).

Allow suitable position (sitting, if not contraindicated).

**R:** The gastrocolic and duodenocolic reflexes stimulate mass peristalsis 2 or 3 times a day, most often after meals.

## Adequate Exercise

Review the current exercise pattern.

Provide for frequent moderate physical exercise (if not contraindicated).

Provide frequent ambulation of hospitalized client when tolerable.

Perform range-of-motion exercises for the client who is bedridden.

Teach exercises for increased abdominal muscle tone (unless contraindicated; Weeks et al., 2000).

- Contract abdominal muscles several times throughout the day.
- Do sit-ups, keeping heels on floor with knees slightly flexed.
- While supine, raise lower limbs, keeping knees straight.

Turn and change positions in bed, lifting hips.

Lift knees alternately to the chest, stretching arms out to side and up over the head.

**R:** Regular physical activity promotes muscle tonicity needed for fecal expulsion. It also increases circulation to the digestive system, which promotes peristalsis and easier feces evacuation.

## Balanced Diet

Review list of foods high in fiber:

| | |
|---|---|
| Fresh fruits and vegetables with skins | Beans (navy, kidney, lima) |
| Bran | Whole-grain breads and cereal |
| Nuts and seeds | Cooked fruits and vegetables |
| Fruit juices | |

Discuss dietary preferences.

Consider any food intolerances or allergies.

Include approximately 800 g of fruits and vegetables (about four pieces of fresh fruit and large salad) for normal daily bowel movement.

Suggest moderate use of bran at first (may irritate GI tract, produce flatulence, cause diarrhea or blockage).

Gradually increase bran as tolerated (may add to cereals, baked goods, and the like). Explain the need for fluid intake with bran.

Suggest 30 to 60 mL daily of a recipe of 2 cups of All Bran cereal, 2 cups of applesauce, and 1 cup of prune juice.

Consider financial limitations (encourage the use of fruits and vegetables in season).

**R:** A daily diet of fiber, 6 to 8 glasses of water, and exercise maintain a normal bowel elimination pattern. In addition, the client must be able to appraise the need to evacuate and establish a toileting routine.

**R:** Diets high in unrefined fibrous food produce large, soft stools that decrease the colon's susceptibility to disease. Diets low in fiber and high in concentrated refined foods produce small, hard stools that increase the colon's susceptibility to disease.

Three tablespoons of bran daily increases dietary fiber by 25% to 40% and eliminates constipation in 60% of individuals (Shua-Haim et al., 1999).

## Adequate Fluid Intake

Encourage intake of at least 2 L (8 to 10 glasses) unless contraindicated.

Discuss fluid preferences.

Set up regular schedule for fluid intake.

Recommend drinking a glass of hot water 30 min before breakfast, which may stimulate bowel evacuation.

Advise avoiding grapefruit juice, coffee, tea, cola, and chocolate drinks as daily fluid intake.

**R:** Sufficient fluid intake, at least 2 L daily, is necessary to maintain bowel patterns and to promote proper stool consistency.

### Optimal Position

Assist the client to normal semi-squatting position to allow optimal use of abdominal muscles and effect of force of gravity.

Assist the client onto the bedpan if necessary; elevate the head of the bed to high Fowler's position or elevation permitted.

Use fracture bedpan for comfort, if preferred.

Stress the avoidance of straining.

Encourage exhaling during straining.

Chart results (color, consistency, amount).

Elevate the legs on a footstool when on the toilet.

**R:** Elevating the legs can increase intra-abdominal pressure (Shua-Haim et al., 1999).

## Eliminate or Reduce Contributing Factors

Administer a mild laxative after oral administration of barium sulfate.*

Assess elimination status while on antacid therapy (may be necessary to alternate magnesium-type antacid with other types).*

Encourage increased intake of high-roughage foods and increased fluid intake as an adjunct to iron therapy (e.g., fresh fruits and vegetables with skins; bran, nuts, and seeds; whole-wheat bread).

Encourage early ambulation, with assistance if necessary, to counter effects of anesthetic agents.

Assess elimination status while the client receives certain narcotic analgesics (morphine, codeine) and alert a physician if the client experiences difficulty with defecation.

Advise the client about medications that cause constipation (e.g., antacids, bismuth, calcium channel blockers, clonidine, levodopa, iron, nonsteroidal anti-inflammatories, opiates, sucrasulfate [Shua-Haim, 1999]).

Discuss laxative abuse (see *Perceived Constipation*).

**R:** Certain fluids act as diuretics: caffeine-containing drinks and grapefruit juice (Weeks, Hubbartt, & Michaels, 2000).

**R:** Laxatives upset a bowel program because they cause much of the bowel to empty and can cause unscheduled bowel movements. With constant use, the colon loses tone and stool retention becomes difficult. Chronic use of bowel aids can lead to problems in stool consistency, which interferes with the scheduled bowel program and bowel management. Stool softeners may not be necessary if diet and fluid intake are adequate. Enemas lead to an overstretched bowel and loss of bowel tone, contributing to further constipation.

## Conduct Health Teaching, as Indicated

Explain the relationship of lifestyle changes to constipation.

Explain interventions that relieve symptoms.

Explain techniques to reduce the effects of stress and immobility.

**R:** Sedentary lifestyle, inadequate fluid intake, inadequate dietary fiber, and stress can contribute to constipation.

---

*May require a primary care provider's order.

## Pediatric Considerations

Discuss some causes of constipation in infants and children (e.g., underfeeding; high-protein, low-carbo-hydrate diet; lack of roughage; dehydration).

If bowel movements are infrequent with hard stools:

• With infants, add corn syrup to feeding or fruit to diet. Avoid apple juice or sauce.
• With children, add bran cereal, prune juice, and fruits and vegetables high in bulk.

Refer cases of persistent constipation for medical evaluation.

Explain to adolescents the effects of fluids, fiber, and exercise on bowel function.

**R:** Several factors contribute to constipation:

• Insufficient roughage or bulk
• A bland diet, too high in dairy products, which results in reduced colonic motility
• Insufficient oral intake of fluids, which allows the normal reabsorption of water from the colon to de-hydrate the feces too much, or dehydration stemming from any activities that increase fluid loss from sweating
• Fecal retention by the child
• Medications (e.g., narcotics or anticonvulsants)
• The child's emotional state

## Maternal Considerations

Explain the risks of constipation in pregnancy and postpartum:

• Decreased gastric motility
• Prolonged intestinal time
• Pressure of enlarging uterus
• Distended abdominal muscles (post)
• Relaxation of intestines (post)

Explain aggravating factors for hemorrhoid development (straining at defecation, constipation, prolonged standing, wearing constrictive clothing).

If woman has a history of constipation, discuss use of bulk-producing laxatives to soften bowels postdelivery.

Assess abdomen (bowel sounds, distention, presence of flatus).

Assess for hemorrhoids and perineal swelling.

Provide relief of rectal or perineal pain.

Instruct the client to take sitz baths and use cool, astringent compresses for hemorrhoids.

**R:** Explaining the causes of constipation during pregnancy and the postpartum period can increase par-ticipation in behaviors that decrease or prevent constipation.

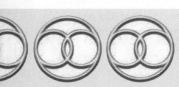

# CONSTIPATION

## ❱ Related to Effects of Immobility on Peristalsis

**NOC**
Bowel Elimination, Hydration, Mobility Level

## ➤ Goal

The client will report improved bowel movements every 2 to 3 days.

### *Indicators:*

• Describe components for effective bowel movements.
• Explain rationale for lifestyle change(s).

**NIC**

Activity Therapy,
Bowel Management,
Constipation:
Impaction
Management Fluid
Management, Health
Education, Nutrition
Management

# ➤ Interventions

## Assess Causative Factors of Immobility

| | |
|---|---|
| Musculoskeletal | Minimal activity |
|   (e.g., fractures, hip replacement) | Trauma (e.g., burns, head injury) |
| Chronic or acute illness | Inappropriate coping mechanisms |
| Physical handicap | Psychosomatic illness |
| Bed rest | Surgery |
| Degenerative joint changes (arthritis) | |

**R:** The specific cause of immobility should be addressed with interventions.

## Eliminate or Reduce Contributing Factors

### Fecal Impaction

If fecal impaction is suspected, perform a digital rectal examination (DRE).

Refer to procedure manual for removal of fecal impaction.

Make the client comfortable and allow rest.
The client may require temporary use of a stool softener or mild cathartic.*
Maintain accurate bowel elimination record.

### Severe Constipation

On the first day, insert a glycerin suppository, wait, and then have the client attempt a bowel movement
  through intermittent straining efforts.
If ineffective, on the second day, insert a glycerin suppository and follow the same routine.
If no results, on the third day, request a prescription for a suppository, which if not effective should be
  followed by an enema.*
To aid in stimulation of reflex emptying, a suppository may be followed in 20 to 30 min by digital
  stimulation of the anal sphincter.
Return to the first-day routine and follow until the pattern is established (may be every 2 to 3 days).

**R:** Manual removal of fecal impaction and the use of suppositories are necessary before a bowel routine
  can begin to establish daily effective habits.

## Conduct Health Teaching, as Indicated

Explain interventions to prevent (e.g., diet, exercise) versus those to treat constipation.
Refer to *Constipation* for additional interventions and rationales.

---

*May require a primary care provider's order.

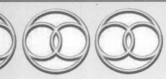

# PERCEIVED CONSTIPATION

## DEFINITION

The state in which an individual self-prescribes the daily use of laxatives, enemas, and/or suppositories to ensure a daily bowel movement

## DEFINING CHARACTERISTICS*

Expectation of a daily bowel movement with the resulting overuse of laxatives, enemas, and suppositories
Expected passage of stool at same time, every day

## RELATED FACTORS

### Pathophysiologic

*Related to faulty appraisal secondary to:*
Obsessive–compulsive disorders      Depression
Deterioration of the CNS

**Situational (Personal, Environmental)**
*Related to inaccurate information secondary to:*
Cultural beliefs                    Family beliefs                    Health beliefs

### ■■■■■ AUTHOR'S NOTE

Refer to Author's Note under *Constipation*.

### ■■■■■ KEY CONCEPTS

Refer to Key Concepts under *Constipation*.

## Focus Assessment Criteria

Refer to Focus Assessment Criteria under *Constipation*.

**NOC**
Bowel Elimination,
Health Beliefs:
Perceived Threat

## ➤ Goal

The client will verbalize acceptance of bowel movement every 1 to 3 days.

### Indicators:

- The client will not use laxatives regularly.
- The client will relate the causes of constipation.
- The client will describe the hazards of laxative use.
- The client will relate an intent to increase fiber, fluid, and exercise in daily life as instructed.

*Adapted from McLane, A. M. & McShane, R. E. (1986). Empirical validation of defining characteristics of constipation: A study of bowel elimination practices of healthy adults. In M. E. Hurley (Ed.). *Classification of nursing diagnosis: Proceedings of the sixth conference*. St. Louis: C. V. Mosby.

**NIC**
Bowel Management,
Health Education,
Behavior
Modification, Fluid
Management,
Nutrition
Management

## ➤ General Interventions

### Assess Causative or Contributing Factors

Cultural/familial belief          Faulty appraisal

### Explain That Bowel Movements Are Needed Every 2 to 3 Days, Not Daily

Be sensitive to the client's beliefs.
Be patient.
**R:** Lifetime habits and beliefs can be corrected with teaching.

## Explain the Hazards of Regular Laxative Use

They provide only temporary relief and can cause disorder.
They promote constipation by interfering with peristalsis.
They can interfere with absorption of vitamins A, D, E, and K.
They can cause diarrhea.
**R:** Regular laxative use can cause an inability to have a bowel movement without laxatives (DiPiro et al., 2001).

## If a Laxative Is Desired, Teach the Client How to Use Bulk-Forming Agents, such as Psyllium Seed or Bran

Start slowly with one half the recommended dose.
Increase the dose gradually over weeks.
**R:** The chronic laxative user must learn dietary modifications and use of bulk-forming laxatives, with the elimination of stimulant laxatives.
Refer to *Constipation* for Interventions to Promote Optimal Elimination and rationales.

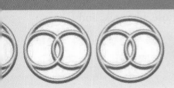

# CONTAMINATION: INDIVIDUAL

**Contamination: Individual**

**Risk for Contamination: Individual**

## DEFINITION

Exposure to environmental contaminants in doses sufficient to cause adverse health effects

## DEFINING CHARACTERISTICS

Defining characteristics are dependent on the causative agent. Causative agents include pesticides, chemicals, biologics, waste, radiation, and pollution.

## Pesticide Exposure Effects

### Pulmonary

Anaphylactic reaction, asthma, irritation to nose and throat, burning sensation in throat and chest, pulmonary edema, shortness of breath, pneumonia, upper airway irritation, dyspnea, bronchitis, pulmonary fibrosis, COPD, bronchiolitis, airway hyperreactivity, and damage to the mucous membranes of the respiratory tract

### Neurologic
Reye's-like syndrome, confusion, anxiety, seizures, decreased level of consciousness, coma, muscle fasciculation, skeletal muscle myotonia, peripheral neuropathy, pinpoint pupils, blurred vision, headache, dizziness, CNS excitation, depression, and paresthesia

### Gastrointestinal
Nausea, vomiting, diarrhea, and flu-like symptoms

### Dermatologic
Chloracne

### Cardiac
Cardiac dysrhythmia, tachycardia, bradycardia, conduction block, and hypotension

### Hepatic
Liver dysfunction

## Chemical Exposure Effects

### Pulmonary
Irritation of nose and throat, dyspnea, bronchitis, pulmonary edema, and cough

### Neurologic
Headache, ataxia, confusion, seizures, lethargy, unconsciousness, coma, lacrimation, ataxia, vertigo, mood changes, delirium, hallucinations, nystagmus, diplopia, psychosis, CNS depression, tremors, weakness, paralysis, memory changes, encephalopathy, hearing loss, Parkinson's-like syndrome, euphoria, narcosis, syncope, and hyperthermia

### Renal
Acetonuria and renal failure

### Gastrointestinal
Hyperglycemia, hypoglycemia, nausea, vomiting, ulceration of the GI tract, and metabolic acidosis

### Dermatologic
Dermatitis; irritation of the skin and mucous membranes; mucosal burns of eyes, nose, pharynx, and larynx; conjunctivitis; hyperpigmentation of skin and nails; and dermal burns

### Immunologic
Altered blood clotting and bone marrow depression

### Reproductive
Shortening of menstrual cycle

### Cardiac
Hypotension and chest pain

### Ophthalmic
Pupil changes, blurred vision, and severe eye pain

### Hepatic
Jaundice, hepatomegaly, hepatitis, corneal irritation, temporary or permanent blindness, and pancreatitis

## Biological Exposure Effects

### Bacteria
Anthrax (Bacillus anthracis): fever, chills, drenching sweats, profound fatigue, minimally productive cough, nausea and vomiting, and chest discomfort

Cholera (*Vibrio cholerae*): profuse watery diarrhea, vomiting, leg cramps, dehydration, and shock

Salmonella (*Salmonella*): fever, abdominal cramps, diarrhea (sometimes bloody), localized infection, and sepsis

E. coli (*Escherichia coli* 0157:H7): severe bloody diarrhea and abdominal cramps; mild or no fever

## Viruses

Smallpox (variola virus): high fever, head and body aches, vomiting, and skin rash with bumps and raised pustules that crust, scab, and form a pitted scar

Ebola hemorrhagic fever (Ebola filovirus): headache, fever, joint and muscle aches, sore throat, and weaknesses followed by diarrhea, vomiting, stomachache, rash, red eyes, and skin rash

Lassa fever (Lassa virus): fever, retrosternal pain, sore throat, back pain, cough, abdominal pain, vomiting, diarrhea, conjunctivitis, facial swelling, proteinuria, and mucosal bleeding

## Toxins

Ricin: respiratory distress, fever, cough, nausea, tightness in chest, heavy sweating, pulmonary edema, cyanosis, hypotension, respiratory failure, hallucinations, seizures, and blood in urine

Staphylococcal enterotoxin B: fever, headache, myalgia, malaise, diarrhea, sore throat, sinus congestion, rhinorrhea, hoarseness, and conjunctivitis

## Radiation Exposure Effects

Oncologic

Skin cancer, thyroid cancer, and leukemia

Immunologic

Impaired response to immunizations, bone marrow suppression, autoimmune diseases

Genetic

DNA mutations, teratogenic effect including smaller head or brain size, poorly formed eyes, abnormally slow growth, and mental retardation

Neurologic

CNS damage, malfunctions of the peripheral nervous system, neuroautoimmune changes, and disturbances in neuroendocrine control

Dermatologic

Burns, skin irritation, dryness, inflammation, erythema, dry or moist desquamation, itching, blistering, and ulceration

Systemic radiation poisoning

Nausea, fatigue, weakness, hair loss, changes in blood chemistries, hemorrhage, diminished organ function, and death

Ophthalmic

Cataracts, degeneration of the macula

Cardiovascular

Changes in cardiovascular control, irregular heartbeat, changes in the electrocardiogram, development of atherosclerosis, hypertension, and ischemia

Pulmonary

Disturbances in respiratory volume, increase in the number of allergic illnesses, atypical cells in the bronchial mucosa

Gastrointestinal

Pathologic changes in the digestive system, inflammation of the duodenum, spontaneously hyperplasic mucous membranes

## Waste Exposure Effects

Coliform bacteria: diarrhea and abdominal cramps

Giardia lamblia (protozoa): diarrhea, abdominal cramps, nausea, and weight loss

Cryptosporidium (protozoa): diarrhea, headache, abdominal cramps, nausea, vomiting, and low fever

Hepatitis A (enteric virus): lassitude, anorexia, weakness, nausea, fever, and jaundice

Helminths (parasitic worms): diarrhea, vomiting, gas, stomach pain, and loss of appetite

Fever

## Pollution Exposure Effects

Pulmonary: coughing, wheezing, labored breathing, pulmonary and nasal congestion, exacerbated allergies, asthma exacerbation, pain when breathing, and lung cancer

Cardiac: chest pain

Neurologic: headaches, developmental delay

Reproductive: reduced fertility

Ophthalmic: eye irritation

# RELATED FACTORS

## Pathophysiologic

Presence of bacteria, viruses, and toxins

Nutritional factors (obesity, vitamin, and mineral deficiencies)

Preexisting disease states

Gender (females have greater proportion of body fat, which increases the chance of accumulating more lipid-soluble toxins than men; pregnancy)

History of smoking

## Treatment-Related

Recent vaccinations

Insufficient or absent use of decontamination protocol

Inappropriate or no use of protective clothing

## Situational

Flooding, earthquakes, or other natural disasters

Sewer-line leaks

Industrial plant emissions; intentional or accidental discharge of contaminants by industries or businesses

Physical factors: climactic conditions such as temperature, wind; geographic area

Social factors: crowding, sanitation, poverty, personal and household hygiene practices, and lack of access to health care

Biological factors: presence of vectors (mosquitoes, ticks, rodents)

Bioterrorism

Occupation

Dietary practices

## Environmental

Contamination of aquifers by septic tanks

Intentional/accidental contamination of food and water supply

Concomitant or previous exposures

Exposure to heavy metals or chemicals, atmospheric pollutants, radiation, bioterrorism, and disaster

Use of environmental contaminants in the home (pesticides, chemicals, radon, tobacco smoke)

Playing in outdoor areas where environmental contaminants are used

Type of flooring surface

## Maturational

Developmental characteristics of children

Children younger than 5 years of age

Older adults

Gestational age during exposure

## ■■■■■■ KEY CONCEPTS

- Bioterrorism is the intentional use of microorganisms or toxins derived from living organisms to cause death or disease in humans, animals, or plants on which we depend (Ashford et al., 2003).
- The time period between exposure and the onset of symptoms may lag from hours to weeks. Nurses need to be familiar with the most likely agents to be used and their consequences (Veenema, 2006).
- Children are often exposed to toxicants through the agricultural and home use of pesticides or through the ingestion of pesticide residues on food or in water. Children are more vulnerable than adults to experiencing delayed effects. Some pesticides may interfere with physiologic processes of the child, including the immune, respiratory, and neurologic systems.

*(continued)*

■■■■■■ **KEY CONCEPTS** *Continued*

- The Environmental Protection Agency (EPA) completed development of a continual review process for pesticides. All pesticide registrations are to be reviewed every 15 years to ensure the protection of public health and the environment (EPA, 2006).
- Indoor pesticide residues can persist for weeks after use, leaving pregnant women at risk, especially in urban areas. In studies of pregnant women living in New York City, 70% to 80% tested positive for pesticide exposure during their pregnancy (Berkowitz et al., 2003).
- The amount and duration of radiation exposure affects the severity or type of health effect. Internal exposure occurs through ingestion of radioactive material (food/water contamination). External exposure occurs through direct contact with radioactive material. The primary health effect from chronic radiation exposure is cancer; however, additional effects include DNA mutations and teratogenic mutations. Acute health effects include burns and radiation poisoning. The symptoms of radiation poisoning vary with the level of exposure and include nausea, fatigue, changes in blood chemistries, hemorrhage, damage to the central nervous system, and eventual death. Children and fetuses are particularly susceptible to the effects of radiation exposure (EPA, 2004).
- Radon enters homes through soil and water. The radon gas decays into particles that get trapped in the lungs. The risk of radon-related lung cancer is particularly elevated for smokers. Although children have been reported to be at greater risk than adults for certain types of cancer from radiation, there are no conclusive data on whether children are at greater risk than adults from radon exposure (EPA, 2008).
- The Air Pollution and Respiratory Health Program tracks indoor and outdoor air quality and associated health effects. Of particular concern is the impact of wildfires, debris fires following natural disasters, carbon monoxide poisoning, and molds (www.cdc.gov/nceh/airpollution/about.htm).
- The World Health Organization (WHO) ranks indoor air pollution as the eighth most important risk factor when considering the global burden of disease. In developing countries, it is the most lethal killer after malnutrition, unsafe sex, and lack of water and sanitation, and is responsible for 1.6 million deaths a year due to pneumonia, chronic respiratory disease, and lung cancer (www.who.int/mediacentre/factsheets/ fs292/en/).
- Contamination of water and food occurs when microorganisms, bacteria, and viruses that live in soil and in the gastrointestinal tract of animals enter the water supply from the direct disposal of waste into streams or lakes or from runoff from wooded areas, pastures, septic tanks, and sewage plants into streams or groundwater.
- Contamination of drinking water sources by sewage can occur from raw sewage overflow, septic tanks, leaking sewer lines, land application of sludge, and partially treated wastewater. Water may also be contaminated by nitrates, metals, toxic materials, and salts (http://extoxnet.orst.edu/faqs/).
- Contamination events may occur as a result of accidents or intentional acts. Biological agents include bacteria, viruses, fungi, and other microorganisms and their associated toxins. They may adversely affect health in several ways ranging from mild, allergic reactions to serious medical conditions, even death. The organisms are widespread in the natural environment and are found in water, soil, plants, and animals (http://www.osha.gov/SLTC/biologicalagents/index.html).
- Exposure to biological agents occurs through direct contact with a hazardous substance, liquid (droplets or aerosols), inhalation of vapors or aerosols, and ingestion. Routes of transmission of infectious agents are contact, droplet, airborne, common vehicle, and vector borne (U.S. Army Medical Research Institute of Infectious Diseases, 2005).
- The mode of transmission of the specific agents will determine the category of isolation precaution used (standard, airborne, droplet, and contact isolation). Isolation precautions are used to reduce and prevent the spread of contamination and to protect health care workers from being exposed (Veenema, 2003).
- Hazardous waste is any waste (liquid, sludge, solid, or gas) that may pose a threat to human health or the environment due to its quantity or characteristics. Industrial and commercial plants and businesses (chemical, electroplating, auto manufacturers, lumber treating, dry cleaners, photo processing, petroleum refineries, and hospitals) generate hazardous waste. Households also produce hazardous waste (pesticides, cleaning agents, paint and solvents, fluorescent light bulbs) (http://www.epa.gov/osw/hazwaste.htm).
- Untreated sewage that ends up in recreational drinking water, in groundwater, and in basements after flooding adversely affects human health and the environment. Each year, swimming in water contaminated by sewage overflows causes 1.8 million to 3.5 million illnesses. Drinking contaminated water causes 500,000 illnesses yearly (http://www.nrdc.org/water/pollution/sewage.asp).

# Focus Assessment Criteria

## Assess for Defining Characteristics

### *Subjective Data*

#### Pesticides, Chemicals, Biologicals
Report of the following:

- Respiratory: difficulty breathing, cough, and flu symptoms
- Gastrointestinal: stomachache, diarrhea, cramping, nausea, and vomiting
- Neurologic: muscle weaknesses and joint and muscle aches
- Dermatologic: skin lesions and pustules
- Unusual liquids, sprays, or vapors at work or home

### *Objective Data*

Neurologic: hallucinations, confusion, seizures, decreased level of consciousness, pupil changes, and blurred vision
Pulmonary: labored breathing and cyanosis
Cardiac: cardiac dysrhythmia, hypertension, and hypotension
Integumentary: skin lesions (rash, pustules, scabs)

#### Radiation
Report of the following:

- History of exposure to radiation
- Pregnancies resulting in birth defects
- Weak muscles and paresthesia
- Skin irritation, itching, blistering, and burns
- Nausea, weakness, and fatigue
- Visual changes
- Irregular heart beat
- Labored breathing
- Abdominal pain and diarrhea

### *Objective Data*

Presence of skin cancer, thyroid cancer, and leukemia
Bone marrow suppression
Birth defects
Confusion, lethargy, and changes to level of consciousness
Skin irritation, burns, erythema, dry or moist desquamation, blistering, and ulceration
Symptoms of radiation sickness: weakness, hair loss, changes in blood chemistries, hemorrhage, and diminished organ function
Cataracts
Irregular heartbeat, changes in the electrocardiogram, and hypertension
Labored breathing and cough
Diarrhea

#### Waste

### *Subjective Data*

Report of the following:

Nausea, abdominal cramps, and anorexia

### *Objective Data*

Diarrhea, weight loss, jaundice, weakness, and fever

#### Pollution

### *Subjective Data*

Report of the following:

Difficulty breathing, lung irritation, chest pain, headaches, and eye irritation

*Objective Data*

Wheezing, shortness of breath, pulmonary or nasal congestion, and developmental delay

## Assess for Related Factors

Refer to Related Factors

**NOC**

Anxiety Level, Fear Level, Grief Resolution, Health Beliefs: Perceived Threat, Immunization Behavior, Infection Control, Knowledge: Health Resources, Personal Safety Behavior, Community Risk Control, Safe Home Environment

➤ **Goal**

Individual adverse health effects of contamination will be minimized.

**NIC**

Community Disaster Preparedness, Environmental Management, Anger Control Assistance, Anxiety Reduction, Grief Work Facilitation, Crisis Intervention, Counseling, Health Education, Health Screening, Immunization/ Vaccination Management, Infection Control, Resiliency Promotion, Risk Identification

➤ **Interventions**

### General Interventions

*Help Individuals Cope with Contamination Incident; Use Groups that Have Survived Terrorist Attacks as a Useful Resource for Victims*

Provide accurate information on risks involved, preventive measures, use of antibiotics, and vaccines.
Assist victims in dealing with feelings of fear, vulnerability, and grief.
Encourage victims to talk to others about their fears.
Assist victims in thinking positively and moving to the future.

**R:** Interventions aimed at supporting a client's coping help the client deal with feelings of fear, helplessness, and loss of control that are normal reactions in a crisis situation.

### Specific interventions

Employ skin decontamination with dermal exposures.
Clinical effects on body systems vary with exposure to specific agents. Monitor carefully and provide supportive care.
Employ appropriate isolation precautions: universal, airborne, droplet, and contact isolation.

**R:** Precautions prevent cross-contamination of other individuals.

*Monitor the Client for Therapeutic Effects, Side Effects, and Compliance with Postexposure Drug Therapy*

**R:** Drug therapy may extend over a long period of time and will require monitoring for compliance as well as for therapeutic and side effects.

*Decontamination Procedure*

Primary decontamination of exposed personnel is agent specific.

• Remove contaminated clothing.
• Use copious amounts of water and soap or diluted (0.5%) sodium hypochlorite.

For secondary decontamination from clothing or equipment of those exposed, use proper physical protection.

**R:** Victims may first require decontamination prior to entering the health facility to receive care in order to prevent the spread of contamination.

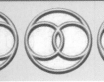

# RISK FOR CONTAMINATION: INDIVIDUAL

## DEFINITION

Accentuated risk of exposure to environmental contaminants in doses sufficient to cause adverse health effects

## RISK FACTORS

See Related Factors under *Contamination: Individual*.

### ■■■■■■ KEY CONCEPTS

See Key Concepts under *Contamination: Individual*.

## Focus Assessment Criteria

### Assess for Risk Factors

Refer to Related Factors under *Contamination: Individual*.

**NOC**
Community Risk Control, Community Health Status, Health Beliefs: Perceived Threat, Knowledge: Health Resources, Knowledge: Health Behavior

## ➤ Goal

The client will remain free of the adverse effects of contamination.

**NIC**
Community Disaster Preparedness Environmental Risk Protection, Environmental Management: Safety, Health Education, Health Screening, Immunization/ Vaccination Management, Risk Identification, Surveillance: Safety

## ➤ Interventions

### General Interventions

#### Provide Accurate Information About Risks Involved and Preventive Measures

Assist to deal with feelings of fear and vulnerability.
Encourage them to talk to others about their fears.

**R:** Interventions aimed at supporting a client's coping help the client deal with feelings of fear, helplessness, and loss of control that are normal reactions in a crisis situation.

### Specific Interventions

#### Conduct Surveillance for Environmental Contamination

Notify agencies authorized to protect the environment of contaminants in the area.
Assist individuals in relocating to safer environment.
Modify the environment to minimize risk.

**R:** Early detection of environmental contamination and modification of the environment will decrease the risk of actual contamination from occurring.

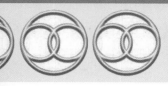

# INEFFECTIVE COPING

**Ineffective Coping**

Defensive Coping
Ineffective Denial
Related to Impaired Ability to Accept Consequences of Own Behavior as Evidenced by Lack of
 Acknowledgment of Substance Abuse/Dependency

## DEFINITION

A state in which a person experiences, or is at risk to experience, an inability to manage internal or environmental stressors adequately due to inadequate resources (physical, psychological, behavioral, and/or cognitive)

## DEFINING CHARACTERISTICS*

### Major (One Must Be Present)

Verbalization of inability to cope or ask for help
*or*
Inappropriate use of defense mechanisms
*or*
Inability to meet role expectations

### Minor (May Be Present)

| | |
|---|---|
| Chronic worry, anxiety | Frequent illnesses |
| Reported difficulty with life stressors | Verbal manipulation |
| Impaired social participation | Inability to meet basic needs |
| Destructive behavior toward self or others | Nonassertive response patterns |
| High incidence of accidents | Change in usual communication pattern |
| | Substance abuse |

### Related Factors

**Pathophysiologic**
***Related to chronicity of condition***
***Related to biochemical changes in brain secondary to:***

| | |
|---|---|
| Bipolar disorder | Personality disorder |
| Chemical dependency | Attention-deficient disorders |
| Schizophrenia | |

***Related to complex self-care regimens***
***Related to neurologic changes in brain secondary to:***

| | |
|---|---|
| Stroke | Multiple sclerosis |
| Alzheimer's disease | End-stage diseases |

***Related to changes in body integrity secondary to:***

| | |
|---|---|
| Loss of body part | Disfigurement secondary to trauma |

***Related to altered affect caused by changes secondary to:***

| | |
|---|---|
| Body chemistry | Intake of mood-altering substance |
| Tumor (brain) | Mental retardation |

---

*Adapted from Vincent, K. G. (1985). The validation of a nursing diagnosis. *Nursing Clinics of North America, 20*, 631–639.

Treatment-Related
*Related to separation from family and home (e.g., hospitalization, nursing home)*
*Related to disfigurement caused by surgery*
*Related to altered appearance from drugs, radiation, or other treatment*

## Situational (Personal, Environmental)

*Related to poor impulse control and frustration tolerance*
*Related to disturbed relationship with parent/caregiver*
*Related to disorganized family system*
*Related to ineffective problem-solving skills*
*Related to increased food consumption in response to stressors*
*Related to changes in physical environment secondary to:*

| | | |
|---|---|---|
| War | Poverty | Natural disaster |
| Homelessness | Relocation | Inadequate finances |
| Seasonal work | | |

*Related to disruption of emotional bonds secondary to:*

| | | |
|---|---|---|
| Death | Institutionalization | Relocation |
| Desertion | Separation or divorce | Orphanage/foster care |
| Jail | Educational institution | |

*Related to unsatisfactory support system*
*Related to sensory overload secondary to:*

| | |
|---|---|
| Factory environment | Urbanization: crowding, noise pollution, excessive activity |

*Related to inadequate psychological resources secondary to:*

| | |
|---|---|
| Poor self-esteem | Helplessness |
| Excessive negative beliefs about self | Lack of motivation to respond |
| Negative role modeling | |

*Related to culturally related conflicts with (specify):*

| | |
|---|---|
| Premarital sex | Abortion |

## Maturational

### Child/Adolescent
*Related to:*

| | | |
|---|---|---|
| Poor impulse control | Panic | Peer rejection |
| Parental substance abuse | Childhood trauma | Parental rejection |
| Inconsistent methods of discipline | Poor social skills | Fear of failure |
| | Repressed anxiety | |

### Adolescent
*Related to inadequate psychological resources to adapt to:*

| | | |
|---|---|---|
| Physical and emotional changes | Sexual awareness | Independence from family |
| Educational demands | Sexual relationships | Career choices |

### Young Adult
*Related to inadequate psychological resources to adapt to:*

| | | |
|---|---|---|
| Career choices | Marriage | Educational demands |
| Parenthood | Leaving home | |

### Middle Adult
*Related to inadequate psychological resources to adapt to:*

| | | |
|---|---|---|
| Physical signs of aging | Problems with relatives | Career pressures |
| Social status needs | Child-rearing problems | Aging parents |

### Older Adult
*Related to inadequate psychological resources to adapt to:*

| | | |
|---|---|---|
| Physical changes | Retirement | Changes in financial status |
| Response of others | Changes in residence | |

## ■■■■■ AUTHOR'S NOTE

*Ineffective Coping* describes a person experiencing difficulty adapting to stressful event(s). Ineffective Coping can be a recent, episodic problem or a chronic problem. Usual effective coping mechanisms may be inappropriate or ineffective, or the person may have a poor history of coping with stressors.

If the event is recent, *Ineffective Coping* may be a premature judgment. For example, a person may respond to overwhelming stress with a grief response such as denial, anger, or sadness, making a *Grieving* diagnosis appropriate.

*Impaired Adjustment* may be more useful than *Ineffective Coping* in the initial period after a stressful event. *Ineffective Coping* and its related diagnoses may be more applicable to prolonged or chronic coping problems, such as *Defensive Coping* for a person with a long-standing pattern of ineffective coping.

## ■■■■■ ERRORS IN DIAGNOSTIC STATEMENTS

1. *Ineffective Coping related to perceived effects of breast cancer on life goals, as evidenced by crying and refusal to talk*
   If the diagnosis of breast cancer was recent, the person's response of crying and refusal to talk would be normal. Thus, the proper diagnosis would be *Grieving related to perceived effects of breast cancer on life goals*. If this response was prolonged with no evidence of "moving on" (e.g., initiation of social activities), *Ineffective Coping* may be appropriate.
2. *Ineffective Coping related to reports of substance abuse*
   Substance abuse is a reportable or observable cue validating a diagnosis. If the person acknowledged the abuse and desires assistance, the diagnosis would be *Ineffective Coping related to inability to manage stressors without drugs*. If the substance abuse was observed but the person denied it or that it was a problem, the diagnosis would be *Ineffective Denial related to unknown etiology, as evidenced by lack of acknowledgment of drug dependency*.

## ■■■■■ KEY CONCEPTS

### Generic Considerations

- Lazarus (1985) defines coping as "constantly changing cognitive and behavioral efforts to manage specific external and/or internal demands that are taxing or exceeding the resources of the person."
- Expectations of mastery encourage maturation and persistence. Expectations of failure induce avoidance behaviors.
- Coping behaviors fall into two broad categories (Lazarus & Folkman, 1984):
  - *Problem-focused.* These are behaviors that attempt to improve the situation through change or taking action. Examples include making an appointment with one's boss to discuss a pay raise, creating and following a schedule for homework, and seeking help.
  - *Emotion-focused:* These are thoughts or actions that relieve emotional distress. They do not alter the situation, but they help the person feel better. Examples include playing basketball, denying anything is wrong, using food to relax, and joking.
- *Minimization* is when the person minimizes the seriousness of a problem. This may be useful as a way to provide needed time for appraisal, but it may become dysfunctional when it precludes appraisal.
- *Projection, displacement,* and *suppression of anger* are when a person attributes anger to or expresses it toward a less threatening person or thing. Doing so may reduce the threat enough to allow the person to deal with it. Distortion of reality and disturbance of relationships may result, which further compound the problem. Suppressed anger may result in stress-related physical symptoms.
- *Anticipatory preparation* is the mental rehearsal of possible consequences or outcomes of behavior or stressful situations. It provides an opportunity to develop perspective as well as to prepare for the worst. It becomes dysfunctional when it creates unmanageable stress, as, for example, in anticipatory mourning.
- *Attribution* is finding personal meaning in the problem. Examples include religious faith, individual belief, fate, and luck. Attribution may offer consolation but becomes maladaptive when a person loses all sense of self-responsibility.
- Addictive behavior is a habitual maladaptive way of coping with stress.

*(continued)*

■■■■■ ■ **KEY CONCEPTS** *Continued*

• According to Miller (2004), people "who have a rigid set or narrow range of coping skills are at more risk for impaired coping because different types of coping strategies are effective in different situations."
• Miller (1983) defines crisis as "the experiencing of an acute situation where one's repertoire of coping responses is inadequate in effecting a resolution of the stress." It usually represents a turning point and a reorganization of some important aspects of a person's psychological structure.
• An individual crisis can be described in four sequential stages: shock, defensive retreat, acknowledgment, and adaptation.
• Selye (1974) defined stress as the nonspecific response of the body to any demand. Responses to stress vary according to personal perceptions. Both positive and negative life events may initiate a stress response.
• Personal and environmental factors influence how a person copes with a disability. Research findings have supported that social support, self-concept, locus of control, and hardiness affect motivation and morale (Miller, 2009).
• Responses to illness, disability, or treatments are influenced by:
  • Attitude toward the event (e.g., punishment, weakness, challenge)
  • Developmental level or age
  • Extent the disability interferes with goal-directed activity and the significance of the goal
• Beck's cognitive theory of depression holds that those with depression process information negatively, even when there is evidence to the contrary. They filter information through a view of the world that is negatively toned, thus leading to thought distortions (Calarco & Krone, 1991). See Table II.4.
• People with chronic mental illness experience low self-esteem and a lack of confidence, competence, and sense of efficacy. Altered perceptions, attention deficits, cognitive confusion, and labile emotions interfere with decision-making, problem solving, and interpersonal relationships (Finkelman, 2000).
• Taylor et al. (2000) have found that the fight-or-flight response is more characteristic of males. Females respond to stress with the tend-and-befriend theory.
• The fight-or-flight response is mediated by catecholamines. The tend-and-befriend response is mediated by oxytocin and endogenous opioids.

## Pediatric Considerations

• Inborn traits, social support, and family coping affect a child's ability to cope (Hockenberry et al., 2009).
• As children mature, they develop and expand their coping strategies.
• In the United States, 3% to 5% of children have attention deficit–hyperactivity disorder (ADHD), with boys outnumbering girls nine to one (American Psychiatric Association [APA], 2000). The symptoms of this developmental disorder change over time. The diagnosis is made when symptoms of inattention or hyperactivity–impulsivity persist for at least 6 months and are maladaptive and inconsistent with developmental level (APA, 2000).

### TABLE II.4  REACTIVE VS. ENDOGENOUS DEPRESSION

| Element | Reactive Depression | Endogenous Depression |
|---|---|---|
| Precipitating event | Identifiable | Unclear |
| Family history | Unrelated | Familial tendency |
| Symptoms | Related to grief and anxiety; worse at night | Seemingly unrelated to events; worse in morning |
| Activity | Diminished motor and cognitive behavior | Agitated, restless |
| Emotion | Client feels sad | Alternates between sadness and manic gaiety |
| Cognitive abilities | May be slightly diminished | Retarded psychomotor performance |
| Orientation | Oriented and responsive to environment | May not be oriented or responsive |
| Treatment | Responds well to counseling and environmental change | May require somatic treatment in addition to counseling |

### Geriatric Considerations

- Miller (2009) identifies six major psychosocial challenges for older adults: (1) retirement, (2) death of friends, (3) chronic illness, (4) relocation of family, (5) disruption of household, and (6) stereotypes associated with the 65th birthday.
- Folkman, Lazarus, Pimley, and Novacek (1987) found that younger subjects reported more stress related to finances and work, whereas older subjects reported stress related to health, home maintenance, and social and environmental issues.
- Anticipation and perceived control over circumstances are predictors of the effects of stress on older adults (Willis, Thomas, Garry, & Goodwin, 1987).
- In older adults, coping is facilitated in those with higher incomes, occupational status, and feelings of self-efficacy. When significant life changes are necessary, however, higher occupational status and feelings of self-efficacy are liabilities, because these people hold an unrealistic view of what is controllable (Simons & West, 1984).
- No one life event has consistently negative effects on an older adult; rather, several events in a short period represent the greatest challenge (Miller, 2009).

### Transcultural Considerations

- Three major components of cultural systems influence responses to illness or chronic disease and a person's ability to make healthful changes in lifestyle: (1) family support systems, (2) coping behaviors, and (3) health beliefs and practices (Andrews & Boyle, 2007).
- In certain cultures, the family plays a critical role in all aspects of the client's life, including rejection or reinforcement of healthy lifestyle changes (Andrews & Boyle, 2007).
- Asian cultures emphasize maintaining harmony and respect. It is not unusual for an Asian client, who sees the nurse as an authority, to agree with all he or she suggests. Agreeing does not mean intended compliance, only good manners. This behavior is opposite to the assertive, questioning behavior emphasized in the dominant U.S. culture (Andrews & Boyle, 2007).
- Some cultures do not have a vocabulary for expressing emotional distress. There may be strong sanctions or taboos against complaining about one's fate.
- Some symptoms that Western medicine would interpret as mental illness are considered normal in other cultures. Visions, hexes, and hearing voices are acceptable in some U.S. subcultures: Appalachian, Asian, African American, Hispanic, and Native American (Flaskerud, 1984).
- East Indian Hindu Americans believe in internal and external forces of control. Uncontrolled psychological factors, such as anger, shame, and envy, make a person more susceptible to disease. They also believe external events or misfortune, such as the wrath of a disease goddess, malevolent spirits of dead ancestors, sins committed in previous lives, or jealous living relatives, cause illness. Hindus wear charms to ward off evil intentions.
- The Chinese culture views mental illness as shameful. Chinese families may wait until a relative's mental illness is unmanageable before seeking Western medicine.

## Focus Assessment Criteria

Ineffective coping can be manifested in various ways. A person or family may respond with a disturbance in another functional pattern (e.g., spirituality, parenting). The nurse should be aware of this and use assessment data to ascertain the dimensions affected.

### Subjective Data

### *Assess for Defining Characteristics*

**Physiologic Stress-Related Symptoms**
*Cardiovascular*

| | |
|---|---|
| Headache | Fainting (blackouts, spells) |
| Chest pain | Palpitations |
| Increased pulse | Increased blood pressure |

*Respiratory*

Shortness of breath     Increased rate and depth of breathing
Smoking history         Chest discomfort (pain, tightness, ache)

*Gastrointestinal*

Nausea               Change in stool
Vomiting             Change in appetite
Abdominal pain      Obesity/frequent weight changes

*Musculoskeletal*

Pain                 Weakness
Fatigue

*Genitourinary*

Menstrual changes    Urinary discomforts (pain, burning, urgency, hesitancy)
Sexual difficulty

*Dermatologic*

Itching              "Sweats"
Rash                Eczema

### Perception of Stressor

How have these stressors affected you?
How are the problems working out?

### Obtain History of Drinking Pattern from the Client or Significant Others (Kappas-Larson & Lathrop, 1993)

What was the date of the last drink?
How much was consumed on that day?
On how many days of the last 30 was alcohol consumed?
What was the average intake?
What was the most you drank?

### Determine the Attitude Toward Drinking by Asking CAGE Questions

Have you ever thought you should *C*ut down your drinking?
Have you ever been *A*nnoyed by criticism of your drinking?
Have you ever felt *G*uilty about your drinking?
Do you drink in the morning (i.e., *E*ye opener; Ewing, 1984)?

### Symptoms of Depression (Depression Guideline Panel, 1993)

Depressed mood most of day, nearly every day
Markedly diminished interest or pleasure in almost all activities most of the day, nearly every day
Significant weight loss/gain
Insomnia/hypersomnia
Psychomotor agitation/retardation
Fatigue (loss of energy)
Impaired concentration (indecisiveness)
Recurrent thoughts of death or suicide

### Coping–Self-Awareness (Finkelman, 2000)

What motivates you to get up in the morning?
If "1" is the worst your problem can be and "10" is your problem solved, where are you today?
What would it take to raise the number?
How would you know it was higher than a "6"?

## Assess for Related Factors

Current/recent stressors (number, type, duration)
Major life events and everyday stresses
Social—financial change, job pressure, marital/family conflicts, role changes, retirement, pregnancy, marriage, divorce, aging, school, and death
Psychological—anxiety, depression, low self-esteem, lack of interpersonal skills, and loneliness
Environmental—moving, hospitalization, loss of privacy, and sensory deprivation/overload

## Objective Data

### *Assess for Defining Characteristics*

**Appearance**

| | |
|---|---|
| Altered affect ("poker" face) | Poor grooming |
| Appropriate dress | Inappropriate dress |

**Behavior**

| | |
|---|---|
| Calm | Sudden mood swings |
| Hostile | Withdrawn |
| Tearful | |

**Cognitive Function**

| | |
|---|---|
| Impaired orientation to time, place, person | Impaired memory |
| Impaired concentration | Impaired judgment |
| Altered ability to solve problems | |

**Abusive Behaviors**

*To Self*

| | |
|---|---|
| Excessive smoking | Reckless driving |
| Excessive alcohol intake | Suicide attempts |
| Excessive food intake | Unsafe sexual practices |
| Drug abuse | |

*To Others*

| | |
|---|---|
| Does not care | Does not communicate |
| Is unwilling to listen | Imposes physical harm on family member |
| Unsafe sexual practices | (bruises, burns, broken bones) |
| Neglects needs of family members | |

*In Children, Attention Difficulties (Johnson, 1995)*

| | |
|---|---|
| Difficulty listening | Speech problems |
| Easily distracted | Reading problems |
| Difficulty concentrating | Oppositional, stubborn |
| Impulsivity | Low frustration |
| Poor judgment | Labile mood |
| Motor hyperactivity | |

For more information on Focus Assessment Criteria, visit http://thepoint.lww.com.

## Goals

**NOC**
Coping, Self-Esteem, Social Interaction Skills

The person will make decisions and follow through with appropriate actions to change provocative situations in the personal environment.

### *Indicators:*

- Verbalize feelings related to emotional state.
- Focus on the present.
- Identify response patterns and the consequences of resulting behavior.
- Identify personal strengths and accept support through the nursing relationship.

## General Interventions

**NIC**
Coping Enhancement, Counseling, Emotional Support, Active Listening, Assertiveness Training, Behavior Modification

### Assess Causative and Contributing Factors (Lyon, 2002)

Refer to Related Factors.

## Establish Rapport

Spend time with the client. Provide supportive companionship.

Avoid being overly cheerful and clichés such as, "Things will get better."

Convey honesty and empathy.

Offer support. Encourage expression of feelings. Let the client know you understand his or her feelings. Do not argue with expressions of worthlessness by saying things such as, "How can you say that? Look at all you accomplished in life."

Offer matter-of-fact appraisals. Be realistic.

Allow extra time for the person to respond.

**R:** The person with a chronic mental illness "must be helped to give up the role of being sick for that of being different" (Finkelman, 2000, p. 99).

## Assess Present Coping Status

Determine the onset of feelings and symptoms and their correlation with events and life changes.

Assess the ability to relate facts.

Listen carefully as the client speaks to collect facts; observe facial expressions, gestures, eye contact, body positioning, and tone and intensity of voice.

**R:** Behavior is disrupted when both needs and goals are threatened.

Determine the risk of the client's inflicting self-harm; intervene appropriately.

Assess for signs of potential suicide:

- History of previous attempts or threats (overt and covert)
- Changes in personality, behavior, sex life, appetite, and sleep habits
- Preparations for death (putting things in order, making a will, giving away personal possessions, acquiring a weapon)
- Sudden elevation in mood

See *Risk for Suicide* for additional information on suicide prevention.

## Assess Level of Depression

Refer depressed people to specialists.

**R:** Severely depressed or suicidal people need environmental controls, usually hospitalization.

## Assist the Client in Developing Appropriate Problem-Solving Strategies

Ask the client to describe previous encounters with conflict and how he or she resolved them.

Evaluate whether his or her stress response is "fight or flight" or "tend and befriend" (Taylor et al., 2008).

Encourage the client to evaluate his or her behavior:

"Did that work for you?" "How did it help?" "What did you learn from that experience?"

Discuss possible alternatives (i.e., talk over the problem with those involved, try to change the situation, or do nothing and accept the consequences).

Assist the client in identifying problems that he or she cannot control directly; help the client to practice stress-reducing activities for control (e.g., exercise, yoga).

Be supportive of functional coping behaviors.

"The way you handled this situation 2 years ago worked well then. Can you do it now?"

Give options; however, leave the decision-making to the client.

**R:** Cognitive interventions help the person regain control over his or her life. They include identifying automatic thoughts and replacing them with positive thoughts (Finkelman, 2000).

Mobilize the client to gradually increase activity:

- Identify activities that were previously gratifying but have been neglected: personal grooming or dress habits, shopping, hobbies, athletic endeavors, and arts and crafts.
- Encourage the client to include these activities in the daily routine for a set time span (e.g., "I will play the piano for 30 minutes every afternoon").

**R:** Depression is immobilizing and the client must make a conscious effort to fight it to recover.

Explore outlets that foster feelings of personal achievement and self-esteem:
• Make time for relaxing activities (e.g., dancing, exercising, sewing, woodworking).
• Find a helper to take over responsibilities occasionally (e.g., sitter).
• Learn to compartmentalize (do not carry problems around with you always; enjoy free time).
• Encourage longer vacations (not just a few days here and there).
• Provide opportunities to learn and use stress management techniques (e.g., jogging, yoga).

**R:** People with chronic mental illness experience low self-esteem and a lack of confidence, competence, and sense of efficacy. Altered perceptions, attention deficits, cognitive confusion, and labile emotions interfere with decision-making, problem solving, and interpersonal relationships (Finkelman, 2000).

Facilitate emotional support from others:
• Seek out people who share a common challenge: establish telephone contact, initiate friendships within the clinical setting, develop and institute educational and support groups.
• Establish a network of people who understand your situation.
• Decide who can best act as a support system (do not expect empathy from people who themselves are overwhelmed with their own problems).
• Make time to share personal feelings and concern with coworkers (encourage expression; frequently people who share the same circumstances help one another).
• Maintain a sense of humor.
• Allow tears.

**R:** Coping effectively requires successful maintenance of many tasks: self-concept, satisfying relationships with other, emotional balance, and stress.

Teach self-monitoring tools (Finkelman, 2000):
• Develop a daily schedule to monitor for signs of improvement or worsening.
• Discuss reasonable goals for present relationships.
• Write down what is done when in control, depressed, confused, angry, and happy.
• Identify activities tried, would like to try, or should do more.
• Create a warning sign checklist that indicates worsening and how to access help.

**R:** Self-monitoring can help the client learn how to observe symptoms and recognize when he or she needs more intensive help (Finkelman, 2000).

## Teach Problem-Solving Techniques

• *Goal setting* is consciously setting time limits on behaviors, which is useful when goals are attainable and manageable. It may become stress-inducing if unrealistic or short-sighted.
• *Information seeking* is learning about all aspects of a problem, which provides perspective and, in some cases, reinforces self-control.
• *Mastery* is learning new procedures or skills, which facilitates self-esteem and self-control (e.g., self-care of colostomies, insulin injection, or catheter care).

**R:** Goals should be realistic and attainable to promote self-esteem and reduce stress.

## Initiate Health Teaching and Referrals, as Indicated

Prepare for problems that may occur after discharge:
• Medications—schedule, cost, misuse, side effects
• Increased anxiety
• Sleep problems
• Eating problems—access, decreased appetite
• Inability to structure time
• Family/significant other conflicts
• Follow-up—forgetting, access, difficulty organizing time

**R:** For depression-related problems beyond the scope of nurse generalists, referrals to an appropriate professional (marriage counselor, psychiatric nurse therapist, psychologist, psychiatrist) will be needed.

Instruct the client in relaxation techniques; emphasize the importance of setting 15 to 20 min aside each day to practice relaxation:

1. Find a comfortable position in a chair or on the floor.
2. Close the eyes.
3. Keep noise to a minimum (only very soft music, if desired).
4. Concentrate on breathing slowly and deeply.
5. Feel the heaviness of all extremities.
6. If muscles are tense, tighten, then relax each one from toes to scalp.

Teach assertiveness skills.
Teach use of cognitive therapy techniques.

**R:** The techniques can effectively reduce stress, which is negatively affecting functioning.

## Pediatric Interventions

If attention disorders are present, explain their etiology and behavioral manifestations to child and caregivers.
Help the child to understand he or she is not "bad" or "dumb."
Establish target behaviors with the child and caregivers.
Avoid repetitive lecturing.

**R:** Interventions focus on helping the child develop self-control and self-respect.
**R:** Children with attention disorders are often very intelligent and do not need repetitive lectures.

Work with parents and teachers to learn more effective behavioral strategies to support success:

• Establish eye contact before giving instructions.
• Set firm, responsible limits.
• Avoid lectures; simply state rules.
• Maintain routines as much as possible.
• Attempt to keep a calm and simple environment.
• Reinforce appropriate behavior with a positive reinforcer (e.g., praise, hug).

**R:** Routine helps to reduce stress for caregivers and child.

Children with attention disorders cannot filter extraneous stimuli and therefore respond to everything, thus losing focus.
Assist the child in improving play with peers (Johnson, 1995):

• Start with short play periods.
• Use simple, concrete games.
• Begin with sympathetic siblings or family members.
• Initially, select a quieter and less demanding peer as playmate.
• Provide immediate and instant feedback (e.g., "I see you are being distracted"; "You are playing nicely").

**R:** Success with peers in play is critical for positive reinforcement and self-esteem.

Initiate health teaching and referrals as needed:

• Provide information about medication therapy if indicated.
• Consult with specialists as needed (e.g., psychological, learning specialists).

## Geriatric Interventions

Assess for risk factors for ineffective coping in older adults (Miller, 2009):

• Inadequate economic resources
• Immature developmental level
• Unanticipated stressful events

*(continued)*

**Geriatric
Interventions**
*Continued*

- Several major events in short period
- Unrealistic goals

**R:** Miller (2009) identifies the following as risk factors for increased stress and poor coping in older adults: diminished economic resources, immature developmental level, unanticipated events, several daily hassles at the same time, several major life events in a short period, high social status, and high feelings of self-efficacy in situations that cannot change.

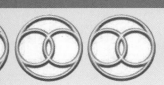

# DEFENSIVE COPING

## DEFINITION

The state in which a person repeatedly presents falsely positive self-evaluation as a defense against underlying perceived threats to positive self-regard

## DEFINING CHARACTERISTICS*

### Major (80%–100%)

Denial of obvious problems/weaknesses
Rationalization of failures
Grandiosity

Projection of blame/responsibility
Hypersensitivity to slight criticism

### Minor (50% to 79%)

Superior attitude toward others
Hostile laughter or ridicule of others
Lack of follow-through or participation
   in treatment or therapy

Difficulty establishing/maintaining relationships
Difficulty testing perceptions against reality

## RELATED FACTORS

See *Chronic Low Self-Esteem*, *Powerlessness*, and *Impaired Social Interaction*.

### ■■■■■ AUTHOR'S NOTE

In selecting this diagnosis, it is important to consider the potentially related diagnoses of *Chronic Low Self-Esteem*, *Powerlessness*, and *Impaired Social Interaction*. They may express how the person established, or why he or she maintains, the defensive pattern.

   *Defensive Coping* is defined by the person's dysfunction and inability to cope over time. It is reinforced if the nurse can establish a correlation between exacerbations and identified stressors. When a defensive pattern is a barrier to effective relationships, *Defensive Coping* is a useful diagnosis.

---

* Source: Norris, J. & Kunes-Connell, M. (1987). Self-esteem disturbance: A clinical validation study. In A. McLane (Ed.). *Classification of nursing diagnoses: Proceedings of the seventh conference*. St. Louis: C. V. Mosby.

■ **KEY CONCEPTS**

- Defensive functioning is the ability to use defense mechanisms to protect the ego from overwhelming anxiety. If defensive mechanisms are overused, they become ineffective or ego-defeating (Mohr, 2007).
- See Key Concepts under *Ineffective Coping*.

**NOC**
Acceptance: Health Status, Coping, Self-Esteem, Social Interaction Skills

➤ **Goal**

The client will report or demonstrate less defensive behavior.

*Indicators:*

- Identify defensive responses.
- Establish realistic goals in concert with caregivers.
- Work effectively toward achieving these goals.

**NIC**
Coping Enhancement, Emotional Support, Self-Awareness Enhancement, Environment Management, Presence, Active Listening

➤ **General Interventions**

### Reduce Demands on the Client If Stress Levels Increase

*Environmental*—Modify the level of or remove environmental stimuli (e.g., noise, activity).
*Interpersonal*—Decrease (or limit) contacts with others (e.g., visitors, other clients, staff) as required.
*Task*—Clearly articulate minimal expectations for activities. Decrease or increase as tolerated.
*Therapeutic*—Structure interactions with staff so the client knows to whom he or she is to talk, when, for how long, and on what topics.
*Strategic*—Identify stressors placing demands on the client's coping resources; develop plans to deal with them. The general goal is to freeze, reduce, or eliminate stress; more specifically, it is to target and deal with those stressors most exacerbating the defensive pattern.
**R:** Increased stress increases defensive coping (Mohr, 2007).

### Establish a Therapeutic Relationship

Maintain a neutral, matter-of-fact tone with a consistent positive regard. Ensure that all staff relate in a consistent fashion, with consistent expectations.

Focus on simple, here-and-now, goal-directed topics when encountering the client's defenses.

Encourage the client to express goals, and then establish agreement with the client in at least one or two areas. (Note that "reflecting-in" statements, such as, "It sounds like you are saying 'x'" *can* produce declarative statements from the client such as, "No, I'm saying '–x,'" which can then be agreed with.)

Do not react to, defend, or dwell on the client's negative projections or displacements; also do not challenge distortions or unrealistic/grandiose self-expressions. Try instead to shift to more neutral, positive, or goal-directed topics.

Disengage or allow the client to disengage from disagreement.

Avoid directive statements. Encourage client-initiated activities.

Avoid control issues; attempt to present positive options to the client, which allows a measure of choice.

Avoid evaluative statements (negative *or* positive). Encourage the client to evaluate self-progress.

To limit maladaptive behaviors, identify for the client those actions that compromise the achievement of established goals.

To promote learning from the client's own actions (i.e., "natural consequences"), identify those actions that have interfered with the achievement of established goals.

Reinforce more adaptive coping patterns (e.g., sublimation, formal problem solving, rationalization) that assist the person in achieving established goals.

Evaluate interactions, progress, and approach with other team members to ensure consistency within the treatment milieu.

**R:** If an ego-support role can be established, it is then possible for the client to begin to learn new, more effective coping strategies. Active stressors continue to elicit and reinforce the established defensive pattern, however, so this effort can be limited by the degree to which the client remains stressed or threatened.

**Promote Dialogue to Decrease the Need to Defend and Permit a More Direct Addressing of Underlying, Related Factors (see *Chronic Low Self-Esteem*)**

Validate the client's reluctance to trust in the beginning. Over time, reinforce the consistency of your statements, responses, and actions. Give special attention to your meeting of (reasonable) requests or your following through with plans and agreements.

Engage the client in diversional, non–goal-directed, noncompetitive activities (e.g., relaxation therapy, games, outings).

Encourage self-expression of neutral themes, positive reminiscences, and so forth.

Encourage other means for self-expression (e.g., writing, art) if verbal interaction is difficult or if this is an area of personal strength.

Listen passively to *some* grandiose or negative self-expression to reinforce your positive regard. If this does not lead to more positive self-expression or activity, then such listening may prove counterproductive.

Establish an ego-support role for yourself by assisting the client in reviewing and examining his interactive patterns with others.

**R:** Interventions should help put the client at ease and focus on self-evaluation (Mohr, 2007).

**R:** Diversional, supportive interactions must be balanced with goal-directed/problem-focused interactions according to the client's tolerance.

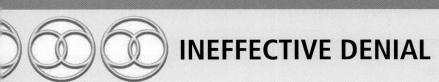

# INEFFECTIVE DENIAL

## DEFINITION

The state in which a person minimizes or disavows symptoms, choices, or a situation to the detriment of his health

## DEFINING CHARACTERISTICS*

### Major (Must Be Present)

Delays seeking or refuses health care attention to the detriment of health
Does not perceive personal relevance of symptoms or danger

### Minor (May Be Present)

Uses home remedies (self-treatment) to relieve symptoms
Does not admit fear of death or invalidism
Minimizes symptoms
Displaces the source of symptoms to other areas of the body
Cannot admit the effects of the disease on life pattern
Makes dismissive gestures or comments when speaking of distressing events
Displaces the fear of effects of the condition
Displays inappropriate affect

---

*Source: Lynch, C. S. & Phillips, M. W. (1989). Nursing diagnosis: Ineffective denial. In R. M. Carroll-Johnson (ed.). *Classification of nursing diagnosis: Proceedings of the eighth conference*. Philadelphia: J. B. Lippincott

# RELATED FACTORS

## Pathophysiologic

*Related to inability to tolerate consciously the consequences of (any chronic or terminal illness) secondary to:*

| | |
|---|---|
| HIV infection | AIDS |
| Cancer | Progressive debilitating disorders (e.g., multiple sclerosis, myasthenia gravis) |

## Treatment-Related

*Related to prolonged treatment with no positive results*

## Situational/Psychological

*Related to inability to tolerate consciously the consequences of:*

| | |
|---|---|
| Loss of a job | Negative self-concept, inadequacy, guilt, loneliness, despair, |
| Financial crisis | sense of failure |
| Smoking | Obesity |
| Loss of spouse/significant other | Domestic abuse |

*Related to physical and emotional dependence on (Varcarolis, 2006):*

| | |
|---|---|
| Alcohol | Cocaine, crack |
| Stimulants | Opiates |
| Cannabis | Barbituates/sedatives |
| Hallucinogens | |

*Related to long-term self-destructive patterns of behavior and lifestyle (Varcarolis, 2006)*
*Related to feelings of increased anxiety/stress, need to escape personal problems, anger, and frustration*
*Related to feelings of omnipotence*
*Related to culturally permissive attitudes toward alcohol/drug use*

## Biologic/Genetic

*Related to family history of alcoholism*

### ■■■■■■ AUTHOR'S NOTE

*Ineffective Denial* differs from denial in response to loss. Denial in response to illness or loss is necessary and beneficial to maintain psychological equilibrium. *Ineffective Denial* is not beneficial when the person will not participate in regimens to improve health or the situation (e.g., denies substance abuse). If the cause is not known, *Ineffective Denial related to unknown etiology* can be used, such as *Ineffective Denial related to unknown etiology as evidenced by repetitive refusal to admit barbiturate use is a problem.*

### ■■■■■■ ERRORS IN DIAGNOSTIC STATEMENTS

See *Ineffective Coping*.

### ■■■■■■ KEY CONCEPTS

- Denial is a set of dynamic processes that protect the person from threats to self-esteem. It is common in the grieving process.
- When action is essential to change a threatening or damaging situation, denial is maladaptive; however, when no action is needed or when the outcome cannot be changed, denial can be positive and can help reduce stress (Lazarus, 1985).
- A strong, intact denial system interferes with the person's realistic perceptions of the consequences (e.g., loss, violence, substance abuse; Boyd, 2005; Tweed, 1989).

*(continued)*

██ ██ ██ ██ ██ **KEY CONCEPTS** *Continued*

- Denial can take several forms:

  Denial of relevance to the person     Denial of immediacy of the threat

  Denial of responsibility     Denial that threat is anxiety-provoking

  Denial of threatening information     Denial of any information

- Denial is a major response in people with addictions. It is the inability to accept one's loss of control over the addictive behavior or severity of the associated consequences (Boyd, 2005).

## Focus Assessment Criteria

See *Ineffective Coping* for general assessment.

If substance abuse is suspected:

## Subjective Data

### Assess for Defining Characteristics

The client will:

- Deny that alcohol/drug use is problematic
- Justify the use of alcohol/drugs
- Blame others for the use of alcohol/drugs

## Objective Data

The person will demonstrate interference in:

### Occupational Functioning

| | |
|---|---|
| Absenteeism | Daytime fatigue |
| Frequent unexplained brief absences | Failed assignments |
| Elaborate excuses | Loss of job |

### Social Functioning

| | |
|---|---|
| Mood swings | Isolation (avoidance of others) |
| Arguments with mate/friends | Violence while intoxicated |
| Traffic accidents/citations | |

### Legal Difficulties

### Physical Functioning

*Alcohol Abuse*

| | |
|---|---|
| Blackout | Liver dysfunction |
| Memory impairment | Gout symptoms |
| Lower extremity paresthesias | Anemia |
| Malnutrition | Gastritis/gastric ulcers |
| Pancreatitis | Cardiomyopathy |

Withdrawal symptoms (e.g., tremors, nausea, vomiting, increased blood pressure and pulse, sleep disturbances, disorientation, hallucinations, agitation, seizures)

*Opiate Abuse*

| | |
|---|---|
| Drowsiness | Impaired memory |
| Slurred speech | Slowed motor movements |
| Pupillary constriction | Malnutrition |
| Skin infections | Respiratory depression |
| Liver disease | Constipation |
| Low testosterone levels | Respiratory infections |
| Gastric ulcers | Decreased response to pain |

Withdrawal symptoms (e.g., tearing, runny nose, gooseflesh, yawning, dilated pupils, mild hypertension, tachycardia, nausea, vomiting, restlessness, abdominal cramps, joint pain)

### Amphetamine and Cocaine Abuse

| | |
|---|---|
| Hyperactivity | Increased alertness |
| Paranoia | |
| Skin infections | Decreased appetite/weight loss |
| Cerebrovascular accident | Increased heart rate |
| Hallucinations | Dilated pupils |
| Cardiac dysrhythmias | Chills |
| Seizures | Nausea and vomiting |
| Respiratory depression | Hepatitis |

### Hallucinogen Abuse

| | |
|---|---|
| Increased heart rate | Tremors |
| Sweating | Incoordination |
| Hallucinations | Blurred vision |
| Flashbacks | |

### Cannabis Abuse

| | |
|---|---|
| Dry mouth | Increased appetite |
| Increased heart rate | Impaired lung structure |
| Conjunctival infection | Sinusitis |

### Barbiturate/Sedative–Hypnotic Abuse

| | |
|---|---|
| Drowsiness | Endocarditis |
| Impaired memory | Pneumonia |
| Cellulitis | Respiratory depression |
| Hepatitis | Signs of intoxication and withdrawal |

For more information on Focus Assessment Criteria, visit http://thepoint.lww.com.

## Goal

**NOC**
Acceptance: Health Status, Anxiety Self- Control, Fear Self-Control, Health Beliefs: Perceived Threat

The client will use alternative coping mechanism instead of denial.

### Indicators:

- Acknowledge the source of anxiety or stress.
- Use problem-focused coping skills.

## General Interventions

**NIC**
Teaching: Disease Process, Anxiety Reduction, Counseling, Active Listening

### Initiate a Therapeutic Relationship

Assess effectiveness of denial.
Avoid confronting the client that he or she is using denial.
Approach the client directly, matter-of-factly, and nonjudgmentally.

**R:** Denial may be valuable in the early stages of coping, when resources are not sufficient to manage more problem-focused approaches (Lazarus, 1985).

## Encourage the Client to Share Perceptions of the Situation (e.g., Fears, Anxieties)

Focus on the feelings shared.
Use reflection to encourage more sharing.

**R:** As denial is reduced, interventions must focus on emerging strong feelings of anxiety and fear.

## When Appropriate, Help the Client with Problem Solving

Attempt to elicit from the client a description of the problem.

**R:** Partial, tentative, or minimal denial allows the client to use problem-focused coping skills while reducing distress (an emotion-focused coping skill; Lazarus, 1985).

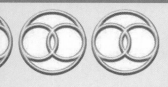

# INEFFECTIVE DENIAL

▶ **Related to Impaired Ability to Accept Consequences of Own Behavior as Evidenced by Lack of Acknowledgment of Substance Abuse/Dependency**

**NOC**
Anxiety Self-Control, Coping, Social Support, Substance Addiction Consequences, Knowledge: Substance Use Control, Knowledge: Disease Process

## Goals

The person will abstain from alcohol/drug use and state recognition of the need for continued treatment.

### Indicators:

- Acknowledge an alcohol/drug abuse problem.
- Explain the psychological and physiologic effects of alcohol or drug use.
- Abstain from alcohol/drug use.
- State recognition of the need for continued treatment.
- Express a sense of hope.
- Use alternative coping mechanisms to cope with stress.
- Have a plan for high-risk situations for relapse.

**NIC**
Coping Enhancement, Anxiety Reduction, Counseling, Mutual Goal Setting, Substance Use Treatment, Support System Enhancement, Support Group

## Interventions

### Assist the Client to Improve Self-Esteem

Be nonjudgmental.

Assist the client to gain an intellectual understanding that this is an illness, not a moral problem.

Provide opportunities to perform successfully; gradually increase responsibility.

Provide educational information about the progressive nature of substance abuse and its effects on the body and interpersonal relationships.

Explain why women are more affected by alcohol (see Key Concepts).

Refer to *Disturbed Self-Esteem* for further interventions.

**R:** The client probably has been reprimanded by many and is distrustful. The nurse's personal experiences with alcohol may increase or decrease empathy for the client.

**R:** Historically, alcoholics have been viewed as immoral and degenerate. Acknowledgment of alcoholism as a disease can increase the client's sense of trust.

### Provide Interventions Appropriate with the Phase of Addictive Behavior Change (Prochasaska, DiClemente, & Norcross, 1992)

#### Precontemplation Phase (Unaware of Problems Related to Addictive Behaviors)

Attempt to raise awareness of the problem and its consequences (e.g., relationships, job, finances).

Discuss the possibility of change.

Explore feelings about making changes.

**R:** If the person does not think the behavior change is important to improved health, he or she is unlikely to initiate the change (Bodenheimer, MacGregor, & Shariffi, 2005).

#### Contemplation Phase (Aware of Addiction-Related Problems and Considering Change, But Ambivalent)

Allow the client to express past successful attempts.

List the advantages and disadvantages for changing and continuing to use.

**R:** If the importance and/or the confidence is low, an action plan with specific behavior changes would not reflect true collaboration.

### *Preparation Phase (Intending to Take Action Within the Next Month or Unsuccessful in the Past Year)*

Initiate referrals to the next most acceptable, appropriate, and effective resource for the client.
Assist the client in making a specific, detailed plan for change and identify barriers.

**R:** The person's level of confidence will increase with success. Goals that are not easily achievable set the person up for failure (Bodenheimer, MacGregor, & Shariffi, 2005).

### *Action Phase (Overtly Involved in Behavioral Changes for at Least One Day)*

Reaffirm the decision to change.
Emphasize successful actions.
Help the client anticipate and prepare for situations that may challenge decisions.

**R:** The person's level of confidence will increase with success. Goals that are not easily achievable set the person up for failure (Bodenheimer, MacGregor, & Shariffi, 2005).

### *Maintenance Phase (Free of Addictive Behavior for More than 6 Months)*

Help the client identify strategies to prevent relapse.
Review reasons why change was made.
Review the benefits gained from change.

**R:** Compliance is increased with targeted interventions depending on the level of motivation present.

## Openly Discuss the Reality of Relapse; Emphasize That Relapse Does Not Mean Failure

After the relapse, help to identify triggers.
Plan an alternative action if triggers are present (e.g., call sponsor, take a walk).
Encourage discussions of relapse with other recovering substance abusers.
Emphasize a "one day at a time" philosophy.

**R:** Relapse must be addressed to increase motivation and to reduce abandoning all attempts to change behavior.

## Assist the Client to Identify and Alter Patterns of Substance Abuse

Explore situations in which the client is expected to use a substance (e.g., after work with friends).
Encourage avoidance of situations in which alcohol/drugs are being used.
Assist the client in replacing drinking/smoking buddies with nonusers. (Alcoholics Anonymous and Narcotics Anonymous are helpful. Each AA/NA group is unique; encourage the client to find a comfortable group for him or her.)
Assist the client in organizing and adhering to a daily routine.
Have the client chart (amount, time, situation) alcohol/drug use (useful with early-stage substance abusers resistant to treatment; Metzger, 1988).

**R:** Alcohol and drug abuse is reinforced by the drug itself (e.g., feelings of being high, increased congeniality, gaining attention) or avoiding unpleasant situations. Treatment approaches must aim at removing identified reinforcers (Smith–DiJulio, 2006).

## Discuss Alternative Coping Strategies

Teach relaxation techniques and meditation. Encourage use when the client recognizes anxiety.
Teach thought-stopping techniques to use during thoughts about drinking/substance use. Instruct client to say vocally or subvocally, "STOP, STOP," and to replace that thought with a positive one. The client must practice the technique and may need assistance in identifying replacements.
Assist the client to anticipate stressful events (e.g., job, family, social situations) in which alcohol/drug use is expected; role-play alternative strategies and teach assertiveness skills.

Teach the client how to handle anger constructively.

**R:** A substance-dependent person sees the substance as a solution to every problem. He or she needs new problem-solving techniques (Smith-DiJulio, 2006).

## Assist the Client in Achieving Abstinence

Assist the client to set short-term goals (e.g., stopping one day at a time).
Assist the client in structured planning:

- Discard supplies.
- Break contact with dealers/users.
- Avoid high-risk places.
- Structure free time.
- Avoid large blocks of time without activities.
- Plan leisure activities not associated with alcohol/drug use.

Assist the client in recognizing stressors that lead to substance abuse (e.g., boredom, interpersonal situations).
Assist the client in evaluating the negative consequences of the behavior. Visualization may be helpful.
When the client denies alcohol/drug use, look for nonverbal clues to substantiate facts (e.g., deteriorating appearance, job performance, social skills).
After you have established a trusting relationship, confront the client's denial.
Discourage the client from trying to correct other problems (e.g., obesity, smoking) during this time.
Do not attempt to probe past history in early abstinence.

**R:** The purpose of the interventions is to assist the client in recognizing and affirming the negative relationship between denial and resulting adverse consequences (health or social; Smith-DiJulio, 2006).

## Initiate Health Teaching and Referral, as Indicated

Refer the client to AA, Alanon, or AlaTeen.
Refer the client to a treatment facility.
Teach the side effects of drug use.
Provide nutritional counseling.

**R:** Participation in a structured treatment program greatly increases the chance of successful recovery from alcoholism. Affording the client direct contact with an expert who can help promotes a sense of hope.

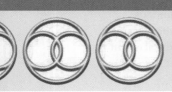

# DECISIONAL CONFLICT

## DEFINITION

The state in which a client/group experiences uncertainty about a course of action when the choice of options involves risk, loss, or challenge to personal life values

## DEFINING CHARACTERISTICS

### Major (80% to 100%)

Verbalized uncertainty about choices
Verbalization of undesired consequences of alternatives being considered

Vacillation between alternatives

Delayed decision making

## Minor (50% to 79%)

Verbalized feeling of distress while attempting a decision

Physical signs of distress or tension (e.g., increased heart rate, increased muscle tension, restlessness) whenever the decision comes within focus of attention

Questioning of personal values and beliefs while attempting to make a decision

# RELATED FACTORS

Many situations can contribute to decisional conflict, particularly those that involve complex medical interventions of great risk. Any decisional situation can precipitate conflict for a client; thus, the examples listed below are not exhaustive, but reflective of situations that may be problematic and possess factors that increase the difficulty.

## Treatment-Related

***Related to risks versus the benefits of (specify test, treatment):***

*Surgery*

| | | |
|---|---|---|
| Tumor removal | Orchiectomy | Mastectomy |
| Cosmetic surgery | Prostatectomy | Joint replacement |
| Amputation | Hysterectomy | Cataract removal |
| Transplant | Laminectomy | Cesarean section |

*Diagnostics*

| | | |
|---|---|---|
| Amniocentesis | X-rays | Ultrasound |

*Chemotherapy*

*Radiation*

*Dialysis*

*Mechanical ventilation*

*Enteral feedings*

*Intravenous hydration*

*Use of preterm labor medications*

*Participation in treatment study trials*

*HIV antiviral therapy*

## Situational

***Related to risks versus the benefits of:***

*Personal*

| | | |
|---|---|---|
| Marriage | Circumcision | Institutionalization (child, parent) |
| Breast vs. bottle feeding | Divorce | Contraception |
| Parenthood | Abortion | Nursing home placement |
| Sterilization | Artificial insemination | Foster home placement |
| In vitro fertilization | Adoption | Separation |
| Transport from rural facilities | | |

*Work/Task*

| | | |
|---|---|---|
| Career change | Business investments | Relocation |
| Professional ethics | | |

***Related to:***

| | |
|---|---|
| Lack of relevant information | Confusing information |

***Related to:***

Disagreement within support systems

Inexperience with decision-making

Unclear personal values/beliefs

Conflict with personal values/beliefs

Resignation

Family history of poor prognosis

Hospital paternalism—loss of control
Ethical dilemmas of:

| Quality of life | Termination of pregnancy |
| Cessation of life-support systems | Organ transplant |
| "Do not resuscitate" orders | Selective termination with multiple-gestation pregnancies |

## Maturational

### *Related to risks versus benefits of:*

*Adolescent*

| Peer pressure | College | Sexual activity |
| Alcohol/drug use | Whether to continue a relationship | Illegal/dangerous situations |
| Career choice | | |
| Use of birth control | | |

*Adult*

| Career change | Relocation | Retirement |

*Older Adult*

| Retirement | Nursing home placement |

## ■■■■■■ AUTHOR'S NOTE

The nurse has an important role in assisting clients and families with making decisions. Because nurses usually do not benefit financially from decisions made regarding treatments and transfers, they are in an ideal position to assist with decisions. Although, according to Davis (1989), "Nursing or medical expertise does not enable health care professionals to know the values of patients or what patients think is best for themselves," nursing expertise does enable nurses to facilitate systematic decision-making that considers all possible alternatives and possible outcomes, as well as individual beliefs and values. The focus is on assisting with logical decision-making, not on promoting a certain decision.

*When people are making a treatment decision of considerable risk, they do not necessarily experience conflict. In situations where the treatment option is "choosing life," individual perception may be one of submitting to fate and be relatively unconflicted. Because of this, nurses must be cautious in labeling patients with the nursing diagnosis of "Decisional Conflict" without sufficient validating cues (Soholt, 1990).*

## ■■■■■■ ERRORS IN DIAGNOSTIC STATEMENTS

1. *Decisional Conflict related to failure of physician to gain permission for mechanical ventilation from family*
   In such a situation, this statement represents an unprofessional and legally problematic approach. Failure of the physician to gain permission for mechanical ventilation would be a practice dilemma necessitating formal reporting to the appropriate parties. Should the family have evidence that the client did not desire this treatment (i.e., a living will), this situation would not be described as *Decisional Conflict*, because there is no uncertainty about a course of action. The nurse should further assess the family for responses fitting other nursing diagnoses, such as *Grieving*.
2. *Decisional Conflict related to uncertainty about choices*
   Uncertainty about choices validates *Decisional Conflict*; it is not a causative or contributing factor. If the client needed more information, the diagnosis would be *Decisional Conflict related to insufficient knowledge about choices and effects*.

## ■■■■■■ KEY CONCEPTS

### Generic Considerations

- An antecedent condition of decision-making is a problem. Problems exist when goals are to be attained and there is uncertainty about an appropriate solution. A problem suggests more than one alternative solution.
- Making a decision is a systematic process—a means, rather than an end. Decision-making is sequential—each step builds on the previous one. Optimal decision-making is more likely when done systematically, but it does not necessarily have to be a rigid, step-by-step process.

*(continued)*

■■■■■ **KEY CONCEPTS** *Continued*

- The logical steps of decision making are well identified in clinical practice. They can be summarized in the following steps:
  3. Defining the problem
  4. Listing the possible alternatives or options
  5. Identifying the probable outcomes of the various alternatives
  6. Evaluating the alternatives based on actual or potential threats to beliefs/values
  7. Making a decision
- People usually are not taught a systematic method for making a decision, so they rely frequently on past experiences and intuition. The intuitive mode of decision-making is characterized by interaction and association among ideas that seem to coexist simultaneously (Soholt, 1990).
- Soholt (1990) identified that the following factors may influence a client when making a health care treatment decision:
  - Reliance on the truth of medical advice
  - Submission to fate when the treatment option is "choosing life"
  - Consideration of values
  - The decision-making process is complicated when there is a need for a rapid decision. Making an intelligent decision during acute stress is difficult, if not impossible. The stress can be enormous if a sense of urgency compounds the decision.
- Jezewski (1993) reported that both intrapersonal and interpersonal conflict occurs when do-not-resuscitate decisions are being made. Intrapersonal conflict results from discord with individual values and life events. The most common interpersonal conflict arises between staff and family members and among family members.
- There are essentially three decision-making models in health care:
  1. *Paternalism*
     - Health care providers make all the decisions regarding client care.
     - Decisions are based on a perceived need to protect the client.
     - Locus of control is external to the client and significant others.
  2. *Consumerism*
     - Health care providers give the client and significant others only the information they request.
     - Decisions are based on the premise that the client knows best.
     - Locus of control is internal for the client and significant others.
  3. *Humanism/Advocacy*
     - Health care providers collaborate with the client and significant others to arrive at a decision.
     - Decisions are based on mutual respect for individual dignity and worth.
     - Locus of control is shared; all participants have an equal role in decision making.
- The most important right that a client possesses is the right of self-determination, or the right to make the ultimate decision concerning what will or will not be done to his or her body. Choice is facilitated when a client is free to make it.
- Not all clients desire the same degree of control over treatment decision-making. The need to play an active, collaborative, or passive role is very individualized and must be assessed carefully.
- Perception of the effect of a treatment on a client's life may be more important in his or her decision than considerations of the medical effectiveness.
- Value conflicts often lead to confusion, indecision, and inconsistency. Decision-making is more complicated when a client's goals conflict with those of significant others. People may decide against their values if the need to please others is greater than the need to please themselves.

One study found that older adults' end-of-life decisions were strongly related to their religiosity and values regarding preservation of life and quality of life (Cicirelli & MacLean, 2000). Those who preferred "to hasten death were less religious and place a higher value on quality of life" (Cicirelli & MacLean, 2000, p. 414). Most of the study group favored hastening death if terminally ill, regardless of religious beliefs (Cicirelli & MacLean, 2000).

### Pediatric Considerations

- In most cases, children do not make major decisions for themselves. A surrogate, usually a parent, must make the decision on the child's behalf.
- A child's ability to understand a situation and make a decision depends on age, developmental level, and past experience. Understanding, however, should not be confused with legal competence.
- As adolescents mature, their ability to analyze problems and make decisions increases.
- Researchers working with children should seek assent from children with a mental age of 7 years or older. Parents must give written, informed consent for the child to participate in the study (Hockenberry & Wilson, 2009).

### Geriatric Considerations

- Decisions are often made for, not with, older adults.
- Barriers to decision-making for older adults include dementia, depression, long-term passivity, and hearing or other communication problems (Miller, 2009).
- Reasons why decision-makers exclude older adults from involvement in decisions that profoundly affect their lives include beliefs that older adults are incompetent, not qualified, or not interested, and the desire to avoid discussion of sensitive topics (e.g., finances, relocation; Miller, 2009).
- Family members making a decision to place an older family member in a long-term facility found information from health care professionals inadequate. Friends who validated the situation were most helpful.

### Transcultural Considerations

- Fatalism is a belief that little can be done to change life events and the best response is submission and acceptance. Americans of Latin, Irish, Appalachian, Filipino, Puerto Rican, and Russian Orthodox origins frequently have this external focus of control (Giger & Davidhizar, 2007).
- Northern European and African Americans have been found to have both internal and external foci of control (Giger & Davidhizar, 2007).
- One study indicated that Mexican-American and Korean-American elders referred end-of-life decisions to family members (Blackhall et al., 1995).

## Focus Assessment Criteria

Decisional conflict is a subjective state that the nurse must validate with the client. The nurse should assess each client to determine his or her level of decision-making within the conflict situation. Some of the same cues may be seen in people with *Hopelessness*, *Powerlessness*, and *Spiritual Distress*.

### Subjective Data

#### *Assess for Defining Characteristics*

**Decision-Making Patterns**
"Tell me about the decision you need to make."
"How would you describe your usual method of making decisions?"
"How involved would you like to be in making the decision?"

**Perception of the Conflict**
"How do you feel when you think about the decision you have to make?"
"Has there been a change in your sleep patterns, appetite, or activity level?"

**Assess for Related Factors**
"Why is this a stressful decision for you?"
"What things make you uncomfortable about deciding?"
"In the past, how did you arrive at decisions that had a positive outcome?"
"What decisions have you made that you felt confident about?"

"When you make a decision, do you do it alone or do you like to involve other people? If so, whom do you consult for advice?"

## Objective Data

### Assess for Defining Characteristics

**Body Language**

| | |
|---|---|
| Posture (rigid) | Facial expression (annoyed, tense) |
| Hands (rigid, wringing) | Eye contact (darting) |

**Motor Activity**

| | |
|---|---|
| Immobile | Pacing |
| Increased | Agitation |

**Affect**

| | |
|---|---|
| Labile | Flat |
| Inappropriate | |

For more information on Focus Assessment Criteria, visit http://thepoint.lww.com.

---

**NOC**

Decision-Making, Information Processing, Participation: Health Care Decisions

## ➤ Goal

The client/group will make an informed choice.

### Indicators:

- Relate the advantages and disadvantages of choices.
- Share fears and concerns regarding choices and responses of others.
- Define what would be most helpful to support the decision-making process.

---

**NIC**

Decision-Making Support, Mutual Goal Setting, Learning Facilitation, Health System Guidance, Anticipatory Guidance, Patient Right Protection, Values Clarification, Anxiety Reduction

## ➤ General Interventions

### Assess Causative/Contributing Factors

Refer to Related Factors.

### Reduce or Eliminate Causative or Contributing Factors

#### Internal

**Lack of Experience With or Ineffective Decision-Making**

Review past decisions and what steps were taken to help the client decide.

Facilitate logical decision-making:

1. Assist the client in recognizing the problem and clearly identifying the needed decision.
2. Generate a list of all possible alternatives or options.
3. Help identify the probable outcomes of the various alternatives.
4. Aid in evaluating the alternatives based on actual or potential threats to beliefs/values.
5. Encourage the client to make a decision.

Encourage significant others to be involved in the entire decision-making process.

Suggest the client use significant others as a sounding board when considering alternatives.

Respect and support the role that the client desires in the decision, whether it is active, collaborative, or passive.

Be available to review the needed decision and the various alternatives.

Facilitate refocusing on the needed decision when the client experiences fragmented thinking during high anxiety.

Encourage the client to take time in deciding.

With adolescents, focus on the present—what will happen versus what will not. Help identify the important things because they do not have extensive past experiences on which to base decisions.

**R:** The role of nurses in situations of interpersonal/intrapersonal conflict reflects a culture broker framework incorporating advocacy, negotiation, mediation, and sensitivity to clients' and families' needs.

**R:** People who are strongly self-directed and have taken past responsibility for health practice are more likely to assume an active role in decision-making.

### Value Conflict (Also Refer to *Spiritual Distress*)

Use values clarification techniques to assist the client in reviewing the parts of his or her life that reflect his or her beliefs.

1. Help the client to identify his or her most prized and cherished activities.
2. Ask reflective statements that lead to further clarification.
3. Review past decisions in which the client needed to publicly affirm opinions and beliefs.
4. Evaluate the stands the client has taken on controversial subjects. Does he or she view them in black-and-white terms, or various shades of gray?
5. Identify values the client is proud of. Rank them in order of importance.

**R:** Every decision is based on consciously or unconsciously held beliefs, attitudes, and values.

Decisional conflict is greater when none of the alternatives is good. Assist the client in exploring personal values and relationships that may affect the decision. Explore obtaining a referral with the client's spiritual leader.

**R:** People are the experts about their life goals and values; therefore, health care professionals need to use a participatory decision-making model.

Encourage the client to base the decision on the most important values.
Support the decision—even if the decision conflicts with your own values.

**R:** Difficult decisions create stress and conflict because values and actions are not congruent. Conflict may lead to fear and anxiety that negatively affect decision-making. External resources become very important for the client in decisional conflict with a low level of self-confidence in making autonomous decisions.

### Fear of Outcome/Response of Others (also refer to *Fear*)

Provide clarification regarding potential outcomes and correct misconceptions.
Explore with the client what the risks of not deciding would be.
Encourage expression of feelings.
Promote self-worth.
Encourage the client to face fears.
Encourage the client to share fears with significant others.
Actively reassure the client that the decision is his or hers to make and that he or she has the right to do so.
Assist the client in recognizing that it is his or her life; if he or she is comfortable with the decision, others will respect the conviction.
Reassure the client that individuality is acceptable.

**R:** The roles of individual values greatly influence the resolution of ethical decision-making dilemmas. Decisional conflict becomes more intense when it involves a threat to status and self-esteem.

## *External*

### Insufficient or Inconsistent Information

Provide information comprehensively and sensitively.
Correct misinformation.
Give concise information that covers the major points when the decision must be made quickly.
Inform the client of his or her right to know.
Enable the client to determine the amount of information that he or she desires.
Encourage verbalization to determine the client's perception of choices.
Ensure that the client clearly understands what is involved in the decision and the various alternatives (i.e., informed choice).

**R:** Information that is valid, relevant, and understandable is required for informed decisions (Oxman, 2004).

Encourage the client to seek second professional opinions regarding health.
Collaborate with other health care members/significant others to determine appropriate timing for truthfulness.

**R:** Mastering content for effective decision-making requires time. Time allows a client to choose the option that provides the most benefit with the least risk.

### Controversy with Support System

Reassure the client that he or she does not have to give in to pressure from others, whether family, friends, or health professionals.
Advocate for the client's wishes if others attempt to undermine his or her ability to make the decision personally.
Identify leaders within the support system and provide information.
Advocate for the client if the family/significant others are excluding him or her from decision-making.
Recognize that the client may become ambivalent about "choosing" when putting the needs of the support system above his or her own.

**R:** Sims, Boland, & O'Neill (1992) interviewed families involved in caregiving and concluded that the process by which a client "frames" a problem is key to understanding decision-making. Values, feelings, and previous experiences significantly influenced caregivers' decision-making.

### Unsatisfactory Health Care Environment

Establish a trusting and meaningful relationship that promotes mutual understanding and caring.
Provide a quiet environment for thought and reduce sensory stimulation.
Allow uninterrupted periods with significant others.
Promote accepting, nonjudgmental attitudes.
Reduce the number of small decisions that the client must make to facilitate focusing on the decision in conflict.

**R:** The role of nurses in situations of interpersonal/intrapersonal conflict reflects a culture broker framework incorporating advocacy, negotiation, mediation, and sensitivity to clients' and families' needs.

## Explore End-of-Life Decisions

Explore with the client and family whether they have discussed and recorded their end-of-life decisions.
Describe the possible future dilemmas when these discussions are avoided.
Instruct client and family to provide directives in the following areas:

- Person to contact in emergency
- Person the client trusts most with personal decisions
- Decision to be kept alive if the client will be mentally incompetent or terminally ill
- Preference to die at home, hospital, or no preference
- Desire to sign a living will
- Decision regarding organ donation
- Funeral arrangements and burial or cremation
- Circumstances (if any) when information should be withheld from the client

Document these decisions and make two copies (retain one and give one to the person who is designated to be the decision-maker in an emergency).
Discuss the purpose of a living will. Provide information when requested. To obtain a copy of your state's living will, write to the Society for the Right to Die, 250 West 57th Street, New York, NY 10107.

**R:** Geary (1987) reported decision conflict for clients in critical care facing life-and-death decisions. Conflicts in client and family religious beliefs and personal values precipitated the difficult decision-making. Taylor (1993) also found conflict in discussions about death and related issues when the client's wishes differed from those of the family.

## Initiate Referrals as Needed

*Refer Families to Social Service for Assistance With Decisions Regarding Care of a Family Member*

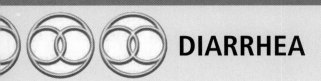

# DIARRHEA

## DEFINITION

The state in which a client experiences or is at risk of experiencing frequent passage of liquid stool or unformed stool

## DEFINING CHARACTERISTICS

### Major (Must Be Present)

Loose, liquid stools and/or
Increased frequency (more than three times a day)

### Minor (May Be Present)

| | |
|---|---|
| Urgency | Cramping/abdominal pain |
| Increased frequency of bowel sounds | Increased fluidity or volume of stools |

## RELATED FACTORS

### Pathophysiologic

*Related to malabsorption or inflammation secondary to:*

| | | |
|---|---|---|
| Colon cancer | Crohn's disease | Gastritis |
| Diverticulitis | Peptic ulcer | Spastic colon |
| Irritable bowel | Celiac disease (sprue) | Ulcerative colitis |

*Related to lactose deficiency, dumping syndrome*
*Related to increased peristalsis secondary to increased metabolic rate (hyperthyroidism)*
*Related to infectious process secondary to:*

| | | |
|---|---|---|
| Trichinosis | Shigellosis | Dysentery |
| Typhoid fever | Cholera | Infectious hepatitis |
| Malaria | Microsporidia | Cryptosporidium |

*Related to excessive secretion of fats in stool secondary to liver dysfunction*
*Related to inflammation and ulceration of gastrointestinal mucosa secondary to high levels of nitrogenous wastes (renal failure)*

### Treatment-Related

*Related to malabsorption or inflammation secondary to surgical intervention of the bowel*
*Related to side effects of (specify):*

| | | |
|---|---|---|
| Thyroid agents | Chemotherapy | Antacids |
| Analgesics | Laxatives | Cimetidine |
| Stool softeners | Iron sulfate | Antibiotics |

*Related to tube feedings*

## Situational (Personal, Environmental)

*Related to stress or anxiety*
*Related to irritating foods (fruits, bran cereals) or increase in caffeine consumption*
*Related to changes in water and food secondary to travel*
*Related to change in bacteria in water*
*Related to bacteria, virus, or parasite to which no immunity is present*

## Maturational

■■■■■■ **AUTHOR'S NOTE**

See *Constipation*.

■■■■■■ **ERRORS IN DIAGNOSTIC STATEMENTS**

1. *Diarrhea related to opportunistic enteric pathogens secondary to AIDS*
   Diarrhea, sometimes chronic, occurs in 60% to 90% of people with AIDS. Prolonged diarrhea represents a collaborative problem: *RC of Fluid/electrolyte/nutritional imbalances related to diarrhea*. Besides cotreating with a physician, the nurse treats other responses to chronic diarrhea (e.g., *Risk for Impaired Skin Integrity*, *Risk for Social Isolation*).

■■■■■■ **KEY CONCEPTS**

### Generic Considerations

- Acute infectious diarrhea is a yearly occurrence for most Americans and is associated with 1 million hospitalizations and about 600 deaths in the U.S. annually (Goodgame, 2006).
- Diarrhea can be acute or chronic. Causes of acute diarrhea include infection, drug reactions, heavy metal poisoning, fecal impaction, and dietary changes. Causes of chronic diarrhea include irritable bowel syndrome, lactose deficiency, colon cancer, inflammatory bowel disease, malabsorption disorders, alcohol, medication side effects, and laxatives.
- Drugs that can induce diarrhea are laxatives, antacids, certain antibiotics (e.g., tetracyclines), certain hypertensives (e.g., reserpine), cholinergics, certain antivirals, and select cardiac agents.
- Diarrhea may occur in 20% of clients receiving broad spectrum antibiotics (Goldman & Ausiello, 2004).
- Rapid transit of feces through the large intestine results in decreased water absorption and unformed, liquid stool. Ongoing diarrhea leads to dehydration and electrolyte imbalance.
- Hyperperistalsis is the motor response to intestinal irritants.
- Diarrhea may be related to an inflammatory process in which the intestinal mucosal wall becomes irritated, resulting in increased moisture content in the fecal masses.

 **Pediatric Considerations**

- Diarrhea in infants is always serious because of their small extracellular fluid reserve. Sudden losses result in circulatory collapse, renal failure, and irreversible acidosis and death (Pillitteri, 2009).
- Oral rehydration therapy is indicated for children with mild diarrhea and normal urine output.
- Signs of severe dehydration are sunken eyes; sunken fontanelles; loss of skin turgor; dry mucous membranes; rapid, thready pulse; cyanosis; rapid breathing; delayed capillary refill; and lethargy.
- Children who live in warm environments with poor sanitation and refrigeration or in crowded, substandard environments are at risk for eating contaminated food.

## Geriatric Considerations

- Clients over 80 years of age have a 3% fatality risk from antibiotic-associated diarrhea (Jabbar & Wright, 2003).
- Age-related loss of elasticity in abdominal muscles and muscle tone in the perineal floor and anal sphincter can cause diarrhea in some older people.
- Refer to the Key Concepts of *Deficient Fluid Volume* related to dehydration.

## Focus Assessment Criteria

Refer to *Constipation*.

**NOC**

Bowel Elimination, Electrolyte & Acid–Base Balance, Fluid Balance, Hydration, Symptom Control

## Goal

The client/parent will report less diarrhea.

### Indicators

- Describe contributing factors when known.
- Explain rationale for interventions.

**NIC**

Bowel Management, Diarrhea Management, Fluid/Electrolyte Management, Nutrition Management, Enteral Tube Feeding

## General Interventions

### Assess Causative Contributing Factors

| | |
|---|---|
| Tube feedings | Dietary indiscretions/contaminated foods |
| Dietetic foods | Food allergies |
| Foreign travel | Medications |

### Eliminate or Reduce Contributing Factors

### *Side Effects of Tube Feeding (Fuhrman, 1999)*

Control the infusion rate (depending on delivery set).
Administer smaller, more frequent feedings.
Change to continuous-drip tube feedings.
Administer more slowly if signs of gastrointestinal intolerance occur.
Control temperature.
If formula has been refrigerated, warm it in hot water to room temperature.
Dilute the strength of feeding temporarily.
Follow the standard procedure for administration of tube feeding.
Follow tube feeding with the specified amount of water to ensure hydration.
Be careful of contamination/spoilage (unused but opened formula should not be used after 24 h; keep unused portion refrigerated).

**R:** High-solute tube feedings may cause diarrhea if not followed by sufficient water.

### *Contaminated Foods (possible sources)*

| | | |
|---|---|---|
| Raw seafood | Shellfish | Excess milk consumption |
| Raw milk | Restaurants | Improperly cooked/stored food |

### *Dietetic Foods: Eliminate Foods Containing Large Amounts of the Hexitol, Sorbitol, and Mannitol that Are Used as Sugar Substitutes in Dietetic Foods, Candy, and Chewing Gum*

### Reduce Diarrhea

Discontinue solids.
Avoid milk (lactose) products, fat, whole grains, fried and spicy foods, and fresh fruits and vegetables.

Gradually add semisolids and solids (crackers, yogurt, rice, bananas, applesauce).

Avoid opiate-containing antidiarrheal drugs with acute infectious diarrhea (e.g., Lomotil, Imodium).

For mild or moderate diarrhea, advise the client to use bismuth subsalicylate (Pepto-Bismol), 30 mL, or 2 tablets every 12 to 1 h, up to 8 doses in 24 h. Avoid in clients with salicylate contraindications.

Instruct the client to seek medical care if blood in stool and fever greater than 101° F.

**R:** Foods with complex carbohydrates (e.g., rice, toast, cereal) facilitate fluid absorption into the intestinal mucosa (Bennett, 2000).

## Replace Fluids and Electrolytes

Increase oral intake to maintain a normal urine specific gravity (light yellow in color).

Encourage liquids (tea, water, apple juice, flat ginger ale).

When diarrhea is severe, use an over-the-counter oral rehydration solution.

Teach the client to monitor the color of urine to determine hydration needs. Increase fluids if urine color is amber or dark yellow.

Caution against the use of very hot or cold liquids.

See *Deficient Fluid Volume* for additional interventions.

**R:** Soft drinks (nondietetic or dietetic) and sport drinks are unsatisfactory for fluid replacement for moderate or severe fluid loss because of their sugar and salt content (Bennett, 2000).

## Conduct Health Teaching as Indicated

Explain the interventions required to prevent future episodes and effects of diarrhea on hydration.

Consult with primary health care provider for prophylactic use of bismuth subsalicylate (e.g., Pepto-Bismol) 30 to 60 mL or 2 tablets qid during travel and 2 days after return; or antimicrobials for prevention of traveler's diarrhea.

**R:** Bismuth subsalicylate (Pepto-Bismol) has been found safe in a variety of diarrheal illnesses and to have antibacterial activity as well. It is also effective in controlling symptoms of traveler's diarrhea (Bennett, 2000).

**R:** Opiate-containing antidiarrheals do not alter the natural cause of the disease and should not be used if invasive pathogens are the cause (Bennett, 2000).

Teach precautions to take when traveling to foreign lands:

- Avoid, salads, milk, fresh cheese, cold cuts, and salsa.
- Drink carbonated or bottled beverages; avoid ice.
- Peel fresh fruits and vegetables.
- Avoid foods not stored at proper temperature.

**R:** Microorganisms can multiply in foods not stored properly and/or washed with contaminated water. Ice can be contaminated.

Explain how to prevent food-borne diseases at home

- Refrigerate all perishable foods.
- Cook all food at high temperature or boil (212° F) for at least 15 min before serving.
- Avoid allowing food to stand at warm temperatures for several hours.
- Caution about foods at picnics in hot summer.

**R:** Improper storage can cause microorganisms to multiply.

- Thoroughly clean kitchen equipment after contact with perishable foods (e.g., meats, dairy, fish).

**R:** Failure to clean equipment used with raw foods can transfer microorganisms to cooked foods.

Explain that a diet primarily made up of dietetic foods containing sugar substitutes (hexitol, sorbitol, and mannitol) can cause diarrhea.

**R:** Sugar substitutes cause rapid small-bowel motility.

Teach the client to gently clean the anal area after bowel movements; lubricants (e.g., petroleum jelly) can protect skin.

**R:** The acidity of diarrheal stools can irritate the anal membranes.

Pediatric
Interventions

## Monitor Fluid and Electrolyte Losses

| | |
|---|---|
| Fluid volume lost | Urine color and output |
| Skin color | Mucous membranes |
| Capillary refill time | |

## Consult with Primary Care Provider If:

| | |
|---|---|
| Diarrhea persists. | Blood or mucus is in stools. |
| Child is lethargic. | Urine output is scanty. |
| Stools suddenly increase. | |
| Child is vomiting. | |

**R:** Children with signs of moderate or severe dehydration should be referred for possible parenteral therapy (Hockenberry & Wilson, 2009).

## Reduce Diarrhea

Avoid milk (lactose) products, fat, whole grains, and fresh fruits and vegetables.
Avoid high-carbohydrate fluids (e.g., soft drinks), gelatin, fruit juices, caffeinated drinks, and chicken or beef broths.

**R:** Fluids high in carbohydrates can worsen diarrhea because of their high osmolarity, which pulls more fluid into the bowel.

## Provide Oral Rehydration

Use oral rehydration solutions (e.g., Pedialyte, Lytren, Ricelyte, Resol [Larson, 2000]).
Determine fluid loss by body weight loss. If less than 5% of total weight is lost, 50 mL/kg of fluids will be needed during the next 3 to 6 hours (Pillitteri, 2009)
For more than a 5% weight loss, consult with the primary care provider for fluid replacement.
Fluids must be given to replace losses and continuing losses until diarrhea improves (Pillitteri, 2009).

**R:** Fluid replacement should be aggressive in infants and very young children.

## Reintroduce Food

Begin with bananas, rice, cereal, and crackers in small quantities.
Gradually return to regular diet (except milk products) after 36 to 48 h; after 3 to 5 days, gradually add milk products (half-strength skim milk to skim milk to half-strength milk (whole or 1%).
Gradually introduce formula (half-strength formula to full-strength formula).

**R:** Small quantities of nonirritating foods will decrease stimulation of the bowel.
**R:** Lactose-containing fluids or foods can worsen diarrhea in some children.

## For Breast-Fed Infants

Continue breast-feeding.
Use oral rehydration therapy if needed.

**R:** Breast-feeding should be continued with fluid replacement therapy. Reduced severity and duration of the illness is attributed to breast milk's low osmolality and antimicrobial effects (Brown, 1991).

## Protect Skin From Irritation with Non–Water-Soluble Cream (e.g., Petroleum Jelly)

**R:** Diarrheal stools are acidic and irritating.

*(continued)*

**Pediatric Interventions**
*Continued*

**Initiate Health Teaching as Needed**

**TEACH PARENTS SIGNS TO REPORT:**

Sunken eyes
Dry mucous membranes
Rapid, thready pulse
Rapid breathing
Lethargy
Diarrhea increases

**R:** Diarrhea in infants and small children can be serious because of their small extracellular fluid reserve. Early signs of hypovolemia needed to be reported to prevent circulatory collapse, renal failure, and irreversible acidosis and death (Pillitteri, 2009).

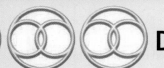

# DISUSE SYNDROME

## DEFINITION

The state in which a client is experiencing or at risk for deterioration of body systems or altered functioning as the result of prescribed or unavoidable musculoskeletal inactivity

## DEFINING CHARACTERISTICS

Presence of a cluster of actual or risk nursing diagnoses related to inactivity:

- *Risk for Impaired Skin Integrity*
- *Risk for Constipation*
- *Risk for Altered Respiratory Function*
- *Risk for Ineffective Peripheral Tissue Perfusion*
- *Risk for Infection*
- *Risk for Activity Intolerance*
- *Risk for Impaired Physical Mobility*
- *Risk for Injury*
- *Powerlessness*
- *Disturbed Body Image*

## RELATED FACTORS (OPTIONAL) (REFER TO AUTHOR'S NOTES)

### Pathophysiologic

*Related to:*
*Decreased Sensorium*
*Unconsciousness*
*Neuromuscular impairment secondary to:*

| | | |
|---|---|---|
| Multiple sclerosis | Muscular dystrophy | Parkinsonism |
| Partial/total paralysis | Guillain-Barré syndrome | Spinal cord injury |

*Musculoskeletal impairment secondary to:*

| | |
|---|---|
| Fractures | Rheumatic diseases |

*End-stage disease*

| | | |
|---|---|---|
| AIDS | Cardiac | Renal |

*Cancer*
*Psychiatric/Mental Health Disorders*
Major depression                          Catatonic state                          Severe phobias

## Treatment-Related

*Related to:*
Surgery (amputation, skeletal)          Mechanical ventilation
Traction/casts/splints                   Invasive vascular lines
Prescribed immobility

## Situational (Personal, Environmental)

*Related to:*
Depression                               Debilitated state
Fatigue                                  Pain

## Maturational

*Related to:*
*Newborn/Infant/Child/Adolescent*
Down syndrome                Risser-Turnbuckle jacket        Legg-Calvé-Perthes disease
Juvenile arthritis           Osteogenesis imperfecta          Autism
Cerebral palsy               Mental/physical disability       Spina bifida
*Older Adult*
Decreased motor agility      Muscle weakness                  Presenile dementia

## ■■■■■ AUTHOR'S NOTE

*Disuse Syndrome* describes a client experiencing or at risk for the adverse effects of immobility. Syndrome nursing diagnoses should not be written as "Risk for," because risk and actual diagnoses are clustered under them. *Disuse Syndrome* identifies vulnerability to certain complications and also altered functioning in a health pattern. As a syndrome diagnosis, its etiology or contributing factor is within the diagnostic label (*Disuse*); a "related to" statement is not necessary. As discussed in Chapter 2, a syndrome diagnosis comprises a cluster of predicted actual or risk nursing diagnoses because of the situation. Eleven risk or actual nursing diagnoses are clustered under *Disuse Syndrome* (see Defining Characteristics).

The nurse no longer needs to use separate diagnoses, such as *Risk for Ineffective Respiratory Function* or *Risk for Impaired Skin Integrity*, because they are incorporated into the syndrome category. If an immobile client manifests signs or symptoms of impaired skin integrity or another diagnosis, however, the nurse should use the specific diagnosis. He or she should continue to use *Disuse Syndrome* so other body systems do not deteriorate.

## ■■■■■ ERRORS IN DIAGNOSTIC STATEMENTS

1. *Disuse Syndrome related to reddened sacral area (3 cm)*
   A reddened sacral area is evidence of *Impaired Skin Integrity*. Thus, the nurse should use two diagnoses: *Impaired Skin Integrity related to effects of immobility, as evidenced by reddened sacral area (3 cm)* and *Disuse Syndrome*.

## ■■■■■ KEY CONCEPTS

### Generic Considerations
- "Immobility is inconsistent with human life." Mobility provides control over the environment; without mobility, the client is at the mercy of the environment (Christian, 1982).
- Prolonged immobility decreases motivation to learn and ability to retain new material. Affective changes are anxiety, fear, hostility, rapid mood shifts, and disrupted sleep patterns (Porth, 2006).

*(continued)*

■■■■■■ **KEY CONCEPTS** *Continued*

- Immobility restricts the ability to seek out sensory stimulation. Conversely, immobile people may be unable to remove themselves from a stressful or noisy environment (Christian, 1982).
- Musculoskeletal inactivity or immobility adversely affects all body systems (Table II.5).
- A muscle loses about 3% of its original strength each day it is immobilized.
- Prolonged immobility adversely affects psychological health, learning, socialization, and ability to cope. Table II.6 illustrates these effects.
- Possible long-term complications in people with traumatic spinal cord injury are pneumonia, atelectasis, autonomic dysreflexia, deep vein thrombosis, pulmonary embolism, pressure ulcers, fractures, and renal calculi (McKinley et al., 1999).

### TABLE II.5 ADVERSE EFFECTS OF IMMOBILITY ON BODY SYSTEMS

| System | Effect |
|---|---|
| Cardiac | Decreased myocardial performance<br>Decreased aerobic capacity<br>Decreased heart rate and stroke volume<br>Decreased oxygen uptake |
| Circulatory | Venous stasis<br>Orthostatic intolerance<br>Dependent edema<br>Decreased resting heart rate<br>Reduced venous return |
| Respiratory | Increased intravascular pressure<br>Stasis of secretions<br>Impaired cilia<br>Drying of sections of mucous membranes<br>Decreased chest expansion<br>Slower, more shallow respirations |
| Musculoskeletal | Muscle atrophy<br>Shortening of muscle fiber (contracture)<br>Decreased strength/tone (e.g., back)<br>Decreased bone density<br>Joint degeneration<br>Fibrosis of collagen fibers (joints) |
| Metabolic/Hemopoietic | Decreased nitrogen excretion<br>Decreased tissue heat conduction<br>Decreased glucose tolerance<br>Insulin resistance<br>Decreased red blood cells<br>Decreased phagocytosis<br>Hypercalcemia<br>Change in circadian release of hormones (e.g., insulin, epinephrine)<br>Anorexia<br>Decreased metabolic rate<br>Obesity<br>Elevated creatine levels |
| Gastrointestinal | Constipation |
| Genitourinary | Urinary stasis<br>Urinary calculi<br>Urinary retention<br>Inadequate gravitational force |
| Integumentary | Decreased capillary flow<br>Tissue acidosis to necrosis |
| Neurosensory | Reduced innervation of nerves<br>Decreased near vision<br>Increased auditory sensitivity |

Caswell, 1993; Porth, 2006; Tyler, 1984; Hockenberry & Wilson, 2009.

## TABLE II.6 PSYCHOSOCIAL EFFECTS OF IMMOBILITY

| | |
|---|---|
| Psychological | Increased tension <br> Negative change in self-concept <br> Fear, anger <br> Rapid mood changes <br> Depression <br> Hostility |
| Learning | Decreased motivation <br> Decreased ability to retain, transfer learning <br> Decreased attention span |
| Socialization | Change in roles <br> Social isolation |
| Growth and development | Dependency |

Porth, 2007; Zubek & McNeil, 1967.

## Pediatric Considerations

- Mobility is essential for physical growth and development and mastery of developmental tasks (Hockenberry & Wilson, 2009)). Restricted movement can thwart achievement of developmental tasks. Refer to Table II.8 in the diagnostic category *Delayed Growth and Development*.
- Physical activity serves as a means of communication and expression for children. Major psychological consequences of immobility include the following:
  - Sensory deprivation, leading to alterations in self-perception and environmental awareness
  - Isolation from peers
  - Feelings of helplessness, frustration, anxiety, and boredom (Wright, 1989; Hockenberry & Wilson 2009)
- Children who are restrained by casts, splints, or straps during the first 3 years of life have more difficulty with language than children with unrestricted activities (Hockenberry and Wilson, 2009).
- Children's responses to immobility may range from active protest to withdrawal or regression (Wright, 1989, Hockenberry & Wilson, 2009).

## Geriatric Considerations

- Aging affects muscle function because of progressive loss of muscle mass, strength, and endurance.
- Age-related changes in joint and connective tissues include impaired flexion and extension movements, decreased flexibility, and reduced cushioning protection for joints.
- Aging slows the response of the central nervous system thus increasing the risk of falls (Miller, 2009).
- After menopause, women experience an accelerated loss of trabecular and cortical bone of 9% to 10% per decade (Miller, 2009).
- Bed rest can cause an average vertical bone loss of 0.9% per week (Maher et al., 1998).

# Focus Assessment Criteria

## Subjective Data

### Assess for Related Factors

Neurologic

Musculoskeletal

Debilitating diseases

History of symptoms (complaints) of pain, muscle weakness, fatigue

Cardiovascular

Respiratory

History of recent trauma or surgery

## Objective Data

### *Assess for Defining Characteristics*

**Dominant Hand**

Right          Left          Ambidextrous

**Motor Function**

| | | | | |
|---|---|---|---|---|
| Right arm | Strong | Weak | Absent | Spastic |
| Left arm | Strong | Weak | Absent | Spastic |
| Right leg | Strong | Weak | Absent | Spastic |
| Left leg | Strong | Weak | Absent | Spastic |

**Mobility**

| | | | |
|---|---|---|---|
| Ability to turn self | Yes | No | Assistance needed (specify) |
| Ability to sit | Yes | No | Assistance needed (specify) |
| Ability to stand | Yes | No | Assistance needed (specify) |
| Ability to transfer | Yes | No | Assistance needed (specify) |
| Ability to ambulate | Yes | No | Assistance needed (specify) |

**Weight Bearing (Assess Both Right and Left Sides)**

Full                    Partial                    As tolerated                    Non–weight bearing

**Gait**

Stable                    Unstable

**Range of Motion of Shoulders, Elbows, Arms, Hips, and Legs**

Full                    Limited (specify)          None

### *Assess for Related Factors*

**Assistive Devices**

| | | |
|---|---|---|
| Crutches | Wheelchair | Cane |
| Prosthesis | Braces | Other |
| Walker | | |

**Restrictive Devices**

| | | |
|---|---|---|
| Cast or splint | Foley | Traction |
| Intravenous line | Braces | Monitor |
| Ventilator | Dialysis | Drain |

**Motivation (as Perceived by Nurse, Reported by the Client, or Both)**

Excellent                    Satisfactory                    Poor

For more information on Focus Assessment Criteria, visit http://thepoint.lww.com.

---

**NOC**

Endurance,
Immobility
Consequences:
Physiological,
Immobility
Consequences:
Psycho-Cognitive,
Mobility Level Joint
Movement

## ➤ Goal _____

The client will not experience complications of immobility.

### *Indicators*

- Intact skin/tissue integrity
- Maximum pulmonary function
- Maximum peripheral blood flow
- Full range of motion
- Bowel, bladder, and renal functioning within normal limits
- Uses of social contacts and activities when possible
- Explain rationale for treatments
- Make decisions regarding care when possible
- Share feelings regarding immobile state

**NIC**
Activity
Therapy, Energy
Management,
Mutual Goal
Settings, Exercise
Therapy, Fall
Prevention, Pressure
Ulcer Prevention,
Body Mechanics
Correction, Skin
Surveillance,
Positioning, Coping
Enhancement,
Decision-Making,
Support Therapeutic
Play

# ➤ General Interventions

## Identify Causative and Contributing Factors

Pain; refer also to *Impaired Comfort*.

Fatigue; refer also to *Fatigue*.

Decreased motivation; refer also to *Activity Intolerance*.

Depression; refer also to *Ineffective Coping*.

## Promote Optimal Respiratory Function

Vary the position of the bed, thus gradually changing the horizontal and vertical position of the thorax, unless contraindicated.

Assist client to reposition, turning frequently from side to side (hourly if possible).

Encourage deep breathing and controlled coughing exercises 5 times every hour.

Teach the client to use a blow bottle or incentive spirometer every hour when awake (with severe neuromuscular impairment, the client also may have to be awakened at night).

For a child, use colored water in the blow bottle; have him or her blow up balloons, soap bubbles, or cotton balls with straw.

Auscultate lung fields every 8 h; increase frequency if breath sounds are altered.

Encourage small, frequent feedings to prevent abdominal distention.

**R:** Bed rest decreases chest expansion and cilia activity and increases mucus retention, increasing risks of pneumonia.

## Maintain Usual Pattern of Bowel Elimination

Refer to *Constipation* for specific interventions.

## Prevent Pressure Ulcers

Use repositioning schedule that relieves vulnerable area most often (e.g., if vulnerable area is the back, the turning schedule would be left side to back, back to right side, right side to left side, and left side to back); post "turn clock" at bedside.

Turn the client or instruct him or her to turn or shift weight every 30 min to 2 h, depending on other causative factors and the ability of the skin to recover from pressure.

Frequency of turning schedule should increase if any reddened areas that appear do not disappear within 1 h after turning.

Position the client in normal or neutral position with body weight evenly distributed.

Keep the bed as flat as possible to reduce shearing forces; limit Fowler's position to only 30 min at a time.

Use foam blocks or pillows to provide a bridging effect to support the body above and below the high-risk or ulcerated area so affected area does not touch the bed surface; do not use foam donuts or inflatable rings because they increase the area of pressure.

Alternate or reduce the pressure on the skin surface with:

| | |
|---|---|
| Foam mattresses | Air mattresses |
| Air-fluidized beds | Vascular boots to suspend heels |

Use enough personnel to lift the client up in bed or a chair rather than pull or slide skin surfaces; use protectors to reduce friction on elbows and heels.

To reduce shearing forces, support feet with a footboard to prevent sliding.

Promote optimum circulation when the client is sitting.

Limit time spent sitting for the client at high risk for ulcer development.

Instruct the client to lift self, using chair arms every 10 min if possible, or assist the client to rise from the chair every 10 to 20 min, depending on risk factors.

Inspect areas at risk for ulcers with each position change:

| | |
|---|---|
| Ears | Occiput |
| Heels | Sacrum |
| Scrotum | Elbows |
| Trochanter | Ischia |
| Scapula | |

Observe for erythema and blanching and palpate for warmth and tissue sponginess with each position change.

Massage nonreddened, vulnerable areas gently with each position change.

**R:** Principles of pressure ulcer prevention include reducing or rotating pressure on soft tissue. If pressure exceeds intracapillary pressure (approximately 32 mm Hg), capillary occlusion causes tissue damage (Porth,2007).

Refer to *Impaired Skin Integrity* for additional interventions and rationale.

## Promote Factors that Improve Venous Blood Flow

Elevate extremity above the level of the heart (may be contraindicated in cases of severe cardiac or respiratory disease).

Ensure the client avoids standing or sitting with legs dependent for long periods.

Consider the use of below-knee elastic stockings to prevent venous stasis.

Reduce or remove external venous compression, which impedes venous flow.

Avoid pillows behind the knees or suggest a bed that is elevated at the knees.

Tell the client to avoid crossing the legs.

Remind the client to change positions, move extremities, or wiggle fingers and toes every hour.

Ensure the client avoids garters and tight elastic stockings above the knees.

Monitor legs for edema, tissue warmth, and redness daily.

**R:** Increased serum calcium resulting from bone destruction caused by lack of motion and weight bearing increases blood coagulability. This, in addition to circulatory stasis, makes the client vulnerable to thrombosis formation (Porth, 2007).

## Maintain Limb Mobility and Prevent Contractures (Maher et al., 1998)

### Increase Limb Mobility

Perform range-of-motion exercises (frequency to be determined by client's condition).

Support extremity with pillows to prevent or reduce swelling.

Encourage client to perform exercise regimens for specific joints as prescribed by physician or physical therapist.

### Position the Client in Alignment to Prevent Complications

Point toes and knees toward ceiling when the client is supine. Keep them flat when in a chair.

Use footboard.

Instruct the client to wiggle toes, point them up and downward, rotate their ankles inward and outward every hour.

**R:** These strategies prevent footdrop, a serious complication of immobility.

Avoid placing pillows under the knee; support calf instead.

Avoid prolonged periods of hip flexion (i.e., sitting position).

To position hips, place rolled towel lateral to the hip to prevent external rotation.

Keep arms abducted from the body with pillows.

Keep elbows in slight flexion.

Keep wrist neutral, with fingers slightly flexed and thumb abducted and slightly flexed.

Change position of shoulder joints during the day (e.g., abduction, adduction, range of circular motion).

**R:** Compression of nerves by casts, restraints, or improper positions can cause ischemia and nerve degeneration. Compression of the peroneal nerve results in footdrop; compression of the radial nerve results in wristdrop.

### Provide or Assist in Range-of-Motion Exercises Every 8 Hours

**R:** Joints without range of motion develop contractures in 3 to 7 days, because flexor muscles are stronger than extensor muscles.

## *Prevent Urinary Stasis and Calculi Formation*

Provide a daily fluid intake of 2000 mL or more (unless contraindicated); see *Deficient Fluid Volume* for specific interventions.

**R:** The peristaltic contractions of the ureters are insufficient when in a reclining position; thus, there is stasis of urine in the renal pelvis. Interventions to maintain hydration prevent hypercoagulability and clot formation and urine concentration of stone-forming elements (Porth, 2007).

Maintain urine pH below 6.0 (acidic) with acid ash foods (cereals, meats, poultry, fish, cranberry juice, apple juice).

Teach client to avoid foods high in calcium and oxalate (*very high):

- Milk, milk products, and cheese
- Bran cereals
- *Spinach, cranberries, plums, raspberries, and gooseberries
- Sardines, shrimp, oysters, legumes, and whole-grain rice

Asparagus, rhubarb, kale, Swiss chard, turnip greens, mustard greens, broccoli, and beet greens
Peanut butter, ripe olives, and chocolate

**R:** Dietary restrictions can reduce the formation of calcium renal calculi.

## Reduce and Monitor Bone Demineralization

Monitor for hypercalcemia.
Serum levels
Nausea/vomiting, polydipsia, polyuria, lethargy
Promote weight-bearing when possible (tilt-table).
Maintain vigorous hydration.
Adults: 2000 mL/day
Adolescents: 3000 to 4000 mL/day

**R:** The upright position improves bone strength, increases circulation, and prevents postural hypotension (Porth, 2007).

## Promote Sharing and a Sense of Well-Being

Encourage the client to share feelings and fears regarding restricted movement.
Encourage the client to wear own clothes, rather than pajamas, and unique adornments (e.g., baseball caps, colorful socks) to express individuality.

## *Reduce the Monotony of Immobility*

Vary daily routine when possible (e.g., give a bath in the afternoon so the client can watch a special show or talk with a visitor during the morning).

## *Include the Client in Planning Daily Schedule*

Allow client to make as many decisions as possible.
Make daily routine as normal as possible (e.g., have the client wear street clothes during the day, if feasible).
Encourage the client to make a schedule for visitors so everyone does not come at once or at inconvenient times.
Spend quality time with the client (i.e., not time that is task oriented; rather, sit down and talk).

## *Be Creative; Vary the Physical Environment and Daily Routine When Possible*

Update bulletin boards, change pictures on the walls, and move furniture within the room.
Maintain a pleasant, cheerful environment (e.g., plenty of light, flowers).
Place the client near a window, if possible.
Provide reading material (print or audio), radio, and television.

Plan an activity daily to give the client something to look forward to; always keep promises.

Discourage the use of television as the primary source of recreation unless it is highly desired.

Consider using a volunteer to spend time reading to the client or helping with an activity.

Encourage suggestions and new ideas (e.g., "Can you think of things you might like to do?").

**R:** Decreased activity reduces social contacts, reduces problem-solving ability, and decreases coping ability and orientation to time. Strategies are focused on increasing visual and auditory stimuli, engaging in decision-making and activities to reduce monotony.

### Pediatric Interventions

## Plan Appropriate Activities for Children

Provide an environment with accessible toys that suit the child's developmental age; ensure they are well within reach.

Encourage the family to bring in the child's favorite toys, including items from nature that will keep the "real world" alive (e.g., goldfish, leaves in fall).

## Use Play Therapy (Pillitteri, 2009)

As an energy release:

- Pounding pegs
- Cut wood with pretend saw
- Pound clay
- Punch a balloon

**R:** Play that releases energy substitutes for the usual hitting, running, and shouting of children.

### AS DRAMATIC PLAY:

- Provide health care equipment as dolls, doll beds, play stethoscopes, IV equipment, syringes, masks, and gowns.
- Allow the child to choose the objects.
- Allow the child opportunities to play and express their feelings.
- Use opportunities to ask the child questions.
- Reflect only what the child expresses.
- Do not criticize.

**R:** Dramatic play allows children to express feelings about illness and treatments.

### AS CREATIVE PLAY:

- Provide opportunities to draw pictures.
- Ask the child to describe the picture.

**R:** Picture drawing may express emotions that the child cannot verbally.

## Vary the Environment

## Transport Child Outside the Room as Much as Possible

**R:** Changes in the environment provide varied stimuli and increased social contact (Hockenberry & Wilson, 2009).

## Engage Child to Participate in Self-Care

Plan daily routine.

Select diet and snacks.

Select clothes (e.g., baseball cap).

## Allow Child to Wear Street Clothes as Soon as Possible

**R:** Increasing self-care activities and decision-making allows expressions of autonomy and individualization (Hockenberry & Wilson 2009).

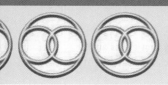

# DEFICIENT DIVERSIONAL ACTIVITY

## DEFINITION

The state in which a client or group experiences or is at risk of experiencing decreased stimulation from, or interest in, leisure activities

## DEFINING CHARACTERISTICS

### Major (Must Be Present)

Observed and/or statements of boredom/depression due to inactivity

### Minor (May Be Present)

Constant expression of:
Hostility unpleasant thoughts/feelings
Flat facial expression
Restlessness/fidgeting

Yawning or inattentiveness
Body language (shifts body away)
Weight loss or gain

## RELATED FACTORS

### Pathophysiologic

*Related to difficulty accessing or participating in usual activities secondary to:*
Communicable disease        Pain

### Situational (Personal, Environmental)

*Related to unsatisfactory social behaviors*
*Related to no peers or friends*
*Related to monotonous environment*
*Related to long-term hospitalization or confinement*
*Related to lack of motivation*
*Related to difficulty accessing or participating in usual activities secondary to:*
Excessive stressful work
Career changes (e.g., new job, retirement)
Immobility
Multiple role responsibilities

No time for leisure activities
Children leaving home ("empty nest")
Decreased sensory perception

### Maturational

**Infant/Child**
*Related to lack of appropriate stimulation toys/peers*

**Older Adult**
*Related to difficulty accessing or participating in usual activities secondary to:*
Sensory/motor deficits      Lack of peer group
Lack of transportation      Limited finances
Fear of crime               Confusion

## ◼◼◼◼◼ AUTHOR'S NOTE

Only the client can express a deficit in diversional activities based on his or her determination that types and amounts of activity are desired. Miller (2009) writes that activities associated with various roles affirm a client's self-concept.

To validate *Deficient Diversional Activity*, explore the etiology of factors amenable to nursing interventions, keeping your main focus on improving the quality of leisure activities. For a client with personality problems that hinder relationships and decrease social activities, *Impaired Social Interactions* is more valid. In this case, focus on helping the client identify behavior that imposes barriers to socialization.

## ◼◼◼◼◼ ERRORS IN DIAGNOSTIC STATEMENTS

1. *Deficient Diversional Activity related to boredom and reports of no leisure activities*
   Boredom and reports of no leisure activities are manifestations, not contributing factors, of the diagnosis. Thus, write the diagnosis as *Deficient Diversional Activity related to unknown etiology, as evidenced by reports of boredom and no leisure activities*.
2. *Deficient Diversional Activity related to inability to sustain meaningful relationships, as evidenced by "no one calls me to go out"*
   In this situation, delay making a formal diagnosis and collect more data to explore more specifically the meaning of "no one calls me to go out." Other diagnoses may be more applicable, such as *Impaired Social Interactions*, *Risk for Loneliness*, and *Ineffective Coping*.

## ◼◼◼◼◼ KEY CONCEPTS

### Generic Considerations

- All human beings need stimulation. In adults, lack of stimulation leads to boredom and depression. In infants and children, it causes "failure to thrive" and may stunt growth severely.
- The relationship between informal activity and life satisfaction is significant. The quality or type of activity is more important than the quantity (Rantz, 1991).
- Boredom paralyzes a client's productivity and causes a feeling of stagnation. It can be a major contributing factor to addictive behaviors (e.g., overeating, drug abuse, alcoholism, smoking).
- The bored client has introspective feelings of being oppressed and trapped, which give rise to conscious or unconscious anger or hostility.
- In recent years, pet therapy has been appreciated increasingly for ill and older clients.

 **Pediatric Considerations**

Children at special risk for deficient diversional activity include the following:
- Those who are bored
- Those who are immobilized
- Those who are hospitalized for long periods
- Those who are isolated to protect themselves or others
- Those who have diminished contact with family, friends, or both
- Age-appropriate activities should be provided to promote mental health and human development. Child life specialists—experts who are certified in early childhood, creative arts, or recreation therapies—provide psychosocial assessment and therapeutic activities in group contexts (they give advice on individual clients, playroom design, and activities). They are available in 98% of pediatric medical–surgical units, working with the multidisciplinary team to provide developmentally appropriate therapy and education to children and aiming to reduce the psychological trauma of illness (Rode, Capitulo, Fishman, & Holden, 1998). Refer to Table II.10 in *Delayed Growth and Development*.
- See also Key Concepts, Pediatric Considerations for *Anxiety and Delayed Growth and Development*.

**Geriatric Considerations**

- Cultural background strongly influences the older client's use of diversional activities because of the value placed on work versus leisure. Older, less educated, rural people tend to place less value on leisure activities.
- In Western society, retirement usually occurs between 62 and 70 years of age. About 80% of men and 90% of women older than 65 years are identified as retired. The lost work role can lead to depression, particularly if the client has engaged in no pre-retirement planning (Miller, 2007).
- Cultivating varied interests and activities throughout life enhances aging (Miller, 2007).
- A change in living arrangements or environment might subject the older adult to a diversional activity deficit. For example, an organic gardener with her own private yard moves to a senior high-rise apartment with no land for a garden. Or an older man who plays the drums moves in with his adult children who have neither the space for his drum set nor the inclination to listen to his drum solos.
- Social isolation resulting from the death of a spouse, lack of transportation, hearing impairment, limited finances, fear of crime, or other physical or psychological disabilities places the older client at risk for diversional activity deficit (Rantz, 1991).
- Volunteer activities provide diversion for 21% of people 55 to 64 years of age and 14% of those 65 years and older. Those 65 years and older volunteered an average of 8 h per week. Reasons cited for not volunteering included transportation difficulties, financial concerns, and age discrimination by some community organizations (Miller, 2007).

## Focus Assessment Criteria

### Subjective Data

#### *Assess for Defining Characteristics*

Perception of the client's current activity level: ask client to rate on a scale of 1 to 10 his or her satisfaction with current diversional activity level (1 = not at all satisfied and 10 = very satisfied).
Past activity patterns (type, frequency): work, leisure
Activities the client desires

### Objective Data

#### *Assess for Related Factors*

**Motivation**

| | |
|---|---|
| Interested | Withdrawn |
| Uninterested | Hostile |

**Any barriers to recreational activities**

**Physical status**

| | |
|---|---|
| Immobility | Pain |
| Altered level of consciousness | Sensory deficits (visual, auditory) |
| Fatigue | Equipment (traction, intravenous [IV] lines) |
| Altered hand mobility | Communicable disease/isolation |

**Psychological/cognitive status**

| | |
|---|---|
| Depression | Lack of knowledge |
| Embarrassment | Fear |

**Socioeconomic Status**

| | |
|---|---|
| Lack of support system | Financial limitations |
| Previous patterns of inactivity | Transportation difficulties |
| Language barrier | |

For more information on Focus Assessment Criteria, visit http://thepoint.lww.com.

**NOC**
Leisure Participation,
Social Involvement

## ➤ Goal

The client will rate that he or she is more satisfied with current activity level.

### Indicators

- Relate methods of coping with anger or depression resulting from boredom.
- Report participation in one enjoyable activity each day.

**NIC**
Recreation Therapy,
Socialization
Enhancement,
Self-Esteem
Enhancement,
Therapeutic Play

## ➤ General Interventions

### Assess Causative Factors

Refer to Related Factors.

### Reduce or Eliminate Causative Factors

#### Monotony

Refer to Interventions, "Reduce the monotony of immobility," under *Disuse Syndrome*.
Provide opportunities for reminiscence individually or in groups (e.g., past trips, hobbies).
Provide music therapy with audiocassette players with lightweight headphones. For group music therapy (Rantz, 1991) the following is recommended:

1. Introduce a topic.
2. Play related music.
3. Develop the topic with discussion.
4. Discuss responses.

**R:** Music therapy can be valuable in relieving boredom, sparking interest, and assisting clients to cope with social problems (Rantz, 1991).

Consider using holistic and complementary therapies (e.g., aromatherapy, pet therapy, therapeutic touch).
For pet therapy (Rantz, 1991), the following is recommended:

- Animals must be well groomed, healthy, and clean.
- Animals should be relaxed with strangers.
- Animals should eliminate before entering the facility.
- Sponsors always should ask the client if he or she likes the type of animal before approaching the client.

**R:** Complementary therapies serve to reduce stress, enhance coping, and foster well-being (Murray, Zentner, & Yakimo, 2009).

#### Lack of Motivation

Stimulate motivation by showing interest and encouraging sharing of feelings and experiences.
Explore fears and concerns about participating in activities.
Discuss likes and dislikes.
Encourage sharing of feelings of present and past experiences.
Spend time with the client purposefully talking about other topics (e.g., "I just got back from the shore. Have you ever gone there?").
Point out the need to "get oneself going" and try something new.
Help the client work through feelings of anger and grief:

- Allow him or her to express feelings.
- Take the time to be a good listener.
- See *Anxiety* for additional interventions.

**R:** Reminiscing, or spending time focusing on significant memories, can be satisfying and stimulating for the bored, ill, confined, or elderly client (Rantz, 1991).

Encourage the client to join a group of possible interest or help. (He or she may have to participate by way of intercom or special arrangement.)
Consider the use of music therapy or reminiscence therapy.

**R:** Membership in a group or a support group can boost self-esteem and self-worth, provide a sense of belonging, and encourage activities that the client otherwise may have avoided. Support groups can often assist those with stressful, costly, or time-consuming problems.

### Inability to Concentrate

Plan a simple daily routine with concrete activities (e.g., walking, drawing, folding linens).
If the client is anxious, suggest solitary, noncompetitive activities (e.g., puzzles, photography).

**R:** Tasks that match the client's concentration and interest can increase contact with reality, promote socialization, and improve self-esteem (Varcarolis, 2006).

## Identify Factors that Promote Activity and Socialization

### Encourage Socialization with Peers and All Age Groups (Frequently Very Young and Very Old Clients Mutually Benefit From Interactions)

### Acquire Assistance to Increase the Client's Ability to Travel

Arrange transportation to activities if necessary.
Acquire aids for safety (e.g., wheelchair for shopping, walker for ambulating in hallways).

### Increase the Client's Feelings of Productivity and Self-Worth

Encourage the client to use strengths to help others and self (e.g., assign him or her tasks to perform in a general project). Acknowledge these efforts (e.g., "Thank you for helping Mr. Jones with his dinner").
Encourage open communication; value the client's opinion ("Mr. Jones, what do you think about _____?").
Encourage the client to challenge himself or herself to learn a new skill or pursue a new interest.
Provide opportunities to interact with nature and animals.
**R:** Exposure to various stimuli can increase social interactions and decrease boredom (Barba et al., 2002).

## Refer to **Social Isolation** for Additional Interventions

**Pediatric Interventions**

Provide an environment with accessible toys that suit the child's developmental age; ensure that they are well within reach.
Keep toys in all waiting areas.
Encourage the family to bring in the child's favorite toys, including items from nature that will help to keep the "real world" alive (e.g., goldfish, leaves in fall).
Consult a child life specialist as indicated.
Refer to the Pediatric Intervention in the Nursing Diagnosis Disuse Syndrome on p. 233 for specifics on how to engage in therapeutic play.

**Geriatric Interventions**

**Explore Interests and the Feasibility of Trying a New Activity (e.g., Mobility)**

**Arrange for Someone to Accompany or Orient the Client During Initial Encounters**
**R:** Change, although a welcome relief from boredom, increases anxiety initially.

**Explore Possible Volunteer Opportunities (e.g., Red Cross, Hospitals)**

**Initiate Referrals, If Indicated**
Suggest joining the American Association of Retired Persons (AARP).
Write local health and welfare council or agencies.
Provide a list of associations with senior citizen activities:

| | | |
|---|---|---|
| YMCA | Sixty Plus Club | Churches |
| XYZ Group (Extra Years of Zest) | Golden Age Club | Young at Heart Club |
| SOS (Senior Outreach Services) | Encore Club | Leisure Hour Group |
| MORA (Men of Retirement Age) | Gray Panthers | |

*(continued)*

**Geriatric Interventions** *Continued*

**R:** Cognitive impairment, musculoskeletal impairment, pain, metabolic abnormality, or sensory deficit may force an older adult to consider modifying long-time leisure activities or developing new activities. For example, a client who likes to cook but has poor eyesight might obtain large-print cookbooks, have a friend write favorite recipes in bold print, or tape-record recipes (Rantz, 1991).

**R:** Change, although a welcome relief from boredom, increases anxiety initially.

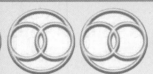

# AUTONOMIC DYSREFLEXIA

**Autonomic Dysreflexia**

**Risk for Autonomic Dysreflexia**

## DEFINITION

The state in which a client with a spinal cord injury at T6 or above experiences or is at risk to experience a potential life-threatening uninhibited sympathetic response of the nervous system to a noxious stimulus

## DEFINING CHARACTERISTICS

### Major (Must Be Present)

Client with spinal cord injury (T6 or above) with:

- Paroxysmal hypertension (sudden periodic elevated blood pressure in which systolic pressure is above 140 mm Hg and diastolic is above 90 mm Hg)
- Bradycardia or tachycardia (pulse rate less than 60 or more than 100 beats/min)
- Profuse diaphoresis (above the injury)
- Red splotches on skin (above the injury)
- Pallor (below the injury)
- Headache (a diffuse pain [dull to pounding] in different portions of the head and not confined to any nerve distribution area)
- Apprehension
- Dilated pupils

### Minor (May Be Present)

Chilling
Conjunctival congestion
Horner's syndrome (pupillary contraction; partial ptosis of the eyelid; enophthalmos; sometimes, loss of sweating over the affected side of the face)
Paresthesia
Response pilomotor (gooseflesh)
Blurred vision
Chest pain
Metallic taste in mouth
Nasal congestion
Penile erection and semen emission

# RELATED FACTORS

## Pathophysiologic

*Related to visceral stretching and irritation secondary to:*

### Gastrointestinal

| | | |
|---|---|---|
| Constipation | Fecal impaction | Acute abdominal condition |
| Gastric ulceration | Hemorrhoids | Anal fissure |

### Urologic

| | | |
|---|---|---|
| Distended bladder | Urinary calculi | Urinary tract infection |

### Cutaneous

| | | |
|---|---|---|
| Pressure ulcers | Burns | Sunburn |
| Insect bites | Ingrown toenails | Blister |

### Reproductive

| | | |
|---|---|---|
| Menstruation | Pregnancy or delivery | Vaginal infection |
| Epididymitis | Uterine contraction | Vaginal dilation |

*Related to fracture*
*Related to stimulation of skin (abdominal, thigh)*
*Related to spastic sphincter*
*Related to deep vein thrombosis*

## Treatment-Related

*Related to visceral stretching secondary to:*
Removal of fecal impaction
Clogged or nonpatent catheter
Visceral stretching and irritation secondary to surgical incision, enemas
Catheterization, enema

## Situational (Personal, Environmental)

*Related to lack of knowledge of prevention or treatment*
*Related to visceral stretching secondary to:*
Boosting
Sexual activity
Menstruation
Pregnancy or delivery
*Related to neural stimulation secondary to immersion in cold water*

■■■■■■ **AUTHOR'S NOTE**

*Autonomic Dysreflexia* represents a life-threatening situation that nurse-prescribed interventions can prevent or treat. Prevention involves teaching the client to reduce sympathetic nervous system stimulation and not using interventions that can cause such stimulation. Treatment focuses on reducing or eliminating noxious stimuli (e.g., fecal impaction, urinary retention). If nursing actions do not resolve symptoms, initiation of medical intervention is critical. When a client requires medical treatment for all or most episodes of dysreflexia, the situation is labeled a collaborative problem: *RC of Dysreflexia*.

■■■■■■ **ERRORS IN DIAGNOSTIC STATEMENTS**

1. *Autonomic Dysreflexia related to paroxysmal hypertension*
   Paroxysmal hypertension is a sign of dysreflexia, not a causative or contributing stimulus. The diagnosis should be restated: *Risk for Autonomic Dysreflexia related to possible reflex stimulation by visceral or cutaneous irritation, as evidenced by (specify)*.
   Clinically, *Risk for Autonomic Dysreflexia* is more descriptive than *Autonomic Dysreflexia*. The client usually is in a potential state, with associated nursing responsibilities of prevention, teaching, and early removal of stimulus.

▪▪▪▪▪▪ **KEY CONCEPTS**

- The autonomic nervous system (sympathetic and parasympathetic) is located in the cerebrum, hypothalamus, medulla, brain stem, and spinal cord. With spinal cord injury, activity below the injury is deprived of the controlling effects from the higher centers. The result is poorly controlled responses (Travers, 1999).
- Stimulation of sensory receptors below a spinal lesion results in sympathetic discharge, mediated by the spinothalamic tract and posterior columns. This reflex stimulation of the sympathetic nervous system causes spasms of the pelvic viscera and arterioles. These spasms cause vasoconstriction below the level of injury. Baroreceptors in the aortic arch and carotid sinus respond to the hypertensive state with superficial vasodilatation, flushing, diaphoresis, and piloerection (gooseflesh) above the level of the spinal lesion (Bennett, 2003).
- Vagal stimulation slows the heart rate, but, because the cord is severed, vagal impulses to dilate vessels are prohibited (Teasell, Arnold, & Delaney, 1996; Porth, 2006).
- Failure to reverse dysreflexia can result in status epilepticus, stroke, and death.
- Uncontrolled hypertension can cause systolic blood pressure to rise as high as 240 to 300 mm Hg (Porth, 2006).
- Three types of stimuli can initiate dysreflexia: visceral distention (e.g., full bladder or rectum), stimulation of pain receptors (e.g., diagnostic procedure, pressure), and visceral contractions (e.g., ejaculation, bladder spasms, uterine contractions; Porth, 2006).
- Eighty-five percent of all clients with quadriplegia experience autonomic dysreflexia some time after spinal shock (Kavchak-Keyes, 2000).

## Focus Assessment Criteria

### Subjective Data

#### *Assess for Defining Characteristics*

**Initial Symptoms**

| | |
|---|---|
| Headache (severe, sudden) | Pallor |
| Sweating (where?) | Dyspnea |
| Chills | Cold extremities |
| Metallic taste in mouth | Pilomotor skin erections (goose bumps) |
| Nasal congestion | Blurred vision |
| Numbness | Other _____ |

#### *Assess for Related Factors*

**History of Dysreflexia, Triggered by:**

| | |
|---|---|
| Bladder distention | Sexual activity |
| Bowel distention | Menstruation |
| Tactile stimulation | Diagnostic study |
| Skin lesion | Pressure |

**Knowledge of Dysreflexia**

| | |
|---|---|
| Cause | Medical treatment |
| Self-treatment | Prevention |

For more information on Focus Assessment Criteria, visit http://thepoint.lww.com.

**NOC**
Neurological Status, Neurological Status: Autonomic, Vital Signs Status

### ➤ Goal

The client/family will respond to early signs/symptoms.

#### *Indicators*

- State factors that cause dysreflexia.
- Describe the treatment for dysreflexia.
- Relate indications for emergency treatment.

**NIC**
Dysreflexia
Management, Vital
Signs Monitoring,
Emergency Care,
Medication
Administration

## ► General Interventions

### Assess for Causative or Contributing Factors

See Related Factors.

### Proceed as Follows If Signs of Dysreflexia Occur

1. Stand or sit the client up.
2. Lower the client's legs.
3. Loosen all the client's constrictive clothing or appliances.

**R:** An upright position and removal of hose increase venous pooling, reduce venous return, and decrease blood pressure (Kavchak-Keyes, 2000; Porth, 2006).

## Check for Distended Bladder

### If the Client Is Catheterized:

1. Check the catheter for kinks or compression.
2. Irrigate the catheter with only 30 mL of saline, very slowly.
3. Replace the catheter if it will not drain.

### If the Client Is Not Catheterized:

1. Insert the catheter using dibucaine hydrochloride ointment (Nupercainal).
2. Remove 500 mL, then clamp for 15 min.
3. Repeat the cycle until the bladder is drained.

**R:** Bladder distension is the most common cause of dysreflexia. Bladder distention can trigger dysreflexia by stimulation of sensory receptors. Nupercainal ointment reduces tissue stimulation. Too rapid removal of urine can result in compensatory hypotension. These interventions aim to reduce cerebral hypertension and induce orthostatic hypotension.

## Check for Fecal Impaction

First apply Nupercainal to the anus and into the rectum for 1 inch (2.54 cm).
Gently check the rectum with a well-lubricated glove using your index finger.
Insert rectal suppository or gently remove impaction.

**R:** Spasms of pelvic viscera and arterioles cause vasoconstriction below the level of injury, producing hypertension and pallor. Afferent impulses triggered by high blood pressure cause vagal stimulation, resulting in bradycardia. Baroreceptors in the aortic arch and carotid sinus respond to the hypertension, triggering superficial vasodilation, flushing, diaphoresis, and headache above the level of cord injury.

## Check for Skin Irritation

Spray the skin lesion that is triggering the dysreflexia with a topical anesthetic agent.
Remove support hose.

**R:** Dysreflexia can be triggered by stimulation (e.g., of the glans penis or skin lesions).

## Continue to Monitor Blood Pressure Every 3 to 5 Min

**R:** Failure to reverse severe hypertension can result in status epilepticus, retinal or intracerebral hemorrhage, and death (Black & DeSantis, 1999; Hickey, 2006).

## Immediately Consult Physician for Pharmacologic Treatment If Hypertension Is Double Baseline or Noxious Stimuli Are Not Eliminated

**R:** Use an antihypertensive agent with rapid onset and short duration while the causes of autonomic dysreflexia (AD) are investigated. Nifedipine and nitrates are the most commonly used agents. Nifedipine used should be in the immediate-release form; sublingual nifedipine may lead to erratic absorption. Other drugs to treat AD with severe symptoms include hydralazine mecamylamine, diazoxide, and phenoxybenzamine. If 2% nitroglycerine ointment is used, 1 inch may be applied to the skin above the level of the spinal cord injury (SCI). For monitored settings, an IV drip of sodium nitroprusside can be used. Nitropaste is also used. Blood pressure is monitored (Hickey, 2003).

## Initiate Health Teaching and Referrals as Indicated

Teach the signs, symptoms, and treatment of dysreflexia to the client and family.

Teach the indications that warrant immediate medical intervention.

Explain situations that trigger dysreflexia (menstrual cycle, sexual activity, elimination).

Teach the client to watch for early signs and to intervene immediately.

Teach the client to observe for early signs of bladder infections and skin lesions (pressure ulcers, ingrown toenails).

Advise consultation with a physician for long-term pharmacologic management if the client is very vulnerable.

Document the frequency of episodes and precipitating factor(s).

Provide printed instructions to guide actions during the crisis or to show to other health care personnel (e.g., dentists, gynecologists; Kavchak-Keyes, 2000).

Advise athletes with high spinal cord injury about the danger of boosting (binding their legs, distending the bladder to increase norepinephrine; McClain et al., 1999).

**R:** Spasms of pelvic viscera and arterioles cause vasoconstriction below the level of injury, producing hypertension and pallor. Afferent impulses triggered by high blood pressure cause vagal stimulation, resulting in bradycardia. Baroreceptors in the aortic arch and carotid sinus respond to the hypertension, triggering superficial vasodilation, flushing, diaphoresis, and headache above the level of cord injury.

**R:** Thorough teaching can help the client and family successfully prevent or treat dysreflexia at home.

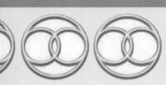

# RISK FOR AUTONOMIC DYSREFLEXIA

## DEFINITION

Refer to *Autonomic Dysreflexia*.

## RISK FACTORS

Refer to *Autonomic Dysreflexia—Related Factors*.

### ▪▪▪▪▪ KEY CONCEPTS

Refer to *Autonomic Dysreflexia*.

## Focus Assessment Criteria

Refer to *Autonomic Dysreflexia—Focus Assessment Criteria*.

## Goal

Refer to *Autonomic Dysreflexia*.

## Interventions

Refer to *Autonomic Dysreflexia*.

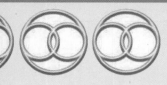

# RISK FOR ELECTROLYTE IMBALANCES
## ◗ Risk for Complications of Electrolyte Imbalances

## DEFINITION (NANDA)

The state in which an individual is at risk for a change in serum electrolyte levels that may compromise health

## RISK FACTORS (NANDA)

Endocrine dysfunction
Diarrhea
Fluid imbalance (e.g., dehydration, water intoxication)
Impaired regulatory mechanisms (e.g., diabetes insipidus, syndrome of inappropriate secretion of antidiuretic hormones)
Renal dysfunction
Treatment-related side effects (e.g., medications, drains)
Vomiting

> **■■■■■■ AUTHOR'S NOTE**
> This new NANDA-I diagnosis is a collaborative problem. Refer to Section 3 for Risk for Complications of Electrolyte Imbalances.

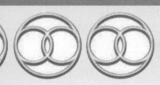

# ENERGY FIELD DISTURBANCE

## DEFINITION

State in which a disruption of the flow of energy surrounding a client's being results in a disharmony of the body, mind, and/or spirit

## DEFINING CHARACTERISTICS

Perception of changes in patterns of the energy flow, such as:

- *Temperature change:* warmth, coolness
- *Visual changes:* image, color
- *Disruption of the field:* vacant, hole, spike, bulge
- *Movement:* wave, spike, tingling, dense, flowing
- *Sounds:* tone, word

# RELATED FACTORS

## Pathophysiologic

*Related to slowing or blocking of energy flows secondary to:*
Illness (specify)     Pregnancy     Injury

## Treatment-Related

*Related to slowing or blocking of energy flows secondary to:*
Immobility          Perioperative experience     Labor and delivery

## Situational (Personal, Environmental)

*Related to slowing or blocking of energy flows secondary to:*
Pain                Fear                Anxiety
Grieving

## Maturational

*Related to age-related developmental difficulties or crises (specify).*

## ■■■■■■ AUTHOR'S NOTE

This diagnosis is unique for two reasons: it represents a specific theory (human energy field theory), and its interventions require specialized instruction and supervised practice. Meehan (1991) recommends the following preparation:

- At least 6 months of professional practice in an acute care setting
- Guided learning by a nurse with at least 2 years of experience
- Conformance with practice guidelines
- Thirty hours of instruction in the theory and practice
- Thirty hours of supervised practice with relatively healthy people
- Successful completion of written and practice evaluations

Some may consider this diagnosis unconventional. Perhaps nurses need to be reminded that there are many theories, philosophies, and frameworks of nursing practice, just as there are many definitions of clients and practice settings. Some nurses practice on street corners with homeless people, whereas others practice in offices attached to their homes. Nursing diagnosis should not represent only mainstream nursing (acute care, long-term care, home health). Rather than criticize a diagnosis as having little applicability, perhaps nurses should celebrate diversity. Fundamentally, nurses are all connected through the quest to improve the condition of individuals, families, groups, and communities.

## ■■■■■■ KEY CONCEPTS

- Therapeutic touch is rooted in Eastern philosophy. The cultural orientation of Western medicine is to conduct research to explain a modality's effects. In the Eastern culture, if something works, research is unnecessary for proof.
- Therapeutic touch is derived from the basic premise that universal life energy sustains all living organisms. Health is defined as the state in which all a client's energies are in harmony or dynamic balance. Health is compromised when there is disequilibrium, blockage, or deficits in energy flow (Macrae, 1988).
- In nursing, the Rogerian conceptual system has provided the foundation for therapeutic touch. This model affirms that energy fields are fundamental units of human beings and their environment (Meehan, 1991).
- "Therapeutic touch is a knowledgeable and purposive patterning of the patient–environmental energy field process" (Meehan, 1991, p. 201). It requires specialized instruction and supervised practice. See the Author's Note for recommended preparation.
- Life-giving, healing energy flows within the universal flow of energy. Such energy, present in all living systems, is composed of intelligence, order, and compassion (Bradley, 1987).

*(continued)*

■■■■■■ **KEY CONCEPTS** *Continued*

- Rogers states that therapeutic touch is an example of how a nurse "seeks to strengthen the coherence and integrity of human and environmental fields and to knowingly participate in the patterning of human and environmental fields for the realization of optimum well-being" (Meehan, 1991).
- In a pilot study, Quinn and Strelkauskas (1993) found that all the recipients of therapeutic touch experienced dramatic increases in all dimensions of positive affect (joy, vigor, contentment, and affection) and dramatic decreases in all dimensions of negative affect (anxiety, guilt, hostility, and depression). They also identified a shift in consciousness during therapeutic touch, which was measured by perception of time. The practitioner and the recipients reported the same time distortions, indicating a shift in consciousness.
- The use of healing touch with critically ill people resulted in no physiologic change before, during, or after therapy; however, recipients experienced significant improvements in relaxation and sleep (Umbreit, 2000).
- An intrinsic relationship may exist between therapeutic touch and the placebo effect. Therapeutic touch may enhance the placebo effect and reduce discomfort and distress (Meehan, 1998).
- Denison (2004) reported that clients with fibromyalgia syndrome reported a decrease in pain with therapeutic touch. Using thermography, there also was an increase in cutaneous skin temperature (Denison, 2004).

## Focus Assessment Criteria

Because assessment of the energy field is quickly followed by the intervention, and reassessment continues throughout, refer to Interventions for assessment.

**NOC**
Spiritual Health

## ➤ Goal

The client will report relief of symptoms after therapeutic touch.

### *Indicators*

- Report increased sense of relaxation.
- Report decreased pain, using a scale of 0 to 10 before and after therapies.
- Have slower, deeper respirations.

**NIC**
Therapeutic Touch,
Spiritual Support,
Presence

## ➤ General Interventions

*Note:* The following phases of therapeutic touch are learned separately but rendered concurrently. Presentation of these interventions is to describe the process for nurses who do not practice therapeutic touch. This discussion may help them to support colleagues who practice therapeutic touch and also to initiate referrals. As discussed before, preparation for therapeutic touch requires specialized instruction, which is beyond the scope of this book. Refer to the reference Nurse Healers Professional Associates International for Standards.

### Prepare the Client and Environment for Therapeutic Touch (TT)

Provide as much privacy as possible.
Explain therapeutic touch and obtain verbal permission to perform it.
Give the client permission to stop the therapy at any time.
Allow the client to assume a comfortable position (e.g., lying on a bed, sitting on a couch).

**R:** Early beliefs regarding therapeutic touch attributed its effects to an energy transfer and exchange between practitioner and recipient (Quinn, 1989). Current beliefs are that the practitioner shifts "consciousness into a state that may be thought of as a 'healing meditation,' facilitates repatterning of the recipient's energy field through the process of resonance, rather than 'energy exchange or transfer'" (Quinn & Strelkauskas, 1993, p. 14).

**R:** The practitioner of therapeutic touch facilitates the flow of healing energy (Umbreit, 2000).

## Shift from a Direct Focus on the Environment to an Inner Focus, Which Is Perceived as the Center of Life within the Nurse (Centering)

**R:** Centering allows the entry of healing (Krieger, 1997).

## Assess the Client by Scanning His or Her Energy Field for Openness and Symmetry (Krieger, 1987)

Move the palms of your hands toward the client, at a distance of 2 to 4 inches over his or her body, from head to feet in a smooth, light movement.

Use calm and rhythmic hand movements.

Sense the cues to energy imbalance (e.g., warmth, coolness, tightness, heaviness, tingling, and emptiness).

**R:** This TT process recognizes what is known and what is felt.

## Facilitate a Rhythmic Flow of Energy by Moving Hands Vigorously From Head to Toe (Unruffling/Clearing)

**R:** Unruffling enhances the energy flows in the healer's system (Krieger, 1997).

## Focus Intent on the Specific Repatterning of Areas of Imbalance and Impeded Flow

## Using Your Hands as Focal Points, Move Them Gently, Sweeping from Head to Feet One Time

Note the energy flow over lower legs and feet.

If the energy flow is not open in this area, continue to move your hands or hold the feet physically to facilitate energy flow.

Briefly shake your hands to dispel congestion from the field if needed.

When therapeutic touch is complete, place your hands over the solar plexus area (just above the waist) and focus on facilitating the flow of healing energy to the client.

Provide the client with an opportunity to rest.

**R:** This corrects energy imbalance (Krieger, 1987).

## Encourage the Client to Provide Feedback

Assess if the client exhibits a relaxation response. Signs include drops of several decibels in voice volume; slower, deeper respirations; audible sign of relaxation; and a peripheral flush perceived on face.

## Document Both the Procedure and the Feedback

**R:** "At the core of the therapeutic touch process is the intent of the practitioner to help the recipient" (Quinn & Strelkauskas, 1993, p. 14). The practitioner focuses entirely on the recipient with unconditional love and compassion. The healer is intentionally motivated to help the recipient, who is willing to accept the change.

**R:** TT can promote feelings of calm, peace, and comfort.

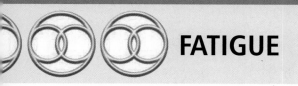

# FATIGUE

## DEFINITION

Self-recognized state in which a client experiences an overwhelming, sustained sense of exhaustion and decreased capacity for physical and mental work that is not relieved by rest

## DEFINING CHARACTERISTICS

### Major (80% to 100%)

Verbalization of an unremitting and overwhelming lack of energy
Inability to maintain usual routines
Verbalization of distress

### Minor (50% to 79%)

| | |
|---|---|
| Perceived need for additional energy to accomplish routine tasks | Increased physical complaints |
| | Emotional ability or irritability |
| Impaired ability to concentrate | Decreased performance |
| Lethargy or listlessness | Sleep disturbances |

## RELATED FACTORS

Many factors can cause fatigue; combining related factors may be useful (e.g., *Related to muscle weakness, accumulated waste products, inflammation, and infections secondary to hepatitis*).

### Bio-Pathophysiologic

*Related to hypermetabolic state secondary to:*

| | | |
|---|---|---|
| Viruses (e.g., Epstein-Barr) | Fever | Pregnancy |

*Related to inadequate tissue oxygenation secondary to:*

| | | |
|---|---|---|
| Chronic obstructive lung disease | Congestive heart failure | Anemia |
| Peripheral vascular disease | | |

*Related to biochemical changes secondary to:*
*Endocrine/Metabolic Disorders*

| | | |
|---|---|---|
| Diabetes mellitus | Pituitary disorders | Acquired immunodeficiency |
| Hypothyroidism | Addison's disease | syndrome (AIDS) |

*Chronic Diseases*

| | | |
|---|---|---|
| Renal failure | Cirrhosis | Lyme disease |

*Related to muscular weakness/wasting secondary to:*

| | | |
|---|---|---|
| Myasthenia gravis | Parkinson's disease | Multiple sclerosis |
| AIDS | Amyotrophic lateral sclerosis | |

*Related to hypermetabolic state, competition between body and tumor for nutrients, anemia, and stressors associated with cancer*
*Related to nutritional deficits or changes in nutrient metabolism secondary to:*

| | | |
|---|---|---|
| Nausea | Side effects of medications | Vomiting |
| Gastric surgery | Diarrhea | Diabetes mellitus |

*Related to chronic inflammatory process secondary to:*

| | | |
|---|---|---|
| AIDS | Cirrhosis | Arthritis |
| Inflammatory bowel disease | Lupus erythematosus | Renal failure |
| Hepatitis | Lyme disease | |

## Treatment-Related

*Biochemical changes secondary to:*
Chemotherapy
Radiation therapy
Side effects of (specify):
*Related to surgical damage to tissue and anesthesia*
*Related to increased energy expenditure secondary to:*
Amputation Gait disorder      Use of walker, crutches

## Situational (Personal, Environmental)

*Related to prolonged decreased activity and deconditioning secondary to:*

| | | |
|---|---|---|
| Anxiety | Social isolation | Fever |
| Nausea/vomiting | Diarrhea | Depression |
| Pain | Obesity | |

*Related to excessive role demands*
*Related to overwhelming emotional demands*
*Related to extreme stress*
*Related to sleep disturbance*

## Maturational

**Child/Adolescent**
*Related to hypermetabolic state secondary to:*
Mononucleosis        Fever
*Related to chronic insufficient nutrients secondary to:*
Obesity                Excessive dieting        Eating disorders
*Related to effects of newborn care on sleep patterns and need for continuous attention*
*Related to hypermetabolic state during first trimester*

## ■■■■■ AUTHOR'S NOTE

Fatigue as a nursing diagnosis differs from acute tiredness. Tiredness is a transient, temporary state (Rhoten, 1982) caused by lack of sleep, improper nutrition, increased stress, sedentary lifestyle, or temporarily increased work or social responsibilities. Fatigue is a pervasive, subjective, drained feeling that cannot be eliminated; however, the nurse can assist the person to adapt to it. Activity intolerance differs from fatigue in that the nurse will assist the person with activity intolerance to increase endurance and activity.

The focus for the person with fatigue is not on increasing endurance. If the cause resolves or abates (e.g., acute infection, chemotherapy, radiation), *Fatigue* as a diagnosis is discontinued and *Activity Intolerance* can be initiated to focus on improving the deconditioned state.

## ■■■■■ ERRORS IN DIAGNOSTIC STATEMENTS

1. *Fatigue related to feelings of lack of energy for routine tasks*
   When a person reports insufficient energy for routine tasks, the nurse performs a focus assessment and collects additional data to determine whether *Fatigue* is appropriate or actually a symptom of another diagnosis, such as *Activity Intolerance, Ineffective Coping, Interrupted Family Processes, Anxiety,* or *Ineffective Health Maintenance*. When acute or chronic conditions cause fatigue, the nurse must determine whether the person can increase endurance (which would call for *Activity Intolerance*) or needs energy conservation techniques to help accomplish desired activities. When fatigue results from ineffective stress management or poor health habits, *Fatigue* or *Activity Intolerance* is not indicated. During data collection to determine contributing factors, the nurse can record the diagnosis as *Possible Fatigue related to reports of lack of energy*. Using a "possible" diagnosis indicates the need for more data collection to rule out or confirm.

## ■■■■■ KEY CONCEPTS

### Generic Considerations

- Fatigue is a subjective experience with physiologic, situational, and psychological components.
- Acute tiredness is an expected response to physical exertion, change in daily activities, additional stress, or inadequate sleep.
- U.S. society values energy, productivity, and vitality. It views those without energy as sluggish or lazy. It views fatigue and tiredness negatively.
- Fatigue can be physical, mental, and motivational. Causes of fatigue are multifactorial. Careful assessment of the causes and interventions to reduce them are critical.
- Fatigue can be manifested in areas of cortical inhibition (Jiricka, 2002; Rhoten, 1982):
  - Decreased attention
  - Slowed and impaired perception
  - Impaired thinking
  - Decreased motivation
  - Decreased performance in physical and mental activities
  - Loss of fine coordination
  - Poor judgment
  - Indifference to surroundings
- Hargreaves (1977) described a high incidence of "fatigue syndrome" in young married women moving to a new town. Contributing factors were increased physical work, changes in support systems, and other stresses in relocation.
- People with rheumatoid arthritis reported that their fatigue was related to joint pain. In addition, clients with flare were observed to awaken more often and take longer to walk and perform activities than nonflare clients and the control group.
- Cancer-related fatigue has been reported in 35% to 100% of cases and is reported to be the most distressing side effect. Stressors contributing to fatigue in clients with cancer are illustrated in Box II.1.
- Women receiving localized radiation to the breast reported that fatigue decreased the second week but increased and reached a plateau after week 4 until 3 weeks after treatment ceased. Fatigue levels did not change significantly on weekends between treatments (Greenberg, Sawicka, Eisenthal, & Ross, 1992).
- When fatigue is a side effect of treatment, it does not resolve when the treatment ends, but gradually lessens over months (Nail & Winningham, 1997).
- Depression slows thought processes and leads to decreased physical activities. Work output decreases, and endurance lessens. The effort to continue activity produces fatigue.
- Anxiety can interfere with thought processes, increase movements, and disturb gastrointestinal function, thus causing fatigue.

### Pediatric Considerations

- Infants and small children cannot express fatigue. The nurse can elicit this information by interviewing the parents and carefully assessing key functional health patterns (e.g., sleep–rest, activity–exercise [which may reveal respiratory difficulties or activity intolerance], and nutrition–metabolic [which may reveal feeding difficulties]).
- Children at risk for fatigue include those with acute or chronic illness, congenital heart disease, exposure to toxins, prolonged stress, or anemia.
- Children depend on parents/caregivers to modify the environment to mitigate effects of fatigue.

### BOX II.1 CONTRIBUTING FACTORS TO FATIGUE IN CLIENTS WITH CANCER

**Pathophysiologic**
Hypermetabolic state associated with active tumor growth
Competition between the body and the tumor for nutrients
Chronic pain
Organ dysfunction (e.g., hepatic, respiratory, gastrointestinal)

**Treatment-Related**
Accumulation of toxic waste products secondary to radiation, chemotherapy
Inadequate nutritional intake secondary to nausea, vomiting
Anemia
Analgesics, antiemetics
Diagnostic tests
Surgery

**Situational (Personal, Environmental)**
Uncertainty about future
Fear of death, disfigurement
Social isolation
Losses (role responsibilities, occupational, body parts, function, appearance, economic)
Separation for treatments

## Maternal Considerations

Fatigue is common in early pregnancy due to increased metabolic requirements. (Pillitteri, 2009)

Gardner reported that levels of fatigue in postpartum women increased at 2 weeks but decreased by 6 weeks. Factors associated with high postpartum fatigue were sleep alterations, additional children, child care problems, less household help, less education, low family income, and young age of mother (Gardner & Campbell, 1991).

## Geriatric Considerations

- The normal effects of aging do not in themselves increase the risk of or cause fatigue. Fatigue in older adults has basically the same etiologies as in younger adults. The difference is that older adults tend to experience more chronic diseases than younger adults. Thus, fatigue in older adults is not the result of age-related factors, but related to such risk factors as chronic diseases and medications.
- Depression is the most common psychosocial impairment in older adults. Depression-related affective disturbances affect 27% of adults in a community-living setting (Miller, 2009).
- Chronic fatigue and diminished energy are functional consequences of late-life depression (Miller, 2009).
- According to Miller (2007), "the activity theory proposed that older adults would remain psychologically and socially fit if they remained active." Participation in activities affirms a person's self-concept.
- Chronic fatigue, reported by approximately 70% of older adults, can result in diminished motor activity and muscle tone. Note that anemia, very common in this population, is another possible contributor to complaints of chronic fatigue (Miller, 2009).

## Focus Assessment Criteria

### Subjective Data

#### Assess for Defining Characteristics

**Description of Fatigue**
Onset
Pattern: morning, evening, transient, unfading
Precipitated by what?
Relieved by rest?

**Effects of Fatigue on:**

| Activities of daily living | Libido | Concentration |
| Mood | Leisure activities | Motivation |

## Assess for Related Factors

Medical Condition (Acute, Chronic; Refer to Key Concepts)

### Nutritional Imbalances

### Treatments

| Chemotherapy | Medication side effects | Radiation therapy |
| Stressors | | |
| Excessive role demands | Financial | Depression |
| Career | Family | |

For more information on Focus Assessment Criteria, visit http://thepoint.lww.com.

---

**NOC**
Activity Tolerance,
Endurance, Energy
Conservation

## ➤ Goals

The person will participate in activities that stimulate and balance physical, cognitive, affective, and social domains.

### Indicators:

- Discuss the causes of fatigue.
- Share feelings regarding the effects of fatigue on life.
- Establish priorities for daily and weekly activities.

---

**NIC**
Energy
Management,
Environmental
Management,
Mutual Goal Setting,
Socialization
Enhancement

## ➤ General Interventions

Nursing interventions for this diagnosis are for people with fatigue regardless of etiology that cannot be eliminated. The focus is to assist the client and family to adapt to the fatigue state.

### Assess Causative or Contributing Factors

If fatigue has related factors that can be treated, refer to the specific Nursing Diagnosis as:
Lack of sleep; refer to Disturbed Sleep Pattern
Poor nutrition; refer to *Imbalanced Nutrition*
Sedentary lifestyle; refer to *Sedentary Lifestyle*
Inadequate stress management; refer to *Stress Overload*
Chronic excessive role or social demands; refer to *Ineffective Coping*

## Explain the Causes of Fatigue (See Key Concepts)

**R:** In many chronic diseases, fatigue is the most common, disruptive, and distressing symptom because it interferes with self-care activities.

## Allow Expression of Feelings Regarding the Effects of Fatigue on Life

Identify difficult activities.
Help the client verbalize how fatigue interferes with role responsibilities.
Encourage the client to convey how fatigue causes frustration.

## Assist the Client to Identify Strengths, Abilities, and Interests

Identify values and interests.
Identify areas of success and usefulness; emphasize past accomplishments.
Use information to develop goals with the client.
Assist the client in identifing sources of hope (e.g., relationships, faith, things to accomplish).
Assist the client in developing realistic short- and long-term goals (progress from simple to more complex; use a "goals poster" to indicate type and time for achieving specific goals).

**R:** Focusing the client on strengths and abilities may provide insight into positive events and lessen the tendency to overgeneralize the severity of disease, which can lead to depression.

## Assist the Client to Identify Energy Patterns

### Instruct the Client to Record Fatigue Levels Every Hour over 24 h; Select a Usual Day

Ask the client to rate fatigue using the Rhoten fatigue scale (0 = not tired, peppy; 10 = total exhaustion). Record the activities during each rating.

### Analyze Together the 24-h Fatigue Levels

Times of peak energy
Times of exhaustion
Activities associated with increasing fatigue

### Explain Benefits of Exercise and Discuss What Is Realistic

**R:** Identifying times of peak energy and exhaustion can aid in planning activities to maximize energy conservation and productivity.

## Explain the Purpose of Pacing and Prioritization

Explore what activities the client views as important to maintain self-esteem.
Attempt to divide vital activities or tasks into components (e.g., preparing menu, shopping, storing, cooking, serving, cleaning up); the client can delegate some parts and retain others.
Plan important tasks during periods of high energy (e.g., prepare all meals in the morning).
Assist client in identifing priorities and to eliminate nonessential activities.
Plan each day to avoid energy- and time-consuming, nonessential decision-making.
Distribute difficult tasks throughout the week.
Rest before difficult tasks and stop before fatigue ensues.

**R:** The client requires rest periods before or after some activities. Planning can provide for adequate rest and reduce unnecessary energy expenditure. Such strategies can enable continuation of most desired activities, contributing to positive self-esteem.

## Teach Energy Conservation Techniques

Modify the environment.

- Replace steps with ramps.
- Install grab rails.
- Elevate chairs 3 to 4 inches.
- Organize kitchen or work areas.
- Reduce trips up and down stairs (e.g., put a commode on the first floor).

Use a taxi instead of driving self.
Delegate housework (e.g., employ a high-school student for a few hours after school).

**R:** Strategies can be utilized to decrease energy used in activities of daily living.

## Promote Socialization with Family and Friends (Dzurec, 2000)

Encourage the client to participate in one social activity, weekly.
Explain that feelings of connectedness decrease fatigue.

**R:** Quality or type of activity reportedly is more important than quantity. Informal activities promoted well-being the most, followed by formal structured activities, and last by solitary activities, which were found to have little or no effect on life satisfaction (Longino & Kart, 1982).

## Explain the Effects of Conflict and Stress on Energy Levels

Teach the importance of mutuality in sharing concerns.
Explain the benefits of distraction from negative events.
Teach and assist with relaxation techniques before anticipated stressful events. Encourage mental imagery to promote positive thought processes.

Allow the client time to reminisce to gain insight into past experiences.

Teach the client to maximize aesthetic experiences (e.g., smell of coffee, feeling warmth of the sun).

Teach the client to anticipate experiences he or she takes delight in each day (e.g., walking, reading favorite book, writing a letter).

**R:** Focusing the client on strengths and abilities may provide insight into positive events and lessen the tendency to overgeneralize the severity of the disease, which can lead to depression (Beck, 1984).

Help the client identify how her or she can help others. Listening to clients' problems, using the computer to access information, and making phone calls

**R:** Reciprocity or returning support to one's support system is vital for balanced and healthy relationships (Tilden & Weinert, 1987). Clients with fatigue have difficulty with reciprocity.

## Provide Significant Others Opportunities to Discuss Feelings in Private Regarding:

Changes in person with fatigue

Caretaking responsibilities

Financial issues

Changes in lifestyle, role responsibilities, and relationships

See *Caregiver Role Strain* for additional strategies for caregivers.

## Initiate Health Teaching and Referrals, as Indicated

Counseling

Community services (Meals On Wheels, housekeeper)

Financial assistance

## Maternal Interventions

Explain the reasons for fatigue in first and third trimesters:

- Increased basal metabolic rate
- Changes in hormonal levels
- Anemia
- Increased cardiac output (third trimester)

Emphasize the need for naps and 8 h of sleep each night.

**R:** Fatigue in the first and third trimesters is normal.

Discuss the importance of exercise (e.g., walking).

**R:** Exercise provides emotional and physical benefits.

For postpartum women, discuss factors that increase fatigue:

| | |
|---|---|
| Labor more than 30 h | Preexisting chronic disease |
| Hemoglobin less than 10 g/dL or postpartum hemorrhage | Episiotomy, tear, or cesarean section |
| Sleeping difficulties | Ill newborn or a congenital anomaly |
| Dependent children at home | Child care problems |
| Unrealistic expectations | No daytime rest periods |

**R:** Explaining the reasons for fatigue can allay fears. Strategies can be discussed to reduce fatigue at home.

## Geriatric Interventions

Consider if chronic fatigue is the consequence of late-life depression.

Refer the client with suspected depression for evaluation.

**R:** Late-life depression causes chronic fatigue and diminishes energy (Miller, 2009).

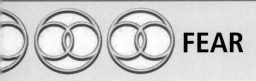

# FEAR

## DEFINITION

State in which an individual or group experiences a feeling of physiologic or emotional disruption related to an identifiable source that is perceived as dangerous

## DEFINING CHARACTERISTICS

### Major (Must Be Present, One or More)

Feeling of dread, fright, apprehension, and/or behaviors of:

- Avoidance
- Narrowing of focus on danger
- Deficits in attention, performance, and control

### Minor (May Be Present)

**Verbal Reports of Panic, Obsessions, Behavioral Acts**

| | | |
|---|---|---|
| Crying | Dysfunctional immobility | Increased questioning/ |
| Compulsive mannerisms | Escape | verbalization |
| Hypervigilance | Aggression | |

**Visceral–Somatic Activity**
*Musculoskeletal*

| | | |
|---|---|---|
| Shortness of breath | Muscle tightness | Fatigue/limb weakness |

*Respiratory*

| | |
|---|---|
| Increased rate | Trembling |

*Cardiovascular*

| | | |
|---|---|---|
| Palpitations | Rapid pulse | Increased blood pressure |

*Skin*

| | | |
|---|---|---|
| Flush/pallor | Sweating | Paresthesia |

*Gastrointestinal*

| | | |
|---|---|---|
| Anorexia | Nausea/vomiting | Diarrhea/urge to defecate |
| Dry mouth/throat | | |

*Central Nervous System (CNS)/Perceptual*

| | | |
|---|---|---|
| Syncope | Irritability | Insomnia |
| Absentmindedness | Lack of concentration | Nightmares |
| Pupil dilation | | |

*Genitourinary*
Urinary frequency/urgency

## RELATED FACTORS

Fear can be a response to various health problems, situations, or conflicts. Some common sources are indicated next.

### Pathophysiologic

*Related to perceived immediate and long-term effects of:*

| | | |
|---|---|---|
| Terminal disease | Long-term disability | Loss of body function or part |
| Cognitive impairment | Disabling illness | Sensory impairment |

## Treatment-Related

*Related to loss of control and unpredictable outcome secondary to:*

| | | |
|---|---|---|
| Hospitalization | Invasive procedures | Surgery and its outcome |
| Radiation | Anesthesia | |

### Situational (Personal, Environmental)
*Related to loss of control and unpredictable outcome secondary to:*

| | | |
|---|---|---|
| Change or loss of significant | Pain | New environment |
| other | New people | Success |
| Divorce | Lack of knowledge | Failure |
| Related to potential loss of income | | |

## Maturational

### Preschool
*Related to:*

| | | |
|---|---|---|
| Not being liked | Strangers | Age-related fears |
| Bodily harm | Being alone | (Dark, strangers, ghosts) |
| Animals | | |
| *Separation from parents, peers* | | |

### School-Age (6 to 12 years)
*Related to:*

| | | |
|---|---|---|
| Being lost | Being in trouble | Thunder, lightning |
| Bad dreams | Weapons | |

### Adolescent
*Related to uncertainty of:*

| | | |
|---|---|---|
| Appearance | Scholastic success | Peer support |

### Adult
*Related to uncertainty of:*

| | | |
|---|---|---|
| Marriage | Job security | Pregnancy |
| Effects of aging | Parenthood | |

### Older Adult
*Related to anticipated dependence:*

| | | |
|---|---|---|
| Prolonged suffering | Financial insecurity | Vulnerability to crime |
| Abandonment | | |

---

■■■■■■ **AUTHOR'S NOTE**

See *Anxiety*.

---

■■■■■ **KEY CONCEPTS**

### Generic Considerations

- Psychological defense mechanisms are distinctly individual and can be adaptive or maladaptive.
- Fear differs from anxiety in that fear is aroused by an identified threat (specific object); anxiety is aroused by a threat that cannot be easily identified (nonspecific or unknown).
- Both fear and anxiety lead to disequilibrium.
- Anger may be a response to certain fears.
- A sense of adequacy in confronting danger reduces fear. Fear disguises itself. The expressed fear may substitute for other fears that are not socially acceptable. Awareness of factors that intensify fears enhances control and prevents heightened feelings. Confronting the safe reality of a situation reduces fear.

*(continued)*

■■■■■ **KEY CONCEPTS** *Continued*

- Fear can become anxiety if it becomes internalized and serves to disorganize instead of becoming adaptive.
- Chronic physical reactions to stressors lead to susceptibility and chronic disease.
- Physiologic responses are manifested throughout the body primarily from the hypothalamus' stimulation of the autonomic and endocrine systems.
- People interpret the degree of danger from a threatening stimulus. The physiologic and psychological systems react with equal intensity (elevations in blood pressure and heart and respiratory rates).
- Fear is adaptive and a healthy response to danger.
- Fear differs from *phobia*, an irrational, persistent fear of a circumscribed stimulus (object or situation) other than having a panic attack (panic disorder) or of humiliation or embarrassment in certain social situations (social phobia) (American Psychiatric Association, 2004).

## Pediatric Considerations

- "Fear is a part of normal development in children. Fear can be a positive adaptive force when it teaches children an awareness of potential danger" (Nicastro & Whetsell, 1999, p. 392).
- Infants and small children experience fear but cannot identify the threat verbally. Verbal (crying, protesting) and nonverbal (kicking, biting, holding back) responses are important indicators of children's fear (Broome, Bates, Lillis, & McGahee, 1990; Hockenberry & Wilson, 2009).
- Fear behaviors are *consistent* and *immediate* on exposure to or mention of a specific stressor; if the response is erratic, the diagnosis more accurately might be anxiety. Refer to Table II.12 in *Delayed Growth and Development* or Key Concepts—Pediatric Considerations in *Anxiety*.
- Fears throughout childhood follow a developmental sequence and are influenced by culture, environment, and parental fears (Hockenberry & Wilson, 2009).
- Fears are most frequent in 8- to 10-year-old children (Nicastro & Whetsell, 1999).
- Main fears of different age groups are as follows (Nicastro & Whetsell, 1999; Hockenberry & Wilson, 2009)
  - *Infants and toddlers (birth to 2 years):* Fears evolve from physical stimuli (e.g., loud noises, separation from parents/caregivers, strangers, sudden movements, animals, certain situations [doctor's office]).
  - *Preschoolers (3 to 5 years):* Fears evolve from real or imagined situations (e.g., injury or mutilation, ghosts, devils, monsters, the dark, bathtub and toilet drains, being alone, dreams, robbers, wild animals, snakes).
  - *School-aged children (6 to 8 years):* Common fears are ghosts, monsters, dark, being alone, thunder, lightning, being lost, kidnapping, guns, and weapons.
  - *School-aged children (9 to 12 years):* Common fears are the dark, being lost or alone, bodily harm, strangers, bad dreams, punishment, grades and tests, and being in trouble.
  - *Adolescents:* Fears may be verbalized and include loss of self-control, disturbance to body image, death, separation from peers, inept social performance, sexuality gossip, AIDS, being alone, and war.
- Fear is a momentary reaction to danger related to a low estimate of one's own power over the situation (Hockenberry & Wilson, 2009).

## Maternal Considerations

The fears and concerns of pregnancy differ for each trimester:

### First Trimester
- Uncertainty about timing of pregnancy
- Uncertainty about her own or her partner's adequacy as parent
- Concerns about material issues (e.g., finances)

### Second Trimester
- Fears diminish as the fetus moves
- Decrease in physical symptoms

### Third Trimester
- Fears for her own well-being and how she will tolerate labor
- Fears for the well-being of the fetus
- Obsessed with labor and delivery

## Geriatric Considerations

Cesarone (1991) clustered the sources of fear in the elderly into five categories:
- Disease, suffering, and falls
- Dependence and abandonment
- Dying
- Illness or death of loved ones
- Miscellaneous reasons (crime, financial insecurity, diagnostic tests)

# Focus Assessment Criteria

## Subjective/Objective Data

### Assess for Defining Characteristics

**Onset**
Have the client tell you a "story" about his or her fearfulness.

**Thought Process and Content**
Are thoughts clear, coherent, logical, confused, or forgetful?
Can the client concentrate or is he or she preoccupied?

**Perception and Judgment**
Does fear remain after the stressor is eliminated?
Is the fear a response to a present stimulus or distorted by past influences?

**Visceral–Somatic Activity**

*Musculoskeletal*

| | | |
|---|---|---|
| Shortness of breath | Muscle tightness | Fatigue/limb weakness |

*Respiratory*

| | |
|---|---|
| Increased rate | Trembling |

*Cardiovascular*

| | | |
|---|---|---|
| Palpitations | Rapid pulse | Increased blood pressure |

*Skin*

| | | |
|---|---|---|
| Flush/pallor | Sweating | Paresthesia |

*Gastrointestinal*

| | | |
|---|---|---|
| Anorexia | Nausea/vomiting | Diarrhea/urge to defecate |
| Dry mouth/throat | | |

*CNS/Perceptual*

| | | |
|---|---|---|
| Syncope | Irritability | Insomnia |
| Absentmindedness | Lack of concentration | Nightmares |
| Pupil dilation | | |

*Genitourinary*
Urinary frequency/urgency

For more information on Focus Assessment Criteria, visit http://thepoint.lww.com.

**NOC**
Anxiety Self-Control,
Fear Self-Control

# Goals

The adult will relate increased psychological and physiologic comfort.

## Indicators

- Show decreased visceral response (pulse, respirations).
- Differentiate real from imagined situations.
- Describe effective and ineffective coping patterns.
- Identify own coping responses.

The child will exhibit or relate increased psychological and physiologic comfort.

## Indicators

- Discuss fears.
- Exhibit less crying.

<table>
<tr><td>

**NIC**

Anxiety
Reduction, Coping
Enhancement;
Presence,
Counseling,
Relaxation Therapy

</td></tr>
</table>

➤ # General Interventions _____

Nursing interventions for *Fear* represent interventions for any client with fear regardless of the etiologic or contributing factors.

## Assess Possible Contributing Factors

Refer to Related Factors.

## Reduce or Eliminate Contributing Factors

### Unfamiliar Environment

Orient client to environment using simple explanations.
Speak slowly and calmly.
Avoid surprises and painful stimuli.
Use soft lights and music.
Remove threatening stimulus.
Plan one-day-at-a-time, familiar routine.
Encourage gradual mastery of a situation.
Provide a transitional object with symbolic safeness (security blanket, religious medal).

**R:** A quiet, calm professional can communicate calm to the client (Varcarolis, 2006).

### Intrusion on Personal Space

Allow personal space.
Move the client away from the stimulus.
Remain with the client until fear subsides (listen, use silence).
Later, establish frequent and consistent contacts; use family members and significant others to stay with the client.
Use touch as tolerated (sometimes holding the client firmly helps him or her maintain control).

**R:** Minimizing environmental stimuli can help reduce escalation of fear (Varcarolis, 2006).

### Threat to Self-esteem

Support preferred coping style when client uses adaptive mechanisms.
Initially, decrease the client's number of choices.
Use simple, direct statements (avoid detail).
Give direct suggestions to manage everyday events (some prefer details; others like general explanations).
Encourage expression of feelings (helplessness, anger).
Give feedback about expressed feelings (support realistic assessments).
Refocus interaction on areas of capability rather than dysfunction.
Encourage normal coping mechanisms.
Encourage sharing common problems with others.
Give feedback of effect the client's behavior has on others.
Encourage the client to face the fear.

**R:** Open, honest dialogue may help initiate constructive problem solving and can instill hope.

## When Intensity of Feelings Has Decreased, Assist with Insight and Controlling Response

### Bring Behavioral Cues into the Client's Awareness

**R:** Severe fear or panic can interfere with concentrating and information processing (Varcarolis, 2006).

*Ask to Write Their Fears in Narrative Form*

> **R:** Writing down one's fears can give insight and control (Crossley, 2003).

## Teach How to Solve Problems

> What is the problem?
> Who or what is responsible?
> What are the options?
> What are the advantages and disadvantages of each option?
> **R:** Open, honest dialogue may help initiate constructive problem solving and can instill hope.

## Initiate Health Teaching and Referrals as Indicated

> Progressive relaxation technique          Reading, music, breathing exercises
> Desensitization, self-coaching             Thought stopping, guided fantasy
> Yoga, hypnosis, assertiveness training
> **R:** These methods can increase control and increase comfort or relaxation.

**Pediatric Interventions**

> ### Participate in Community Functions to Teach Parents Age-Related Fears and Constructive Interventions (e.g., Parent–School Organizations, Newsletters, Civic Groups
>
> Provide child opportunities to talk and write about fears and to learn healthy outlets for anger or sadness, such as play therapy.
>
> Acknowledge illness, death, and pain as real; refrain from protecting children from the reality of existence; encourage open, honest sharing that is age-appropriate.
>
> Never make fun of the child. Share with child that these fears are okay.
>
> Fear of imaginary animals and intruders (e.g., "I don't see a lion in your room, but I will leave the light on for you, and, if you need me again, please call.")
>
> Fear of parent being late (establish a contingency plan [e.g., "If you come home from school and Mommy is not here, go to Mrs. S next door."]).
>
> Fear of vanishing down a toilet or bathtub drain:
>
> - Wait until child is out of the tub before releasing the drain.
> - Wait until child is off the toilet before flushing.
> - Leave toys in bathtub and demonstrate how they do not go down the drain.
>
> Fear of dogs and cats:
>
> - Allow child to watch a child and a dog playing from a distance.
> - Do not force child to touch the animal.
>
> Fear of death (see Key Concepts for *Grieving*)
> Fear of pain (see *Pain* under Pediatric Interventions)
> Refusal to go to sleep:
>
> - Establish a realistic hour for retiring.
> - Contract for a reward if the child is successful.
> - Do not sleep with the child or take the child to the parent's room.
>
> Discuss with parents the normality of fears in children; explain the necessity of acceptance and the negative outcomes of punishment, shaming, or of forcing the child to overcome the fear.
>
> Provide the child with the opportunity to observe other children cope successfully with the feared object.
>
> - Demonstrate strength and self-confidence.
> - Take child's hand and gently guide into shallow water.
> - Allow child to watch you pet a dog.
>
> *(continued)*

Pediatric
Interventions
*Continued*

**R:** Strategies focus on accepting the child's fear, providing an explanation, if possible, or some form of control The more successfully a child handles a fearful situation, the more confidence and less vulnerability the child feels (Nicastro & Whetsell, 1999).

**R:** Desensitization by gradually facing a fearsome object or situation is effective with most children (Hockenberry & Wilson, 2009).

Maternal
Interventions

Provide opportunities to express fears during each trimester.

**R:** Fears and concerns change with each trimester. Refer to Key Concepts—Maternal Considerations for specifics.

Provide opportunities for expectant father to share his concerns and fears.

**R:** Expectant fathers are concerned about changes in the relationship with their partner, their competence as a provider, and meeting the newly evolving expectations of the mother.

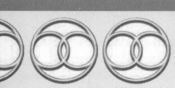

# DEFICIENT FLUID VOLUME

## DEFINITION

State in which a client who can take fluids (not NPO) experiences or is at risk of experiencing dehydration

## DEFINING CHARACTERISTICS

### Major (Must Be Present, One or More)

Insufficient oral fluid intake
Negative balance of intake and output

Dry skin/mucous membranes
Weight loss

### Minor (May Be Present)

Increased serum sodium
Concentrated urine or urinary frequency

Thirst/nausea/anorexia
Decreased urine output or excessive urine output

## RELATED FACTORS

### Pathophysiologic

***Related to excessive urinary output***
Uncontrolled diabetes
Diabetes insipidus (inadequate antidiuretic hormone)
***Related to increased capillary permeability and evaporative loss from burn wound (nonacute)***
***Related to losses secondary to:***
Fever or increased metabolic rate
Abnormal drainage
Wound
Excessive menses

Peritonitis
Diarrhea

## Situational (Personal, Environmental)

> *Related to vomiting/nausea*
> *Related to decreased motivation to drink liquids secondary to:*
> Depression  Fatigue
> *Related to fad diets/fasting*
> *Related to high-solute tube feedings*
> *Related to difficulty swallowing or feeding self secondary to:*
> Oral or throat pain    Fatigue
> *Related to extreme heat/sun/dryness*
> *Related to excessive loss through:*
> Indwelling catheters  Drains
> *Related to insufficient fluids for exercise effort or weather conditions*
> *Related to excessive use of:*
> Laxatives or enemas  Diuretics, alcohol, or caffeine

## Maturational

> **Infant/Child**
> *Related to increased vulnerability secondary to:*
> Decreased fluid reserve and decreased ability to concentrate urine

> **Older Adult**
> *Related to increased vulnerability secondary to:*
> Decreased fluid reserve and decreased sensation of thirst

### ■■■■■■ AUTHOR'S NOTE

*Deficient Fluid Volume* frequently is used incorrectly to describe people who are NPO, in hypovolemic shock, or experiencing bleeding. This author recommends its use only when a client has insufficient oral fluid intake but can drink. If the client cannot drink or needs intravenous therapy refer to the collaborative problems in Section 3: Risk for Complications of Hypovolemia and Risk for Complications of Electrolyte Imbalances

   Should *Deficient Fluid Volume* be used to represent such clinical situations as shock, renal failure, or thermal injury? Most nurses would agree that these are collaborative problems to report to the physician for collaborative treatments.

### ■■■■■■ ERRORS IN DIAGNOSTIC STATEMENTS

1. *Risk for Deficient Fluid Volume related to increased capillary permeability, protein shifts, inflammatory process, and evaporation secondary to burn injuries*
   This diagnosis does not represent a situation for which nurses could prescribe interventions with achievable outcomes (e.g., "Client will have stable vital signs and adequate urine output [0.5 to 1.0 mL/kg]"). Because both nurse- and physician-prescribed interventions are needed to accomplish this outcome, this situation is actually the collaborative problem *RC of Fluid/Electrolyte Imbalance* with the nursing goal of "The nurse will monitor to detect fluid and electrolyte imbalances."
2. *Deficient Fluid Volume related to effects of NPO status*
   Managing fluid balance in an NPO client is a nursing responsibility involving both nurse- and physician-prescribed interventions. Thus, this situation is best described as *RC of Fluid/Electrolyte Imbalance*. If the nurse wants to specify etiology, he or she can write *RC of Fluid/Electrolyte Imbalance related to NPO state*. This usually is not necessary, however.

   When a client can drink but is not drinking sufficient amounts, *Deficient Fluid Volume related to decreased desire to drink fluids secondary to fatigue and pain* may apply.

## ■ KEY CONCEPTS

### Generic Considerations

- Table II.7 shows average intake and output over 24 h for an adult. Ingested and excreted water and electrolytes (sodium, potassium, chloride) influence fluid balance.
- The two main causes of deficient fluid volume are inadequate fluid intake and increased fluid and electrolyte losses (e.g., gastrointestinal, urinary, skin, third-space [edema]).
- Vomiting or gastric suctioning results in fluid, potassium, and hydrogen losses.
- The thirst sensation primarily regulates fluid intake. The kidneys' ability to concentrate urine primarily regulates fluid output.
- Urine specific gravity reflects the kidneys' ability to concentrate urine; the range of urine specific gravity varies with the state of hydration and the solids to be excreted. (Specific gravity is elevated with dehydration, signifying concentrated urine.) Normal values are 1.010 to 1.025. Diluted values are less than 1.010. Concentrated values are greater than 1.025.
- People at high risk for fluid imbalance include the following:
  - Those taking medication for fluid retention, high blood pressure, seizures, or "anxiety" (tranquilizers)
  - Those with diabetes, cardiac disease, excessive alcohol intake, malnourishment, obesity, or gastrointestinal distress
  - Adults older than 60 years and children younger than 6 years of age (decreased sensation of thirst)
  - Those who are confused, depressed, comatose, or lethargic (no sensation of thirst)
  - Athletes unaware of the need to replace electrolytes as well as fluids
- Excessive fluid and electrolyte loss can be expected during:

  Fever or increased metabolic rate    Climate extremes (heat/dryness)
  Extreme exercise or diaphoresis    Excessive vomiting or diarrhea
  Burns, tissue insult, fistulas
- Fluid balance maintenance is a major concern for all athletes competing in hot climates. The following is true for both men and women (Maughan, Leiper, & Shirreffs, 1997):
- Drinking large volumes of plain water will inhibit thirst and promote a diuretic response.
- To maintain hydration during extreme exercise, high levels of sodium (as much as 50 to 60 mmol) and possibly some potassium to replace losses in sweat are needed.
- Palatability of drinks is important to stimulate intake and ensure adequate volume replacement.
- Because adequate hydration greatly affects athletic performance, the goal should be to be hydrated *at the beginning* of exercise and to maintain hydration as well as possible thereafter, focusing on replacing salt loss as well as water.

## Pediatric Considerations

Infants are vulnerable to fluid loss because of the following:
- They can lose more water rapidly because their bodies have a higher proportion of water.
- More fluid is in the extracellular space, from where it is lost more easily.
- They have a greater metabolic turnover of water.
- Homeostatic regulation (i.e., renal function) is immature.
- They have a greater surface area relative to body mass

### TABLE II.7 AVERAGE INTAKE AND OUTPUT IN AN ADULT FOR A 24-HOUR PERIOD

| Intake | | Output | |
|---|---|---|---|
| Oral liquids | 1,300 mL | Urine | 1,500 mL |
| Water in food | 1,000 mL | Stool | 200 mL |
| Water produced by metabolism | 300 mL | Insensible | |
| **Total** | 2,600 mL | Lungs | 300 mL |
| | | Skin | 600 mL |
| | | **Total** | 2,600 mL |

Metheny N. (2000). *Fluid and electrolyte balance: Nursing considerations* (4th ed.). Philadelphia: Lippincott Williams & Wilkins.

## Geriatric Considerations

- A general decrease in thirst with aging puts older adults at risk for not drinking sufficient fluids to maintain adequate hydration.
- Older adults are more susceptible to fluid loss and dehydration because of (Sansevero, 1997, Bennett, 2000):
  - Decreased percentage of total body water
  - Decreased renal blood flow and glomerular filtration
  - Impaired ability to regulate temperature
  - Decreased ability to concentrate urine
  - Increased physical disabilities (decrease access to fluids)
  - Self-limiting of fluids for fear of incontinence
  - Diminished thirst sensation
- About 75% of fluid intake in older adults occurs between 6 AM and 6 PM (Miller, 2009).
- Cognitive impairments can interfere with recognition of cues of thirst.
- Dehydration, defined as diminished total body water content, is the most common fluid and electrolyte disturbance among older adults. Because it is associated with morbidity and mortality rates, careful screening and prevention in primary care settings are essential.
- Dehydration in nursing home residents is a complex problem that requires a comprehensive approach, including facility-wide involvement and use of checklists to ensure adequate hydration (Zembruski, 1997).

## Focus Assessment Criteria

### Subjective Data

*Assess for Defining Characteristics*

Decreased thirst

*Assess for Related Factors*

Refer to Related Factors.

### Objective Data

*Assess for Defining Characteristics*

**Present Weight/Usual Weight**
Weight loss (How much? Since when?)
Fluid intake (amounts, type, *last 2 to 48 h*)
Mucosa (lips, gums) (dry)
Skin Moisture (dry or diaphoretic)          Color (pale or flushed)
Tongue (furrowed/dry)                        Fontanelles of infants (depressed)
   Eyeballs (sunken)
Tachycardia

**Urine Output**
Amount (varied; very large or minimal amount)
Color (amber; very dark or very light; clear? cloudy?)
Specific gravity (increased or decreased)
Odor

*Assess for Related Factors*

**Abnormal or Excessive Fluid Loss**
Liquid stools                        Vomiting or gastric suction
Diuresis or polyuria                   (e.g., fistulas, drains)
Abnormal or excessive drainage        Diaphoresis
Fever                                Loss of skin surfaces (e.g., healing burns)

**Decreased Fluid Intake Related to:**

Fatigue

Depression/disorientation

Physical limitations (e.g., cannot hold glass)

Decreased level of consciousness

Nausea or anorexia

For more information on Focus Assessment Criteria, visit http://thepoint.lww.com.

---

**NOC**

Electrolyte and Acid/
Base Balance, Fluid
Balance, Hydration

## ➤ Goal

The client will maintain urine specific gravity within normal range.

### Indicators

- Increase fluid intake to a specified amount according to age and metabolic needs.
- Identify risk factors for fluid deficit and relate need for increased fluid intake as indicated.
- Demonstrate no signs and symptoms of dehydration.

---

**NIC**

Fluid/Electrolyte
Management, Fluid
Monitoring

## ➤ General Interventions

## Assess Causative Factors

### Prevent Dehydration in High-Risk Clients (see Key Concepts)

Monitor client intake; ensure at least 2,000 mL of oral fluids every 24 h. Offer fluids that are desired hourly.

Teach the client to avoid coffee, tea, grapefruit juice, sugared drinks, and alcohol.

**R:** Large amounts of sugar, alcohol, and caffeine act as diuretics that increase urine production and may cause dehydration.

Monitor output; ensure at least 5 mg/kg per h.

**R:** Monitoring of output will help to evaluate hydration status early.

Weigh the client daily in the same clothes, at the same time. A 2% to 4% weight loss indicates mild dehydration; 5% to 9% weight loss indicates moderate dehydration.

**R:** To monitor weight effectively, weights should be measured at the same time on the same scale with the same clothes.

Monitor urine and serum electrolytes, blood urea nitrogen, osmolality, creatinine, hematocrit, and hemoglobin.

**R:** These laboratory studies will reflect hydration status.

For older people scheduled to fast before diagnostic studies, advise them to increase fluid intake 8 h before fasting.

**R:** This will reduce the risks of dehydration.

Review the client's medications. Do they contribute to dehydration (e.g., diuretics)? Do they require increased fluid intake (e.g., lithium)?

**R:** Certain medications can contribute to dehydration.

**R:** Output may exceed intake, which already may be inadequate to compensate for insensible losses.

## Initiate Health Teaching, as Indicated

Give verbal and written directions for desired fluids and amounts.

Include the client/family in keeping a written record of fluid intake, output, and daily weights.

Provide a list of alternative fluids (e.g., ice cream, pudding).

Explain the need to increase fluids during exercise, fever, infection, and hot weather.

Teach the client/family how to observe for dehydration (especially in infants, elderly) and to intervene by increasing fluid intake (see Subjective and Objective Data for signs of dehydration).

**R:** Careful monitoring after discharge will be needed for at-risk clients.

*For Athletes*

Stress the need to hydrate before and during exercise, preferably with a high–sodium-content beverage. (Refer to *Hyperthermia* for additional interventions.)

## Pediatric Interventions

### To Increase Fluid Intake, Offer:

- Appealing fluids (popsicles, frozen juice bars, snow cones, water, milk, Jell-O); let the child help make them
- Use unusual containers (colorful cups, straws)
- A game or activity (e.g., on a chart, have the child cross out the number of cups he or she drank each day)

Read a book to the child and have him or her drink a sip when turning a page, or have a tea party.
Have child take a drink when it is his or her turn in a game.
Set a schedule for supplementary liquids to promote the habit of in-between–meal fluids (e.g., juice or Kool-Aid at 10 AM and 2 PM each day).
Decorate straws.
Let the child fill small cups with a syringe.
Make a progress poster; use stickers or stars to indicate fluid goals met.

**R:** A variety of age-appropriate strategies can be used to increase fluid intake.

Older children usually respond to the challenge of meeting a specific intake goal.
Rewards and contracts are also effective (e.g., a sticker for drinking a certain amount).
Young children usually respond to games that integrate drinking fluids.

### For Fever in Children Younger Than 5 Years
Work to attain a temperature below 101° F (38.4° C) with medication (acetaminophen or ibuprofen) only. Instruct parents to closely follow instructions for age.

**R:** Aspirin is not to be used in children with fevers due to its association with Reye's syndrome.

Overdose of these medications can cause liver toxicity.
Dress children in lightweight pajamas, and infant in diapers only.

**R:** Overdressing increases the child's temperature and does not prevent trembling (Pillitteri, 2009).

Should a seizure occur; instruct the parents to:

- Not give oral medications.
- Place cool washcloths on forehead, axillary, and groin areas.
- Transport the child to the emergency room.

**R:** Seizures can occur with high fevers (102° to 104° F); immediate medical evaluation is needed.

### For Fluid Replacement, Refer to Pediatric Interventions Under Diarrhea

## Geriatric Interventions

Monitor for signs of dehydration, dizziness, weakness, mucous membrane, and intake versus output.

**R:** The elderly are at high risk for dehydration due to decreased thirst sensation, decreased fluid volume, and decreased ability to concentrate urine (Bennett, 2000).

Avoid caffeine, alcohol, and high sugar foods and drinks.

**R:** Large amounts of sugar, alcohol, and caffeine act as diuretics that increase urine production and may cause dehydration.

Explain to the client the need to drink fluids and to use a system for reminding himself or herself not to rely on thirst.

*(continued)*

**Geriatric Interventions** *Continued*

Incorporate strategies to prompt fluid intake:

- Fill a large pitcher of water in the morning to monitor intake.
- Drink an extra glass of water with medications.
- In care facilities, structure a schedule with a beverage cart with choices.

**R:** Strategies that include verbal prompting and choices of fluids will increase fluid intake. Elders who live alone need help to design prompts that will remind them to drink.

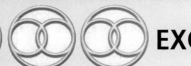

# EXCESS FLUID VOLUME

## DEFINITION

State in which a client experiences or is at risk of experiencing intracellular or interstitial fluid overload

## DEFINING CHARACTERISTICS

### Major (Must Be Present, One or More)

Edema (peripheral, sacral)    Taut, shiny skin

### Minor (May Be Present)

Intake greater than output    Shortness of breath    Weight gain

## RELATED FACTORS

### Pathophysiologic

*Related to compromised regulatory mechanisms secondary to:*
Renal failure (acute or chronic)    Systemic and metabolic abnormalities
Endocrine dysfunction    Lipedema

*Related to portal hypertension, lower plasma colloidal osmotic pressure, and sodium retention secondary to:*
Liver disease    Cirrhosis    Ascites
Cancer

*Related to venous and arterial abnormalities secondary to:*
Varicose veins    Phlebitis    Infection
Peripheral vascular disease    Immobility    Trauma
Thrombus    Lymphedema    Neoplasms

### Treatment-Related

*Related to sodium and water retention secondary to:*
Corticosteroid therapy
*Related to inadequate lymphatic drainage secondary to:*
Mastectomy

### Situational (Personal, Environmental)

*Related to excessive sodium intake/fluid intake*

*Related to low protein intake:*

Fad diets                                    Malnutrition

*Related to dependent venous pooling/venostasis secondary to:*

Standing or sitting for          Immobility          Tight cast or bandage
   long periods

*Related to venous compression from pregnant uterus*

## Maturational

Older Adult

*Related to impaired venous return secondary to increased peripheral resistance and decreased efficiency of valves*

## AUTHOR'S NOTE

*Excess Fluid Volume* frequently is used incorrectly to describe pulmonary edema, ascites, or renal failure. These are all collaborative problems that should not be renamed as *Excess Fluid Volume. Refer to Section 3 for Collaborative Pproblems related to renal failure, pulmonary edema, and hepatic dysfunction.* This diagnosis represents a situation for which nurses can prescribe if the focus is on peripheral edema. Nursing interventions center on teaching the client or family how to minimize edema and protect tissue.

## ERRORS IN DIAGNOSTIC STATEMENTS

1. *Risk for Excess Fluid Volume related to left-sided mastectomy*
   For this diagnosis, the nurse would institute strategies to reduce edema and teach the client how to manage it. Thus, the nurse would write the diagnosis as *Risk for Excess Fluid Volume related to lack of knowledge of techniques to reduce edema secondary to compromised lymphatic function.* If edema were present, the nurse might use *Risk for Impaired Physical Mobility related to effects of lymphedema on motion.*

2. *Excess Fluid Volume related to portal hypertension and decreased colloid osmotic pressure secondary to cirrhosis*
   This diagnosis requires frequent monitoring, electrolyte replacement, diuretic therapy, dietary restrictions, and plasma expander therapy. These interventions call for three collaborative problems: (1) *RC of Hepatic Dysfunction,* (2) *RC of Negative nitrogen balance,* and (3) *RC of Hypokalemia.* Because edema predisposes skin to injury and breakdown, the nurse also could use *Risk for Impaired Skin Integrity related to vulnerability of skin secondary to edema.*

## KEY CONCEPTS

### Generic Considerations

- See *Deficient Fluid Volume.*
- Edema results from the accumulation of fluid in the interstitial compartment of the extravascular space. Without intervention, edema can progress to further tissue damage and permanent swelling.
- Determining the underlying cause is essential to identifying specific interventions.
- Peripheral edema should be classified as unilateral or bilateral. *Unilateral* usually results from venous and arterial abnormalities, lymphedema, infection, trauma, and neoplasms. *Bilateral* usually results from congestive heart failure, systemic and metabolic abnormalities, endocrine dysfunction, lipedema, and pregnancy (Terry, O'Brien, & Kerstein, 1998).
- People with cardiac pump failure are at high risk for excesses in both vascular and tissue fluids (i.e., pulmonary and peripheral edema). Pulmonary edema is a medical emergency.

 **Maternal Considerations**

Increased estrogen levels during pregnancy cause water retention of 6 to 8 L to supply tissue needs for water and electrolytes.

**Geriatric Considerations**

Older adults are prone to stasis edema of the feet and ankles as a result of increased vein tortuosity and dilatation and decreased valve efficiency (Miller, 2007).

## Focus Assessment Criteria

### Subjective Data

#### *Assess for Defining Characteristics*

**History of Symptoms**
*Complaints of:*
Shortness of breath          Weakness/fatigue          Weight gain
Edema
*Onset/duration*

#### *Assess for Related Factors*

See Related Factors.

### Objective Data

#### *Assess for Defining Characteristics*

**Signs of Fluid Overload**
*Pulse (bounding or dysrhythmic)*
*Respirations*
  Rate (tachypnea)          Lung sounds (rales or rhonchi)
  Quality (labored or shallow)
*Blood pressure (elevated)*
*Edema*
Press thumb for at least 5 s into the skin, and note any remaining indentations.
Rate edema according to the following scale:

- None = 0
- Trace = +1
- Moderate = +2
- Deep = +3
- Very deep = +4

Note degree and location (feet, ankles, legs, arms, sacral, generalized).
*Weight gain (weigh daily on the same scale, at the same time)*
*Neck vein distention (distended neck veins at 45-degree elevation of head may indicate fluid overload or decreased cardiac output)*
For more information on Focus Assessment Criteria, visit http://thepoint.lww.com.

**NOC**
Electrolyte Balance,
Fluid Balance,
Hydration

## Goals

The client will exhibit decreased edema (specify site).

### Indicators

- Relate causative factors.
- Relate methods of preventing edema.

**NIC**
Electrolyte
Management, Fluid
Management, Fluid
Monitoring, Skin
Surveillance

## ➤ General Interventions

### Identify Contributing and Causative Factors

Refer to Related Factors.

### Reduce or Eliminate Causative and Contributing Factors

#### Improper Diet

Assess dietary intake and habits that may contribute to fluid retention.
Be specific; record daily and weekly intake of food and fluids.
Assess weekly diet for inadequate protein or excessive sodium intake.

- Discuss likes and dislikes of foods that provide protein.
- Teach the client to plan a weekly menu that provides protein at an affordable price.
- Teach the client to decrease salt intake.
- Read labels for sodium content.
- Avoid convenience and canned and frozen foods.
- Cook without salt; use spices (lemon, basil, tarragon, mint) to add flavor.
- Use vinegar in place of salt to flavor soups, stews, etc. (e.g., 2 to 3 teaspoons of vinegar to 4 to 6 quarts, according to taste).

Ascertain whether the client may use salt substitute (caution that he or she must use the exact substitute prescribed).

**R:** High-sodium intake leads to increased water retention. High-sodium foods include salted snacks, bacon, cheddar cheese, pickles, soy sauce, processed lunchmeats, monosodium glutamate (MSG), canned vegetables, ketchup, and mustard. Some over-the-counter drugs, such as antacids, also are high in sodium.

#### Dependent Venous Pooling

Assess for evidence of dependent venous pooling or venous stasis.
Encourage alternating periods of horizontal rest (legs elevated) with vertical activity (standing); this may be contraindicated in congestive heart failure.

- Keep the edematous extremity elevated above the level of the heart whenever possible (unless contraindicated by heart failure).
- Keep the edematous arms elevated on two pillows or with IV pole sling.
- Elevate the legs whenever possible, using pillows under them (avoid pressure points, especially behind the knees).
- Discourage leg and ankle crossing.

**R:** These strategies reduce venous stasis.

Reduce constriction of vessels.

- Assess clothing for proper fit and constrictive areas.
- Instruct the client to avoid panty girdles/garters, knee-highs, and leg crossing and to practice elevating the legs when possible.

Consider using antiembolism stockings or Ace bandages; measure the legs carefully for stockings/support hose.*
Measure circumference of the calf and thigh. Consider both measurements in choosing stockings, matching measurements with a size requirement chart that accompanies the stockings.

- Apply stockings while lying down (e.g., in the morning before arising).
- Check extremities frequently for adequate circulation and evidence of constrictive areas.

---

*May require a primary care professional's order.

**R:** Edema inhibits blood flow to the tissue, resulting in poor cellular nutrition and increased susceptibility to injury. Compression stockings increase venous return.

## Venous Pressure Points

Assess for venous pressure points associated with casts, bandages, and tight stockings.

- Observe circulation at edges of casts, bandages, and stockings.
- For casts, insert soft material to cushion pressure points at the edges.

Check circulation frequently.
Shift body weight in the cast to redistribute weight within (unless contraindicated).

- Encourage client to do this every 15 to 30 min while awake to prevent venostasis.
- Encourage wiggling of fingers or toes and isometric exercise of unaffected muscles within the cast.
- If the client cannot do this alone, assist him or her at least hourly to shift body weight.

**R:** These strategies increase circulation and venous return.

See *Impaired Physical Mobility*.

## Inadequate Lymphatic Drainage

Keep the extremity elevated on pillows.

- If the edema is marked, the arm should be elevated, *but not in adduction* (this position may constrict the axilla).
- The elbow should be higher than the shoulder.
- The hand should be higher than the elbow.

Measure blood pressure in the unaffected arm.
Do not give injections or start IV fluids in the affected arm.
Protect affected limb from injury.
Teach the client to avoid using strong detergents, carrying heavy bags, holding cigarettes, injuring cuticles or hangnails, reaching into hot ovens, wearing jewelry or a wristwatch, or using Ace bandages.
Advise the client to apply lanolin or a similar cream, often daily, to prevent dry, flaky skin.
Encourage the client to wear a Medic-Alert tag engraved with *Caution: lymphedema arm—no tests/no needle injections*.
Caution the client to visit a physician if the arm becomes red, swollen, or unusually hard.
After a mastectomy, encourage range-of-motion (ROM) exercises and use of the affected arm to facilitate development of a collateral lymphatic drainage system (explain that lymphedema often decreases within 1 month, but that the client should continue massaging, exercising, and elevating the arm for 3 to 4 months after surgery).

**R:** Compromised lymph drainage compromises the body defenses against infection. Trauma to tissue can increase lymphedema.

## Immobility/Neurologic Deficit

Plan passive or active ROM exercises for all extremities every 4 h, including dorsiflexion of the foot to massage veins.
Change the client's position at least every 2 h, using the four positions (left side, right side, back, abdomen), if not contraindicated (see *Impaired Skin Integrity*).
If the client must remain in high Fowler's position, assess for edema of buttocks and sacral area; help the client shift body weight every 2 h to prevent pressure on edematous tissue.

**R:** Contracting skeletal muscles increases lymph flow. Exercise increases muscle efficiency.

## Protect Edematous Skin from Injury

Inspect skin for redness and blanching.
Reduce pressure on skin areas; pad chairs; use knee-high stockings and footstools.
Prevent dry skin.

- Use soap sparingly.
- Rinse off soap completely.
- Use a lotion to moisten skin.

See *Impaired Skin Integrity* for additional information on preventing injury.

**R:** Edema inhibits blood flow to the tissues, resulting in poor cellular nutrition and increased susceptibility to injury.

## Initiate Health Teaching and Referrals, as Indicated

Give clear verbal and written instructions for all medications: what, when, how often, why, side effects; pay special attention to drugs that directly influence fluid balance (e.g., diuretics, steroids).

Write down instructions for diet, activity, and use of Ace bandages, stockings, and so forth.

Have the client demonstrate the instructions.

With severe fluctuations in edema, have the client weigh himself or herself every morning and before bedtime daily; instruct the client to keep a written record of weights. For less severe illness, the client may need to weigh himself or herself daily only and record the weight.

Caution the client to call a physician for excessive edema/weight gain (greater than 2 lb/day) or increased shortness of breath at night or on exertion. Explain that these signs may indicate early heart problems and may require medication to prevent them from worsening.

Consider home care or visiting nurses referral to follow at home.

Provide literature concerning low-salt diets; consult with a dietitian if necessary.

**R:** Home management of edema will require specific instructions and monitoring.

**Maternal Interventions**

Explain the cause of edema of ankles and fingers.

**R:** Increased estrogen levels cause fluid retention.

Advise the client to limit salt intake moderately (e.g., eliminate processed meats, chips) and to maintain water intake of 8 to 10 glasses daily unless contraindicated.

**R:** Sodium is important to maintain adequate circulatory blood volume. A health care professional should supervise restrictions.

Consult with an advanced practice nurse or physician if client has elevated blood pressure, proteinuria, facial puffiness, sacral or pitting edema, or weight gain of more than 2 lb in 1 week.

**R:** A medical evaluation is needed.

**R:** During pregnancy, possible causes of edema are peripheral arterial vasodilation, sodium and water retention, decreased thirst threshold, the enlarging uterus increasing capillary pressure on the lower extremities, and changes in the renin–angiotensin–aldosterone system (Davis, 1996).

Advise the client to avoid reclining on her back, sitting for prolonged periods without elevating feet, or standing for prolonged periods (Davis, 1996).

Instruct the client to lie on the left side for short periods several times a day and to take a warm tub bath daily.

**R:** Lying on the left side removes weight of the gravid uterus from the vessels, increases venous return to heart, and improves renal function. Research findings have suggested that rest periods in water (i.e., baths) instead of bed rest may better reduce edema during pregnancy.

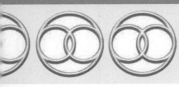

# RISK FOR IMBALANCED FLUID VOLUME

## DEFINITION (NANDA)

State in which a client is at risk to experience a decrease, increase, or rapid shift from one to the other of intravascular, interstitial, and/or intracellular fluid. This refers to body fluid loss, gain, or both.

## RISK FACTORS (NANDA)

Major invasive procedures scheduled
Others need to be developed (NANDA, 2002)

### ■■■■■■ AUTHOR'S NOTE

This diagnosis can represent several clinical conditions, such as edema, hemorrhage, dehydration, and compartmental syndrome. If the nurse is monitoring a client for imbalanced fluid volume, labeling the specific imbalance as a collaborative problem, such as hypovolemia, compartment syndrome, increased intracranial pressure, gastrointestinal bleeding, or postpartum hemorrhage, would be more useful clinically. For example, most intraoperative clients would be monitored for hypovolemia. If the procedure was neurosurgery, then cranial pressure also would be monitored. If the procedure were orthopedic, compartment syndrome would be addressed. Refer to Section 3 for specific collaborative problems and interventions.

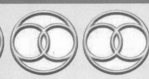

# DYSFUNCTIONAL GASTROINTESTINAL MOTILITY

## ▶ Risk for Complications of Paralytic Ileus

## DEFINITION (NANDA)

The state in which a client is experiencing increased, decreased, ineffective, or lack of peristaltic activity within the gastrointestinal system.

## DEFINING CHARACTERISTICS (NANDA)

Absence of flatus
Abdominal cramping or pain
Abdominal distention
Accelerated gastric emptying
Bile-colored gastric residual
Change in bowel sounds (e.g., absent, hypoactive, hyperactive)
Diarrhea
Dry stool difficulty passing stools
Hard stools
Increased gastric residual Nausea
Regurgitation, vomiting

## RELATED FACTORS (NANDA)

Aging
Anxiety
Enteral feedings
Food intolerance (e.g., gluten lactose)
Immobility
Ingestion of contaminates (e.g., food, water)
Malnutrition
Pharmaceutical agents (e.g., narcotics/opiates, antibiotics, laxatives, anesthesia)
Prematurity, sedentary lifestyle
Surgery

### ■■■■■■ AUTHOR'S NOTE

This new NANDA-I diagnosis is too broad for clinical usefulness. It represents collaborative problems and also some nursing diagnoses as Diarrhea, Constipation. Refer to Section 3 for more specific collaborative problems as Risk for Complications of Gastrointestinal Dysfunction, Risk for Complications of Paralytic Ileus, and Risk for Complications for GI Bleeding.

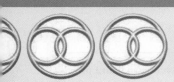

# RISK FOR DYSFUNCTIONAL GASTROINTESTINAL MOTILITY

## ▶ Risk for Complications of Gastrointestinal Dysfunction

## DEFINITION (NANDA)

The state in which an individual is a risk for increased, decreased, ineffective, or lack of peristaltic activity within the gastrointestinal system.

## RISK FACTORS (NANDA)

Abdominal Surgery
Aging
Anxiety
Change in food
Change in water
Decreased gastrointestinal circulation
Diabetes mellitus
Food intolerance (gluten, lactose)
Gastroesophageal reflux disease (GERD)
Immobility
Infection (e.g., bacteria parasitic, viral)
Pharmaceutical agents (e.g., antibiotics, laxatives, narcotics/opiates, proton pump inhibitors)
Prematurity
Sedentary lifestyle
Stress
Unsanitary food

■■■■■■ **AUTHOR'S NOTES**

This newly accepted NANDA-I diagnosis is too broad for clinical use. This diagnosis represents some collaborative problems as Risk for Complications of Gastrointestinal Dysfunction, Risk for Complications of GI Bleeding, Risk for Complications of Paralytic Ileus and nursing diagnoses such as Risk for Diarrhea, Risk for Constipation, and Risk for Infection. Refer to Section 3.

Examine the risk factors in the client and determine if the focus of nursing interventions are prevention; if yes, use Risk for Infection, Risk for Diarrhea, or Risk for Constipation. If the focus is to monitor gastrointestinal function for complications that require medical and nursing interventions use a collaborative problem as Risk for Complications of _____ (specify)

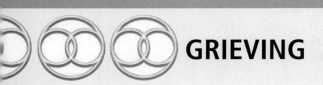

# GRIEVING

**Grieving**

**Anticipatory Grieving***
**Complicated Grieving**

## DEFINITION

State in which a client or family experiences a natural human response involving psychosocial and physiologic reactions to an actual or perceived loss (person, object, function, status, or relationship)

## DEFINING CHARACTERISTICS

### Major (Must Be Present)

The client reports an actual or perceived loss (person, object, function, status, or relationship) with varied responses such as:

| | | |
|---|---|---|
| Denial | Suicidal thoughts | Guilt |
| Crying | Anger | Sorrow |
| Despair | Longing/searching behaviors | Inability to concentrate |
| Delusions | Phobias | Anergia |
| Hallucinations | Feelings of worthlessness | |

## RELATED FACTORS

Many situations can contribute to feelings of loss. Some common situations follow.

### Pathophysiologic

***Related to loss of function or independence secondary to:***

| | | |
|---|---|---|
| Neurologic | Digestive | Cardiovascular |
| Respiratory | Sensory | Renal |
| Musculoskeletal | Trauma | |

### Treatment-Related

***Related to losses associated with:***

Long-term dialysis   Surgery (e.g., mastectomy)

_____

*This diagnosis is not currently on the NANDA list but has been included for clarity or usefulness.

## Situational (Personal, Environmental)

*Related to the negative effects and losses secondary to:*

| | | |
|---|---|---|
| Chronic pain | Death | Terminal illness |

*Related to losses in lifestyle associated with:*

| | | |
|---|---|---|
| Childbirth | Child leaving home | Marriage |
| Divorce | Separation | |

*Related to loss of normalcy secondary to:*

| | | |
|---|---|---|
| Handicap | Illness | Scars |

## Maturational

*Related to changes attributed to aging:*

| | | |
|---|---|---|
| Friends | Function | Occupation |
| Home | | |

*Related to loss of hope, dreams*

### AUTHOR'S NOTE

*Grieving, Anticipatory Grieving,* and *Complicated Grieving* represent three types of responses of individuals or families experiencing a loss. *Grieving* describes normal grieving after a loss and participation in grief work. *Anticipatory Grieving* describes engaging in grief work before an expected loss. *Complicated Grieving* represents a maladaptive process in which grief work is suppressed or absent or a client exhibits prolonged exaggerated responses. For all three diagnoses, the goal of nursing is to promote grief work. In addition, for *Complicated Grieving,* the nurse directs interventions to reduce excessive, prolonged, problematic responses.

In many clinical situations, the nurse expects a grief response (e.g., loss of body part, death of significant other). Other situations that evoke strong grief responses are sometimes ignored or minimized (e.g., abortion, newborn death, death of one twin or triplet, death of illicit lover, suicide, loss of children to foster homes, or adoption).

### ERRORS IN DIAGNOSTIC STATEMENTS

1. *Complicated Grieving related to excessive emotional reactions (crying, anger) to recent death of son*
   Response to loss is highly individualized. Regardless of severity, no response to acute loss should be labeled "dysfunctional." *Complicated Grieving* is characterized by a sustained or prolonged detrimental response; this diagnosis cannot be validated until 18 to 24 months after the loss. The nurse should reword this diagnosis as *Grieving related to recent death of son, as evidenced by emotional responses of anger and profound sadness.*
2. *Anticipatory Grieving related to perceived effects of spinal cord injury on life goals*
   Using *Anticipatory Grieving* here focuses on anticipated, not actual losses. Because this client is grieving for both actual and anticipated losses, the nurse should rewrite this as *Grieving related to actual or anticipated losses associated with recent spinal cord injury.*

### KEY CONCEPTS

#### Generic Considerations

- U.S. culture is devoted to youth and life. Even though death surrounds each person, society views it as pertaining to someone else. Society today has been called "death defying," failing to recognize and confront the realities of death and grief.
- Caregivers must recognize that their attitudes and beliefs about death, dying, and grief significantly influence their care of people experiencing loss.
- Loss can occur without death; when a person experiences any loss (object, relationship), grief and mourning ensue.
- Bereavement is the event: the loss, the death, the divorce, health, and body part.
- Grief is the emotional feeling: anger, frustration, loneliness, sadness, guilt, and regret related to the perception of the loss.

*(continued)*

### ■■■■■■■ **KEY CONCEPTS** *Continued*

- Mourning is the behavioral response and process of resolving the grief; mourning has a beginning, the loss, and it can have an ending, the resolution.
- The flowing tasks of grieving have been identified by Worden (2002) and can assist the nurse in identifying the client's current progression in the grief process:
  - Task 1: To accept the reality of loss
  - Task 2: To feel the pain of grief
  - Task 3: To adjust to an environment in which the deceased is missing
  - Task 4: To emotionally relocate the deceased and move on with life
- The normal grief process may include the following (Worden, 2002):

Feelings:

| | |
|---|---|
| Numbness; shock | Anger, frustration, irritation, misdirected hostility |
| Sadness | Fear |
| Loneliness | Relief |
| Guilt | Yearning |
| Helplessness; out of control | |

Physical sensations:

| | |
|---|---|
| Depersonalization—"Nothing seems real" | Shakiness, edginess |
| Lack of energy, weakness | Dry mouth, increased perspiration |
| Stomach hollowness, "butterflies" | Headache |
| Chest or throat pain or tightness, breathlessness | Same physical symptoms as the deceased |

Thoughts:

| | |
|---|---|
| Disbelief—"This isn't really happening" | Anger—"Why did it happen? It's not fair." |
| Forgetfulness, confusion | Guilt—"If only _____." "I wish _____." |
| Preoccupation or obsessive thinking about the deceased | Forging ahead—"I have to make changes/decisions now." |
| Suicide—"Life has no meaning" | Dread–fear of one's own or another's death |
| Paranormal experiences—sense of "presence" of the deceased, dreams, etc. | Finality—"Things will never be the same." |

Behaviors:

| | |
|---|---|
| Sleeping and appetite disturbances | Yelling |
| Crying, sighing | Increased alcohol/drug/nicotine intake |
| Absent-minded behavior | Activities regarding the deceased—calling out, visiting or avoiding places or objects that remind the survivor of the deceased, talking to the deceased (pictures/ashes). |
| Searching behavior—expecting the deceased | |
| Social withdrawal | |
| Change in work performance—tardiness, leaving early or working late, etc. | |

Shock and disbelief:

- Research findings have refuted the notion that grief is neat, orderly, linear, and completed at an arbitrary point (Boyd, 2001).
- Terminal illness with its concurrent treatments and progression produces many losses:
  - Loss of function (all systems/roles)
  - Loss of financial independence
  - Change in appearance
  - Loss of friends/social support or systems/other relationships
  - Loss of self-esteem
  - Loss of self
- Divorce poses many losses for the partners and their families: roles, relationships, homes, possessions, finances, control, routines, and patterns.

*(continued)*

■■■■■■ **KEY CONCEPTS** *Continued*

- When men lose their spouses, they respond as if they have lost a part of themselves, whereas women respond as if they been deserted or abandoned (Bateman, 1999).
- Disenfranchised grief occurs when social stigma is associated with a death or illness (e.g., suicide, AIDS); the person may be alone, emotionally isolated, or fearful of public expressions of grief (Bateman, 1999).
- Complex social issues of morality, sexuality, contagion, and shame associated with AIDS-related losses interfere with the healing process of bereavement (Mallinson, 1999).
- Gay men who have experienced multiple AIDS-related losses (e.g., loss of friends and community, disintegrating family structures and social networks) may receive little understanding from heterosexuals (Mallinson, 1999).

## Pediatric Considerations

- Children respond to death depending on developmental stage and response of significant others:
  - *Younger than 3 years:* Cannot comprehend death and fear separation
  - *3 to 5 years of age:* View illness as punishment for real or imagined wrongdoing; have little concept of death as final because of immature concept of time; may view death as a kind of sleep; may believe they caused the event (magical thinking, e.g., by bad thoughts about person)
  - *6 to 10 years of age:* Begin to fear death; attempt to give meaning to the event (e.g., devil, ghost, God); associate death with mutilation and punishment; can feel responsibility for the event; may still believe it happens only to other people.
  - *10 to 12 years of age:* Usually have an adult concept of death (inevitable, irreversible, universal); attitudes greatly influenced by reactions of parents and others; very interested in post-death services and rituals; grief may interfere with child's development of identity.
- *Adolescence:* Have a mature understanding of death; may suffer from guilt and shame; least likely to accept death, particularly their own (Hockenberry & Wilson, 2009).
- "The death of a child is emotionally, psychologically, and physically the most painful experience that one can encounter and is often philosophically unintelligible in today's society" (Vickers & Carlisle, 2000, p. 12).

## Maternal Considerations

- The death of a fetus or infant presents multiple stresses for the family.
- Birth of a child with a congenital anomaly creates emotional difficulties for the parents, their relationship with the child, and family functioning.

## Geriatric Considerations

- Grief in older adults often is related to losses within the self, such as changes in roles or body image or decreased body function. These losses sometimes are less easily accepted than is the loss of a significant other (Miller, 2009).
- Many cultures document the death of a mate as the most stressful life event. Increasing longevity brings increased potential for 50 years or more of marriage to the same spouse, with concomitantly greater effects of the loss of that spouse. The spouse may be the older client's only close family member and social contact.
- There seems to be some support for extending traditional bereavement periods to at least 24 months for older adults who have lost a spouse. Of greater influence than the loss of a significant other is the loss of a crucial relationship that provides meaning to the client's life. Even in young widows, the estimate of adjustment period has been extended, based on research showing movement at the 24-month mark from high distress to low distress (as measured on the Goldberg General Health Questionnaire) (Caserta, Lund, & Dimond, 1985).

- Bereavement is a risk factor for suicide. Older adults commit about 25% of all suicides. Suicide attempts are less frequent in older adults; however, the rate of attempted to successful suicide increases to 4:1 after 60 years of age, compared with 20:1 in those younger than 40 years. Men older than 65 years have the highest incidence of suicide; men 65 to 74 years of age have 30.4 suicides per 100,000; men 75 to 84 years of age have 42.3 suicides per 100,000; and men older than 85 years have 50.6 suicides per 100,000 (Miller, 2009).
- Death of a pet can be significant for an isolated older client and can result in a grieving process.
- Reminiscence therapy or life review can help integrate losses. Frequently, older adults use reminiscence to move through Erikson's eighth developmental stage, Ego Integrity versus Despair (Miller, 2009).
- Social supports, strong religious beliefs, and good prior mental health are resources that decrease psychosocial and physical dysfunction (Miller, 2009).

## Transcultural Considerations

- Mourning, a behavioral response to death or loss, is culturally determined.
- "Even if bereavement is regarded as a universal stressor, the magnitude of the stress and its meaning to the individual varies significantly cross-culturally" (Andrews & Hansen, 2004, p. 96). The dominant U.S. culture assumes that the death of a child is more stressful than that of an older relative.
- Puerto Ricans believe that a person's spirit is not free to enter the next life if he or she has left something unsaid before death. Heightened grieving may occur if closure has not been achieved, such as through sudden death.
- Hispanics sometimes express grief with seizure-like behavior, hyperkinetic episodes, aggression, or stupor. This syndrome is called *elliptic*.
- The degree of mourning in the Chinese culture depends on the mourner's closeness to and the importance of the deceased person.
- Grief work for Haitians frequently includes taking on symptoms of the deceased person's last illness (Giger & Davidhizar, 2009).

# Focus Assessment Criteria

## Subjective Data

### Assess for Defining Characteristics

**Present Interactions Between or Among Family Members**
Adults
Children
Maturational level       Understanding of crisis      Degree of participation
Knowledge of expected grief reactions
Relationship to ill or deceased client

**Expressions of**
Ambivalence      Anger      Denial
Depression       Fear       Guilt

**Report of**
Gastrointestinal disturbances          Insomnia          Preoccupation with sleep
Fatigue (decreased or increased)       Inability to carry out work, self-care, social responsibility

### Assess for Related Factors

**Family**
Previous coping patterns for crisis
Quality of the relationship of the ill or deceased client with each family member
Position or role responsibilities of the ill or deceased client
Sociocultural expectations for bereavement
Religious expectations for bereavement

**Individual Family Members**
Previous experiences with loss or death (as child, adolescent, or adult)
Did family share their grief?
Did they practice any particular religious or cultural rituals associated with bereavement?

## Objective Data

### Assess for Defining Characteristics

**Normative**

| | | |
|---|---|---|
| Shock | Disbelief, denial | Withdrawal |
| Anger | Preoccupation | Crying |
| Hopelessness | Sorrow | Sadness |

**Pathologic Pattern (Profound; Progressively Worsened Responses) (Subjective, Objective)**

| | | |
|---|---|---|
| Anger | Isolation | Hallucinations |
| Denial | Obsession | Suicidal thoughts |
| Despair | Delusions | Inability to go back to pre- |
| Substance abuse | Regression | bereavement functioning |

For more information on Focus Assessment Criteria, visit http://thepoint.lww.com.

| | |
|---|---|
| **NOC**<br>Coping, Family Coping, Grief Resolution, Psychosocial Adjustment: Life Change | ➤ **Goals** _____<br><br>The client will express his or her grief.<br>Grief will be freely expressed.<br><br>### Indicators:<br><br>• Describe the meaning of the death or loss to him or her.<br>• Share his or her grief with significant others. |
| **NIC**<br>Family Support, Grief Work Facilitation, Coping Enhancement, Anticipatory Guidance, Emotional Support | ➤ **General Interventions** _____<br><br>### Assess for Factors that May Delay Grief Work |

| | | |
|---|---|---|
| Unavailable or no support system | Dependency | Previous emotional illness |
| Uncertain loss (e.g., missing child) | Inability to grieve | Early object loss |
| Failure to grieve for past loss | Personality structure | |
| Nature of relationship | Multiple losses | |

## Reduce or Eliminate Factors, If Possible

### Promote a Trust Relationship

Promote feelings of self-worth through one-on-one or group sessions.
Allow for established time to meet and discuss feelings.
Communicate clearly, simply, and to the point.
Never try to lessen the loss (e.g., "She didn't suffer long"; or "You can have another baby").
Use feedback to assess what the client and family are learning.
Offer support and reassurance.
Create a therapeutic milieu (convey that you care).
Establish a safe, secure, and private environment.
Demonstrate respect for the client's culture, religion, race, and values.
Provide privacy but be careful not to isolate the client or family inadvertently.
Provide a presence of simply "being" with the bereaved.

**R:** Grief work cannot begin until the client acknowledges the loss. Nurses can encourage this acknowledgment by engaging in open, honest dialogue, providing the family an opportunity to view the dead person, and recognizing and validating the grief (Vanezis & McGee, 1999).

> **R:** *Life review* is a process by which a dying client reminisces about the past, especially unresolved conflicts, in an attempt to resolve them. It also provides an opportunity for the client to evaluate successes and failures.

## Support Grief Reactions

Explain grief reactions: shock and disbelief, developing awareness, and resolution.
Describe varied acceptable expressions:

- Elated or manic behavior as a defense against depression
- Elation and hyperactivity as a reaction of love and protection from depression
- Various states of depression
- Various somatic manifestations (weight loss or gain, indigestion, dizziness)

Assess for past experiences with loss (e.g., losses in childhood and later life).

> **R:** Anger is often perceived as negative; however, it can energize behavior, facilitate expression of negative feelings, and help defend against threats (Boyd, 2001).
>
> **R:** Silent presence and use of touch can covey acceptance of crying.
>
> **R:** Acknowledging that grief responses are expected and normal can support an anxious grieving client.

## Determine Whether Family Has Special Requests Regarding Viewing the Deceased (Vanezis & McGee, 1999)

Respect their requests.
Prepare them for any body changes.
Remove all equipment; change soiled linen.
Support their request (e.g., holding, washing, touching, kissing).

## Promote Family Cohesiveness

Support the family at its level of functioning.
Encourage self-exploration of feelings with family members.
Explain the need to discuss behaviors that interfere with relationships.
Recognize and reinforce the strengths of each family member.
Encourage family members to evaluate their feelings and support one another.

> **R:** Death of a child can put extreme strain on a marriage (Pallikkathayil & Flood, 1991).

## Promote Grief Work with Each Response

### Denial
Recognize that response is useful and necessary.
Explain the use of denial by one family member to the other members.
Do not push client to move past denial without emotional readiness.

### Isolation
Convey acceptance by acknowledging grief.
Create open, honest communications to promote sharing.
Reinforce the client's self-worth by providing privacy.
Encourage client/family to increase social activities (e.g., support groups, church groups) gradually.
Prepare client/family that they may experience avoidance from some friends and family who may not be comfortable with their situation of loss or their grief responses.
Encourage client/family to let significant others know their needs (e.g., support, privacy, permission to share their experience).

### Depression
Reinforce the client's self-esteem.
Identify the level of depression and develop the approach accordingly.
Use empathic sharing; acknowledge grief ("It must be very difficult").
Identify any indications of suicidal behavior (frequent statements of intent, revealed plan).
See *Risk for Self-Harm* for additional information.

**Anger**

Distinguish between the client's general anger and the use of anger in the bereavement process.

Explain to the family that anger serves to try to control one's environment more closely because of an inability to control loss.

Stress that the illness or death did not result from being bad or because the well child wished it.

**R:** Mourners who were very busy with the practical and necessary caregiving tasks of the dying client may not address the impending loss and, therefore, are at risk for delayed grieving response (Stuart & Sundeen, 2002).

**R:** Acknowledging that grief responses are expected and normal can support an anxious grieving client.

**R:** Helping the client identify perceptions of dying and death can provide opportunities to examine their accuracy.

## Identify Clients at High Risk for Complicated Grieving Reactions

Identify clients at high risk for complicated grief reactions:

- Length of relationship: more than 55 years, less than 5 years; consider significance and quality of relationship to the survivor
- Medical issues: pending treatments or surgeries; history of acute or chronic illness
- Mental health history or treatment: outpatient counseling/follow-up; psychiatric medications (depression, anxiety, sleep, etc); psychiatric hospitalizations; suicide attempts; suicidal ideations
- Substance abuse: alcohol or drug abuse treatment
- Suicidality: in family history, suicidal ideation or potential for it
- Family dynamics: alliances, conflicts
- Children: 17 years or younger, either in home or with significant relationship to deceased (e.g., grandparent who lived in the same home)
- Multiple losses: deaths, moves, retirement, divorce
- Traumatic death: circumstances of death, sudden or unexpected, as perceived by bereaved
- Isolation: geographical, social, emotional

**R:** Sudden death or suicide is catastrophic. Interventions focus on helping survivors with valid perceptions of the event, and, in suicide, shame and embarrassment (Mohr, 2007).

**R:** Interventions must begin immediately after a completed suicide, because those left behind experience guilt, rejection, and disillusionment.

## Teach the Client/Family Signs of Pathologic Grieving, Especially Those at Risk

Prolonged hallucinations

Continued searching for the deceased (frequent moves/relocations)

Delusions

Isolation

Egocentricity

Overt hostility (usually toward a family member)

**R:** Mourners who were very busy with the practical and necessary caregiving tasks of the dying person may not address the impending loss and, therefore, are at risk for delayed grieving response (Stuart & Sundeen, 2002).

**R:** Secrecy related to suicide impedes grief work because it thwarts open discussion (Boyd, 2001).

## Promote Physical Well-Being: Nutrition, Sleep-Rest, Exercise for Survivors of Suicide

Encourage them to see a primary care professional.

Elicit their interpretation of the event. Clarify distortions.

Discuss plans for the funeral and notification of friends and relatives.

Discuss the hazards of secrecy.

Allow for expression of guilt, rage, and blame (e.g., of professionals).

Follow up with telephone contacts to family.

Refer all survivors to counseling, especially those at high risk (surviving children; those with inadequate support; those who respond with blaming, scapegoating, or secrecy).

**R:** Secrecy related to suicide impedes grief work because it thwarts open discussion (Boyd, 2001).

## Provide Health Teaching and Referrals, as Indicated

### Teach the Client and Family Signs of Resolution

Grieving client no longer lives in the past but is future oriented and establishes new goals.
Grieving client redefines relationship with the lost object/person.
Grieving client begins to resocialize.

### Identify Agencies that May Be Helpful (e.g., Community Agencies, Religious Groups)

Pediatric Interventions

### Explain What Caused the Death
Clarify child's perceptions.
Openly clarify that the child did not cause the death.

**R:** Children need to feel the joys and sorrows of life to begin to incorporate both in their lives appropriately (Boyd, 2001; Kübler-Ross, 1975).
**R:** Children of parents who commit suicide are at increased risk for future psychopathology and depression and for suicide as a coping measure (Boyd, 2001).

### Openly Discuss Possible Responses
"Sometimes when someone dies we feel bad if we said or did something bad to them."
"Sometimes we feel glad we didn't die and then feel bad because _____ did."
"When someone dies, we can become afraid that we may die also."
"I remember when _____ said or did _____. What do you remember?"

### Explain Rituals (e.g., Read Children's Book on Death)
**R:** Children can be encouraged to communicate symbolically through writing, telling stories, or drawing pictures.

### Assist Family with the Decision About the Child Attending the Funeral and Determine If the Following Are Present (Boyd, 2001):
• Child has a basic understanding of death and good coping skills.
• Child is not afraid of adults' emotional responses.
• The ethnic group approaches death openly (e.g., children commonly attend funerals).
• A familiar adult who is coping well with his or her own grief is available to monitor the child's needs.
• Child expresses a desire to attend and has a basic understanding of what will happen.

### Explore the Child's Modified Involvement in Funeral Activities (e.g., Visit Funeral Home Before Guests Come, Attend After-Service Gathering)
**R:** Children need to be included in grief rituals based on their developmental level or "they may feel abandoned and left to face their fear alone" (Bateman, 1999, p. 144).

### Allow Child to Grieve at Own Pace. Give Adolescents Permission to Grieve Openly. Consider a Sibling Support Group, If Indicated
**R:** Children can feel rejected or unloved if parents or significant others fail to offer emotional support and nurturing because of their own grief (Hockenberry & Wilson, 2009).
**R:** Siblings of deceased children may experience guilt, anger, jealousy, and fear (Hockenberry & Wilson, 2009).

Maternal
Interventions

### Assist Parents of a Deceased Infant, Newborn, or Fetus with Grief Work (Mina, 1985; Hockenberry & Wilson, 2009)

**PROMOTE GRIEVING**

Use baby's name when discussing the loss.

Allow parents to share the hopes and dreams they had for the child.

Provide parents with access to a hospital chaplain or religious leader of their choice.

Encourage parents to see and to hold their infant to validate the reality of the loss.

Design a method to communicate to auxiliary departments that the parents are in mourning (e.g., rose sticker on door, chart).

Prepare a memory packet wrapped in a clean baby blanket (photograph [Polaroid], ID bracelet, footprints with birth certificate, lock of hair, crib card, fetal monitor strip, infant's blanket). Encourage them to take the memory packet home. If they prefer not to, keep the packet on file in case they change their minds later.

Encourage parents to share the experience with their other children at home (refer to pertinent literature for consumers).

Provide for follow-up support and referral services (e.g., support group) after discharge.

**R:** Researchers have found that 100% of parents who held their deceased babies reported positive experiences. Parents who did not hold their infants reported problems with resolution of the grief process.

**R:** In a study, 80% of the parents who did not hold their deceased infants reported it was the decision of a health care professional (Ransohoff-Adler & Berger, 1989).

### Assist Others to Comfort Grieving Parents

Stress the importance of openly acknowledging the death.

If the baby or fetus was named, use the name in discussions.

Never try to lessen the loss with discussions of future pregnancies or other healthy siblings.

Send sympathy cards. Create a remembrance (e.g., plant a tree).

Be sensitive to the gravity of the loss for both the mother and father.

**R:** Fetal/infant death is sometimes viewed as less traumatic than the death of others.

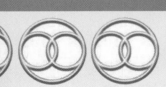

# ANTICIPATORY GRIEVING*

## DEFINITION

State in which a client/group experiences reactions in response to an expected significant loss

## DEFINING CHARACTERISTICS

### Major (Must Be Present)

Expressed distress at potential loss

### Minor (May Be Present)

| | | |
|---|---|---|
| Change in sleep patterns | Denial | Change in social patterns |
| Change in communication patterns | Guilt | Anger |
| Decreased libido | Sorrow | Change in eating habits |

*This diagnosis has been replaced by NANDA with Grieving. It has been included here for clarity and usefulness.

## RELATED FACTORS

See *Grieving*.

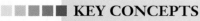

## KEY CONCEPTS

See *Grieving*.

## Focus Assessment Criteria

See *Grieving*.

**NOC**
See also *Grieving*

### ➤ Goal

Grief reactions will be freely expressed.

### Indicators:

- Participate in decision-making for the future.
- Share concerns with significant others.

**NIC**
See also *Grieving*

### ➤ General Interventions

#### Assess for Causative and Contributing Factors of Anticipated or Potential Loss

| | | |
|---|---|---|
| Terminal illness | Body image changes | Self-esteem changes |
| Separation (divorce, hospitalization, marriage, relocation, job) | Aging | Socioeconomic status |
| | Role changes | Impending retirement |

#### Assess Individual Response

| | | |
|---|---|---|
| Denial | Shock | Rejection |
| Anger | Bargaining | Depression |
| Isolation | Guilt | Helplessness/hopelessness |
| Fear | Sadness | Anxiety |

#### Encourage the Client to Share Concerns

Use open-ended questions and reflection ("What are your thoughts today?" "How do you feel?").
Acknowledge the value of the client and his or her grief by using touch, sitting with him or her, and verbalizing your concern ("This must be very difficult," "What is most important to you now?").
Recognize that some people may choose not to share their concerns, but convey that you are available if they desire to do so later ("What do you hope for?").

#### Assist the Client and Family to Identify Strengths

"What do you do well?"
"What are you willing to do to address this issue?"
"Is religion a source of strength for you?"
"Do you have close friends?"
"Whom do you turn to in times of need?"
"What does this person do for you?"

#### Promote Integrity of the Client and Family by Acknowledging Strengths

"Your brother looks forward to your visit."
"Your family is so concerned for you."

## Support the Client and Family with Grief Reactions

Prepare them for grief reactions.
Explain grief reactions.
Focus on the current situation until the client or family indicates the desire to discuss the future.

## Promote Family Cohesiveness

### *Identify Availability of a Support System*

Meet consistently with family members.
Identify family member roles, strengths, and weaknesses.

### *Identify Communication Patterns within the Family Unit*

Assess positive and negative feedback, verbal and nonverbal communication, and body language.
Listen and clarify messages being sent.

### *Provide for the Concept of Hope*

Supply accurate information.
Resist the temptation to give false hope.
Discuss concerns willingly.

### *Promote Group Decision-Making to Enhance Group Autonomy*

Establish consistent times to meet with the client and family.
Encourage members to talk directly with and to listen to one another.

## Promote Grief Work with Each Response

### *Denial*

Initially support and then strive to increase development of awareness (when client indicates readiness).

### *Isolation*

Listen and spend designated time consistently with client and family.
Offer the client and family opportunity to explore their emotions.
Reflect on past losses and acknowledge loss behavior (past and present).

### *Depression*

Begin with simple problem solving and move toward acceptance.
Enhance self-worth through positive reinforcement.
Identify level of depression and indications of suicidal behavior or ideas.
Be consistent and establish times daily to speak with client and family.

### *Anger*

Support crying as a release of this energy.
Listen to and communicate concern.
Encourage concerned support from significant others as well as professionals.

### *Guilt*

Listen and communicate concern.
Promote more direct expression of feelings.
Explore methods to resolve guilt.

### *Fear*

Help the client and family to recognize the feeling.
Explain that fear is a normal aspect of grieving.
Explore attitudes about loss, death, and so forth.
Explore methods of coping.

### Rejection

Allow for verbal expression of this feeling to diminish the emotional strain.
Recognize that expression of anger may cause rejection by significant others.

## Provide for Expression of Grief

### Encourage Emotional Expressions of Grieving

### Caution the Client About Use of Sedatives and Tranquilizers, Which May Prevent or Delay Expressions

### Encourage Verbalization by Clients of All Age Groups and Families

Support family cohesiveness.
Promote and verbalize strengths of the family group.

### Encourage the Client and Family to Engage in Life Review

Focus and support the social network relationships.
Reevaluate past life experiences and integrate them into a new meaning.
Convey empathic understanding.
Explore unfinished business.

## Identify Potential Complicated Grieving Reactions

| | | |
|---|---|---|
| Suicidal indications | Delusions | Hallucinations |
| Difficulty crying | Difficulty controlling crying | Phobias |
| Obsessions | Isolation | Conversion hysteria |
| Agitated depression | Restrictions of pleasure | Delay in grief work |
| Intense reaction (longer than 12 to 18 months with few signs of relief) leading to hopelessness/helplessness | Loss of control of environment | |

## Provide Health Teaching and Referrals, as Indicated

### Refer the Client With Potential for Dysfunctional Grieving Responses for Counseling (Psychiatrist, Nurse Therapist, Counselor, Psychologist)

### Explain What to Expect:

| | | |
|---|---|---|
| Sadness | Rejection | Feelings of aloneness |
| Anger | Guilt | Labile emotions |
| Fear | | |

### Teach the Client and Family Signs of Resolution

Grieving client no longer lives in the past but establishes new goals for life.
Grieving client redefines relationship with the lost object/person.
Grieving client begins to resocialize.

### Teach Signs of Complicated Responses and Referrals Needed

Defenses used in uncomplicated grief work that become exaggerated or maladaptive responses
Persistent absence of any emotion
Prolonged intense reactions of anxiety, anger, fear, guilt, and helplessness

### Identify Agencies that May Enhance Grief Work:

Self-help groups        Widow-to-widow groups    Parents of deceased children
Single-parent groups Bereavement groups

**R:** The knowledge that no further treatment is warranted and that death is imminent may give rise to feelings of powerlessness, anger, profound sadness, and other grief responses. Open, honest discussions can help the client and family members accept and cope with the situation and their response to it.

**R:** Research validates that professional interventions and professionally supported voluntary and self-help services are capable of reducing the risk of psychiatric and psychoanalytic disorders resulting from bereavement (Boyd, 2001).

**R:** Home care of a dying relative can provide the family with choice and control, reduce feelings of helplessness, and promote effective grieving after death (Vickers & Carlisle, 2000).

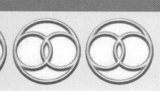

# COMPLICATED GRIEVING

## DEFINITION

State in which a client or group experiences prolonged unresolved grief and manifests in functional impairments

## DEFINING CHARACTERISTICS

### Major (Must Be Present, One or More)

Unsuccessful adaptation to loss          Prolonged denial, depression
Delayed emotional reaction               Inability to assume normal patterns of living
Grief avoidance                          Yearning

### Minor (May Be Present)

Social isolation or withdrawal           Inability to develop new relationships/interests
Inability to restructure life after loss Rumination
Self-blame                               Verbalizes persistent painful memories

## RELATED FACTORS

See *Grieving*.

## ◼◼◼◼◼ KEY CONCEPTS

### Generic Considerations

- Unresolved grief may be difficult to determine because the grief experience has no clearly defined end point, nor is there a "right way" to grieve (Varcarolis, 2002). Some people do experience factors that interfere with the natural progress of grief work and, therefore, its resolution. Rando (1984) outlines seven variations of unresolved grief:
  - *Absent grief:* as if the death never occurred
  - *Inhibited grief:* can mourn only certain aspects of the loss
  - *Delayed grief:* cannot experience grief at the time of loss (e.g., mourner feels he or she cannot deal with grief at the time of loss: "I must be strong for my children now.")
  - *Conflicted grief:* often associated with a previous dependent or ambivalent relationship
  - *Chronic grief:* ongoing intense grief reaction, sometimes serves to keep the deceased "alive" through grief
  - *Unanticipated grief:* cannot grasp the full implications of loss; extreme bewilderment, anxiety, self-reproach, and depression
  - *Abbreviated grief:* often confused with unresolved grief, this shortened but normal form of grief might occur when significant grief work has been done before the loss
  - *Disenfranchised grief:* usually associated with a socially unacceptable or negated loss (e.g., suicide, AIDS)

*(continued)*

■ ■ ■ ■ ■ ■ **KEY CONCEPTS** *Continued*

* Unresolved grief is a pathologic response of prolonged denial of the loss or a profound psychotic response. Examples include the following:
  * Refusal to remove possessions of deceased after a reasonable time
  * Lasting loss of normal patterns of social behavior
  * Progressively deeper regression and depression
  * Progressively deeper isolation
  * Somatic manifestations (prolonged)
  * Obsessions and phobias
  * Delusions and hallucinations
  * Attempted suicide
* Predisposing factors attributed to *Complicated Grieving* are as follows (Bateman, 1999; Worden, 1991):
  * A socially unspeakable or negated loss (e.g., suicide, AIDS-related death)
  * New feelings of dependency and neediness associated with the loss
  * History of depressive illness or previous complicated grief reactions
  * Sudden, uncertain, or overcomplicated circumstances surrounding the loss
  * A highly ambivalent, narcissistic, or dependent relationship with the deceased
* Rando (1984) describes the social factors that can contribute to unresolved grief as social negation of the loss (e.g., abortion, newborn, death of twin, death of frail elderly parent) and socially defined as inappropriate to discuss (e.g., death of lover, suicide).

## Focus Assessment Criteria

See *Grieving*.

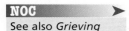
See also *Grieving*

## Goal

The client will verbalize intent to seek professional assistance.

### Indicators:

* Acknowledge the loss.
* Acknowledge an unresolved grief process.

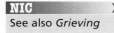
See also *Grieving*

## General Interventions

### Assess for Causative and Contributing Factors

Unavailable (or lack of) support system
History of dependency on deceased
History of a difficult relationship with the lost person or object
Multiple past losses
Ineffective coping strategies
Unexpected death
Expectations to "be strong"

**R:** The more dependent the person was on the deceased person, the more difficult the resolution (Varcarolis, 2006).
**R:** Unresolved conflicts disrupt successful grief work (Varcarolis, 2006).

## Promote a Trust Relationship

Implement the General Interventions under *Grieving*.

## Support the Client and the Family's Grief Reactions

Implement the General Interventions under *Grieving*.

## Promote Family Cohesiveness

Implement the General Interventions under *Grieving*.

Slowly and carefully identify the reality of the situation (e.g., "After your husband died, who helped you most?").

**R:** People with few supportive relationships have more difficulty grieving (Varcarolis, 2006).

## Promote Grief Work with Each Response

Explain the use of denial by one family member to the other members.

Do not force the client to move past denial without emotional readiness.

### Isolation

Convey a feeling of acceptance by allowing grief.

Create open, honest communications to promote sharing.

Reinforce the client's self-worth by allowing privacy.

Encourage the client/family gradually to increase social activities (e.g., support or church groups).

### Depression

Implement the General Interventions under *Grieving*.

### Anger

Understand that this feeling usually replaces denial.

Explain to the family that anger serves to try to control one's environment more closely because of inability to control loss.

Encourage verbalization of the anger.

See *Anxiety* for additional information for anger.

### Guilt/Ambivalence

Acknowledge the client's expressed self-view.

Role play to allow the client to "express" to dead person what he or she wants to say or how he or she feels.

Encourage the client to identify positive contributions/aspects of the relationship.

Avoid arguing and participating in the client's system of shoulds and should nots.

Discuss the client's preoccupation with him and attempt to move verbally beyond the present.

### Fear

Focus on the present and maintain a safe and secure environment.

Help the client to explore reasons for a meaning of the behavior.

Consider alternative ways of expressing his or her feelings.

**R:** Unresolved conflicts disrupt successful grief work (Varcarolis, 2006).

**R:** People with few supportive relationships have more difficulty grieving (Varcarolis, 2006).

**R:** Risk of death is greater in men than in women during the first 6 months of conjugal bereavement. Changes in health behavior patterns, such as nutrition, alcohol use, smoking, and decreased physical activity levels, may contribute to this increased mortality rate.

## Provide Health Teaching and Referrals, as Indicated

## Teach the Client and the Family Signs of Resolution

Grieving client no longer lives in the past but is future oriented and establishing new goals.

Grieving client redefines the relationship with the lost object/person.

Grieving client begins to resocialize; seeks new relationships, experiences.

## Teach the Client/Family to Recognize Signs of Pathologic Grieving, Especially for People Who Are at Risk, and to Seek Professional Counseling:

| Continued searching for deceased | Prolonged depression | Denial |
|---|---|---|
| Living in past | Prolonged hallucinations | Delusions |
| Isolation | Egocentricity | Overhostility |

**R:** Unresolved conflicts disrupt successful grief work (Varcarolis, 2006).

## Identify Agencies that May Be Helpful:

| Support groups | Mental health agencies | Religious groups |
|---|---|---|
| Psychotherapists | Grief specialists | |

**R:** Risk of death is greater in men than in women during the first 6 months of conjugal bereavement. Changes in health behavior patterns, such as nutrition, alcohol use, smoking, and decreased physical activity levels, may contribute to this increased mortality rate (Kaprio & Koskenvuo, 1987).

**R:** People with few supportive relationships have more difficulty grieving (Varcarolis, 2006).

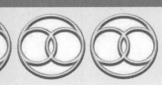

# DELAYED GROWTH AND DEVELOPMENT

**Delayed Growth and Development**

Risk for Delayed Development
Risk for Disproportionate Growth
Adult Failure to Thrive

## DEFINITION

State in which a client has, or is at risk for, impaired ability to perform tasks of his or her age group or impaired growth

## DEFINING CHARACTERISTICS

### Major (Must Be Present, One or More)

Inability or difficulty performing skills or behaviors typical of his or her age group (e.g., motor, personal/social, language/cognition; Table II.8)
*and/or*
Altered physical growth: weight lagging behind height by two standard deviations; pattern of height and weight percentiles indicate a drop in pattern

### Minor (May Be Present)

Inability to perform self-care or self-control activities appropriate for age (see Table II.8)
Flat affect, listlessness, decreased responses, slow social responses, limited signs of satisfaction to caregiver, limited eye contact, difficulty feeding, decreased appetite, lethargy, irritability, negative mood, regression in self-toileting, regression in self-feeding (see Focus Assessment Criteria)
Infants: watchfulness, interrupted sleep pattern

## RELATED FACTORS

### Pathophysiologic

***Related to compromised physical ability and dependence secondary to:***

| Congenital heart defects | Repeated acute or chronic illness | Acute illness |
|---|---|---|
| Cerebral damage | Congestive heart failure | Cerebral palsy |

# TABLE II.8  AGE-RELATED DEVELOPMENTAL TASKS

| Developmental Tasks/Needs | Parental Guidance | Implications for Nursing |
|---|---|---|
| **Birth to 1 Year** | | |

*Personal/Social*
Learns to trust and anticipate satisfaction
Sends cues to mother/caretaker
Begins understanding self as separate from others (body image)

*Motor*
Responds to sound
Social smile
Reaches for objects
Begins to sit, creep, pull up, and stand with support
Attempting to walk

*Language/Cognition*
Learns to signal wants/needs with sounds, crying
Begins to vocalize with meaning (two-syllable words: Dada, Mama)
Comprehends some verbal/nonverbal messages (no, yes, bye-bye)
Learns about words through senses

*Fears*
Loud noises
Falling

Encourage parent to respond to cry, meet infant's need *consistently*
Teach parent not to be afraid of spoiling infant with too much attention
Talk and sing to child; hold and cuddle often
Provide variety of stimulation
Allow infant to feed self (cereal, etc.)
Do not prop bottle

*Toys*
Brightly colored crib toys, mobiles
Stuffed toys of varied textures
Music boxes

*Safety*
Be aware of rapidly changing locomotive ability (e.g., childproof kitchen, stairways; small objects within reach; tub safety)

Encourage parent to participate in care:
  Bathing
  Feeding
  Holding
Teach parent guidance information
Provide ongoing stimulation while confined through use of toys, mirrors, mobiles, music
Hold, speak to infant, maintain eye contact
Investigate crying
Do not restrain

---

| **1 to 3 Years** | | |

*Personal/Social*
Establishes self-control, decision-making, self-independence (autonomy)
Extremely curious, prefers to do things himself
Demonstrates independence through negativism
Very egocentric: believes he controls the world
Learns about words through senses

*Motor*
Begins to walk and run well
Drinks from cup, feeds self
Develops fine motor control
Climbs
Begins self-toileting

*Language/Cognition*
Has poor time sense
Increasingly verbal (4- to 5-word sentences by age 3½)
Talks to self/others
Misconceptions about cause/effect

*Fears*
Loss/separation from parents
Darkness
Machines/equipment
Intrusive procedures

Provide child with peer companionship
Allow for brief periods of separation under familiar surroundings
Practice safety measures that guard against child's increased motor ability and curiosity (poisoning, falls)
Tell the truth
Disciplining child for violation of safety rules:
  Running in street
  Touching electrical wires
Allow child some control over fears:
  Favorite toy
  Night light
Allow exploration within safe limits
Explain as simply as possible why things happen
Allow child to explain why he thinks things are happening
Correct misconceptions
Include child in domestic activities when possible:
  Dusting
  Cleaning spoons
Discuss differences in opinions (between parents) in front of child
Do not threaten child with what will happen if he does not behave
Always follow through with punishment

*Toys*
Manipulative toys
Puzzles
Bright-colored, simple books
Large-muscle devices (gym sets, etc.)
Music (songs, records)

Allow child to take liquids from a cup (including medicines)
Allow child to perform some self-care tasks:
  Wash face and arms
  Brush teeth
Expect resistant behavior to treatments; reinforce treatments, not punishments
Use firm, direct approach and provide child with choices only when possible
Restrain child when needed
Explain to parents methods for disciplining child:
  Slap hand once (for dangerous touching, [e.g., stove])
  Sit in chair for 2 min (if child gets up, put him back and reset timer)
Explain the need for consistency
Allow expression of fear, pain, displeasure
Assign consistent caregiver
Let child play with simple equipment (stethoscope)
Provide materials for play (favorite toy)
Be honest about procedure
Praise child for helping you:
  Holding still
  Holding the Band-Aid
Give child choices whenever possible
Tell child he can cry or squeeze your hand, but you expect him to hold still
Have parents present for procedures when at all possible
Explore with child his fantasies of the situation:
  Use play therapy
  Explain the procedure immediately beforehand if short (e.g., injection) and when appropriate if longer or intrusive (e.g., x-ray, IV insertion)
Follow home routines when possible

*(continued)*

## TABLE II.8 AGE-RELATED DEVELOPMENTAL TASKS (Continued)

| Developmental Tasks/Needs | Parental Guidance | Implications for Nursing |
|---|---|---|
| **3 to 5 Years** | | |
| *Personal/Social* <br> Attempts to establish self as like his parents, but independent <br> Explores environment on his own initiative <br> Boasts, brags, has feelings of indestructibility <br> Family is primary group <br> Peers increasingly important <br> Assumes sex roles <br> Aggressive <br><br> *Motor* <br> Locomotion skills increase, and coordinates easier <br> Rides tricycle/bicycle <br> Throws ball, but has difficulty catching <br><br> *Language/Cognition* <br> Egocentric <br> Language skills flourish <br> Generates many questions: how, why, what? <br> Simple problem solving; uses fantasy to understand, problem solve <br><br> *Fears* <br> Mutilation <br> Castration <br> Dark <br> Unknown <br> Inanimate, unfamiliar objects | Teach parents to listen to child's fears, feelings <br> Encourage hugs, touch as expressions of acceptance <br> Provide simple explanations <br> Limit stimulation from television to avoid intense material <br> Focus on positive behaviors <br> Allow child to help as much as possible <br> Provide child with regular contact with other children (e.g., nursery school) <br> Explain that television, movies are make-believe <br> Practice definite limit-setting behavior <br> Offer child choices <br> Allow child to express anger verbally but limit motor aggression ("You may slam a door but you may not throw a toy") <br> Discipline (examples): <br>　Sit in chair 5 minutes <br>　Forbid a favorite pastime (no bicycle riding for 2 h) <br> Be consistent and firm <br> Teach safety precautions about strangers <br><br> *Toys and Games* <br> "Make-believe" play (play house, toy models, etc.) <br> Simple games with others, books, puzzles, coloring | Encourage expressing of fears <br> Reinforce reality of body image <br> Encourage self-care, decision-making when possible <br> Involve parents in teaching <br> Provide peer stimulation <br> Limit physical restraint <br> Provide play opportunities for acting out fantasy, story-telling <br> Explain to child how he can cooperate (e.g., hold still), and expect that he will <br> Use play therapy to allow child free expression <br> Explain all procedures: <br>　Use equipment if possible; allow therapeutic play <br>　Encourage child to ask questions <br>　Tell child the exact body parts that will be affected <br>　Use models, pictures <br> Explain when procedure will occur in relation to daily schedule (e.g., after lunch, after bath) |
| **5 to 11 Years** | | |
| *Personal/Social* <br> Learns to include values and skills of school, neighborhood, peers <br> Peer relationships important <br> Focuses more on reality, less on fantasy <br> Family is main base of security and identity <br> Sensitive to reactions of others <br> Seeks approval, recognition <br> Enthusiastic, noisy, imaginative, desires to explore <br> Likes to complete a task <br> Enjoys helping <br><br> *Motor* <br> Moves constantly <br> Physical play prevalent (sports, swimming, skating, etc.) <br><br> *Language/Cognition* <br> Organized, stable thought <br> Concepts more complicated <br> Focuses on concrete understanding <br><br> *Fears* <br> Rejections, failures <br> Immobility <br> Mutilation <br> Death | Teach appropriate foods needed each day; provide choices <br> Encourage interaction outside home <br> Include cooking and cleaning in home activities <br> Teach safety (bicycle, street, playground equipment, fire, water, strangers) <br> Maintain limit-setting and discipline <br> Prepare child for bodily changes of pubescence and provide with concrete sex education information (late childhood) <br> Expect fluctuations between immature and mature behavior <br> Respect peer relationships but do not compromise your values (e.g., "But, Mom, all the other girls are wearing makeup!") <br> Promote responsibility, contribution to family (e.g., duties for helping, etc.) <br> Promote exploration and development of skills (e.g., joining clubs, sports, hobbies, etc.) <br><br> *Toys and Games* <br> Group games, board games, art activities, crafts, video games, reading | Promote family and peer interactions (e.g., visiting, telephone) <br> Explain all procedures and impact on body <br> Encourage questioning, *active* participation in care <br> Be direct about explanation of procedures (e.g., body part involved, use anatomic names, pictures, etc.); explain step by step <br> Be honest <br> Reassure child that he is liked <br> Provide privacy <br> Involve parents but make direction of care the child's decision <br> Reason and explain <br> Encourage continuance of school work, activities if condition permits (e.g., homework, contact with classmates) <br> Encourage continuance of hobbies, interests |

*(continued)*

## TABLE II.8  AGE-RELATED DEVELOPMENTAL TASKS (Continued)

| Developmental Tasks/Needs | Parental Guidance | Implications for Nursing |
|---|---|---|
| **11 to 15 Years** | | |

*Personal/Social*

| | | |
|---|---|---|
| Family values continue to be significant influence<br>Peer group values have increasing significance<br>Early adolescence: outgoing and enthusiastic<br>Emotions are extreme: mood swings, introspection<br>Sexual identity fully mature<br>Wants privacy/independence<br>Develops interests not shared with family<br>Concern with physical self<br>Explores adult roles<br><br>*Motor*<br>Well developed<br>Rapid physical growth<br>Secondary sex characteristics<br><br>*Language/Cognition*<br>Plans for future career<br>Able to abstract solutions and solve problems in future tense<br><br>*Fears*<br>Mutilation<br>Disruption in body image<br>Rejection from peers | Encourage independent problem solving, decision-making within established values<br>Be available<br>Compliment child's achievements<br>Listen to interests, likes, dislikes without passing judgment<br>Respect privacy<br>Allow independence while maintaining safety limits<br>Provide concrete information about sexuality, function, bodily changes<br>Teach about:<br>  Auto safety<br>  Drug abuse<br>  Alcohol hazards<br>  Tobacco hazards<br>  Mechanical safety<br>  Sexuality relations<br>  Dating<br><br>*Games/Interests*<br>Intellectual games<br>Reading<br>Arts, crafts, hobbies<br>Video games<br>Problem-solving games<br>Computers | Respect privacy<br>Accept expression of feelings<br>Direct discussions of care and condition to child<br>Ask for opinions, allow input into decisions<br>Be flexible with routines; explain all procedures/treatments<br>Encourage continuance of peer relationships<br>Listen actively<br>Identify impact of illness on body image, future functioning<br>Correct misconceptions<br>Encourage continuance of schoolwork, hobbies, interests |

Malabsorption syndrome · Congenital neurologic defects · Cystic fibrosis

Congenital anomalies of extremities · Gastroesophageal reflux · Prolonged pain · Muscular dystrophy · Inadequate nutritional intake

## Treatment-Related

***Related to separation from significant others or school, or inadequate sensory stimulation secondary to:***

Confinement for ongoing treatment · Prolonged, painful treatment · Traction or casts

Repeat or prolonged hospitalizations · Prolonged bed rest · Isolation from disease

## Situational (Personal and Environmental)

***Related to parental stressor secondary to:***

Insufficient knowledge

Change in usual environment

Separation from significant others (parents, primary caretaker)

School-related conflicts

Loss of significant other

Loss of control over environment (established rituals, activities, established hours of contact with family)

Related to inadequate, inappropriate parental support (neglect, abuse)

Related to inadequate sensory stimulation (neglect, isolation)

## Maturational

**Infant–Toddler (Birth to 3 Years)**

***Related to limited opportunities to meet social, play, or educational needs secondary to:***

Separation from parents/
    significant others
Inadequate parental support
Inability to communicate (e.g., deafness)

Restriction of activity secondary to (specify)
Inability to trust significant other
Multiple caregivers

### Preschool Age (4 to 6 Years)
***Related to limited opportunities to meet social, play, or educational needs secondary to:***
Loss of ability to communicate          Lack of stimulation
Lack of significant other
***Related to loss of significant other (death, divorce)***
***Related to loss of peer group***
***Related to removal from home environment***

### School Age (6 to 11 Years)
***Related to loss of significant others***
Peer group  Strange environment

### Adolescent (12 to 18 Years)
***Related to loss of independence and autonomy secondary to (specify):***
***Related to disruption of peer relationships***
***Related to disruption of body image***
***Related to loss of significant others***

## ▪▪▪▪▪ AUTHOR'S NOTE

Specific developmental tasks are associated with various age groups (e.g., to gain autonomy and self-control [e.g., toileting] from 1 to 3 years of age and to establish lasting relationships from 18 to 30 years of age). An adult's failure to accomplish a developmental task may cause or contribute to a change in functioning in a functional health pattern (e.g., *Impaired Social Interactions, Powerlessness*). Because nursing interventions focus on altered functioning rather than achievement of past developmental tasks, the diagnosis *Delayed Growth and Development* has limited uses for adults. It is most useful for a child or adolescent experiencing difficulty achieving a developmental task.

## ▪▪▪▪▪ ERRORS IN DIAGNOSTIC STATEMENTS

1. *Delayed Growth and Development related to inability to perform toileting self-control appropriate for age (4 years)*
   Inability to perform toileting self-control is not a contributing factor but a diagnostic cue. The nurse should rewrite the diagnosis as Delayed Growth and Development related to unknown etiology, as evidenced by inability to perform toileting self-control appropriate for age (4 years). The use of "unknown etiology" directs nurses to collect more data on reasons for the problem.
2. *Delayed Growth and Development related to mental retardation secondary to Down syndrome*
   When *Delayed Growth and Development* is used to describe a client with mental or physical impairment, what is the nursing focus? What client goals would nursing interventions achieve? If physical impairments represent barriers to achieving developmental tasks, the nurse can write the diagnosis as *Risk for Delayed Growth and Development related to impaired ability to achieve developmental tasks (specify—e.g., socialization) secondary to disability*. For a child with mental impairment, the nurse should determine what functional health patterns are altered or at high risk for alteration and amenable to nursing interventions and address the specific problem (e.g., *Toileting Self-Care Deficit*).

## ▪▪▪▪▪ KEY CONCEPTS

### Generic Considerations

- *Development* can be defined as the patterned, orderly, lifelong changes in structure, thought, or behavior that evolve from maturation of physical and mental capacity, experiences, and learning. It results in a new level of maturity and integration. *Growth* refers to an increase in body size, function, and complexity of body cell content (Hockenberry & Wilson, 2009). For *Delayed Growth and Development*, growth and development are synonymous, because any disruption that does not affect development most likely results in *Imbalanced Nutrition*.

*(continued)*

■■■■■■ **KEY CONCEPTS** *Continued*

- The following assumptions concerning development are relevant (Hockenberry & Wilson, 2009):
  - Growth and development is most rapid in the early stages of life.
  - Childhood is the foundation period that establishes the basis for successful or unsuccessful development throughout life.
  - Growth and development are continuous and occur in spurts, not straight and upward.
  - Development follows a definable, predictable, and sequential pattern.
  - Critical periods exist when development is rapid and the client's ability to respond to stressors is limited.
  - Growth proceeds in a cephalocaudal, proximodistal direction.
  - Development proceeds from simple to complex.
  - Development occurs in all components of a client (i.e., motor, intellectual, personal, social, language).
  - Development results from biologic, maturational, and client learning.
- Often, development is defined in terms of stages or levels (e.g., Erikson's and Piaget's theories). In addition, development may be defined in terms of tasks that must be accomplished. A *developmental task* is a growth responsibility at a particular point in life. Achievement of the task leads to success with later tasks. Various influences affect development, either by accelerating or slowing down the process. Physiologic disruptions, through either genetic malfunction or insult from illness, may potentially alter development, temporarily or permanently. Psychological and social influences also may alter development positively or negatively. Altered development in a child is particularly critical because it may establish a foundation that then remains faulty for life. Because of the rapid acceleration of development in childhood, several critical periods exist (Hockenberry & Wilson, 2009).

## Focus Assessment Criteria

See Table II.8 for descriptions of appropriate developmental milestones/behaviors for each age group, as well as information for nursing interventions and parental guidance.

## Subjective Data

Data should be verified with primary caregiver.

### *Assess for Defining Characteristics*

Developmental level: behaviors listed under developmental tasks (see Table II.8) may be assessed through direct observation or the report of a parent/primary caregiver. The Denver Developmental Screening Tool (DDST) may be used for children younger than 6 years.

### *Assess for Related Factors*

**Current Nutritional Patterns**

| | |
|---|---|
| Diet recall for past 24 h (from parent or child, type of food, amounts) | Parental/child knowledge of nutrition |
| | Diet history |
| | Height/weight at birth |
| Intake pattern | Child's reaction to eating, feeding |

**Physiologic Alterations**

| | |
|---|---|
| Any nausea, vomiting, diarrhea | Allergies |
| Food intolerances | Dysphagia |
| Fatigue | |

**Parental Attitudes**

What are the parents' expectations for the child?
What are the parents' feelings about being parents?
What is the parents' approach to care and discipline of the child?
How do the parents feel about the home situation?
How do the parents feel about child's illness, treatments/hospitalization?
Assess family functioning with an appropriate assessment tool.

### Stressors in the Environment

Illness in family

History of illness or conflict in
    family hospitalization of child

Child's behavior/success in school

Child's peer/sibling relationships

## Objective Data

### *Assess for Defining Characteristics*

#### General Appearance

Cleanliness, grooming

Eye contact

Facial responses

Response to stimulation

Mood (e.g., crying, elated)

#### Response/Interaction With Parent

Spontaneous, happy when
    comforted by parent

Response to procedures, strangers

Reaction when separated

#### Nutritional Status

Height/weight (compare to norms)

Frontal/occipital circumference (also see Focus Assessment Criteria under *Imbalanced Nutrition: Less Than Body Requirements*)

#### Bowel and Bladder Control Personal/Social

Language/cognition

Motor activity: assess for achievement of developmental skills in appropriate age group (see Table II.8)

#### Developmental Level (see Behaviors Described Under Developmental Tasks, Table II.8)

For more information on Focus Assessment Criteria, visit http://thepoint.lww.com.

---

**NOC**
Child Development
(specify age)

## ➤ Goal

The child will demonstrate increased age-appropriate behaviors.

### Indicators (specify for age):

- Socialization
- Language
- Motor skills
- Self-care
- Cognitive skills

---

**NIC**
Development
Enhancement,
Parenting
Promotion, Infant/
Child Care

## ➤ General Interventions

### Assess Causative or Contributing Factors

Refer to Related Factors.

### Teach Parents Age-Related Developmental Tasks and Anticipatory Guidance Information (See Table II.8)

### Carefully Assess Child's Level of Development in All Areas of Functioning by Using Specific Assessment Tools (e.g., Brazelton Assessment Table, DDST)

### Provide Opportunities for an Ill Child to Meet Age-Related Developmental Tasks (See Implications for Nursing in Table II.8 to Assist with Designing Interventions)

## Birth to 1 Year

Increase stimulation by using various-colored toys in crib (e.g., mobiles, musical toys, stuffed toys of varied textures) and frequently holding and speaking to the infant.

Hold the infant while feeding him or her slowly and in a relaxed environment.

Provide rest periods before feeding.

Observe mother and child during interaction, especially feeding.

Investigate crying promptly and consistently.

Assign a consistent caregiver.

Encourage parental visits, calls, and, if possible, involvement in care.

Provide buccal experience (i.e., thumb, pacifier) if the infant desires.

Allow the infant's hands and feet to be free, if possible.

## 1 to 3 Years

Assign a consistent caregiver.

Encourage self-care activities (e.g., self-feeding, self-dressing, and bathing).

Reinforce word development by repeating words the child uses, naming objects, and speaking to the child often.

Provide frequent periods of play with peers and various toys (puzzles, books with pictures, manipulative toys, trucks, cars, blocks, and bright colors).

Demonstrate all procedures on a doll before you do them to the child.

Provide a safe area where the child can move around.

Encourage parental visits, calls, and, if possible, involvement in care.

Provide comfort measures after painful procedures.

## 3 to 5 Years

Encourage self-care: self-grooming, self-dressing, mouth care, hair care.

Provide frequent playtime with others and various toys (e.g., models, musical toys, dolls, puppets, books, mini-slides, wagons, tricycles).

Read stories aloud. Ask for verbal responses and requests.

Say words for equipment, objects, and people; ask the child to repeat them.

Allow time for individual play and exploration of play environment.

Encourage parental visits, calls, and, if possible, involvement in care.

Monitor and use television as a means of helping the child understand time (e.g., "After Sesame Street, your mother will come.").

## 5 to 11 Years

Talk with the child about care provided.

Request input from the child (e.g., diet, clothes, routine).

Allow the child to dress in clothes instead of pajamas.

Provide periods of interaction with other children.

Provide craft projects that the child can complete each day or week.

Continue schoolwork at intervals each day.

Praise positive behaviors.

Read stories and provide several independent games, puzzles, books, video games, and art projects.

Introduce the child by name to people on the unit.

Encourage visits with or telephone calls from parents, siblings, and peers.

## 11 to 15 Years

Speak frequently with child about feelings, ideas, and concerns over condition or care.

Provide an opportunity for interaction with others of the same age.

Identify an interest or a hobby that the unit can support, and support it daily.

Allow the health care facility routine to be altered to suit the child's schedule.

Allow the child to wear his or her own clothes if possible.

Involve the child in decisions about his or her care.

Provide an opportunity for involvement in several activities (e.g., reading, video games, movies, board games, art, and trips outside or to other areas).

Encourage visits or telephone calls from parents, siblings, and peers.

**R:** All dimensions of growth and development have a predictable, definite sequence. New behaviors or biologic parts evolve from those previously established. Each stage is affected by those before and influences those that follow (Hockenberry & Wilson, 2009).

**R:** Of the range of physiologic, psychological, and social influences that may affect development, many exist within the context of illness and wellness care, and nurses often encounter them as they provide care to children. As a result, nursing interventions should be designed with particular developmental information and tasks as the basis. As part of such care, nurses also must consider the influence of the primary caregiver or parent figure on the child's development. Parents essentially control most psychological and social influences in the early years of childhood. By virtue of the child's dependence on parents, these influences can modify development (Hockenberry & Wilson, 2009).

## Initiate Health Teaching and Referrals, When Indicated

Provide anticipatory guidance for parents regarding constructive handling of developmental problems and support of developmental process (see Table II.8 and *Impaired Parenting*).

Refer the family to the appropriate agency for counseling or follow-up treatment of abuse, parent–child conflict, chemical dependency, and so forth (see *Disabled Family Coping*).

Refer the family to the appropriate agency for structured, ongoing stimulation program (e.g., schooling) when functioning is likely to be impaired permanently.

Refer the family to community programs specific to contributing factors (e.g., Women, Infants, and Children Program [WIC], social services, family services, counseling).

Provide a list of parent support groups (e.g., Down Syndrome Awareness, Muscular Dystrophy Association, National Epilepsy Association).

**R:** Illness, hospitalization, separation from family, conflict, or inadequate parental support, as well as specific pathophysiologic processes that interfere with growth, may ultimately affect a child's development. The nurse must support both family and child in ensuring continuance of the child's developmental processes throughout the illness if optimal recovery is to be achieved. In addition, the nurse must seek to stimulate as well as to maintain the child's unique developmental level to promote optimal recovery. Stimulation of the developmental process may occur through parental support or teaching, referral, or direct intervention (see also *Impaired Parenting*).

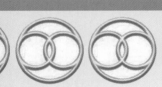

# RISK FOR DELAYED DEVELOPMENT

## DEFINITION

State in which a client is at risk for an impaired ability to perform tasks (social or self-regulating behavior, cognitive, language, gross, or fine motor skills) of his or her age group

## RISK FACTORS

Refer to *Delayed Growth and Development*—Related Factors.

## Goal

The child/adolescent will continue to demonstrate appropriate behavior.

**Indicators (Specify for Age):**

- Self-care
- Social skills
- Language
- Cognitive skills
- Motor skills

## General Interventions

Refer to *Delayed Growth and Development*.

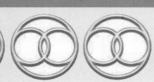

# RISK FOR DISPROPORTIONATE GROWTH

## DEFINITION

State in which a client is at risk for impaired growth (above the 97th percentile or below the third percentile for age)

## Risk Factors

Refer to *Delayed Growth and Development*—Related Factors.

## Goal

The child/adolescent will continue to demonstrate age-appropriate growth.

**Indicators:**

- Height
- Weight
- Head circumference

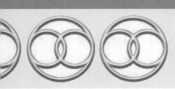

# ADULT FAILURE TO THRIVE

## DEFINITION

State in which a client experiences insidious and progressive physical and psychosocial deterioration characterized by limited coping and diminished resilience

## DEFINING CHARACTERISTICS

### Major (Must Be Present, One or More)

Declining physical functioning        Social withdrawal        Declining cognitive function

| Self-care deficit | Depression | Apathy |
| Weight loss | Anorexia | Loss of interest in pleasurable activities |
| Denial of symptoms | Loneliness | Giving up |

## RELATED FACTORS

The cause of failure to thrive in adults (usually older adults) is unknown (Kimbal & Williams-Burgess, 1995; Murray, Zentnrer, & Yakimo, 2009). Researchers have identified some possible contributing factors, listed below.

### Situational (Personal, Environmental)

*Related to diminished coping abilities*
*Related to limited ability to adapt to effects of aging*
*Related to loss of social skills and resultant social isolation*
*Related to loss of social relatedness*
*Related to increasing dependency and feelings of helplessness*

## ■■■■■ ERRORS IN DIAGNOSTIC STATEMENTS

1. *Adult Failure to Thrive related to dementia*
   Dementia does not cause *Adult Failure to Thrive*, but actually represents a response of the condition. Because the cause is uncertain, the nurse may find *Adult Failure to Thrive related to unknown etiology* clinically useful.

## ■■■■■ KEY CONCEPTS

### Generic Considerations

• Failure to thrive is a "complex presentation of symptoms causing gradual decline in physical and cognitive function that occurs without immediate explanation" (Murray, Zentner, & Yakimo, 2009).
• People not predisposed to failure to thrive (Felten, 2000; Haight et al., 2002; Wagnil & Young, 1990):
  • Have pride
  • Help others
  • Have family support
  • Are perseverant and self-reliant
  • Have experienced hardships
  • Have cultural, spiritual, and religious values
  • Regularly enhance their self-care activities
• Older adults who cannot cope with changes after a stressful life event will feel unprotected, empty, and lonely (Newbern & Krowchuk, 1994).
• "Interaction with the environment is as critical to thriving as a human being at the end of life as at the beginning" (Newbern & Krowchuk, 1994, p. 844).
• Older adults overwhelmed by a sense of helplessness and hopelessness give up.
• Failure to thrive implies that the older adult *should* thrive despite chronic illness and age-related changes. It is not a normal part of aging (Kimball & Williams-Burgess, 1995).
• Resilience is a combination of abilities and characteristics that allow an individual to bounce back and/or cope successfully in spite of significant stress or adverse events (Tusaie & Dyer, 2004).

## Focus Assessment Criteria

Assessing and diagnosing *Adult Failure to Thrive* requires evaluation for new pathology, or, if a condition is under treatment, a thorough functional assessment (physical, cognitive) and evaluation of the client's strengths and coping patterns (Kimball & Williams-Burgess, 1995). Focus assessment for these areas can be found under other nursing diagnoses in this book, such as:

• Self-Care Ability—refer to *Self-Care Deficit Syndrome*
• Cognition—refer to *Confusion*

- Coping—refer to *Ineffective Coping*
- Socialization—refer to *Risk for Loneliness*
- Nutrition—refer to *Imbalanced Nutrition*

For more information on Focus Assessment Criteria, visit http://thepoint.lww.com.

**NOC**

Physical Aging, Psychological Adjustment: Life Change, Will to Live

## ➤ Goal

The client will participate to increase functioning.

### *Indicators:*

- Increase social relatedness.
- Maintain or increase present weight.

**NIC**

Coping Enhancement, Hope Instillment, Spiritual Support, Social Enhancement Family Support, Referral

## ➤ General Interventions

### Consult with a Therapist to Evaluate Client for Depression.

**R:** Depression has been identified in 52% of homebound elderly.

### Assess for Malnutrition, Renal Failure, Dementia, and Dehydration.

**R:** Malnutrition, dehydration, and other conditions can cause cognitive impairments.

## Promote Socialization (Refer to **Risk for Loneliness**).

Attempt to identify one activity that provides enjoyment.
Provide opportunities to increase social relatedness, such as music therapy, recreation therapy, and reminiscence therapy.
Engage in useful and meaningful conversations about likes, dislikes, interests, hobbies, and work history.
Speak as one adult to another. Use average volume, appropriate eye contact, and slow rate of speech.
Encourage the client to be as independent as possible.

**R:** "Interaction with the environment is as critical to thriving as a human being at the end of life as at the beginning" (Newbern & Krowchuk, 1994, p. 844).
**R:** Loss of independence and reciprocity negatively affects self-esteem (Newbern & Krowchuk, 1994).

## Assist Client to Adapt to Changes:

- Elicit unpleasant experiences and promote discussion of them.
- Encourage reminiscing about strengths and successes.
- Validate that adaptation to these changes is difficult.

**R:** Interventions that focus on strengths may help restore self-worth and reduce stress (Murray, Zentner, & Yakimo, 2009).

## Provide Respect and Promote Sharing:

- Pay attention to what the client is saying.
- Pick out meaningful comments and continue talking.
- Call the client by name and introduce yourself each time you make contact; use touch if welcomed.

**R:** Acknowledgment of feelings will increase the client's dignity. Interventions attempt to reverse feelings of uselessness.

## Advise the Family of the Condition and the Need to Monitor Social Interactions for Cognitive Changes and Nutrition.

**R:** Family involvement should improve the elderly client's life (Gosline, 2003).

## Institute Health Teaching and Referrals, as Indicated (e.g., Consult with Home Health Agency for a Home Assessment).

Advise on the need to go outside the house at least weekly, if possible (Kono et al., 2004). Refer also to *Chronic Confusion* for additional interventions.

**R:** Homebound elderly and those with gaps in care have higher rates of depression (Piette, 2005).

For specific problems, refer to other nursing diagnoses, such as *Imbalanced Nutrition*, *Self-Care Deficits*, *Ineffective Coping*, *Confusion*, and *Risk for Loneliness*.

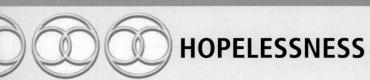

# HOPELESSNESS

## DEFINITION

A sustained subjective emotional state in which a person sees no alternatives or personal choices available to solve problems or to achieve what is desired and cannot mobilize energy on own behalf to establish goals

## DEFINING CHARACTERISTICS

### Major (Must Be Present, One or More)

Expresses profound, overwhelming, sustained apathy in response to a situation perceived as impossible. States "My future seems dark to me" (Yip & Chang, 2006).

**Physiologic**

Slowed responses to stimuli
Increased sleep

Lack of energy

**Emotional**
*Person Feels:*

They don't get the breaks and there is no reason to believe they will in the future
Lack of meaning or purpose in life
Sense of loss and deprivation
Demoralized

Incompetent or trapped
Unable to seek good fortune, luck, God's favor
Empty or drained
Helpless

*Person Exhibits:*

Passivity and lack of involvement in care
Decreased affect
"Giving up–given up complex"
Lack of responsibility for decisions and life
Isolating behaviors
Negative present and future comments

Decreased verbalization
Lack of ambition, initiative, and interest
Inability to accomplish anything
Slowed thought processes
Demoralization
Fatigue

**Cognitive**

Focus on past and future, not here and now
Decreased flexibility in thought processes
Rigidity (e.g., all-or-none thinking)
Lack of imagination and wishing capabilities
Inability to identify or accomplish desired objectives and goals
Inability to plan, organize, make decisions, or problem-solve

Inability to recognize sources of hope
Suicidal thoughts

## Minor (May Be Present)

**Physiologic**

| | |
|---|---|
| Anorexia | Weight loss |

**Emotional**
*Person Feels:*

| | |
|---|---|
| A lump in the throat | Tense |
| Discouraged | Overwhelmed (just "can't . . .") |
| At the end of his or her rope | Loss of gratification from roles and relationships |
| Vulnerable | |

*Person Exhibits:*

| | |
|---|---|
| Poor eye contact | Decreased motivation |
| Sighing | Regression |
| Resignation | Depression |

# COGNITIVE

Decreased ability to integrate information received
Loss of time perception (past, present, and future)
Decreased ability to recall from the past
Inability to communicate effectively
Distorted thought perceptions and associations or confusion
Unreasonable judgment

# RELATED FACTORS

## Pathophysiologic

Any chronic or terminal illness (e.g., heart disease, kidney disease, cancer, acquired immunodeficiency syndrome [AIDS]) can cause or contribute to hopelessness.
*Related to impaired ability to cope secondary to the following:*
Failing or deteriorating physiologic condition
New and unexpected signs or symptoms of previous disease process
Prolonged pain, discomfort, and weakness
Impaired functional abilities (walking, elimination, eating, dressing, bathing, speaking, writing)

## Treatment-Related

*Related to:*
Prolonged treatments (e.g., chemotherapy, radiation) that cause pain, nausea, and discomfort
Treatments that alter body image (e.g., surgery, chemotherapy)
Prolonged diagnostic studies
Prolonged dependence on equipment for life support (e.g., dialysis, respirator)
Prolonged dependence on equipment for monitoring bodily functions (e.g., telemetry)

## Situational (Personal, Environmental)

*Related to:*
Prolonged activity restriction (e.g., fractures, spinal cord injury, imprisonment)
Prolonged isolation (e.g., infectious diseases, reverse isolation for suppressed immune system)
Abandonment by, separation from, or isolation from significant others (parents, spouse, children)
Inability to achieve valued goals in life (marriage, education, children)
Inability to participate in desired activities (walking, sports, work)
Loss of something or someone valued (spouse, children, friend, financial resources)

Prolonged caretaking responsibilities (spouse, child, parent)
Exposure to long-term physiologic or psychological stress
Loss of belief in transcendent values/God
Ongoing, repetitive losses in community related to AIDS
Repetitive nature disasters (hurricanes, tornadoes, flooding, fires)
Prolonged exposure to violence and war

## Maturational

### Child

Loss of caregiver
Rejection, abuse or abandonment
  by caregivers
Loss of bodily functions

Loss of trust in significant other
Loss of autonomy related to illness (e.g., fracture)
Inability to achieve developmental tasks
  (trust, autonomy, initiative, industry)

### Adolescent

Loss of significant other (peer, family)
Change in body image
Inability to achieve developmental task (role identity)

Rejection by family
Loss of bodily functions

### Adult

Impaired bodily functions, loss of body part
Loss of job, career
Inability to achieve developmental tasks
  (intimacy, commitment, productivity)

Impaired relationships (separation, divorce)
Loss of significant others (death of spouse, child)
Miscarriage
Abortion

### Older Adult

Sensory deficits
Cognitive deficits
Loss of significant others, things
  (generativity)

Motor deficits
Loss of independence
Inability to achieve developmental tasks

## ▪▪▪▪▪ AUTHOR'S NOTE

*Hopelessness* describes a person who sees no possibility that his or her life will improve and maintains that no one can do anything to help. *Hopelessness* differs from *Powerlessness* in that a hopeless person sees no solution or no way to achieve what is desired, even if he or she feels in control. In contrast, a powerless person may see an alternative or answer, yet be unable to do anything about it because of lack of control or resources. Sustained feelings of powerlessness may lead to hopelessness. Hopelessness is commonly related to grief, depression, and suicide. For a person at risk for suicide, the nurse also should use the diagnosis *Risk for Suicide*.

## ▪▪▪▪▪ ERRORS IN DIAGNOSTIC STATEMENTS

### Hopelessness related to AIDS

This diagnostic statement does not describe a situation the nurse can treat. The statement should include specific factors the person has identified as overwhelming, as in the following diagnostic statement: *Hopelessness related to recent diagnosis of AIDS and rejection by parents.*

■■■■■■ **KEY CONCEPTS**

## Generic Considerations

### HOPE

- Hope is an unconscious cognitive behavior that energizes and allows a person to act, achieve, and use crisis as an opportunity for growth. It activates motivation and defends against despair (Korner, 1970). It has been defined as any expectation greater than zero for achieving a given goal (Stotland, 1969). Hope is a "common human experience in that it is a way of propelling self towards envisioned possibilities in everyday encounters with the world" (Parse, 1990).
- Early childhood experiences influence a person's ability to hope. A trusting environment promotes hope.
- Hope is related to faith because many people experience hope by recognizing their reliance on higher powers to restore meaning and purpose to their lives.
- Plummer (1988) found high indices of hope in people who have a relationship with a higher being, participate in religious services, and can control their immediate environment. Spiritual practices provide a source of hope.
- Watson (1979) has identified hope as both a curative and a "carative" factor in nursing. Hope, with faith and trust, provides psychic energy to draw on to aid the curative process.
- Researchers have observed that hope prolongs life in critical survival conditions, whereas loss of hope often results in death (Korner, 1970).
- Kübler-Ross (1975) observed that those who expressed hope coped more effectively during their difficult dying periods. She also noted that death occurred soon after these people stopped expressing hope.
- A person's level of hope relates directly to his or her level of coping. Christman (1990) found uncertainty and less hope to be associated with adjustment problems during radiation therapy.
- According to Hickey (1986), hope enables the living to continue and the dying to die better.
- Notwotny (1989) identified six dimensions of hope: confidence in outcome, possibility of a future, relating to others, spiritual beliefs, emergence from within, and active involvement.
- Owen (1989) found hopeful clients with cancer able to set goals, be optimistic, redefine the future, find meaning in life, feel peaceful, and give out or use energy.
- Miller (1989) studied 60 critically ill clients to determine hope-inspiring strategies:
  - Thinking to buffer threatening perceptions
  - Using positive thinking
  - Feeling that life has meaning and growth results from crises
  - Engaging in beliefs and practices that enable transcendence of suffering
  - Receiving from caregivers a constructive view, expectations of client's ability to manage difficulty, and confidence in therapy
  - Sustaining relationships with loved ones
  - Perceiving that knowledge and actions can affect outcomes
  - Having desired activities and outcomes to attain
  - Other specific behaviors that thwart despair, including distraction and humor
- Researchers have found significant correlations between perceived level of control and hope and information seeking.
- Theorists have postulated that hope is a powerful resource that can promote wound healing through the electrochemical reaction that affects the autonomic, endocrine, and immune systems (Jackson, 1993).
- Hopeful people engage in health-promoting lifestyles and self-care.

### HOPELESSNESS

- Hopelessness is an emotional state in which a person feels that life is too much or impossible. A person without hope sees no possibility that life will improve and no solutions. He or she believes that no one can do anything to help. Hopelessness is related to despair, helplessness, doubt, grief, apathy, sadness, depression, and suicide. It is present and past oriented and a deenergizing state.
- Researchers have observed that hope reflected in clients' drawings is related directly to health improvement, whereas lack of hope is related to disease recurrence. Thus, nurses should help clients to find their resources of hope.
- Cancer has been predicted significantly in people based on identifying hopelessness in their lives before diagnosis. Therefore, terminal illness may lead to hopelessness, or a state of hopelessness may contribute to terminal illness.

*(continued)*

■■■■■ **KEY CONCEPTS** *Continued*

- Hopelessness results in three basic categories of feeling:
  - Sense of the impossible: what a person feels compelled to do, he or she cannot; thus, he or she feels trapped
  - Overwhelmed: the person perceives tasks and others as too big and difficult to handle and self as small
  - Apathy: the person has no goals or sense of purpose
- Hopeless people lack internal resources and strengths (e.g., autonomy, self-esteem, integrity). Regardless of age, they reach outside for help because their internal resources are depleted.
- Everyone's life has some degree of hopelessness. It occurs in various forms and is more common and usual than reported (e.g., we all must die; hoping for anything else is hopeless).
- Hopelessness is observed most often in people who are rigid and inflexible in their thoughts, feelings, and actions.
- People may have ideals that are hopeless in reality (e.g., not to die, trusting everyone, all people always act appropriately).
- Engel (1989) identified the "giving up–given up" complex as having five characteristics:
  - Experiencing the feeling of giving up as helplessness or hopelessness
  - Having a depreciated image of self
  - Experiencing a sense of loss of gratification from relationships or roles
  - Feeling disruption
  - Reactivating memories of earlier periods of giving up
- Engel proposed that this state of coping activates neurally regulated biologic emergency patterns, which may decrease the capacity to fight off pathogenic processes. Therefore, the "giving up–given up" complex is a contributing factor to disease.
- Often, when internal and external resources are exhausted, a person relies on his or her relationship with God for hope. The person may feel more secure placing hope in God than in others or self. Hoping in God may not mean an abrupt end to the crisis, but it may give a sense of God's control of circumstances and ability to provide support during this time. Meaning and purpose for life and suffering may be found in a client's relationship with God and the knowledge of His control. Hope for a client's future may depend on his or her perception of a promise of eternal fellowship with God that continues after life on earth ends. With this eternal relationship comes the belief in God's promise to end all suffering and restore harmonious relationships—with God, self, and others (Jennings, 1997).
- Hope and hopelessness are not mutually exclusive. Hope is not the complete absence of hopelessness (LeGresley, 1991).
- Hopelessness can be found in the gay community in response to multiple AIDS-related losses, such as loss of friends and community and disintegrating family structures and social networks. These losses are unending and repetitive and receive little understanding from many heterosexuals (Mallinson, 1999).

**R:** Instilling hope as a nursing intervention was found to increase hope, self-esteem and decrease depression in veterans (Tollett & Thomas, 1995).

**R:** Hope was found to have profound effects on coping for HIV-positive persons (Kylma, 2005) and spinal cord–injured clients (Davies, 1993; Lohne & Severinsoon, 2006).

 **Pediatric Considerations**

**R:** Ninety-four percent of parents with children with cancer followed up at a university center were found to have feelings of hopelessness (Bayat, Erdem, & Kuzucu, 2008).
- Consistent nurturing, trustworthiness, and achievement of hoped-for things and events nurture hope in children.
- Families of children with life-threatening diseases may feel hopeless and become dysfunctional. The nurse may need to identify dysfunctional family interactions, use strategies from family therapy, or make appropriate referrals.
- Hinds (1984) introduced a definition of hope for teens through the use of grounded theory methodology: the degree to which an adolescent believes that a personal tomorrow exists.

- To become an adult, the adolescent must first achieve hopefulness. Hinds, Martin, and Vogel (1987) found that adolescents with cancer progress through four sequential, self-sustaining phases to cope and achieve hopefulness:
  - Cognitive discomfort
  - Distraction
  - Cognitive comfort
  - Personal competence
- These phases have implications for nurses planning appropriate strategies to assist adolescents to achieve hopefulness.
- Hinds (1987) identified that adolescent hopefulness differs from adult hopefulness in that adolescents experience a wider range or greater intensity of hopefulness. In addition, they usually focus on hope for others and believe in the value of forced effort—that is, identifying an area of hope and fostering it.
- Nursing interventions that have been found to influence hopefulness in adolescents include truthful explanations, doing things with them, nursing knowledge of survivors, caring behaviors, focusing on the future, competency, and conversing about less sensitive areas. In addition, humor has been identified as promoting cognitive distraction and facilitating hope. Nursing interventions that inhibit cognitive distraction, (e.g., focusing on nursing tasks and on negative adolescent behaviors) promote hopelessness (Hinds, Martin, & Vogel, 1987).

## Geriatric Considerations

- Older adults are at risk for hopelessness because of the many psychosocial and physiologic changes that accompany normal aging, which often are perceived as losses. Older adults also have decreased energy, and energy is necessary for hopefulness.
- Healthy coping in older adults is related to acquiring developmental resources in later adulthood. Older adults must learn to give up less useful operations and acquire more effective resources to deal with age-related life changes (Reed, 1986).
- Stressors for older adults are unique and differ from those of other age groups. They include changes in personal care, longing for absent children or grandchildren, fear of being a victim of crime, and fear of being taken advantage of by the "system." The nurse may be able to assist older clients to identify stressors and locate resources to prevent hopelessness.
- **R:** Empowerment and instillation of hope in older patients with chronic heart failure was found to be a means by which to promote successful adjustment to the disease process (Yu, Lee, Kwong, Thompson, & Woo, 2008).

## Transcultural Considerations

- Nurses who subscribe to the dominant U.S. culture may misinterpret cultural differences related to values, expectations, and loci of control (Leininger, 1978).
- Hopelessness focuses on an inability to achieve goals, which is future oriented. The concept of hopelessness may not be relevant to cultures that are not future oriented.
- Interventions for hopelessness vary among cultures.
- Disease (in cancer) perceived as hopelessness in certain cultures may be taboo to discuss and delay early detection and treatment.

## Focus Assessment Criteria

Hopelessness is a subjective emotional state that the nurse must validate with the client. The nurse must assess emotional and cognitive areas carefully to infer that the client is experiencing hopelessness. Some of these same cues may be seen in people with diagnoses of *Social Isolation, Powerlessness, Disturbed Self-Concept, Spiritual Distress,* or *Ineffective Coping.* The nurse can use the Herth Hope Scale to determine the level of hope in adults of various ages and with different levels of illness (Herth, 1993).

## Subjective Data

### Assess for Defining Characteristics

#### Activities of Daily Living

Exercise: amount, type

Sleep: time, amount, quality

Hobbies: self-interest activities

Self-care participation: grooming habits

Appetite: eating habits

#### Energy and Motivation

Is the client exhausted, tired?

Does he or she have any goals or desires?

Does the client believe he or she can achieve goals?

Does the client feel overwhelmed?

Does he or she express an interest in any activities?

Can the client solve day–to-day typical problems?

#### Meaning and Purpose in Life

What does this client value most in life? Why?

What does this client describe as his or her purpose or role in life?

Is this purpose or role fulfilled?

Are perceptions of his or her meaning and purpose realistic or achievable?

What kind of relationship does he or she have with God or a higher being?

Does this relationship give meaning or purpose to his or her life?

What does this illness mean to the person?

#### Choice or Control in Situations

What does the client perceive to be his or her most difficult problem? Why?

What does he or she believe is the solution? Is this solution realistic?

Is his or her perception of the problem distorted? If so, how?

Has the client considered or tried other alternatives?

Does this client believe he or she has any control in the situation?

How flexible or rigid are this client's thought processes?

#### Future Options

What does the client believe the future will bring? Negative or positive things?

What does he or she see as worth living for?

How does the future look to this client?

How does this client perceive his or her present illness? Its effect on his or her life? Its effect on his or her relationships?

How does this person perceive current treatments for his or her illness? Promising, or stressful and useless?

Can this client describe something to which he/she is looking forward to happening?

Does this client recognize any sources of hope?

What does he or she want most in life?

Does this client have suicidal thoughts? If so, refer to *Risk for Suicide*.

### Assess for Related Factors

#### Presence of Illness or Treatment

Chronic, prolonged, deteriorating, and exhausting.

#### Significant Relationships

Whom does this client perceive as the most significant other?

What is this client's current relationship with this significant other?

Has divorce or death of a spouse, child, sibling, friend, or pet occurred recently?

Has this client moved away from or been rejected by significant others?

## Objective Data

### *Assess for Defining Characteristics*

General appearance:
Grooming
Posture
Interaction with others
Involvement in self-care activities

Eye contact
Speed of activities

For more information on Focus Assessment Criteria, visit http://thepoint.lww.com.

**NOC**
Decision-Making,
Depression Control,
Hope, Quality of Life

## ➤ Goals

The client will:

- Demonstrate increased energy, as evidenced by an increase in activities (e.g., self-care, exercise, hobbies).
- Express desirable expectations for the near future. Describe one's own meaning and purpose in life.
- Demonstrate initiative, self-direction, and autonomy in decision-making. Demonstrate effective problem-solving strategies.
- Redefine the future, setting realistic goals with expectation to meet these goals.
- Exhibit peace and comfort with situation.

### *Indicators:*

- Shares suffering openly and constructively with others.
- Reminisces and reviews life positively.
- Considers values and the meaning of life.
- Expresses optimism about the present.
- Practices energy conservation.
- Develops, improves, and maintains positive relationships with others.
- Participates in a significant role.
- Expresses spiritual beliefs.

**NIC**
Hope Instillation,
Values Classification,
Decision-Making
Support, Spiritual
Support, Support
System Enhancement

## ➤ General Interventions

### Assist Client to Identify and Express Feelings

Listen actively, treat the client as an individual, and accept his or her feelings.

Convey empathy to promote verbalization of doubts, fears, and concerns.

Validate and reflect impressions with the person. It is important to realize that clients with cancer often have their own reality, which may differ from the nurse's.

Encourage expressions of how hope is uncertain and areas in which hope has failed the client.

Assist the client in recognizing that hopelessness is part of everyone's life and demands recognition. The client can use it as a source of energy, imagination, and freedom to consider alternatives. Hopelessness can lead to self-discovery.

Assist the client to understand that he or she can deal with the hopeless aspects of life by separating them from the hopeful aspects. Help the client to identify and to acknowledge areas of hopelessness. Help the client to distinguish between the possible and impossible.

The nurse mobilizes a client's internal and external resources to promote hope. Assist clients to identify their personal reasons for living that provide meaning and purpose to their lives.

**R:** This gives the client permission to talk and explore his or her life, which is a hopeful intervention (Kylma, 2005).

## Assess and Mobilize the Client's Internal Resources (Autonomy, Independence, Rationality, Cognitive Thinking, Flexibility, Spirituality)

### *Emphasize Strengths, Not Weaknesses*

## Compliment the Client on Appearance or Efforts as Appropriate

## Promote Motivation

Identify reasons for living to inspire hope.

Identify areas of success and usefulness; emphasize past accomplishments. Use this information to develop goals with the client.

Assist the client in identifing things he or she has fun doing and perceives as humorous. Such activities can serve as distractions to discomfort and allow the client to progress to cognitive comfort (Hinds, Martin and Vogel, 1987).

Assist the client in identifing sources of hope (e.g., relationships, faith, things to accomplish).

Assist the client in adjusting and developing realistic short- and long-term goals (progress from simple to more complex; may use a "goals poster" to indicate type and time for achieving specific goals). Attainable expectations promote hope.

Teach the client to monitor specific signs of progress to use as self-reinforcement.

Encourage "means–end" thinking in positive terms (i.e., "If I do this, then I'll be able to . . .").

Foster lightheartedness and the sharing of uplifting memories.

**R:** It is important to recognize constructive possibilities in adults living with HIV/AIDS to promote a life worth living and to recognize a glimmer of hope. Otherwise, one becomes stuck and sinks to a narrowing existence, focusing on the impossible, and loses a future perspective (Kylma, 2005).

**R:** "Lightheartedness," humor, and uplifting memories were found to foster hope in terminally ill people.

## Assist the Client with Problem Solving and Decision-Making

Respect the client as a competent decision-maker; treat his or her decisions and desires with respect.

Encourage verbalization to determine the client's perception of choices.

Clarify the client's values to determine what is important.

Correct misinformation.

Assist the client in identifying those problems he or she cannot resolve to advance to problems he or she can. In other words, assist the client to move away from dwelling on the impossible and hopeless and to begin to deal with realistic and hopeful matters.

Assess the client's perceptions of self and others in relation to size. (People with hopelessness often perceive others as large and difficult to deal with and themselves as small.) If perceptions are unrealistic, assist the client to reassess them to restore proper scale.

Promote flexibility. Encourage the client to try alternatives and take risks.

**R:** If a person recognizes and deals with hopelessness imaginatively; movement, growth, and resourcefulness can result. Rigidity never overcomes hopelessness.

**R:** Motivation is essential to recovering from hopelessness. The client must determine a goal even if he or she has low expectation of achieving it. The nurse is the catalyst to encourage the client to take the first step to identify a goal. Then, the client must create another goal.

## Assist Client to Learn Effective Coping Skills

Assist the client with setting realistic, attainable short- and long-term goals.

Teach the importance of mutuality in sharing concerns.

Teach the value of confronting issues.

Allow the client time to reminisce to gain insight into past experiences.

**R:** Self-reports of mental well-being in 914 prisoners revealed a decrease in sense of hopelessness as the number of minutes spent in exercise increased (Cashin, Potter, & Butler, 2008).

Explain the benefits of distraction from negative events.

Teach and assist with relaxation techniques before anticipated stressful events.

Encourage mental imagery to promote positive thought processes.

Teach the client to "hope to be" the best person possible today and to appreciate the fullness of each moment.

Teach the client to maximize aesthetic experiences (e.g., smell of coffee, back rub, feeling warmth of the sun, or a breeze) that can inspire hope.

Teach the client to anticipate experiences he or she delights in daily (e.g., walking, reading favorite book, writing a letter).

Assist the client to express spiritual beliefs (Jennings, 1997).

Teach the client ways to conserve and generate energy through moderate physical exercise.

Encourage music therapy, aromatherapy, and message with essential oils to improve the client's physical and mental status.

**R:** Music therapy, aromatherapy, and massage with essential oils were found to help the client learn to release stress and express feelings to adapt to current life and face the impact of illness with a positive attitude (Ye & Yeh, 2007).

**R:** People can cope with a part of life they view as hopeless if they realize that other factors in life are hopeful. For example, a person may realize he or she may never walk again but will be able to go home, be with grandchildren, and move around. Therefore, hopelessness can lead to the discovery of alternatives that provide meaning and purpose in life. It is essential to keep hopelessness out of the way of hope.

**R:** Loss of control of life in diseases, such as epilepsy can result in negative thoughts leading to learned hopelessness unless the necessary interventions needed to challenge negative thoughts about situations that one cannot control are provided (Wagner, Smith, Ferguson, Horton, & Wilson, 2008).

## Assess and Mobilize the Client's External Resources (Significant Others, Health Care Team, Support Groups, God or Higher Powers)

### Family or Significant Others

Involve the family and significant others in plan of care.

Encourage the client to spend increased time or thoughts with loved ones in healthy relationships.

Teach the family members their role in sustaining hope through supportive, positive relationships.

Discuss the client's attainable goals with family.

**R:** Maintaining family role responsibilities is essential for hope and coping. In addition, hope is essential for families of the critically ill to facilitate coping and adjustment.

Empower patients who have chronic disease by instilling hope through the bolstering of support systems.

**R:** Clients who live alone with no family support were found to have more symptoms of hopelessness.

Convey hope, information, and confidence to the family because they will convey their feelings to the client.

Use touch and closeness with the client to demonstrate to the family its acceptability (provide privacy).

Herth (1993) found the following strategies to foster hope in caregivers of terminally ill people:

- *Cognitive reframing*—positive self-talk, praying/meditating, and envisioning hopeful images (this may involve letting go of expectations for things to be different)
- *Time refocusing*—focusing less on the future and more on living one day at a time
- *Belief in a power greater than self*—empowering the caregiver's hope
- *Balancing available energy*—listening to music or other favorite activities to empower the caregiver's hope through uplifting energy

**R:** Hope is related to help from others, in that a client believes external resources may be supportive when his or her internal resources and strengths seem insufficient to cope (i.e., a family or significant other is often a source of hope) (Benzeiw & Berg, 2005).

**R:** Hope maintained by family members has a contagious effect on clients.

### Health Care Team

Develop positive, trusting nurse–client relationship by:

| | |
|---|---|
| Answering questions | Touching |
| Respecting client's feelings | Providing comfort |
| Providing consistent care | Being honest |
| Following through on requests | Conveying positive attitude |

Convey attitude of "We care too much about you to let you just give up," or "I can help you."

Hold conferences and share the client's goals with staff.

Share advances in technology and research for treatment of diseases.

Have available a list of laughter resources (e.g., books, films).

**R:** The health care team must be hopeful if the client is to be hopeful; otherwise, the client views efforts of the team as a waste of time.

Provide nurses and caregivers support in times of disaster.

**R:** A study of 41 school nurses revealed uncertainty and a sense of hopelessness in caring for a sudden influx of students with no medical records during Hurricane Katrina and Rita (Breussard, Myers, & Meaux, 2008).

### Support Groups

Encourage the client to share concerns with others who have had similar problem or disease and positive experiences from coping effectively with it.

Provide information on self-help groups (e.g., "Make today count"—40 chapters in the United States and Canada; "I can cope"—series for clients with cancer; "We Can Weekend"—for families of clients with cancer).

**R:** Isolation, concurrent losses, and poorly controlled symptom management hinder hope.

**R:** Hopelessness was found to be a predictor of suicide.

### God or Higher Powers

Assess the client's belief support system (value, past experiences, religious activities, relationship with God, meaning and purpose of prayer; refer to *Spiritual Distress*).

Create an environment in which the client feels free to express spirituality.

Allow the client time and opportunities to reflect on the meaning of suffering, death, and dying.

Accept, respect, and support the client's hope in God.

**R:** Clients with enhanced psycho-spiritual well-being were found to cope more effectively by finding meaning and purpose in the lived experience (Lin & Bauer-Wu, 2003; Jennings, 1997). Hope was found to be positively correlated with spiritual well-being in women with breast cancer.

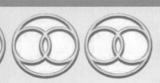

# RISK FOR COMPROMISED HUMAN DIGNITY

## DEFINITION (NANDA)

At risk for actual or perceived loss of respect and honor

### ■■■■■■ AUTHOR'S NOTE

*Risk for compromised human dignity* was accepted by NANDA I in 2006. This diagnosis as approved is problematic. Most of the risk factors listed are defining characteristics (signs/symptoms), not risk factors,, for example, perceived dehumanizing treatment, perceived humiliation, exposure of the body, perceived invasion of privacy, perceived intrusion by clinical personnel, and disclosure of confidential information. This author has deleted the proposed risk factors and has added others.

This nursing diagnosis presents a new application for nursing practice. All clients are at risk for this diagnosis. Providing respect and honor to all clients, families, and communities is a critical core element of professional nursing. Prevention of compromised human dignity must be a focus of all nursing interventions. It is the central concept of a caring profession.

*(continued)*

■■■■■■ **AUTHOR'S NOTE** *Continued*

This diagnosis can also apply to prisoners, who as part of their penalty will be deprived of some rights, for example, privacy and movement. Prisoners, however, should always be treated with respect and not be tortured or humiliated. Nurses have the obligation to honor and "do no harm" in all settings in which they practice.

This author recommends that this diagnosis be developed and integrated into a Standard Care of the Nursing Department for all clients and families. The outcomes and interventions apply to all individuals, families, and groups. This Department of Nursing Standards of Practice could also include *Risk for Infection*, *Risk for Infection Transmission*, *Risk for Falls*, and *Risk for Compromised Family Coping*.

## RISK FACTORS

### Situational (Personal, Environmental)

Related to multiple factors associated with hospitalization, institutionalization, supervised group living environments, or any health care environment

Examples of factors are:

• Unfamiliar procedures
• Intrusions for clinical procedures
• Multiple, unfamiliar personnel
• Assistance needed for personal hygiene
• Painful procedures
• Unfamiliar terminology

Related to the nature of restrictions and environment of incarceration

■■■■■■ **ERRORS IN DIAGNOSTIC STATEMENTS**

**Risk for Compromised Human Dignity related to perceived dehumanizing treatments.**
This diagnosis represents actual compromised human dignity, not an at-risk diagnosis. This situation should be examined, investigated, and reported to the appropriate authority in the agency for immediate action.

■■■■■■ **KEY CONCEPTS**

• Can a nurse maintain and defend the dignity of a client or a group if she or he cannot maintain and defend her or his own dignity?
• "Dignity is a slippery concept, most easily understood when it has been lost" (Reed et al., 2003). Nurses have a responsibility and commitment to protect and preserve client dignity (Walsh & Kownake, 2002).
• Dignity exists when an individual is "capable of exerting control or choice over his or her behavior, surroundings, and the way he or she is treated by others. He or she should be capable of understanding information and making decisions. He or she should feel comfortable with his or her physical and psychosocial status quo" (Mairis, 1994, p. 952).
• The ability to maintain dignity is dependent on one's ability in the presence of the threat to keep intact one's beliefs about oneself (Haddock, 1994).
• People are like other people, like some other people, like no other people (Allport, 1961, cited in Haddock, 1994).
• "Dignity is the ability to feel important and valuable in relation to others, in contexts which are perceived as threatening. Dignity is a dynamitic subjective belief but also has a shared meaning among humanity. Dignity is striven for and its maintenance depends on one's ability to keep intact the boundary containing beliefs about oneself and the extent of the threat. Context and possession of dignity within oneself affects one's ability to maintain or promote the dignity of another" (Haddock, 1996, p. 930).
• To have dignity is to have control over oneself. The effects of loss of dignity are emotional distress, humiliation, and embarrassment (Walsh & Kawanko, 2002; Mairis, 1994).
• Protecting dignity is acknowledgement of humanity in people, alive or dead, rather than treating them as inanimate objects (Haddock, 1996). When people are helpless or unconscious, preserving their dignity is of the utmost priority (Mairis, 1994).

# Focus Assessment

A focus assessment is not needed for this nursing diagnosis. Any client or group who is in any health care facility—for example, hospitals, ambulatory settings, private office, and long-term facility or certain facilities such as residential homes, group homes, jails, and prisons—is at risk for compromised human dignity. *Risk for Compromised Human Dignity* is related to multiple negative factors associated with the procedures and environment of a health care facility.

**NOC**
Abuse Protection, Comfort Level, Dignified Dying, Information Processing, Knowledge: Illness Care, Self-esteem, Spiritual Well-Being

# ➤ Goals

The client will report respectful and considerate care.

## Indicators:

Respect for privacy
Consideration of emotions
Anticipation of feelings
Given options and control
Asked for permission
Given explanations
Minimization of body part exposure
No involvement of unnecessary personnel during stressful procedures

**NIC**
Patient Rights Protection, Anticipatory Guidance, Counseling, Emotional Support, Preparatory Sensory Information, Family Support, Humor, Mutual Goal Setting, and Teaching: Procedure/Treatment, Touch

# ➤ Interventions

## Determine If the Agency Has a Policy for Prevention of Compromised Human Dignity (Note: This Type of Policy or Standard May Be Titled Differently)

**R:** Agency policies can assist the nurse when problematic situations occur; however, the moral obligation to protect and defend the dignity of clients or groups does not depend on the existence of a policy.

## Review the Policy: Does It Include (Walsh & Kowanko, 2002):

• Protection of privacy and private space
• Acquiring permission continuously
• Providing time for decision-making
• Advocating for the client

## Ensure that There Are Clear Guidelines Regarding the Number of Personnel (e.g., Students, Nurses, Physicians, Residents, Interns) that Can Be Present When Confidential and/or Stressful Information Is Discussed

**R:** This type of policy can project a philosophy for an institution for moral, respectful care and for expectations for personnel to be moral and caring.

## Reduce Exposure of the Client's Body with the Use of Drapes and Limit the Gaze of Others Who Are Not Needed

**R:** Clients have reported being exposed as their central concern of humiliation, along with high levels of indignity (Walsh & Kowanko, 2002).

## Provide Care to Each Client and Family as You Would Expect or Demand for Your Family, Partner, Child, Friend, or Colleague

**R:** Setting this personal standard can spur you to defend the client/group, especially when they do not belong to the same socioeconomic group as you.

When Performing a Procedure, Engage the Client in a Conversation; Act As If the Situation Is Matter-of-Fact for You in Order to Reduce Embarrassment; Use Humor If Appropriate; Talk to the Client Even If He or She Is Unresponsive

**R:** Clients reported that when in embarrassing situations that were unavoidable (e.g., a bowel or bladder accident), a nurse who was matter-of-fact and made them feel at ease with small talk or humor (Walsh & Kowanko, 2002).

## Explain the Procedure to the Client During Painful or Embarrassing Procedures and Explain What He or She Will Feel

**R:** Clients reported that they did not like being rushed and needed time to understand the upcoming procedure.

## Determine If Unnecessary Personnel Are Present Before a Vulnerable or Stressful Event Is Initiated (e.g., Code or a Painful or Embarrassing Procedure) Advise Them that They Are Not Needed

**R:** Protecting the dignity and privacy of individual also includes unconscious or deceased clients (Mairis, 1994).

## Allow the Client an Opportunity to Share His or Her Feelings After a Difficult Situation and Maintain Privacy for the Client's Information and Emotional Responses

**R:** Allowing the client to share his or her feelings can help him or her maintain or regain dignity. Recognition of the client as a living, thinking, and experiencing human being enhances dignity (Walsh & Kowanko, 2002).

## Role-Model and Advocate to Maintain Client Dignity After Death

**R:** Role-modeling considerate and respectful care can assist others to a heightened awareness and encourage them to perform this care themselves.

## Discuss with Involved Personnel an Incident that Was Disrespectful to a Client or Family and Report Any Incident that May Be a Violation of a Client's Dignity to the Appropriate Person

**R:** Professionals have a responsibility to practice ethically and morally and to address situations and personnel that compromise human dignity.

## Engage in a Dialogue with the Client and Family Regarding Their Preemptions of the Present Plan of Care, and Decisions that May Need to Be Explained

**R:** "Extremes measures, when futile, were an infringement of the basic respect for the dignity innate in being a person" (Walsh & Kowanda, 2002, p. 146).

## When Extreme Measures That Are Futile Are Planned for or Are Being Provided for a Client, Refer to *Moral Distress*

## "Practice Expecting that Honoring and Protecting the Dignity of a Client/Group Is NOT A VALUE BUT A WAY OF BEING"

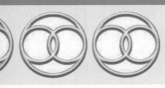 # DISORGANIZED INFANT BEHAVIOR

## DEFINITION

The degree to which an infant has reached his or her organizational threshold and no longer is maintaining self, as reflected in his or her use of varying physiologic, postural, or state strategies, and as reflected across all subsystems of behavioral adaptation (i.e., autonomic, motor, state, and attention–interaction systems)

## DEFINING CHARACTERISTICS (VANDENBERG, 1990; HOCKENBERRY & WILSON, 2009)

### Autonomic System

**Cardiac**
Increased rate

**Respiration**

| | | |
|---|---|---|
| Pauses | Tachypnea | Gasping |

**Color Changes**

| | | |
|---|---|---|
| Paling around nostrils | Perioral duskiness | Mottling |
| Cyanosis | Grayness | Flushing/ruddiness |

**Visceral**

| | | |
|---|---|---|
| Hiccuping | Straining as if actually producing a bowel movement | Grunting |
| Spitting up | | Gagging |

**Motor**

| | | |
|---|---|---|
| Seizures | Sneezing | Tremoring/startling |
| Yawning | Twitching | Sighing |
| Coughing | | |

### Motor System

**Fluctuating Tone**
*Flaccidity of*

| | | |
|---|---|---|
| Trunk | Face | Extremities |

**Hypertonicity**

| | | |
|---|---|---|
| Extending legs | Arching | Saluting |
| Splaying fingers | Airplaning | Extending tongue |
| Sitting on air | Fisting | |

**Hyperflexions**

| | | |
|---|---|---|
| Trunk | Fetal tuck | Extremities |

**Frantic Diffuse Activity**

### State System (Range)

Difficulty maintaining state control
Difficulty in transitions from one state to another

**Sleep**

| | | |
|---|---|---|
| Twitches | Whimpers | Makes sounds |
| Grimaces | Makes jerky movements | Fusses in sleep |
| Has irregular respirations | | |

Awake

| Eyes floating | Panicky, worried, dull look | Glassy eyes |
| Weak cry | Strain, fussiness | Irritability |
| Staring | Abrupt state changes | Gaze aversion |

## Attention–Interaction System

Attempts at engaging behaviors elicit stress.
Impaired ability to orient, attend, engage in reciprocal social interactions
Difficulty consoling

# RELATED FACTORS

## Pathophysiologic

*Related to immature or altered central nervous system (CNS) secondary to:*

| Prematurity | Infection | Prenatal exposure to cocaine |
| Hyperbilirubinemia | Congenital anomalies | Decreased oxygen saturation |
| Hypoglycemia | Perinatal factors | |

*Related to nutritional deficits secondary to:*

| Reflux | Swallowing problems | Colic |
| Feeding intolerance | Emesis | Poor Suck/Swallow coordination |

*Related to excess stimulation secondary to:*

| Pain | Hunger | Oral hypersensitivity |
| Temperature variation | Environmental stimuli | |

## Treatment-Related

*Related to excess stimulation secondary to:*

| Invasive procedures | Restraints | Chest physical therapy |
| Movement | Noise (e.g., prolonged alarm, | Feeding |
| Lights | voices, environment) | Tubes, tape |
| Medication administration | | |

*Related to inability to see caregivers secondary to eye patches*

## Situational (Personal, Environmental)

*Related to unpredictable interactions secondary to multiple caregivers*
*Related to imbalance of task touch and consoling touch*
*Related to decreased ability to self-regulate secondary to:*

| Sudden movement | Noise |
| Disrupted sleep–wake cycles | Fatigue |

■■■■■■ **AUTHOR'S NOTE**

This diagnosis describes an infant who has difficulty regulating and adapting to external stimuli. This difficulty is from immature neurobehavioral development and increased environmental stimuli associated with neonatal units. When an infant is overstimulated or stressed, he or she uses energy to adapt, which depletes the supply of energy available for physiologic growth. The goal of nursing care is to assist the infant to conserve energy by reducing environmental stimuli, allowing the baby sufficient time to adapt to handling, and providing sensory input appropriate to the infant's physiologic and neurobehavioral status.

■■■■■■ **KEY CONCEPTS**

### Generic Considerations

- Als (1986) explained that an infant's primary route of communication of competency and efforts at self-regulation is through behavioral indices.

*(continued)*

■■■■■■ **KEY CONCEPTS** *Continued*

- Infant behavior is a continual interaction with the environment by means of five subsystems (Blackburn, 1993; Merenstein & Gardner, 1998; Yecco, 1993):
    - *Autonomic/physiologic*—regulation of respiration, color, and visceral functions (e.g., gastrointestinal, swallowing)
    - *Motor*—regulation of tone, posture, activity level, specific movement patterns of the extremities, head, trunk, and face
    - *State/organizational*—the range, transition between, and quality of states of consciousness (e.g., sleep to arousal, awake to alert, crying)
    - *Attention–interactive*—ability to orient and to focus on sensory stimuli (e.g., faces, sounds, objects) and to take in cognitive, social, and emotional information
    - *Self-regulatory*—maintenance of the integrity and balance of the other subsystems, smooth transitions between states, and relaxation among subsystems
- In full-term infants, these systems function smoothly and are synchronized and regulated with ease. Less mature or ill infants, however, can tolerate only one activity at a time. Loss of control results in instability or disorganization in one or more subsystems (Blackburn, 1993). The defining characteristics represent signs of the instability.
- Premature infants must adapt to the extrauterine environment with underdeveloped body systems, usually in a neonatal intensive care unit (NICU; Merenstein & Gardner, 1998).
- Although mortality and morbidity rates have been reduced greatly in high-risk infants, these babies experience various neurobehavioral problems. These problems have been labeled as *the new morbidities of low-birth-weight infants* and include hyperexcitability, language problems, attention-deficit disorders, higher-order cognitive problems, and schooling problems (Blackburn, 1993).
- The six stages of CNS development are dorsal induction, ventral induction, proliferation and neurogenesis, neuron migration, organization, and myelinization. The first three occur completely before the 4th month of gestation. The last three stages continue until development is complete. The *migration stage* involves the movement of millions of cells from their point of origin in the periventricular region to their terminal location within the cerebral cortex and cerebellum. The *organization stage* peaks from 6 months' gestation to 1 year after birth. The *myelinization stage* peaks from 8 months' gestation to 1 year after birth. Myelinization insulates individual nerve fibers to facilitate specificity of connections, increases the number of alternative pathways, and increases the speed of transmission (Blackburn, 1993).
- Neurologic dysfunctions resulting from neurologic underdevelopment include the following (Blackburn, 1993):

| | |
|---|---|
| Sparse myelin | Long refractory period |
| Weak transmission | Decreased inhibitory potential |
| Decreased ability to use various systems | Slow nerve conduction |
| Slow synaptic conduction | Inability to sustain high firing rates |
| Incomplete cell differentiation | Decreased ability to process impulses for cell-to-cell communication |

- These limitations result in the following behavior characteristics of immature infants (Blackburn, 1993; Merenstein & Gardner, 1998):

| | |
|---|---|
| Irregular state of regulation | Increased and decreased tone |
| Deficits in primitive reflexes | Easy exhaustion |
| Irritability (difficult to soothe) | Inability to inhibit |
| Jerky movements | Low arousal |
| Difficulty sustaining alertness | Poor coordination |
| Altered autonomic regulation | Uncoordinated posture/movements |

- For too long, researchers believed that newborns could not perceive, respond to, or remember pain. Findings have validated, however, that newborns do feel and express pain. Williamson and Williamson (1983) found that infants who received local anesthesia for circumcision cried less and had less variation in heart rate and higher oxygen saturation compared with infants who did not have a local anesthetic.
- Loudness of sound is measured in decibels (db). Adult speech is recorded at about 45 to 50 db. Sound levels in infant incubators have been reported to be 50 to 80 db. Hearing loss in adults has been associated with levels above 80 to 85 db (Blackburn, 1993).
- Incidence of sensorineural hearing impairment is 4% in low-birth-weight infants and 13% in very-low-birth-weight infants (Thomas, 1989).

## Focus Assessment Criteria

Experts recommend three assessment tools for neurobehavioral function: the Brazelton Neonatal Behavioral Assessment Scale (NBAS) for healthy, full-term newborns; Assessment of Preterm Infant Behavior (APIB) for preterm newborns; and NIDCAP (Newborn Individualized Developmental Care and Assessment Program). All tools require training in their use.

## Objective Data

### Assess for Defining Characteristics.
*Autonomic System*
Respirations (see Defining Characteristics)
Color changes (see Defining Characteristics)
Visceral (see Defining Characteristics)
Motor (see Defining Characteristics)

*Motor System (Fluctuating Tone)*
Flaccid trunk, extremities, face (see Defining Characteristics)
Hypertonic (see Defining Characteristics)
Hyperflexions (see Defining Characteristics)
Frantic, diffuse activity (see Defining Characteristics)

*State System (Range)*
Sleep

| | | |
|---|---|---|
| Twitches | Jerky movements | Grimaces |
| Whimpers | Fussiness | |

Awake

| | | |
|---|---|---|
| Lack of coordination | Glassy eyes | Unfocused eyes |
| Staring | Panicked look | Weak cry |

Irritability
*Abrupt state changes*

*Attention–Interaction System*
Imbalance of withdrawal versus engaging behaviors
Impaired ability to orient, engage in reciprocal interactions, attend
Difficulty consoling
For more information on Focus Assessment Criteria, visit http://thepoint.lww.com.

**NOC**
Neurologic Status, Preterm Infant Organization, Sleep, Comfort Level

## ➤ Goal

The infant will demonstrate increase signs of stability.

### Indicators

• Exhibit smooth, stable respirations; pink, stable color; consistent tone; improve posture; calm, focused alertness; well-modulated sleep; responsive to authority, visual and social stimuli.
• Demonstrate self-regulatory skills as sucking, hand to mouth, hand holding, position changes.

The parent(s)/caregiver(s) will describe techniques to reduce environmental stress in agency, at home, or both.

• Describe situations that stress infant.
• Describe signs/symptoms of stress in infant.

**NIC**
Environmental
Management,
Neurologic
Monitoring, Sleep
Enhancement,
Newborn Care,
Parent Education:
Newborn Positioning

## ➤ General Interventions

See Related Factors.

## Reduce or Eliminate Contributing Factors, If Possible.

### Pain

Observe infant before touching him or her.

Document infant's baseline behavioral manifestations.

Observe for responses different from baseline that have been associated with neonatal pain responses (Bozzette, 1993):

- Facial responses (open mouth, brow bulge, grimace, chin quiver, nasolabial furrow, taut tongue)
- Motor responses (flinch, muscle rigidity, clenched hands, withdrawal)

If unsure whether behavior indicates pain, but you suspect pain, consult with physician for an analgesic trial. Evaluate infant's response.

Aggressively manage obvious pain stimuli (e.g., postsurgical, lack of feeding, painful procedures, hyperglycemia; Merenstein & Gardner, 1998):

- Consult with physician for an analgesic.
- Provide an analgesic before painful procedures.
- Consider topical analgesia for frequent painful procedures (eg, heelstick, venipuncture).

When administering analgesics (Merenstein & Gardner, 1998):

- Reduce initial dose and monitor respiratory response cautiously.
- Determine optimal dose and interval.
- Monitor when pain breaks through.
- Determine if infant appears comfortable after the dose.
- When indicated, wean infant slowly over a period of days from the drug. Assess response to withdrawal. Consult with physician to manage withdrawal symptoms if indicated.

**R:** "If care providers are unsure whether a behavior indicates pain, and if there is a reason to suspect pain, an analgesic trial can be diagnostic as well as therapeutic" (Acute Pain Management Guideline Panel, 1992a, p. 12).

## Disrupted 24-h Diurnal Cycles

Evaluate the need for and frequency of each intervention.

Consider 24-h caregiving assignment and primary caregiving to provide consistent caregiving throughout the day and night for the infant from the onset of admission. This is important in terms of responding to increasingly more mature sleep cycles, feeding ability, and especially emotional development.

Consider supporting the infant's transition to and maintenance of sleep by avoiding peaks of frenzy and overexhaustion; continuously maintaining a calm, regular environment and schedule; and establishing a reliable, repeatable pattern of gradual transition into sleep in prone and side-lying positions in the isolette or crib.

**R:** Intervention to facilitate motor-sleep-wake organization improves behavioral organization.

## Feeding Experience

Observe and record infant's readiness for participation with feeding.

**Hunger Cues**
Transitioning to drowsy or alert state
Mouthing, rooting, or sucking
Bringing hands to mouth
Crying that is not relieved with pacifier or non-nutritive sucking alone

**Physiologic Stability**
Look for regulated breathing patterns, stable color, and stable digestion.
Promote nurturing environment in support of coregulatory feeding experience.

Decrease environmental stimulation.

Provide comfortable seating (be especially sensitive to the needs of postpartum mothers: e.g., soft cushions, small stool to elevate legs, supportive pillows for nursing).

Encourage softly swaddling the infant to facilitate flexion and balanced tone during feeding.

Explore feeding methods that meet the goals of both infant and family (e.g., breastfeeding, bottle-feeding, gavage).

**R:** Preterm infants may have difficulty or demonstrate disorganization in the progression of their feeding behaviors (e.g., readiness, availability of hunger cues) and gastrointestinal motility (e.g., esophageal motility, intestinal motility, gastric emptying time).

**R:** Individualized developmental care can cause an earlier transition to full oral feedings (Als et al., 2003).

## Support the Infant's Self-Regulatory Efforts

When administering painful or stressful procedures, consider actions to enhance calmness.

Support the flexed position with another caregiver.

Provide opportunities to suck while shielding the infant from other stresses.

Consider the efficient execution of necessary manipulations while supporting the infant's behavioral organization.

Consider *unhurried* reorganization and stabilization of the infant's regulation (e.g., position prone, give opportunities to hold onto caregiver's finger and suck, encase trunk and back of head in caregiver's hand, provide inhibition to soles of feet).

Consider removing extraneous stimulation (e.g., stroking, talking, shifting position) to institute restabilization. Consider spending 15 to 20 min after manipulation; over time, the infant's self-regulatory abilities will improve, making the caregiver's intervention less important.

Consider supporting the infant's transition to and maintenance of sleep by avoiding peaks of frenzy and overexhaustion; by continuously maintaining a calm, regular environment and schedule; and by establishing a reliable, repeatable pattern of gradual transition into sleep in prone and side-lying positions in the isolette or crib.

Consider initiating calming on the caregiver's body and then transferring the baby to the crib as necessary. For other infants, this may be too arousing, and transition is accomplished more easily in the isolette with the provision of steady boundaries and encasing without any stimulation.

Critical review of use of the automatic swing may be indicated for irritable infants. For some infants, it leads to momentary quieting, but not necessarily to increased internal regulatory control over time.

Soothing, gentle instrumental music or the parent's voice is comforting for some infants during transition to sleep.

A nonstimulating sleep space with minimal exciting visual targets, social inputs, and so forth, may need to be made available to facilitate relaxation before sleep. A regularly implemented sleep routine helps many infants.

**R:** When a premature newborn is ill, the combination of an immature CNS, exposure to inappropriate and unexpected patterned sensory input, and multiple caregivers leads to disorganization and imbalance of the behavioral indices to regulation.

**R:** Individualized interventions are implemented to increase organized behavior.

## Reduce Environmental Stimuli

### Noise (Merenstein & Gardner, 1998; Thomas, 1989)

Do not tap on incubator.

Place a folded blanket on top of the incubator if it is the only work surface available.

Slowly open and close porthole.

Pad incubator doors to reduce banging.

Use plastic instead of metal waste cans.

Remove water from ventilator tubing.

Speak softly at the bedside and only when necessary.

Slowly drop the head of the mattress.

Eliminate radios.

Close doors slowly.

Position the infant's bed away from sources of noise (e.g., telephone, intercom, unit equipment).

Consider the following methods to reduce unnecessary noise in the NICU:

Perform rounds away from the bedsides.

Adapt large equipment to eliminate noise and clutter.

Alert staff when the decibel level in the unit exceeds 60 db (e.g., by a light attached to a sound meter). Institute quiet time for 10 min to lower noise.

Move more vulnerable infants out of unit traffic patterns.

**R:** Noise levels in NICUs are hazardous because of potential damage to the cochlea with subsequent hearing loss, and because of arousal effects on infants who cannot inhibit their responses. Noise interferes with sleep, increases heart rate, and leads to vasoconstriction (Blackburn, 1993). The infant expends energy he or she needs to grow and to supply the brain with glucose and oxygen (Thomas, 1989).

**R:** Thomas (1989) found that NICUs have a loud, continuous pattern of background noise. In addition, peak noises over the continuous noise level can raise the decibel level 10-fold. Examples of peak noises are monitor alarms (67 db), NICU radios (62 db), opening of plastic sleeves (67 db), tappings of hoods (70 db), and sinks (66 db).

## Lights

Use full-spectrum instead of white light at bedside. Avoid fluorescent lights.

Cover cribs, incubators, and radiant warmers completely during sleep and partially during awake periods.

Install dimmer switches, shades, and curtains. Avoid bright lights.

Shade infants' eyes with a blanket tent or cutout box.

Avoid visual stimuli on cribs.

Shield eyes from bright procedure lights. Avoid patches unless for phototherapy.

**R:** When a premature newborn is ill, the combination of an immature CNS, exposure to inappropriate and unexpected patterned sensory input, and multiple caregivers leads to disorganization and imbalance of the behavioral indices to regulation.

## Position Baby in Postures that Permit Flexion and Minimize Flailing

Consider gentle, *unhurried* reorganization and stabilization of infant's regulation by supporting the infant in softly tucked prone position, giving opportunities to hold onto caregiver's finger and suck, encasing trunk and back of head in caregiver's hand, and providing inhibition to soles of feet.

Use the prone/side-lying position.

Avoid the supine position.

Swaddle baby, if possible, to maintain flexion.

Create a nest using soft bedding (eg, natural sheepskin, soft cotton, flannel).

Avoid oversized diapers to allow you to perceive normal hip alignment.

Avoid tension on lines or tubing.

**R:** Developmentally correct handling and positioning can decrease stress, conserve energy, and enhance normal development (Aida & Snider, 2003).

## Reduce the Stress Associated with Handling

When moving or lifting the infant, contain him or her with your hands by wrapping or placing rolled blankets around his or her body.

Maintain containment during procedures and caregiving activities.

Handle slowly and gently. Avoid stroking.

Initiate all interactions and treatments with one sense stimulus at a time (e.g., touch), then slowly progress to visual, auditory, and movement.

Assess child for cues for readiness, impending disorganization, or stability; respond to cues.

Support minimal disruption of the infant's own evolving 24-h sleep–wake cycles.

Use PRN instead of routine suctioning or postural drainage.

Use minimal adhesive tape. Remove any carefully.

**R:** Stress reduction will conserve energy, promote comfort, and enhance adaption.

**R:** Stroking preterm infants who are unstable results in decreased levels of oxygen saturation (Harrison et al., 1996).

## Reduce Disorganized Behavior During Active Interventions and Transport

Have a plan for transport, with assigned roles for each team member.

Establish behavior cues of stress on this infant with the primary nurse before transport.

Minimize sensory input:

- Use calm, quiet voices.
- Shade the infant's eyes from light.
- Protect infant from unnecessary touch.

Support the infant's softly tucked postures with your hands and offer something to grasp (your finger or corner of a soft blanket or cloth).

Swaddle the infant or place him or her in a nest made of blankets.

Ensure that the transport equipment (e.g., ventilator) is ready. Warm mattress or use sheepskin.

Carefully and smoothly move the infant. Avoid talking, if possible.

Consider conducting caregiving routines while parent(s) or designated caregiver hold infant, whenever possible.

Reposition in 2 to 3 hours or sooner if infant behavior suggests discomfort.

**R:** Interventions seek to reduce stimuli to prevent a disorganized response.

## Engage Parents in Planning Care

Encourage them to share their feelings, fears, and expectations.

Consider involving parents in creating the family's developmental plan

My strengths are:      These things stress me:

Time-out signals:      How you can help me:

Teach caregivers to continually observe the changing capabilities to determine the appropriate positioning and bedding options, e.g., infant may fight containment (Hockenberry & Wilson, 2009).

**R:** Anticipatory guidance and support can prevent overstimulation of their infant.

## Initiate Health Teaching and Referrals as Indicated

### *Review the Following Information Relating to Growth and Development of the Infant and Family in Anticipatory Guidance for Home*

**Health Concerns**

| | | |
|---|---|---|
| Feeding | Hygiene | Illness |
| Infection | Safety | Temperature |
| Growth and development | | |

**State Modulation**

| | |
|---|---|
| Appropriate stimulation | Sleep–wake patterns |

**Parent–Infant Interaction**

| | | |
|---|---|---|
| Behavior cues | Signs of stress | |
| *Infant's environment* | | |
| Animate, inanimate stimulation | Playing with infant | Role of father and siblings |

**Parental Coping and Support**

| | | |
|---|---|---|
| Support network | Challenges | Problem solving |

### *Discuss Transition to Community Supports (Nursing Respite, Social and Civic Groups, Religious Affiliations)*

### *Refer for Follow-Up Home Visits*

**R:** Teach parents to identify interventions that will support optimal growth and development for their infant.

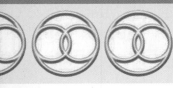

# RISK FOR DISORGANIZED INFANT BEHAVIOR

## DEFINITION

State in which the neonate is at risk for an alteration in integration and modulation of the physiologic and behavioral systems of adaptation (autonomic, motor, state, organizational, self-regulatory, and attentional–interactional)

## RISK FACTORS

Refer to Related Factors.

## RELATED FACTORS

Refer to *Disorganized Infant Behavior*.

## Focus Assessment Criteria

Refer to *Disorganized Infant Behavior*.

## General Interventions

Refer to *Disorganized Infant Behavior*.

---

# RISK FOR INFECTION

## DEFINITION

State in which a person is at risk to be invaded by an opportunistic or pathogenic agent (virus, fungus, bacteria, protozoa, or other parasite) from endogenous or exogenous sources

## RISK FACTORS

See Related Factors.

## RELATED FACTORS

Various health problems and situations can create favorable conditions that would encourage the development of infections.* Some common factors follow.

### Pathophysiologic

*Related to compromised host defenses secondary to:*

| | | |
|---|---|---|
| Cancer | *Altered or insufficient leukocytes* | Arthritis |
| Respiratory disorders | *Periodontal disease* | Renal failure |
| Hematologic disorders | Hepatic disorders | Diabetes mellitus |

---

*See Key Concepts.

Acquired immunodeficiency syndrome (AIDS)
*Alcoholism*
*Immunosuppression*
*Immunodeficiency secondary to: specify*
***Related to compromised circulation secondary to:***

| | | |
|---|---|---|
| Lymphedema | Obesity | Peripheral vascular disease |

## Treatment-Related

***Related to a site for organism invasion secondary to:***

| | | |
|---|---|---|
| Surgery | Invasive lines | Dialysis |
| Intubation | Total parenteral nutrition | Enteral feedings |

***Related to compromised host defenses secondary to:***
Radiation therapy
Organ transplant
Medication therapy (specify; e.g., chemotherapy, immunosuppressants)

## Situational (Personal, Environmental)

***Related to compromised host defenses secondary to:***

| | | |
|---|---|---|
| History of infections | Malnutrition | Prolonged immobility |
| Stress | Increased hospital stay | Smoking |

***Related to a site for organism invasion secondary to:***

| | |
|---|---|
| Trauma (accidental, intentional) | Postpartum period |
| Bites (animal, insect, human) | Thermal injuries |
| Warm, moist, dark environment (skin folds, casts) | |

***Related to contact with contagious agents (nosocomial or community acquired)***

## Maturational

### Newborns
***Related to increased vulnerability of infant secondary to:***

**HIV positive mother**

| | |
|---|---|
| Lack of maternal antibodies (dependent on maternal exposures) | Lack of normal flora |
| | Immature immune system |
| Open wounds (umbilical, circumcision) | |

### Infant/Child/Adolescent
***Related to increased vulnerability secondary to:***

| | |
|---|---|
| Lack of immunization | Multiple sex partners |

### Older Adult
***Related to increased vulnerability secondary to:***

| | | |
|---|---|---|
| Diminished immune response | Debilitated condition | Chronic diseases |

■■■■■■ **AUTHOR'S NOTE**

All people are at risk for infection. Secretion control, environmental control, and hand washing before and after client care reduce the risk of transmission of organisms. Included in the population at risk for infection is a smaller group at high risk for infection. *Risk for Infection* describes a person whose host defenses are compromised, thus increasing susceptibility to environmental pathogens or his or her own endogenous flora (e.g., a person with chronic liver dysfunction or with an invasive line). Nursing interventions for such a person focus on minimizing introduction of organisms and increasing resistance to infection (e.g., improving nutritional status). For a person with an infection, the situation is best described by the collaborative problem *RC of Sepsis*.

*Risk for Infection Transmission* describes a person at high risk for transferring an infectious agent to others. Some people are at high risk both for acquiring opportunistic agents and for transmitting infecting organisms, warranting the use of both *Risk for Infection* and *Risk for Infection Transmission*.

## ERRORS IN DIAGNOSTIC STATEMENTS

1. *Risk for Infection related to progression of sepsis secondary to failure to treat infection*
   Sepsis is a collaborative problem, not a nursing diagnosis. This person is not at risk for infection; rather, he or she requires medical and nursing interventions to treat the sepsis and prevent septic shock.

2. *Risk for Infection related to direct access to bladder mucosa secondary to Foley catheter and lack of staff knowledge of aseptic technique*
   If the staff's lack of knowledge of aseptic technique is valid, the nurse should proceed with reporting the situation to nursing management in an incident report. Adding this to a nursing diagnosis statement would be legally and professionally inadvisable. Nurses never should use nursing diagnostic statements to criticize a client, group, or member of the health team or to expose unsafe or unprofessional practices or behavior. Nurses must use other organizational channels of communication for these purposes.

## KEY CONCEPTS

### Generic Considerations

- Resistance to infection depends on the host's immune response (*susceptibility*), dose of the infecting agent, and virulence of the organism. Factors influencing the host's immune response include the following:
  - Anatomic barriers—each system has specific lines of defenses.
  - Therapies—pose a threat to normal lines of defense by either invasiveness or alteration of body function.
  - Developmental and heritable factors—factors that negatively affect the person's immune system function (e.g., newborn status; agammaglobulinemia).
  - Hormonal factors—males are more vulnerable to infection than are females; pregnancy increases the female's vulnerability; steroid therapy increases vulnerability in both sexes.
  - Age—includes both extremes (immaturity or degeneration of immune system).
  - Nutrition—influences protein synthesis and phagocytosis, decreasing the body's vulnerability to infection.
  - Fever—hyperthermia may inhibit the growth of organisms; hypothermia may decrease the effects of the fever.
  - Secretions such as mucus, saliva, and skin secretions—contain substances that are bactericidal, decreasing the risk of infection and colonization.
  - Endotoxins, a product of some gram-negative bacteria—have a limited ability to kill other bacteria or increase a person's resistance to some infections.
  - Interference—the interaction between two distinct organisms that are parasitizing the host leads to interference, in which one remains dominant and the other is suppressed.
- The inflammatory response consists of (1) activation of leukocytes, (2) plasma proteins, which localize and phagocytize the infectious process, and (3) increased blood and lymph flow, which dilutes and flushes out toxic materials; this process causes a local increase in temperature.
- Phagocytosis is the process by which parasites are removed by engulfment and digestion.

### Host Defenses

Specific host defenses of each system that influence the immune response include the following:

#### CENTRAL NERVOUS SYSTEM (CNS)

Because the most common route for both bacterial and viral infections of the CNS is the hematogenous route, blood host defenses play an important primary role.

*Cutaneous*

- Skin provides a first line of defense against organisms, both anatomically and chemically.
- Sweat glands and sebaceous glands do not allow overgrowth of bacteria.
- The acid pH of the skin does not allow pathogenic organisms to grow or survive on the skin for any length of time.
- The flushing and lysozyme actions of tears control eye infections. The lacrimal duct flushes out organisms and deposits them in the nasopharynx.

#### BLOOD

- Circulating blood is the major vehicle for transporting internal defense mechanisms.
- The febrile response is associated with the circulation of pyrogens to the hypothalamus.

*(continued)*

■■■■■■ **KEY CONCEPTS** *Continued*

### GENITOURINARY TRACT

- Anatomic structure eliminates easy ascent of perineal microorganisms into the bladder.
- Mucous layer allows entrapment of organisms and engulfment by bladder cells.
- The pH and osmolality of urine prevent bacterial multiplication.
- The ability to empty the bladder completely eliminates stasis of invading organisms and allows continual flushing.

### RESPIRATORY TRACT

- The nares entrap most foreign matter on the mucous membranes as a result of turbulence caused by the turbinates and hairs.
- The mucociliary transport system consists of cilia and mucus, which remove additional matter passing to the upper and lower bronchi.
- Lysozymes and immunoglobulin A (IgA), a secretion of phagocytes, are found in nasal secretions and assist in the prevention of colonization.
- Particles reaching as far as the alveoli can be removed through the expulsive action of sneezing and coughing, and the gag reflex.
- Phagocytosis occurs in the alveoli, with the macrophages used as a major defense mechanism.

### GASTROINTESTINAL TRACT

- A mucous layer traps ingested microbes in the epithelium of the gastrointestinal (GI) tract.
- Gastric acids kill most organisms.
- Peristalsis aids in the removal of organisms.
- Intestinal secretions contain antibody (IgA), bile salts, lysozyme, glycolipids, and glycoproteins that prevent proliferation and adherence.
- Normal gut flora interact to restrict over proliferation.

### WOUNDS

- Skin provides a first line of defense; the opening of the skin, either surgically or traumatically, potentiates infection.
- A wound essentially closes within 24 h, eliminating the risk of direct inoculations of organisms.
- Wound infections rely on the capabilities of other host defenses to assist in healing.
- Risk factors associated with wound infections depend on (1) endogenous factors such as the presence of confounding factors, skin preparation, and the use of prophylactic antibiotics; and (2) exogenous factors such as the preoperative scrub, barrier techniques, airborne contamination, environmental disinfection, wound care, and the condition of the wound at the time of closure.
- Wounds are at risk for infection owing to the following factors:
  - Sutures and staples, unlike tape, create their own wounds, act like drains, and cause their own inflammatory response.
  - Drains provide a site for microorganism entry.
  - The incidence of infection in clients who are not shaved or clipped is 0.9%. It increases to 1.4% with electric shaving, 1.7% with clipping, and 2.5% with razor shaving (Kovach, 1990).

### SEXUALLY TRANSMITTED DISEASE/INFECTIONS

- The high prevalence of risky sexual behavior among teenagers contributes to the high rates of sexually transmitted infections and pregnancy (Centers for Disease Control and Prevention, 2005).
- Since 2005, gonorrhea rates of infection have risen 5.5%: Chlamydia rates of infection have risen 5.6%; Syphilis has increased by 13.8%
- Adolescents perceive themselves as low risk, however as many as 50% are sexually active (CDC, 2005)
- Older adults are at risk for sexuallity transmitted disease/infections including HIV because of little or no condom use due to low or no risk for pregnancy due to menopause.

## Pediatric Considerations

- Congenital infections, those acquired in utero, usually result from exposure to such viruses as cytomegalovirus, rubella, hepatitis B, herpes simplex, herpes zoster, varicella, and Epstein-Barr. Nonviral agents also may cause some infections, such as toxoplasmosis, syphilis, tuberculosis, trypanosomiasis, HIV and malaria.
- Congenital bacterial infections may arise from bacterial organisms that travel to the fetus through the placenta. The fetus also may become infected by organisms that reach the amniotic cavity through the mother's cervix.
- Fetal skin and mucous membranes, intervillous placenta spaces, the umbilical cord, and respiratory airways (through aspiration) provide other avenues of infection.
- Approximately 80% of all childhood illnesses are infections, with respiratory infections occurring two to three times as often as other illnesses combined (Hockenberry & Wilson, 2009).
- In general, acute illness is less frequent in children younger than 6 months, increases from then until 3 or 4 years of age, and then gradually decreases throughout childhood.
- According to Kliegman (1990), newborns are at increased risk for infections. By the time a child is a toddler, production of antibodies is well established. Phagocytosis is much more efficient in toddlers than in infants.
- Children who attend day care centers are at increased risk for infections caused by *Shigella*, rotavirus, *Haemophilus influenzae* type b, and hepatitis A.
- Good hygiene, optimal nutrition, immunizations, and strict sanitary practices can reduce the incidence of infectious disease during childhood.
- Perinatal transmission of HIV occurs in utero, intrapartum, or after delivery through breastfeeding.
- Twenty percent to 50% of infants born to untreated HIV-positive women will contract the virus and develop AIDS in the first year of life. Perinatal HIV transmission can be reduced to 2% with antiviral treatment of the pregnant woman beginning with the 14th week of pregnancy, and her newborn for 6 weeks after birth (CDC, 2007).
- Without treatment the prenatal infection rate is 25% (CDC, 2007).
- Perinatally inflicted children have a more rapid progression of the disease because of the immaturity of their immune system.

## Geriatric Considerations

- A slower rate of epidermal proliferation causes injured skin to take twice as long to heal in older adults.
- Older adults also have compromised dermal immunologic responses because of a reduced number of Langerhans cells and reduced microcirculation (Miller, 2009).
- In older adults, the lung's alveolar surface and elastic recoil are slightly decreased, and gas exchange in lower lung regions is decreased (Miller, 2009).
- Age-related changes in respiratory function do not significantly increase risk for infection. Rather, non–age-related risk factors, such as smoking and exposure to occupational toxins, increase risk.
- Studies have shown 5% to 20% of residents in long-term care facilities to have infections. The most frequent are those of the urinary tract, respiratory system, and skin and soft tissues (usually pressure ulcers; Miller, 2009).
- The increased susceptibility of older adults to infections is multifactorial (either host factors or environmental). Host factors include underlying diseases, invasive treatment modalities, indiscriminate use of antibiotics, malnutrition, dehydration, impaired mobility, and incontinence. Environmental factors in institutions include limited surveillance for infection, crowded areas, cross-contamination, and delay in early detection.
- Skin and urinary tract colonization is a greater problem in older than in younger clients. Changes in immune competence with aging increase susceptibility to fungal, viral, and mycobacterial pathogens (Miller, 2009).
- Older adults do not exhibit the usual signs of infection (fever, chills, tachypnea, tachycardia, leukocytosis) but, instead, present with anorexia, weakness, change in mental status, normothermia, or hypothermia (Miller, 2009).

## Transcultural Considerations

- The incidence of tuberculosis in American Indians is seven to 15 times that of non-Indians. African-Americans have an incidence three times that of white Americans. Urban American Jews are the most resistant to tuberculosis.
- Susceptibility to disease may also be environmental or a combination of genetic, psychosocial, and environmental factors (Giger & Davidhizar, 2009).
- The incidence of HIV in the US population is 53% in male to male (MM) transmission, 12% in IV drug use (IDU), 4% in MM and IDU, and 31% in heterosexual persons. The incidence in Afro-Americans is 45% (Hall, Song, Rhodes et al., 2008).
- American Indians and Alaskan natives have twice the reported rate of gonorrhea and syphilis than other Americans (Giger & Davidhizar, 2009).
- Patient education regarding safe sex in many religions is difficult because according to the Torah, the Bible, and other "holy books," homosexuality is an abomination and premarital sexual activity is not permitted (Giger & Davidhizar, 2009).

# Focus Assessment Criteria

## Subjective Data

### Assess for Related Factors

**Does the person complain of the following::**
Previous infections
Pain or swelling (generalized, localized)
Hemoptysis
Productive, prolonged cough
Chest pain associated with other criteria
Systemic symptoms

| | | |
|---|---|---|
| Fever, continuous or intermittent | Easy fatigability | Chills |
| Loss of appetite | Night sweats | Weight loss |

**History of recent travel**
Within United States
Outside United States

**History of exposure to infectious diseases**
Airborne (most childhood infections result from communicable diseases [e.g., chickenpox, tuberculosis])
Vector-borne and other vector-associated infections (malaria, plague)
Vehicle-borne and other food- and water-borne infections (hepatitis A, salmonellas)
Contact spread (most common type of exposure)
Direct (person to person)
Indirect (e.g., by instruments, clothing, and so forth)
Contact droplet (e.g., pneumonias, colds)

**History of risk factors associated with infections**
See Related Factors

## Objective Data

### Assess for Related Factors

Presence of wounds
  Surgical
  Burns
  Invasive devices (tracheostomy, intravenous [IV], drains)
  Self-induced
Temperature, abnormal
Nutritional deficiency

For more information on Focus Assessment Criteria, visit http://thepoint.lww.com.

## ➤ Goal

The person will report risk factors associated with infection and precautions needed.

### Indicators

- Demonstrate meticulous hand washing technique by the time of discharge.
- Describe methods of transmission of infection.
- Describe the influence of nutrition on prevention of infection.

## ➤ General Interventions

### Identify Clients at High Risk for Nosocomial Infections (Owen & Grier, 1987)

### Use Appropriate Universal Precautions for All Body Fluids

Wash hands before and after all contact with client or specimen.

**R:** Hand washing is one of the most important means to prevent the spread of infection.

Handle the blood of all clients as potentially infectious.
Wear gloves for potential contact with blood and body fluids.
Handle all linen soiled with blood or body secretions as potentially infectious.
Process all laboratory specimens as potentially infectious.

**R:** Gloves provide a barrier from contact with infectious secretions and excretions.

Place used syringes immediately in a nearby impermeable container; do not recap or manipulate he needle in any way! Use retractable needle syringes when possible.

**R:** Needlesticks can transmit infectious blood.

Wear protective eyewear and mask if splatter with blood or body fluids is possible (e.g., bronchoscopy, oral surgery).

**R:** Eye coverings protect the eyes from accidental exposure to infectious secretions present; gowns prevent soiling of clothes if contact with secretions/excretions is likely. Wear mask for tuberculosis and other respiratory organisms. (HIV is not airborne.)
**R:** Masks prevent transmission by aerosolization of infectious agents if oral mucosal lesions are present.
**R:** Universal precautions reduce contact with contagious substances.

### Consider Those with the Following Factors at High Risk for Delayed Wound Healing:

| | | |
|---|---|---|
| Malnourishment | Tobacco use | Obesity |
| Anemia | Diabetes | Cancer |
| Corticosteroid therapy | Renal insufficiency | Hypovolemia |
| Hypoxia | Surgery >3 h | Night or emergency surgery |
| Zinc, copper, magnesium deficiency | Immune system compromise | |

**R:** Intervention can be implemented to control or influence the degree of risk associated with predictors and confounding factors (Owen & Grier, 1987).

### Use Universal Precautions

### Reduce Client's Susceptibility to Infection

Encourage and maintain caloric and protein intake in diet (see *Imbalanced Nutrition*).
Assess client for adequate immunizations against childhood diseases, bacterial infections (e.g., pneumonia, *Haemophilus influenzae*), and other viral infections (e.g., influenza). (Refer to Altered Health Maintenance in Section 3.)

Administer prescribed antimicrobial therapy within 15 min of schedule.

**R:** Antibiotics administered at proper intervals ensure maintenance of therapeutic levels.

Minimize length of stay in hospital

**R:** Limiting exposure nosocomial organisms.

Observe for superinfection in clients receiving antimicrobial therapy.

**R:** Subtle changes in vital signs may be early signs of sepsis, particularly fever.

## Reduce Entry of Organisms into Clients (Owen & Grier, 1987)

### Surgical Wound

Monitor temperature every 4 h; notify physician if temperature is greater than 100.8°F.
Assess wound site every 24 h and during dressing changes; document any abnormal findings.
Evaluate all abnormal laboratory findings, especially culture/sensitivities and complete blood count (CBC).

**R:** Wound healing by primary intention requires a dressing to protect it from contamination until the edges seal (usually 24 h). Wound healing by secondary intention requires a dressing to maintain adequate hydration; the dressing is not needed after wound edges seal.

Assess nutritional status to provide adequate protein and caloric intake for healing.

**R:** To repair tissue, the body needs increased protein and carbohydrate intake and adequate hydration for vascular transport of oxygen and wastes.

### Urinary Tract

Evaluate all abnormal laboratory findings, especially cultures/sensitivities and CBC.
Assess for abnormal signs and symptoms after any urologic procedure, including frequency, urgency, burning, abnormal color, and odor.
Monitor client's temperature at least every 24 h for elevation; notify physician if temperature is greater than 100.8°F.
Encourage fluids when appropriate.
Use aseptic technique when emptying any urinary drainage device; keep bag off the floor, but below bladder or clamped during transport.
Reassess need for indwelling urinary catheter daily.

**R:** Urinary catheters provide a site for microorganism entry.

### Circulatory

Assess all invasive lines every 24 h for redness, inflammation, drainage, and tenderness.
Monitor client's temperature at least every 24 h; notify physician if greater than 100.8°F.
Maintain aseptic technique for all invasive devices, changing sites, dressings, tubing, and solutions per policy schedule.
Evaluate all abnormal laboratory findings, especially cultures/sensitivities and CBC.

**R:** Invasive lines provide a site for organism entry. Interventions focus on prevention and identification of early signs of infection.
Assess client's nutritional status.

**R:** Healing requires adequate protein and caloric intake

### Respiratory Tract

Evaluate risk for infection after any instrumentation of the respiratory tract for at least 48 h after procedure.
Monitor temperature at least every 8 h and notify physician if greater than 100.8°F.
Evaluate sputum characteristics for frequency, purulence, blood, odor.
Evaluate sputum and blood cultures, if done, for significant findings.

Assess lung sounds every 8 h or PRN.

If client has abdominal/thoracic surgery, instruct before surgery on importance of coughing, turning, and deep breathing.

Prompt to cough and deep breathe hourly.

If client has had anesthesia, monitor for appropriate clearing of secretions in lung fields.

Evaluate need for suctioning if client cannot clear secretions adequately.

Assess for risk of aspiration, keeping head of bed elevated 30 degrees unless otherwise contraindicated

Ensure optimal pain management

**R:** Individuals with pain, post-anesthesia, compromised ability to move, and those with ineffective cough are at risk for infection due to pooling of respiratory secretions.

## Protect the Client with Immune Deficiency from Infection

Place client in private room.

Instruct client to ask all visitors and personnel to wash their hands before approaching.

Limit visitors when appropriate.

Screen all visitors for known infections or exposure to infections.

Limit invasive devices to those that are necessary.

Teach client and family members signs and symptoms of infection.

Evaluate client's personal hygiene habits.

**R:** Persons with compromised immune systems are more vulnerable to infection.

## Initiate Health Teaching and Referrals, as Indicated

Instruct client and family regarding the causes, risks, and communicability of the infection.

Have family demonstrate use of equipment or treatment procedure

Collaborate with nurse epidemiologist on needs of client and family.

**R:** Familites and caregivers must use precautions with blood and body fluids from all clients to protect themselves from exposure to all potentially infectious organisms

**R:** Proper use of equipment and treatment procedures are needed to prevent infection and injury.

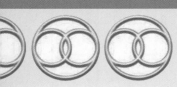

# RISK FOR INFECTION TRANSMISSION*

**Risk for Infection Transmission**

**Related to Lack of Knowledge of Reducing the Risk of Transmitting the AIDS Virus**

## DEFINITION

The state in which an individual is at risk for transferring an opportunistic or pathogenic agent to others

## RISK FACTORS

Presence of risk factors (see Related Factors).

## RELATED FACTORS

### Pathophysiologic

*Related to:*

Colonization with highly antibiotic-resistant organism

*This diagnosis is not currently on the NANDA list but has been included for clarity or usefulness.

Airborne transmission exposure (sneezing, coughing, spitting)

Contact transmission exposure (direct, indirect, contact droplet)

Vehicle transmission exposure (food, water, contaminated drugs or blood, contaminated sites (IV, catheter)

Vector-borne transmission exposure (animals, rodents, insects)

## Treatment-Related

*Related to exposure to a contaminated wound*
*Related to devices with contaminated drainage:*
Urinary, chest, endotracheal tubes
Suction equipment

## Situational (Personal, Environmental)

*Related to:*
Unsanitary living conditions (sewage, personal hygiene)
Areas considered high risk for vector-borne diseases (malaria, rabies, bubonic plague)
Areas considered high risk for vehicle-borne disease (hepatitis A, *Shigella*, *Salmonella*)
Exposures to sources of infection as:

* Intravenous/intranasal/intradermal drug use (sharing of needles, drug paraphernalia (straws)
* Contaminated sex toys
* Multiple sex partners
* Natural disaster (e.g., flood, hurricane)
* Disaster with hazardous infectious material

## Maturational

Newborn
*Related to birth outside hospital setting in uncontrolled environment*
*Related to exposure during prenatal or perinatal period to communicable disease through mother*

## ▪▪▪▪▪▪ KEY CONCEPTS

### Generic Considerations

* To spread an infection, three elements are required (Figure II.1):
  * A source of infecting organism
  * A susceptible host
  * A means of transmission for the organism
* Sources of infecting organisms include the following:
  * Clients, personnel, and visitors with acute disease, incubating infection, or colonized organisms without apparent disease
  * Client's own endogenous flora (autogenous infection)
  * Inanimate environment, including equipment and medications
* Susceptibility of the host varies according to:
  * Immune status
  * Ability to develop a commensal relationship with the infecting organism and become an asymptomatic carrier
  * Preexisting diseases
* Means of transmission for the organism include one or more of the following:
  * Contact transmission, the most frequent method of transferring organisms, can be divided into three subgroups:
    * Direct contact—involves direct physical transfer between a susceptible host and an infected or colonized person
    * Indirect contact—involves the exchange of organisms between a host and contaminated objects, usually inanimate

*(continued)*

■■■■■■ **KEY CONCEPTS** *Continued*

- Droplet contact—involves an infected person transferring organisms into the conjunctivae, nose, or mouth of a susceptible host by coughing, sneezing, or talking. Droplets travel no more than 3 feet.
- Vehicle route transmission infections are spread through means such as:
  - Food (e.g., hepatitis A, Salmonella)
  - Water (e.g., Legionella)
  - Drugs (e.g., IV-contaminated products)
  - Blood (e.g., hepatitis B, hepatitis C, HIV)
- Airborne infections are disseminated by droplet nuclei (residue of evaporated droplets that may remain suspended in the air for long periods) or dust particles in the air containing the infectious agent.
- Vector-borne infections are spread through vectors such as animals or insects.
- Universal body substance precautions require precautions with all blood and body fluids. Those clients with a suspected or confirmed medical diagnosis indicative of an infectious disease process, however, need documentation with a comprehensive plan of care for that infection or potential infection. The nursing diagnosis Risk for Infection Transmission can be used to document specific universal precaution practices.

### Human Immunodeficiency Virus (HIV)

- The cause of AIDS is a retrovirus labeled human immunodeficiency virus (HIV). Transmission is by exposure to contaminated semen, vaginal fluids, or blood.
- HIV infection has a latency or incubation period of 18 months to 5 years. During this period, the person transmits disease through sexual activity or through contaminated blood or body fluids

HIV destroys the body's T and B lymphocytes, thus making the host susceptible to a select group of diseases (Table II.9).

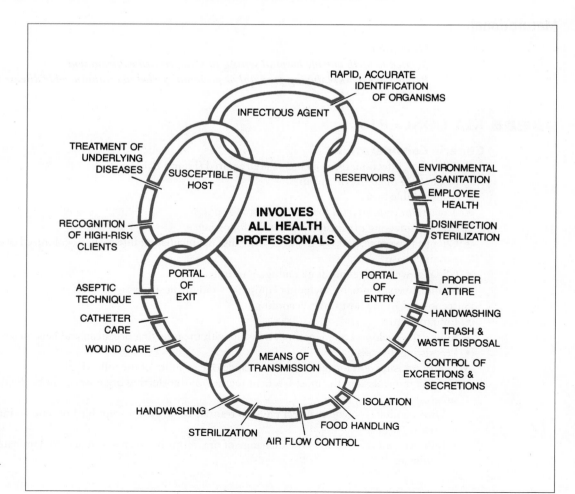

**FIGURE II.1**
Breaking the chain of infection. (Adapted from the APIC Starter Kit with permission from the Association for Professionals in Infection Control and Epidemiology. Washington, DC, copyright APIC, 1978.)

## TABLE II.9  MOST FREQUENT INFECTIONS AND NEOPLASMS IN ACQUIRED IMMUNODEFICIENCY SYNDROME (AIDS)

| Problem | Site |
| --- | --- |
| **AIDS-Related Complex** | |
| *Candida albicans* | Mouth (thrush), throat |
| Herpes simplex | Mucocutaneous; may be severe |
| Herpes zoster | Disseminated; may be severe |
| Lymphadenopathy | Generalized (always more than one lymph node) |
| Fevers | Usually greater than 100° F; persistent over months |
| Diarrhea | No organisms recovered, or conventional organisms recovered |
| Weight loss | Progressive and sustained |
| Night sweats | Characteristically severe and drenching; persistent and sustained over months |
| Thrombocytopenia | Often accompanied by petechia; may be severe and life threatening |
| Human immunodeficiency virus (HIV) encephalopathy | Clinical findings of disabling cognitive or motor dysfunction in absence of concurrent illness or condition other than HIV infection |
| HIV wasting syndrome | Profound, in the absence of concurrent illness or condition other than HIV infection |
| **Infections** | |
| *Candida albicans* | Mouth (thrush); throat |
| *Cryptococcus neoformans* | Central nervous system (CNS); pulmonary; disseminated |
| *Pneumocystis carinii* | Pneumonia |
| *Toxoplasma gondii* | CNS |
| *Histoplasma gondii* | CNS |
| *Cryptosporidium* | Intestine; diarrhea |
| Cytomegalovirus | Retinas; intestine; pulmonary; disseminated |
| Herpes simplex | Mucocutaneous; severe |
| Herpes zoster | Disseminated; severe |
| HIV dementia | CNS, disseminated |
| Progressive multifocal leukoencephalopathy | CNS |
| *Mycobacterium avium-intracellulare* | Disseminated |
| *Mycobacterium tuberculosis* | Pulmonary; tuberculosis (TB) |
| **Neoplasms** | |
| Kaposi's sarcoma | Skin; disseminated |
| Burkitt's lymphoma | Lymphatic system |
| Non-Hodgkin's lymphoma | Lymphatic system |
| Mycosis fungoides | Skin (dermal lymphoma) |

## Pediatric Considerations

- Infections in newborns can be acquired transplacentally or transcervically. They can occur before, during, or after birth.
- Children are at greater risk for transmission of disease because of the following factors:
  - Close contact with other children
  - Frequency of infectious disease in children
  - Lack of hygienic habits (e.g., not washing hands after toileting or before eating)
  - Frequent hand-to-mouth activity, increasing risk for infection and reinfection (e.g., pinworms)

## Focus Assessment Criteria

Refer to *Risk for Infection*.

**NOC**
Infection Status, Risk Control, Risk Detection

## ➤ Goal

The client will describe the mode of transmission of disease by the time of discharge.

### *Indicators:*

- Relate the need to be isolated until noninfectious (e.g., TB)
- Relate factors that contribute to the transmission of the infection

• Relate methods to reduce or prevent infection transmission
• Demonstrate meticulous hand washing

**NIC**
Teaching: Disease
Process, Infection
Control Infection
Protection

## General Interventions

### Identify People Who Are Susceptible Hosts Based on Focus Assessment for Risk for Infection and History of Exposure

### Identify the Mode of Transmission Based on Infecting Agent

Airborne
Contact:

• Direct
• Indirect
• Contact droplet

Vehicle-borne
Vector-borne

**R:** To prevent transmission of infection, the mode of transmission (i.e., airborne, contact, vehicle-borne, or vector-borne) must be known. For example tuberculosis is spread airborne by coughing, sneezing, and spitting.

## Reduce the Transfer of Pathogens

Isolate clients with airborne communicable infections (Table II.10).
Secure appropriate room assignment depending on the type of infection and hygienic practices of the infected client.
Use universal precautions to prevent transmission to self or other susceptible host.

**R:** Nurses must use precautions with blood and body fluids from all clients to protect themselves from exposure to HIV and hepatitis B and C.

## Initiate Health Education and Referrals as Indicated and Discuss the Mode of Transmission of Infection with the Client, Family, and Significant Others

**R:** Practices to prevent infection transmission must be continued after discharge.

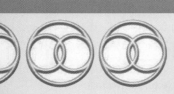

# RISK FOR INFECTION TRANSMISSION

## ▶ Related to Lack of Knowledge of Reducing the Risk of Transmitting HIV

**NOC**
Infection Status,
Risk Control, Risk
Detection

## Goal

The client will relate practices that reduce the transmission of HIV.

### Indicators:

• Describe the causes of AIDS and factors contributing to its transmission.
• Describe how to disinfect equipment.

## TABLE II.10  AIRBORNE COMMUNICABLE DISEASES

| Disease | Apply Airborne Precautions for How Long | Comments |
|---|---|---|
| Anthrax, inhalation | Duration of illness | Promptly report to infection control office. |
| Chickenpox (varicella) | Until all lesions are crusted | Immune person does not need to wear a mask. Exposed susceptible clients should be placed in a private special airflow room on STOP SIGN alert status beginning 10 days after initial exposure until 21 days after last exposure. Report to epidemiology. |
| Diphtheria, pharyngeal | Until two cultures from both nose and throat taken at least 24 h after cessation of antimicrobial therapy are negative for *Corynebacterium diphtheriae* | Promptly report to epidemiology. |
| Epiglottis, due to *Haemophilus influenzae* | For 24 h after cessation of antimicrobial therapy | Report to epidemiology. |
| Erythema infectiosum | For 7 days after onset | Report to epidemiology. |
| Hemorrhagic fevers | Duration of illness | Call epidemiology office immediately. Physician may call the State Health Department and Centers for Disease Control and Prevention for advice about management of a suspected case. |
| Herpes zoster (varicella zoster), disseminated | Duration of illness | Localized; does not require STOP SIGN. |
| Lassa fever | Duration of illness | Call epidemiology office immediately. |
| Marburg virus disease | | Physician may call the State Health Department and Centers for Disease Control and Prevention for advice about management of a suspected case. |
| Measles (rubeola) | For 4 days after start of rash, except in immunocompromised patients, for whom precautions should be maintained for duration of illness | Immune people do not need to wear a mask. Exposed susceptible clients should be placed in a private special air flow room on STOP SIGN alert status beginning the 5th day after exposure until 21 days after last exposure. |
| Meningitis *Haemophilus influenzae* known or suspected | For 24 h after start of effective antibiotic therapy | Call epidemiology to report. |
| *Neisseria meningitidis* (meningococci) known or suspected | For 24 h after start of effective antibiotic therapy | Promptly report to epidemiology. |
| Meningococcal pneumonia | For 24 h after start of effective antibiotic therapy | Promptly report to epidemiology. |
| Meningococcemia | For 24 h after start of effective antibiotic therapy | Consult with epidemiology. |
| Multiply resistant organisms | Until culture negative or as determined by epidemiology | Consult with epidemiology. |
| Mumps (infectious parotitis) | For 9 days after onset of swelling | People with history do not need to wear a mask. Call epidemiology office to report. |
| Pertussis (whooping cough) | For 7 days after start of effective therapy | Call epidemiology to report. |
| Plague, pneumonic | For 3 days after start of effective therapy | Promptly report to epidemiology. |
| Pneumonia, *Haemophilus* in infants and children any age | For 24 h after start of effective therapy | Call epidemiology. |
| Pneumonia, meningococcal | For 24 h after start of effective antibiotic therapy | Promptly report to epidemiology. |
| Rubella (German measles) | For 7 days after onset of rash | Immune people do not need to wear a mask. Promptly report to epidemiology. |
| Tuberculosis, bronchial, laryngeal, pulmonary, confirmed or suspect | Clients are not considered infectious if they meet all these criteria: Adequate therapy received for 2–3 weeks Favorable clinical response to therapy Three consecutive negative sputum smear results from sputum collected on different days | Call epidemiology to report; prompt use of effective antituberculosis drugs is the most effective means of limiting transmission. |
| Varicella (chickenpox) | Until all lesions crusted over | See chickenpox. |

*Source:* Centers for Disease Control and Prevention. www.cdc.gov.

**NIC**
Teaching: Disease
Process, Infection
Control Infection
Protection, Sexual
Counseling, Behavior
Management: Sexual
Behavior

# ➤ Interventions

## Identify Susceptible Individuals

| | | |
|---|---|---|
| Homosexual practices | Bisexual practices | Intravenous/intranasal/ |
| Blood transfusions | Multiple sexual partners | intradermal drug users |
| before 1985 | with sexually transmitted diseases | |
| High-risk behaviors | Health care workers | |
| Tattoo by unlicensed persons | First responders (police, rescue | |
| | workers, ambulance, firefighters) | |

## Counsel Susceptible Individuals to Be Tested for HIV

**R:** Some high-risk behaviors can be eliminated. Professional in high-risk situations must practice universal precautions.

Testing can provide baseline data and can help can predict onset of infection, enabling the client to receive medications.

## Discuss the Mode of Transmission of the Virus.

Unprotected vaginal, anal, or oral sex with infected hosts or infected sex toys
Unprotected sex with infected person
Sharing intravenous needles and syringes; intranasal drug paraphernalia
Contact of infected fluids with broken skin or mucous membrane
Breastfeeding, perinatal transmission

**R:** HIV is transmitted by sexual contact, by contact with infected blood, body fluid and blood products, and perinatally (from mother to fetus).

## Use Appropriate Universal Precautions for All Body Fluids

Wash hands before and after all contact with client or specimen.

**R:** Hand washing is one of the most important means to prevent the spread of infection.

Handle the blood of all clients as potentially infectious.
Wear gloves for potential contact with blood and body fluids.
Handle all linen soiled with blood or body secretions as potentially infectious.
Process all laboratory specimens as potentially infectious.

**R:** Gloves provide a barrier from contact with infectious secretions and excretions.

Place used syringes immediately in a nearby impermeable container; do not recap or manipulate he needle in any way! Use retractable needle syringes when possible.

**R:** Needlesticks can transmit infectious blood.

Wear protective eyewear and mask if splatter with blood or body fluids is possible (e.g., bronchoscopy, oral surgery).

**R:** Eye coverings protect the eyes from accidental exposure to infectious secretions present; gowns prevent soiling of clothes if contact with secretions/excretions is likely. Wear mask for tuberculosis and other respiratory organisms. (HIV is not airborne.)
**R:** Masks prevent transmission by aerosolization of infectious agents if oral mucosal lesions are present.
**R:** Universal precautions reduce contact with contagious substances.

## Reduce the Risk of Transmission of HIV

Explain low-risk sexual behaviors:

• Mutual masturbation
• Massage

Vaginal intercourse with condom

**R:** The risk in sexually transmitted infections is prevented with abstinence. Activities that do not include penile, vaginal anal, or oral contact carry low or no risk. Transmission is reduced by condom use and limiting partners.

Explain other risks:

- Alcohol and drug use
- Sex aides
- Multiple partners

**R:** Alcohol and drug use reduce the client's ability to make safe decisions regarding sexual activity. The risk of acquiring HIV increases as the number of partners increase.

Explain the risk of ejaculate contact with broken skin or mucous membranes (oral, anal).

**R:** These measures aim to prevent contact of body fluids with mucous membranes.

Teach client to use condoms of latex rubber, not "natural membrane"; teach appropriate storage to preserve latex. Avoid spermicides with nonoxynol-9.
Explain the need for water-based lubricants to reduce prophylactic breaks. Avoid petroleum-based lubricants, which dissolve latex.
Explain that a condom with a spermicide may provide additional protection by decreasing the number of viable HIV particles.

**R:** Nonoxynol-9 spermicides may increase the risk of HIV transmission. Natural membrane condoms do not prevent transfer of infected fluids.

## Teach the Client How to Disinfect Equipment at Home (Needles, Syringes, Drug Paraphernalia, Sex Aids)

Wash under running water.
Fill or wash with household bleach.
Rinse well with water.

**R:** Exposure to disinfecting agents rapidly inactivates HIV. Household bleach solution (dilute 1:10 with water) is an inexpensive choice.

## Provide Facts to Dispel Myths Regarding HIV Transmission

The AIDS virus is not transmitted by mosquitoes, swimming pools, clothes, eating utensils, telephones, toilet seats, or close contact (e.g., at work, school).
Saliva, sweat, tears, urine, and feces do not transmit HIV.
AIDS cannot be contracted during blood donations.
Blood for transfusions is tested to reduce substantially the risk of contracting the AIDS virus.

**R:** Dispelling myths and correcting misinformation can reduce anxiety and allow others to interact more normally with the client.

## Initiate Health Teaching and Referrals as Indicated

Emphasize the need to be careful about sex partners (past sexual partners, experimentation with drugs).
Provide the community and schools with facts regarding AIDS transmission, and dispel myths.
In case of acute exposure to HIV (e.g., sexual assault, needlestick, break in barrier with HIV-infected person), immediately refer to health care facility for immediate initiation of postexposure prophylaxis of antiviral therapy.

**R:** Protocols for exposure to body fluids possibly contaminated with HIV are available in all health care facilities.

Educate clients and families about the chain of infection and precautions needed both in the hospital and at home.

**R:** It is advisable that family members and others caring for or coming into contact with the client take simple precautions.

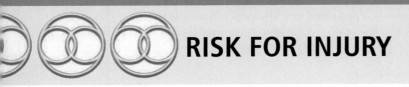

# RISK FOR INJURY

**Risk for Injury**

    Related to Lack of Awareness of Environmental Hazards
    Related to Lack of Awareness of Environmental Hazards Secondary to Maturational Age
    Related to Vertigo Secondary to Orthostatic Hypotension
Risk for Aspiration
Risk for Falls
Risk for Poisoning
Risk for Suffocation
Risk for Trauma
Risk for Perioperative Positioning Injury

## DEFINITION

State in which a client is at risk for harm because of a perceptual or physiologic deficit, a lack of awareness of hazards, or maturational age

## RISK FACTORS

Presence of risk factor (see Related Factors).

## RELATED FACTORS

### Pathophysiologic

*Related to altered cerebral function secondary to hypoxia*
Related to syncop
Related to vertigo or dizziness
*Related to impaired mobility secondary to:*
Cerebrovascular accident    Arthritis Parkinsonism
Related to loss of limb
Related to impaired vision
Related to hearing impairment
*Related to fatigue*
*Related to orthostatic hypotension*
*Related to vestibular disorders*
*Related to lack of awareness of environmental hazards secondary to:*
Confusion
*Related to tonic–clonic movements secondary to:*
Seizures

### Treatment-Related

*Related to prolonged bed rest*
*Related to effects of (specify) or sensorium*
Examples:

| | | |
|---|---|---|
| Sedatives | Diuretics | Vasodilators |
| Phenothiazine | Antihypertensives | Psychotropics |
| Hypoglycemics | Pain medications | Muscle relaxants |

*Related to casts/crutches, canes, walkers*

## Situational (Personal, Environmental)

*Related to decrease in or loss of short-term memory*
*Related to faulty judgment secondary to:*

| | | | |
|---|---|---|---|
| Stress | Alcohol, drugs | Dehydration | Depression |

*Related to household hazards (specify)*

| | | |
|---|---|---|
| Unsafe walkways | Stairs | Unsafe toys |
| Slippery floors | Inadequate lighting | Faulty electric wires |
| Bathrooms (tubs, toilets) | Improperly stored poisons | |

*Related to automotive hazards*
Lack of use of seat belts or child seats
Mechanically unsafe vehicle
*Related to fire hazards*
*Related to unfamiliar setting (hospital, nursing home)*
*Related to improper footwear*
*Related to inattentive caretaker*
*Related to improper use of aids (crutches, canes, walkers, wheelchairs)*
*Related to history of accidents*
*Related to unstable gait*

## Maturational

Infant/Child
*Related to lack of awareness of hazards*

Older Adult
*Related to faulty judgments, secondary cognitive deficits*
*Related to sedentary lifestyle and loss of muscle strength*

### ■■■■■■ AUTHOR'S NOTE

This diagnosis has five subcategories: *Risk for Aspiration, Poisoning, Suffocation Poisoning,* and *Trauma.* Interventions to prevent poisoning, suffocation, falls, and trauma are included under the general category *Risk for Injury.* Should the nurse choose to isolate interventions only for prevention of poisoning, suffocation, or trauma, then the diagnosis *Risk for Poisoning, Risk for Suffocation, Risk for Falls,* or *Risk for Trauma* would be useful.

Nursing interventions related to *Risk for Injury* focus on protecting a client from injury and teaching precautions to reduce the risk of injury. When the nurse is teaching a client or family safety measures to prevent injury but is not providing on-site protection (as in the community or outpatient department, or for discharge planning), the diagnosis *Risk for Injury related to insufficient knowledge of safety precautions* may be more appropriate.

### ■■■■■■ ERRORS IN DIAGNOSTIC STATEMENTS

1. *Risk for Injury: Hemorrhage related to abnormal blood profile secondary to cirrhosis*
   This diagnosis does not represent a situation that a nurse can prevent, but one that he or she monitors and co-manages with physicians as the collaborative problem *RC of Hemorrhage related to altered clotting factors.* Refer to Section 3, Manual of Collaborative Problems, for additional interventions.

### ■■■■■■ KEY CONCEPTS

#### Generic Considerations

- Injury is the fourth leading cause of death in the general population (40.1 deaths per 100,000) and the leading cause of death in children and young adults.
- Health education activities that focus on fire safety, home safety, water safety, seat belt use, motor vehicle safety, cardiopulmonary resuscitation (CPR) training, poison control, and first aid can reduce the rate of accidents (Clemen-Stone, Eigasti, & McGuire, 2002).
- Table II.11 lists common sources of poisoning in the home.

*(continued)*

■■■■■■ **KEY CONCEPTS** *Continued*

### Orthostatic Hypotension

- Postural hypotension refers to a sudden drop in blood pressure of 20 mm Hg or more for at least 1 min when standing.
- Studies have shown that postprandial hypotension occurs in about one third of healthy adults 1 h after eating breakfast and lunch (Lipsitz & Fullerton, 1986).
- Postural hypotension can affect quality of life if it contributes to falls or fear of falling. It also can precipitate stroke and myocardial infarction (Porth, 2006).

## Pediatric Considerations

- Injury is the leading cause of death in people 1 to 19 years of age (Hockenberry & Wilson, 2009).
- Six leading types of death are traffic accidents, drowning, burns and fires, chokings, poisonings, and falls (Hockenberry & Wilson, 2009).
- Each year, car crashes injure and kill more children than do any disease. Used properly, safety seats and belts protect children in crashes and help save lives (National Safety Council, 2007).
- Injury accounts for 72% of total fatalities among late adolescents (15 to 19 years of age), the pediatric age group at highest risk for injury mortality (National Safety Council, 2007).
- Between 70% and 80% of infants will use a walker, usually between 5 and 12 months of age. Of them, 30% to 40% will have an accident (American Medical Association [AMA] Board of Trustees, 1991). Most walker accidents are minor; however, serious trauma from head injuries, lacerations, and burns occurs occasionally. Nurses should counsel parents on the risk of injury from use of infant walkers (AMA Board of Trustees, 1991).
- Children should be taught early (2 years of age) and reminded constantly about rules for streets, playground equipment, fires, water (pools, bathtubs), animals, and strangers.
- Swimming programs that use total submersion put infants at risk for water intoxication, hypothermia, and bacterial infections. In addition, infants may learn to fear the water.
- Children 1 to 3 years of age are at greatest risk to be scalded by hot water. More than one third of children 3 to 8 years of age are burned while playing with matches. When a fire strikes, young children need help to escape (Hockenberry & Wilson, 2009).
- For children younger than 3 years, choking is the fourth leading cause of accidental death.
- Toddlers are at highest risk for poisoning. Children are poisoned by medications as well as by common household items (e.g., plants, makeup, cleaning products).
- For children 1 to 4 years of age, the leading cause of accidental death and serious injury is falls in the home (Hockenberry & Wilson, 2009).

### TABLE II.11 POISONOUS SUBSTANCES AROUND THE HOUSE

**Drugs**

| | | | |
|---|---|---|---|
| Aspirin | Cough medicines | Laxatives | Tranquilizers |
| Vitamins | Oral contraceptives | Barbiturates | Acetaminophen |

**Petroleum Products**

| | | | |
|---|---|---|---|
| Cleaning Agents | Soaps and polishes | Disinfectants | Drain cleaners |

**Poisonous plants**

| | | | |
|---|---|---|---|
| Amaryllis | Iris | Philodendron | Azalea |
| Jack-in-the-pulpit | Poinsettia | Baneberry | Jerusalem cherry |
| Poison hemlock | Belladonna | Jimsonweed | Poison ivy |
| Bittersweet | Lily of the valley | Pokeweed | Bloodroot |
| Marijuana | Potato leaves | Castor-bean plant | Mistletoe |
| Rhododendron | Climbing nightshade | Morning glory | Rhubarb leaves |
| Daffodil | Mountain laurel | Schefflera | Devil's ivy |
| Mushrooms | Tomato leaves | Dieffenbachia | Oleander |
| Wisteria | Foxglove | Peace lily | Yew |
| Holly | | | |

**Miscellaneous**

| | | | |
|---|---|---|---|
| Baby powder | Cosmetics | Lead paint | |

## Geriatric Considerations

- Falls are more frequent in older adults, and the mortality, dysfunction, disability, and need for medical services that result are greater than in younger age groups. Unintentional injury, a category including falls, motor vehicle collisions, and burns, is the seventh leading cause of death in older adults, and the incidence of falls represents more than 60% of that category.
- Fall-related complications are the leading cause of death in clients age 65 or older (Miller, 2009).
- The risk of dying in one year after a hip fracture is 18% to 33% (Miller, 2009).
- Approximately 25% of hospital admissions for older adults are directly related to falling; 47% of these people are admitted to long-term–care facilities (Miller, 2009).
- "Fallaphobia" refers to fears related to a client's loss of confidence to perform activities without falling. These fears actually increase the risk for falling, and the client eventually becomes housebound (Miller, 2009).
- A fall-free existence is not always possible for some people. Increased independence and mobility may be an important and valuable trade-off for increased risk of falling. Collaboration among client, family, and team members helps arrive at the decision of a less restricted environment.
- With age comes some loss of the postural control system. To not fall, a client must be able to keep his or her center of gravity over an adequate base, as well as to rapidly process and respond to sensory information (Baumann, 1999).
- Older adults frequently lack muscle strength in lower extremities and have insufficient torque in their ankles (Baumann, 1999).
- Regular walking, as little as 60 min twice a week, can improve sensory function, balance, stability, hip flexion strength, hip extension, and dorsiflexion, all of which can reduce falls (Schoenfelder, 2000).
- The following factors increase the risk for falls in older adults (Miller, 2009; Murray, Zentner, & Yakimo, 2009):
  - History of falls
  - Sensory–motor deficits (e.g., vision, hearing, hemianopia [loss of half of visual field], paresis, aphasia)
  - Gait instability
  - Improper footwear or foot problems (corns, bunions, calluses)
  - Postural hypotension, especially with complaints of dizziness
  - Confusion (persistent or acute)
  - Incontinence, urinary urgency
  - Cardiovascular disease affecting cerebral perfusion and oxygenation: dysrhythmias, syncopal episodes, congestive heart failure, fibrillation
  - Kinesthetic changes, changes in postural reflexes, or sway
  - Neurologic disease affecting movement or judgment: cerebrovascular accident with impulsivity; Parkinsonism; moderate Alzheimer's disease; seizure disorder; vertigo
  - Orthopedic disorders or devices affecting movement or balance: casts, splints, slings, prostheses, recent surgery, severe arthritis
  - Medications affecting blood pressure or level of consciousness: psychotropics, sedatives, analgesics, diuretics, antihypertensives, antidepressants, antibiotics medication change, more than five drugs
  - Agitation, increased anxiety, and emotional lability
  - Excess ingestion of alcohol
  - Willfulness, uncooperativeness
  - Situational factors: new admission, room change, roommate change

## Focus Assessment Criteria

This entire assessment is indicated only when the client is at high risk for injury because of personal deficits, alterations (e.g., mobility problems), or maturational age. In households without such a family member, the functional assessment of the individual can be deleted with the focus on the environment.

## Subjective Data

These consist of the client's physical capabilities (as reported by client or caretaker).

### Assess for Risk Factors

**Vision**
Corrected (date of last prescription)

Complaints of

| | | |
|---|---|---|
| Blurriness | Difficulty focusing | Loss of side vision |
| Inability to adjust to darkness | | |

### Hearing

| | |
|---|---|
| Need to read lips | Use of hearing aid |
| Inadequate | (condition, batteries) |

### Thermal/Tactile

Altered sense of hot/cold

### Mental Status

Drowsy
Confused
Oriented to time, place, events
Complaints of:

| | |
|---|---|
| Vertigo | Orthostatic hypotension |

Altered sense of balance
Cognitive stage (immature reasoning/judgment)

### Mobility

*Reports of:*

| | | |
|---|---|---|
| Feeling lightheaded, dizzy | Losing balance | Difficulty standing, sitting |
| Wandering | Falling or almost falling | |

*Ability to ambulate:*

| | | |
|---|---|---|
| Around room | Around house | Up and down stairs |
| Outside house | | |

*Ability to travel:*

| | |
|---|---|
| Drive car (date of last reevaluation) | Use public transportation |

*Devices:*

| | | |
|---|---|---|
| Cane | Walker | Condition of devices |
| Wheelchair | Prosthesis | Competence in their use |

*Shoes/slippers:*

| | | |
|---|---|---|
| Condition | Nonskid soles | Fit |

*Abilities related to developmental milestones:*

| | | |
|---|---|---|
| Turning over | Climbing | Sitting |
| Crawling | Standing | Walking |

### Miscellaneous

*Drug therapy:*

| | | |
|---|---|---|
| Type | Dosage | Storage |
| Labeling | Ability to self-medicate safely | |

*Communication Ability:*

| | | |
|---|---|---|
| Write | Use telephone | Make needs known |

Contact emergency assistance
*Support system/primary caregiver*
*Help available from relatives, friends, neighbors, club, and church contacts*
*History of "blackouts"*
*Urinary frequency or incontinence*

## Objective Data

### *Assess for Related Factors*

**Blood Pressure (left, right, sitting/lying more than 5 min, 1 min after standing)**

**Gait**

| | | |
|---|---|---|
| Steady | Requires aids | Unsteady |

**Strength**

| | |
|---|---|
| Can stand on one leg | Can sit-stand-sit |

### Cognitive Processes

| | | |
|---|---|---|
| Can communicate needs | Can interact | History of wandering (witnessed and |
| Can understand cause and effect | | reported by others) |

### Presence of

| | | |
|---|---|---|
| Anger | Withdrawal | Depression |
| Faulty judgment | | |

### Ability for Self-Care Activities

| | | |
|---|---|---|
| Dress and undress | Bathe | Groom self |
| Feed self | Reach toilet | |

## Assess for Risk Factors in the Home

### Safety

| | | |
|---|---|---|
| Toilet facilities | Water supply | Heating |
| Sewage | Ventilation | Garbage disposal |

### Safety of Walkways (Inside and Outside)

*Sidewalks (uneven, broken)*
*Stairs (inside and outside):*

| | | |
|---|---|---|
| Broken steps | Lighting | No hand rails |
| Protection for children | | |

*Halls:*

| | |
|---|---|
| Cluttered | Poor lighting |

### Electrical Hazards

No outlet covers
Cords frayed and unanchored
Outlets overloaded; accessible to children; near water
Switches too far from bedside

### Inadequate Lighting

| | | |
|---|---|---|
| At night | Outdoors | To bathroom at night |

### Unsafe Floors

| | | |
|---|---|---|
| Even or uneven | Highly polished | Rugs not anchored |

### Kitchen Hazards

Pot handles not turned inward
Stove (grease or flammable objects on stove)
Refrigerator (improperly stored food; inadequate temperatures)

### Toxic Substances

Stored in food containers; not properly labeled; accessible to children
Medications kept beyond date of expiration
Poisonous household plants

### Fire Hazards

Matches/lighters accessible to children
No fire extinguishers
Improper storage of corrosives, combustibles
Lack of furnace maintenance
No fire escape plan, no fire extinguishers
Emergency telephone numbers not accessible (fire, police)

### Hazards for Children in Nursery

Cribs near drapery cords
Cribs with wide slat openings
Plastic bags
Pillows in crib
Unattended without crib rails up

Space between mattress and crib rails
Unattended on changing table
Pacifier hung around infant's neck
Propped bottle placed in infant's crib
Toys with pointed edges, removable parts

### Hazards for Children in Household

Accessible medications, lighters, matches, and cleaning products
Objects with lead paint
Poisonous plants (see Table II.11)
Open windows with loose or no screens
Plastic bags
Furniture with glass or sharp corners
Open doorways, stairways

### Outdoor Hazards for Children

| | | |
|---|---|---|
| Porches without rails | Play area without fence | Backyard pools |
| Domestic/wild animals | Poisonous plants | |

For more information on Focus Assessment Criteria, visit http://thepoint.lww.com.

**NOC**

Risk Control, Safe Home Environment, Falls Occurrence, Fall Prevention Behavior

## ➤ Goal

The client will relate fewer or no injuries.

### Indicators:

- Identify factors that increase risk for injury.
- Relate intent to use safety measures to prevent injury (e.g., remove or anchor throw rugs).
- Relate intent to practice selected prevention measures (e.g., wear sunglasses to reduce glare).
- Increase daily activity, if feasible.

**NIC**

Fall Prevention, Environmental Management: Safety, Health Education, Surveillance: Safety, Risk Identification

## ➤ General Interventions

### Refer to Related Factors

### *Reduce or Eliminate Causative or Contributing Factors, If Possible*

#### Unfamiliar Surroundings

Orient each client to surroundings on admission; explain the call system, and assess client's ability to use it.
Closely supervise the client during the first few nights to assess safety.
Use a night-light.
Encourage the client to request assistance during the night.
Teach about side effects of certain drugs (e.g., dizziness, fatigue).
Keep bed at lowest level during the night.
Consider use of a movement detection monitor, if needed.

**R:** An unfamiliar environment and problems with vision, orientation, mobility, and fatigue can increase risk of falling.

#### Impaired Vision

Provide safe illumination and teach client to:

- Ensure adequate lighting in all rooms, with soft light at night.
- Have a light switch easily accessible, next to the bed.
- Provide background light that is soft.

Teach the client how to reduce glare:

- Avoid glossy surfaces (e.g., glass, highly polished floors).

- Use diffuse rather than direct light; use shades that darken the room.
- Turn the head away when switching on a bright light.
- Wear sunglasses or hats with brims, or carry umbrellas, to reduce glare outside.
- Avoid looking directly at bright lights (e.g., headlights).

Teach the client or family to provide sufficient color contrast for visual discrimination and to avoid green and blue:

- Color-code edges of steps (e.g., with colored tape).
- Avoid white walls, dishes, and counters.
- Avoid clear glasses (i.e., use smoked glass).
- Choose objects colored black on white (e.g., black phone).
- Avoid colors that merge (e.g., beige switches on beige walls).
- Paint doorknobs bright colors.

**R:** Visual difficulty because of glare is often responsible for falls in older adults, who have increased susceptibility to glare. Incandescent (nonfluorescent) lighting produces less glare and therefore provides better illumination for older clients.

### Decreased Tactile Sensitivity
Teach preventive measures:

- Assess temperature of bath water and heating pads before use.
- Use bath thermometers.
- Assess extremities daily for undetected injuries.
- Keep the feet warm and dry and skin softened with emollient lotion (lanolin, mineral oil).

**R:** Loss of sensation in the limbs can increase the risk of burns and undetected injuries.

See *Ineffective Peripheral Tissue Perfusion* for additional interventions.

### Orthostatic Hypotension
See *Risk for Injury Related to Vertigo Secondary to Orthostatic Hypotension* for additional interventions.

### Decreased Strength/Flexibility
Perform ankle-strengthening exercises daily (Schoenfelder, 2000):

- Stand behind a straight chair, with feet slightly apart.
- Slowly raise both heels until body weight is on the balls of the feet; hold for a count of 3 (e.g., 1 Mississippi, 2 Mississippi, 3 Mississippi).
- Do 5 to 10 repetitions; increase repetitions as strength increases.

Walk at least two or three times a week.

- Use ankle exercises as a warm-up before walking.
- Begin walking with someone at side, if needed, for 10 min.
- Increase time and speed according to capabilities.

**R:** Ankle strengthening and a walking program can improve balance, increase ankle strength, improve walking speed, decrease falls and fear of falling, and increase confidence in performing activities of daily living (Schoenfelder, 2000).

### Hazardous Environmental Factors
Teach the client to:

- Eliminate throw rugs, litter, and highly polished floors.
- Ensure nonslip surfaces in bathtub or shower by applying commercially available traction tapes.
- Install handgrips in bathroom.
- Install railings in hallways and on stairs.
- Remove protruding objects (e.g., coat hooks, shelves, light fixtures) from stairway walls.

Instruct staff to:

- Keep side rails on bed in place and bed at the lowest position when the client is left unattended.
- Keep the bed at the lowest position with wheels locked when stationary.

- Teach the client in the wheelchair to lock and unlock the wheels.
- Ensure that client's shoes or slippers have nonskid soles.

**R:** Goals to prevent or manage falls focus on reducing their likelihood by minimizing environmental hazards and strengthening individual competence to resist falls and fall-related injury.

If Cognitively Impaired, Refer to *Wandering*.

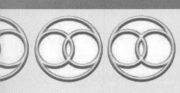

# RISK FOR INJURY
## ❱ Related to Lack of Awareness of Environmental Hazards

**NOC**
Safe Home Environment, Risk Control, Parenting: Infant/Toddler/ Early Childhood/ Middle Childhood, Adolescent Safety

## ➤ Goal

The parent or family will identify and reduce environmental hazards.

### *Indicators:*

- Teach children safety habits.
- Safely store hazardous items.
- Repair hazards as needed.
- Remove environmental hazards when possible.
- Install safety measures (e.g., locks, rails).

**NIC**
Area Restriction, Surveillance: Safety, Environmental Management: Safety, Home Maintenance Assistance, Risk Identification, Teaching: Infant, Toddler Safety

## ➤ Interventions

### Identify Situations that Contribute to Accidents

Unfamiliar setting (homes of others, hotels)
Peak activity periods (meal preparation, holidays)
New equipment (bicycle, chain saw, lawn mower, snow blower)
Lack of awareness of or disregard for environmental hazards (reckless driving)

**R:** Injury is the fourth leading cause of death in the general population and the leading cause of death in children and young adults (Clemen Stone et al., 2005).

## Reduce or Eliminate Hazardous Situations

### *Teach About New Equipment*

Teach the client to read directions completely before using a new appliance or piece of equipment.
Determine the limitations of the equipment.
Unplug and turn off any appliance that is not functioning before examining it (e.g., lawn mower, snow blower, electric mixer).

**R:** Unfamiliarity with equipment can cause injuries.

### *Review Unsafe Practices*

**Automobiles**
Driving a mechanically unsafe vehicle
Not using or misusing seat restraints
Driving after drinking alcohol or drugs
Driving with unrestrained babies and children in the car

Driving at excessive speeds
Driving without necessary visual aids
Driving with unsafe road or road crossing conditions
Not using or misusing necessary headgear for motorcyclist
Allowing children to ride in the front seat of the car
Backing up without checking the location of small children
Warming a car in a closed garage

### Flammables
Igniting gas leaks
Delayed lighting of gas burner or oven
Experimenting with chemicals or gasoline
Using unscreened fires, fireplaces, or heaters
Inadequately storing combustibles, matches, or oily rags
Smoking in bed or near oxygen
Buying highly flammable children's toys or clothing
Playing with fireworks or gunpowder
Playing with matches, candles, cigarettes, or lighters
Wearing plastic aprons or flowing clothing around an open flame

### Kitchen
Allowing grease waste to collect on stoves
Wearing plastic aprons or flowing clothing around an open flame
Using cracked glasses or dishware
Using improper canning, freezing, or preserving methods
Storing knives uncovered
Keeping pot handles facing front of stove
Using thin or worn pot holders or oven mitts
Placing stove controls on front
Using dishes that have lead in them

### Bathroom
Keeping the medicine cabinet unlocked
Not having grab rails in the bathtub
Not having nonskid mats or emery strips in the bathtub
Maintaining poor lighting in the bathroom and hallways
Improperly placing electrical outlets

### Chemicals and Irritants
Improperly labeling medication containers
Keeping medications in containers other than the original ones
Maintaining poor illumination at the medicine cabinet
Improperly labeling containers of poisons and corrosive substances
Keeping expired medications that dangerously decompose
Storing toxic substances in accessible areas (e.g., under the sink)
Storing corrosives (e.g., lye) inadequately
Having contact with intense cold
Being overexposed to sun, sunlamps, or heating pads

### Lighting and Electrical
Using uncovered outlets
Using unanchored electrical wires
Overloading electrical outlets
Overloading fuse boxes
Using faulty electrical plugs, frayed wires, or defective electrical appliances
Maintaining inadequate lighting over landings and stairs
Maintaining inaccessible light switches (e.g., bedside)
Using machinery or appliances without prior instruction

**R:** Specific instructions can reduce the rate of accidents and injury (Clemen-Stone et al., 2005).

## Initiate Health Teaching and Referral, as Indicated

### Teach Measures to Prevent Car Accidents

Frequently reevaluate the ability to drive.
Wear good-quality sunglasses (gray or green) to reduce glare.
Keep windshields clean and wipers in good condition.
Place mirrors on both sides of the car.
Stop periodically to stretch and to rest eyes.
Know the effects of medications on driving ability.
Do not smoke while driving or drive after drinking.
Do not use a cellular phone while driving.

### Teach Measures to Prevent Pedestrian Accidents

Allow enough time to cross streets.
Wear garments that reflect light (beige, white) at night.
Wait to cross on the sidewalk, not the street.
Look both ways.
Do not rely solely on green traffic lights to provide safe crossing (right turn on red light may be legal, or driver may disobey traffic regulations).

### Teach Measures to Prevent Burns

Equip the home with a smoke alarm system and check its function each month.
Have a handheld fire extinguisher.
Set thermostats for water heater to provide warm, but not scalding, water.
Use baking soda or a lid cover to smother a kitchen grease fire.
Do not wear loose-fitting clothing (e.g., robes, nightgowns) when cooking.
Do not smoke when sleepy.
Ensure that portable heaters are safely used.
Provide health teaching and referrals as indicated.

**R:** Accidents occur more frequently:

- During the initial period of hospitalization and between 6:00 and 9:00 PM
- During peak activity periods (meals, playtime)
- In unfamiliar surroundings
- With adequate lighting
- At holidays
- On vacation
- During home repairs

**R:** Injury prevention requires anticipation and recognition of where safety measures are applicable. Passive strategies provide automatic protection without choice (e.g., air bags, product design). Active strategies require persuasion through teaching or legislation to practice safety measures (Hockenberry & Wilson, 2009).

### Refer Clients with Motor or Sensory Deficits for Assistance in Identifying Environmental Hazards

Local fire company
Community nursing agency
Accident-prevention information (see References/Bibliography)

### Refer to Physical Therapist for Evaluation of Gait

**Pediatric Interventions**

### Teach Parents Basic Safety Measures and Assessments

Instruct parents to expect frequent changes in infants' and children's abilities and to take precautions (e.g., an infant who suddenly rolls over for the first time might be on a changing table unattended).

Discuss the necessity of constantly monitoring small children.

Provide information to assist parents in selecting a babysitter:

- Determine previous experiences and knowledge of emergency measures.
- Observe interaction of sitter with child (e.g., have sitter arrive 30 min before you are ready to leave).

Teach parents to expect children to mimic them and to teach what children can do with or without supervision.

- Tell the child to ask you before attempting a new task.

Explain and expect compliance with certain rules (depending on age) concerning:

Streets          Fire                    Playground equipment
Animals       Water (pools, bathtubs)   Strangers
Bicycles

Role-play with children to assess understanding of the problem.

- "You're walking home. A strange man pulls up in a car near you. What do you do?"
- "While walking past a barbecue, your dress catches on fire. What do you do?"

## Identify Situations That Contribute to Accidents

### Bicycles, Wagons, Skateboards, and Skates

No reflectors or lights          Not in single file
Riding a too-large bicycle       No training wheels
Use of skateboards or skates     Lack of knowledge of the rules of the road
  in heavily traveled areas      Lack of helmet, protective pads

Safe riding area for young children (not in street)

**R:** Every day, more than 1,000 children are injured, and one dies, in bicycle accidents. School-aged children are at greatest risk. One third of children treated in emergency rooms for bicycle accidents have head injuries. Use of bicycle helmets could reduce the incidence of these injuries.

**R:** Prevention strategies to decrease serious injuries resulting from skateboarding include warnings against skateboard use by children younger than 5 years of age, prohibition of skateboards on streets and highways, and the promotion of use of helmets and other protective gear (Hockenberry & Wilson, 2009).

### Water and Pools

Discourage use of flotation or swim aids (water wings, tubs) with children who cannot swim.
Teach safe water behavior:

No running, pushing            No jumping on others
No swimming alone              No playful screaming for help
No diving in water less        No swimming after meals
  than 8 feet deep             No excessive alcohol use
Keep sharp objects out of the pool
No swimming during electrical storms
Enclose the pool:

- Use a 5- to 12-foot fence.
- Use a fence that children cannot climb.
- Use self-locking gates with an alarm system.

Remove the pool cover completely.

Avoid free-floating pool covers.

Teach safe diving and sliding techniques:

- Allow diving only from diving boards.
- Discourage running dives.
- Teach to steer upward with hands and head.
- Descend pool slide sitting with feet first.

Have lifesaving equipment at poolside (life preserver, rope, or hook).

Learn CPR and how to respond to accidental submersion:

- Remove the child from the water.
- If spinal injury is suspected, immobilize on a board and apply a cervical collar.
- Clear airway of debris.
- If the client is unresponsive, place on side if vomiting occurs.
- Remove wet clothes, dry, and cover with blankets (including head).
- Begin CPR and continue until help arrives.

**R:** Drowning is the second leading cause of death from injury during childhood. Children younger than 4 years of age are at especially high risk (National Safety Council, 2000).

**R:** Many near-drownings take place while a parent is supervising the child but has a momentary lapse of attention (Hockenberry & Wilson, 2009).

**R:** Effective swimming depends on intellectual as well as physical maturity. Organized swimming lessons may give parents a false sense of security that their child "can swim."

## Miscellaneous

Unsupervised contact with animals and poisons in the environment (plants, pool chemicals, pills)

Obstructed passageways

Unsafe window protection in home with young children

Guns or ammunition stored in unlocked fashion

Large icicles hanging from roof

Icy walkways

Glass sliding doors that look open when closed

Low-strung clothesline

Discarded or unused refrigerators or freezers without removed doors

## Infants and Toddlers

### Household

Pillows in crib

Staircases without stair gates

Crib mattresses that do not fit snugly

Cribs with slat openings that allow the child's body to fall through, catching the head

Glass or sharp-edged tables

Porches and decks without railings

Poisonous plants (see Table II.11)

Furniture painted with lead paint

Unsupervised bathing

Open windows

Propped bottle in crib

### Toys

| | | |
|---|---|---|
| Sharp edges | Balloons | Easily breakable parts |
| Lollipops | Removable small pieces | Pacifier around neck |

*Miscellaneous*

Child unattended in a shopping cart
Child unattended in a car
Cribs, walkers, or high chairs with movable parts that trap the child (e.g., springs)
Put the child in a car safety seat in the back seat only

## Assist Parents to Analyze an Accident

What happened?
How did it happen?
Where, when did it happen?
Why did the accident happen?

**R:** Analysis of an accident may prevent recurrence.

Teach the Heimlich maneuver for choking on an object or piece of food.

**R:** This procedure creates an artificial cough that forces air and the foreign object out of the child's airway.

## Teach Poison Prevention

Instruct parents how to "childproof" the home.
Instruct parents to keep poisons and corrosive substances in tightly closed, carefully marked containers in locked closets.
Instruct parents to avoid taking medications in front of children.
Parents should discard unused supplies of medications and keep needed medications in a locked, inaccessible medicine closet.
Parents should be taught how to administer antidotes for specific toxic substances, if advised by the Poison Control Center.
Parents should also have the phone number of the Poison Control Center in a convenient place.
Refer individuals to the local poison control center for "Mr. Yuk" poison warning stickers and advice on emergency procedures; teach the child what a "Mr. Yuk" sticker means.
Instruct parents to have two doses of ipecac syrup for each child in the house. Instruct parents to call the Poison Control Center before using. Post the telephone number in the kitchen.

**R:** Poisoning is common in toddlers. They put everything into their mouths.

## Initiate Health Teaching and Referrals, as Indicated

Assist the family in evaluating environmental hazards in the home and when visiting others.
Install specially designed locks to prevent children from opening closets where combustible, corrosive, or flammable materials or medications are stored.
Instruct parents to use socket covers to prevent accidental electrical shocks to children.
Teach parents about the hazards of lead paint ingestion and how to identify "pica" in a child.
Refer parents to public health department if lead paint screening is necessary.
Encourage the use of childproof caps.
Advise parents to avoid storing dangerous substances in containers ordinarily used for foods.

**R:** All environmental hazards cannot be removed. Strategies that include supervision and education of parents can reduce accidents (Clemen-Stone et al., 2005).
**R:** Analysis of an accident may prevent recurrence.
**R:** Injury prevention requires anticipation and recognition of where safety measures are applicable. Passive strategies provide automatic protection without choice (e.g., air bags, product design). Active strategies require persuasion through teaching or legislation to practice safety measures.
**R:** Prevention strategies to decrease serious injuries resulting from skateboarding include warnings against skateboard use by children younger than 5 years of age, prohibition of skateboards on streets and highways, and the promotion of use of helmets and other protective gear.

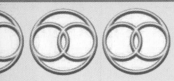

# RISK FOR INJURY

▶ **Related to Lack of Awareness of Environmental Hazards Secondary to Maturational Age**

**NOC**
Risk Control, Fall
Revention Behavior

➤ **Goals** _____

- The child/adolescent will be free from injury from potentially hazardous factors identified in the hospital environment.
- The family will reinforce and demonstrate safe practices in the hospital.

**NIC**
Refer to *Risk for Injury*

➤ **Interventions** _____

### Protect the Infant/Child From Injury in the Hospital by Controlling Age-Related Hazards

#### Infant (1 to 12 Months)

Ensure that the infant can be identified by an identification band and a tag on his or her crib.

Do not shake powder directly on an infant; rather, place powder in the hand and then on infant's skin. Keep powder out of an infant's reach.

Keep unsafe toys out of reach (e.g., buttons, beads, balloons, broken toys, sharp-edged toys, other small toys).

Use mitts to prevent an infant from removing catheters, eye patches, intravenous (IV) infusions, dressings, and feeding tubes, as needed.

Keep side rails up in locked position when the child is in the crib.

Pad side rails if an infant can move out of bed or is at risk for seizures.

Use a cool-mist vaporizer.

Do not use an infant walker.

Ascertain identity of all visitors.

Use a firm mattress that fits crib snugly.

Do not feed honey to infants younger than 12 months because of the danger of botulism.

Fasten safety straps on infant seats, swings, highchairs, and strollers.

Do not allow bottles to be propped. The infant should be held with his or her head upright.

Do not place pillows in the crib.

Place one hand over the child while weighing, changing diapers, and so forth, to keep him or her safe.

Do not allow an infant to wear pacifier on a string around the neck.

Check bathwater to make sure the temperature is appropriate. Never leave an infant alone while bathing! Support the small infant's head out of the water.

Check the temperature of formula, especially if you have heated it in the microwave.

Position the crib away from the bedside stand, infusion pumps, and so forth, to prevent the child from reaching unsafe objects (e.g., suction machine, electrical outlets, flowers, dials on infusion pump).

Do not allow parents to smoke or drink hot beverages in an infant's room.

Do not offer the child foods that must be chewed or are small enough to occlude the airway (e.g., nuts, popcorn, hard candy, whole hot dogs). Forks and knives are not appropriate utensils for infants.

Discard syringes, needles, med packets, and plastic bags safely.

Protect the feet of the infant who can walk with shoes or slippers.

Transport the infant safely to other areas of the hospital (e.g., x-ray, laboratory).

Remind parents to have an approved car seat in their automobile to transport the child home.

*Assess each unique situation for risk for injury to the infant. Inform parents of the infant's risk for injury.*

### Early Childhood (13 Months to 5 Years)

Ensure that the young child is identifiable by name band and name tag on the crib.

Keep the side rails up in locked position when the child is in the crib—top and bottom compartments; use side rails on youth beds.

Monitor child at all times when eating, bathing, playing, and toileting.

Keep cleaning agents, sharp items, and plastic bags out of reach.

Secure the thermometer while taking temperature (use rectal or axillary method with toddler, oral method when child is old enough not to bite down on thermometer) or use an infrared instant thermometer in the ear canal.

Assess for loose teeth, and document findings on records.

Check the temperature of the bathwater before immersing the child.

Use electric beds with extreme caution. For example, children may get their fingers caught or get under the bed and be at risk for a crushing injury.

Position the crib/bed away from the bedside stand, infusion pumps, flowers, and so forth, to prevent child from reaching unsafe objects.

Keep the child safe when mobile:

- Protect the child's feet with shoes or slippers when ambulating.
- Keep the bathroom and closet doors firmly shut.
- Check any tubing attached to the child to prevent kinking or dislodgment.
- Apply safety straps when the child is in the high chair or stroller or on a cart.
- Transport the child safely to other areas of the hospital (e.g., x-ray).
- Use mitts to prevent the child from removing catheters, eye patches, IV infusion, dressings, and feeding tubes, as needed.
- Place one hand over the child when weighing, changing diapers, and so forth, to prevent falls.

Do not call medications "candy."

Do not permit the child to chew gum or eat hard candy, nuts, whole hot dogs, or fish with bones.

Set limits. Enforce and repeat what the child can do in the hospital and areas he or she can go.

Provide age-appropriate, safe toys (see manufacturer's guidelines).

Do not allow parents to smoke or drink hot beverages in the child's room.

Feed the child in a quiet environment; ensure that he or she sits while eating, to prevent choking.

Remind parents to have an approved car seat in the automobile to transport the child home.

Ascertain identity of all visitors.

*Assess each unique situation for risk for injury to the young child. Inform parents of the young child's risk for injury.*

## School-Aged/Adolescent (6 to 12 Years/13 to 18 Years)

Ensure that the child or adolescent can be identified by a name band and a tag on his or her bed. School-aged children may claim to be someone else as a joke, not realizing the danger of this.

Assess for loose teeth; document findings on records.

Assess for self-care deficits and activity intolerance, because the school-aged child or adolescent may not ask for help when ambulating, bathing, toileting, and so forth.

Apply safety straps when transporting by cart or wheelchair.

Set limits. Enforce and repeat what the child can do and areas he or she can go in the hospital.

Provide age-appropriate activities. Supervise therapeutic play closely. Do not allow the child to use syringes as squirt guns.

Do not allow parents to smoke or drink hot beverages in the child's room.

Encourage the child or adolescent to wear a Medic-Alert necklace or bracelet, if appropriate. Encourage the child to carry identification in a wallet or purse.

Remind the child to wear his or her seat belt in the car when discharged.

Discourage smoking and use of illicit drugs, including alcohol.

*Assess each unique situation for risk for injury to the school-age child or adolescent. Inform parents of their child's risk for injury.*

**R:** The nurse should assess each child's unique risk of potential for injury. This includes the child with sensory or motor deficits and developmental delay. Environmental changes, such as hospitalization, visiting relatives' homes, and celebrating holidays, pose special hazards for children (Hockenberry & Wilson, 2009).

**R:** To protect children from injury, caretakers must be aware of the age-related behavioral characteristics that increase the child's vulnerability to injury (Hockenberry & Wilson, 2009).

**R:** Anatomically, children are more susceptible to head injuries because of their large head, to liver and spleen trauma because these organs are larger, and to being thrown more easily (in a car) because of their small, light bodies (Hockenberry & Wilson, 2009).

**R:** Infants explore the environment through taste and touch.

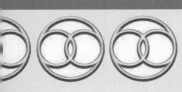

# RISK FOR INJURY

▶ **Related to Vertigo Secondary to Orthostatic Hypotension**

**NOC**
Refer to *Risk for Injury*

## ➤ Goal

The client will relate fewer episodes of dizziness or vertigo.

### Indicators:

- Identify situations that cause vertigo.
- Relate methods of preventing sudden decreases in cerebral blood flow.
- Demonstrate maneuvers to change position and avoid sudden drop in cerebral pressure.

**NIC**
Refer to *Risk for Injury*

## ➤ Interventions

### Identify Contributing Factors

Cardiovascular disorders (hypertension, cerebral infarct, anemia, dysrhythmias)

Fluid or electrolyte imbalances

Peripheral neuropathy, Parkinson's disease

Diabetes

Certain medications (antihypertensives, anticholinergics, barbiturates, vasodilators, tricyclic antidepressants, levodopa, nitrates, monoamine oxidase inhibitors, phenothiazine)

Alcohol use

Age 75 years or older

Prolonged bed rest

Surgical sympathectomy

Valsalva maneuver during voiding (Miller, 2009)

Arthritis (spurs on cervical vertebrae)

### Assess for Orthostatic Hypotension

Take bilateral brachial pressures with the client supine.

If the brachial pressures are different, use the arm with the higher reading and take the blood pressure immediately after the client stands up quickly. Report differences to the physician.

Ask the client to describe sensations (e.g., lightheaded, dizzy).

Assess skin and vital signs.

**R:** Use of the arm with the higher pressure gives a more accurate assessment of the blood pressure.

### Teach the Client Techniques to Reduce Orthostatic Hypotension

Change positions slowly.

Move from lying to an upright position in stages.

1. Sit up in bed.
2. Dangle first one leg, then the other over the side of the bed.
3. Allow a few minutes before going on to each step.
4. Gradually pull oneself from a sitting to a standing position.
5. Place a chair, walker, cane, or other assistive device nearby to use to steady oneself when getting out of bed.

Sleep with the head of the bed elevated up to 30 degrees.
During day, rest in a recliner rather than in bed.
Avoid prolonged standing.
Avoid stooping to pick something up from the floor; use an assistive device available from an orthotics department or a self-help store.

**R:** Prolonged bed rest increases venous pooling which reduces circulation to the brain. Gradual position change allows the body to compensate for venous pooling (Porth, 2006).

Evaluate the possible effectiveness of waist-high stockings.

- Wrap the legs from below the toes to the top of thigh with elastic compression bandages. Check compression effectiveness before purchase.
- Put stockings on in the morning before getting out of bed if compression is advised.
- Avoid sitting for long periods.
- Remove stockings when supine.

**R:** Compression stockings can reduce venous pooling.

## Encourage the Client to Increase Daily Activity, If Permissible

Discuss the value of daily exercise.
Establish an exercise program.

**R:** Exercise increases circulation and energy levels, decreases stress and the process of osteoporosis, and contributes to overall well-being.

## Teach the Client to Avoid Dehydration and Vasodilation

Replace fluids during periods of excess fluid loss (e.g., hot weather).
Minimize diuretic fluids (e.g., coffee, tea, cola).
Minimize alcohol consumption.
Avoid sources of intense heat (e.g., direct sun, hot showers, baths, electric blankets).
Avoid taking nitroglycerin while standing.

**R:** Adequate hydration is necessary to prevent decreased circulating volume. Certain fluids are diuretics and reduce body fluids. Heat and alcohol can cause vasodilatation.

## Teach the Client to Reduce Postprandial Hypotension (Miller, 2009)

Take antihypertensive medications after meals rather than before.
Eat small, frequent meals.
Remain seated or lie down after meals.

**R:** Studies have shown that in healthy older adults, blood pressure is reduced by 20 mm Hg within 1 h of eating the morning or afternoon meal. This is thought to result from an impaired baroreflex compensatory response to splanchnic blood pooling during digestion (Miller, 2009).

## Institute Environmental Safety Measures (Refer to Risk for Injury Related to Lack of Awareness of Environmental Hazards)

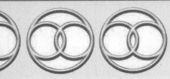

# RISK FOR ASPIRATION

## DEFINITION

State in which a client is at risk for entry of secretions, solids, or fluids into the tracheobronchial passages

## RISK FACTORS

### Pathophysiologic

***Related to reduced level of consciousness secondary to:***

| | | |
|---|---|---|
| Presenile dementia | Parkinson's disease | Seizures |
| Head injury | Alcohol- or drug-induced | Anesthesia |
| Cerebrovascular accident | Coma | |

Related to depressed cough/gag reflexes

***Related to increased intragastric pressure secondary to:***

| | | |
|---|---|---|
| Lithotomy position | Obesity | Enlarged uterus |
| Ascites | | |

***Related to impaired swallowing or decreased laryngeal and glottic reflexes secondary to:***

| | | |
|---|---|---|
| Achalasia | Muscular dystrophy | Scleroderma |
| Cerebrovascular accident | Esophageal strictures | Parkinson's disease |
| Myasthenia gravis | Debilitating conditions | Guillain-Barré syndrome |
| Catatonia | Multiple sclerosis | |

Related to tracheoesophageal fistula

***Related to impaired protective reflexes secondary to:***

| | |
|---|---|
| Facial/oral/neck surgery or trauma | Paraplegia or hemiplegia |

### Treatment-Related

***Related to depressed laryngeal and glottic reflexes secondary to:***

| | | |
|---|---|---|
| Tracheostomy/endotracheal tube | Sedation | Tube feedings |

***Related to impaired ability to cough secondary to:***

| | |
|---|---|
| Wired jaw | Imposed prone position |

### Situational (Personal, Environmental)

***Related to inability/impaired ability to elevate upper body***
***Related to eating when intoxicated***

### Maturational

**Premature**
***Related to impaired sucking/swallowing reflexes***

**Neonate**
***Related to decreased muscle tone of inferior esophageal sphincter***

**Older Adult**
***Related to poor dentition***

### ■■■■■■ AUTHOR'S NOTE

*Risk for Aspiration* is a clinically useful diagnosis for people at high risk for aspiration because of reduced level of consciousness, structural deficits, mechanical devices, and neurologic and gastrointestinal disorders. People with swallowing difficulties often are at risk for aspiration; the nursing diagnosis *Impaired Swallowing* should be used to describe a client with difficulty swallowing who also is at risk for aspiration. *Risk for Aspiration* should be used to describe people who require nursing interventions to prevent aspiration, but do not have a swallowing problem.

## ■■■■■■ ERRORS IN DIAGNOSTIC STATEMENTS

1. *Risk for Aspiration related to bronchopneumonia*
   This diagnostic statement does not direct the nurse to the risk factors that could be reduced. If the nurse were monitoring and co-managing bronchopneumonia, the correct statement would be the collaborative problem *RC of Bronchopneumonia*.
2. *Risk for Aspiration related to difficulty swallowing*
   Difficulty swallowing is validation for *Impaired Swallowing*; thus, *Impaired Swallowing* would be correct. Nursing measures also would include prevention of aspiration.

## ■■■■■■ KEY CONCEPTS

### Generic Considerations

- Swallowing is a complicated mechanism with three stages:
- The *voluntary stage* is the moving of the food from the palate to the pharynx.
- The *pharyngeal stage* is automatic.
- The soft palate is pulled up to close the posterior nares.
- Palatopharyngeal folds on the sides of the pharynx constrict to permit passage of properly masticated food.
- The epiglottis swings backward over the larynx opening to prevent aspiration into the trachea.
- Relaxation of the hypopharyngeal sphincter stretches the opening of the esophagus.
- Rapid peristaltic wave forces food into the upper esophagus.
- The *esophageal stage* moves the food from the pharynx to the stomach by peristaltic movements controlled by vagal reflexes.
- Central nervous system (CNS) depression interferes with the protective mechanism of the sphincters.
- Nasogastric and endotracheal tubes cause incomplete closure of the esophageal sphincters and depress the gag and cough reflexes.
- Clients with debilitating conditions who aspirate are at high risk for aspiration pneumonia.
- The volume and characteristics of the aspirated contents influence morbidity and mortality. Food particles can cause mechanical blockage. Gastric juice erodes alveoli and capillaries and causes chemical pneumonitis.

### Pediatric Considerations

- A proportionately oversized airway diameter in infants and small children increases the risk of aspiration of foreign objects (Hockenberry & Wilson, 2009).
- Children, especially toddlers, have a natural curiosity, seek attractive objects, and frequently put things in their mouth. Children cannot comprehend danger to self or others.
- Common household objects and food items that are aspirated include balloons (toy rubber balloons are the leading cause of choking deaths from children's products), baby powder, hot dogs, candy, nuts, grapes, and small batteries.
- Children with certain congenital anomalies (e.g., tracheoesophageal fistula, cleft palate, gastroesophageal reflux) are at greater risk for aspiration.

## Focus Assessment Criteria

### Subjective Data

#### Assess for Related Factors

History of a problem with swallowing or aspiration
Presence or history of: (see Pathophysiologic Related Factors)

### Objective Data

#### Assess for Related Factors

Ability to swallow, chew, feed self

Neuromuscular impairment:

- Decreased/absent gag reflex
- Decreased strength on excursion of muscles involved in mastication
- Perceptual impairment
- Facial paralysis

Mechanical obstruction:

- Edema
- Tracheostomy tube
- Tumor

Perceptual patterns/awareness
Level of consciousness
Condition of oropharyngeal cavity
Nasal regurgitation
Hoarseness
Aspiration
Coughing 1 or 2 s after swallowing
Dehydration
Apraxia
For more information on Focus Assessment Criteria; visit http://thepoint.lww.com.

## Goal

**NOC**
Aspiration Control

The client will not experience aspiration.

### Indicators:

- Relate measures to prevent aspiration.
- Name foods or fluids that are high risk for causing aspiration.

The parent will reduce opportunities for aspirations

### Indicators:

- Remove small objects from child' reach.
- Inspect toys for removable small objects.
- Discourage the child from putting objects in his or her mouth

## General Interventions

**NIC**
Aspiration Precautions, Airway Management, Positioning, Airway Suctioning

### Assess Causative or Contributing Factors

Refer to Related Factors.

### Reduce the Risk of Aspiration in:

#### Clients with Decreased Strength, Decreased Sensorium, or Autonomic Disorders

Maintain a side-lying position if not contraindicated by injury.
If the client cannot be positioned on the side, open the oropharyngeal airway by lifting the mandible up and forward and tilting the head backward. (For a small infant, hyperextension of the neck may not be effective.)
Assess for position of the tongue, ensuring it has not dropped backward, occluding the airway.
Keep the head of the bed elevated, if not contraindicated by hypertension or injury.
Maintain good oral hygiene. Clean teeth and use mouthwash on cotton swab; apply petroleum jelly to lips; removing encrustations gently.
Clear secretions from mouth and throat with a tissue or gentle suction.
Reassess frequently for obstructive material in mouth and throat.

Reevaluate frequently for good anatomic positioning.
Maintain side-lying position after feedings.

**R:** Regurgitation is often silent in people with decreased sensorium or depressed mental states.

Positions are maintained to reduce aspiration.

**R:** Increased intragastric pressure can contribute to regurgitation and aspiration. Causes include bolus tube feedings, obstructions, obesity, pregnancy, and autonomic dysfunction.

### Tracheostomy or Endotracheal Tubes

Inflate cuff:

- During continuous mechanical ventilation
- During and after eating
- During and 1 h after tube feedings
- During intermittent positive-pressure breathing treatments

Suction every 1 to 2 h and PRN.

**R:** Tracheostomy tubes interfere with the synchrony of the glottic closure. Inadequate cuff inflation provides a path for aspirate.

### Gastrointestinal Tubes and Feedings

Confirm that tube placement has been verified by radiography or aspiration of greenish fluid.
Confirm that tube position has not changed since it was inserted and verified.
Elevate the head of the bed for 30 to 45 min during feeding periods and 1 h after to prevent reflux by use of reverse gravity.
Aspirate for residual contents before each feeding for tubes positioned gastrically.
Administer feeding if residual contents are less than 150 mL (intermittent), or administer feeding if residual is no greater than 150 mL at 10% to 20% of hourly rate (continuous).
Regulate gastric feedings using an intermittent schedule, allowing periods for stomach emptying between feeding intervals.

**R:** Verifying correct placement of feeding tubes is done most reliably by radiography. Aspiration of green-colored fluid or gastric aspirant with a pH of 6.5 or lower is also reliable. Verifying placement by instilling air and simultaneously auscultating or by aspirating non-green fluid has proven inaccurate.

### For an Older Adult with Difficulties Chewing and Swallowing (See Impaired Swallowing)

### Initiate Health Teaching and Referrals, as Indicated

Instruct the client and family on causes and prevention of aspiration.
Have the family demonstrate tube-feeding technique.
Refer the family to a community nursing agency for assistance at home.
Teach the client about the danger of eating when under the influence of alcohol.
Teach the Heimlich or abdominal thrust maneuver to remove aspirated foreign bodies.

**R:** The risk of aspiration increases after discharge due to less supervision.

Pediatric
Interventions

**For Newborns with Cleft Lip, Palate, or Both**

Position infant's head upright.

**R:** All newborns have poor muscle tone of the cardiac sphincter of the esophagus, thus causing regurgitation easily (Hockenberry & Wilson, 2009).

Use a special feeding device for infants with cleft lip/cleft palate such as a cleft lip/cleft palate nurser, the Haberman Feeder, or a gravity flow nipple.

*(continued)*

**Pediatric Interventions**
*Continued*

If nipple feeding is unsuccessful, use a rubber-tipped syringe to deposit the formula on the back of the tongue.

**R:** These infants cannot apply enough suction to use normal nipples.

Observe for signs to stop feeding momentarily, such as elevated eyebrows and wrinkled forehead. Do not position the nipple through the cleft.

**R:** These signs indicate distress.

Position the nipple so it is compressed by the infant's tongue and existing palate.

Apply gentle counterpressure on the base of the bottle to assist the infant with tongue and palate control of the milk flow.

**R:** Gentle pressure at the base of bottle assists the infant with tongue and palate control.

Burp frequently because of excessive air swallowing.

**R:** Excessive air swallowing necessitates frequent burping.
**R:** Sucking is important for muscle development for later speech development (Hockenberry & Wilson, 2009).

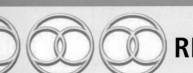

# RISK FOR FALLS

## DEFINITION

State in which a client has increased susceptibility to falling

## RISK FACTORS

Presence of risk factors (see Risk Factors for *Risk for Injury*).

## ■■■■■ AUTHOR'S NOTE

This new nursing diagnosis can be used to specify a client at risk for falls. If the client is at risk for various types of injuries (e.g., a cognitively impaired client), the broader diagnosis *Risk for Injury* is more useful.

## ■■■■■ ERRORS IN DIAGNOSTIC STATEMENTS

1. *Risk for Falls related to inadequate supervision*
   This diagnosis represents a legally inappropriate statement. Even if it is true, the diagnosis should be rewritten as *Risk for Falls related to inability to identify environmental hazards as a result of dementia*.

## ■■■■■ KEY CONCEPTS

Refer to *Risk for Injury*.

## Focus Assessment Criteria

Refer to *Risk for Injury*.

| NOC | ➤ **Goals** |
|---|---|
| Refer to Risk for Injury | |

The client will relate controlled falls or no falls.

### *Indicators:*

- Relate the intent to use safety measures to prevent falls.
- Demonstrate selective prevention measures.

| NIC | ➤ **General Interventions** |
|---|---|
| Refer to Risk for Injury | |

Orient to environment and safety measures:

- Location of the bathroom.
- Bed controls and call bell
- Leave the bathroom light on
- Remove obstacles to the bathroom
- Evaluate if side rails are hazardous
- Keep the bed position at low
- Instruct the client to wear nonslip shoes

**R:** Orientation to the environment may reduce accidents. Getting out of bed at night to go to the bathroom may be more safe with no side rails and bed at low position.

## Identify Clients Who Are at High Risk for Falling for All Personnel

- Sticker on headboard
- Brightly colored arm band
- Sign on door
- "Red Slipper Program"

Specific programs to alert staff to high-risk clients are effective.

## For Those Cognitively Impaired Clients

Place an alarm pad on the bed.

**R:** An alarm pad alerts staff that the client is attempting to leave the bed.

Clients can be place in small groups with intense, focused supervision.

**R:** Studies show that clients with dementia fall twice as much as others. Intense supervision is effective in preventing falls.

## Ensure Proper Use of Assistive Devices

Consult with physician therapist.

**R:** Expert instruction is needed to ensure proper equipment and use.

## Engage the Client in Exercise Routines

Assess the client' fear of falling.
Encourage group classes if feasible (e.g. T'ai chi, water classes).
Provide opportunities for exercise walking.
Engage in exercises specifically to improve gait, balance, and ankle strength.

**R:** The elderly experience decreased range of motion of arms, decreased muscle strength and endurance, and decreased joint flexion (knee, hip, foot). Their gait is less controlled and their ability to recover if unbalanced is compromised (Miller, 2009).

Initiate Health Teaching and Referrals as needed.
Refer the client to Home Health Nursing Agency for a home assessment.
Ensure that family are aware of issues related to safety and risk for falls.
Refer to *Risk for Injury*.

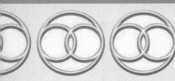

# RISK FOR POISONING

**DEFINITION**

State in which a client is at risk of accidental exposure to or ingestion of drugs or dangerous substances

**RISK FACTORS**

Presence of risk factors (see Risk Factors for *Risk for Injury*).

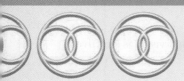

# RISK FOR SUFFOCATION

**DEFINITION**

Risk for Suffocation: state in which a client is at risk for smothering and asphyxiation

**RISK FACTORS**

Presence of risk factors (see Risk Factors for *Risk for Injury*).

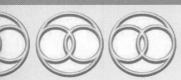

# RISK FOR TRAUMA

**DEFINITION**

State in which a client is at risk of accidental tissue injury (e.g., wound, burns, fracture)

**RISK FACTORS**

Presence of risk factors (see Risk Factors for *Risk for Injury*).

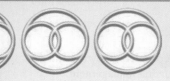

# RISK FOR PERIOPERATIVE POSITIONING INJURY

## DEFINITION

Risk for Perioperative Positioning Injury: state in which a client is at risk for harm as a result of positioning requirements for surgery and loss of usual protective responses secondary to anesthesia

## RISK FACTORS

Presence of risk factors (see Related Factors).

## RELATED FACTORS

### Pathophysiologic

*Related to increased vulnerability secondary to:*

| | | |
|---|---|---|
| Chronic disease | Radiation therapy | Renal, hepatic dysfunction |
| Cancer | Osteoporosis | Infection |
| Thin body frame | Compromised immune system | |

*Related to compromised tissue perfusion secondary to:*

| | | |
|---|---|---|
| Diabetes mellitus | Cardiovascular disease | Peripheral vascular disease |
| Anemia | Hypothermia | History of thrombosis |
| Ascites | Dehydration | Edema |

*Related to vulnerability of stoma during positioning*
*Related to preexisting contractures or physical impairments secondary to:*

Rheumatoid arthritis    Polio

### Treatment-Related

*Related to position requirements and loss of usual sensory protective responses secondary to anesthesia\**
*Related to surgical procedures of 2 hours or longer*
*Related to vulnerability of implants or prostheses (e.g., pacemakers) during positioning*

### Situational (Personal, Environmental)

*Related to compromised circulation secondary to:*

| | | |
|---|---|---|
| Obesity | Pregnancy | Cool operating suite |
| Tobacco use | Infant status | Elder status |

### Maturational

*Related to increased vulnerability to tissue injury secondary to:*

<!-- -->

■■■■■■ **AUTHOR'S NOTE**

This diagnosis focuses on identifying the vulnerability for tissue, nerve, and joint injury resulting from required positions for surgery. The addition of *perioperative positioning* to *Risk for Injury* adds etiology to the label.

If a client has no preexisting risk factors that make him or her more vulnerable to injury, this diagnosis could be used with no related factors because they are evident. If related factors are desired, the statement could read *Risk for Perioperative Positioning Injury related to position requirements for surgery and loss of usual sensory protective measures secondary to anesthesia.*

When a client has preexisting risk factors, the statement should include these—for example, *Risk for Perioperative Positioning Injuries related to compromised tissue perfusion secondary to peripheral arterial disease.*

---

\*This risk factor is always present and may be deleted from the diagnostic statement.

### ░░▪▪▪▪ ERRORS IN DIAGNOSTIC STATEMENTS

1. *Risk for Perioperative Positioning Injury related to inadequate protective measures*
   These related factors are legally problematic. Even if inadequate protective measures are a problem, they must not be included in the diagnostic statement. Instead, this problem should be referred to nursing management.

### ░░▪▪▪▪ KEY CONCEPTS

#### Generic Considerations

- The physiologic effects of positioning for surgical procedures vary with the specific position. Overall, positioning affects the cardiovascular, respiratory, neurologic, musculoskeletal, and integumentary systems.
- Prolonged immobility diminishes the pulmonary capillary blood flow volume. Positional pressure on the ribs or the diaphragm's ability to force abdominal contents downward limits lung expansion.
- Anesthesia causes peripheral blood vessels to dilate, resulting in hypotension, and decreases blood return to heart and lungs. Prolonged immobility causes pooling in vascular beds.
- People with obesity are at increased risk for injury from surgical positions as a result of the following:
  - Lifting them into position is difficult.
  - Massive tissue and pressure areas need extra padding.
  - The mechanics of manipulating adipose tissue may prolong length of surgery.
  - Recovery period may be prolonged because adipose tissue retains fat-soluble agents and slows elimination of agents.
  - Venous stasis decreases circulation, and adipose tissue has a poor blood supply.
  - Anesthesia causes the less normal defenses to protect against excessive manipulation.

 **Geriatric Considerations**

Osteoarthritis, loss of subcutaneous fat, decreased peripheral circulation, and wasted flaccid muscles can contribute to injury or trauma to bones, joints, nerves, and skin when on the operating table (Martin, 2000).

## Focus Assessment Criteria

### Subjective Data

#### *Assess for Preexisting Risk Factors*

Refer to Related Factors.

### Objective Data

#### *Assess for Presurgical Risk Factors*

Skin
Temperature (cool, warm)
Color (pale, dependent erythema, flushed, cyanotic, brown discolorations)
Ulcerations (size, location, description of surrounding tissue)

Bilateral Pulses (Radial, Posterior Tibial, Dorsalis Pedis)
Rate, rhythm
Volume
+0 = Absent, nonpalpable
+1 = Thready, weak, fades in and out
+2 = Present but diminished
+3 = Normal, easily palpable
+4 = Aneurysmal

Paresthesia (Numbness, Tingling, Burning)

Edema (Location, Pitting)

Capillary Refill (Normal Less Than 3 Seconds)

Range of Motion (Normal, Compromised)

Current Muscle or Joint Pain
0 = No pain; 10 = Worst pain
For more information on Focus Assessment Criteria, visit http://thepoint.lww.com.

**NOC**
Circulation Status,
Neurologic Status,
Tissue Perfusion:
Peripheral

## ➤ Goal

The client will have no neuromuscular damage or injury related to the surgical position.

### Indicators:

- Padding is used as indicated for procedure.
- Limbs are secured when at risk.
- Limbs are flexed when indicated.

**NIC**
Positioning
Intraoperative,
Surveillance, Pressure
Management

## ➤ General Interventions

### Determine Whether the Client Has Preexisting Risk Factors (Refer to Risk Factors); Communicate Findings to Surgical Team

#### Before Positioning, Assess and Document:

Range-of-motion ability                     Physical abnormalities (skin, contractions)
External/internal prostheses or implants    Neurovascular status
Circulatory status

### Advise If Any Preexisting Factors Exist and Determine If the Position Will Be Arranged Before or After Anesthesia

**R:** Documentation of all visible abnormalities is critical before surgery. Tissue and skin can be injured by excessive pressure or bruised by hitting a hard surface. People more vulnerable to pressure injuries are the very young; older adults; those who are dehydrated, very thin, or obese; and those undergoing more than 2 h of immobility.

### Discuss with the Surgeon the Surgical Position Desired

### Move the Client from the Transport Stretcher to the Operating Room (OR) Bed.

Have a minimum of two people with their hands free (e.g., not holding an IV bag).
Explain the transfer to the client. Lock all wheels on the stretcher and bed.
Ask the client to move slowly to the OR bed. Assist during the move. Do not pull or drag the client.
When the client is on the OR bed, attach a safety belt a few inches above the knees with a space of three fingerbreadths.
Check that legs are not crossed and that feet are slightly separated and not over the edge.
Do not leave the client unattended.

**R:** These strategies reduce injury from shearing and trauma.

### Always Ask the Anesthesiologist or Nurse Anesthetist for Permission Before Moving or Repositioning an Anesthetized Client

**R:** If repositioning is necessary after induction, lifting, rather than rolling or pulling, the client prevents shearing forces and friction. Shearing occurs when the dermal layers stay fixed because of the friction between linen and skin, and tissues attached to bony structures move with the weight of the torso. Tissue layers slide on each other, resulting in the kinking or stretching of subcutaneous blood vessels, thus obstructing blood flow to and from areas (Porth, 2006).

## Reduce Vulnerability to Injury (Soft Tissue, Joint, Nerves, Blood Vessels)

Align the neck and spine at all times.

Gently manipulate the joints. Do not abduct more than 90 degrees.

Do not let limbs extend off the OR bed. Reposition slowly and gently.

Use a draw-sheet above the elbows to tuck in arms at the side or abduct arm on an arm board with padding.

**R:** Anesthetic agents interfere with normal vasodilatation and constriction, thus reducing perfusion to bony prominences or compressed or dependent limbs.

## Protect Eyes and Ears from Injury

Use padding or a special headrest to protect ears, superficial nerves, and blood vessels of the face if the head is on its side.

Ensure that the ear is not bent when positioned.

If needed, protect eyes from abrasions with an eye patch or shield.

**R:** Excessive pressure of position, equipment, or surgery can injure the face and eyes. Excessive pressure to the eyes can cause thrombosis of the central renal artery. Eyes should be kept closed and lubricated to prevent drying and scratching.

## Depending on the Surgical Position Used, Protect Vulnerable Areas; Document Position and Protection Measures Used (Rothrock, 2003)

### Supine

Pad the calcaneus, sacrum, coccyx, olecranon process, scapula, ischial tuberosity, and occiput.

Keep the arms at side, palms down or abducted on an arm board.

Protect the head and ears if the head is turned to the side.

### Trendelenburg

Use a well-padded shoulder brace over the acromion process, not soft tissue, and away from the neck.

### Reverse Trendelenburg

Use a padded footboard.

### Jack-Knife (Modified Prone)

Use padded arm boards at correct heights to allow elbows to bend comfortably.

Place a soft pillow under the down ear.

Cushion hips and thighs with large pillows.

Cushion breasts.

Cushion male genitalia in natural position.

Use a large pillow under the lower legs and ankles to raise the toes off the bed.

Use additional padding on the shoulder girdle, olecranon, anterosuperior iliac spine, patella, and dorsum of the foot.

Apply a safety strap across the thighs.

### Prone

Position two large body rolls longitudinally from the acromioclavicular joint to the iliac crest.

Refer to jack-knife for additional information.

### Laminectomy

After induction of anesthesia, at least six people help roll the client from the stretcher to the OR bed onto the laminectomy brace.

Keep body aligned.

Protect limbs from torsion.

Place rolled towels in axillary regions.

Follow precautions for jack-knife.

### Lithotomy

Prepare stirrups with padding.

Have two people simultaneously and slowly raise the client's legs with slight rotation of the hips. Gently position the knees slightly flexed.

Position the client's buttocks about 1 inch over the end of the table.

Use a small lumbar pad and extra padding in the sacral area.

Cover the legs with cotton boots.

Position arms on arm boards or loosely over abdomen, supported with a sheet.

### Fowler

Position the neck in straight alignment.

Use a padded footboard.

Support the knees with a pillow.

Cross the arms loosely over the abdomen and tape them on the pillow.

### Sims (Lateral)

Position the client on the side with arms extended on double arm boards.

Flex the lower leg.

Use a small pillow under the head.

Use a rolled towel in the axillary area of the downside arm.

Elevate and pad the flank.

Flex the lower leg and place a long pillow the length of the leg to the groin.

Use a 4-inch strip of adhesive tape attached to one side of the table, over the iliac crest and to the other side.

Protect ankles and feet from pressure.

Protect male genitalia, female breasts, and ear as for jack-knife position.

**R:** Prolonged positioning can cause mechanical pressure on peripheral and superficial nerves. Hyperextension (greater than 90-degree angle) of a limb of an anesthetized client can cause nerve injuries (Rothrock, 2003):

- Hyperextension of the arm on an arm board can injure the brachial plexus (in the arm). Improper positioning of the brace also can injure the brachial plexus.
- Ulnar nerve injuries occur when an elbow slips off the mattress and is compressed between the table and the medial epicondyle.
- Radial nerve injuries occur when the nerve is compressed between the client and the table surface or from striking the table.
- Saphenous and peroneal nerve damage occurs with the use of stirrups with lithotomy—compression of the peroneal nerve against the stirrups or of the saphenous nerve between the metal popliteal knee support stirrup and the medial tibial condyle.

**R:** Anesthesia and muscle relaxants cause the loss of the normal protective range-of-motion limitations (e.g., muscles stretch and strain, causing joint, tendon, or ligament injuries).

**R:** Anesthetic agents interfere with normal vasodilation and constriction, thus reducing perfusion to bony prominences or compressed or dependent limbs. Padding protects bony prominences and limbs from injury.

## If Feasible, Ask the Client If He or She Feels Pain, Burning, Pressure, or Any Discomfort After Positioning

**R:** This can direct the nurse to assess the area.

## Continually Assess that Team Members Are Not Leaning on the Client, Especially Limbs

## Ensure that the Head Is Lifted Slightly Every 30 Min

## Slowly Reposition or Return the Client to Supine Position After Certain Surgical Positions (e.g., Trendelenburg, Lithotomy, Reverse Trendelenburg, Jack-Knife, Lateral)

**R:** Positions are changed slowly to prevent severe hypotension.

## Assess Skin Condition When Surgery Is Over; Document Findings; Inform Postanesthesia Nurses of Any Preexisting Risk Factors That Increase Postoperative Vulnerability

## Continue to Assess and to Relieve Pressure to Vulnerable Areas Postoperatively

**R:** The OR nurse is continuously assessing and reporting abnormal data to the appropriate professionals to relieve pressure to vulnerable areas.

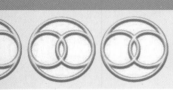

# LATEX ALLERGY RESPONSE

**Latex Allergy Response**

Latex Allergy Response, Risk for

## DEFINITION

State in which a person experiences an immunoglobulin E (IgE)-mediated response to latex

## DEFINING CHARACTERISTICS

### Major (Must be Present)

Positive skin or serum test to natural rubber latex (NRL) extract.

### Minor

Allergic conjunctivitis    Urticaria    Rhinitis
Asthma

## RELATED FACTORS

### Biopathophysiologic

*Related to hypersensitivity*
*Response to the protein component of natural rubber latex*

## ◼◼◼◼◼ KEY CONCEPTS

### Generic Considerations

- Natural rubber latex (NRL) has been used widely in many products for more than 100 years. The first case of immediate hypersensitivity to latex was reported in 1979 (Reddy, 1998).
- Use of latex gloves and condoms has increased dramatically since 1985. The increase in total exposure to latex has led to more people with latex sensitivity (Reddy, 1998).

*(continued)*

■■■■■■ **KEY CONCEPTS** *Continued*

- Risk groups for *Latex Allergy* are health care workers; rubber industry workers; people with spina bifida, history of barium enema, history of indwelling catheter, repeated catheterizations, urogenital abnormalities, or history of repeated or prolonged surgeries or mucous membrane exposure to latex; and people with atopic history or history of food allergy (banana, avocado, mango, kiwi, passion fruit, chestnut, melon, tomato, celery).
- Some reactions to latex products are delayed immunologic responses caused by chemical irritants used in the manufacture of latex gloves. This is a type IV allergic reaction, which is not a true latex allergy (Kleinbeck et al., 1998). A true latex allergy (type I reaction) occurs shortly after exposure to the proteins in NRL (Kleinbeck et al., 1998).

## Focus Assessment Criteria

### Subjective Data

#### Assess for Defining Characteristics

**History of Swelling, Itching, Sneezing, Itchy Throat, Watery Eyes, or Redness of Skin or Mucous Membranes upon Exposure to Any of the Following:**

| | | |
|---|---|---|
| Dental work | Condom use | Blowing up a balloon |
| Adhesive tape | Rubber cement | Elastic underwear |
| Rubber gloves | Shoes | Tennis racket |
| Golf grip | | Garden hose |

**Personal History of Any of the Following:**

| | | |
|---|---|---|
| Asthma | Urticaria | Contact dermatitis |
| Conjunctivitis | Eczema | Rhinitis |
| Anaphylactic reaction | | |

**Allergies to Any of the Following:**

| | | |
|---|---|---|
| Avocado | Passion fruit | Peach |
| Chestnut | Tomato | Banana |
| Mango | Raw potato | Kiwi |
| Papaya | | |

**History of Adverse Reaction or Complication to Surgery**
Positive diagnostic testing (e.g., antilatex IgE).

#### Assess for Risk Factors

Occupation with frequent contact with latex in the present or past?
History of surgeries, urinary catheterizations, barium enema (before 1992)
Congenital abnormalities; spina bifida
For more information on Focus Assessment Criteria, visit http://thepoint.lww.com.

---

NOC
Immune
Hypersensitivity
Control

➤ ## Goal

The client will report no exposure to latex.

### Indicators:

- Describe products of NRL.
- Describe strategies to avoid exposure.

---

NOC
Allergy
Management,
Latex Precautions,
Environmental Risk
Protection

➤ ## General Interventions

### Assess for Causative and Contributing Factors (Refer to Focus Assessment)

## Eliminate Exposure to Latex Products

### Use Nonlatex Alternative Supplies

Clear disposable amber bags
Silicone baby nipples
2 × 2 gauze pads with silk tape in place of adhesive bandages
Clear plastic or Silastic catheters
Vinyl or neoprene gloves
Kling-like gauze
**R:** Nonlatex items are sometimes available.

## Protect from Exposure to Latex

Cover the skin with cloth before applying the blood pressure cuff.
Do not allow rubber stethoscope tubing to touch the client.
Do not inject through rubber parts (e.g., heparin locks); use syringe and stopcock.
Change needles after each puncture of rubber stopper.
Cover rubber parts with tape.

## Teach Which Products Are Commonly Made of Latex

### Health Care Equipment

Natural latex rubber gloves, powdered or unpowdered, including those labeled "hypoallergenic"

| | | |
|---|---|---|
| Blood pressure cuffs | Stethoscopes | Tourniquets |
| Electrode pads | Airways, endotracheal tubes | Syringe plunges, bulb syringes |
| Masks for anesthesia | Rubber aprons | Catheters, wound drains |
| Injection ports | Tops of multidose vials | Adhesive tape |
| Ostomy pouches | Wheelchair cushions | Briefs with elastic |
| Pads for crutches | Some pre-filled syringes | |

### Office/Household Products

| | | |
|---|---|---|
| Erasers | Rubber bands | Dishwashing gloves |
| Balloons | Condoms, diaphragms | Baby bottle nipples, pacifiers |
| Rubber balls and toys | Racquet handles | Cycle grips |
| Tires | Hot water bottles | Carpeting |
| Shoe soles | Elastic in underwear | Rubber cement |

## Initiate Health Teaching as Indicated

Explain the importance of completely avoiding direct contact with all NRL products.
Advise that a client with a history of a mild skin reaction to latex is at risk for anaphylaxis.
Instruct the client to wear a Medic-Alert bracelet stating "Latex Allergy" and to carry autoinjectable epinephrine.
Instruct the client to warn all health care providers (e.g., dental, medical, surgical) of allergy.

**R:** Any exposure (tactile, inhaled, ingested) can precipitate an anaphylactic reaction.

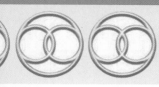

# RISK FOR LATEX ALLERGY RESPONSE

## DEFINITION

State in which a person is at risk for experiencing an immunoglobulin E (IgE)-mediated allergic response to latex.

## RISK FACTORS

### Biopathophysiologic

*Related to history of atopic eczema*
*Related to history of allergic rhinitis*
*Related to history of asthma*

### Treatment-Related

*Related to frequent urinary catheterizations*
*Related to frequent rectal impaction removal*
*Related to frequent surgical procedures*
*Related to barium enema (before 1992)*

### Situational (Personal, Environmental)

*Related to*
History of food allergy to banana, kiwi, avocado, tomato, raw potato, peach, chestnuts, mango, papaya, passion fruit
History of allergy to gloves, condoms, and so forth
Frequent occupational exposure to Natural Rubber Latex (NRL), such as:

| | | |
|---|---|---|
| Workers making NRL products | Food handlers | Greenhouse workers |
| Health care workers | Housekeepers | |

## Generic Considerations

Refer to *Latex Allergy Response.*

## Focus Assessment Criteria

Refer to *Latex Allergy Response.*

**NOC**
Immune
Hypersensitivity
Control

## ➤ Goals

Refer to *Latex Allergy Response.*

**NIC**
Allergy
Management,
Latex Precautions,
Environmental Risk
Rrotection

## ➤ General Interventions

Refer to *Latex Allergy Response.*

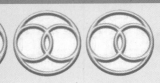

# RISK FOR IMPAIRED LIVER FUNCTION

▶ **Risk for Complications of Hepatic Dysfunction**

## RISK FACTORS

- Hepatotoxic medications (e.g., acetaminophen, statins)
- HIV co-infection
- Substance abuse (e.g., alcohol, cocaine)
- Viral infection (e.g., hepatitis A, hepatitis B, hepatitis C, Epstein-Barr virus)

■■■■■■■ **AUTHOR'S NOTE**

This new diagnosis represent a situation that requires collaborative intervention with medicine. This author recommends the collaborative problem Risk for Complications of Hepatic Dysfunction be used instead. Refer to Section 3 for interventions. Students should consult with their faculty for advice on the use of Risk for Impaired Liver Function or Risk for Complications of Hepatic Dysfuction.

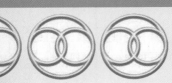

# RISK FOR LONELINESS

## DEFINITION

State in which a person is at risk for experiencing discomfort associated with a desire or need for more contact with others

## RISK FACTORS

See Related Factors.

## RELATED FACTORS

### Pathophysiologic

*Related to fear of rejection secondary to:*
Obesity
Cancer (disfiguring surgery of head or neck, superstition from others)
Physical handicaps (paraplegia, amputation, arthritis, hemiplegia)
Emotional handicaps (extreme anxiety, depression, paranoia, phobias)
Incontinence (embarrassment, odor)
Communicable diseases (acquired immunodeficiency syndrome [AIDS], hepatitis)
Psychiatric illness (schizophrenia, bipolar affective disorder, personality disorders)
*Related to difficulty accessing social events secondary to:*
Debilitating diseases  Physical disabilities

### Treatment-Related

*Related to therapeutic isolation*

## Situational (Personal, Environmental)

*Related to insufficient planning for retirement*
*Related to death of a significant other*
*Related to divorce*
*Related to disfiguring appearance*
*Related to fear of rejection secondary to:*

| | |
|---|---|
| Obesity | Hospitalization or terminal illness (dying process) |
| Extreme poverty | Unemployment |

*Related to moving to another culture (e.g., unfamiliar language)*
*Related to history of unsatisfactory social experiences secondary to:*

| | | |
|---|---|---|
| Drug abuse | Unacceptable social behavior | Alcohol abuse |
| Delusional thinking | Immature behavior | |

*Related to loss of usual means of transportation*
*Related to change in usual residence secondary to:*

| | |
|---|---|
| Long-term care | Relocation |

## Maturational

### Child
*Related to protective isolation or a communicable disease*

### Older Adult
*Related to loss of usual social contacts secondary to:*
Retirement Death of (specify) Relocation
Loss of driving ability

■■■■■■ **AUTHOR'S NOTE**

*Risk for Loneliness* was added to the NANDA list in 1994. Currently, *Social Isolation* is also on the NANDA list. *Social Isolation* is a conceptually incorrect diagnosis because it does not represent a response but a cause. *Loneliness* and *Risk for Loneliness* better describe the negative state of aloneness.

Loneliness is a subjective state that exists whenever a person says it does and perceives it as imposed by others. Social isolation is *not* the voluntary solitude necessary for personal renewal, nor is it the creative aloneness of the artist or the aloneness—and possible suffering—a person may experience from seeking individualism and independence (e.g., moving to a new city, going away to college).

■■■■■■ **ERRORS IN DIAGNOSTIC STATEMENTS**

1. *Loneliness related to inability to engage in satisfying personal relationships since death of wife 1 year ago*
   When a person fails to resume activities or to renew or to initiate social relationships after the death of a spouse, the nurse should suspect *Complicated Grieving*. Prolonged social isolation after a death is a cue for unresolved grief. The nurse should conduct a focus assessment to identify other cues, such as prolonged denial, depression, or other evidence of unsuccessful adaptation to the loss. Until additional data are confirmed, the diagnosis *Possible Complicated Grieving related to failure to resume or initiate relationships after wife's death 1 year ago* would be appropriate.
2. *Loneliness related to multiple sclerosis*
   Using multiple sclerosis as a related factor clusters all people with this condition as socially isolated and for the same reasons. This not only violates the uniqueness of each person but also does not specify how a nurse can intervene. If mobility and incontinence problems are present but no data support social isolation, the nurse can record the diagnosis as *Risk for Loneliness related to mobility and incontinence problems secondary to multiple sclerosis.*

■■■■■■ **KEY CONCEPTS**

### Generic Considerations
- Loneliness is an affective statement involving an awareness of being apart from others with an accompanying vague need for them.

*(continued)*

■■■■■■ **KEY CONCEPTS** *Continued*

- Loneliness differs from aloneness, solitude, and grief. *Aloneness* refers to being without company (not necessarily a negative state). *Solitude* involves being alone with a positive affective state. *Grief* is a response to traumatic loss (Hillestad, 1984).
- Social isolation can result in intense feelings of loneliness and suffering. Suffering associated with social isolation is not always visible. To diagnose this state, nurses must first be able to identify those at risk.
- The lonely or isolated person often aggravates his or her condition by suffering alone. Lonely people tend to shun one another. They may resign themselves to their situation and never seek companionship or help. They may deny their feelings. Illness, whether physical or psychiatric, may be the only legitimate way a socially isolated person can get attention.
- Lonely people are preoccupied with self, are hypervigilant to threats, and tend to interpret social cues as hostile.
- Loneliness may become part of a person's self-image. Although ego dystonic, he or she may find the state familiar, so that fear of the social risks may outweigh the discomfort level to overcome loneliness.
- The lonely often see the rest of the world (including health care providers) as a socially interactive milieu. They usually are not exposed to others who suffer from loneliness and so believe that their pain is unique. As a result, they tend to resent nurses, who seem to enjoy what lonely people see as unobtainable.
- A person cannot focus on meeting social needs until he or she has met more basic ones (shelter, food, safety; Maslow, 1968).
- Human immunodeficiency virus (HIV)-negative gay men may experience multiple ongoing loss of friends that causes them to suffer alone because of associated stigma (Mallinson, 1999).

## Pediatric Considerations

- Children at high risk for social isolation include the chronically ill or disabled, terminally ill, and disfigured, and their siblings.
- A child in protective isolation or with a communicable disease may not understand the rationale for separation from others.
- Gay or lesbian teenagers often suffer emotional isolation and lack access to information specific to their needs (e.g., they are at increased medical risk for sexually transmitted diseases, substance use, and violence; Bidwell & Deisher, 1991).

## Geriatric Considerations

- "Resources valued by this society include knowledge, skills, power, and position, and the elderly may be ignored because they no longer have these in their control. This lack of control is noted in at least two contrasting views of the elderly. Some view the elderly as free to relax and enjoy freedom from worries and responsibilities. Others see the elderly as being slow and worthless, having nothing to contribute to society. In neither of these views is the older person seen as a contributing member of society" (Elsen & Blegen, 1991, p. 519).
- Family roles become altered and stressed when parents become dependent on their children and children begin to assume traditional parental tasks or decision making. To help older adults meet affiliative needs and increase satisfaction with social encounters, it is suggested that small groups (rather than large, noisy crowds) be formed to promote interaction and that one or two meaningful relationships (confidantes) be encouraged.
- Factors increasing social isolation in older adults include hearing impairment, limited mobility, fatigue, caregiving responsibilities, inability to drive, mental or psychosocial impairments, and separation from spouse, friends, and/or relatives by death, illness, or physical distance (Miller, 2009).
- Impaired ability to drive from impaired vision, financial hardship, musculoskeletal functioning, or central nervous system functioning can increase an older adult's social isolation and dependency on others (Miller, 2009).
- Sensory deficits rate highest on the list of problems in the older adult with the potential to cause social isolation (Miller, 2009).

# Focus Assessment Criteria

## Subjective Data

### Assess for Related Factors

**Social Resources (Support)**

"Who lives with you?"

"About how many times did you talk to someone—friends, relatives, or others—on the telephone in the past week (either you called them or they called you)?" If subject has no telephone, ask, "How many times during the past week did you spend some time with someone who does not live with you; that is, you went to see them, or they came to visit you, or you went out to do things together?"

To whom does the person turn in time of need?

Does the client rely on friends or neighbors for such things as meals and transportation?

"Do you see your relatives and friends as often as you want to, or are you somewhat unhappy about how little you see them?"

If institutionalized: "In the past year, about how often did you leave here to visit your family or friends for weekends or holidays or to go on shopping trips or outings, or are most of your friends here in the institution with you?"

**Desire for More Human Contact**

What kind of relationships would he or she like? (Same sex or opposite sex? Same age? Someone with same situational or maturational problem?)

Can the person make the effort to meet new people and go to new places?

What kind of group activities does he or she most enjoy? (Travel? Religious service or activity?)

Has divorce or death (of spouse, child, sibling, friend, pet) occurred recently?

**Barriers to Social Contacts**

Does the person lack knowledge of resources available, where to meet others, how to initiate conversation with strangers?

Is client housebound? (Illness or incapacity—lack of mobility on steps or curbs—and weather hazards can physically isolate older adults, as can loss of usual transportation, living in dangerous area, and lack of access to public transportation.)

Are there changes in the person's sensory ability (tactile sense, hearing, visual acuity, ability to write letters)?

**Change in Living Arrangement**

Has the person moved recently (to nursing home, child's home, apartment, strange location)?

## Objective Data

### Assess for Related Factors

**Aesthetic Problems**

Mutilating surgery    Extreme obesity    Odor (e.g., ulcerating tumor)
Incontinence

**Personality Problems**

Does this person lack certain social skills or have personality features (e.g., aggression, egocentricity, racism, sexism, complaining, critical, problem drinker) that may discourage others from befriending him or her?

For more information on Focus Assessment Criteria, visit http://thepoint.lww.com.

**NOC**
Loneliness, Social Involvement

## ➤ Goal

The person will report decreased feelings of loneliness.

### Indicators

- Identify the reasons for his or her feelings of isolation.
- Discuss ways to increase meaningful relationships.

**NIC**
Socialization
Enhancement,
Spiritual Support,
Behavior
Modification: Social
Skills, Presence,
Anticipatory
Guidance

## ➤ General Interventions

The nursing interventions for various contributing factors that might be associated with *Risk for Loneliness* are very similar.

### Identify Causative and Contributing Factors (Refer to Related Factors)

### Reduce or Eliminate Causative and Contributing Factors

Promote social interaction.

Support the person who has experienced a loss as he or she works through grief (see *Grieving*).

Encourage person to talk about feelings of loneliness and their causes.

Encourage development of a support system or mobilize person's existing family, friends, and neighbors to form one.

Discuss the importance of high-quality, rather than high-quantity, socialization.

Refer to social skills teaching (see *Impaired Social Interaction*).

Offer feedback on how the person presents himself or herself to others (see *Impaired Social Interaction*).

**R:** Longino and Karl (1982) reported that type and quality of social interactions are more important than quantity. Informal activities promote well-being more than do formal, structured activities.

### *Decrease Barriers to Social Contact*

Help identify transportation options.

Determine available transportation in the community (public, church-related, volunteer).

Determine if person must learn how to use alternative transportation. Help desensitize client to fear/ stigma of using public transportation.

Assist with the development of alternative means of communication for people with compromised sensory ability (e.g., amplifier on phone, taped instead of written letters; see *Impaired Communication*).

Assist with management of aesthetic problems (e.g., consult enterostomal therapist if ostomy odor is a problem; teach client with cancer to control odor of tumors by packing area with yogurt or pouring in buttermilk, then rinsing well with saline solution).

**R:** Functional ability of the senses strongly influences a person's perception of the world, behavior, and treatment from others. A person with visible deficits may be shunned.

Refer to *Impaired Urinary Elimination* for specific interventions to control incontinence.

### *Identify Strategies to Expand the World of the Isolated*

Senior centers and church groups

Volunteer assignments (e.g., hospital, church)

Foster grandparent programs

Adult day care centers

Retirement communities

House sharing, group homes, community kitchens

Adult education classes, special interest courses

Pets

Regular contact to diminish the need to obtain attention through a crisis (e.g., suicidal gesture)

Psychiatric day hospital or activity program

**R:** Older adults are at high risk for loneliness because they often have fewer natural opportunities to be among others. Retirement from work, difficulty securing transportation, health problems that restrict visiting, sensory deficits that make communication laborious or frustrating, or isolation from the mainstream in institutions (hospitals or nursing homes) can significantly limit natural interpersonal encounters

### *Implement the Following for People with Poor or Offensive Social Skills*

Refer to *Impaired Social Interactions*

### *Discuss the Anticipatory Effects of Retirement; Assist with Planning*

Prepare for ambivalent feelings and short-term negative effects on self-esteem.

**R:** In our society working people have a higher status that non-working ones. Reitrement rquires coping with a change in social status (Miller, 2009)

### *Discuss Those Factors that Contribute to Successful Retirement (Santock, 2004; Murray, Zentner, & Yakimo, 2009)*

*Stable health status*
*Adequate income and health benefits*
*Active in community, church or professional organizations*
*Higher education level and ability to pursue new goal /activities*
*Extended social network, family friends,colleagues*
*Satisfied with life before retirement*
*Satisfied with living arrangements*
Plan to ensure adequate income.
Decrease time at work the last 2 to 3 years (e.g., shorter days, longer vacations).
Cultivate friends outside work.
Develop routines at home to replace work structure.
Rely on others rather than spouse for leisure activities.
Cultivate realistic leisure activities (energy, cost).
Engage in community or church programs or professional organizations.

**R:** "Retirement is a significant life event that requires preplanning and realistic expectation of life changes" (Stanley & Beare, 1994, p. 365).

## Initiate Referrals, as Indicated

Community-based groups that contact the socially isolated
Self-help groups for clients isolated because of specific medical problems (e.g., Reach to Recovery, United Ostomy Association)
Wheelchair groups
Psychiatric consumer rights associations

**R:** Chronic illness can contribute to social isolation because of lack of energy, decreased mobility, discomforts, fear of exposure to pathogens, and distancing by previous friends who are uncomfortable with the ill person's disabilities or the stigma associated with psychiatric problems (Miller, 2009).
**R:** Community resources and support groups can provide ongoing long-term assistance.

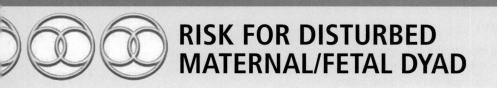

# RISK FOR DISTURBED MATERNAL/FETAL DYAD

## DEFINITION (NANDA)

At risk for disruption of the symbiotic maternal/fetal dyad as a result of comorbid or pregnancy-related conditions

## RISK FACTORS (NANDA)

Complications of pregnancy (e.g., premature rupture of membranes, placenta previa or abruption, late prenatal care, multiple gestations)

Compromised oxygen transport (e.g., anemia, cardiac disease, asthma, hypertension, seizures, premature labor, hemorrhage)

Impaired glucose metabolism (e.g., diabetes, steroid use)

Physical abuse

Substance abuse (e.g., tobacco, alcohol, drugs)

Treatment-related side effects (e.g., medications, surgery, chemotherapy)

### ▪▪▪▪▪ AUTHOR'S NOTE

This new NANDA-I nursing diagnosis represents numerous situations or factors that can compromise the pregnant woman and/or the fetus. The primary responsibility of nursing is to monitor the status of the mother, fetus, and pregnancy and to collaborate with medicine for monitoring (e.g., electronic fetal, Doppler, laboratory tests) and treatments.

Refer to Section 3 under Risk for Complications of Maternal/Infant Dyad, for interventions for this generic Collaborative problem or for more specific collaborative problems such as:

- Risk for Complications of Preterm Labor
- Risk for Complications of Non-Assuring Fetal Status
- Risk for Complications of Prenatal Bleeding
- Risk for Pregnancy-Associated Hypertension
- Risk for Complications of Postpartum Hemorrhage

For example if a pregnant woman is using cocaine, the collaborative problem, Risk for Complications of Maternal-Fetal Dyad secondary to cocaine use, would be valid because cocaine contributes to preterm labor and fetal complications. In another situation such as placenta previa, Risk for Complications of Prenatal Bleeding would be valid. In addition, some Nursing Diagnoses may be valid as Ineffective Denial, Disabled Family Coping.

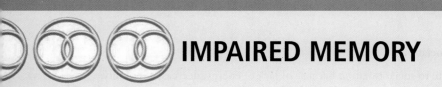

# IMPAIRED MEMORY

## DEFINITION

State in which a person experiences a temporary or permanent inability to remember or recall bits of information or behavioral skills

## DEFINING CHARACTERISTICS

### Major (Must Be Present, One or More)

Observed or reported experiences of forgetting

Inability to determine if a behavior was performed

Inability to learn or retain new skills or information

Inability to perform a previously learned skill

Inability to recall factual information

Inability to recall recent or past events

## RELATED FACTORS

### Pathophysiologic

***Related to central nervous system changes secondary to:***

Degenerative brain disease      Lesion      Head injury

Cerebrovascular accident

*Related to reduced quantity and quality of information processed secondary to:*

| | | |
|---|---|---|
| Visual deficits | Hearing deficits | Poor physical fitness |
| Fatigue | Learning habits | Intellectual skills |
| Educational level | | |

*Related to nutritional deficiencies (e.g., vitamins C and B12, folate, niacin, thiamine)*

## Treatment-Related

*Related to effects of medication (specify) on memory storage*

## Situational (Personal, Environmental)

*Related to self-fulfilling expectations*
*Related to excessive self-focusing and worrying secondary to:*

| | | |
|---|---|---|
| Grieving | Anxiety | Depression |

*Related to alcohol consumption*
*Related to lack of motivation*
*Related to lack of stimulation*
*Related to difficulty concentrating secondary to:*

| | | |
|---|---|---|
| Stress | Pain | Distractions |
| Lack of intellectual stimulation | Sleep disturbances | |

### ■■■■■ AUTHOR'S NOTE

This diagnosis is useful when the person can be helped to function better because of improved memory. If the person's memory cannot be improved because of cerebral degeneration, this diagnosis is not appropriate. Instead, the nurse should evaluate the effects of impaired memory on functioning, such as *Self-Care Deficits* or *Risk for Injury*. The focus of interventions for these nursing diagnoses would be improving self-care or protection, not improving memory.

### ■■■■■ KEY CONCEPTS

#### Generic Considerations

- Memory is a continuum of processing. It ranges from shallow to deep levels, and the duration of particular memories depends on the depths of processing (Miller, 2009).
- There are three stages of memory (Miller, 2009):
  - *Sensory memory*—awareness of information obtained through vision, hearing, taste, smell, and touch, which lasts only a few seconds
  - *Short-term memory*—working memory, contains small amounts of information (e.g., a telephone number)
  - *Long-term memory*—memory bank; can be retrieved whenever it is needed
- Memory function worries people more than any other cognitive function. When an older person forgets, it is interpreted as a sign of disease; when a younger person forgets, it is attributed to too many things being on one's mind.
- The most notable deficit in the first stage of Alzheimer's disease is the loss of recent memory (Maier-Lorentz, 2000).

### Geriatric Considerations

- Short-term memory shows a slight decline with aging (Miller, 2009).
- Benign senescent forgetfulness involves minor degrees of memory loss; it is not progressive and does not produce dysfunction in daily living (Kane et al., 1994).
- If memory deficits progress and affect other areas of intellectual functioning, dementia should be considered.

## Focus Assessment Criteria

Acquire from client and significant others.

### Subjective Data

### *Assess for Defining Characteristics*

Remote events: "Where were you born?" "Where did you go to grade school?" "What was your first job?" "When were you married?"

Recent past events: "Do you live with anyone?" "Do you have any grandchildren?" "What are the names of your grandchildren?" "When was the last time you went to the doctor?"

Immediate memory, retention: State three unrelated facts and ask the person to repeat the information immediately and again after 5 min.

Immediate memory, general grasp, and recall: Have the person read a short story and then summarize the information.

Immediate memory, recognition: Ask a multiple-choice question and ask the person to choose the correct answer.

Ability to remember:

| | | |
|---|---|---|
| Self-care activities | To shop for necessities | To take medications |
| Appointments | To pay bills | |

For more information on Focus Assessment Criteria, visit http://thepoint.lww.com.

---

**NOC**
Cognitive Orientation, Memory

➤ ## Goal

The person will report increased satisfaction with memory.

### *Indicators*

- Identify three techniques to improve memory.
- Relate factors that deter memory.

---

**NIC**
Reality Orientation, Memory Training, Environmental Management

➤ ## General Interventions

### Discuss the Person's Beliefs About Memory Deficits.

Correct misinformation.
Explain that negative expectations can result in memory deficits.

**R:** Many personal and environmental factors, such as level of education and expectations, influence memory significantly. For example, if society expects older people to be forgetful, it can be become a self-fulfilling prophecy.

**R:** Memory problems can be related to many factors, e.g., CNS pathology, nutritional deficiencies, low literacy, sensory deficits, stress, pain, or depression.

### If the Person Has Difficulty Concentrating, Explain the Favorable Effects of Relaxation and Imagery.

**R:** When concentration is difficult, relaxation and imagery have improved memory and learning (Miller, 2009).

### Teach the Person Two or Three of the Following Methods to Improve Memory Skills (Maier-Lorentz, 2000; Miller, 2009):

Write things down (e.g., use lists, calendars, notebooks).
Use auditory cues (e.g., timers, alarm clocks) in conjunction with written cues.
Use environmental cues (e.g., you might remove something from its usual place, then return it to its normal location after it has served its purpose as a reminder).

Have specific places for specific items; keep items in their proper place (e.g., keep keys on a hook near the door).

Put reminders in appropriate places (e.g., place shoes to be repaired near the door).

Use visual images ("A picture is worth a thousand words"). Create a picture in your mind when you want to remember something; the more bizarre the picture, the more likely it is you will remember.

Use active observation—pay attention to details around you, and be alert to the environment.

Make associations or mental connections (e.g., "Spring ahead and fall back" for changing clocks to and from daylight savings time).

Make associations between names and mental images (e.g., Carol and Christmas carol).

Rehearse items you want to remember by repeating them aloud or writing them on paper.

Use self-instruction—say things aloud (e.g., "I'm putting my keys on the counter so I remember to turn off the stove before I leave").

Divide information into small chunks that can be remembered easily (e.g., to remember an address or a zip code, divide it into groups ["seven hundred sixty, fifty-five"]).

Organize information into logical categories (e.g., shampoo and hair spray, toothpaste and mouthwash, soap and deodorant).

Use rhyming cues (e.g., "In 1492, Columbus sailed the ocean blue").

Use first-letter cues and make associations (e.g., to remember to buy carrots, apples, radishes, pickles, eggs, and tea bags, remember the word *carpet*).

Make word associations (e.g., to remember the letters of your license plate, make a word, such as "camel" for CML).

Search the alphabet while focusing on what you're trying to remember (e.g., to remember that someone's name is Martin, start with names that begin with "A" and continue naming names through the alphabet until your memory is jogged for the correct one).

Make up a story to connect things you want to remember (e.g., if you have to go to the cleaners and post office, create a story about mailing a pair of pants).

**R:** If one wants to improve one's memory, both the intent to remember and the knowledge about techniques for remembering are needed (Miller, 2009).

## When Trying to Learn or Remember Something:

Minimize distractions.

Do not rush.

Maintain some form of organization of routine tasks.

Carry a note pad or calendar or use written cues.

**R:** Memory impairment can be improved when information is meaningful and logical rather than abstract.

## When Teaching (Miller, 2004):

Determine if there are barriers to learning, e.g., stress, alcohol, pain, depression, low literacy.

Eliminate distractions.

Present information as concretely as possible.

Use practical examples.

Allow learner to pace the learning.

Use visual, auditory aids.

Provide advance organizers; outlines, written cues.

Encourage use of aids.

Make sure glasses are clean and lights are soft white.

Correct wrong answers immediately.

Encourage verbal responses.

Try to organize self-care activities in the same order and same time each day.

**R:** Simple, direct teaching strategies with visual prompts can increase learning and retention.

**Geriatric Interventions**

Provide accurate information about age-related changes.
Explain the difference between age-related forgetfulness and dementia.

**R:** Providing accurate information can allay fears. Clients and family members may equate any memory problems with Alzheimer's disease.

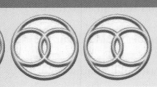

# IMPAIRED PHYSICAL MOBILITY

**Impaired Physical Mobility**

Impaired Bed Mobility
Impaired Walking
Impaired Wheelchair Mobility
Impaired Transfer Ability

## DEFINITION

State in which a client experiences or is at risk of experiencing limitation of physical movement but is not immobile

## DEFINING CHARACTERISTICS
## (LEVIN, KRAINOVITCH, BAHRENBURG, & MITCHELL, 1989)

### Major (80% to 100%)

Compromised ability to move purposefully within the environment (e.g., bed mobility, transfers, ambulation)
Range-of-motion (ROM) limitations

### Minor (50% to 80%)

Imposed restriction of movement
Reluctance to move

## RELATED FACTORS

### Pathophysiologic

*Related to decreased strength and endurance secondary to:*
Neuromuscular impairment
Autoimmune alterations (e.g., multiple sclerosis, arthritis)
Nervous system diseases (e.g., Parkinson's disease, myasthenia gravis)
Respiratory conditions (e.g., COPD)
Muscular dystrophy
Partial paralysis (spinal cord injury, stroke)
Central nervous system (CNS) tumor
Trauma
Cancer
Increased intracranial pressure
Sensory deficits

Musculoskeletal impairment
Fractures
Connective tissue disease (systemic lupus erythematosus)
Cardiac conditions
*Related to joint stiffness or contraction secondary to:*

| | |
|---|---|
| Inflammatory joint disease | Post joint-replacement surgery |
| Degenerative joint disease | Degenerative disc disease |

*Related to edema*

## Treatment-Related

*Related to external devices (casts or splints, braces, intravenous [IV] tubing)*
*Related to insufficient strength and endurance for ambulation with (specify):*

| | | |
|---|---|---|
| Prosthesis | Crutches | Walker |

## Situational (Personal, Environmental)

*Related to:*

| | | |
|---|---|---|
| Fatigue | Motivation | Pain |
| Obesity | Dyspnea | |

## Maturational

**Children**
*Related to abnormal gait secondary to:*

| | |
|---|---|
| Congenital skeletal deficiencies | Congenital hip dysplasia |
| Legg-Calvé-Perthes disease | Osteomyelitis |

**Older Adult**
*Related to decreased motor agility*
*Related to muscle weakness*

## ■■■■■■ AUTHOR'S NOTE

*Impaired Physical Mobility* describes a client with limited use of arm(s) or leg(s) or limited muscle strength. Nurses should not use this diagnosis to describe complete immobility; in this case, *Disuse Syndrome* is more applicable. Limitation of physical movement also can be the etiology of other nursing diagnoses, such as *Self-Care Deficit* and *Risk for Injury*. Nursing interventions for *Impaired Physical Mobility* focus on strengthening and restoring function and preventing deterioration. If the client can exercise but does not, refer to *Sedentary Lifestyle*. If the client has no limitations in movement but is deconditioned and has reduced endurance, refer to *Activity Intolerance*.

## ■■■■■■ ERRORS IN DIAGNOSTIC STATEMENTS

1. *Impaired Physical Mobility related to traumatic amputation of left arm*
   Listing traumatic amputation of the left arm as a related factor does not describe the problem. Rather, the diagnostic statement should reflect how the loss has affected functioning. A more appropriate diagnosis might be *Self-Care Deficit: Feeding related to insufficient knowledge of adaptations needed secondary to loss of left arm.*
2. *Impaired Physical Mobility related to limited muscle strength secondary to cerebrovascular accident (CVA)*
   Limited muscle strength is a sign of *Impaired Physical Mobility*, not a related factor. Related factors should represent direction for nursing intervention, as reflected in the diagnosis *Impaired Physical Mobility related to insufficient knowledge of techniques needed to increase motor function secondary to upper motor neuron damage.*

## ■■■■■■ KEY CONCEPTS

### Generic Considerations

• According to Miller (2009), mobility is one of the most significant aspects of physiologic functioning because it greatly influences the maintenance of independence.

*(continued)*

■■■■■■ **KEY CONCEPTS** *Continued*

- Activity, mobility, and flexibility are integral to a person's lifestyle. Compromised mobility seriously affects self-concept and lifestyle.
- The four ROM categories are passive, active assistive, active, and active resistive (Addams & Clough, 1998).
  - *Passive ROM* is movement of the client's muscles by another person with the client's help.
  - *Active assistive ROM* is active contraction of a muscle with assistance by an external force such as a therapist, mechanical appliance, or the uninvolved extremity.
  - *Active ROM* is active contraction of a muscle against the force of gravity, such as straight leg lifts.
  - *Active resistive ROM* is active contraction of a muscle against resistance, such as weights.
- Isometric exercises are when muscles contract or tense without joint movement. They are contraindicated for people with cardiac conditions because they increase left ventricular function. When done, muscles should be tensed for 5 to 15 s (Pellino et al., 1998).
- *Ambulation* is a complex, three-dimensional activity involving the legs, pelvis, trunk, and upper extremities. *Gait* is a complex movement involving the musculoskeletal, neurologic, and cardiovascular systems. Cognitive factors such as mentation and orientation are critical for safe ambulation (Addams & Clough, 1998).

## Pediatric Considerations

See *Disuse Syndrome*.

## Geriatric Considerations

- About 10% of noninstitutionalized older adults report some limitation in mobility; of institutionalized older adults, more than 90% are dependent in at least one activity of daily living (Miller, 2009). Mobility problems are often the reason for nursing home admission or extensive in-home care. Assessment of mobility determines the extent of functional impairment as a result of disease or disability.
- Effects of immobility are particularly dangerous in older adults. Muscle weakness, atrophy, and decreased endurance occur quickly, and biochemical and physiologic effects such as nitrogen loss and hypercalciuria are important to consider (Porth, 2007). Permanent functional loss is more likely with prolonged immobility, and older adults also are vulnerable to new morbidity such as pneumonia, pressure sores, falls and fracture, osteoporosis, incontinence, confusion, and depression. Every effort toward prevention and mobilization should be made (Miller, 2009).
- Age-related changes in joint and connective tissue impair flexion and extension movements, decrease flexibility, and reduce cushioning protection for joints (Miller, 2009).

## Focus Assessment Criteria

### Subjective Data

#### Assess for Defining Characteristics

**History of Symptoms (Complaints of):**
Pain
Muscle weakness
Dyspnea
Fatigue
Attributed to?    Amount of time out of bed
Induced by?       Amount of time sleeping or resting

#### Assess for Related Factors

**History of Systemic Disorders**
*Neurologic:*

| | | |
|---|---|---|
| Head trauma | CVA | Multiple sclerosis |
| Increased intracranial pressure | Polio | Guillain-Barré syndrome |

| Myasthenia gravis | Spinal cord injury | Tumor |
|---|---|---|
| Birth defect | | |

*Cardiovascular:*

| Myocardial infarction | Congenital heart anomaly | Congestive heart failure |
|---|---|---|

*Musculoskeletal:*

| Osteoporosis | Arthritis | Fractures |
|---|---|---|

*Respiratory:*

| COPD | Pneumonia | Dyspnea on exertion |
|---|---|---|
| Orthopnea | | |

*Debilitating diseases:*

| Cancer | Renal disease | Endocrine disease |
|---|---|---|

### History of Symptoms That Interfere with Mobility:

| Onset | Frequency | Duration |
|---|---|---|
| Precipitated by what? | Location | Relieved by what? |
| Description | Aggravated by what? | |

### History of Recent Trauma or Surgery

### Current Drug Therapy

## Objective Data

### Assess for Defining Characteristics

*Dominant hand*

*Motor function*

| Right arm | Strong | Weak | Absent | Spastic |
|---|---|---|---|---|
| Left arm | Strong | Weak | Absent | Spastic |
| Right leg | Strong | Weak | Absent | Spastic |
| Left leg | Strong | Weak | Absent | Spastic |

*Mobility:*

| Ability to turn self | Yes | No | Assistance needed (specify) |
|---|---|---|---|
| Ability to sit | Yes | No | Assistance needed (specify) |
| Ability to stand | Yes | No | Assistance needed (specify) |
| Ability to get up | Yes | No | Assistance needed (specify) |
| Ability to transfer | Yes | No | Assistance needed (specify) |
| Ability to ambulate | Yes | No | Assistance needed (specify) |

Weight-bearing (assess both right and left sides)

| Full | As tolerated | Partial | Non–weight-bearing |
|---|---|---|---|

Gait

| Stable | Unstable |
|---|---|

Assistive devices

| Crutches | Wheelchair | Cane | Prosthesis |
|---|---|---|---|
| Braces | Walker | Other | |

Restrictive devices:

| Cast or splint | Foley | Traction | IV |
|---|---|---|---|
| Braces | Monitor | Ventilator | Dialysis |
| Drain | | | |

Range of motion (neck, shoulders, elbows, arms, spine, hips, legs)

| Full | Limited (specify) | None |
|---|---|---|

### Assess for Related Factors

**Endurance (see *Activity Intolerance* for Additional Information)**

*Assess*

Resting pulse, blood pressure, and respirations

Blood pressure, respirations, and pulse immediately after activity

Pulse every 2 min until pulse returns to within 10 beats of resting pulse

After activity, assess for indicators of hypoxia (showing intensity, frequency, or duration of activity must be decreased or discontinued) as follows:

*Blood pressure:*

| | |
|---|---|
| Failure of systolic rate to increase | Increase in diastolic of 155 mm Hg |

*Respirations:*

| | | |
|---|---|---|
| Excessive rate increases | Decrease in rate | Dyspnea |
| Irregular rhythm | | |

*Cerebral and other changes:*

| | | |
|---|---|---|
| Confusion | Pallor | Weakness |
| Change in equilibrium | Incoordination | Cyanosis |

### Peripheral Circulation

Capillary refill time (normal, less than 3 s)
Skin color, temperature, and turgor
Peripheral pulses (rate, quality)

| | | |
|---|---|---|
| Brachial | Posterior tibial | Radial |
| Popliteal | Femoral | Pedal |

### Motivation (as Perceived by Nurse and/or Stated by the Client)

| | | |
|---|---|---|
| Excellent | Satisfactory | Poor |

For more information on Focus Assessment Criteria, visit http://thepoint.lww.com.

---

**NOC**
Ambulation, Joint Movement, Mobility, Fall Prevention Behavior

## ➤ Goal

The client will report increased strength and endurance of limbs.

### Indicators:

- Demonstrate the use of adaptive devices to increase mobility.
- Use safety measures to minimize potential for injury.
- Describe rationale for interventions.
- Demonstrate measures to increase mobility.
- Evaluate pain and quality of management

---

**NIC**
Exercise Therapy: Joint Mobility, Exercise Promotion: Strength Training, Exercise Therapy: Ambulation, Positioning, Teaching: Prescribed Activity/Exercise, Fall Prevention

## ➤ General Interventions

### Assess Causative Factors

Refer to Related Factors.

### Consult with Physical Therapy for Evaluation and Development of a Mobility Plan

**R:** Physical therapists are professional experts on mobility.

## Promote Optimal Mobility and Movement

### Promote Motivation and Adherence (Addams & Clough, 1998)

Explain the problem and the objective of each exercise.
Establish short-term goals. Ensure that initial exercises are easy and require minimal strength and coordination.
Progress only if the client is successful at the present exercise.
Provide written instructions for prescribed exercises after demonstrating and observing return demonstration.
Document and discuss improvement specifically (e.g., can lift leg 2 inches higher).

**R:** Mobility is one of the most significant aspects of physiologic functioning because it greatly influences maintenance of independence (Miller, 2009). Motivation can be increased if short-term goals are accomplished.

**R:** Promoting the client's feelings of control and self-determination may improve compliance with the exercise program.

Evaluate level of motivation and depression. Refer to a specialist as needed.

**R:** Effective management of pain and depression is sometimes necessary. Inadequate pain relief may be a primary factor leading to depression in some people, but depression should not be discounted as a secondary feature of pain. Depression may require aggressive management, including drugs and other therapies.

### Increase Limb Mobility and Determine Type of ROM Appropriate for the Client (Passive, Active Assistive, Active, Active Resistive)

Perform passive or active assistive ROM exercises (frequency determined by client's condition):

* Teach the client to perform active ROM exercises on unaffected limbs at least four times a day, if possible.
* Perform passive ROM on affected limbs. Do the exercises slowly to allow the muscles time to relax, and support the extremity above and below the joint to prevent strain on joints and tissues.
* During ROM, the client's legs and arms should move gently to within his or her pain tolerance; perform ROM slowly to allow the muscles time to relax.
* For passive ROM, the supine position is most effective. The client who performs ROM himself or herself can use a supine or sitting position.
* Do ROM daily with bed bath or three or four times daily if there are specific problem areas. Try to incorporate into activities of daily living.

Support extremity with pillows to prevent or reduce swelling.
Medicate for pain as needed, especially before activity* (see *Impaired Comfort*).
Apply heat or cold to reduce pain, inflammation, and hematoma (after 48 h).*
Apply cold to reduce swelling after injury (usually first 48 h).*
Encourage the client to perform exercise regimens for specific joints as prescribed by physician, nurse practitioner, or physical therapist (e.g., isometric, resistive).

**R:** Active ROM increases muscle mass, tone, and strength and improves cardiac and respiratory functioning. Passive ROM improves joint mobility and circulation.

### Position in Alignment to Prevent Complications

Use a footboard.

**R:** This measure prevents foot drop.

Avoid prolonged sitting or lying in the same position.

**R:** This prevents hip flexion contractures.

Change the position of the shoulder joints every 2 to 4 h.

**R:** This helps to prevent shoulder contractures.

Use a small pillow or no pillow when in Fowler's position.

**R:** This prevents flexion contracture of neck.

Support the hand and wrist in natural alignment.

**R:** This prevents dependent edema and flexion contractures of the hand.

If the client is supine or prone, place a rolled towel or small pillow under the lumbar curvature or under the end of the rib cage.

---

*May require a primary care professional's order.

**R:** This prevents flexion or hyperflexion of lumbar curvature.

Place a trochanter roll or sandbags alongside the hips and upper thighs.

**R:** This presents external rotation of the femur and hips.

If the client is in the lateral position, place pillow(s) to support the leg from groin to foot, and use a pillow to flex the shoulder and elbow slightly. If needed, support the lower foot in dorsal flexion with a sandbag.

**R:** These measures prevent internal rotation and adduction of the femur and shoulder and prevent foot drop.

For upper extremities:

- Arms abducted from the body with pillows
- Elbows in slight flexion
- Wrist in a neutral position, with fingers slightly flexed, and thumb abducted and slightly flexed
- Position of shoulder joints changed during the day (e.g., adduction, abduction, range of circular motion)

**R:** These positions prevent contractures.

## Maintain Good Body Alignment When Mechanical Devices Are Used

### Traction Devices
Assess for correct position of traction and alignment of bones.
Observe for correct amount and position of weights.
Allow weights to hang freely, with no blankets or sheets on ropes.
Assess for changes in circulation; check pulse quality, skin temperature, color of extremities, and capillary refill (should be less than 3 s).
Assess for feelings of numbness, tingling, and/or pain).
Assess for changes in mobility (ability to flex/extend unaffected joints).
Assess for signs of skin irritation (redness, ulceration, blanching).
Assess skeletal traction pin sites for loosening, inflammation, ulceration, and drainage; clean pin insertion sites (procedure may vary with type of pin and physician's order).
Encourage isometrics* and prescribed exercise program.

### Casts
Assess for proper fit of cast (should not be too loose or too tight).
Assess circulation to the encased area every 2 h (color and temperature of skin, pulse quality, capillary refill less than 2 s).
Assess for changes in sensation of extremities every 2 h (numbness, tingling, pain).
Assess motion of uninvolved joints (ability to flex and extend).
Assess for skin irritation (redness, ulceration, or complaints of pain under the cast).
Keep the cast clean and dry; do not allow sharp objects to be inserted under the cast; petal rough edges with adhesive tape; place soft cotton under edges that seem to be causing pressure points.
Allow cast to air dry while resting on pillows to prevent dents.
Observe the cast for areas of softening or indentation.
Exercise joints above and below the cast if allowed (e.g., wiggle fingers and toes every 2 h).
Assist with prescribed exercise regimens and isometrics of muscles enclosed in casts.*
Keep extremities elevated after cast application to reduce swelling.

### Braces
Assess for correct positioning of braces.
Observe for signs of skin irritation (redness, ulceration, blanching, itching, pain).
Assist with exercises as prescribed for specific joints.
Have the client demonstrate correct application of the brace.

### Prosthetic devices

---

*May require a primary professional's order.

Observe for signs of skin irritation of the stump before applying prosthetic device (stump should be clean and dry; Ace bandage should be rewrapped and securely in place).

Have the client demonstrate correct application of the prosthesis.

Assess for gait alterations or improper walking technique.

Proceed with health teaching, if indicated.

### Ace bandages

Assess for correct position of Ace bandage.

Apply Ace bandage with even pressure, wrapping from distal to proximal portions, and making sure that the bandage is not too tight or too loose.

Observe for bunching of the bandage.

Observe for signs of irritation of skin (redness, ulceration, excessive tightness).

Rewrap Ace bandage twice daily or as needed, unless contraindicated (e.g., if the bandage is a postoperative compression dressing, it should be left in place).

When wrapping lower extremity, leave the heel exposed, using a figure-8 technique.

### Slings

Assess for correct application; sling should be loose around the neck and should support the elbow and wrist above the level of the heart.

Remove slings for ROM.*

Note: Some mechanical devices may be removed for exercises, depending on the nature of the injury or type and purpose of the device. Consult with the physician to ascertain when the client may remove the device.

**R:** Compression of nerves by casts, braces, other mechanical devices, or improper positioning can cause ischemia and nerve degeneration (Porth, 2006).

**R:** Frequent assessments of circulation, pressure points, and skin conditions can detect problems early to prevent complications.

## Provide Progressive Mobilization

Assist the client slowly to a sitting position.

Allow the client to dangle legs over the side of the bed for a few minutes before standing.

Limit time to 15 min, three times a day, the first few times out of bed.

Increase time out of bed, as tolerated, by 15-min increments.

Progress to ambulation with or without assistive devices.

If the client cannot walk, assist him or her out of bed to a wheelchair or chair.

Encourage ambulation for short, frequent walks (at least three times daily), with assistance if unsteady.

Increase lengths of walks progressively each day.

**R:** Prolonged bed rest and decreased blood volume can cause a sudden drop in blood pressure (orthostatic hypotension) as blood returns to peripheral circulation. Gradual progression to increased activity reduces fatigue and increases endurance.

**R:** Researchers have shown that early mobilization has better outcomes than bed rest after an injury, a medical procedure, or as treatment of a medical condition.

## Encourage Use of Affected Arm When Possible

Encourage the client to use affected arm for self-care activities (e.g., feeding self, dressing, brushing hair).

For post-CVA neglect of upper limb, see *Unilateral Neglect*.

Instruct the client to use the unaffected arm to exercise the affected arm.

Use appropriate adaptive equipment to enhance the use of arms:

- Universal cuff for feeding in clients with poor control in both arms and hands
- Large-handled or padded silverware to assist clients with poor fine-motor skills
- Dishware with high edges to prevent food from slipping
- Suction-cup aids to prevent sliding of plate

Use a warm bath to alleviate early-morning stiffness and improve mobility.

---

*May require a primary professional's order.

Encourage the client to practice handwriting skills, if able.
Allow time to practice using affected limb.
Determine if other factors are interfering with mobility

- If the pain is interfering with mobility, refer to *Acute* or *Chronic Pain*.
- If depression is interfering with mobility, refer to *Ineffective Individual Coping*.
- If fatigue is interfering with mobility, refer to *Fatigue*.

**R:** Specific strategies are implemented to increase use of affected arm and motivation.

## Teach Methods of Transfer from Bed to Chair or Commode and to Standing Position

Refer to Impaired Transfer Ability for interventions

## Teach the Client How to Ambulate with Adaptive Equipment (e.g., Crutches, Walkers, Canes)

Instruct client in weight-bearing status.
Observe and teach the use of:

### Crutches
Do not exert pressure on axilla; use hand strength.
Type of gait varies with client's diagnosis.
Measure crutches 2 to 3 inches below axilla and tips 6 inches away from feet.

### Walkers
Use arm strength to support weakness in lower limbs.
Gait varies with the client's problems.

### Prostheses (teach about the following):
Stump wrapping before application of the prosthesis
Application of the prosthesis
Principles of stump care
Importance of cleaning the stump, keeping it dry, and applying the prosthesis only when the stump is dry
Teach client safety precautions:

- Protect areas of decreased sensation from extremes of heat and cold.
- Practice falling and how to recover from falls while transferring or ambulating.
- For decreased perception of lower extremity (post-CVA "neglect"), instruct the client to check where limb is placed when changing positions or going through doorways; also check to make sure both shoelaces are tied, that affected leg is dressed with trousers, and that pants are not dragging.
- Instruct people who are confined to a wheelchair to shift position and lift up buttocks every 15 min to relieve pressure; maneuver curbs, ramps, inclines, and around obstacles; and lock wheelchairs before transferring

Practice proper positioning, ROM (active or passive), and prescribed exercises.
Practice climbing stairs if client's condition permits.
Refer to physical therapy for continued structured physical therapy.

**R:** Ambulatory aids must be used correctly and safely to ensure effectiveness and prevent injury.

## Initiate Health Teaching and Referrals, as Indicated

Home health nurse and physical therapist.

**R:** This will ensure an assessment to determine if inpatient, outpatient, or home rehabilitation is indicated.

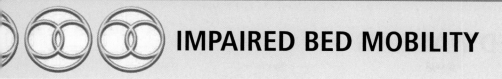

# IMPAIRED BED MOBILITY

## DEFINITION

State in which a client experiences, or is at risk of experiencing, limitation of movement in bed

## DEFINING CHARACTERISTICS

Impaired ability to turn side to side
Impaired ability to move from supine to sitting to supine
Impaired ability to "scoot" or reposition self in bed
Impaired ability to move from supine to prone or prone to supine
Impaired ability to move from supine to long sitting or long sitting to supine

### ■■■■■■ AUTHOR'S NOTE

*Impaired Bed Mobility* may be a clinically useful diagnosis when a client is a candidate for rehabilitation to improve strength, range of motion, and movement. The nurse can consult with a physical therapist for a specific plan. This diagnosis is inappropriate for an unconscious or terminally ill client.

## RELATED FACTORS

Refer to *Impaired Physical Mobility*.

### ■■■■■■ KEY CONCEPTS

Refer to *Impaired Physical Mobility*.

## Focus Assessment Criteria

Refer to *Impaired Physical Mobility*.

**NOC**
Ambulation Joint Movement, Mobility, Fall Prevention Behavior

## ➤ Goals

Refer to *Impaired Physical Mobility*.

**NIC**
Exercise Therapy: Joint Mobility, Exercise Promotion: Strength Training, Exercise Therapy: Ambulation, Positioning, Teaching: Prescribed Activity/Exercise, Prosthesis Care

## ➤ General Interventions

Refer to *Impaired Physical Mobility*.

# IMPAIRED WALKING

## DEFINITION

State in which a client experiences, or is at risk of experiencing, limitation in walking

## DEFINING CHARACTERISTICS

Impaired ability to climb stairs
Impaired ability to walk required distances
Impaired ability to walk on an incline
Impaired ability to walk on uneven surfaces
Impaired ability to navigate curbs

## RELATED FACTORS

Refer to *Impaired Physical Mobility*.

## ■■■■■■ KEY CONCEPTS

Refer to *Impaired Physical Mobility*.

## Focus Assessment Criteria

Refer to *Impaired Physical Mobility*.

**NOC**
Refer to *Impaired Physical Mobility*

## ➤ Goal

The client will increase walking distances (specify distance goal).

### Indicators:

• Demonstrate safe mobility.
• Use mobility aids correctly.

**NIC**
Refer to *Impaired Physical Mobility*

## ➤ General Interventions

### Explain that Safe Ambulation Is a Complex Movement Involving the Musculoskeletal, Neurologic, and Cardiovascular Systems and Cognitive Factors Such as Mentation and Orientation

**R:** A client who is deconditioned needs a progressive exercise program.

### Consult with a Physical Therapist for Evaluation and Planning Prior to Initiation

**R:** Physical therapy consultation is imperative to prevent injury and to maintaining weight-bearing limitations.

Ascertain that client is:

• Using ambulatory aids (e.g., cane, walker, crutches) correctly and safely:
  • Wears well-fitting shoes

- Can ambulate on inclines, uneven surfaces, and up and down stairs
- Is aware of hazards (e.g., wet floors, throw rugs)

**R:** Evaluation is needed to prevent injury to tissue structures and falls.

Refer to *Impaired Physical Mobility*.

## Provide Progressive Mobilization If Indicated

Assist the client slowly to a sitting position.
Allow the client to dangle legs over the side of the bed for a few minutes before standing.
Limit the time to 15 min, three times a day, the first few times out of bed.
Increase time out of bed, as tolerated, by 15-min increments.
Progress to ambulation, with or without assistive devices.
Encourage ambulation for short frequent walks (at least three times daily), with assistance if unsteady:

- Increase lengths of walks progressively each day.
- Evaluate the client's response to ambulation.

Refer to *Activity Intolerance* if needed.
Refer to *Activity Intolerance* and *Risk for Falls*.

**R:** Researchers have shown that early mobilization has better outcomes than bed rest after an injury, a medical procedure, or as treatment of a medical condition (Allen et al., 1999; Ebell, 2005).

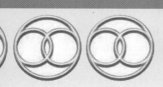

# IMPAIRED WHEELCHAIR MOBILITY

## DEFINITION

State in which a client experiences or is at risk for experiencing difficulty with wheelchair mobility and safety

## DEFINING CHARACTERISTICS

Impaired ability to operate manual or power wheelchair on an even or uneven surface
Impaired ability to operate manual or powered wheelchair on an incline
Impaired ability to operate the wheelchair on curbs

## RELATED FACTORS

Refer to *Impaired Physical Mobility*.

## ■■■■■ KEY CONCEPTS

Refer to *Impaired Physical Mobility*.

## Focus Assessment Criteria

Refer to *Impaired Physical Mobility*.

**NOC**
Ambulation:
Wheelchair, Fall
Prevention Behavior

## ➤ Goal

The client will report satisfactory, safe wheelchair mobility.

### Indicators:

- Demonstrate safe use of the wheelchair.
- Demonstrate safe transfer to the wheelchair.
- Demonstrate pressure relief and safety principles.

**NIC**
Exercise Therapy:
Ambulation,
Exercise therapy:
Balance, Exercise
Promotion: Joint
Mobility, Exercise
Promotion: Strength
Training, Muscle
Control, Positioning:
Wheelchair, Fall
Prevention

## ➤ General Interventions

### Consult with Physical Therapy for a Collaborative Plan

**R:** The specialists should direct the plan in collaboration with nursing.

### If Signs of Pressure Occur, Tefer to a Physical Therapist for Evaluation of Wheelchair Seat

**R:** Sitting-acquired pressure ulcers can be caused by immobility cushion stiffness and shape (Wound, Ostomy, and Continence, Nursing Society, 2003).

Avoid doughnut-type cushions and sheepskin.

**R:** Doughnut-type cushions increase pressure on surrounding tissues (Defloor & Grypdonck, 1999).

## Instruct on Methods to Shift Weight

- Instruct the client to stand briefly and shift weight when in the wheelchair.
- Instruct the client to manually tilt the chair backward 45° to 150° for 3 to 5 min hourly
- Instruct the client while sitting to lean toward one side of the chair and forward. The client should push himself or herself up with the hands on armrests to lift the buttocks.
- Instruct the client to put the feet on the floor, not the footrests while sitting.

**R:** Maneuvers that provide pressure relief prevent capillary occlusion from continued unrelieved pressure (Minke, 2000).

## Refer to Physical Therapy for Instruction on Using the Wheelchair on Flat Surfaces, Curbs, in Elevators, etc.

**R:** Specialists should be consulted to improve confidence and to prevent injuries.

## Refer to Home Health Nurse for Evaluation of Home Environment

**R:** Wheelchair accessibility and other barriers to safe wheelchair use need to be assessed. Research has reported falls with sustained injuries and failure to make home modifications in a home with a person in a wheelchair (Berg et al., 2002).

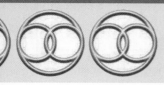

# IMPAIRED TRANSFER ABILITY

## DEFINITION

State in which a client experiences or is at risk for experiencing difficulty with transfer to and from the wheelchair

## DEFINING CHARACTERISTICS

Impaired ability to transfer from bed to chair and chair to bed
Impaired ability to transfer on or off a toilet or commode
Impaired ability to transfer in and out of tub or shower
Impaired ability to transfer between uneven levels
Impaired ability to transfer from chair to car or car to chair
Impaired ability to transfer from chair to floor or floor to chair
Impaired ability to transfer standing to floor or floor to standing

## RELATED FACTORS

Refer to *Impaired Physical Mobility*.

## ▰▰▰▰▰ KEY CONCEPTS

Refer to *Impaired Physical Mobility*.

## Focus Assessment Criteria

Refer to *Impaired Physical Mobility*.

**NOC**
Transfer
Performance, Fall
Prevention Behavior

## ➤ Goal

The client will demonstrate transfer to and from the wheelchair.

### Indicators:

- Identify when assistance is needed.
- The client will demonstrate ability to transfer in varied situations (e.g., toilet, bed, car, chair, uneven levels).

**NIC**
Positioning:
Wheelchair, Fall
Prevention

## ➤ General Interventions

### Consult and Refer to a Physical Therapist to Evaluate the Client's Ability to Transfer:

- Consider weight, strength, movement ability, tolerance to position changes, balance, motivation, cognition
- Use of manual transfer or device-assisted lift.
- Consider staff ratio to clients

**R:** A consultation with a physical therapist is needed to create a care plan for this client under Impaired Transfer Ability.

## Proceed with Established Plan to Transfer:

Before transferring the client, assess the number of personnel needed for assistance.

The client should transfer toward the unaffected side.

Position the client on the side of the bed. His or her feet should be touching the floor, and he or she should be wearing stable shoes or slippers with nonskid soles.

For getting in and out of bed, encourage weight-bearing on the uninvolved or stronger side.

Lock the wheelchair before the transfer. If using a regular chair, be sure it will not move.

Instruct the client to use the arm of the chair closer to him or her for support while standing.

Place your arm around the client's rib cage and keep the back straight, with knees slightly bent.

Tell the client to place his or her arms around your waist or rib cage, *not the neck*.

Support client's legs by bracing his with yours. (While facing the client, lock his or her knees with your knees.)

Instruct clients with hemiplegia to pivot on the uninvolved foot.

**R:** Specific instructions and sufficient staff can prevent injury to the client and staff.

## For Clients with Lower Limb Weakness or Paralysis, a Sliding Board Transfer May Be Used

The client should wear pajamas so he or she will not stick to the board.

The client needs good upper extremity strength to be able to slide the buttocks from the bed to the chair or wheelchair. (Wheelchairs should have removable arms.)

When the client's arms are strong enough, he or she should progress to a sitting transfer without the board, if he or she can lift the buttocks enough to clear the bed and chair seat.

If the client's legs give out, guide him or her gently to the floor and *seek additional assistance*.

**R:** A complex assessment is needed to determine whether a slide-board transfer is needed (Hoeman, 2002).

Consult and refer client and family to home health nurses for a home evaluation and to access resources for discharge.

**R:** The incidence of injuries and falls at home with clients in wheelchairs has been found to be at 37% (Berg et al., 2002).

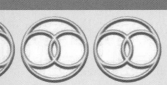

# NEONATAL JAUNDICE

## ▶ Risk for Complications of Hyperbilirubinemia

## DEFINITION

The state in which there is a yellow-orange tint of the neonate's skin and mucous membranes that occurs after 24 hours of life as a result of unconjugated bilirubin in the circulation

## DEFINING CHARACTERISTICS

Abnormal blood profile (hemolysis; total serum bilirubin greater than 2 mg/dL: inherited disorder; total serum bilirubin in high-risk range on age in hour-specific nomogram)

Abnormal skin bruising

Yellow-orange skin

Yellow sclera

## RELATED FACTORS

Abnormal weight loss in breastfeeding newborn; 15% in term infant)
Feeding pattern not well established
Infant experiences difficulty making transition to extrauterine life
Neonate age 1 to 7 days
Stool (meconium) passage delayed

 **AUTHOR'S NOTE**

This new NANDA-I diagnosis is a collaborative problem that requires a laboratory test for diagnosis and treatment from medicine and nursing. Refer to Section 3 to Risk for Complications of Hyperbilirubinemia for neonates at risk for or experiencing hyperbilirubinemia.

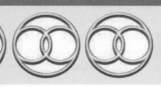

# NONCOMPLIANCE

## DEFINITION

State in which a client or group desires to comply but factors are present that deter adherence to health-related advice given by health professionals

## DEFINING CHARACTERISTICS

### Major (Must Be Present, One or More)

Verbalization of noncompliance or nonparticipation or confusion about therapy
*and/or*
Direct observation of behavior indicating noncompliance

### Minor (May Be Present)

Missed appointments
Partially used or unused medications
Persistence of symptoms
Progression of disease process
Undesired outcomes (postoperative morbidity, pregnancy, obesity, addiction, regression during rehabilitation)

## RELATED FACTORS

### Pathophysiologic

***Related to impaired ability to perform tasks because of disability secondary to:***
Poor memory                                    Motor and sensory deficits
***Related to increasing disease-related symptoms despite adherence to advised regimen***

### Treatment-Related

***Related to:***
Side effects of therapy                        Past unsuccessful experiences with advised regimen
Impersonal aspects of referrals                Nontherapeutic environment
Financial cost of therapy                      Complex, unsupervised, prolonged therapy

## Situational (Personal, Environmental)

*Related to barriers to access secondary to:*

Mobility problems    Transportation problems    Financial issues

Inclement weather    Lack of child care

*Related to concurrent illness of a family member*

Nonsupportive family, peers, or community

*Related to barriers to care secondary to homelessness*

*Related to change in employment status*

*Related to change in health insurance coverage*

*Related to barriers to comprehension secondary to:*

Cognitive deficits    Anxiety    Visual deficits

Fatigue    Hearing deficits    Decreased attention span

Poor memory    Motivation

## ■ AUTHOR'S NOTE

Compliance depends on various factors, including motivation, perception of vulnerability, and beliefs about controlling or preventing illness; environment; quality of health instruction; and ability to access resources (cost, accessibility). The diagnosis *Noncompliance* describes a client desiring to comply but prevented from doing so by certain factors (e.g., lack of understanding, inadequate finances, overly complex instructions). The nurse must attempt to reduce or eliminate these factors to ensure successful interventions. A new nursing diagnosis—Risk-Prone Health Behavior—can also be useful to describe a client who is having difficulty modifying behaviors in response to a change in health status.

The process of *informed consent* protects a client's right to self-determination. Informed consent has three conditions: the client must be capable of giving consent, understand the advantages and disadvantages of consent, and not be coerced (Cassells & Redman, 1989). When a client refuses to comply with advice or instructions, it is important for the nurse to assess for and validate the presence of all required elements for informed consent. The nurse is cautioned against using *Noncompliance* to describe a client who has made an informed autonomous decision not to comply. As Cassells and Redman (1989) state, "Human dignity is respected by granting individuals the freedom to make choices in accordance with their own values." When a client must change habits or lifestyle or perform certain activities to manage a health problem, *Risk for Ineffective Self-Health Management* is very useful.

## ■ ERRORS IN DIAGNOSTIC STATEMENTS

1. *Noncompliance related to reports of not following low-salt diet and resulting increased edema*

The above factors would not have caused or contributed to noncompliance. Rather, they represent evidence. If the reason for noncompliance is unknown, *Noncompliance related to unknown etiology, as evidenced by reports of (specify)* would be appropriate.

When the reasons are identified, the nurse must determine whether these factors can be reduced or eliminated. If the client has made an informed decision not to follow the prescribed diet, *Noncompliance* may not be the correct nursing diagnosis. Perhaps the nurse and client could examine the prescribed diet. Is it realistic? What is the probability that compliant behavior will improve quality of life?

## ■ KEY CONCEPTS

### Generic Considerations

- Compliance is a positive behavior that clients exhibit when moving toward mutually accepted therapeutic goals.
- Compliance should be viewed on a continuum rather than as separate states of compliance or noncompliance.
- Partnerships between health care provider and client involve choices and compromises. Some clients desire a passive role, whereas others want complete autonomy.
- Compliance involves a behavioral change. Which the following can influence positively?
  - Initial and continuing trust in the health care professional

*(continued)*

■■■■■■ **KEY CONCEPTS** *Continued*

- Reinforcement from significant others
- Perception of own susceptibility to the disease
- Perception that the disease is serious
- Evidence that compliance helps control symptoms or the disease
- Tolerable side effects
- Less interference with daily activities of client or significant others
- More benefit than harm provided by therapy
- Positive sense of self
- The following factors hinder compliance (Hussey & Gilliland, 1989):
  - Inadequate explanation
  - Disagreement between client and provider
  - Long duration of therapy
  - High complexity or expense of regimen
  - Great number and severity of side effects
- Motivation, "the pre- and post-decisional processes which guide the initiation and maintenance of health behaviors," is important for nurses to act on (Fleury, 1992, p. 229). Aspects of motivation to consider include the following:
  - What does the prescribed health behavior change mean to the client?
  - What environmental factors may interfere with the new behavior?
  - What future events may challenge the client's motivation?
  - How will personal values affect the client's ability to remain motivated?
- *Self-efficacy*, the client's beliefs about his or her ability to adopt, perform, and maintain a healthy behavior change, also has been shown to contribute to long-term compliance. The nurse can evaluate a client's self-efficacy with questions such as:
  - How many days per week do you think you can take a walk?
  - At what interval do you feel comfortable enough to breastfeed your baby?
  - How often do you think you can check your sugar?
- Noncompliance that follows a period of compliant behavior is termed *relapse*. It usually happens when nonsupportive environmental influences overcome the client's desire to perform the newly adopted behavior. Causes of relapse can be any of the related factors already listed.
- When evaluating noncompliance related to medication, the nurse must consider the following factors that may affect drug absorption, metabolism, effectiveness, side effects, and excretion: body weight, age, time of administration, route of administration, genetic factors, basal metabolic rate, interactions with other drugs and foods, presence of organ disease (e.g., liver, kidneys), altered body chemistry (e.g., hypokalemia), and infection. For example, serum theophylline levels are diminished in a client who smokes cigarettes.

### Pediatric Considerations

- Transfer of responsibility for self-care of a child with chronic illness is difficult when noncompliance increases risks to the child, anxiety to the parents, and costs to the family. The child should progress gradually to self-care to increase self-confidence and reduce overdependence (Hockenberry & Wilson, 2009).
- Compliance is lower during adolescence, when following a regimen competes with self-consciousness and concerns over peer reactions (Whatley, 1991).
- Following a particular treatment regimen can be difficult and trying for an ill child and family. For example, certain drugs may affect behavior, alertness, or school performance (Scipien, Chard, Howe, & Barnard, 1990).

### Geriatric Considerations

Factors influencing noncompliance in older adults are functional deficits, complicated regimens, costs, inconvenience, and side effects that decrease functional status (e.g., strength, alertness).

**Transcultural Considerations**

Refer to Transcultural Considerations under *Impaired Communication* and *Ineffective Health Maintenance*.

## Focus Assessment Criteria

### Subjective Data

#### *Assess for Defining Characteristics*

Unacceptable side effects of therapy

| | | |
|---|---|---|
| Unpleasant taste | Pain | Difficulty swallowing |
| Too expensive | Time-consuming | Inconvenient |

Does a family member report any of the above problems?

What does the client want from the nurse or physician?

#### *Assess for Related Factors*

**What Is the Client's General Health Motivation?**

Does the client seek help as needed?

Does the client intend to make advised lifestyle alterations?

Does the client accept the diagnosis?

**What Is the Client's Perception of His or Her Present State of Health?**

Does the client consider self to be generally well?

Does the client fear a specific illness?

Does the client believe his or her illness is severe?

**How Does the Client View the Advised Treatment Regimen? (e.g., Does It Make Personal Sense?)**

*Situations that interfere with prescribed behavior*

| | | |
|---|---|---|
| Family demands | Travel (hotels, restaurants) | Stress |
| Lack of transportation | Occupations | Denial |

### Objective Data

#### *Assess for Defining Characteristics*

**Evidence of Noncompliance**

Persistence of symptoms

Problems with medications (pill count, serum drug levels)

Progression of disease

Missed appointments

#### *Assess for Related Factors*

**Obstacles to Self-Care**

| | | |
|---|---|---|
| Inability to read | Musculoskeletal deficits | Immaturity |
| Cognitive deficits | Memory lags | Pain |

**Evidence of Obstacles in Caregiving Environment**

| | |
|---|---|
| Long waiting period | Hurried atmosphere |

**NOC**
Adherence Behavior, Compliance Behavior, Symptom Control, Treatment Behavior: Illness/ Injury

## ➤ Goal

The client will report a desire to change or initiate change.

### Indicators:

- Describe the reasons for the suggested regimen.
- Identify the barriers to adhering to the regimen.

**NIC**
Health Education, Self-Modification Assistance, Self-Responsibility Facilitation, Coping Enhancement, Decision-Making Support, Health System Guidance, Mutual Goal Setting, Teaching: Disease Process, Teaching: Prescribed Medication

## ➤ General Interventions

### Determine the Client's Understanding of:

Presence of or risk for health problem (prognosis, disability)
Vulnerability to problem
Prevention or treatment measures available
Effectiveness of preventive measures
Effectiveness of treatment measures

**R:** Lack of understanding of the health problem, complications, and the client's own vulnerability contribute to noncompliance.

### Explore the Client's Feelings Regarding:

Past attempts at compliance
Present concerns regarding prevention or treatment modalities:

- Confidence in his or her ability to make changes
- *Self-efficacy*, the client's beliefs about his or her ability to adopt, perform, and maintain a healthy behavior change, also has been shown to contribute to long-term compliance.

## Encourage Positive Thinking About New Health-Related Behaviors

### Collaborate With the Client to Set Goals

Short-term goals are most useful.
Be flexible.
Be realistic, considering each client's uniqueness.
Avoid imposing your goals for client.

### Consider Using an Agreement, a Written Statement of Expected Behaviors

Initially, use short-term contracts with family member, coworker, friend, or nurse.
For the longer term, self-contracts work well; the client finds his or her own rewards and reinforces his or her own positive behavior changes.

**R:** Establishing a consensual regimen and goals validates that the client is the decision maker and the health care professional is the adviser.

## Self-Monitoring Is Useful to Determine Positive and Negative Influences on Compliance

Daily records
Charts
Diary of progress or symptoms, clinical values (e.g., blood pressure), or dietary intake

**R:** Involving the client in decision-making places some responsibility on him or her to make sure the plan works, promoting compliance with treatment.
**R:** Agreements involve a commitment to make changes and to be accountable for choices.

## Review Present Medication Therapy (Prescribed and Over-the-Counter)

Discuss present therapy (names, dosages, time taken, side effects). Do not ask, "Are you taking your medications?" Ask:

- "What medications did you take today? Yesterday?"
- "What time of day is it difficult for you to take your medications?"
- "Are there times when you decide not to take one of the doses?"

Determine the client's understanding of the need for medication:

- Emphasize lifelong therapy when indicated (e.g., hypertension, diabetes mellitus).
- Explain the complications of unmanaged disease.

Identify possible adverse interactions among drugs (consult a pharmacist).
Commit to work with the client to reduce or eliminate side effects (e.g., change agents or dose).
Help the client identify a reminder to take the medication (e.g., brushing teeth at night, daily favorite TV show, watch timer).
Ask the client to call the primary provider with problems rather than stopping the medication.
Emphasize that unavoidable side effects are still better than the consequences of no therapy (e.g., stroke, blindness, renal failure).

**R:** Lack of understanding regarding reasons for drug therapy and options available contributes to noncompliance. Open discussions about side effects can encourage the client to report problems before discontinuing treatment.

## Medications for HIV

Address the benefits of antiviral medications and the risks of nonadherence with HIV medications.
Emphasize that HIV/AIDS can be a chronic disease.
Describe the actions of the medications on the virus.
Explain and track CD4 and viral load counts.
Explain how resistance to medications occurs (e.g., missed doses).
Design a system and schedule with the client that will decrease missed doses.
Advise the client, if he or she is regularly missing doses, to stop all HIV medications and to call the nurse.

**R:** Missing one or two doses of HIV medications a week can cause resistance to the medications and subsequent failure.

## Help to Reduce Side Effects

Address side effects that may occur and encourage the client to report them for evaluation.
Specify the difference between side effects and adverse events.

**R:** Warning clients of possible side effects can reduce the anxiety. Side effects are signs and symptoms that can usually be managed if they occur. Adverse events are serious and usually require discontinuation of the medicine.

For gastric irritation, administer the drug with milk or food; yogurt may be advisable (unless contraindicated).
For drowsiness, administer the medication at bedtime or late in the afternoon; consult the primary provider for dose reduction.
For leg cramps (hypokalemia), increase foods high in potassium (e.g., oranges, raisins, tomatoes, bananas).
For other side effects, consult pertinent references.
Use long-acting intramuscular preparations whenever possible; this includes some antibiotics and antipsychotic medications.
Suggest the use of combination pills if available.
When appropriate, be sure client is taking the fewest medications possible (check dosages to provide the largest dose available in the fewest number of drugs).
To decrease the frequency of oral medications, suggest longer-acting drug preparations, such as such transdermal patch (e.g., nitroglycerin).

R: Some barriers to compliance can be eliminated with specific teaching.

Management of side effects can increase adherence.

## If Indicated, Focus on Emotional Responses that Interfere with Compliance (e.g., Situational Anxiety, Depression, Denial, Relationship Problems)

## Initiate Health Teaching and Referrals, as Indicated

Encourage prescription of generic drugs for people with financial concerns. Determine if the client needs assistance.

Access specific pharmaceutical assistance programs at www.pparx.org/ or www.rxasst.org/.

When expensive equipment is involved for treatments at home, make appropriate referrals to social workers and local agencies.

R: Financial barriers are often barriers to compliance

Teach the importance of adhering to the prescribed regimen.

Provide written drug information tailored to the client's needs. Include drug names, dosages, number of tablets to take and when, purpose of drugs, potential side effects and adverse reactions, and directions for relief of side effects.

Offer praise for honesty about compliance and for sharing reasons. For example:

• "I'm glad you told me that you stopped taking Motrin because it made your stomach hurt. Now I understand why your hands still ache. Let's talk about ways we can get you some comfort."
• "It's good that you told me about your stopping the blood pressure pills. That explains your headaches and higher pressure today. Let's discuss how those pills made you feel."

At discharge from the hospital or outpatient setting, provide the written name and phone number of whom to call with concerns about prescribed drug regimen.

R: Involving the client in decision-making places some responsibility on him or her to make sure the plan works, promoting compliance with treatment.

R: Ways that assistance can be accessed after discharge must be addressed.

## Pediatric Interventions

Talk with the child to help him or her understand the need for the treatment and likely problems if it is not followed.

Keep the information short, simple, and concrete; speak on the family's/child's level.

Introduce important information first.

Emphasize visible benefits of compliance.

Attempt to minimize side effects and/or teach how to manage side effects.

Design a reminder system with child and family (checklist); write down simple instructions in steps.

Avoid being punitive; instead, problem-solve with the family to improve compliance.

R: Strategies to improve compliance must include the child and caregivers in the home (Hockenberry & Wilson, 2009).

Discuss how the child can participate in self-care according to developmental level (Wysocki & Wayne, 1992):

• Put stars on the child's chart when exercises are completed.
• Draw up insulin.
• Select food choices.
• Establish accountability for the child or family members.

Discuss conflicts (see *Impaired Parenting*).

Elicit problems in compliance and possible solution or compromises

R: Compliance increases when expectations, responsibilities, and consequences are discussed ((Hockenberry & Wilson, 2009).

*(continued)*

**Pediatric Interventions**
*Continued*

Use age-related behavioral strategies:

- Earning tokens or stickers
- Written agreements with positive reinforcers
- Disciplinary techniques (e.g., time-out for young children, withholding privileges for older children)

**R:** Attempts to engage the child in some aspect of self-care can increase independence, initiative, and self-confidence (Wysocki & Wayne, 1992).

**R:** Agreements are an effective method with older children when they are involved in defining the rules of the agreement.

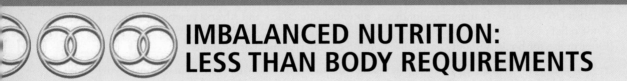

# IMBALANCED NUTRITION: LESS THAN BODY REQUIREMENTS

**Imbalanced Nutrition: Less Than Body Requirements**

Related to Anorexia Secondary to (Specify)
Related to Difficulty or Inability to Procure Food
Altered Dentition
Impaired Swallowing
Ineffective Infant Feeding Pattern

## DEFINITION

Less Than Body Requirements: state in which a client who is not NPO experiences or is at risk of experiencing reduced weight related to inadequate intake or metabolism of nutrients for metabolic needs

## DEFINING CHARACTERISTICS

### Major (Must Be Present, One or More)

The client who is not NPO reports or is found to have food intake less than the recommended daily allowance (RDA) with or without weight loss
*and/or*
Actual or potential metabolic needs in excess of intake with weight loss

### Minor (May Be Present)

Weight 10% to 20% or more below ideal for height and frame
Triceps skinfold, mid-arm circumference, and mid-arm muscle circumference less than 60% Standard measurement
Muscle weakness and tenderness
Mental irritability or confusion
Decreased serum albumin
Decreased serum transferrin or iron-binding capacity
Sunken fontanel in infant

## RELATED FACTORS

### Pathophysiologic

*Related to increased caloric requirements and difficulty in ingesting sufficient calories secondary to:*

| | | |
|---|---|---|
| Burns (postacute phase) | Cancer | Infection |
| Trauma | Chemical dependence | |
| GI complications/deformities | AIDS | |

*Related to dysphagia secondary to:*

| | | |
|---|---|---|
| Cerebrovascular accident (CVA) | Muscular dystrophy | Amyotrophic lateral sclerosis |
| | Cerebral palsy | Neuromuscular disorders |
| Parkinson's disease | Cleft lip/palate | |
| Möbius syndrome | | |

*Related to decreased absorption of nutrients secondary to:*

| | |
|---|---|
| Crohn's disease | Lactose intolerance |
| Necrotizing enterocolitis | Cystic fibrosis |

*Related to decreased desire to eat secondary to altered level of consciousness*

*Related to self-induced vomiting, physical exercise in excess of caloric intake, or refusal to eat secondary to anorexia nervosa*

*Related to reluctance to eat for fear of poisoning secondary to paranoid behavior*

*Related to anorexia, excessive physical agitation secondary to bipolar disorder*

*Related to anorexia and diarrhea secondary to protozoal infection*

*Related to vomiting, anorexia, and impaired digestion secondary to pancreatitis*

*Related to anorexia, impaired protein and fat metabolism, and impaired storage of vitamins secondary to cirrhosis*

*Related to anorexia, vomiting, and impaired digestion secondary to GI malformation or necrotizing enterocolitis*

*Related to anorexia secondary to gastroesophageal reflux*

### Treatment-Related

*Related to protein and vitamin requirements for wound healing and decreased intake secondary to:*

| | |
|---|---|
| Surgery | Surgical reconstruction of mouth |
| Radiation therapy | Medications (chemotherapy) |
| Wired jaw | |

*Related to inadequate absorption as a medication side effect of (specify):*

| | | |
|---|---|---|
| Colchicine | Neomycin | Pyrimethamine |
| *Para*-aminosalicylic acid | Antacid | |

*Related to decreased oral intake, mouth discomfort, nausea, and vomiting secondary to:*

| | | |
|---|---|---|
| Radiation therapy | Tonsillectomy | Chemotherapy |

### Situational (Personal, Environmental)

*Related to decreased desire to eat secondary to:*

| | | |
|---|---|---|
| Anorexia | Social isolation | Depression |
| Nausea and vomiting | Stress | Allergies |

*Related to inability to procure food (physical limitation or, financial or transportation problems)*

*Related to inability to chew (damaged or missing teeth, ill-fitting dentures)*

*Related to diarrhea secondary to (specify)*

### Maturational

**Infant/Child**

*Related to inadequate intake secondary to:*

Lack of emotional/sensory stimulation

Lack of knowledge of caregiver

Inadequate production of breast milk

*Related to malabsorption, dietary restrictions, and anorexia secondary to:*

| | | | |
|---|---|---|---|
| Celiac disease | Lactose intolerance | Necrotizing enterocolitis | Cystic fibrosis |
| GI malformation | Gastroesophageal reflux | | |

*Related to sucking difficulties (infant) and dysphagia secondary to:*

| | |
|---|---|
| Cerebral palsy | Cleft lip and palate |

*Related to inadequate sucking, fatigue, and dyspnea secondary to:*

| | |
|---|---|
| Congenital heart disease | Viral syndrome |
| Hyperbilirubinemia | Prematurity |
| Respiratory distress syndrome | Developmental delay |

## AUTHOR'S NOTE

Nurses usually are the primary diagnosticians and prescribers for improving nutritional status. Although *Imbalanced Nutrition* is not a difficult diagnosis to validate, interventions for it can challenge the nurse.

Many factors influence food habits and nutritional status: personal, family, cultural, financial, functional ability, nutritional knowledge, disease and injury, and treatment regimens. *Imbalanced Nutrition: Less Than Body Requirements* describes people who can ingest food but eat an inadequate or imbalanced quality or quantity. For instance, the diet may have insufficient protein or excessive fat. Quantity may be insufficient because of increased metabolic requirements (e.g., cancer, pregnancy) or interference with nutrient use (e.g., impaired storage of vitamins in cirrhosis).

The nursing focus for *Imbalanced Nutrition* is assisting the client or family to improve nutritional intake. Nurses should not use this diagnosis to describe people who are NPO or cannot ingest food. They should use the collaborative problems *RC of Electrolyte Imbalance* or *RC of Negative Nitrogen Balance* to describe those situations.

## ERRORS IN DIAGNOSTIC STATEMENTS

1. *Imbalanced Nutrition: Less Than Body Requirements related to insulin deficiency, altered consciousness, and hypermetabolic state*

   This diagnosis represents a client with diabetes experiencing diabetic ketoacidosis. In such a situation, nursing responsibility focuses on two major problems: managing the ketoacidosis with the physician and teaching the client and family how to prevent future episodes. The first is described by the collaborative problem *RC of Ketoacidosis*, for which the nurse would be responsible for monitoring for physiologic instability, initiate timely interventions, and evaluate the client's response. The nurse would investigate the second problem, described by the nursing diagnosis *Possible Ineffective Self-Health Management related to adherence to diabetic diet and insufficient knowledge of adaptation needed when sick*, after the client was stable.

2. *Imbalanced Nutrition: Less Than Body Requirements related to parenteral therapy and NPO status*

   This diagnosis represents a situation with which nurses are intricately involved (parenteral therapy). From a nutritional perspective, however, what interventions do nurses prescribe to improve the nutritional status of an NPO client? Parenteral nutrition in a client who is NPO influences several actual or potential responses that nurses treat, representing both nursing diagnoses, such as *Risk for Infection* and *Impaired Comfort*, and the collaborative problems *RC of Hypo/hyperglycemia* and *RC of Negative Nitrogen Balance*.

## KEY CONCEPTS

### Generic Considerations

- For proper metabolic functioning, the body requires adequate carbohydrates, protein, fat, vitamins, minerals, electrolytes, and trace elements. Figure II.2 depicts the Food Pyramid developed by the United States Department of Agriculture. It recommends daily servings of five food groups. The sixth group—fats, oils, and sweets—should be eaten sparingly and should not exceed 30% of total calorie intake.
- Overall, 54.9% of adult Americans are overweight (15% over ideal weight for height); 18% to 25% of adolescents are overweight. The rate for children is 25% to 30% (Dudek, 2006).

*(continued)*

## ■■■■■■ KEY CONCEPTS *Continued*

- Obesity is a risk factor for hypertension; type 2 diabetes mellitus; coronary artery disease; cancer of the breast, endometrium, cervix, ovary, colon, rectum, prostate, gallbladder, and biliary tract; and joint and foot disorders (Dudek, 2006).
- Studies report that U.S. women consume insufficient iron, calcium, and vitamins A and C.
- Americans eat half of the fiber requirement and 20% more fat than needed (Dudek, 2001).
- The National Research Council (1989) compiled the dietary recommendations outlined in Box II.2.
- Factors influencing nutrient requirements include age, activity, gender, health status (presence of disease, injuries), and nutrient metabolism (storage, absorption, use, excretion).
- Factors influencing nutrient intake include personal (appetite, chewing and swallowing ability, functional ability, psychological status, culture) and structural (socialization, finances, ability to obtain and prepare food, kitchen facilities, transportation; Miller, 2009).
- Drugs can reduce nutrient intake by altering the following (White & Ashworth, 2000):
  - Appetite (e.g., metformin, digoxin, paroxetine)
  - Absorption (e.g., neomycin, cimetidine)
  - Metabolism (e.g., metformin, isoniazid, phenytoin)
- The body requires a minimum level of nutrients for health and growth. During the life span, nutritional needs vary, as indicated in Table II.12 (Dudek, 2006; Hockenberry & Wilson, 2009).
- Table II.13 shows the basal metabolic index (BMI) for height.
- The client with cancer experiences disease- and treatment-related nutritional problems:

*Disease-Related:*

| | | |
|---|---|---|
| Malabsorption | Diarrhea | Constipation |
| Anemia | Protein deficits | Fatigue |

*Treatment-Related:*

| | | |
|---|---|---|
| Stomatitis | Diarrhea | Nausea and vomiting |
| Anorexia | Fatigue | |

## Pediatric Considerations

- Changes in nutritional needs characterize each growth period (see Table II.13).
- Non-adolescent children should not be put on diets. The goal for growing children is to maintain, not lose, weight. Healthy food choices of fruit, vegetables, and low-fat snacks (e.g., pretzels) can replace foods high in salt, fats, and sugar. Refer to *Ineffective Health Maintenance* for specific interventions for weight loss.
- Children at special risk for inadequate nutritional intake include those with:
  - Congenital anomalies (e.g., tracheoesophageal fistula, GI malformation, cardiac or neurologic anomalies)
  - Prematurity, developmental delay, and intrauterine growth retardation
  - Inborn errors of metabolism (e.g., phenylketonuria)
  - Gastroesophageal reflux
  - Malabsorption disorders
  - Developmental disorders (e.g., cerebral palsy)
  - Chronic illness (e.g., cystic fibrosis, chronic infections, diabetes)
  - Accelerated growth rates (e.g., prematurity, infancy, adolescence)
  - Parents who have inadequate attachment
- Parents must follow sound feeding practices to prevent nutritional deficits in their infants (Hockenberry & Wilson, 2009):
  - Feeding the infant breast milk or iron-fortified formula for the first year
  - Adding solid foods by 5 to 6 months of age
  - Assessing the infant's cues for burping or satiety
  - Holding the infant during feeding versus propping the bottle
  - Selecting foods appropriate to the infant's physiologic and motor development
  - Preparing formula correctly
    Cheek and chin support while nippling for premature, developmentally delayed or orally compromised infants

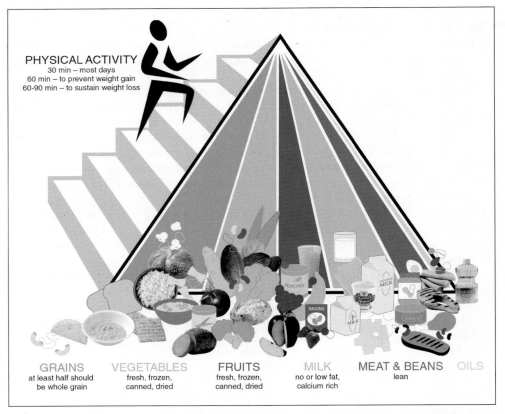

FIGURE II.2 USDA food pyramid. (U.S. Department of Agriculture, Center for Nutrition Policy and Promotion, April 2005, CNPP-15.)

### BOX II.2 DIETARY RECOMMENDATIONS OF THE NATIONAL RESEARCH COUNCIL REPORT

Reduce total fat intake to 30% or less of calories; saturated fatty acid intake to less than 10% of kilocalories; and cholesterol to less than 300 mg daily.*

Drink 8–10 glasses of water or noncaffeinated beverages.

Increase intake of starches and other complex carbohydrates.

Maintain protein intake at moderate levels.[†] Increase dry beans, fish.

Increase fiber intake to 25–35 g daily.

Eat 2–4 servings of fruit daily.

Eat 3–5 servings of vegetables daily.

Limit total daily intake of salt (sodium chloride) to 6 g or less.[‡]

Maintain adequate calcium and iron intake.

Avoid taking dietary supplements in excess of the recommended daily allowance (RDA) in any one day.

Balance food intake and physical activity to maintain appropriate body weight.

For those who drink alcoholic beverages, limit consumption to the equivalent of less than 1 oz of pure alcohol in a single day.[§]

[*]The intake of fat and cholesterol can be reduced by substituting fish, poultry without skin, lean meats, and low-fat or nonfat dairy products for fatty meats and whole-milk dairy products; by choosing more vegetables, fruits, cereals, and legumes; and by limiting oils, fats, egg yolks, and fried and other fatty foods.

[†]Meet at least the RDA for protein, do not exceed twice the RDA.

[‡]Limit the use of salt in cooking, and avoid adding it to food at the table. Salty, highly processed salty, salt-preserved, and salt-pickled foods should be consumed sparingly.

[§]The Committee does not recommend alcohol consumption. One ounce of pure alcohol is the equivalent of two cans of beer, two small glasses of wine, or two average cocktails.

National Research Council, Committee on Diet and Health of Food and Nutrition Board. (1989). Diet and health: Implications for reducing chronic disease risk. *Nutrition Reviews, 47,* 142–149; *Food guide pyramid: A guide to daily food choices.* Leaflet No. 572. Washington, DC: US Department of Agriculture; Dudek, S.G. (2006). *Nutrition essentials for nursing practice.* (5th ed.) Philadelphia: Lippincott Williams & Wilkins.

## TABLE II.12 AGE-RELATED DAILY NUTRITIONAL REQUIREMENTS

| Age | Daily Nutritional Requirements |
|---|---|
| **Infants** | 100–120 kcal/kg/day for growth |
| Newborn | 12–18 oz formula or breast milk |
| 2–3 months | 20–30 oz formula or breast milk |
| 4–5 months | 25–35 oz formula or breast milk; strained vegetables and fruits; egg yolks |
| 6–7 months | 28–40 oz formula or breast milk; above solids, plus meat, finger foods |
| 8–11 months | 24 oz formula or breast milk; three regular meals, chopped table food |
| 1–2 years | 24 oz formula or breast milk; 100 cal/kg same as 8–11 months |
| **Children** | |
| Preschool (3–5 years) | 90 cal/kg; 1.2g/kg protein |
| | Basic food groups |
| | Calcium 800 mg |
| School (6–12 years) | 80 cal/kg; 1.2 g/kg protein |
| | Basic food groups (as preschool) |
| |     1.5–2 g calcium |
| |     400 units vitamin D |
| |     1.5–3 L water |
| Adolescent (13–17 years) | 2,200–2,400 cal for girls |
| | 3,000 cal for boys |
| | Basic food groups (as preschool) |
| |     50–60 g protein |
| |     1,200–1,500 mg calcium (to age 25) |
| |     400 units vitamin D |
| **Adults** | 1,600–3,000 calorie range (based on physical activity, emotional state, body size, age, and individual metabolism) |
| | Basic food groups |
| | Refer to Figure II.2 |
| | Men need increased protein, ascorbic acid, riboflavin, and vitamins E and $B_6$ |
| | Women need the above and also increased iron, calcium, and vitamins A and $B_{12}$ |
| Pregnant women (2nd and 3rd trimesters) | Daily calorie requirement |
| |     11–15 years, 2,500 |
| |     16–22 years, 2,400 |
| |     23–50 years, 2,300 |
| | Increase protein 10 g or 1 serving meat |
| | 1.2–3.5 g calcium |
| | Increase vitamins A, B, and C |
| Lactating women | 30–60 mg iron |
| | 2,500–3,000 cal (500 over regular diet) |
| | Basic food groups |
| |     4 servings protein |
| |     5 servings dairy |
| |     4+ servings grain |
| |     5+ servings vegetables |
| |         2+ servings vitamin C-rich |
| |         1+ green leafy |
| |         2+ others |
| | Fluids 2–3 qt (1 qt milk) |
| | Increase in vitamin A, C, niacin |
| Over 65 years | Basic food groups (same as adult) |
| | Caloric requirements decrease with age (1,600–1,800 for women, 2,000–2,400 for men), but dependent on activity, climate, and metabolic needs |
| | Ensure intake of essential amino acids, fatty acids, vitamins, elements, fiber, and water |
| | 60 mg ascorbic acid |
| | 40–60 mg protein |
| | 1,200 mg calcium (1,500 mg for women not taking estrogen) |
| | 10 mg iron |

## TABLE II.13 BODY MASS INDEX

Locate the height of interest in the left-most column and read across the row for that height to the weight of interest. Follow the column of the weight up to the top row that lists the BMI. BMI of 19–24 is the healthy weight range, BMI of 25–29 is the overweight range, and BMI of 30 and above is in the obese range. 40 or above is considered extreme obesity.

| BMI | 19 | 20 | 21 | 22 | 23 | 24 | 25 | 26 | 27 | 28 | 29 | 30 | 31 | 32 | 33 | 34 | 35 |
|-----|----|----|----|----|----|----|----|----|----|----|----|----|----|----|----|----|----|
| **Height** | | | | | | | *Weight in Pounds* | | | | | | | | | | |
| 4'10" | 91 | 96 | 100 | 105 | 110 | 115 | 119 | 124 | 129 | 134 | 138 | 143 | 148 | 153 | 158 | 162 | 167 |
| 4'11" | 94 | 99 | 104 | 109 | 114 | 119 | 124 | 128 | 133 | 138 | 143 | 148 | 153 | 158 | 163 | 158 | 173 |
| 5' | 97 | 102 | 107 | 112 | 118 | 123 | 128 | 133 | 138 | 143 | 148 | 153 | 158 | 163 | 158 | 174 | 179 |
| 5'1" | 100 | 106 | 111 | 116 | 122 | 127 | 132 | 137 | 143 | 148 | 153 | 158 | 164 | 169 | 174 | 180 | 185 |
| 5'2" | 104 | 109 | 115 | 120 | 126 | 131 | 136 | 142 | 147 | 153 | 158 | 164 | 169 | 175 | 180 | 186 | 191 |
| 5'3" | 107 | 113 | 118 | 124 | 130 | 135 | 141 | 146 | 152 | 158 | 163 | 169 | 175 | 180 | 186 | 191 | 197 |
| 5'4" | 110 | 116 | 122 | 128 | 134 | 140 | 145 | 151 | 157 | 163 | 169 | 174 | 180 | 186 | 192 | 197 | 204 |
| 5'5" | 114 | 120 | 126 | 132 | 138 | 144 | 150 | 156 | 162 | 168 | 174 | 180 | 186 | 192 | 198 | 204 | 210 |
| 5'6" | 118 | 124 | 130 | 136 | 142 | 148 | 155 | 161 | 167 | 173 | 179 | 186 | 192 | 198 | 204 | 210 | 216 |
| 5'7" | 121 | 127 | 134 | 140 | 146 | 153 | 159 | 166 | 172 | 178 | 185 | 191 | 198 | 204 | 211 | 217 | 223 |
| 5'8" | 125 | 131 | 138 | 144 | 151 | 158 | 164 | 171 | 177 | 184 | 190 | 197 | 203 | 210 | 216 | 223 | 230 |
| 5'9" | 128 | 135 | 142 | 149 | 155 | 162 | 169 | 176 | 182 | 189 | 196 | 203 | 209 | 216 | 223 | 230 | 236 |
| 5'10" | 132 | 139 | 146 | 153 | 160 | 167 | 174 | 181 | 188 | 195 | 202 | 209 | 216 | 222 | 229 | 236 | 243 |
| 5'11" | 136 | 143 | 150 | 157 | 165 | 172 | 179 | 186 | 193 | 200 | 208 | 215 | 222 | 229 | 236 | 243 | 250 |
| 6' | 140 | 147 | 154 | 162 | 169 | 177 | 184 | 191 | 199 | 206 | 213 | 221 | 228 | 235 | 242 | 250 | 258 |
| 6'1" | 144 | 151 | 159 | 166 | 174 | 182 | 189 | 197 | 204 | 212 | 219 | 227 | 235 | 242 | 250 | 257 | 265 |
| 6'2" | 148 | 155 | 163 | 171 | 179 | 186 | 194 | 202 | 210 | 218 | 225 | 233 | 241 | 249 | 256 | 264 | 272 |
| 6'3" | 152 | 160 | 168 | 176 | 184 | 192 | 200 | 208 | 216 | 224 | 232 | 240 | 248 | 256 | 264 | 272 | 279 |
| | | | Healthy Weight | | | | | Overweight | | | | | | Obese | | | |

Source: Evidence Report of Clinical Guidelines on the Identification, Evaluation, and Treatment of Overweight and Obesity in Adults, 1998. NIH/National Heart, Lung, and Blood Institute (NHLBI).

Use of specialized nipple for infants with cleft lip/palate and Möbius syndrome when bottle feeding Elevate infant's head during and immediately after feeding
- The frequent eating of fast food (high in salt, sugar, and fat) and the increasing rate of obesity in children has created a problem that needs specific interventions (Hockenberry & Wilson, 2009).

## Maternal Considerations

- Nutritional needs change during pregnancy (refer to Table II.12).
- Recommendations for total weight gain during pregnancy vary. Women underweight before pregnancy should gain 28 to 40 lb; women at a desirable weight, 25 to 35 lb; women who are moderately overweight, 15 to 25 lb; women who are very overweight (BMI greater than 29), 15 lb (Pilliteri, 2003).
- Dieting during pregnancy may result in insufficient maternal intake to provide the fetus with the necessary energy for growth. The fetus depends on the mother's dietary intake for growth and development, taking only iron and folate from maternal stores.

## Geriatric Considerations

- In general, older adults need the same kind of balanced diet as any other group, but fewer calories. Diets of older clients, however, tend to be insufficient in iron, calcium, and vitamins. The combination of long-established eating patterns, income, transportation, housing, social interaction, and the effects of chronic or acute disease influence nutritional intake and health (Miller, 2009).
- The decreased energy needs of many older adults require a change in nutrient intake:

| | 25 to 50 years of age | 50 years or older |
|---|---|---|
| Carbohydrates | 60% | 55% |
| Protein | 10% | 20% |
| Fat | 30% | 25% |
| Kcal/day | | |
| Women | 2,200 | 1,900 |
| Men | 2,900 | 2,300 |

- People taking diuretics must be observed closely for adequate hydration (intake and output) and electrolyte balance, especially sodium and potassium. Potassium-rich foods should be included regularly in the diet.
- Iron-deficiency anemia usually occurs over time and may be related to chronic diseases and insufficient dietary iron. Increasing the intake of foods rich in vitamin C, folic acid, and dietary iron can improve the conditions necessary for optimal absorption of iron. Iron supplementation is often necessary.

## Transcultural Considerations

- Many cultures have used diet for centuries to treat specific diseases, promote health during pregnancy, foster growth and development in children, and prolong life (Andrews & Boyle, 2008).
- Some cultures view health as a state of balance among the body humors (blood, phlegm, black bile, and yellow bile). In this framework, a humoral imbalance that causes excessive dryness, cold, hot, or wetness leads to illness. For example, an upset stomach is believed to result from eating too many foods identified as cold. Foods, herbs, and medicines are classified as hot or cold or wet or dry. They are used to restore the body to its natural balance. For example, bananas are classified as a cold food, whereas cornmeal is a hot food (Andrews & Boyle, 2008).
- Adult lactose intolerance has been reported among most populations, affecting 94% of Asians, 90% of African blacks, 79% of American Indians, 75% of American blacks, 50% of Mexican Americans, and 17% of American whites (Overfield, 1985).
- Nutritional practices can be categorized as beneficial, neutral, or harmful. Beneficial and neutral practices should be encouraged. Harmful practices should be approached with sensitivity and their detrimental effects explained (Andrews & Boyle, 2008).
- Group dining, which is encouraged in some settings (e.g., rehabilitation, long-term, mental health), may be in conflict with certain cultures (e.g., women eating with men; Andrews & Boyle, 2009).
- Maintaining a kosher diet for a Jewish client is possible even if the agency does not have a kosher kitchen. Fish with fins or scales will meet dietary requirements. Dairy products are also possible. Paper plates with disposable utensils should be used so that meat and milk dishes are not mixed (Giger & Davidhizar, 2009).

# Focus Assessment Criteria

## Subjective Data

### Assess for Defining Characteristics

**Usual intake**
*Diet recall for 24 h*
Is this the usual intake pattern?
Is intake of the basic five food groups sufficient?
Is fluid intake sufficient?

### Assess for Related Factors

**Appetite (usual, changes)**
*Dietary patterns*
Food/fluid dislikes, preferences, and taboos
Religious dietary practices
Frequency of fast food consumption

**Activity level**
Occupation, exercise (type, frequency)

### Food procurement/preparation (who):

| Functional ability | Kitchen facilities | Transportation |
|---|---|---|
| Income adequate for food needs | | |

### Knowledge of nutrition

Five basic food groups
Recommended intake of carbohydrates, fats, and salt
Relationship of activity and metabolism

### Physiologic risk factors

Neurologic impairment
Chronic illness (renal failure, chronic obstructive pulmonary disease [COPD], human immunodeficiency
    virus [HIV], liver disease)
Malabsorption
Inflammatory bowel disease

### Psychosocial conditions

| Alcohol abuse | Drug use | Household status |
|---|---|---|
| Isolation | Depression | Institutionalization |

### Medications (prescribed, over-the-counter)

*Reports of:*

| Allergies | Dysphagia | Nausea |
|---|---|---|
| Indigestion | Vomiting | Chewing problems |
| Anorexia | Constipation | Fatigue |
| Diarrhea | Sore mouth | Pain |

## Objective Data

## Assess for Defining Characteristics

### General

| Appearance | Muscle mass | Fat distribution |
|---|---|---|
| Hair | Skin | Nails |
| Height | Weight | Body mass index |
| Mouth | Teeth | Edema |

### Anthropometric measurements

| Mid-arm circumference | Triceps skinfold | Mid-arm muscle circumference |
|---|---|---|

### Laboratory studies

| Decreased serum prealbumin | Decreased serum transferrin |
|---|---|

## Assess for Related Factors

### Ability to chew, swallow, and feed self

Parent's knowledge of nutrition for infant or child
Infant suck/swallow/breathe coordination
For more information on Focus Assessment Criteria, visit http://thepoint.lww.com.

---

**NOC**
Nutritional Status,
Teaching: Nutrition,
Symptom Control

➤ ## Goal

The client will ingest daily nutritional requirements in accordance with activity level and metabolic needs.

### Indicators:

• Relate importance of good nutrition.
• Identify deficiencies in daily intake.
• Relate methods to increase appetite.

**NIC**
Nutrition
Management,
Weight Gain
Assistance,
Nutritional
Counseling

## ➤ General Interventions

### Explain the Need for Adequate Consumption of Carbohydrates, Fats, Protein, Vitamins, Minerals, and Fluids

**R:** Nutrients provide energy sources, build tissue, and regulate metabolic processes.

### Consult with a Nutritionist to Establish Appropriate Daily Caloric and Food Type Requirements for the Client

**R:** Consultation can help ensure a diet that provides optimal caloric and nutrient intake.

### Discuss with the Client Possible Causes of Decreased Appetite

**R:** Factors such as pain, fatigue, analgesic use, and immobility can contribute to anorexia. Identifying a possible cause enables interventions to eliminate or minimize it.

### Encourage the Client to Rest Before Meals

**R:** Fatigue further reduces an anorectic client's desire and ability to eat.

### Offer Frequent, Small Meals Instead of a Few Large Ones; Offer Foods Served Cold

**R:** Even distribution of total daily caloric intake helps prevent gastric distention, possibly increasing appetite.

### With Decreased Appetite, Restrict Liquids with Meals and Avoid Fluids 1 h Before and After Meals

**R:** Restricting fluids with meals helps prevent gastric distention.

### Encourage and Help the Client to Maintain Good Oral Hygiene

**R:** Poor oral hygiene leads to bad odor and taste, which can diminish appetite.

### Arrange to Have High-Calorie and High-Protein Foods Served at the Times that the Client Usually Feels Most Like Eating

**R:** Presenting high-calorie and high-protein food when the client is most likely to eat increases the likelihood that he or she will consume adequate calories and protein.

### Take Steps to Promote Appetite

Determine the client's food preferences and arrange to have them provided, as appropriate.
Eliminate any offensive odors and sights from the eating area.
Control any pain and nausea before meals.
Encourage the client's support people to bring permitted foods from home, if possible.
Provide a relaxed atmosphere and some socialization during meals.

**R:** Diet planning focuses on avoiding nutritional excesses. Reducing fats, salt, and sugar can reduce the risk of heart disease, diabetes, certain cancers, and hypertension.

### Give the Client Printed Materials Outlining a Nutritious Diet that Includes the Following:

High intake of complex carbohydrates and fiber
Decreased intake of sugar, salt, cholesterol, total fat, and saturated fats
Alcohol use only in moderation
Proper caloric intake to maintain ideal weight

**R:** Self-help materials can be used at home for reinforcement.

**Pediatric Interventions**

Teach parents the following regarding infant nutrition:

- Adequate infant feeding schedule and weight gain requirements for growth: 100 to 120 kcal/kg/day for growth
- Proper preparation of infant formula
- Proper storage of breast milk and infant formula
- Proper elevation of infant's head during and immediately after feedings
- Proper chin/cheek support techniques for orally compromised infants
- The age-related nutritional needs of their children (consult an appropriate textbook on pediatrics or nutrition for specific recommendations).

Discuss the importance of limiting snacks high in salt, sugar, or fat (e.g., soda, candy, chips) to limit risks for cardiac disorders, obesity, and diabetes mellitus. Advise families to substitute healthy snacks (e.g., fresh fruits, plain popcorn, frozen fruit juice bars, fresh vegetables).

Assist families in evaluating their nutritional patterns.

Discuss strategies to make meals a social event and to avoid struggles (Dudek, 2006; Hockenberry & Wilson, 2009).

Allow the child to select one type of food he or she does not have to eat.

Provide small servings (e.g., one tablespoon of each food for every year of age).

Make snacks as nutritiously important as meals (e.g., hard-boiled eggs, raw vegetable sticks, peanut butter/crackers, fruit juices, cheese, and fresh fruit).

Offer a variety of foods.

Encourage all members to share their day.

Involve the child in monitoring healthy eating (e.g., create a chart where the child checks off intake of healthy foods daily).

Replace passive television watching with a group activity (e.g., Frisbee tossing, biking, walking).

Address strategies to improve nutrition when eating fast foods:

- Drink skim milk.
- Avoid French fries.
- Choose grilled foods.
- Eat salads and vegetables.
- Substitute quick, nutritious fast meals (e.g., frozen dinners).

**R:** Nutritional requirements vary greatly for each age group. Periods of accelerated physical growth (e.g., infancy, puberty) may necessitate doubling iron, calcium, zinc, and protein intake (Hockenberry & Wilson, 2009).

**R:** During periods of slow growth (e.g., preschool, elementary school), appetite is diminished (Dudek, 2006).

**R:** Increasing healthy snacks reduces the pressure for the child to eat a certain amount at mealtime.

**R:** Family nutritional patterns are the primary influence on the development of food habits (e.g., unhealthy snacks, excessive television watching; Dudek, 2006).

**Maternal Interventions**

Teach the importance of adequate calorie and fluid intake while breastfeeding in relation to breast milk production

Explain physiologic changes and nutritional needs during pregnancy (see Table II.12).

Discuss the effects of alcohol, caffeine, and artificial sweeteners on the developing fetus.

Explain the different nutritional requirements for pregnant girls 11 to 18 years of age, pregnant young women 19 to 24 years of age, and women older than 25 years.

Determine if a woman needs more calories because of daily activity.

**R:** Explanations about metabolic changes can increase awareness of nutritional requirements.

**R:** Studies have shown that alcohol consumption (two to four drinks/day) can cause low–birth-weight babies. Larger amounts cause fetal alcohol syndrome.

*(continued)*

**Maternal Interventions**
*Continued*

**R:** Studies have shown caffeine to have few effects on pregnancy outcome, but moderation is recommended (Dudek, 2006).

**R:** Consumption of artificial sweeteners during pregnancy has not been found to be contraindicated, but moderation is suggested (Dudek, 2006).

**R:** Adolescent girls need increased nutritional intake because of their own accelerated growth, and pregnancy increases the requirements even more (Dudek, 2006).

**R:** Resting caloric needs for pregnant women differ according to age (Pilliteri, 2003):

- 28.5 kcal/kg for 11 to 14 years
- 24.9 kcal/kg for 15 to 18 years
- 23.3 kcal/kg for 19 to 24 years
- 21.9 kcal/kg for 25 to 50 years

**R:** More calories are needed depending on activity level (Pilliteri, 2003). Multiply resting caloric needs by:
- 1.5 for light activity
- 1.6 for moderate activity
- 1.9 for heavy activity

**Pediatric Interventions**

## Determine the Client's Understanding of Nutritional Needs with:

Aging    Medication use    Illness    Activity

## Assess If Any Factors Interfere with Procuring or Ingesting Foods (Miller, 2009)

Anorexia from medications, grief, depression, or illness

Impaired mental status leading to inattention to hunger or selecting insufficient kinds/amounts of food

Impaired mobility or manual dexterity (paresis, tremors, weakness, joint pain, or deformity)

Voluntary fluid restriction for fear of urinary incontinence

Small frame or history of undernutrition

Inadequate income to purchase food

Lack of transportation to buy food or facility to cook

New dentures or poor dentition

Dislike of cooking and eating alone

Client regularly eats alone

Client has more than 2 alcoholic drinks daily

## Explain Decline in Sensitivity to Sweet and Salty Tastes

## If Indicated, Consult with Home Health Nurse to Evaluate Home Environment (e.g., Cooking Facilities, Food Supply, Cleanliness)

## Access Community Agencies as Indicated (e.g., Nutritional Programs, Community Centers, Home-Delivered Grocery Services)

**R:** With age, nutritional requirements do not diminish, but overall caloric needs do. High-quality, nutritious foods are very important (Miller, 2009).

**R:** Multiple factors can interfere with access or ingestion of food. Strategies to improve nutrition should address specific factors (Dudek, 2006).

**R:** Older adults can consume excessive salt and sugar to compensate for loss of sensitivity to these tastes (Miller, 2009).

**R:** A home assessment may provide valid data in cases of suspected nutritional problems (Miller, 2009).

**R:** Certain medications or illnesses may require an adjustment in diet (e.g., potassium, sodium, fiber).

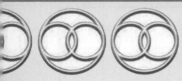

# IMBALANCED NUTRITION: LESS THAN BODY REQUIREMENTS

## ▶ Related to Anorexia Secondary to (Specify)

**NOC**
Nutritional Status

### ➤ Goal

The client will increase oral intake as evidenced by (specify).

### *Indicators:*

- Describe causative factors when known.
- Describe rationale and procedure for treatments.

**NIC**
Nutrition Management, Nutrition Monitoring: Weight Gain Assistance, Nutritional Counseling

### ➤ Interventions

### Assess Causative Factors

### Refer to Related Factors

### Reduce or Eliminate Contributing Factors, If Possible

### *Diminished Sense of Taste or Smell*

Explain to the client the importance of consuming adequate nutrients.

Teach the client to use spices (e.g., lemon juice, mint, cloves, basil, thyme, cinnamon, rosemary, bacon bits) to help improve the taste and aroma of food.

Teach protein sources that the client may find more acceptable than red meat:

- Eggs and dairy products
- Poultry
- Fish
- Marinated meat (in wine, vinegar)
- Soy products (tofu)

Chopped- or ground-meat protein sources may be more acceptable.

Mixing protein and vegetables may be more acceptable.

Refer to meals as "snacks" to make them sound smaller.

**R:** Strategies to stimulate appetite and increase the nutrition in food consumed are used.

### *Social Isolation*

Encourage the client to eat with others (meals served in the dining room or group area at the local meeting place such as the community center or by church groups).

Provide daily contact through phone calls by the support system.

See *Risk for Loneliness* for additional interventions.

**R:** For most people, meals are social events. Loneliness at meals can reduce the incentive to prepare nutritious meals.

### *Noxious Stimuli (Pain, Fatigue, Odors, Nausea, and Vomiting)*

#### Pain

Plan care so unpleasant or painful procedures do not take place before meals.

Schedule pain relief medications so optimal relief without drowsiness is achieved at mealtime.

Provide a pleasant, relaxed atmosphere for eating (no bedpans in sight; no rushing); try a "surprise" (e.g., flowers with meal).

**R:** Arrange to decrease or eliminate pain and painful procedures near mealtimes.

### Fatigue

Teach or assist the client in resting before meals.

Teach the client to expend minimal energy in food preparation (cook large quantities and freeze several meals at a time; request assistance from others).

**R:** Fatigue will decrease appetite and interfere with the effort needed to eat.

### Odor of food

Teach the client to avoid cooking odors—frying foods, brewing coffee—if possible (take a walk; select foods that can be eaten cold).

Suggest using foods that require little cooking during periods of anorexia.

**R:** The smell of cooking foods can increase nausea and anorexia.

### Nausea and vomiting

Refer to *Nausea Nursing Diagnosis*

## See Impaired Swallowing for Additional Interventions

### Promote Foods That Stimulate Eating and Increase Protein Consumption (Foltz, 1997)

Maintain good oral hygiene (brush teeth, rinse mouth) before and after eating.

**R:** Maintaining good oral hygiene before and after meals decreases microorganisms that can cause foul taste and odor, inhibiting appetite.

Offer frequent small feedings (six per day plus snacks). Restrict fluids with meals.

**R:** Small feedings and fluid restrictions with meals can help to prevent gastric distention which can decrease appetite.

Practice relaxation techniques prior to meals.

To stimulate appetite:

- Try a different food choice.
- Avoid sight and smell of food prior to eating.
- Eat sour foods.
- Eat cold foods.
- Use a straw.
- Increase seasoning.
- Use plastic utensils.
- Try a small amount of alcohol.

**R:** Attempts to vary the taste and texture can improve appetite.

To increase intake, teach the client to:

- Arrange to serve the highest protein/calorie nutrients when the client feels most like eating (e.g., if chemotherapy is in the early morning, serve food in the late afternoon).
- Eat dry foods (toast, crackers) on arising.
- Try salty foods, if permissible.
- Avoid overly sweet, rich, greasy, or fried foods.
- Try clear, cool beverages. Sip slowly through a straw.
- Try whatever the client feels can be tolerated.
- Eat small portions low in fat. Eat more frequently.
- Review high-calorie versus low-calorie foods. Avoid empty-calorie foods (e.g., soda).
- Encourage significant others to bring in favorite home foods.
- Try commercial supplements available in many forms (liquids, powder, pudding); keep switching brands until some are found that are acceptable to the client in taste and consistency.

**R:** Varied techniques should be attempted to increase intake of nutritious foods and beverages.

Teach techniques for home food preparation to client and family:

- Add powdered milk or egg to milkshakes, gravies, sauces, puddings, cereals, meatballs, or milk to increase protein and calorie content.
- Add blended foods or baby foods to meat juices or soups.
- Use fortified milk (i.e., 1 cup of instant nonfat milk to 1 qt of fresh milk).
- Use milk or half-and-half cream instead of water when making soups and sauces; soy formulas also can be used.
- Add cheese or diced meat.
- Add cream cheese or peanut butter to toast, crackers, or celery sticks.
- Add extra butter or margarine to soups, sauces, or vegetables.
- Spread butter on toast while hot.
- Use mayonnaise (100 cal/T) instead of salad dressing.
- Add sour cream or yogurt to vegetables or as dip.
- Use whipped cream (60 cal/T).
- Add raisins, dates, nuts, and brown sugar to hot or cold cereals.
- Have extra food (snacks) easily available.

**R:** Certain measures can increase the nutritional content of foods even when intake is limited.

## Initiate Health Teaching and Referrals, as Indicated

Dietitian for meal planning | Psychiatric therapy when indicated
Community meal centers | Support groups for clients with anorexia

**R:** Resources in the community can assist the client and family.

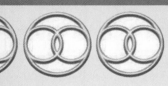

# IMBALANCED NUTRITION: LESS THAN BODY REQUIREMENTS

## ▶ Related to Difficulty or Inability to Procure Food

Altered ability to procure food is the inability to acquire food because of physical, economic, or sociocultural barriers.

**NOC**
Nutritional Status

➤ **Goal**

The client will identify a method to acquire food on a regular schedule.

### Indicators:

- Describe causative factors when known.
- Relate importance of good nutrition.

**NIC**
Nutritional
Counseling,
Nutrition
Management,
Teaching: Individual,
Family, Referral,
Environmental
Management

➤ **Interventions**

## Assess Causative Factors

Inadequate economic resources to obtain adequate nutrition
Sociocultural barriers
Physical inability to procure food related to health problem such as COPD, CVA, or quadriplegia

## Reduce or Eliminate Contributing Factors, If Possible

### *Inadequate Economic Resources*

Assess the client's eligibility for food stamps or other government-funded programs for low-income groups; consult with social services.

Suggest cooperatives or local farmers' markets for shopping.

Buy foods and meats on sale and freeze; use cheaper cuts and tenderize.

Suggest foods that are low in cost and high in nutrients; decrease use of prepackaged or prepared items:

- Beans and legumes as protein sources
- Powdered milk (alone or mixed half and half with whole milk)
- Seasonal foods when plentiful

Encourage growing a small garden or participating in a community plot.

Freeze or can fruits and vegetables in season (refer to county agricultural agent for information on canning and freezing).

### *Sociocultural Barriers*

Introduce the client to locally available foodstuffs; instruct in their preparation.

Suggest substitutions of locally available foodstuffs for those to which the client is accustomed.

Refer the client to adult education home economics classes for food preparation.

Assist the client to recognize and use additional outlets and sources of food (grocery stores, meat and fruit markets).

Encourage peer group meetings among people of similar backgrounds to allow learning and exchange of ideas.

Acquaint the client with ethnic food store locations, if available.

### *Physical Deficits*

Promote alternative methods of food procurement and preparation:

- Support systems of people willing to purchase or prepare food for client or take him or her to the store
- Supermarkets that deliver
- Meals on Wheels or similar service
- Homemaker
- Group housing
- Door-to-store bus service

Teach the client or others to cook enough for six meals at once and freeze; make own complete "frozen dinners."

Aid the client to plan daily activities that allow enough energy for shopping and cooking; such as suggesting rest periods before, during (if needed), and after activity.

**R:** People who are impaired either physically or cognitively should receive the necessary support and supervision in selecting foods and self-feeding. Activities needed to procure food depend on skills of cognition, balance, mobility, manual dexterity, and all five senses (Miller, 2009).

## Teach Techniques for Meal Planning and Preparation for One

Buy small cans of food (they may seem more expensive, but spoiled food is costly).

When buying fruit, select three stages of ripeness (ripe, medium ripe, green).

Family-sized packages of meat or fresh vegetables can be broken down and frozen.

When buying in large quantity, make soups and stews with the extra.

Use powdered instead of fresh milk in recipes.

Buy fresh milk in pints or quarts.

Store large-quantity items (rice, flour, corn meal, dry milk, cereal) in glass jars. Place tightly sealed jars in the freezer for one night to kill any organisms and their eggs.

Experiment with stir-frying vegetables (e.g., Chinese cabbage, celery) in a little chicken broth.

If freezer space is available, prepare four to six times as much as you need and freeze in individual portions, dating the packages.

Store half a loaf of bread well wrapped in the freezer. (It will become stale in the refrigerator.)

Buy large bags of frozen vegetables, use small amounts, and reclose bags with twist ties.

Finely chop and freeze fresh herbs (parsley, dill, basil) in small freezer bags. Flatten so small portions can be broken off after freezing.

Buy large quantities of meat and freeze in foil wrap (not freezer paper).

**R:** People with difficulty preparing meals can be assisted in reducing daily preparation time through specific planning (Mahan & Arlin, 1996).

## Initiate Health Teaching and Referrals, as Indicated

Refer the client to social worker, occupational therapist, or visiting nurse, as needed.

Refer the client to local extension office for information on vegetable gardening, community gardens, and techniques of freezing and canning foods.

Refer the client to a dietitian for meal planning.

**R:** Nurses must be familiar with available local resources so they can initiate referrals (Miller, 2009).

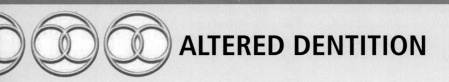

# ALTERED DENTITION

## DEFINITION (NANDA)

A disruption in tooth development/eruption patterns or structural integrity of individual teeth

## DEFINING CHARACTERISTICS (NANDA)

Excessive plaque

Halitosis

Toothache

Excessive calculus

Malocclusion or tooth misalignment

Premature loss of primary teeth

Missing teeth or complete absence

Asymmetric facial expression

Crown or root caries

Tooth enamel discoloration

Loose teeth

Incomplete eruption for age (may be primary or permanent teeth)

Tooth fracture(s)

Erosion of enamel

## ■■■■■■■ AUTHOR'S NOTE

*Altered Dentition* describes a multitude of problems with teeth. It is unclear how nurses or any health care professional would use this diagnosis. If the client had caries, abscesses, misaligned teeth, or malformed teeth, the nurse would refer the client to a dental professional. If the tooth problem is affecting comfort or nutrition, *Impaired Comfort* or *Imbalanced Nutrition* would be the appropriate nursing diagnosis, not *Altered Dentition*.

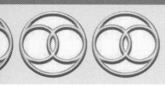

# IMPAIRED SWALLOWING

## DEFINITION

State in which a person has abnormal functioning of the swallowing mechanism associated with deficits in oral, pharyngeal, or esophageal structure or function

## DEFINING CHARACTERISTICS

### Major (Must Be Present, One or More)

Observed evidence of difficulty in swallowing
*and/or*
Stasis of food in oral cavity

Coughing before a swallow

Coughing after food or fluid intake

Choking

Gagging

### Minor (May Be Present)

Nasal-sounding voice

Drooling

Slurred speech

Vomiting

Regurgitation

Lack of chewing

## Related Factors

### Pathophysiologic

*Related to decreased/absent gag reflex, mastication difficulties, or decreased sensations secondary to:*

Cerebral palsy

Muscular dystrophy

Poliomyelitis

Parkinson's disease

Guillain-Barré syndrome

Myasthenia gravis

Amyotrophic lateral sclerosis

CVA

Neoplastic disease affecting brain

Right or left hemispheric brain damage

Cranial nerve damage (V, VII, IX, X, XI)

*Related to tracheoesophageal tumors, edema*
*Related to irritated oropharyngeal cavity*
*Related to decreased saliva*

### Treatment-Related

*Related to surgical reconstruction of the mouth, throat, jaw, or nose*
*Related to decreased consciousness secondary to anesthesia*
*Related to mechanical obstruction secondary to tracheostomy tube*
*Related to esophagitis secondary to radiotherapy*

### Situational (Personal, Environmental)

*Related to fatigue*
*Related to limited awareness, distractibility*

### Maturational

**Infants/Children**
*Related to decreased sensations or difficulty with mastication*
*Related to poor suck/swallow/breathe coordination*

**Older Adult**
*Related to reduction in saliva, taste*

■■■■■ **AUTHOR'S NOTE**

See *Imbalanced Nutrition: Less Than Body Requirements.*

■■■■■ **ERRORS IN DIAGNOSTIC STATEMENTS**

See *Imbalanced Nutrition: Less Than Body Requirements.*

■■■■■ **KEY CONCEPTS**

### Generic Considerations

- Swallowing has an intellectual as well as a physical component.
- The swallowing process occurs in three stages with select cranial nerve involvement (Porth, 2007).
  - *Stage 1*—Oral: Food is placed in oral cavity, the lips close, and swallowing is initiated as a reflex. The tongue maneuvers the food, and the soft palate and uvula close off the nasopharynx.
  - *Stage 2*—Pharyngeal: The food passes the anterior fossa arches and triggers the swallow reflex. The tongue prevents the food from returning to the oral cavity by elevation and contraction of the soft palate. Pharyngeal peristalsis begins, causing the food to move downward.
  - *Stage 3*—Esophageal: Pharyngeal peristalsis pushes the food downward. The larynx elevates and the crico-pharyngeal muscles relax, allowing the food to move from the pharynx into the esophagus. The larynx wave pushes the food down the esophagus to the stomach.
- Cranial nerves V, VII, IX, X, and XI are involved in swallowing.
- Impairment of cranial nerve function can cause the following swallowing problems:
  - Trigeminal (V)—loss of sensation and ability to move mandible
  - Facial (VII)—Increased salivation; inability to pucker lips, pouching of foods
  - Glossopharyngeal (IX)—diminished taste sensation, salivation, and gag reflex
  - Vagus (X)—decreased peristalsis, decreased gag reflex
  - Hypoglossal (XI)—poor tongue control, poor movement of food to the throat
- A cough reflex is essential for rehabilitation, but a gag reflex is not.
- Do not confuse the ability to chew with the ability to swallow. See also *Imbalanced Nutrition: Less Than Body Requirements.*

## Focus Assessment Criteria

### Subjective Data

#### Assess for Defining Characteristics

History of problem with swallowing

- Onset
- History of nasal regurgitation, hoarseness, choking, or coughing

Problem foods or liquids
Non-problem foods or liquids

#### Assess for Related Factors

| | | |
|---|---|---|
| CVA | Parkinson's disease | Multiple sclerosis |
| Brain lesions | Head trauma | Tracheoesophageal tumors |
| Oral surgery | | |

## Objective Data

### Assess for Defining Characteristics

Decreased or absent swallowing, cough, or gag reflex
Poor coordination of tongue
Observed choking or coughing with food or fluid

### Assess for Related Factors.

| | | |
|---|---|---|
| Facial muscle weakness | Impaired use of tongue | Chewing difficulties |
| Decreased saliva production | Thick secretions | Impaired cognition |

For more information on Focus Assessment Criteria, visit http://thepoint.lww.com.

**NOC**
Aspiration Control,
Swallowing Status

## ➤ Goal

The person will report improved ability to swallow.

### Indicators

The person and/or family will

- Describe causative factors when known.
- Describe rationale and procedures for treatment.

**NIC**
Aspiration
Precautions,
Swallowing Therapy,
Surveillance,
Referral, Positioning

## ➤ General Interventions

### Assess for Causative or Contributing Factors

#### Refer to Related Factors

Consult with a speech therapist for an evaluation and recommended plan of care.

**R:** A speech pathologist has the expertise needed to perform the dysphagia evaluation.

Alert all staff that client has impaired swallowing.

**R:** Alerting all staff can reduce the risk of aspiration.

## Reduce or Eliminate Causative/Contributing Factors in People with:

### Mechanical Impairment of Mouth

Assist client with moving the bolus of food from the anterior to the posterior part of mouth. Place food in the posterior mouth where swallowing can be ensured, using:
A syringe with a short piece of tubing attached
A glossectomy spoon
Soft, moist food of a consistency that can be manipulated by the tongue against the pharynx, such as gelatin, custard, or mashed potatoes
Prevent/decrease thick secretions with:

- Artificial saliva
- Papain tablets dissolved in mouth 10 min before eating
- Meat tenderizer made from papaya enzyme applied to oral cavity 10 min before eating
- Frequent mouth care
- Increase fluid intake to 8 glasses of liquid (unless contraindicated)

Check medications for potential side effects of dry mouth/decreased salivation
Use of Haberman or comparable nipple when bottle feeding for infant with cleft lip/palate and Möbius syndrome

**R:** Decreased secretions and dry mouth can deter swallowing.

## *Muscle Paralysis or Paresis*

Establish a visual method to communicate at bedside to staff that client is dysphagic.

Plan meals when client is well rested; ensure that reliable suction equipment is on hand during meals. Discontinue feeding if client is tired.

If indicated, use modified supraglottic swallow technique (Emick-Herring & Wood, 1990).

1. Position the head of the bed in semi- or high Fowler's position, with the neck flexed forward slightly and chin tilted down.
2. Use cutout cup (remove and round out one third of side of foam cup).
3. Take bolus of food and hold in strongest side of mouth for 1 to 2 s. Then immediately flex the neck with chin tucked against chest.
4. Without breathing, swallow as many times as needed.
5. When mouth is emptied, raise chin and clear throat.

Offer highly viscous foods (e.g., mashed bananas, potatoes, gelatin, gravy) first.

Offer thick liquids (e.g., milkshakes, slushes, nectars, cream soups).

Establish a goal for fluid intake.

If drooling is present, use a quick-stretch stimulation just before and toward the end of each meal (Emick-Herring & Wood, 1990):

• Digitally apply short, rapid, downward strokes to edge of bottom lip, mostly on affected side.
• Use a cold washcloth over finger for added stimulation.

If a bolus of food is pocketed in the affected side, teach client how to use tongue to transfer food or apply external digital pressure to cheek to help remove the trapped bolus (Emick-Herring & Wood, 1990).

**R:** Poor tongue control with impaired oral sensation allows food into affected side.

## *Impaired Cognition or Awareness*

### General

Remove feeding tube during training if increased gag reflex is present.

Concentrate on solids rather than liquids, because liquids usually are less well tolerated.

Minimize extraneous stimuli while eating (e.g., no television or radio, no verbal stimuli unless directed at task).

Have person concentrate on task of swallowing.

Have person sit up in chair with neck slightly flexed.

Instruct person to hold breath while swallowing.

Observe for swallowing and check mouth for emptying.

Avoid overloading mouth, because this decreases swallowing effectiveness.

Give solids and liquids separately.

Progress slowly. Limit conversation.

Provide several small meals to accommodate a short attention span.

### Person with aphasia, or left hemispheric damage

Demonstrate expected behavior.

Reinforce behaviors with simple, one-word commands.

### Person with apraxia, or right hemispheric damage

Divide task into smallest units possible.

Assist through each task with verbal commands.

Allow to complete one unit fully before giving next command.

Continue verbal assistance at each eating session until no longer needed.

Incorporate written checklist as a reminder to person.

Note: Person may have both left and right hemispheric damage and require a combination of the above techniques.

**R:** A confused client needs repetitive, simple instructions.

## Reduce the Possibility of Aspiration

Before beginning feeding, assess that the client is adequately alert and responsive, can control the mouth, has cough/gag reflex, and can swallow own saliva.

**R:** Impaired reflexes and fatigue increase the risk of aspiration.

Have suction equipment available and functioning properly.
Position client correctly:

- Sit client upright (60 to 90 degrees) in chair or dangle his or her feet at side of bed if possible (prop pillows if necessary).
- Client should assume this position 10 to 15 min before eating and maintain it for 10 to 15 min after finishing eating.
- Flex client's head forward on the midline about 45 degrees to keep esophagus patent.
- Keep infant's head elevated during and immediately after feedings

**R:** Upright position uses the force of gravity to aid downward motion of food and decreases the risk of aspiration.

Keep client focused on task by giving directions until he or she has finished swallowing each mouthful:

- "Take a breath."
- "Move food to middle of tongue."
- "Raise tongue to roof of mouth."
- "Think about swallowing."
- "Swallow."
- "Cough to clear airway."
- Reinforce voluntary action.

**R:** A confused client needs repetitive, simple instructions.

Avoid straws and thin fluids

**R:** Straws and thin fluids hasten transit time and increase the risk of aspiration.

Start with small amounts and progress slowly as person learns to handle each step:

- Ice chips
- Eyedropper partly filled with water
- Whole eyedropper filled with water
- Juice in place of water
- ¼ teaspoon semisolid food
- ½ teaspoon semisolid food
- 1 teaspoon semisolid food
- Pureed or commercial baby foods
- One half cracker
- Soft diet
- Regular diet; chew food well

**R:** Small amounts of fluid with progressive increases can reduce aspiration. Thicker fluids have a slower transit time and allow more time to trigger the swallow reflex.

For client who has had a CVA, place food at back of tongue and on side of face he or she can control:

- Feed slowly, making certain client has swallowed the previous bite.
- Some clients do better with foods that hold together (e.g., soft-boiled eggs, ground meat and gravy).

If the above strategies are unsuccessful, consultation with a physician may be necessary for alternative feeding techniques such as tube feedings or parenteral nutrition.

**R:** Avoid foods that do not form a bolus (e.g., sticky foods, pureed foods, applesauce, dry foods) or do not stimulate the swallowing reflex (e.g., thin liquids).

## Initiate Health Teaching and Referrals, as Indicated

### *Teach Exercises to Strengthen (Grober, 1984):*

**Lips and facial muscles**
Alternate a tight frown with a broad smile with lips closed.
Puff out cheeks with air and hold.
Blow out of pursed lips.
Practice pronouncing *u, m, b, p, w.*
Suck hard on a popsicle.

**Tongue**
Lick a popsicle or lollipop.
Push tip of tongue against roof of mouth and floor.
Count teeth with tongue.
Pronounce *la, la, la; ta, ta, ta; d; n; z; s.*
Explain to client and significant others rationale for treatment and how to proceed with it.

**R:** Exercise can strengthen muscles to improve chewing and tongue movement of bolus to back of mouth to stimulate swallowing reflex (Porth, 2006).

See *Impaired Oral Mucous Membranes.*
See *Imbalanced Nutrition: Less Than Body Requirements.*

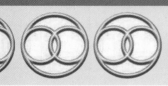

# INEFFECTIVE INFANT FEEDING PATTERN

## DEFINITION

State in which an infant (birth to 9 months) demonstrates an impaired ability to suck or coordinate the suck/swallow response, resulting in inadequate oral nutrition for metabolic needs

## DEFINING CHARACTERISTICS

### Major (Must Be Present, One or More)

Inability to initiate or sustain an effective suck; inability to coordinate sucking, swallowing, and breathing
Actual metabolic needs in excess of oral intake with weight loss or need for enteral feeding supplement

### Minor (May Be Present)

Inconsistent oral intake (volume, time interval, duration)
Oral motor developmental delay
Tachypnea with increased respiratory effort
Regurgitation or vomiting after feeding

## RELATED FACTORS

### Pathophysiologic

*Related to increased caloric need secondary to:*

| | |
|---|---|
| Body temperature instability | Growth needs |
| Tachypnea with increased respiratory effort | Wound healing |
| | Major organ system disease or failure |
| Infection | Cleft lip/palate |
| Möbius syndrome | |

*Related to muscle weakness/hypotonia secondary to:*

| | | |
|---|---|---|
| Malnutrition | Congenital defects | |
| Prematurity | Major organ system disease or failure | Hyperbilirubinemia |
| Acute/chronic illness | Neurologic impairment/delay | |
| Lethargy | | |

## Treatment-Related

*Related to hypermetabolic state and increased caloric needs secondary to:*

| | |
|---|---|
| Surgery | Painful procedures |
| Cold stress | Sepsis |

*Related to muscle weakness and lethargy secondary to:*

Medications

Muscle relaxants (antiseizure medications, paralyzing agents in past, sedatives, narcotics)

Sleep deprivation

*Related to oral hypersensitivity*

*Related to previous prolonged NPO state*

## Situational (Personal, Environmental)

*Related to inconsistent caretakers (feeders)*

*Related to lack of knowledge or commitment of caretaker (feeder) to special feeding needs or regimen*

*Related to presence of noxious facial stimuli or absence of oral stimuli*

*Related to inadequate production of breast milk*

### ◼◼◼◼◼ AUTHOR'S NOTE

*Ineffective Infant Feeding Pattern* describes an infant with sucking or swallowing difficulties. This infant experiences inadequate oral nutrition for growth and development, which is exacerbated when caloric need increases, as with infection, illness, or stress. Nursing interventions assist infants and their caregivers with techniques to achieve nutritional intake needed for weight gain. In addition, the goal is for the intake eventually to be exclusively oral.

Infants with sucking or swallowing problems who have not lost weight need nursing interventions to prevent weight loss. *Ineffective Infant Feeding Pattern* is clinically useful for this situation.

### ◼◼◼◼◼ ERRORS IN DIAGNOSTIC STATEMENTS

1. *Risk for Ineffective Infant Feeding Pattern related to inconsistent oral intake with or without weight loss.* Inconsistent oral intake is a defining characteristic for *Ineffective Infant Feeding Pattern*, not *Risk for Ineffective Infant Feeding Pattern*. *Ineffective Infant Feeding Pattern* may not be useful as a risk nursing diagnosis because this actual diagnosis exists whenever an infant has sucking or suck/swallow response difficulties, whether mild or severe. The diagnosis would be appropriate as *Ineffective Infant Feeding Pattern related to (specify contributing factors, e.g., lethargy) as evidenced by inconsistent oral intake.*

### ◼◼◼◼◼ KEY CONCEPTS

- There are two goals for the infant with an ineffective feeding pattern:
  - The infant will receive adequate and appropriate calories (carbohydrate, protein, fat) for age with weight gain at a rate consistent with an individualized plan based on age and needs. Infant caloric intake of 100-120 kcal/kg/day for growth.
  - The infant will take all feedings orally.
- For an infant with an ineffective feeding pattern (with or without a demonstrable oral motor impairment), conversion from a catabolic state to an anabolic state with consistent weight gain from appropriate calories is a prerequisite for goal attainment.
- Identification of contributing physiologic factors assists in evaluating and adapting the feeding plan. For example, fever increases caloric needs; mechanical ventilation can decrease caloric needs; infants with impaired renal function or fluid retention can experience weight gain without meeting nutritional metabolic needs; dysfunction in major organ systems or infection affects feeding patterns adversely and increases caloric needs.

*(continued)*

■■■■■■ **KEY CONCEPTS** *Continued*

- Some infants with oral motor impairment or weakness feed adequately by mouth when their metabolic need for calories is normal. But in cases of increased caloric need (e.g., congestive heart failure, infection, major organ system dysfunction, wound healing, malnutrition), they cannot take in adequate calories by increasing their volume intake sufficiently because of their ineffective feeding skills. Intervention with these infants is based on providing adequate calories, promoting oral feeding skills, and decreasing (if possible) caloric needs.
- Knowledge of normal infant feeding patterns is necessary to promote effective feeding patterns. For example, a quiet, awake state is ideal for feeding; non-nutritive sucking preceding nutritive sucking can enhance feeding behaviors; and there is a relation between sucking–swallowing–gastric emptying–bowel emptying during feeding. Over time, each infant develops an effective unique feeding pattern.
- For newborns, a lactation specialist should explore with mothers options to promote breast-feeding (either by using previously pumped breast milk or feeding directly from the breast). Many infants who initially have oral motor delays or lack of coordination of suck and swallow can successfully breast-feed with appropriate early intervention.
- High-calorie formulas (up to 32 cal/oz) or calorie-enhanced breast milk can be administered safely to most infants, provided the preparation is consistent with the child's age and needs. For example, concentrating formula to increase calories can increase the protein load disproportionately; therefore, additives (carbohydrate or fat) are often used to increase calories safely. The appropriate use of high-calorie formulas can reduce the target volume/day goal for an infant, making it easier to attain the goal of total oral feedings. Serum protein, albumin, and renal function need to be assessed periodically when high-calorie formulas are used.
- Adapting equipment and feedings for alterations in oral intake. Use of Haberman nipple or comparable for infants with cleft lip/palate or Möbius syndrome. Rice cereal for thinking of feeding for infants with Gastroesophageal reflux. Use of cheek/chin support for orally compromised infants.
- Enteral feedings may be required initially to ensure adequate caloric intake, weight gain, and anabolic state. Identifying a total plan for feeding from the beginning that includes both enteral and oral feeding (and oral stimulation if feeding is not possible) is instrumental in promoting the goal of total oral feeding. Infants who are exclusively enterally fed in the first months of life, with no effort to develop oral feeding skills, can become behaviorally disinterested in oral feeding and may remain enterally fed indefinitely.

## Generic Considerations

# Focus Assessment Criteria

## Subjective and Objective Data

### *Assess for Defining Characteristics*

**General**
Current weight and height
Weight gain daily/weekly goal
Calorie/kg daily goal

**Feeding history**
Previous oral feeding pattern (volume, time interval, duration)
Previous enteral feeding pattern (continuous or bolus, volume, time interval, duration)
Gastrointestinal tolerance of feedings (oral, enteral, emesis, stool pattern)

### *Assess for Related Factors*

Presence/absence of noxious stimuli to face and mouth (including NG/NJ feedings, endotracheal intubation, oral or nasopharyngeal suction, nasal cannula oxygen)

**Physiologic factors**
Hyperthermia or hypothermia
Oral motor developmental delay
Infection
Gastroesophageal reflux
Congestive heart failure

Colic

Prematurity

Prolonged NPO state with or without enteral feedings

Neurologic dysfunction

Elevated body temperature

Increased respiratory rate and effort

Strength and coordination of non-nutritive sucking

Strength and coordination of nutritive sucking

Impaired sleep patterns

Irritability

Lethargy

For more information on Focus Assessment Criteria, visit http://thepoint.lww.com.

**NOC**

Muscle Function, Nutritional Status, Swallowing Status

## ➤ Goal

The infant will receive adequate nutrition for growth appropriate to age and need.

### Indicators

- Parent demonstrates increasing skill.
- Parent identifies techniques that increase effective feeding.

**NIC**

Nonnutritive Swallowing, Swallowing Therapy, Aspiration, Precautions, Bottle Feeding, Parent Education: Infant

## ➤ General Interventions

### Assess the Infant's Feeding Pattern and Nutritional Needs

Assess volume, duration, and effort during feeding; respiratory rate and effort; signs of fatigue.

Assess past caloric intake, weight gain, trends in intake and output, renal function, fluid retention.

Identify physiologic risk factors.

Identify physiologic ability to feed:

- Can infant stop breathing when sucking and swallowing?
- Does infant gasp or choke during feedings?
- What happens to oxygen level, heart rate, and respiratory rate when sucking/swallowing?
- Does the infant need rest periods? How long? Are there problems in initiating sucking/swallowing again?

Assess nipple-feeding skills:

- Does the infant actively suck with a bottle?
- Does the infant initiate a swallow in coordination with suck?
- Does the infant coordinate sucking, swallowing, and breathing?
- Is the feeding completed in a reasonable time?

**R:** Identification of ineffective feeding patterns should be based on systematic assessment of the infant, in collaboration with other professionals. Behaviors that are cues to feeding dysfunction include ineffective coordination of suck/swallow/breathing, low energy or stamina, poor ability or inability to initiate sucking, disorganized rhythm in suck/swallow pattern, inadequate neurobehavioral control, and difficulty shifting back and forth from non-nutritive sucking and nutritive sucking.

Collaborate with clinical dietitian to set calorie, volume, and weight gain goals.

**R:** Close collaboration with a clinical dietitian to assess, plan, set, and evaluate calorie goals, weight gain goals, calorie distribution, and formula preparation is necessary for infants at risk.

Collaborate with occupational therapist, speech therapist to identify oral motor skills and planned intervention, if needed.

**R:** Close collaboration with a professional skilled in the assessment of infant oral motor skills (e.g., occupational therapist, speech therapist) is necessary to assess, plan, intervene, and evaluate progress toward appropriate oral motor skills in infants with oral motor impairment.

Collaborate with parent(s) about effective techniques used with this infant or other children, temperament, and responses to environmental stimuli.

**R:** Close collaboration with parents from the beginning about identified needs, negotiation of priorities, and development of interventions is crucial to establishing effective feeding patterns in the infant and strengthening the infant–parent relationship.

## Provide Specific Interventions to Promote Effective Oral Feeding (Hockenberry & Wilson, 2009)

Ensure a quiet, calm dim environment.
Eliminate painful procedures prior to feeding.

**R:** Calm, quiet, dim environments offer less distraction; attempt to decrease the negative effects of painful or very stimulating experiences shortly before or after feedings by timing them.

Ensure uninterrupted sleep periods.

**R:** Efforts to promote sleep and reduce energy expenditure (primarily by controlling environmental stimuli) can substantially improve the infant's strength and stamina during feeding.

Encourage non-nutritive sucking not in response to noxious stimuli.
Ensure nutritive sucking for an identified period
Control adverse environmental stimuli and noxious stimuli to face and mouth.

**R:** Non-nutritive sucking (pacifier) should not be used exclusively to comfort infants during or after painful procedures or exposure to noxious stimuli. In addition, care and attention to reducing noxious stimuli to the face and mouth (type, frequency, intensity) should be initiated long before attempts to feed orally begin.

Specific interventions for facilitating feeding are as follows:

* Choose nipple according to individual needs and successes; assess effects of changes in formula/breast milk temperature and thickness.
* Position infant semi-upright, with trunk approximately 45 to 60 degrees. (Do not use a "head-back" position because it makes swallowing and sucking coordination more difficult.)
* Stroke infant's lips, cheeks, and tongue before feeding.
* Support cheeks and chin to encourage adequate suck
* Use non-nutritive sucking before feeding to promote an awake and alert state.
* Use fingers to provide inward and forward support for infant's cheeks during feeding.
* Provide support for the base of the tongue (by placing fingers halfway between the chin and the throat, the nurse can provide a slight upward lift under the base of the tongue); *do not* provide strong upward pressure; steady support is most helpful; avoid moving fingers because it may interfere with the infant's own tongue movements.

Implement specific interventions for oral motor delays (position, equipment, jaw/mouth manipulation).
Promote consistency in approach to feeding.

**R:** Environmental factors, including light, noise, inconsistent caretakers (feeders), and noxious stimuli, contribute significantly to ineffective feeding patterns.

The following actions hinder, not help, feeding:

* Twisting or turning the nipple
* Moving the nipple up, down, around in the mouth
* Putting the nipple in and out of the mouth
* Putting pressure on the jaw or moving the infant's jaw up and down
* Placing the infant in a head-back position
* Caregiver anxiousness and impatience
* Promote sleep and reduce unnecessary energy expenditure.

**R:** For infants with demonstrable oral motor impairment, early intervention with an identified consistent approach to promoting oral feeding (equipment, body position, jaw and mouth manipulation, volume, time interval, duration) is essential for goal attainment.

Refer to *Risk for Aspiration* for interventions for feeding an infant with cleft lip and/or palate.

### Establish Partnership with Parent(s) in All Stages of Plan.

Create a supportive environment for the parents to have the primary role in providing feeding-related intervention, when they are present. Whenever possible, nurses use the parents' approach when a parent is not present. In addition, when parents are not present, nurses can support the parents' role by imitating their approach to the infant, and communicate the infant's responses to the parents at a later time.

**R:** An infant who receives adequate calories will be more able physically to eat orally; if parents support and value the way calories are delivered and recognize milestones toward the goal, the child will be more likely to receive adequate calories after discharge. In addition, interactions will be more rewarding for both infant and parent during the intervention period.

### Negotiate and Identify Plans for Discharge with Parents and Incorporate into the Overall Feeding Plan; Provide Ongoing Information About Special Needs and Assist Parents to Establish Needed Resources (Equipment, Nursing Care, Other Caretakers) When Needed

**R:** Establishing parents as essential participants in the feeding plan gives them a role, place, and reason to be present so they can develop a closer relationship with the child.

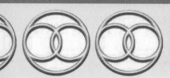

# IMBALANCED NUTRITION: MORE THAN BODY REQUIREMENTS

## DEFINITION

More Than Body Requirements: State in which a person experiences or is at risk of experiencing weight gain related to an intake in excess of metabolic requirements

## DEFINING CHARACTERISTICS

### Major (Must Be Present, One or More)

Overweight (weight 10% over ideal for height and frame), or
Obese (weight 20% or more over ideal for height and frame)
Triceps skinfold greater than 15 mm in men and 25 mm in women

### Minor (May Be Present)

Reported undesirable eating patterns
Intake in excess of metabolic requirements
Sedentary activity patterns

## RELATED FACTORS

### Pathophysiologic

*Related to altered satiety patterns secondary to (specify)*
*Related to decreased sense of taste and smell*

## Treatment-Related

*Related to altered satiety secondary to:*
Medications (corticosteroids, antihistamines, estrogens)
Radiation (decreased sense of taste and smell)

## Situational (Personal, Environmental)

*Related to risk to gain more than 25 to 30 lb when pregnant*
*Related to lack of basic nutrition knowledge*

## Maturational

**Adult/Older Adult**
*Related to decreased activity patterns, decreased metabolic needs*

### ■■■■■ AUTHOR'S NOTE

Using this diagnosis to describe people who are overweight or obese places the focus of interventions on nutrition. Obesity is a complex condition with sociocultural, psychological, and metabolic implications. When the focus is primarily on limiting food intake, as with many weight-loss programs, the chance of permanent weight loss is slim. To be successful, a weight-loss program must focus on behavior modification and lifestyle changes.

The nursing diagnosis *Imbalanced Nutrition: More Than Body Requirements* does not describe this focus. Rather, *Ineffective Health Maintenance related to intake in excess of metabolic requirements* better reflects the need to increase metabolic requirements through exercise and decreased intake. For some people who desire weight loss, *Ineffective Coping related to increased eating in response to stressors* could be useful in addition to *Ineffective Health Maintenance*.

The nurse should be cautioned against applying a nursing diagnosis for an overweight or obese person who does not want to participate in a weight-loss program. Motivation for weight loss must come from within. Nurses can gently and expertly teach the hazards of obesity but must respect a person's right to choose, the right of self-determination.

*Imbalanced Nutrition: More Than Body Requirements* does have clinical usefulness in people at risk for or who have experienced weight gain because of pregnancy, taste or smell changes, or medications (e.g., corticosteroids).

### ■■■■■ ERRORS IN DIAGNOSTIC STATEMENTS

1. Imbalanced Nutrition: More Than Body Requirements related to excessive calorie intake and sedentary lifestyle
   As discussed in the Author's Note, *Imbalanced Nutrition* does not describe the complex nature of obesity or overweight conditions. Obesity is not a nutritional problem but a problem with coping and lifestyle choices. *Ineffective Health Maintenance* and *Ineffective Coping* are more useful diagnoses for the focus of nursing interventions.
2. Imbalanced Nutrition: More Than Body Requirements related to reports of gaining 50 lb with first pregnancy
   A report of gaining 50 lb during first pregnancy should prompt the nurse to initiate a focus assessment to explore other variables. For example, the nurse could ask, "What do you think contributed to your weight gain during your first pregnancy?" "What was the pattern of weight gain during each trimester?" The nurse also should discuss the difference between dieting during pregnancy versus a diet not excessive in simple carbohydrates or fat. After additional data collection, the following diagnosis possibly could prove valid: *Risk for Imbalanced Nutrition: More Than Body Requirements related to lack of knowledge of nutrition and exercise needed during pregnancy and history of 50-lb weight gain during previous pregnancy*.

### ■■■■■ KEY CONCEPTS

#### Generic Considerations

- Certain medications (e.g., steroids, antihistamines, androgens, antipsychotics, hyperglycemics antidepressants) can cause weight gain (Archangelo & Peters, 2006).
- Medications that can affect taste include amphetamines, clofibrate, lithium, griseofulvin, methicillin, phenindione, phenytoin, and probucol (Dudek, 2006).

## Focus Assessment Criteria

See *Imbalanced Nutrition: Less Than Body Requirements*.

**NOC**
Nutritional Status,
Weight Control

## ➤ Goal

The person will describe why he or she is at risk for weight gain.

### Indicators

• Describe reasons for increased intake with taste or olfactory deficits.
• Discuss the nutritional needs during pregnancy.
• Discuss the effects of exercise on weight control.

**NIC**
Nutritional
Management,
Weight
Management,
Teaching: Individual,
Behavioral
Modification,
Exercise Promotion

## ➤ General Interventions

### Refer to Related Factors

### Explain the Effects of Decreased Sense of Taste and Smell on Perception of Satiety After Eating. Encourage Client to:

Evaluate intake by calorie counting, not feelings of satiety.
If not contraindicated, season foods heavily to satisfy decreased sense of taste. Experiment with seasonings (e.g., dill, basil).
When taste is diminished, concentrate on food smells.

**R:** People with altered smell or taste may consume more food in an attempt to satisfy their taste (Dudek, 2006).

### Explain the Rationale for Increased Appetite Owing to Use of Certain Medications (e.g., Steroids, Androgens)

**R:** The ability to lose weight while undergoing corticosteroid therapy likely depends on limiting sodium intake and maintaining reasonable caloric intake.

### Discuss Nutritional Intake and Weight Gain During Pregnancy

See Key Concepts under *Imbalanced Nutrition: Less Than Body Requirements*.

### Assist Client to Decrease Calorie Intake

Request that client write down all the food he or she ate in the past 24 h.
Instruct client to keep a diet diary for 1 week that specifies the following:

• What, when, where, and why eaten
• Whether he or she was doing anything else (e.g., watching television, cooking) while eating
• Emotions before eating
• Others present (e.g., snacking with spouse, children)

Review the diet diary to point out patterns (e.g., time, place, emotions, foods, persons) that affect food intake.
Review high- and low-calorie food items.

**R:** Strategies focus on increasing client's awareness of actions that contribute to excessive food intake.

### Teach Behavior Modification Techniques to Decrease Caloric Intake

Eat only at a specific spot at home (e.g., the kitchen table).
Do not eat while performing other activities.
Drink an 8-oz glass of water immediately before a meal.
Decrease second helpings, fatty foods, sweets, and alcohol.

Prepare small portions, just enough for one meal, and discard leftovers.
Use small plates to make portions look bigger.
Never eat from another person's plate.
Eat slowly and chew food thoroughly.
Put down utensils and wait 15 s between bites.
Eat low-calorie snacks that must be chewed to satisfy oral needs (e.g., carrots, celery, apples).

**R:** Strategies to assist a person initiate a change in eating patterns and exercise patterns will focus on why, where, and what is eaten and methods to reduce intake and increase activity.

### Instruct Client to Increase Activity Level to Burn Calories

Use the stairs instead of elevators.
Park at the farthest point in parking lots and walk to buildings.
Plan a daily walking program with a progressive increase in distance and pace.
Note: Urge client to consult with a primary provider before beginning any exercise program.

**R:** Increased activity promotes weight loss.

### Initiate Referral to a Community Weight Loss Program (e.g., Weight Watchers), if Indicated

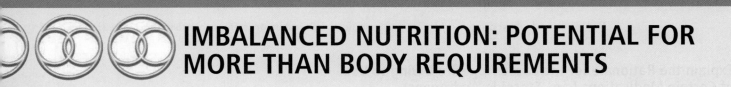

# IMBALANCED NUTRITION: POTENTIAL FOR MORE THAN BODY REQUIREMENTS

## DEFINITION

State in which a person is at risk of experiencing an intake of nutrients that exceeds metabolic needs

## DEFINING CHARACTERISTICS

Reported or observed obesity in one or both parents
Rapid transition across growth percentiles in infants or children
Reported use of solid food as major food source before 5 months of age
Observed use of food as reward or comfort measure
Reported or observed higher baseline weight at beginning of each pregnancy
Dysfunctional eating patterns

### ■■■■■■ AUTHOR'S NOTE

This nursing diagnosis is similar to *Risk for Imbalanced Nutrition: More Than Body Requirements*. It describes a person who has a family history of obesity, is demonstrating a pattern of higher weight, or has had a history of excessive weight gain (e.g., previous pregnancy). Until clinical research differentiates this diagnosis from other currently accepted diagnoses, use *Risk for Ineffective Health Maintenance* to direct teaching to assist clients and families to identify unhealthy dietary patterns.

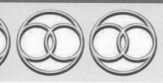

# POST-TRAUMA SYNDROME

**Post-Trauma Syndrome**

Risk for Post-Trauma Syndrome
Rape Trauma Syndrome

## DEFINITION

State in which a person experiences a sustained painful response to one or more overwhelming traumatic events that have not been assimilated

## DEFINING CHARACTERISTICS

### Major (Must Be Present, One or More)

*Re-experience of the traumatic event, which may be identified in cognitive, affective, and/or sensory motor activities for more than 1 month such as:*
Flashbacks, intrusive memories
Repetitive dreams/nightmares
Excessive verbalization of the traumatic event(s)
Survival guilt or guilt about behavior required for survival
Painful emotion, self-blame, shame, or sadness
Vulnerability or helplessness, anxiety, or panic
Fear of repetition, death, or loss of bodily control
Angry outbursts/rage, startle reaction
Hyperalertness or hypervigilance
Persistent avoidance of stimuli
Exaggerated startle response
Avoidance of thoughts, feelings or conversations associated with trauma
Sleep disturbances

### Minor (May Be Present)

Psychic/Emotional Numbness
Impaired interpretation of reality, impaired memory
Confusion, dissociation, or amnesia
Vagueness about the traumatic event(s)
Narrowed attention or inattention/daze
Feeling of numbness, constricted affect
Feeling detached/alienated
Reduced interest in significant activities
Altered Lifestyle
Submissiveness, passiveness, or dependency
Self-destructiveness (e.g., alcohol/drug abuse, suicide attempts, reckless driving, illegal activities)
Thrill-seeking activities
Difficulty with interpersonal relationships
Development of phobia regarding trauma
Avoidance of situations or activities that arouse recollection of the trauma
Social isolation/withdrawal, negative self-concept
Sleep disturbances, emotional disturbances
Irritability, poor impulse control, or explosiveness
Loss of faith in people or the world, feeling of meaninglessness in life
Chronic anxiety or chronic depression
Somatic preoccupation/multiple physiologic symptoms

# RELATED FACTORS

## Situational (Personal, Environmental)

*Related to traumatic events of natural origin, including*

| | | |
|---|---|---|
| Floods | Earthquakes | Volcanic eruptions |
| Storms | Avalanches | Epidemics |
| Other natural disasters | | |

*Related to traumatic events of human origin, such as*

| | | |
|---|---|---|
| Concentration camp confinement | Serious car accidents | Assault |
| Torture | Rape | Bombing |
| Large fires | Witnessing violence | Terrorist attacks |
| Wars | Airplane crashes | |

*Related to industrial disasters (nuclear, chemical, or other life-threatening accidents)*

■■■■■■ **AUTHOR'S NOTE**

*Post-Trauma Syndrome* represents a group of emotional responses to a traumatic event of either natural origin (e.g., floods, volcanic eruptions, earthquakes) or human origin (e.g., war, rape, torture). The emotional responses (e.g., guilt, shame, fear, anger) interfere with interpersonal relationships and can precipitate self-destructive behavior (e.g., substance abuse, suicide). The nurse may find it necessary to use additional diagnoses when specific interventions are indicated (e.g., *Compromised Family Coping, Risk for Self-Harm*).

The diagnosis *Rape Trauma Syndrome* was described in 1975 as encompassing an acute phase of disorganization and a long-term phase of reorganization. Based on the most recent definition of syndrome nursing diagnoses as a cluster of associated nursing diagnoses, this diagnosis does not represent a syndrome and would be more accurately labeled *Rape Trauma Response*. The inclusion of causative or contributing factors with this category is unnecessary, because the etiology is always rape. Thus, the nurse omits the second part of the diagnostic statement; however, he or she can add the client's report of the rape to the statement. For example, *Rape Trauma Syndrome as evidenced by the report of a sexual assault and sodomy on June 22 and multiple facial bruises* (refer to ER record for description).

■■■■■■ **ERRORS IN DIAGNOSTIC STATEMENTS**

### Post-Trauma Response related to expressions of survival guilt and recurring nightmares of auto accident

Survival guilt and nightmares of a traumatic event represent possible manifestations of post-trauma response, not related factors. The nurse should restate the diagnosis as *Post-Trauma Response related to auto accident, as evidenced by recurring nightmares and expressions of survival guilt.*

■■■■■■ **KEY CONCEPTS**

### Generic Considerations

- Trauma is defined in terms of the subjective experience of an event that cannot be dealt with or assimilated in the usual way. Traumatic situations differ from ordinary experiences in that they involve realistic danger of physiologic or psychological destruction, which could mobilize fear of death. A traumatic event may affect only one person or many people at once. It may be of human origin (e.g., rape, wars) or natural origin (e.g., avalanches, volcanoes).
- In general, traumatic events of natural origin are less severe or long lasting than are those of human origin. Those of human origin are often perceived as resulting from indifference, negligence, or malice.
- Horowitz (1986a, 1986b) conceptualized these phenomena and postulated a phasic tendency in human responses to traumatic events.
  - The initial response to trauma is to survive and to function in the immediate life-threatening situation by using all resources.
  - The powerful coping method of "numbing" reduces psychological and emotional effects.

*(continued)*

■■■■■■ **KEY CONCEPTS** *Continued*

- In an attempt to master the traumatic experience, intrusive recollection or reenactment of the trauma erupts into conscious awareness.
- There is a pattern of oscillation between "numbing" and intrusive reactions peculiar to each person.
- Gradually, the person works through the trauma by using a broader perception and rationale for the event and the aftermath.
- Finally, the person assimilates such an experience into a meaningful whole congruent with basic beliefs and values.
- Severity of trauma is associated with intensity, duration, and frequency. It involves a complex interaction of environmental conditions and the person's subjective experiences, such as degree of warning, threat to life, exposure to the grotesque, bereavement, displacement, and moral conflict about the role of the survivor.
- Individual characteristics, such as early childhood experience, developmental phase, and character strength, may affect the outcome of responses to trauma.
  - The current trauma may reactivate unresolved childhood conflicts.
  - Age can be a crucial factor, because trauma can interrupt a stage of human development.
  - Individual coping resources are important when a person confronts a traumatic situation, and they influence the effectiveness of adaptation.

## Pediatric Considerations

- A child's response to trauma depends on the nature and the extent of the trauma, developmental age, and response of significant others (Hockenberry & Wilson, 2009).
- Children can experience post-traumatic stress symptoms after a friend or acquaintance is killed (Pfefferbaum et al., 2000).
- Child abuse includes neglect and physical, emotional, and sexual abuse affecting 3 million children in the United States.

# Focus Assessment Criteria

## Subjective and Objective Data

### *Assess for Defining Characteristics*

#### History of the Trauma*
Exposure to a very stressful, disturbing situation (see *Related Factors*)
List all traumas, including dates and duration.

#### The Person's Responses to the Traumatic Event(s)
Thoughts, feelings, or actions that he or she believes have been different since the traumatic experience, to assess signs and symptoms of reexperiencing or numbing responses
Changes in general lifestyle or pattern since the traumatic event(s), to assess any readjustment difficulties

#### Observe or Consult with Family Members or Other Appropriate People, As Possible
Excessive verbalization of the traumatic events
Preoccupation with trauma reminders, such as sorting through pictures or other trauma-related objects
Use of denial, distortion, minimization, exaggeration, disavowal, fantasy, or avoidance
Evidence of indifference or dissociation to stimuli (questions, noise, activities around him or her)
Sudden or significant behavioral/personality changes since the traumatic event

---

*The purpose of securing a history is to substantiate evidence of trauma and not to explore details of trauma. This should be done in an appropriate therapy session.

**NOC**
Abuse Recovery,
Coping, Fear Control

## ➤ Goals

The person will assimilate the experience into a meaningful whole and go on to pursue his or her life, as evidenced by goal setting.

### *Indicators*

- Report a lessening of re-experiencing the trauma or numbing symptoms.
- Acknowledge the traumatic event and begin to work with the trauma by talking about the experience and expressing feelings such as fear, anger, and guilt.
- Identify and make connection with support persons/resources.

**NIC**
Counseling,
Anxiety Reduction,
Emotional Support,
Family Support,
Support System
Enhancement,
Coping
Enhancement, Active
Listening, Presence,
Grief Work,
Facilitation, Referral

## ➤ General Interventions

### Determine If the Person Has Experienced a Traumatic Event.

During the interview, secure a quiet room where there will be no interruptions but easy access to other staff in case of management problems.

Be aware that talking about a traumatic experience may cause significant discomfort to the person.

If the person becomes too anxious, discontinue the assessment and help the person to regain control of the distress or provide other appropriate interventions.

**R:** Short-term crisis intervention should begin as soon as victims are identified.

### Document the Person's Responses

**R:** Careful recording of psychological responses assists in documenting progress in therapy, planning treatment, or identifying those at greatest risk. Behavior can differ among individuals. Feelings can be fast and furious or slow, trancelike, mixed, or clear (Charron, 1998).

### Evaluate the Severity of the Responses and Effects on Current Functioning.

### Assist Client to Decrease Extremes of Reexperiencing or Numbing Symptoms.

Provide a safe, therapeutic environment where the person can regain control.

Reassure the person that others who have experienced such traumatic events often experienced these feelings/symptoms.

Stay with the person and offer support during an episode of high anxiety (see *Anxiety* for additional information).

Assist client to control impulsive acting-out behavior by setting limits, promoting ventilation, and redirecting excess energy into physical exercise or activity (e.g., walking, jogging). (See *Risk for Self-Harm* and *Risk for Violence* for additional information.)

Recognize that psychic/emotional numbness provides a cushion.

Provide techniques to reduce anxiety, e.g., progressive relaxation, deep breathing.

**R:** Attempts to decrease extreme symptoms can help person regain some control.

**R:** Interventions that focus on helping the person cope can reduce powerlessness (Charron, 1998).

### Assist Client to Acknowledge and Begin to Work Through the Trauma by Discussing the Experience and Expressing Feelings Such as Fear, Anger, and Guilt.

Provide a safe, structured setting.

Explain that talking about the traumatic event may intensify the symptoms (e.g., nightmares, flashbacks, painful emotions, numbness).

Assist person to proceed at an individual pace.

Listen attentively with empathy and an unhurried manner.

**R:** Providing immediate and ongoing empathy and support prepares victims for referral to more in-depth psychological counseling. Main issues in the acute stage are being in control, fear of being left alone, and having someone to listen.

Assist client to talk about trauma, to understand what has occurred, and to validate the reality of personal involvement.

Help client to express feelings associated with the traumatic event and to become aware of the link between the experience and anger, depression, or anxiety.

Assist client to differentiate reality from fantasy and to look back and talk about the areas of his or her life that have changed.

Recognize and support cultural and religious values in dealing with the traumatic event.

**R:** Assisting the person to recall and clarify the event puts that event in perspective and helps prevent repression. Victims need to work through trauma at their own pace.

**R:** Anxiety management offers one way to maintain some control over their bodies (Boyd, 2005).

## Assist Client to Identify and Make Connections with Support People and Resources.

Help client to identify his or her strength and resources.

Explore available support system.

Assist client to make connections with support and resources according to his or her needs.

Assist client to resume old activities and begin some new ones.

**R:** Providing immediate and ongoing empathy and support prepares victims for referral to more in-depth psychological counseling. Main issues in the acute stage are being in control, fear of being left alone, and having someone to listen.

## Assist Family/Significant Others.

Assist them to understand what is happening to the victim.

Encourage expression of their feelings.

Provide counseling sessions or link them with appropriate community resources, as necessary.

**R:** Strategies focus on assisting significant others identify how they can be most helpful to prevent victim isolation, which can lead to withdrawal.

## Provide Nursing Care Appropriate to Each Person's Traumatic Experience and Needs. (See **Rape Trauma Syndrome** for Additional Information, If Relevant.)

## Provide or Arrange Follow-Up Treatment in Which Person can Continue to Work Through the Trauma and to Integrate the Experience into a New Self-Concept.

**R:** Follow-up counseling and long-term support therapy in the community should be arranged. Postponing professional help lengthens the time reactions persist and can lengthen recovery.

**Pediatric Interventions**

Assist children to understand and to integrate the experience in accordance with their developmental stage.

Assist them to describe the experience and to express feelings (e.g., fear, guilt, rage) in safe, supportive places, such as play therapy sessions.

Provide accurate information and explanations in terms child can understand.

Provide family counseling to promote understanding of the child's needs

Refer to a specialist for on-going therapy.

**R:** Play therapy, such as writing, drawing, telling stories, or playing with dolls, should be offered so children can act out, express feelings, and communicate their experience safely.

**R:** Counseling for the parents and child will be needed to assist with evaluating the trauma and assimilating the experience into their lives.

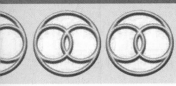

# RISK FOR POST-TRAUMA SYNDROME

## DEFINITION

State in which a client experiences a sustained painful response to one or more overwhelming traumatic events that have not been assimilated

## RISK FACTORS

Refer to Related Factors in *Post-Trauma Syndrome*.

## Goal

The client will continue to function appropriately after the traumatic event.

*Indicators:*

- Identify signs or symptoms that necessitate professional consultation.
- Express feelings regarding traumatic event.

## General Interventions

Refer to *Post-Trauma Syndrome*.

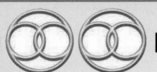

# RAPE TRAUMA SYNDROME

## DEFINITION

State in which a client experiences a forced, violent sexual assault (vaginal or anal penetration) against his or her will and without his or her consent. The trauma syndrome that develops from this attack or attempted attack includes an acute phase of disorganization of the victim and family's lifestyle and a long-term process of reorganization of lifestyle (Burgess, 1995).

## DEFINING CHARACTERISTICS

### Major (Must Be Present)

Reports or evidence of sexual assault.

### Minor (May Be Present)

If the victim is a child, parents may experience similar responses.

**Acute Phase**
*Somatic Responses*
*Physical trauma (bruises, soreness)*
Gastrointestinal irritability (nausea, vomiting, anorexia, diarrhea)
Genitourinary discomfort (pain, pruritus, vaginal discharge)
Skeletal muscle tension (spasms, pain, headaches, sleep disturbances)

*Psychological Responses*
*Overt*
- Crying, sobbing
- Joking, laughing
- Volatility, anger
- Confusion, incoherence, disorientation

*Ambiguous reaction*
- Confusion, incoherence, disorientation
- Masked facies
- Calm, subdued appearance
- Shock, numbness, confusion, or disbelieving

Distractibility and difficulty making decisions

*Emotional Reaction*
- Fear—of being alone or that the rapist will return (a child victim fears punishment, repercussions, abandonment, rejection)
- Denial, shock, humiliation, and embarrassment
- Desire for revenge; anger
- Guilt, shame, and self-blame
- Fatigue

*Sexual Responses*
Mistrust of men (if victim is a woman)
Change in sexual behavior

## Long-Term Phase (Varcarolis, Carlson, & Shoemaker, 2006)

Any response of the acute phase may continue if resolution does not occur. In addition, the following reactions can occur 2 or more weeks after the assault.

*Psychological Responses*
*Intrusive thoughts* (anger toward assailant, flashbacks of the traumatic event, dreams, insomnia)
Increased motor activity (moving, taking trips, staying some other place)
Increased emotional lability (intense anxiety, mood swings, crying spells, depression)
Fears and phobias (of indoors, or outdoors, where the rape occurred, of being alone, of crowds, of sexual encounters (with partner or potential partners)

## ■■■■■■ AUTHOR'S NOTE
See *Post-Trauma Syndrome.*

## ■■■■■■ ERRORS IN DIAGNOSTIC STATEMENTS
See *Post-Trauma Syndrome.*

## ■■■■■■ KEY CONCEPTS
### Generic Considerations
- Estimates are that more than 200,000 cases of rape are reported in the United States yearly (RAINN, 2002).
- Experts report a decrease in rape from 1993 to 2002 by 60% and attribute this to tougher sentences, "three-strike" laws, and more assertive young women who report the crime (RAINN, 2002; Varcarolis, Carson, & Shoemaker, 2006).
- Rape is a crime using sexual means to humiliate or degrade the victim. Someone commits sexual acts against a nonconsenting person. Rape violates the victim's right of privacy, sense of security, safety, and well-being.
- Rape is a crime that health care providers must report. Estimates are that only 4 of 10 rapes are reported (Symes, 2000; Carson & Smith-DiJulio, 2006).
- Our past culture (and some cultures today) supported that (Heinrich, 1987).

*(continued)*

■■■■■■ **KEY CONCEPTS** *Continued*

- A woman's rightful place in society is to fulfill man's destiny.
- Women are property of men and responsible for retaining value. (Therefore, women who allow themselves to get raped are bad.)
- Women are important to men, as symbols of their power and status and as prizes of prowess.
- Some myths about rape include the following (Heinrich, 1987):
  - The rapist is a sexually unsatisfied man who cannot control his urges.
  - Rape is a one-time incident, representing a momentary lapse in judgment.
  - Rapists are strangers.
  - The victim provokes the rape.
  - Only promiscuous women get raped.
  - Rapes happen to women out alone at night. If a woman stays home, she will be safe.
  - Women cannot be raped against their will—they can avoid rape by resistance.
  - Most rapes involve black men and white women.
  - Women respect men for overpowering them; they may even enjoy the rape.
  - Rapists are mentally ill or retarded and, therefore, not responsible for their acts.
- Victims, families, society, and caregivers who subscribe to these myths may not view themselves as victims or recognize the criminality of rape, may not seek help, or may be denied supportive interventions (Heinrich, 1987).
- Rapists can be divided into three broad categories (Petter & Whitehill, 1998):
  - Power rapists (55% of sexual assaults): they attack persons near their age and use intimidation and minimal violence to control. The attack is premeditated.
  - Anger rapists (40% of sexual assaults): they target the very young or elderly. They use extreme force and restraints, resulting in physical injury.
  - Sadistic rapists (5% of sexual assaults): the attack is premeditated. They derive erotic satisfaction from torturing.
- Burgess (1995) categorized three main types of rape:
  - *Rape:* Sex without consent in which the assailant uses confidence, coercion, or violence.
  - *Accessory to sex:* Survivors collaborate in a secondary manner with the sexual activity, and consent or lack of consent is from cognitive or personality development. (Mentally retarded people and children are susceptible.)
  - *Sex-stress situation:* Sex is agreed on initially, but then one party decides not to go through with it, usually because of exploitation, but this change of heart is not heeded.
- Rape occurs in all age groups, races, and educational and economic groups (Carlson & Smith-DiJulio, 2006).
- Male rape victims (including homosexuals) are unlikely to report the rape but are most likely to experience symptoms of rape trauma syndrome (Carlson & Smith-DiJulio, 2006).
- "Many child and adult survivors of sexual assaults never report the crime or seek help" (Symes, 2000, p. 30).
- Survivors of sexual assault are more likely to attempt suicide, experience an eating disorder, be sexually assaulted again, and have substance abuse, depressive episodes, and anxiety disorders (Symes, 2000).

## Transcultural Considerations

- The battered woman may come from a culture that accepts domestic violence and may be isolated by cultural dynamics that do not permit her to seek assistance. Additionally, language barriers may interfere with her ability to call 911 or learn about her rights or legal options (American Bar Association, 2004).
- Regardless of the culture of the victim, the professional nurse has an obligation to report injuries and to protect the victim. In situations of spousal rape with no visible injuries, the victim should be informed of options available.

## Pediatric Considerations

- The female adolescent is particularly at risk for sexual assault; estimates are that more than 50% of rape victims are between 10 and 19 years of age (Hockenberry & Wilson 2009).
- Statuary rape is when the victim is unable to legally give consent because of age (age varies from state to state), mental deficiencies, psychosis, or altered state of consciousness (sleep, drugs, illness, alcohol) (Hockenberry & Wilson, 2009).
- The assailant of a child is most likely someone the child knows, and the assaults usually have occurred for some time within the child's own home or neighborhood.
- Adolescents, particularly boys, are more prone to attempt suicide in the aftermath of rape.
- Acquaintance rape is very prevalent among college-age women and is believed to be underrecognized and underreported.
- Greater emotional distress and long-term effects have been reported when a child knew and trusted the abuser.
- Adolescent girls frequently underreport acquaintance rape because they believe they may have contributed to the act in some way (e.g., alcohol use).
- Drug-facilitated sexual assaults are caused by slipping a drug in a drink. "Date rape" drugs are Rohypnol, gammahydroxybutyrate (GHB), Burundanga, datura, and ketamine. They cause disinhibition, passivity, relaxation of muscles, and amnesia (Smith, 1999: Varcarolis, Carson, & Shoemaker, 2006).

## Maternal Considerations

Refer to *Disabled Family Coping—Domestic Violence*.

## Geriatric Considerations

- Only 7% of elder abuse cases are reported and of these cases less than 1% were sexual abuse (Teaster, Dugar, Mendiondo, & Otto, 2005).
- Residents of nursing homes are the most vulnerable to abuse. The failure to address the problem of sexual abuse may be the result of the incomprehensibility of sexual assault of nursing home residents and generalized negative attitudes or hostility toward older and cognitively impaired persons (Burgess et al., 2000).
- Burgess found that, of 20 nursing home victims of sexual assault, 11 died within 1 year of the assault. These victims are not equipped physically, constitutionally, or psychologically to defend themselves or to cope with the aftermath (Burgess et al., 2000).
- Elder abuse may include physical and sexual abuse, psychological abuse, neglect, exploitation, and medical abuse (Goldstein, 2005).

## Focus Assessment Criteria

### Subjective Data (Must Be Recorded)

#### *Assess for Defining Characteristics*

**History of the Undesired Sexual Activity (Child, Adolescent, Adult)***
Time and place of event
Identity or description of assailant
Sexual contact (type, amount, coercion, weapon)
Witnesses, if any
Activities that may alter evidence (changing clothes, bathing, urinating, douching)

---

*The purpose of securing a history is to substantiate evidence of trauma and not to explore details of trauma. This should be done in an appropriate therapy session.

Sexual history

| | | |
|---|---|---|
| Date of last menses | Contraceptive use | Menstrual history |
| Date of last sexual contact | History of venereal disease | |

### Response to the Assault During Acute Phase

*Assess client and family for (refer to Defining Characteristics for specific responses):*

| | |
|---|---|
| Overt behaviors | Ambiguous reactions |
| Somatic reactions | Emotional reactions |

*Assess child for:*

Understanding of the event

Knowledge of the identity of the molester

Possibility of previous assaults

*Assess parents, spouse, others for:*

| | | |
|---|---|---|
| Understanding of the event | Ability to help victim cope | Ability to cope |

### Response to the Assault During Long-Term Phase

Assess the client for psychological reactions. Refer to Defining Characteristics for specific responses.

## Objective Data

## Assess for Injury (Ecchymoses, Lacerations, Abrasions)

Gastrointestinal system (mouth, anus, abdomen)

Skeletal muscle system

Genitourinary system

## Assess the Emotional Responses

| | | |
|---|---|---|
| Crying | Detachment | Hysteria |
| Composure | Withdrawal | |

## Assess for Change in Behavior in the Cognitively Impaired (Burgess et al., 2000)

| | | |
|---|---|---|
| Avoidance behavior with males | Staying near nurses' station | Lying in fetal position |
| Fear of men | Withdrawal behavior | |

For more information on Focus Assessment Criteria, visit http://thepoint.lww.com.

---

**NOC**
Abuse Protection,
Abuse Recovery,
Coping

## ➤ Goals

The client will return to pre-crisis level of functioning.

The child will express feelings concerning the assault and the treatment.

The parents, spouse, or significant other will return to pre-crisis level of functioning.

### Indicators:

*Short-term goals*

- Share feelings.
- Describe rationale and treatment procedures.
- Identify members of support system and use them appropriately.

*Long-term goals*

- Report sleeping well.
- Report return to former eating pattern.
- Report occasional somatic reactions or none.
- Demonstrate calmness and relaxation.

**NIC**
Abuse Protection Support, Coping Enhancement, Rape-Trauma Treatment, Support Group, Anxiety Reduction, Presence, Emotional Support, Calming Technique, Active Listening, Family Support, Grief Work Facilitation

## ➤ General Interventions

### Assist the Client in Identifing Major Concerns (Psychological, Medical, Legal) and Perception of Help Needed

**R:** The sooner intervention begins with a rape victim, the less psychological damage she or he will incur. Many victims try to suppress the memory of the assault, so postponing counseling even 1 day may weaken their pursuit of follow-up care. Immediate contact with a counselor may overcome this reluctance.

### *Explain the Care and Examination*

Provide interventions in an unhurried manner.
Do not leave the client alone.
Help the client to meet personal needs (bathing *after* examination and evidence has been acquired).
Explain every detail before acting and secure permission.

**R:** Because the client's right to deny or consent has been violated it is important to seek permission for care (Heinrich, 1987). The goal is to establish a safe and empathetic environment.

## *Explain the Legal Issues and Police Investigation (Heinrich, 1987)*

## *Promote a Trusting Relationship*

Stay with the client during acute stage or arrange for other support.
Brief the client on police and hospital procedures during acute stage.
Explain that the choice to report the rape is the victim's. Explore pros and cons of reporting.

**R:** Improved emotional outcomes have been reported by victims that have reported the crime.

Explain the need to collect specimens for future possible court use.
If this is the client's first pelvic examination, explain the position and the instruments. Explain each step prior to intervention. Have another nurse support the client through the exam.

**R:** The evidentiary examination is especially distressing because it can be reminiscent of the assault (Ledray, 2001).

If the police interview is permitted:

* Negotiate with the victim and police for an advantageous time.
* Explain to the victim what kind of questions will be asked.
* Remain with the victim during the interview; do not ask questions or offer answers.

If the officer is insensitive, intimidating, or offensive, or asks improper questions, discuss this with the officer in private. If the behavior continues, use proper channels and make a complaint.

**R:** The medical–legal examination serves to assess the condition of the victim and to gather documentary evidence. It consists of a general examination; oral, pelvic, and rectal examinations; a culture for sperm and sexually transmitted diseases; serum pregnancy test; blood typing; and a drug and alcohol screen. Obvious debris is placed in separate envelopes. Dried sperm is collected. The victim's pubic hair and head hair are combed, and samples are placed in separate envelopes. Fingernail scrapings are placed in separate envelopes for each hand (Heinrich, 1987).

Initiate play therapy with a child to explain treatments and allow the child to express feelings.

**R:** The child's reaction depends on age, degree of physical trauma, relation to the assailant, and parental (caretaker) reaction.

Play therapy should be an integral part of the treatment regimen for children. The child can act out the assault with dolls of the appropriate sex. Puppets are also beneficial for play therapy (Hockenberry & Wilson, 2009).

## *Whenever Possible, Provide Crisis Counseling within 1 h of Rape*

Ask permission to contact the rape crisis counselor.

Be flexible and individualize the approach according to the victim's needs.

Observe the victim's behavior carefully and record objective data.

Encourage the victim to verbalize thoughts, feelings, or perceptions of the event.

Discuss treatment as victim; express empathy.

Assess the victim's verbal style (expressive, controlled).

Discuss with the victim previous coping mechanism.

Explore available support systems; involve significant others if appropriate.

Assess stress tolerance.

Reassure the victim about the manner in which she or he reacted.

Explore with the victim her or his strengths and resources.

Convey confidence in the victim's ability to return to prior level of functioning.

Assist the victim in decision-making and problem solving; involve the victim in own treatment plan.

Help restore the victim's dignity by calmly exploring together basis for feelings.

Reassure the victim that rape trauma victims often experience these feelings/symptoms: fear of rapist or death, guilt, loss of control, shame, short attention span, anger, anxiety, phobias, depression, flashbacks, embarrassment, and eating/sleeping pattern disturbances.

Respect the victim's rights; honor wishes to restrict unwanted visitors; offer privacy when appropriate.

Explain to the victim that this experience will disrupt her or his life, and that feelings that occurred during acute phase may recur; encourage the victim to proceed at her or his own pace.

Explain any papers that need to be signed.

Briefly counsel family and friends at their level.

Share the immediate needs of the victim for love and support.

Encourage the victim to express feelings and ask questions.

**R:** Crisis counseling can provide accurate information and ongoing assessment of emotional state (Carlson & Smith-DiJulio, 2006).

**R:** Rape crisis centers provide rape victims and significant others with information concerning the medical examination, police interrogation, and court procedures; they provide escort service to hospital, police department, and courts; and they provide information about counseling.

## Fulfill Medical–Legal Responsibilities by Documentation (Ledray, 2001)

Consult with a sexual assault nurse examiner (SANEs) or clinicians who are specially trained to address the needs of a sexually assault survivor.

If in the emergency room, consult The Emergency Nurses Association position statement on the role of the nurse in collecting medical and legal evidence at http://www.ena.org/about/posirtion/forensicevidence.asp.

### *Document*

History of rape (date, time, place)

Nature of injuries, use of force, weapons used, threats of violence or retribution, restraints used

Nature of assault (fondling, oral, anal, vaginal penetration, ejaculation, use of condom)

Post-assault activities (douching, bathing/showering, gargling, urinating, defecating, changing clothes, eating, or drinking)

Present state (use of drugs, alcohol)

Medical history, immunization status (tetanus, hepatitis A, B), gynecologic history (last menstrual period, last voluntary intercourse, using a birth control method)

Emotional state and mental status

Examination findings, smears/cultures taken, blood tests, evidence collected, and photographs (if appropriate)

Document what evidence is delivered and when and to whom

**R:** Providing accurate information about the medical–legal procedures and their relevance can reduce feelings of physical intrusion and loss of control.

## Explain the Risks of Sexually Transmitted Infections (Ledray, 2001; Centers for Disease Control and Prevention, 2008)

Sexually transmitted diseases (specimens, blood tests)

| | | |
|---|---|---|
| Gonorrhea | Human immunodeficiency virus (HIV) | Trichomoniasis |
| Syphilis | Hepatitis B, A, C | Chlamydia |

Consult with protocol or physician/nurse practitioner for prophylaxis for:

Chlamydia    HIV    Trichomoniasis    Gonorrhea

**R:** Certain sexually transmitted infections (STIs) can be treated with medications to eliminate pathogens. The Centers for Disease Control and Prevention recommend HIV post-exposure prophylaxis if begun within 48 hours (2008).

Vaccinate individuals if needed for tetanus and Hepatitis A, B.

**R:** An assault outdoors carries the risk for tetanus infection. Hepatitis A and B can be transmitted via body fluids.

Determine if the victim is a risk for pregnancy and, if at risk, explain emergency contraceptive pills (ECP).

- No contraceptive use
- No surgical sterilization
- Postmenopausal

# Eliminate or Reduce Somatic Symptomatology

## Gastrointestinal Irritability

### Anorexia
Offer small, frequent feedings.
Provide appealing foods.
Record intake.
Refer to *Imbalanced Nutrition* if anorexia is prolonged.

### Nausea
Avoid gas-forming foods.
Restrict carbonated beverages.
Observe for abdominal distention.
Offer antiemetic per physician's order.

## Genitourinary Discomfort

### Pain
Assess for quality and duration.
Monitor intake and output.
Inspect urine and external genitalia for bleeding.
Listen attentively to the victim's description of pain.
Give pain medication per physician's order (see *Impaired Comfort*).

### Discharge
Assess amount, color, and odor of discharge.
Allow the victim time to wash and change garments after initial examination has been completed.

### Itching
Encourage bathing in cool water.
Avoid use of detergent soaps.
Avoid touching the area causing discomfort.

## Skeletal Muscle Tension

### Headaches
Avoid any sudden change of the victim's position.
Approach the victim calmly.

Slightly elevate the bed (unless contraindicated).
Discuss pain-reducing measures that have been effective in the past.

### Fatigue
Assess present sleeping patterns if altered (see *Disturbed Sleep Pattern*).
Discuss precipitating factors for sleep disturbance; try to eliminate them, if possible.
Provide frequent rest periods throughout the day.
Avoid interruptions during sleep.
Avoid stress-producing situations.

### Emotional Responses
Provide an emotionally secure environment.
Discuss the victim's daily routines and adhere to them as much as possible.
Avoid any sudden movements, and approach the victim in a calm manner.
Provide frequent quiet periods throughout the day.

## Generalized Bruising and Edema

Avoid constrictive garments.
Handle affected body parts gently.
Elevate affected body part if edema is present.
Apply a cool, moist compress to the edematous area for the first 24 h, then a warm compress after 24 h.
Encourage the victim to verbalize discomfort.
Record any bruises, lacerations, edema, or abrasions.

**R:** The interventions for rape trauma syndrome are listed for usefulness under the varied responses for each victim; minimize any further trauma.

## Proceed with Health Teaching to Victim and Family

Before the victim leaves the hospital, provide a card with information about follow-up appointments and names and telephone numbers of local crisis and counseling centers.
Plan a home visit or telephone call.
Arrange for legal or pastoral counseling, if appropriate.
Recommend and make referrals to a psychotherapist, mental health clinic, citizen action or community group advocacy-related service.

**R:** Some long-term problems can be prevented if the victim's family and friends recognize symptoms as normal (Adams & Fay, 1989). Responses of others can help or hinder recovery greatly. Significant others may also face a crisis and the need for recovery (Adams & Fay, 1989).

## Teach Management of Discomforts:

Gastrointestinal irritability: explain that the side effects of emergency contraceptive pills (ECP) are nausea and vomiting.
Genitourinary discomfort: advise against scratching the area causing discomfort.
Skeletal muscle tension:
• Explain potential causes of discomfort.
• Explain measures that may help release tension.
• Teach relaxation methods.

**R:** Detailed written follow-up instructions are given because the victim cannot assimilate the information at this time.
Follow-up counseling provides support over time and may lessen the intrapsychic effects of the rape (Carson & Smith-DiJulio, 2006).

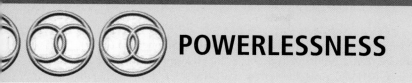

# POWERLESSNESS

## DEFINITION

State in which an individual or group perceives a lack of personal control over certain events or situations that affects outlook, goals, and lifestyle

## DEFINING CHARACTERISTICS

### Major (Must Be Present)

Overt or covert (anger, apathy) expressions of dissatisfaction over inability to control a situation (e.g., work, illness, prognosis, care, recovery rate) that is negatively affecting outlook, goals, and lifestyle
A sense of worthlessness, being trapped in a negative life situation, and emotional suffering.

### Minor (May Be Present)

*Lack of information-seeking behaviors*

| | | |
|---|---|---|
| Unsatisfactory dependence on others | Passivity | Resignation |
| | Apathy | Anxiety |
| Acting-out behavior | Anger | Depression |
| Violent behavior | Feelings of alienation | Sense of vulnerability |

### Related Factors

**Pathophysiologic**

Any disease process, acute or chronic, can cause or contribute to powerlessness. Some common sources are as follows.

*Related to inability to communicate secondary to stroke, Guillain-Barré syndrome, intubation*

*Related to inability to perform activities of daily living secondary to, stroke, cervical trauma, myocardial infarction, or pain, for example*

*Related to inability to perform role responsibilities secondary to surgery, trauma, or arthritis*

*Related to progressive debilitating disease secondary to, multiple sclerosis, terminal cancer, or AIDS, for example*

*Related to substance abuse*

*Related to cognitive distortions secondary to depression*

**Situational (Personal, Environmental)**

*Related to change from curative status to palliative status*

*Related to feeling of loss of control and lifestyle restrictions secondary to (specify)*

*Related to overeating patterns*

*Related to personal characteristics that highly value control (e.g., internal locus of control)*

*Related to effects of hospital or institutional limitations*

*Related to elevated fear of disapproval*

*Related to consistent negative feedback*

*Related to long-term abusive relationship*

**Maturational**

*Adolescent*

*Older Adult*

*Related to multiple losses secondary to aging (e.g., retirement, sensory deficits, motor deficits, money, significant others)*

## AUTHOR'S NOTE

Powerlessness is a feeling that all people experience to varying degrees in various situations. Stephenson (1979) described two types of powerlessness. *Situational powerlessness* occurs in a specific event and is probably short-lived. *Trait powerlessness* is more pervasive, affecting general outlook, goals, lifestyle, and relationships. The nursing diagnosis *Powerlessness* may be more useful clinically when describing a client experiencing trait rather than situational powerlessness.

Hopelessness differs from powerlessness in that a hopeless client sees no solution to problems or no way to achieve what is desired, even if he or she feels in control. A powerless client may see an alternative or answer yet is unable to do anything about it because of perception of lack of control and resources. Prolonged powerlessness may lead to hopelessness.

## ERRORS IN DIAGNOSTIC STATEMENTS

### Powerlessness Related to Hospitalization

Hospitalization evokes varied responses in people and families, including anxiety, fear, and powerlessness. If the hospitalization is expected to be short, the diagnosis of *Anxiety related to unfamiliar environment, loss of usual routines, and invasion of privacy* may be useful to describe situational powerlessness. If the hospitalization is a readmission for a continuing problem, *Powerlessness* may be more appropriate to describe trait powerlessness. The nurse should restate the diagnosis as *Powerlessness related to readmission for pulmonary infection and effects of illness on career and marriage.*

## KEY CONCEPTS

### Generic Considerations

- A client's response to loss of control depends on the meaning of the loss, individual coping patterns, personal characteristics (psychological, sociologic, cultural, spiritual), and response of others.
- When a client does not expect to be able to control outcomes, attention to and retention of information are poor.
- Powerlessness is very closely related to, but not synonymous with, the concept of external versus internal locus of control. Locus of control is a rather stable personality trait, whereas powerlessness is situationally determined.
- People with an internal locus of control believe they can affect outcomes by actively manipulating themselves or the environment. Examples of internal behavior are participating in regular exercise, acquiring printed literature about a new diagnosis, or learning assertiveness skills.
- People with external locus of control believe that outcomes are outside their control and attribute what happens to them to others or to fate. Examples of external behavior are losing weight because of fear of a professional's response and blaming others for his present position (e.g., depression, anger).
- Internally controlled people motivate themselves, whereas externally controlled people usually need others to motivate them. Young children are usually internally controlled but can learn to be externally controlled. For example, a child can learn to keep a record of the nutrients needed daily and his intake of them to help him understand the concept of good nutrition and to encourage him to take responsibility for his eating patterns.
- People with an internal locus of control may experience the loss of decision-making ability more profoundly than those with an external locus of control. Clients with external locus of control seem to be more prone to develop powerlessness.
- Powerlessness is part of a continuum with hopelessness and helplessness.
- Younger adults tend to cope more effectively with uncontrollable situations if positive past experiences have been present, and if high income and high occupational status are present.

### Pediatric Considerations

- Hospitalized children commonly experience powerlessness.
- Differentiating *Powerlessness* from *Anxiety* and *Fear* may be difficult, especially in children. Refer to Key Concepts, Pediatric Considerations under *Anxiety* and *Fear*.

- Children with a more positive self-concept and a higher perceived ability to control their own health were more likely to adhere to treatments (Burkhart & Rayens, 2005).

## Geriatric Considerations

- Older adults are at high risk for powerlessness because multiple losses (previous roles, family, health, and functioning) may accompany the aging process. The added stressors of illness and institutionalization only compound feelings of powerlessness (O'Heath, 1991). Miller describes seven sources of power: physical strength and reserve, psychological stamina and support network, positive self-concept, energy, knowledge, motivation, and belief system (Miller, 1983).
- A source of power is gained by being able to control one's own life; however, this can be derailed by powerlessness experienced in negative client–nurse relationships (Oudshoorn, Ward-Griffin, & McWilliam, 2007).
- Personality traits, various effects of diseases, and environmental conditions affect powerlessness. For older adults, disease states might restrict mobility. Changes in environment (e.g., relocating to an extended care facility) can remove opportunities for decision-making and autonomy. Institutional policy may require physical or chemical restraints for certain agitated behaviors (Miller, 2009).
- Late-life changes in role, resources, and responsibility can contribute to feelings of loss of control.
- Extensive interactions with caregivers, rather than peers, can lead to a sense of powerlessness. This has implications for the older client, who, with an increased chance of multiple chronic illnesses, might be in the sick role for an extended period (Lambert & Lambert, 1981; Miller, 2009).
- In the elderly, perceived control over desirable outcomes is linked to high emotional well-being; conversely, perceived control by others is an emotional risk factor.

## Transcultural Considerations

- The diagnosis of *Powerlessness* can be problematic with clients from various cultures. In Latin cultures, the concept of fatalism (e.g., what will be will be) may be a challenge to a nurse who is trying to initiate a lifestyle change for better health (Andrews & Boyle, 2008; Giger & Davidhizar, 2009).
- Appropriate language interaction, inclusion of client and family, and healthcare provider's ability to show respect and compassion can prevent many healthcare related problems encountered by immigrants with poor language skills (Garrett, Dickson, Young, & Whelan, 2008).
- The powerlessness associated with fatalism is accepted, and this usually does not constitute a problem for the client.
- Preferences for involvement in health care decision-making are in part related to national health policy and communication.

## Focus Assessment Criteria

Because powerlessness is subjective, the nurse must validate with the client all inferences concerning the client's feelings of powerlessness. The nurse assesses each client to determine his or her usual level of control and decision-making and the effects that losing elements of control has had. To plan effective interventions, the nurse must determine whether the client usually seeks to change his or her own behaviors to control problems, or whether he or she expects others or external factors to control problems.

## Subjective Data

### Assess for Defining Characteristics

#### Decision-Making Patterns
"How would you describe your usual method of making decisions (career, financial, health care)?"
Make them alone
Consult with others for advice (who?)
Allow others to make them for me (spouse? children? others?)

#### Individual and Role Responsibilities
Ask what responsibilities the client had:

- As a school child and adolescent?
- At home?
- At work?
- In community and religious organizations?

## Assess for Related Factors

### Perception of Control

"How would you describe your ability—high, moderate, fair, or poor—to control or cure your present health problem (e.g., diabetes mellitus, aphasia, activity intolerance, obesity)?"

"To what do you attribute your (high, moderate, fair, poor) ability to control?"

Preventive measures

| | | | |
|---|---|---|---|
| Good nutrition | Stress management | Weight control | Exercise program |
| Others | | | |
| Physician | Significant others | Nurse | |
| Peer group | | | |
| No control | | | |
| Fate | Luck | Chance | |

## Objective Data

## Assess for Defining Characteristics

### Participation in Grooming and Hygiene Care (When Indicated)

| | |
|---|---|
| Actively seeks involvement | Requires encouragement |
| Reluctant to participate | Refuses to participate |

### Information-Seeking Behaviors

Actively seeks information and literature from others concerning condition

Requires encouragement to ask questions

Refuses to receive information

Expresses lack of interest

### Response to Limits Placed on Decision-Making and Self-Control Behaviors

| | |
|---|---|
| Acceptance | Increases attempts to exercise control |
| Apathy | Depression |
| Attempts to circumvent limits | Anger |
| Ignores limits | Withdrawal |

### Nonverbal Language

| | |
|---|---|
| Posture | Tone of voice |
| Eye contact | Gestures |

For more information on Focus Assessment Criteria, visit http://thepoint.lww.com.

---

**NOC**

Depression Control, Health Beliefs, Health Beliefs: Perceived Control, Participation: Health Care Decisions

## ► Goal

The client will verbalize ability to control or influence situations and outcomes.

### Indicators:

- Identify factors that the client can control.
- The client will make decisions regarding his or her care, treatment, and future when possible.

**NIC**
Mood Management,
Teaching: Individual,
Decision-Making
Support, Self-
Responsibility
Facilitation, Health
System Guidance,
Spiritual Support

## ➤ General Interventions

### Assess for Causative and Contributing Factors

Lack of knowledge

Previous inadequate coping patterns (e.g., depression; for discussion, see *Ineffective Coping related to depression*)

Insufficient decision-making opportunities

### Eliminate or Reduce Contributing Factors, If Possible

#### *Lack of Knowledge*

Increase effective communication between client and health care provider.

Explain all procedures, rules, and options to the client; avoid medical jargon. Help the client anticipate situations that will occur during treatments (provides reality-oriented cognitive images that bolster a sense of control and coping strategies).

Allow time to answer questions; ask the client to write questions down so he or she does not forget them.

Provide a specific time (10 to 15 min) per shift that the client knows can be used to ask questions or discuss subjects as desired.

Anticipate questions/interest and offer information. Help the client to anticipate events and outcomes.

While being realistic, point out positive changes in the client's condition, such as serum enzymes decreasing after myocardial infarction or surgical incision healing well.

**R:** People with chronic illness require adjustments to make sense of the disease, accept the prognosis, and move forward with living with the condition (Yu, Lee, Kwong, Thompson, & Woo, 2008). People with a sense of hope, self-control, direction, purpose, and identity are better able to meet the challenges of their disease.

Be an active listener by allowing the client to verbalize concerns and feelings; assess for areas of concern.

Designate one nurse to be responsible for a 24-h plan of care, and provide opportunities for the client and family to identify with this nurse.

**R:** Powerlessness can be ameliorated by implementing coping strategies and by having consistent and reliable nursing care (Carroll, 2007).

If contributing factors are pain or anxiety, provide information on how to use behavioral control techniques (e.g., relaxation, imagery, deep breathing).

**R:** Feelings of powerlessness and helplessness are closely associated with incurable diseases (Neufeld, Harrison, Stewart, & Hughes, 2008)

### *Provide Opportunities for the Client to Control Decisions and to Identify Personal Goals of Care*

Allow the client to manipulate surroundings, such as deciding what is to be kept where (shoes under bed, picture on window).

If the client desires, and as hospital policy permits, encourage the client to bring personal effects from home (e.g., pillows, pictures).

Keep needed items within reach (call bell, urinal, tissues).

Do not offer options if there are none (e.g., a deep intramuscular [IM] Z-track injection must be rotated). Offer options that are personally relevant.

Discuss daily plan of activities and allow the client to make as many decisions as possible about it.

Increase decision-making opportunities as the client progresses.

Respect and follow the client's decision if you have given him options.

Record the client's specific choices on care plan to ensure that others on staff acknowledge preferences ("dislikes orange juice," "takes showers," "plan dressing change at 7:30 AM before shower").

Keep promises.

Provide opportunity for the client and family to express feelings.

Provide opportunities for the client and family to participate in care.

Be alert for signs of paternalism/maternalism in health care providers (e.g., making decisions for clients).

Plan a care conference to allow staff to discuss methods of individualizing care; encourage each nurse to share at least one action that she or he discovered a particular person liked.

Shift emphasis from what one cannot do to what one can do.

Set goals that are short-term, behavioral, practical, and realistic (walk 5 more feet every day; then in 1 week, client can walk to the television room).

Provide daily recognition of progress.

Praise gains/achievements.

Assist in identifying factors that are controllable and those that are not. Assist in accepting what cannot be changed and altering what can.

Emphasize positive aspects when the client becomes focused on fears of the worst (reduces fear by shifting perspective and allowing the client to regain control).

Allow the client to experience outcomes that result from his own actions.

**R:** People with chronic illness require adjustments to make sense of the disease, accept the prognosis, and move forward with living with the condition (Yu, Lee, Kwong, Thompson, & Woo, 2008). People with a sense of hope, self-control, direction, purpose, and identity are better able to meet the challenges of their disease.

**R:** Changing passivity into active decision-making plays an important role in reducing anxiety associated with powerlessness (Corradi, 2007).

## Monitor a Client with External Locus of Control to Encourage Participation

Have the client keep a record (e.g., food intake for 1 week; weight loss chart; exercise program; type and frequency of medications taken).

Use telephone or e-mail contact to monitor the client if feasible.

Provide explicit written directions (e.g., meal plans; exercise regimen—type, frequency, duration; speech practice lessons—for aphasia).

Teach significant others methods to manipulate behaviors, if appropriate.

Provide reward for each goal reached.

**R:** Create a learning environment that assists the client to identify self-management strategies that are meaningful to him or her.

## Assist the Client in Deriving Power from Other Sources

Give permission to use other power sources to both client and significant others (e.g., prayer, stress reduction techniques)

Self-help groups

Support groups

Offer referral to religious leader

Provide privacy and support for other measures the client may request (e.g., meditation, imagery, special rituals)

**R:** Self-help groups that focused on empowerment issues assisted participants in the direction of valuable progress toward recovery (Stang & Mittelmark, 2008).

**R:** The client can be empowered through an enhanced educational experiences and opportunities to share their fears and concerns (Johansson, Salantera, & Katajisto, 2007).

**R:** Setting realistic goals can increase motivation and hope.

**R:** Self-concept can be enhanced when clients actively engage in decisions regarding health and lifestyle.

# Initiate Health Teaching and Referrals as Indicated (Social Worker, Psychiatric Nurse/Physician, Visiting Nurse, Religious Leader, Self-Help Groups)

## Evaluate the Situation with the Client

Once the outcome criteria have been accomplished or feelings of powerlessness are diminishing, discuss the process used to relieve powerlessness. Explain how factors contributed to the powerlessness, review why certain strategies were effective, and discuss how the client will manage feelings of powerlessness in the future.

Advocate within the system to eliminate policies and routines that contribute to powerlessness.

**R:** Self-concept can be enhanced when clients actively engage in decisions regarding health and lifestyle.

**Pediatric Interventions**

Provide opportunities for the child to make decisions (e.g., set time for bath, hold still for injection). Engage the child in play therapy before and after a traumatic situation (refer to *Delayed Growth and Development* for specific interventions for age-related development needs).

**R:** The goals of nursing interventions to treat powerlessness include modifying the environment to resemble the child's home and providing opportunities for acceptable control Children can gain mastery over stressful situations by participating in play activities while ill or hospitalized (Hockenberry & Wilson, 2009).

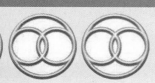

# INEFFECTIVE PROTECTION

**Ineffective Protection**

Impaired Tissue Integrity
Impaired Skin Integrity
Risk for Impaired Skin Integrity
Related to the Effects of Pressure, Friction, Shear, Maceration
Impaired Oral Mucous Membrane
Risk for Impaired Oral Mucous Membrane
Related to Inadequate Oral Hygiene or Inability to Perform Oral Hygiene

## DEFINITION

State in which a client experiences a decrease in the ability to guard against internal or external threats, such as illness or injury

## DEFINING CHARACTERISTICS

### Major (Must Be Present, One or More)

| | | |
|---|---|---|
| Deficient immunity | Impaired healing | Altered clotting |
| Maladaptive stress response | Neurosensory alterations | Pressure ulcers |

### Minor (May Be Present)

| | | |
|---|---|---|
| Chills | Insomnia | Perspiration |
| Fatigue | Dyspnea | Anorexia |
| Cough | Weakness | Itching |
| Immobility | Restlessness | Disorientation |
| Pressure sores | | |

### ■■■■■ AUTHOR'S NOTE

This broad diagnosis describes a client with compromised ability to defend against microorganisms, bleeding, or both because of immunosuppression, myelosuppression, abnormal clotting factors, or all these. Use of this diagnosis entails several potential problems.

*(continued)*

■■■■■■ **AUTHOR'S NOTE** *Continued*

The nurse is cautioned against substituting *Ineffective Protection* for an immune system compromise, acquired immunodeficiency syndrome (AIDS), disseminated intravascular coagulation, diabetes mellitus, or other disorders. Rather, the nurse should focus on diagnoses describing the client's functional abilities that are or may be compromised by altered protection, such as *Fatigue*, *Risk for Infection*, and *Risk for Social Isolation*. The nurse also should address the physiologic complications of altered protection that require nursing and medical interventions for management, identifying appropriate collaborative problems.

For example, the nurse could use *Ineffective Protection* in each of these three cases: Mr. A, who has leukemia, leukopenia, and no evidence of infection; Mr. B, who is experiencing sickle cell crisis; and Mr. C, who has AIDS. The problem is that this diagnosis does not describe the specific focus of nursing but describes situations in which more specific responses can be diagnosed. For Mr. A, the nursing diagnosis of *Risk for Infection related to compromised immune system* would apply. For Mr. B., the collaborative problem *RC of Sickle Cell Crisis* best describes his situation, which the nurse monitors and manages using physician- and nurse-prescribed interventions. The nursing diagnosis *Risk for Infection* and the collaborative problem *RC of Opportunistic Infections* would apply for Mr. C.

As these examples show, in most cases, the nursing diagnosis *Risk for Infection* and selected collaborative problems prove more clinically useful than *Ineffective Protection*.

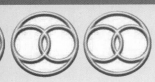

# IMPAIRED TISSUE INTEGRITY

## DEFINITION

State in which a client experiences or is at risk for damage to the integumentary, corneal, or mucous membranous tissues of the body

## DEFINING CHARACTERISTICS

### Major (Must Be Present)

Disruptions of corneal, integumentary, or mucous membranous tissue or invasion of body structure (incision, dermal ulcer, corneal ulcer, oral lesion)

### Minor (May Be Present)

| | | |
|---|---|---|
| Lesions (primary, secondary) | Dry mucous membrane | Edema |
| Leukoplakia | Erythema | Coated tongue |

## RELATED FACTORS

### Pathophysiologic

*Related to inflammation of dermal–epidermal junctions secondary to:*

*Autoimmune alterations:*

| | |
|---|---|
| Lupus erythematosus | Scleroderma |

*Metabolic and endocrine alterations:*

| | | |
|---|---|---|
| Diabetes mellitus | Jaundice | Hepatitis |
| Cancer | Cirrhosis | Thyroid dysfunction |
| Renal failure | | |

*Bacterial:*

| | | |
|---|---|---|
| Impetigo | Folliculitis | Cellulitis |

*Viral:*

| Herpes zoster [shingles] | Herpes simplex | Gingivitis |
| AIDS | | |

*Fungal:*

| Ringworm [dermatophytosis] | Athlete's foot | Vaginitis |

**Related to decreased blood and nutrients to tissues secondary to:**

*Diabetes mellitus:*

| Peripheral vascular | Anemia | Cardiopulmonary disorders |
|   alterations | Venous stasis | Arteriosclerosis |

**Nutritional alterations:**

| Obesity | Emaciation | Dehydration |
| Malnutrition | Edema | |

## Treatment-Related

**Related to decreased blood and nutrients to tissues secondary to:**

| Therapeutic extremes | NPO status | Surgery |
|   in body temperature | | |

**Related to imposed immobility secondary to sedation**

**Related to mechanical trauma**

Therapeutic fixation devices

| Wired jaw | Casts | Traction |
| Orthopedic devices/braces | | |

**Related to effects of radiation on epithelial and basal cells**

**Related to effects of mechanical irritants or pressure secondary to:**

| Inflatable or foam donuts | Tourniquets | Footboards     Restraints |
| Dressings, tape, solutions | External urinary catheters | Nasogastric (NG) tubes |
| Endotracheal tubes | Oral prostheses/braces | Contact lenses |

## Situational (Personal, Environmental)

**Related to chemical trauma secondary to:**

| Excretions | Secretions | Noxious agents/substances |

**Related to environmental irritants secondary to:**

| Radiation–sunburn | Humidity | Bites (insect, animal) |
| Poisonous plants | Temperature | Parasites |
| Inhalants | | |

**Related to the effects of pressure of immobility secondary to:**

| Pain | Fatigue | Motivation |
| Cognitive, sensory, or motor deficits | | |

**Related to inadequate personal habits (hygiene/dental/dietary/sleep)**

**Related to impaired mobility secondary to (specify)**

**Related to thin body frame**

## Maturational

**Related to dry, thin skin and decreased dermal vascularity secondary to aging**

■■■■■ **AUTHOR'S NOTE**

*Impaired Tissue Integrity* is the broad diagnosis under which the more specific diagnoses of *Impaired Skin Integrity* and *Impaired Oral Mucous Membranes* fall. Because tissue is composed of epithelium, connective tissue, muscle, and nervous tissue, *Impaired Tissue Integrity* correctly describes some pressure ulcers that are deeper than the dermis. *Impaired Skin Integrity* should be used to describe disruptions of epidermal and dermal tissue only. (Refer to p. 590 for definitions of stages.)

*(continued)*

## AUTHOR'S NOTE *Continued*

When a pressure ulcer is stage IV, necrotic, or infected, it may be more appropriate to label the diagnosis a collaborative problem, such as *Risk for Complications of Stage IV Pressure Ulcer*. This would represent a situation that a nurse manages with physician- and nurse-prescribed interventions. When a stage II or III pressure ulcer needs a dressing that requires a physician's order in an acute-care setting, the nurse should continue to label the situation a nursing diagnosis because it would be appropriate and legal for a nurse to treat the ulcer independently in other settings (e.g., in the community).

If a client is immobile and multiple systems are threatened (respiratory, circulatory, musculoskeletal as well as integumentary), the nurse can use *Disuse Syndrome* to describe the entire situation. If a client is at risk for damage to corneal tissue, the nurse can use a diagnosis such as *Risk for Impaired Corneal Tissue Integrity related to corneal drying and lower lacrimal production secondary to unconscious state*.

## ERRORS IN DIAGNOSTIC STATEMENTS

1. *Impaired Skin Integrity related to surgical removal of skin/tissues*
   *Impaired Skin Integrity* should not be used as a new label for surgical incisions, tracheostomies, or burns. Surgical incisions disrupt the skin's protective mechanism, increasing vulnerability to microorganism invasion; a more clinically useful diagnosis would be *Risk for Infection related to surgical incision*.
2. *Impaired Skin Integrity related to fecal diversion*
   The nurse should not rename fecal diversions such as colostomy or ileostomy with the nursing diagnosis *Impaired Skin Integrity*. Instead, the nurse should assess the client's actual or potential responses to the surgical procedure that the nurse can treat. For example, the skin around an ostomy is at risk for erosion from effluent, calling for *Risk for Impaired Skin Integrity related to chemical irritation of effluent on adjacent skin*. If the adjacent skin exhibits lesions from irritants (chemical or mechanical), *Impaired Skin Integrity related to exposure to ostomy effluent, as evidenced by a 2-cm ulcer left midline of stoma* would be appropriate.

## KEY CONCEPTS

### Generic Considerations

- At any given time, more than 1 million Americans are estimated to have pressure ulcers. Pressure ulcer incidence ranges from 2.7% to 29.5% in acute care settings, as high as 41% in critical care populations, and from 2.4% to 23% in skilled nursing facilities and nursing homes (Maklebust & Sieggreen, 2006).
- Tissues are groupings of specialized cells that unite to perform specific functions. The human body is composed of four basic types of tissue: epithelial, connective (including skeletal tissue and blood), muscle, and nervous.
- The external covering of the body is composed of epithelial tissue, called the integument. Wherever the body exposes large openings to the outside (e.g., the mouth), its outer covering changes from integument to an inner lining called the mucous membrane. Each layer of the integument has its counterpart in a complete mucous membrane. The integument includes both the skin and the subcutaneous tissue.
- The skin is a complex organ consisting of two layers: the outer epidermis and the deeper dermis. The epidermis is approximately 0.04 mm thick, and the dermis is about 0.5 cm thick (Porth, 2007).
- The epidermis functions as a barrier to protect inner tissues (from injury, chemicals, organisms); as a receptor for a range of sensations (touch, pain, heat, cold); as a regulator of body temperature through radiation (giving off heat), conduction (transfer of heat), and convection (movement of warm air molecules away from the body); as a regulator of water balance by preventing water and electrolyte loss; and as a receptor for vitamin D from the sun (Maklebust & Sieggreen, 2006).
- A water-soluble mitotic inhibitor called *chalone* depresses epidermal regeneration. Chalone levels are high during daytime stress and activity and lower during sleep. Therefore, healing is promoted during rest and sleep (Maklebust & Sieggreen, 2006).

*(continued)*

■■■■■■ **KEY CONCEPTS** *Continued*

- Beneath the avascular epidermis lies the highly vascularized dermis. The dermis contains epithelial tissue, connective tissue, muscle, and nervous tissue. The dermis is rich in collagen, which imparts toughness to the skin. Hair follicles extend into the dermis and serve as islands of cells for rapid reepithelialization of minor wounds. Sweat glands in the dermis contribute to control of body water and temperature. Small muscles within the dermis serve to produce goose pimples. Specialized dermal nerve endings for pain, touch, heat, and cold cannot be replaced once destroyed (Maklebust & Sieggreen, 2006).
- The subcutaneous tissue, which lies beneath the dermis, stores fat for temperature regulation and contains the remainder of the sweat glands and hair follicles (Porth, 2007).
- The skin's responses to antigens are capillary dilation (erythema), arteriole dilation (flare), and increased capillary permeability (wheal), which all contribute to localized edema, spasms, and pruritus.
- Causes of tissue destruction can be mechanical, immunologic, bacterial, chemical, or thermal. Mechanical destruction includes physical trauma and surgical incision. Immunologic destruction occurs as an allergic response. Bacterial destruction results from an overgrowth of organisms. Chemical destruction results when a caustic substance contacts unprotected tissue. Thermal destruction occurs when tissue is exposed to temperature extremes that are incompatible with cell life (Maklebust & Sieggreen, 2006).

## Wound Healing

- Wound healing is a complex sequence of events initiated by injury to the tissues. The components are coagulation of bleeding, inflammation, epithelialization, fibroplasia and collagen metabolism, collagen maturation, scar remodeling, and wound contraction.
- A wound must be considered in relation to the entire client. Major factors that affect wound healing are nutrition, vitamins, minerals, anemia, blood volume and tissue oxygenation, steroids and anti-inflammatory drugs, diabetes mellitus, chemotherapy, and radiation.
- Wound healing requires the following intrinsic factors (Dudek, 2006):
  - Increased protein–carbohydrate intake sufficient to prevent negative nitrogen balance, hypoalbuminemia, and weight loss
  - Increased daily intake of vitamins and minerals
  - Vitamin A, 10,000 to 50,000 IU
  - Vitamin $B_1$, 0.5 to 1.0 mg/1,000 diet calories
  - Vitamin $B_2$, 0.25 mg/1,000 diet calories
  - Vitamin $B_6$, 2 mg
  - Niacin, 15 to 20 mg
  - Vitamin $B_{12}$, 400 mg
  - Vitamin C, 75 to 300 mg
  - Vitamin D, 400 mg
  - Vitamin E, 10 to 15 IU
  - Traces of zinc, magnesium, calcium, copper, manganese
- Vitamin K indirectly aids in healing wounds by assisting in the prevention of hematoma formation, and subsequently reducing infection (Porth, 2007).
- Adequate oxygen supply and the blood volume and ability to transport it.

## Pediatric Considerations

- A newborn commonly exhibits normal skin variations, such as mongolian spots, milia, and stork bites, which can be upsetting to parents but are clinically insignificant.
- Several common skin conditions affect children in specific age groups. These include atopic, seborrheic, and diaper dermatitis in infancy and acne in adolescence.
- Infants and young children have a thin epidermis and require special protection from the sun.

## Geriatric Considerations

- Elastin, which gives the skin flexibility, elasticity, and tensile strength, decreases with age. It is found in tissues associated with body movement, such as the walls of major blood vessels, heart, lungs, and skin (Boynton et al., 1999). The decreased turgor results in dry, wrinkled skin.
- Collagen, found in all connective tissue, such as blood, lymph, and bone, binds together and supports other tissues. The extracellular matrix of connecting tissue is composed primarily of collagen and elastin, and approximately 80% of the dermis consists of collagen. With aging, skin strength decreases owing to age-related loss of collagen from the dermis and the degeneration of the elastic properties of the remaining collagen.
- Some older adults exhibit shiny, loose, thin, transparent skin, primarily on the backs of the hands and the forearms. Subcutaneous fat decreases with aging, reducing the cushioning of bony prominences and putting older adults at increased risk for pressure ulcers.
- Aging causes diminished immunocompetence and decreased angiogenesis, which delays wound healing (Boynton et al., 1999).
- Age-related decreases in sebum secretion and the number of sebaceous glands cause drier, coarser skin that is more prone to fissures and cracks.
- In older adults, cells are larger and proliferate more slowly, fibroblasts decrease in number, and dermal vascularity decreases. All these factors contribute to slower wound healing.
- With aging, the thermal threshold for sweating increases and the sweat output decreases.
- Aging nails become dull, brittle, and thickened owing to decreased blood supply to the nailbed. Splitting of the nails can occur, increasing the risk of infection. Thickening of the toenails causes the distal portion of the nail to lift from the nailbed; debris collection creates a risk of fungal infection.

## Transcultural Considerations

- The darker the client's skin, the more difficult it is to assess for changes in color. A baseline must be established in daylight or with at least a 60-watt bulb. Baseline skin color should be assessed in areas with the least amount of pigmentation (e.g., palms of hands, soles of feet, underside of forearms, abdomen, and buttocks; Weber & Kelley, 2003).
- All skin colors have an underlying red tone. Pallor in black-skinned people is seen as an ashen or gray tone. Pallor in brown-skinned people appears as a yellowish-brown color. Pallor can be assessed in mucous membranes, lips, nailbeds, and conjunctiva of the lower eyelids (Andrews & Boyle, 2008).
- Assessment of capillary refill time can be done on the second or third finger, lips, or earlobes (Andrews & Boyle, 2008).
- To assess for rashes and skin inflammations in dark-skinned people, the nurse should rely on palpation for warmth and induration, not observation (Giger & Davidhizar, 2009).
- Mongolian spots are dark-blue or black areas of pigmentation seen on the skin of black, Asian, Native American, or Mexican American newborns. They are often mistaken for bruises. By adulthood, they are lighter but still visible (Giger & Davidhizar, 2009).
- Some folk remedies may be misdiagnosed as injuries. Three folk practices of Southeast Asians leave marks on the body that can be taken for signs of violence or abuse. *Cao gio* is rubbing of the skin with a coin to produce dark blood or ecchymotic strips; it is done to treat colds and flu-like symptoms. *Bat gio* is skin pinching on the temples to treat headaches or on the neck for a sore throat; if petechiae or ecchymoses appear, the treatment is a success. *Poua* is the burning of the skin with the tip of a dried weed like grass; it is believed the burning will cause the noxious element that causes the pain to exude (Andrews & Boyle, 2008).

# Focus Assessment Criteria

## Subjective Data

### Assess for Related Factors

**History of Symptoms**
Onset
Precipitated by what?
Relieved by what?
Frequency?

### History of Exposure (If Allergy Is Suspected)
Carrier of contagious disease
Chemicals, paints, cleaning agents, plants, and animals
Heat or cold

### Medical, Surgical, and Dental History; Use of Tobacco, Alcohol
Current Drug Therapy
What drugs? How often? When was last dose taken?
Effects on symptoms?

### Factors Contributing to the Development or Extension of Tissue Destruction (Assess for):
*Skin deficits:*

| | | |
|---|---|---|
| Dryness | Thinness | Edema |
| Excessive perspiration | Obesity | Aging skin |

*Mucous membrane deficits:*

| | | |
|---|---|---|
| Mouth pain | Oral lesions or ulcers | Bleeding gums |
| Oral plaque | Coated tongue | Dryness |

*Corneal deficits:*

| | | |
|---|---|---|
| Absence of blink reflex | Excessive tearing | Ptosis |
| Contact lens wear | Diminished tearing | Sensory deficits |

*Impaired oxygen transport:*
Edema
Anemia
Peripheral vascular disorders

| | | |
|---|---|---|
| Arteriosclerosis | Venous stasis | Cardiopulmonary disorders |

*Chemical/mechanical irritants:*

| | | |
|---|---|---|
| Radiation | Contact lenses | Casts, splints, braces |
| Oral prostheses | Incontinence (feces, urine) | |

*Nutritional deficiencies:*

| | | |
|---|---|---|
| Protein | Vitamin | Mineral and trace elements |

Dehydration
*Systemic disorders:*
Refer to Related Factors (Pathophysiologic).
*Sensory deficits:*

| | | |
|---|---|---|
| Decreased level of consciousness | Neuropathy | Visual or taste alterations |
| | Brain or cord injury | Confusion |

*Immobility:*

## Objective Data

## *Assess for Defining Characteristics*

### Skin

| | | |
|---|---|---|
| Color | Texture | Turgor |
| Vascularity | Moisture | Temperature |

Lesions:

| | | |
|---|---|---|
| Type | Shape | Location |
| Size | Distribution | Drainage |

Color
Circulation
Do capillaries refill within 3 s after blanching?
Does erythema subside within 30 min after pressure is removed?
Edema
Note degree and location
Palpate over bony prominences for sponginess (indicates edema)

## *Oral Mucous Membrane*

Refer to Focus Assessment Criteria for *Impaired Oral Mucous Membrane*.
For more information on Focus Assessment Criteria, visit http://thepoint.lww.com.

**NOC**
Tissue Integrity

➤ # Goal

The client will demonstrate progressive healing of tissue.

### *Indicators:*

• Participate in risk assessment.
• Express willingness to participate in prevention of pressure ulcers.
• Describe etiology and prevention measures.
• Explain rationale for interventions.

**NIC**
Teaching: Individual,
Surveillance

➤ # General Interventions

## Identify Causative/Contributing Factors

Refer to Related Factors.

## Reduce Contributing Factors to Mechanical Irritants to Skin

Encourage highest degree of mobility to avoid prolonged periods of pressure.
For neuromuscular impairment:

• Teach the client/significant other appropriate measures to prevent pressure, shear, friction, maceration.
• Teach the client to recognize early signs of tissue damage.
• Change the client's position at least every 2 h around the clock.
• Use a 30-degree lateral side-lying position.
• Frequently supplement full-body turns with minor shifts in body weight.

Keep client clean and dry.
Reduce environmental sources of pressure (drains, tubes, dressings).
Avoid stripping of epidermis when removing adhesives.
Use pressure-dispersing devices as appropriate.
Limit semi-Fowler's position in high-risk clients (limit elevation of head of bed to less than 30 degrees).
Avoid use of knee gatch on bed.
Use lift sheet to reposition the client.
Install an overhead trapeze to allow the clients increased mobility.
Use cornstarch to reduce friction and moisture.

**R:** Principles of pressure ulcer prevention include reducing or rotating pressure on soft tissue. If pressure on soft tissue exceeds intracapillary pressure (approximately 32 mm Hg), capillary occlusion and resulting hypoxia can cause tissue damage. The greater the duration of immobility, the greater the likelihood of the development of small vessel thrombosis and subsequent tissue necrosis (Smeltzer, Bare, Hinkle, & Cheever, 2008).

**R:** Exercise and mobility increase blood flow to all areas.

**R:** Keeping the bed as flat as possible (lower than 30 degrees) and supporting the feet with a footboard help prevent shear, the pressure created when two adjacent tissue layers move in opposition. If a bony prominence slides across the subcutaneous tissue, the subepidermal capillaries may become bent and pinched, resulting in decreased tissue perfusion.

## Reduce Causative Factors, If Possible

For casts:

• Monitor common pressure sites in relationship to cast application.
• Apply padding over bony prominence.
• Keep cast edges smooth and away from skin surfaces.
• Inspect for loose plaster and shifting of padding.

**R:** Prolonged pressure of the cast on neurovascular structures and other body parts can cause necrosis, pressure sores, and nerve palsies.

**R:** Padding over bony prominences is essential to prevent pressure ulcers.

**R:** Rough or improperly bent plaster edges may cause damage to surrounding skin by friction. When an extremity is not elevated properly, cast edges press into the skin and cause pain.

**R:** Loose plaster or wrinkled padding can irritate skin under casts.

## Protect Skin Around Feeding Tubes or Endotracheal Tubes with a Protective Barrier

Change skin barrier when loose or leaking.
Instruct to report discomforts.

**R:** An NG tube can irritate skin and mucosa. Gastric juices can cause severe skin breakdown.

## Teach How to Reduce Mechanical Irritation with Contact Lens Use

Have client review care of lens.
If irritation occurs:

- Remove the contact lens.
- Clean the lens with proper solution.
- Check for tears or chips.
- Reinsert the lens after rewetting.

**R:** Emphasize the need to follow disinfection procedures strictly, to rinse the case daily and air dry, and to replace the case every 3 to 6 months.

**R:** Contact lenses are foreign bodies; teaching should focus on prevention of infection and irritation.

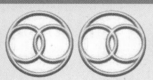

# IMPAIRED SKIN INTEGRITY

▶ **Risk for Impaired Skin Integrity**

## DEFINITION

State in which a client experiences or is at risk for damage to the epidermal and dermal tissue

## DEFINING CHARACTERISTICS

### Major (Must Be Present)

Disruptions of epidermal and dermal tissue.

### Minor (May Be Present)

| | | |
|---|---|---|
| Denuded skin | Erythema | Pruritus |
| Lesions (primary, secondary) | | |

## RELATED FACTORS

See *Impaired Tissue Integrity*.

## Focus Assessment Criteria

See *Impaired Tissue Integrity*.

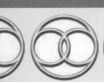

# RISK FOR IMPAIRED SKIN INTEGRITY

**NOC**
Tissue Integrity:
Skin and Mucous
Membrane

➤ **Goal**

The client will demonstrate skin integrity free of pressure ulcers (if able).

*Indicators:*

- Participate in risk assessment.
- Express willingness to participate in prevention of pressure ulcers.
- Describe etiology and prevention measures.

**NIC**
Pressure
Management,
Pressure Ulcer Care,
Skin Surveillance,
Positioning

➤ **General Interventions**

### Use a Formal Risk Assessment Scale to Identify Individual Risk Factors in Addition to Activity and Mobility Deficits (e.g., The Braden Scale, Worton Score [AHCPR, 1992]); Refer to Focus Assessment

### Attempt to Modify Contributing Factors to Lessen the Possibility of a Pressure Ulcer Developing

*Incontinence of Urine or Feces*

Determine the etiology of the incontinence.

Maintain sufficient fluid intake for adequate hydration (approximately 2,500 mL daily, unless contraindicated); check oral mucous membranes for moisture and check urine specific gravity.

Establish a schedule for emptying the bladder (begin with every 2 h).

If the client is confused, determine what his or her incontinence pattern is and intervene before incontinence occurs.

Explain problem to the client; secure his or her cooperation for the plan.

When incontinent, wash the perineum with a liquid soap that does not alter skin pH.

Apply a protective barrier to the perineal region (incontinence film barrier spray or wipes).

Check the client frequently for incontinence when indicated.

For additional interventions, refer to *Impaired Urinary Elimination*.

**R:** Maceration is a mechanism by which the tissue is softened by prolonged wetting or soaking. If the skin becomes waterlogged, the cells are weakened and the epidermis is easily eroded. Bowel incontinence is more damaging than urinary incontinence, due to the additional digestive enzymes found in stool. Care must be taken to prevent excoriation (Wilkinson & Van Leuven, 2007).

*Immobility*

Encourage range-of-motion exercises and weight-bearing mobility, when possible, to increase blood flow to all areas.

Promote optimal circulation when in bed:

- Use repositioning schedule that relieves vulnerable area most often (e.g., if the vulnerable area is the back, the turning schedule would be left side to back, back to right side, right side to left side, and left side to back); post "turn clock" at bedside.
- Turn or instruct the client to turn or shift weight every 30 min to 2 h, depending on other causative factors and the ability of the skin to recover from pressure.
- Increase frequency of the turning schedule if any reddened areas that appear do not disappear within 1 h after turning.
- Place the client in normal or neutral position with body weight evenly distributed. Use 30-degree laterally inclined position when possible.
- Keep the bed as flat as possible to reduce shearing forces; limit semi-Fowler's position to only 30 min at a time.
- Use foam blocks or pillows to provide a bridging effect to support the body above and below the high-risk or ulcerated area so the affected area does not touch the bed surface. Do not use foam donuts or inflatable rings because these increase the area of pressure.
- Alternate or reduce the pressure on the skin with an appropriate support surface.
- Suspend heels off bed surface.
- Use enough personnel to lift the client up in bed or a chair rather than pull or slide skin surfaces.

Have the client wear a long-sleeved top and socks to reduce friction on elbows and heels.
To reduce shearing forces, support the feet with a footboard to prevent sliding.
Promote optimal circulation when the client is sitting.

- Limit sitting time for the client at high risk for ulcer development.
- Instruct the client to lift self using chair arms every 10 min, if possible, or assist the client in rising up off the chair at least every hour, depending on risk factors present.
- Do not elevate the legs unless calves are supported, to reduce the pressure over the ischial tuberosities.
- Pad the chair with pressure-relieving cushion.

Inspect areas at risk of developing ulcers with each position change.

| | | |
|---|---|---|
| Ears | Elbows | Occiput |
| Trochanter* | Heels* | Ischia |
| Sacrum | Scapula | Scrotum |

Observe for erythema and blanching and palpate for warmth and tissue sponginess with each position change.
Do not rub reddened areas. To avoid damaging the capillaries, do not perform massage.

**R:** Pressure is a compressing downward force on a given area. If pressure against soft tissue is greater than intracapillary blood pressure (approximately 32 mm Hg), the capillaries can be occluded, and the tissue can be damaged as a result of hypoxia.

**R:** Shear is a parallel force in which one layer of tissue moves in one direction and another layer moves in the opposite direction. If the skin sticks to the bed linen and the weight of the body makes the skeleton slide down inside the skin (as with semi-Fowler's positioning), the subepidermal capillaries may become angulated and pinched, resulting in decreased perfusion of the tissue (Porth, 2007).

**R:** Friction is the physiologic wearing away of tissue. If the skin is rubbed against the bed linens, the epidermis can be denuded by abrasion.

## Malnourished State

Consult a dietitian.
Increase protein and carbohydrate intake to maintain a positive nitrogen balance; weigh the client daily and determine serum albumin level weekly to monitor status.
Ascertain that daily intake of vitamins and minerals is maintained through diet or supplements (see Key Concepts for recommended amounts).
See *Imbalanced Nutrition: Less Than Body Requirements* for additional interventions.

**R:** Adequate nutrition (protein, vitamins, minerals) is vital for healing wounds, preventing infection, preserving immune function, and minimizing loss of strength (Maklebust & Sieggreen, 2006).

---

*Areas with little soft tissue over a bony prominence are at greatest risk.

### Sensory Deficit

Inspect the client's skin daily because he or she will not experience discomfort.
Teach the client or family to inspect the skin with a mirror.

**R:** A pressure-reducing surface must not be able to be fully compressed by the body. To be effective, a support surface must be capable of first being deformed and then redistributing the weight of the body across the surface. Comfort is not a valid criterion for determining adequate pressure reduction. A hand check should be performed to determine if the product is effectively reducing pressure. The palm is placed under the pressure-reducing mattress; if the client can feel the hand or the caregiver can feel the client, the pressure is not adequate (AHCPR, 1992; Bergstrom et al., 1994).

## Initiate Health Teaching, as Indicated

Instruct the client and family in specific techniques to use at home to prevent pressure ulcers.
Consider the use of long-term pressure-relieving devices for permanent disabilities.

**R:** Pressure reduction is the one consistent intervention that must be included in all pressure ulcer treatment plans.

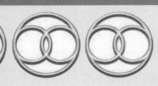

# IMPAIRED SKIN INTEGRITY

## ▶ Related to the Effects of Pressure, Friction, Shear, and Maceration

**NOC**
See *Impaired Skin Integrity*

### ➤ Goal

The client will demonstrate progressive healing of dermal ulcer.

### Indicators:

- Identify causative factors for pressure ulcers.
- Identify rationale for prevention and treatment.
- Participate in the prescribed treatment plan to promote wound healing.

**NIC**
See *Impaired Skin Integrity*

### ➤ General Interventions

### Identify the Stage of Pressure Ulcer Development (AHCPR, 1992)

Stage I: Nonblanchable erythema of intact skin
Stage II: Ulceration of epidermis and/or dermis
Stage III: Ulceration involving subcutaneous fat
Stage IV: Extensive ulceration penetrating muscle, bone, or supporting structure

## Reduce or Eliminate Factors that Contribute to the Extension of Pressure Ulcers

## Refer to **Risk for Impaired Skin Integrity Related to Immobility**

## Prevent Deterioration of the Ulcer

Wash reddened area gently with mild soap, rinse area thoroughly to remove soap, and pat dry.
Avoid massage of bony prominence to stimulate circulation.
Protect the healthy skin surface with one or a combination of the following:

- Apply a thin coat of liquid copolymer skin sealant.
- Cover the area with moisture-permeable film dressing.
- Cover the area with a hydrocolloid wafer barrier and secure with strips of 1-inch tape; leave in place for 2 to 3 days.
- Wound healing occurs most efficiently with the following extrinsic factors (Maklebust & Sieggreen, 2000):
  - Humidity affects the rate of epithelialization and the amount of scar formation. A moist environment provides optimal conditions for rapid healing.
  - When wounds are left uncovered, epidermal cells must migrate under the scab and over the fibrous tissue below. When wounds are semi-occluded and the surface of the wound remains moist, epidermal cells migrate more rapidly over the surface.
  - Appropriate use of dressings may promote a moist wound. Use of semi-occlusive film dressings or hydrocolloid barrier wafers mechanically protect and properly humidify wounds that are epidermal or dermal. These dressings bathe the wound in serous exudate and do not adhere to the wound surface when they are removed. A physician's order may be required.

Increase dietary intake to promote wound healing:

- Initiate calorie count. Consult a dietitian.
- Increase protein and carbohydrate intake to maintain a positive nitrogen balance. Weigh daily and determine serum albumin level weekly to monitor status.
- Ascertain that client maintains daily intake of vitamins and minerals through diet or supplements (see Key Concepts for recommended amounts).
- See *Imbalanced Nutrition: Less Than Body Requirements* for additional interventions.

**R:** Wound healing occurs most efficiently with the following extrinsic factors (Maklebust & Sieggreen, 2006):

- Humidity affects the rate of epithelialization and the amount of scar formation. A moist environment provides optimal conditions for rapid healing.
- When wounds are left uncovered, epidermal cells must migrate under the scab and over the fibrous tissue below. When wounds are semi-occluded and the surface of the wound remains moist, epidermal cells migrate more rapidly over the surface.
- Appropriate use of dressings may promote a moist wound. Use of semi-occlusive film dressings or hydrocolloid barrier wafers mechanically protect and properly humidify wounds that are epidermal or dermal. These dressings bathe the wound in serous exudate and do not adhere to the wound surface when they are removed. A physician's order may be required.

**R:** Wound healing requires increased protein–carbohydrates intake to prevent weight loss and increased intake of vitamins and minerals (Dudek, 2006).

## Devise a Plan for Pressure Ulcer Management Using Principles of Moist Wound Healing (Maklebust & Sieggreen, 2006)

Assess the status of pressure ulcer (Bates-Jensen, 1999).*
Assess the size—measure the longest and widest wound surface.
Assess depth:

- No break in skin
- Abrasion or shallow crater
- Deep crater
- Necrosis
- Involved tendon, joint capsule
- Assess edges.
- Attached
- Not attached
- Fibrotic

*Areas with little soft tissue over a bony prominence are at greatest risk.

Assess undermining:

- Less than 2 cm
- 2 to 4 cm
- Greater than 4 cm
- Tunneling

Assess necrotic tissue type (color, consistency, adherence) and amount.

Assess exudate type and amount.

Assess surrounding skin color.

Check for any peripheral edema and induration.

Assess for granulation tissue.

Assess for epithelialization.

Débride necrotic tissue (collaborate with physician).

Flush ulcer base with sterile saline solution. Avoid use of harsh antiseptic solutions.

Protect granulating wound bed from trauma and bacteria. Insulate wound surface.

Cover pressure ulcer with a sterile dressing that maintains a moist environment over the ulcer base (e.g., film dressing, hydrocolloid wafer dressing, moist gauze dressing). Do not occlude ulcers on immunocompromised patients.

Avoid the use of drying agents (heat lamps, Maalox, Milk of Magnesia).

Monitor for clinical signs of wound infection.

Measure the pressure ulcer weekly to determine progress of wound healing.

**R:** Rationales for topical treatment (Maklebust & Sieggreen, 2006) are as follows:

- Remove necrotic tissue, which delays wound healing by prolonging the inflammatory phase.
- Cleanse wound bed to decrease bacterial count. Bacterial counts above 105 may produce infection by overwhelming the host.
- Obliterate dead space in the wound, which prevents premature closure and abscess formation.
- Absorb excess exudate, which macerates surrounding skin and increases the risk of infection in the wound bed.
- Maintain a moist wound surface, which promotes cellular migration. Dry wound surfaces delay epithelialization secondary to difficult cellular migration.
- Insulate the wound surface; this enhances blood flow and increases epidermal migration.
- Protect the healing wound from trauma and bacterial invasion. Open wounds are vulnerable to abrasion, contamination, drying, and shear mechanisms.

## Consult With Nurse Specialist or Physician for Treatment of Necrotic, Infected, or Deep Pressure Ulcers

**R:** Surgical debridement may be needed.

## Initiate Health Teaching and Referrals, as Indicated

Instruct the client and family on care of ulcers.

Teach the client importance of good skin hygiene and optimal nutrition.

Refer the client to a community nursing agency if additional assistance at home is needed.

**R:** Wound healing occurs most efficiently with the following extrinsic factors (Maklebust & Sieggreen, 2006):

- Humidity affects the rate of epithelialization and the amount of scar formation. A moist environment provides optimal conditions for rapid healing.
- When wounds are left uncovered, epidermal cells must migrate under the scab and over the fibrous tissue below. When wounds are semi-occluded and the surface of the wound remains moist, epidermal cells migrate more rapidly over the surface.
- Appropriate use of dressings may promote moist wound. Use of semi-occlusive film dressings or hydrocolloid barrier wafers mechanically protect and properly humidify wounds that are epidermal or dermal. These dressings bathe the wound in serous exudate and do not adhere to the wound surface when they are removed. A physician's order may be required.

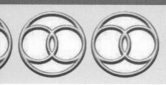

# IMPAIRED ORAL MUCOUS MEMBRANE

## DEFINITION

State in which a person experiences or is at risk for disruptions in the oral cavity

## DEFINING CHARACTERISTICS

### Major (Must Be Present)

Disrupted oral mucous membranes

### Minor (May Be Present)

- Color changes—erythema, pallor, white patches, lesions and ulcers
- Moisture changes—increased or decreased saliva
- Cleanliness changes—debris, malodor, discoloration of the teeth
- Mucosal integrity changes—difficulty swallowing, decreased taste, difficulty weaning
- Perception changes—difficulty swallowing, decreased taste, difficulty wearing dentures, burning, pain, and change in voice quality.

## RELATED FACTORS

### Pathophysiologic

*Related to inflammation secondary to:*

Diabetes mellitus         Periodontal disease         Oral cancer
Infection

### Treatment-Related

*Related to drying effects of:*

NPO more than 24 h

Radiation to head or neck

Prolonged use of steroids or other immunosuppressives and other medications including opioids, antidepressants, phenothiazines, antihypertensives, antihistamines, diuretics and sedatives.

Use of antineoplastic drugs

Oxygen therapy

Mouth breathing

Blood and marrow stem cell transplant

*Related to mechanical irritation secondary to:*

Endotracheal tube         NG tube

### Situational (Personal, Environmental)

*Related to chemical irritants secondary to:*

Acidic foods         Drugs         Noxious agents
Alcohol              Tobacco       High sugar intake

*Related to mechanical trauma secondary to:*

Broken or jagged teeth   Ill-fitting dentures   Braces

*Related to malnutrition*

*Related to inadequate oral hygiene*

*Related to lack of knowledge of oral hygiene*

## ▪▪▪▪▪ AUTHOR'S NOTE

See *Impaired Tissue Integrity*.

## ▪▪▪▪▪ ERRORS IN DIAGNOSTIC STATEMENTS

See *Impaired Tissue Integrity*.

## ▪▪▪▪▪ KEY CONCEPTS

### Generic Considerations

- Oral health directly influences many activities of daily living (eating, fluid intake, breathing) and interpersonal relations (appearance, self-concept, communication).
- Many oral diseases begin quietly and are painless until significant involvement has taken place.
- Common causes of decreased salivation are dehydration, anemia, radiation treatment to head and neck, vitamin deficiencies, removal of salivary glands, allergies, and side effects of drugs (e.g., antihistamines, anticholinergics, phenothiazine, narcotics, chemotherapy).
- Mucosal damage usually occurs 7–14 days after the start of radiation and 3–9 days after the start of chemotherapy.
- The National Cancer Institute (2008) estimates that 40% of chemotherapy patients, 80% of stem cell transplant patients and 100% of radiation to the head and neck will developed oral mucositis.
- Consequences of mucositis include increased mortality risk, delaying treatment, increased need for nutritional support, increased fatigue and bleeding, increased infection risk, pain, and decreased quality of life.
- When the mucosa is damaged, the treatment includes the principles of wound management; moisture, cleansing, and promoting healing.
- Alcohol and tobacco are chronic irritants to oral mucosa and may lead to oral carcinoma.
- Stomatitis is synonymous with oral mucositis.
- Stomatitis and mucositis denote inflammation and ulceration of the oral cavity. Mucositis refers to any oral mucosal inflammation, regardless of cause. It may progress from dry, red, inflamed, cracked areas to open sores of the mucosa and bleeding ulcers anywhere in the mouth, esophagus, vagina, or rectum. Mucous membranes are highly susceptible to toxicity because of their rapidly proliferating cells. Persons exposed to multiple therapies or who have predisposing risk factors such as poor oral hygiene, dental caries, and tobacco or alcohol use are more likely to develop mucositis.
- Chemotherapy or direct radiation also can cause xerostomia, which is a decrease in the quality and quantity of saliva (NCI, 2008).
- The Cochrane Review (2007) showed that allopurinol, certain mouthwashes, granulocyte macrophage colony stimulating factor, immunoglobins or human placenta extract may relieve or cure ulcers caused by cancer treatments. The review also showed that benzydamine, sulcrafate, chlorhexidine and magic mouthwash was not effective in relieving or curing ulcer caused by cancer treatments.
- Palifermin, a keratinocyte growth factor, may prevent chemotherapy-induced oral mucositis for patients with a hematologic malignancy receiving a stem cell transplant. Another advantage is that Palifermin reduces the incidence and duration of the mucositis (Clarkson, 2005).

 **Pediatric Considerations**

- Oral candidiasis (thrush) is common in newborns. It can be acquired by person-to-person transmission, from a maternal vaginal infection during delivery, or from use of contaminated nipples or other articles (Hockenberry & Wilson, 2009).
- Teething may cause discomfort and make gums appear red and swollen.

## Geriatric Considerations

- Age-related changes in oral mucosa include loss of elasticity, atrophy of epithelial cells, and diminished blood supply to connective tissue (Miller, 2009).
- Dry mouth and vitamin deficiencies in older adults increase vulnerability to oral ulcerations and infection (Miller, 2009).
- Older adults commonly exhibit increased saliva viscosity and diminished saliva quantity (Miller, 2009).

# Focus Assessment Criteria

## Subjective Data

### Assess for Defining Characteristics

Refer to Defining Characteristics

### Assess for Related Factors

Refer to Related Factors

## Objective Data and Physical Assessment

Use a standardized oral assessment/measurement tool.

Gather equipment to use to assess oral cavity. Equipment includes a good light source, tongue blade, nonsterile gloves, and gauze to retract the tongue and suction equipment if needed. Systemically examine oral cavity for change in oral mucosa, moisture level, cleanliness, presence of ulcers or lesions, integrity of lips, and quality of speech and voice.

### Assess for Defining Characteristics

#### Lips

| | | |
|---|---|---|
| Color | Cracks | Blisters |
| Fissures | Ulcers/lesions | Bleeding |
| Edema | | |

#### Tongue

| | | |
|---|---|---|
| Color | Masses | Cracks, dryness |
| Ulcers | Edema | Bleeding |
| Lesions | Exudates | Hairy extensions |
| Blisters | | |

#### Oral Mucosa (gums, floor of mouth, inner cheeks, palate)

| | | |
|---|---|---|
| Color | Moisture | Bleeding |
| Plaques | Swelling (along gum line) | Ulcers |
| Saliva | | |
| Watery | Absent | Thick |
| Color | | |

#### Teeth

| | | |
|---|---|---|
| Sharp edges | Looseness | Chips |
| Missing teeth | Cracks | Plaque or debris |

#### Dentures/Prosthetics

| | | |
|---|---|---|
| Condition | Fit | Sharp edges |
| Cracks | Loose parts | Chips |
| Gingiva | Color | Edema |
| Bleeding | Swallowing | Ability to swallow |
| Pain | Voice | Difficulty to talk |
| Deeper raspy voice | | |

For more information on Focus Assessment Criteria, visit http://thepoint.lww.com.

➤ **Goal**

The person will be free of oral mucosa irritation or exhibit signs of healing with decreased inflammation.

### Indicators

- Describe factors that cause oral injury.
- Demonstrate knowledge of optimal oral hygiene.

➤ **General Interventions**

## Assess for Causative or Contributing Factors

Refer to Related Factors.

## Teach Preventive Oral Hygiene to Clients at Risk for Development of Mucositis

### Refer to Impaired Oral Mucous Membrane Related to Inadequate Oral Hygiene for Specific Instructions on Brushing and Flossing

**Instruct Client to:**
Perform the regimen including brushing, flossing, rinsing, and moisturizing, after meals and before sleep.
Avoid mouthwashes with alcohol content, lemon/glycerin swabs, or prolonged use of hydrogen peroxide.
Rinse mouth with saline or saline and bicarbonate solution.
Apply lubricant to lips every 2 h and PRN (e.g., lanolin, A&D ointment).
Inspect mouth daily for lesions and inflammation and report alterations.
Avoid foods that are spicy, salty, hot, rough, or acidic.
Report following symptoms: temperature greater than 101° F, new lesions or sores in mouth, bleeding from gums, difficulty swallowing or inability to take in fluids, and pain in the mouth.
Keep mouth clean and moist.

**R:** Factors that contribute to oral diseaseinclude inadequate hygiene and dry mucous membranes.

### Consult with Physician for Possible Need of Prophylactic Antifungal or Antibacterial Agent for Immunocompromised Clients at Risk for Mucositis (NCCN, 2008)

Instruct client to see a dentist 2 to 3 weeks before therapy begins for diagnosis and treatment of infections and to ensure adequate time for healing.
Consult with dentist for a regimen of daily fluoride treatments and oral hygiene.
Instruct client to see a dentist during treatment as needed and 2 months after treatment.
Refer any suspicious oral lesions to health care provider for culture to identify organism.
Administer antibiotics, antifungals or antivirals as prescribed.
Monitor temperature every four hours and report abnormal readings to health care provider.
Replace toothbrush after treatment of suspected or documented oral infection.

**R:** Dental disease is a reservoir of infections and requires careful management by knowledgeable professionals.

### Promote Healing and Reduce Progression of Mucositis

Inspect oral cavity three times daily with tongue blade and light; if mucositis is severe, inspect mouth every 4 h.
Ensure that oral hygiene regimen is done every 1–2 h while awake and every 4 h during the night.
Use normal saline solution as a mouthwash.
Floss teeth only once in 24 h.
Omit flossing if bleeding is excessive

**R:** Systematically applied protocols may significantly decrease the incidence, severity, and duration of oral problems (ONS, 2007).

**R:** Salt and soda rinses are effective and the least costly selection for the prevention of treatment of mucositis. Foam brushes are not equal to toothbrushes for removing plaque and bacteria for cavity prevention. The effectiveness of mouthwash preparations over normal saline has not been supported in the literature (ONS, 2007).

**R:** Proper hydration must be maintained to liquefy secretions and prevent drying of oral mucosa.

## Reduce Oral Pain and Maintain Adequate Food and Fluid Intake

Assess person's ability to chew and swallow.

Administer mild analgesic every 3 to 4 h as ordered by physician.

Instruct client to:

- Avoid commercial mouthwashes, citrus fruit juices, spicy foods, extremes in food temperature (hot, cold), crusty or rough foods, alcohol, mouthwashes with alcohol.
- Eat bland, cool foods (sherbets).
- Drink cool liquids every 2 h and PRN.

Consult with dietitian for specific interventions.

Refer to *Impaired Nutrition: Less Than Body Requirements related to anorexia* for additional interventions.

Consult with physician for an oral pain relief solution.

- Xylocaine Viscous 2% oral, swish and expectorate every 2 h and before meals. (If throat is sore, the solution can be swallowed; if swallowed, Xylocaine produces local anesthesia and may affect the gag reflex.) The dose of the viscous xylocaine is not to exceed 25 ml per day (NCCN, 2008).
- Gelclair is a concentrated gel that provides a protective barrier. Requires frequent applications because of limited duration. Prophylaxis is not recommended.
- Topical morphine provides a reduction in pain severity and duration of pain. If the morphine is in an alcohol-based formula it may cause burning.

**R:** Proper hydration must be maintained to liquefy secretions and prevent drying of oral mucosa.

**R:** Dry oral mucosa causes discomfort and increases the risk of breakdown and infection.

## Initiate Health Teaching and Referrals, as Indicated

Teach person and family the factors that contribute to stomatitis and its progression.

Teach diet modifications to reduce oral pain and to maintain optimal nutrition.

Have client describe or demonstrate home care regimen.

**R:** The frequency of oral health maintenance varies according to a person's health status and self-care ability. All clients should have their teeth and mouths cleaned at least once after meals and at bedtime. High-risk clients (e.g., NG tubes, cancer, poorly nourished) should have oral assessments daily. Clients in chronic care settings should have oral assessment at least once a week.

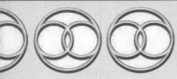

# RISK FOR IMPAIRED ORAL MUCOUS MEMBRANE

▶ **Related to Inadequate Oral Hygiene or Inability to Perform Oral Hygiene**

## ➤ Goal

The person will demonstrate integrity of the oral cavity.

### Indicators

- Be free of harmful plaque to prevent secondary infection.
- Be free of oral discomfort during food and fluid intake.
- Demonstrate optimal oral hygiene.

## ➤ General Interventions

### Assess for Causative or Contributing Factors

Refer to Related Factors

### Discuss the Importance of Daily Oral Hygiene and Periodic Dental Examinations

Explain the relationship of plaque to dental and gum disease.
Evaluate person's ability to perform oral hygiene.
Allow person to perform as much oral care as possible.

**R:** Plaque, microbial flora found in the mouth, is the primary cause of dental cavities and periodontal disease. Daily removal of plaque through brushing and flossing can help prevent dental decay and disease.

## Teach Correct Oral Care

### Have Person Sit or Stand Upright Over Sink (If He or She Cannot Get to a Sink, Place an Emesis Pan Under the Chin or Have Suction Setup at Bedside)

### Remove and Clean Dentures and Bridges Daily

Brush dentures daily with a denture brush or stiff, hard toothbrush inside and outside; rinse in cool water before replacing.
Patients who are intubated, unconscious or have severe mucositis should not have dentures replaced into mouth. Store dentures in a cleaning solution and change solution daily to prevent bacterial growth.
Have family discard any ill-fitting dentures.

**R:** Unclean or ill-fitting dentures can contribute to infection.

### Floss Teeth (Every 24 h)

With a piece of dental floss approximately 25 inches long, floss each tooth by wrapping the floss around the second and third fingers of each hand.
Begin with the back teeth; insert the floss between each tooth gently to avoid injuring the gum.
Wrap floss around tooth, making a C, and gently pull floss up and down over the back of each tooth.
Repeat this in reverse to floss the front of the tooth.
Remove the floss either by pulling straight up or by releasing one end and pulling the floss through. (Minor bleeding may occur.)

Rinse.

Floss holders can make flossing easier. (Back teeth cannot be reached with a floss holder.)

**R:** Flossing removes plaque from gum line.

### Brush Teeth (After Meals and Before Sleep)

Use a soft bristled toothbrush (avoid hard brushes) with a nonabrasive toothpaste with Fluoride or sodium bicarbonate (1 tsp in 8 oz of water; may be contraindicated in people with sodium restrictions). Air dry toothbrush between uses.

Brush back and forth or in a small circle, starting at the back of the mouth and brushing one or two teeth at a time.

Gently brush tongue and inner sides of cheeks.

Rinse with normal saline or sterile water for 30 seconds.

Apply moisturizer to lips and inside of mouth.

**R:** Daily removalof plaque can prevent dental disease.

### Inspect Mouth for Lesions, Sores, or Excessive Bleeding

## Perform Oral Hygiene on Person Who Is Unconscious or at Risk for Aspiration as Often as Needed

### Preparation

Gather equipment: soft-bristled toothbrush, toothpaste, cup of water, suction set-up, yankauer, light source, emesis basin, towel, wash cloth, and gloves.

Tell person what you are going to do.

Turn person on the side, supporting the back with a pillow (protect bed with an absorbent pad).

Place a tongue blade or bite block if necessary to keep mouth open.

Wear gloves to protect self.

### Brushing Procedure

For people with their own teeth, brush following the procedure outlined above. Use sodium bicarbonate (1 tsp:8 oz water), or normal saline solution (may be contraindicated in people with sodium restrictions).

Place emesis basin against patient's mouth and use the yankauer to suction secretions from the mouth.

For people with dentures, remove dentures and clean as above. Leave dentures out for people who are semicomatose and store in water (in denture cup).

Do not use toothettes.

Use a bulb syringe to rinse mouth; aspirate rinse with suction or use an aspirating toothbrush.

Move tongue blade or bite block if necessary, for access to other areas; do not put fingers on tops or edges of teeth.

Brush tongue and inner cheek tissue gently.

Pat mouth dry and apply lip lubricant and mouth moisturizer.

## Perform Oral Hygiene on Patients Who Are Intubated and/or Mechanically Ventilated

Gather equipment: same as for unconscious patient.

Position patient head of bed (HOB) > 30 degrees unless medically contraindicated.

Brush teeth, tongue and gums as described above twice a day.

Swab oral cavity every 2 hours and as needed with normal saline or mouth rinse solution.

Use oral chlorhexadine gluconate (0.12%) rinse twice a day for patients undergoing cardiac surgery with health care providers' written order. Further studies are needed for other patient population (Fournier, Dubois, & Pronnier, 2005).

Apply mouth moisturize to mouth and lips.

Remove excess oral secretions by using the yankauer suction.

**R:** Factors that contribute to oral disease are excessive use of alcohol and tobacco, microorganisms, inadequate nutrition (quantity, quality), inadequate hygiene, and trauma (NG tubes, ill-fitting dentures, sharp-edged teeth, sharp-edged prostheses, improper use of cleaning devices.

**R:** Oral health is influenced by microorganisms that grow in the plaque. With ventilators the microorganisms can transfer to the lungs and cause ventilator-associated pneumonia (Munro & Grap, 2004; Berry, Davidson, & Masters, 2007).

**R:** The NCCN (2008) and CDC (2003) recommends that BMSCT patients should receive dental evaluation and treatment before treatment. Oral care should include daily flossing, brushing teeth with a soft-bristled toothbrush at least twice a day, and using toothettes if cannot tolerate the toothbrush, and oral rinses 4–6 times a day with normal saline, sterile water, or sodium bicarb.

**R:** Toothettes do not remove the plaque compared to a toothbrush (Luoma, Martin, & Pearson, 2002; Berry et al., 2007).

## Initiate Health Teaching and Referrals, as Indicated

### *Identify Clients Who Need Toothbrush Adaptations to Perform Own Mouth Care*

For clients with difficulty closing hands tightly, refer to occupational therapy.

For clients with limited hand mobility, enlarge toothbrush handle with a sponge hair roller, wrinkled aluminum foil, or a bicycle handlebar grip attached with a small amount of plaster of Paris.

For clients with limited arm movement, extend handle of standard toothbrush by attaching handle of an old toothbrush (after cutting off bristle end) to a new toothbrush with strong cord or plastic cement, or by attaching toothbrush to a plastic rod. (The toothbrush can be curved by gently heating and then bending it.)

### *Refer Clients with Tooth and Gum Disorders to a Dentist*

Pediatric Interventions

**Teach Parents to:**

Provide their child with fluoride supplements if not present in concentrations over 0.7 parts per million (ppm) in drinking water.

Avoid taking tetracycline drugs during pregnancy or giving them to children younger than 8 years.

Refrain from putting an infant to bed with a bottle of juice or milk.

Provide child with safe objects for chewing during teething.

Replace toothbrushes frequently (every 3 months).

Schedule dental checkups every 6 months after 2 years of age.

Supervise and assist preschool child with brushing and flossing in front of mirror:

* Talk to child when brushing.
* "Ask child to 'tweet like a bird' to brush front teeth and 'roar like a lion' to brush back teeth" (Hockenberry & Wilson, 2009).
* Incorporate brushing and flossing teeth into bedtime rituals.

**Teach Child:**

Why tooth care is important

To avoid highly sugared liquids, foods, and chewing gum

To drink water and extra fluid

To brush teeth using fluoride toothpaste

**R:** The objective of oral hygiene is to remove plaque, which causes decay and periodontal disease (Berry et al., 2007).

**R:** Flossing removes plaque from gum line.

**R:** Fluoride makes enamel more resistant to caries by decreasing the effects of acid on surface (NCCN, 2007).

Maternal Interventions

Stress the importance of good oral hygiene and continued dental examinations. Advise woman to increase intake of vitamin C.

Remind client to advise dentist of her pregnancy.

Explain that gum hypertrophy and tenderness are normal during pregnancy.

**R:** Gum hypertrophy, tenderness, and bleeding during normal pregnancy may be the result of vascular swelling called *epulis of pregnancy* (Pillitteri, 2009).

Geriatric
Interventions

### Explain High-Risk Age-Related Factors (Miller, 2009)

| | |
|---|---|
| Degenerative bone disease | Diminished oral blood supply |
| Dry mouth | Vitamin deficiencies |

**R:** Age-related changes and nutritional deficiencies increase vulnerability to oral ulcerations and infection (Miller, 2009; NCCN, 2007).

### Explain that Some Medications Cause Dry Mouth

| | | |
|---|---|---|
| Laxatives | Antibiotics | Antidepressants |
| Anticholinergics | Analgesics | Iron sulfate |
| Cardiovascular medications | | |

**R:** Dry mouth contributes to tissue injury.

### Determine Any Barriers to Dental Care

| | | |
|---|---|---|
| Financial | Mobility | Dexterity |
| Lack of knowledge | | |

**R:** Barriers to dental care can be reduced or eliminated.

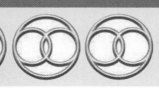

# RELOCATION STRESS [SYNDROME]

**Relocation Stress [Syndrome]**

**Related to Changes Associated with Health Care Facility Transfers or Admission to Long-Term–Care Facility**

## DEFINITION

State in which a client experiences physiologic and/or psychological disturbances as a result of transfer from one environment to another

Other terms found in the literature that describe relocation stress include admission stress, postrelocation crisis, relocation crisis, relocation shock, relocation trauma, transfer stress, transfer trauma, translocation syndrome, and transplantation shock.

## DEFINING CHARACTERISTICS*

### Major (80% to 100%)

Responds to transfer or relocation with:

| | | |
|---|---|---|
| Loneliness | Depression | Anger |
| Apprehension | Anxiety | Increased confusion (older adult population) |

### Minor (50% to 79%)

| | |
|---|---|
| Change in former eating habits | Decrease in self-care activities |
| | Decrease in leisure activities |

---

*Harkulich, J. & Bruggler, C. (1988). *Nursing Diagnosis–translocation syndrome: Expert validation study.* Partial funding granted by the Peg Schlitz Fund, Delta Ix Chapter, Sigma Theta Tau International; Barnhouse, A. (1987). *Development of the nursing diagnosis of translocation syndrome with critical care patients.* Unpublished master's thesis, Kent State University, Kent, OH.

Change in former sleep patterns   Gastrointestinal disturbances
Increased verbalization of needs
Demonstration of dependency   Need for excessive reassurance
Demonstration of insecurity   Restlessness
Demonstration of lack of trust   Withdrawal
Vigilance   Allergic symptoms
Weight change
Sad affect
Unfavorable comparison of posttransfer to pretransfer staff
Verbalization of being concerned/upset about transfer
Verbalization of insecurity in new living situation

## RELATED FACTORS

### Pathophysiologic

**Related to compromised ability to adapt to changes secondary to:**
Decreased physical health status
Physical difficulties
Decreased psychosocial health status
Increased/perceived stress before relocation
Depression
Decreased self-esteem

### Situational (Personal, Environmental)

Related to insufficient finances
*Related to high degree of changes secondary to admission to a care facility*
*Related to:*
Loss of social and familial ties
Abandonment
Change in relationship with family members
*Related to little or no preparation for the impending move*

### Maturational

#### School-Aged Children and Adolescents
*Related to losses associated with moving secondary to:*
Fear of rejection, loss of peer group or school-related problems
Decreased security in new adolescent peer group and school

#### Older Adult
Related to the need to be closer to family members for assistance
Related to admission to a care facility

## ■ ■ ■ ■ ■ ■ AUTHOR'S NOTE

NANDA has accepted *Relocation Stress* as a syndrome diagnosis. It does not fit the criterion for a syndrome diagnosis, which is a cluster of actual or risk nursing diagnoses as defining characteristics. The defining characteristics associated with *Relocation Stress* are observable or reportable cues consistent with *Relocation Stress*, not *Relocation Stress Syndrome*. The author recommends deleting "Syndrome" from the label.

Relocation represents a disruption for all parties involved. It can accompany a transfer from one unit to another, or from one facility to another. It can involve a permanent move to a long-term–care facility or new home. The relocation disturbs all age groups involved. When physiologic and psychological disturbances compromise functioning, the nursing diagnosis *Relocation Stress [Syndrome]* is appropriate.

The optimal nursing approach to relocation stress is to initiate preventive measures using *Risk for Relocation Stress* as the diagnosis.

## ■■■■■ ERRORS IN DIAGNOSTIC STATEMENTS

### Relocation Stress related to apprehension and sadness associated with impending family move

Apprehension and sadness are appropriate responses for children involved in a family move. Adolescents specifically are very disrupted because of peer relationships. Apprehension and sadness are not related factors but manifestations. The nurse should write the diagnosis as *Relocation Stress related to perceived negative effects of family move as evidenced by statements of apprehension and sadness.*

## ■■■■■ KEY CONCEPTS

### Generic Considerations

- The process of relocation represents a transition for all involved parties (Miller, 1995; Puskar, 1986).
- Annually, 20% of all people in the United States either choose or are forced to relocate (Puskar & Rohay, 1999).
- Relocation stress can accompany any type of move. Types include previous home to new home (house, apartment); home to college; home to institution (hospital, long-term–care nursing facility); institution to home (especially after an extended illness); moves within an institution (from one bed to another in the same room; from one room to another on the same unit/floor; from one room to another on different units/floors); and moves between institutions (hospital to long-term–care facility or one long-term nursing care facility to another) (Davies & Nolan, 2004).
- Relocation stress typically occurs shortly before and after the move. Not all relocated people experience relocation stress, because the related factors are not present to the same degree in all those experiencing relocation.
- When a move results from a husband's change of employment, a relocated husband often finds satisfaction with his new job. The relocated wife seeks new neighbors, friends, home, and community activities as a primary source of satisfaction. If previously employed, she often feels isolated over the unavailability of jobs in the new environment (Puskar, 1990). Relocated wives who coped well demonstrated active behaviors (problem solving, support seeking from family and friends, volunteer activities); wives who coped poorly showed passive behaviors (eating, sleeping, crying, watching television, becoming angry at self and others; Puskar, 1990).
- Relocation stress has been compared to separation anxiety as a result of separation from monitors and nurse and physician surveillance, which results in an inability to cope.
- Houser (1974) reported the following in a study of 12 clients transferred from a coronary care unit: 6 of 12 people required readmission for cardiovascular complications, and 5 of the 6 had a high anxiety rating when transferred. Those who did not discuss their feelings were most likely to experience complications after transfer. After instituting a program aimed at reducing transfer stress, clients had fewer complications, and observed complications were less dangerous than those that the control group experienced.
- The incidence of psychophysiologic responses to relocation stress was higher for clients transferred during the afternoon and evening than for those transferred in the morning (Lethbridge et al., 1976).
- In their study of 177 clients with myocardial infarction in six hospitals, Minckley et al. (1979) found that:
  - The duration for which the client had been notified of the transfer was related inversely to the need for reassurance.
  - Clients with abnormal blood pressure readings on admission to the coronary care unit were at higher risk for negative effects of transfer.
  - Women had more physiologic indicators of stress with relocation than did men.
  - Clients as well as families were found to be very anxious about transfer from an intensive care unit (ICU) (Mitchell, Courtney, & Coyer, 2003).
  - Clients who are more dependent are more likely to experience negative effects with relocation than clients who are less dependent (Adshead et al., 1991).

 **Pediatric Considerations**

- When families need to relocate, their social attachment systems may be disrupted, thus producing slight changes in health status, daily functioning, and loneliness (Puskar, 1986).

- Because of age and maturation, children of different ages experience relocation in different ways.
- A relocated child's stress and frustration may lead to aggression, withdrawal, and deterioration in schoolwork, which may lead to future adjustment problems if the child is not well socialized in the new environment.
- Relocated children and adults may experience pains of past separations, which may arouse feelings of insecurity (Puskar & Dvorsak, 1991).
- When relocated, toddlers and preschoolers often demonstrate changes in eating and sleeping patterns along with minor disabilities (Puskar & Dvorsak, 1991).
- Relocated adolescent boys may experience more difficulties with peers (diminished contact, rejection, teasing, meanness) in the new environment (Vernberg, 1990). Relocated adolescent girls, however, may verbalize more stress and loneliness.
- During interviews of 15 parents of premature infants transferred between Level 1, 2, and 3 nurseries and home, Gibbins and Chapman (1996) documented the following parental responses:
  - Sources of parental stress included lack of information about their infants' condition and events of the transfer between units and discharge home, insecurity about their own comfort in a new unit, inconsistencies in care within the different nurseries, and dependency on particular caregivers within the neonatal intensive care unit (NICU).
  - Parents had ambivalent feelings about transfer from a NICU (Level 3 nursery) to an intermediate care unit (Level 2 nursery). Parents also became more judgmental about the NICU care near the time of transfer to the Level 2 nursery and rationalized the transfer from the NICU.
  - Forty-one mothers of infants transferred from a tertiary-care NICU to a community hospital nursery reported mild to moderate stress with the transfer and perceived the transfer as fairly positive. The higher the mothers viewed the quality of the transfer, the less stress they reported with this transfer (Flanagan et al., 1996).

## Geriatric Considerations

- Older adults have three types of moves (Longino & Bradley, 2006):
  - Voluntary move to a desirable geographic area
  - Move closer to family because of widowhood and moderate disability
  - Move to an institution because of health problems
- Older adults move from their family home (Johnson & Tripp-Reimer, 2001; Miller 2009)
- Loss of spouse
- Chronic conditions and declining functional abilities
- Lack of available assistive services
- Lack of caregiver
- Cognitive impairments
- Psychiatric illness
- Change in neighborhood (e.g. unsafe, socially isolated)
- Reactions to relocation are related to the client's psychological resources before the move and the move's context. Findings from older women relocating to an independent location, but not their own private home, were as follows:
  - Women with a greater ability to manage the world to meet their needs, as well as with more pressure to relocate and more prerelocation autonomy, were less sad and aggravated after the move than was expected.
  - Women with less autonomy or personal growth before the move were less sad after the move than was expected if they also experienced many unexpected gains, such as ease in making friends and opportunities for involvement in activities (Smider et al., 1996).
  - Relocating rural older adults frequently identified perceived choice, environmental predictability, and social support from family, residential neighbors, and friends as factors associated with positive adjustment (Armer, 1996).
- Positive appraisal of relocation to a nursing home is associated with positive morale; a negative appraisal is associated with negative morale.
- Highly educated nursing home residents have been found to view relocation more negatively than less educated residents (Gass et al., 1992).

- Nursing home residents' views of relocation and later adaptation are reported to be related to psychological and physical health, prior and new support systems, morale, and functional independence (Beirne et al., 1995; Gass et al., 1992; Davies & Nolan, 2004).
- Living in a nursing home has been shown to be a cause of suicide in older adults. The client at risk for suicide when relocating to a nursing home is depressed and hopeless, with decreased life satisfaction and psychological well-being, as well as anger at the loss of control over his or her own life.
- Lack of a confidante in a nursing home has been correlated with suicidal ideation. High self-esteem, arthritis, and a mean age of 85 years also have been found to be significant indicators of suicide risk in older adults in nursing homes (Haight, 1995).
- The greatest incidence of relocation stress typically occurs shortly before and up to 3 months after the move (Beirne et al., 1995; Reinardy, 1995).
- In a study conducted by Rodgers (1997), the process of nursing home placement began with families recognizing and ultimately accepting the need to admit their loved ones to a nursing home. Concerns over safety provided a means to justify, rather than an initial incentive to seek, the placement.
- Relocated long-term–care residents with a diagnosis of cognitive impairment demonstrated decreased self-care and withdrawal 3 months after relocation.
- Long-term–care residents very familiar with their environments (median length of stay of 36 months) were more prone to falls after a secondary relocation than those residents with a shorter length of stay (24 months; Lander et al., 1997).
- Some minimal familiarity with a nursing home before relocation (e.g., having driven by it over the years; Reed et al., 2003) or viewing a video about the facility (Kaisik & Ceslowitz, 1996) made the move less threatening for older people. Also, proximity of a nursing home to the resident's previous home assisted residents in feeling continuity with their previous lifestyle and in developing new relationships with other residents from the same geographic area (Reed et al., 2003).
- An older couple experiences complex changes in their roles, relationships, life structure (routine, activities, and so forth), time management, support systems, and self-esteem when one spouse is admitted to a nursing home.
- In a study of nursing home rehabilitation after acute rehabilitation, clients had favorable outcomes under the care of the same shared group of therapists between the two settings (Kosasih et al., 1998).
- Residents whose admission to a long-term–care facility was unplanned experienced a longer phase of being overwhelmed (focus on self, emotional response, crying, and loneliness) than residents with a planned admission.

## Transcultural Considerations

- Relocation stress is a transcultural phenomenon that occurs in all age groups. Of 33 nurses practicing in China, 100% reported that relocation stress exists; 23 nurses from 12 different countries also reported that relocation stress exists (Harkulich & Brugler, 1991).
- Israeli adolescents were found to experience relocation stress after moving.
- Children from Sweden experiencing a 1-year international relocation significantly reduced their leisure activities, experienced a loss of identity, and developed a more negative attitude toward international assignments after the move. They also demonstrated significant increases in atopic sensitization and subjective symptoms of allergies, including dry skin, eczema, and prickling sensations after 1 year in the foreign country (Anderzén et al., 1997).
- Relocation did not pose adverse psychological effects when children from Armenia were relocated after a major earthquake. They were found to have similar levels of post-traumatic stress disorder and depression as children who remained in the disaster area.
- In her Soviet Jewish resettlement experience, Hulewat (1996) identified three control concepts to address when families relocate internationally: stages of resettlement (splitting, actual migration, arrival in new home, decompensation, and transgenerational stage); cultural styles and psychological dynamics of the population being resettled; and individual family dynamics based on the ability to tolerate cultural dissonance and to manage the tasks necessary to proceed through the resettlement stages.
- Cultural beliefs regarding family obligations influence a client's relocation to a long-term–care facility. For example, Lee (1997) reported that Chinese older adults view caregiving as part of family duty. Therefore, many of them equate admission to a residential care home with family rejection, powerlessness, and a devalued sense of self.

# Focus Assessment Criteria

## Subjective Data

### Assess for Defining Characteristics

**The Relocated Client Complains of:**

| | |
|---|---|
| Dissatisfaction with new environment | Increased family conflicts |
| | Loneliness |
| Problems adjusting | Loss of control |
| Feelings of insecurity | Anger at loss of control over own life |
| Anger toward people responsible for placement | |

**Changes in:**

| | |
|---|---|
| Sleep patterns | Nutritional intake |
| Socialization | Cognition |
| Orientation | |

### Assess for Related Factors

**History of:**

One or more changes in environment in the last 3 months
Multiple moves in the last 5 years
Traumatic experiences after previous moves
Being in the same environment for more than 40 years

**Risk Factors**

Moderate to severe confusion/disorientation
Perceived poor health
Lack of support/family/friends/staff
Low self-esteem
Functional deterioration
Involuntary move
Communication difficulties
Lack of continuity of care
Expression of dissatisfaction with life
Lack of preparation for move(s)
Lack of choices or input on the part of the relocating client
Multiple chronic illnesses
Lack of familiarity with nursing home before relocation
Nursing home location far from previous residence

## Objective Data

### Assess for Defining Characteristics

| | | |
|---|---|---|
| Change in weight | Sleep problems | Change in eating patterns |
| Increased medical visits | Change in cognition | Decline in self-care activities |

For more information on Focus Assessment Criteria, visit http://thepoint.lww.com.

---

**NOC**
Anxiety Self-Control, Coping, Loneliness, Psychosocial Adjustment: Life Change, Quality of Life

# ▶ Goals

The client/family will:

• Report adjustment to the new environment with minimal disturbances.

### Indicators:

• Share in decision-making activities regarding the new environment.
• Express concerns regarding the move to a new environment.
• Verbalize one positive aspect of the relocation.
• Establish new bonds in the new environment.
• Become involved in activities in the new environment.

**NIC**
Anxiety
Reduction, Coping
Enhancement,
Counseling, Family
Involvement
Promotion,
Support System
Enhancement,
Anticipatory
Guidance, Family
Integrity Promotion,
Transfer, Relocation
Stress Reduction

## ➤ General Interventions

### Encourage Each Family Member to Share Feelings About the Move

Provide privacy for each client.

Encourage family members to share feelings with one another.

Discuss the possible and different effects of the move on each family member.

Inform parents regarding potential changes in children's conduct with relocation, such as regression, withdrawal, acting-out, and changes with eating (breast/bottle-feeding).

Instruct parents to obtain all pertinent documents regarding children's medical/dental history (e.g., immunizations, communicable diseases, dental work).

Allow for some ritual(s) when leaving the old environment. Encourage reminiscing, which will bring closure for many family members.

**R:** Many researchers report that relocation stress is preventable (Lander et al., 1997; Loehner et al., 2004).

## Teach Parents Techniques to Assist Their Children with the Move

Remain positive about the move before, during, and after, accepting that the child may not be optimistic.

Explore various options with children on how to communicate with friends/families in previous environment. Children's relationships with friends in the previous community are very important, especially for "peer reassurance" after relocation.

Keep regular routines in the new environment; establish them as soon as possible.

Acknowledge the difficulty of peer losses with the adolescent.

Join the organizations to which the child previously belonged (e.g., Scouts, sports).

Assist children to focus on similarities between old and new environments (e.g., clubs, Scouts, church groups).

Plan a trip to school during a class and lunch period to reduce fear of unknown.

Allow children some choices regarding room arrangements, decorating, and the like.

Ask teacher or counselor at the new school to introduce the adolescent to a student who recently relocated to that school.

Allow children to mourn their losses as a result of the move.

**R:** Children need early notification, predictability, and decision-making opportunities when an upcoming relocation is planned.

## Assess the Following Areas When Counseling a Relocated Adolescent

Perceptions About the Move

Concurrent Stressors

Usual and Present Coping Skills

Support (Family, Peers, and Community)

**R:** The adolescent has a developmental task of becoming independent, which is challenged with relocation (Puskar & Rohay, 1999).

**R:** Peer networks are important during adolescence because the relocated adolescent needs additional parental and peer reassurance.

## Initiate Health Teaching and Referrals, as Indicated

Alert the family to the possible need for counseling before, during, or after the move.

Furnish a written directory of relevant community organizations such as area churches, children's groups, Parents Without Partners, senior citizens' groups, and Welcome Wagon or other local new-neighbor groups.

Instruct the family about appropriate community services.

Consult the school nurse regarding school programs for new students.

**R:** Early relocation planning is paramount in ensuring a smooth transfer for all involved individuals.

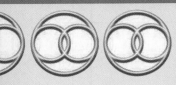

# RELOCATION STRESS [SYNDROME]

## ▶ Related to Changes Associated with Health Care Facility Transfers or Admission to Long-Term–Care Facility

**NOC**
See also Relocation Stress, Adaptation to New Environment

### ➤ Goals

The client will:

• Describe realistic expectations of the new environment.

### Indicators:

• Participate in decision-making activities regarding the new environment.
• Voice concerns regarding the move to a new environment.
• Describe realistic expectations of the new environment.

**NIC**
See also Relocation Stress

### ➤ General Interventions

#### Provide Family and Client with the Relocation or Transfer Plans as Soon as Possible

Elicit discussions with concerns and questions

**R:** All staff members must be aware of and alert to the complex process of relocation for both the client and family before proactively decreasing stress factors.

**R:** The most important strategy for families and individuals when transferring from an ICU was information prior to the actual transfer (Mitchell, Courtney, & Coyer, 2003).

#### Assess for Factors that May Contribute to Relocation Stress (See Related Factors and Focus Assessment Criteria)

#### Reduce or Eliminate Causative and Contributing Factors

#### Environmental Differences Between Old and New Settings/ Minimal Continuity of Care in a New Environment

Design a program to prepare relocated residents and staff for the move, orienting them to the physical layout many times until they feel familiar with the new environment.

Initially maintain theclient on thesame activity level and diet through pretransfer and posttransfer units.

Transfer the client to similar, proximal area when possible.

Wean any monitoring equipment gradually before transfer.

Transfer all client's items with the client, such as mobility aids, eyeglasses, hearing aids, dentures, prostheses, and belongings.

Transfer the client during daytime hours.

Maintain people in familiar groups at mealtimes and in living arrangements.

Allow time for discussions regarding living spaces in old and new environments.

Gradually decrease nursing attention before ICU transfer, when possible.

**R:** The most important strategy for families and individuals when transferring from an ICU was information prior to the actual transfer (Mitchell, Courtney, & Coyer, 2003). There should be a visible, gradual transition from critical-care monitoring to usual nursing-unit monitoring to reduce fears.

**R:** Open communication with older adults both before and after a move is necessary, assessing their experiences with change and adjustment, coping history and style, and decisional control.

## Involuntary Relocation/Lack of Control in Decision-Making

Offer decision-making opportunities throughout the relocation experience.

Promote the client's input regarding the new environment when possible, such as use of decorations and arrangement of furniture.

Present transfer from a critical-care unit as an indicator of improvement.

Inform the hospitalized client of signs of daily progress.

Transfer the client in an unhurried manner.

Establish mutual goals before relocation to a nursing home.

Provide opportunities for questions/answers with relocation preparation.

Hold regular staff/resident meetings after relocation, encouraging new members to be involved with the facility's rules and regulations (Wilson, 1997).

**R:** Wilson (1997) and Meacham and Brandriet (1997) found older adults made an effort to protect their significant others by hiding their feelings about relocation and attempting to maintain a sense of normalcy. Therefore, it is critical for new residents to develop trusting relationships with others to discuss the stressors of relocation.

Include parents in the care of their hospitalized premature infant as much as possible.

Promote the use of support systems both inside and outside the hospital for parents of hospitalized infants.

**R:** Parents of children facing transfer from the ICU to a general unit who were given a verbal explanation 1 to 2 h before the transfer had significantly less anxiety than parents who were informed immediately before the transfer (Miles, 1999).

## Reduce the Physiologic Effects of Relocation

### Assess Before Relocation:

| | | |
|---|---|---|
| Blood pressure, temperature | Respiratory function | Orientation |
| Signs of infection | Level of discomfort | |

**R:** Adaptation to relocation can negatively affect physical status, leading to increased morbidity and mortality.

### Identify the Client at High Risk for Selected Physiologic Responses

Musculoskeletal/neurologic deficits
Advanced age
Cardiovascular disorders
Changes in orientation
Cardiovascular complications (e.g., ischemia, dysrhythmias)

**R:** Clients with abnormal blood pressure readings on admission to the coronary care unit were at higher risk for negative effects of transfer. Women had more physiologic indicators of stress with relocation than did men (Minckley et al., 1979).

### Prevent or Reduce Confusion

### Refer to Confusion for Additional Interventions

## Promote Integration After Transfer into a Long-Term–Care Nursing Facility

Allow as many choices as possible regarding physical surroundings and daily routines.
Encourage the client or family to bring familiar objects from the client's home.
Orient to the physical layout of the environment.
Introduce relocated clients to new staff and fellow residents.
Encourage interaction with other people in the new facility.
Assist the client in maintaining previous interpersonal relationships.
Clearly state smoking rules and orient the client to areas where smoking is permitted.

Promote the development or maintenance of a relationship with a confidante.

Reestablish normal routines, while initially increasing staffing and lighting, when a large number of long-term–care residents are involved in a secondary relocation.

Assist nursing home residents to meet people from their previous geographic area.

Arrange frequent contacts by a volunteer or staff member with each newly admitted resident. Also, match a successfully relocated resident with the new resident to begin the networking process.

**R:** Older adults may use a variety of coping strategies, ranging from aggressive anger to passive resignation, when relocated to a nursing home. Any nursing interventions related to relocation stress should reflect the resident's effective coping strategies.

**R:** Residents who were allowed choice regarding room location and favorite objects had an increased sense of control and less stress (Mitchell, 1999).

## Initiate Health Teaching and Referrals, as Indicated

Prepare the client for relocation.

Notify the client about relocation as early as possible to increase the predictability of his or her reaction.

Provide ongoing and structured teaching regarding:

- Characteristics of new environment
- Staff capabilities
- Mechanisms for continuity of care
- Rationale for relocation and less constant professional attention when applicable
- Expectations of the client in the new environment
- Any increasing stages of activity/independence

Include the family in teaching.

Offer information about positive health habits and resources during illness.

Make appropriate professional referrals as needed, as well as suggesting a telephone monitoring system such as "Lifeline."

**R:** Open communication with older adults both before and after a move is necessary, assessing their experiences with change and adjustment, coping history and style, and decisional control.

Refer relocated families to community agencies related to newcomers and to mental health agencies when at risk for relocation stress syndrome.

**R:** With the influx of people who have chronic mental illness into the community, it is important that their needs and problems be assessed accurately so interventions and services that ensure successful relocation and adjustment can be planned and implemented.

Assess the perceptions of parents of hospitalized infants regarding an upcoming transfer and their interest in related information.

Maintain at least daily communication with parents about their hospitalized infant (e.g., condition, timing of transfer, mechanisms for continuity of care between the pre- and posttransfer nurseries) and their concerns.

Suggest that parents of hospitalized infants visit the nursery where their child will be transferred before the event.

Develop and use a mechanism for a thorough exchange of information between pre- and posttransfer nurseries.

**R:** Parents of preterm infants want to protect their child during hospitalization in addition to wanting to receive information about each new environment where their child will be transferred (Gibbins & Chapman, 1996).

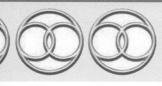

# RISK FOR COMPROMISED RESILIENCE

## DEFINITION (NANDA)

The state in which a client is at risk for decreased ability to sustain a pattern of positive responses to an adverse situation or crisis

## RISK FACTORS (NANDA)

Chronicity of existing crises
Multiple coexisting adverse situations
Presence of additional new crisis (e.g., unplanned pregnancy, death of spouse, loss of job, illness, loss of housing, death of family member

■■■■■■ AUTHOR'S NOTE

This new NANDA-I diagnosis is not a response but an etiology of a coping problem. Resilience is a strength that can be taught and nurtured in children. Resilient individuals and families can cope in adverse situations and crises. They problem-solve and adapt their functioning to the situation. For example, when a mother of a family of five had to undergo chemotherapy, the family formulated a plan together to divide the responsibilities previously managed by the mother.

When a client or family has is experiencing a chronic, multiple adverse situation or a new crisis, refer to *Risk for Ineffective Coping*. In situations involving the loss of family member, significant other, or friend, refer to *Grieving* for Key Concepts, Goals, and Interventions/Rationale.

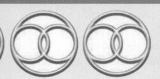

# RISK FOR INEFFECTIVE RESPIRATORY FUNCTION

**Risk for Ineffective Respiratory Function***

Dysfunctional Ventilatory Weaning Response
Risk for Dysfunctional Ventilatory Weaning Response
Ineffective Airway Clearance
Ineffective Breathing Patterns
Impaired Gas Exchange
Inability to Sustain Spontaneous Ventilation

## DEFINITION

State in which a client is at risk of experiencing a threat to the passage of air through the respiratory tract and/or to the exchange of gases ($O_2$–$CO_2$) between the lungs and the vascular system

## RISK FACTORS

Presence of risk factors that can change respiratory function (see Related Factors).

---

*This diagnosis is not currently on the NANDA list but has been included for clarity or usefulness.

## RELATED FACTORS

### Pathophysiologic

*Related to excessive or thick secretions secondary to:*

| | | |
|---|---|---|
| Infection | Inflammation | Allergy |
| Cardiac or pulmonary disease | Smoking | |

*Related to immobility, stasis of secretions, and ineffective cough secondary to:*

Diseases of the nervous system (e.g., Guillain-Barré syndrome, multiple sclerosis, myasthenia gravis)

Central nervous system (CNS) depression/head trauma

Cerebrovascular accident (stroke)

Quadriplegia

### Treatment-Related

*Related to immobility secondary to:*

Sedating effects of medications, drugs or chemicals (specify)

Anesthesia, general or spinal

*Related to suppressed cough reflex secondary to (specify)*

*Related to effects of tracheostomy (altered secretions)*

### Situational (Personal, Environmental)

*Related to immobility secondary to:*

| | | |
|---|---|---|
| Surgery or trauma | Fatigue | Pain |
| Perception/cognitive impairment | Fear | Anxiety |

*Related to extremely high or low humidity*

For infants, related to placement on stomach for sleep

Exposure to cold, laughing, crying, allergens, smoke

■■■■■■ **AUTHOR'S NOTE**

Nursing's many responsibilities associated with problems of respiratory function include identifying and reducing or eliminating risk (contributing) factors, anticipating potential complications, monitoring respiratory status, and managing acute respiratory dysfunction.

The author has added *Risk for Ineffective Respiratory Function* to describe a state that may affect the entire respiratory system, not just isolated areas, such as airway clearance or gas exchange. Allergy and immobility are examples of factors that affect the entire system; thus, it is incorrect to say *Impaired Gas Exchange related to immobility*, because immobility also affects airway clearance and breathing patterns. The nurse can use the diagnoses *Ineffective Airway Clearance* and *Ineffective Breathing Patterns* when nurses can definitely alleviate the contributing factors influencing respiratory function (e.g., ineffective cough, stress).

The nurse is cautioned not to use this diagnosis to describe acute respiratory disorders, which are the primary responsibility of medicine and nursing together (i.e., collaborative problems). Such problems can be labeled *RC of Acute hypoxia* or *RC of Pulmonary edema*. When a client's immobility is prolonged and threatens multiple systems—for example, Integumentary, musculoskeletal, vascular, as well as respiratory—the nurse should use *Disuse Syndrome* to describe the entire situation.

■■■■■■ **ERRORS IN DIAGNOSTIC STATEMENTS**

1. *Ineffective Breathing Patterns related to respiratory compensation for metabolic acidosis*
   This diagnosis represents the respiratory pattern associated with diabetic ketoacidosis. Related nursing responsibilities would include monitoring, early detection of changes, and rapid initiation of nursing and medical interventions. This does not represent a situation for which nurses diagnose and are accountable to prescribe treatment. Rather, the collaborative problem *RC of Ketoacidosis* represents the nursing accountability for the situation.

*(continued)*

## ERRORS IN DIAGNOSTIC STATEMENTS *Continued*

2. *Ineffective Airway Clearance related to mucosal edema and loss of ciliary action secondary to thermal injury*
   After sustaining burns of the upper airway, a client is at risk for pulmonary edema and respiratory distress. This potentially life-threatening situation requires both nurse- and physician-prescribed interventions. The collaborative problem *RC of Respiratory secondary to thermal injury* would alert nurses that close monitoring for respiratory complications and management if they occur are indicated.

3. *Ineffective Airway Clearance related to decreased cough and gag reflexes secondary to anesthesia*
   The nursing focus for the above problem is on preventing aspiration through proper positioning and good oral hygiene, not on teaching effective coughing. Thus, the nurse should restate the diagnosis as *Risk for Aspiration related to decreased cough and gag reflexes secondary to anesthesia.*

## KEY CONCEPTS

### Generic Considerations

- Ventilation requires synchronous movement of the walls of the chest and abdomen. With *inspiration*, the diaphragm moves downward, the intercostal muscles contract, the chest wall lifts up and out, the pressure inside the thorax lowers, and air is drawn in. *Expiration* occurs as air is forced out of the lungs by the elastic recoil of the lungs and the relaxation of the chest and diaphragm. Expiration is diminished in older adults and those with chronic pulmonary disease, increasing the likelihood of $CO_2$ retention.
- Pulmonary function depends on:
  - Adequate perfusion (passage of blood through pulmonary vessels)
  - Satisfactory diffusion (movement of oxygen and carbon dioxide across alveolar capillary membrane)
  - Successful ventilation (exchange of air between alveolar spaces and the atmosphere)
- Oxygenation depends on the ability of the lungs to deliver oxygen to the blood and on the ability of the heart to pump enough blood to deliver the oxygen to the microcirculation of the cells.
- With pulmonary dysfunction, pulmonary function tests (PFTs) are essential to determine the nature and extent of dysfunction caused by obstruction, restriction, or both. Airway resistance causes *obstructive* defects. A limitation in chest wall expansion causes *restrictive* defects. *Mixed* defects are a combination of obstructive and restrictive problems.
- Although arterial blood gases and oxygen saturation studies are very helpful in diagnosing problems with oxygenation, *vital signs* and *mental function* are key guides to determining the seriousness of the problem. (Some clients can tolerate oxygen problems better than others can.)
- The effects of insufficient oxygenation (hypoxia or hypoxemia) on vital signs are as follows:

| Vital Sign | Early Hypoxia/Hypoxemia | Late Hypoxia/Hypoxemia |
|---|---|---|
| Blood pressure | Rising systolic/falling diastolic | Falling |
| Pulse | Rising, bounding, arrhythmic | Falling, shallow, arrhythmic |
| Pulse pressure | Widening | Widened/narrowed |
| Respirations | Rapid | Slowed/rapid |

- The effects of insufficient oxygenation on mental function are as follows:

| Early Hypoxia/Hypoxemia | Late Hypoxia/Hypoxemia |
|---|---|
| Irritability | Seizures |
| Headache | Coma or brain tissue swelling |
| Confusion | |
| Agitation | |

- A cough ("the guardian of the lungs") is accomplished by closure of the glottis and the explosive expulsion of air from the lungs by the work of the abdominal and chest muscles. Although most coughing serves a beneficial purpose, the following may be signs of a medical problem requiring medical intervention:
  - Coughs lasting longer than 2 weeks or associated with high fever
  - Coughs consistently triggered by something (may actually be allergic bronchial asthma)
  - Barking cough, especially in a child
  - Breath holding can result in a Valsalva maneuver: a marked increase in intrathoracic and intra-abdominal pressure, with profound circulatory changes (decreased heart rate, cardiac output, and blood pressure).

*(continued)*

■ ■ ■ ■ ■ ■ **KEY CONCEPTS** *Continued*

- The terms *tachypnea*, *hyperpnea*, *hyperventilation*, *bradypnea*, *hypoventilation*, and *hypopnea* are frequently confused.
  - *Tachypnea:* rapid, shallow respiratory rate
  - *Hyperpnea:* rapid respiratory rate with increased depth
  - *Hyperventilation:* increased rate or depth of respiration causing alveolar ventilation that is above the body's normal metabolic requirements
  - *Bradypnea:* slow respiratory rate
  - *Hypoventilation:* decreased rate or depth of respiration, causing a minute alveolar ventilation that is less than the body's requirements
  - *Hypopnea:* under breathing; slower and/or shallower than normal (Venes, 2006)
- Hypoxia and hypoxemia contribute to increased intracranial pressure, brain swelling, brain damage, and shock. Oxygen demand is greater during febrile illness, exercise, pain, and physical and emotional stress.
- Low-flow $O_2$ should be delivered to people with a history of chronic $CO_2$ retention because their drive to breathe is hypoxia. Administer only enough $O_2$ to maintain $PaO_2$ at adequate levels for the client (usually 50 to 60 mm Hg) (Grif-Alspach, 2006).
- Suctioning and instillation of saline should not be used routinely; rather, their use should be based on assessment of individual needs (Chulay, 2005; Halm & Krisko-Hagel, 2008).
- Use the following as clinical indicators of need for endotracheal suctioning (Chulay, 2005):
  - Secretions in artificial airway
  - Frequent or sustained coughing with or without increased respiratory rate
  - Adventitious breath sounds on auscultation (rhonchi, or upper airway gurgles)
  - Increased peak airway pressure
  - Decreasing pulse oximetry readings ($SpO_2$, $Sao_2$, $PaO_2$)
  - Sudden onset of respiratory distress whenever airway patency is questioned
- Instillation of normal saline does not thin secretions and is not recommended (Chulay, 2005; Halm & Krisko-Hagel, 2008).
- Although endotracheal suctioning is associated with several significant complications, insufficiently frequent or inadequate suction also carries substantial risks. Maintain a delicate balance to minimize all complications.
- The nurse can reduce the risk of hypoxemia by using the following (Change, 1995):
  - Oxygen saturation and cardiac rhythm monitors during and immediately after suctioning
  - Intermittent suction for less than 15 s (prolonged, continuous suction causes microatelectasis and decreases arterial $O_2$ levels) (Chulay, 2005).
  - Hyperinflation (increasing tidal volume to 112 times preset ventilation volume using a resuscitation bag or the sigh function of the ventilator)
  - Preoxygenation (administering oxygen before suctioning)
  - Hyperoxygenation (administering oxygen at greater oxygen concentrations than the preset ventilator level)
  - Hyperventilation (increasing the respiratory rate without changing tidal volume)
  - The use of harmonicas by pulmonary therapists to help people with lung disease exercise their lungs and learn how to control breathing during acute dyspnea shows promising results. Clients not only have fun, but they also improve their ability to control their breathing and maximize lung function.
- Nicotine is one of the most toxic and addicting of all poisonous substances. Education, preventive health practices, interventions to enhance tobacco cessation, nicotine dependence treatment, and relapse prevention should be standard nursing practice.\* Nurses must be persistent in helping their clients to stop smoking by encouraging efforts to quit as often as needed (in many cases, at each client encounter). Refer to *Ineffective Health Maintenance related to Insufficient Knowledge of Effects of Tobacco Use*.

---

\*American Academy of Medical–Surgical Nursing Position Statement on Tobacco Use. Accessed from http://www.medsurgnurse.org on December 5, 2000.

 **Pediatric Considerations**

- The characteristics of normal respiration in the newborn differ from those of older infants and children (Hockenberry, Wilson, Winklestein, & Kline, 2009).

- Respirations are irregular and abdominal; to be accurate, count respirations for 1 full minute.
- The rate is between 30 and 50 breaths/min.
- Periods of apnea, lasting less than 15 s, may occur.
- Obligate nasal breathing occurs through the first 3 weeks of life.
- Characteristics of the respiratory system of the infant and young child include the following:
  - Abdominal breathing continues until the child is about 5 years of age.
  - Retractions are observed more often with respiratory illness because of increased chest wall compliance. Respiratory insufficiency may develop quickly in children (Hunsberger, 1989).
- Smaller airway diameter increases the risk of obstruction.
- Infants and small children swallow sputum when it is produced.
- Janson-Bjerklie et al. (1987) found that younger asthmatics appear to experience more intense dyspnea than older people at a given level of airway obstruction.
- Huckabay and Daderian (1989) noted that pediatric clients who were given a choice in the selection of the color of water in blow bottles performed significantly more breathing exercises than those who were not given a choice.
- Studies show that the past common practice of placing infants on their stomach for sleep increases the incidence of sudden infant death syndrome (SIDS), making placement on back or side a safer option. Refer to *Risk for Sudden Infant Death Syndrome*.

## Maternal Considerations

- Increased levels of estrogen and progesterone increase tidal volume by decreasing pulmonary resistance (Pillitteri, 2009).
- During pregnancy, oxygen consumption increases by 14%: half is for fetus development and the rest is for other increased needs (e.g., uterus, breasts; Pillitteri, 2009).

## Geriatric Considerations

- Age-related changes in the respiratory system have little effect on function in healthy adults unless they interact with risk factors such as smoking, immobility, or compromised immune system (Miller, 2009).
- The following age-related changes in the respiratory system are typical (Miller, 2009):
  - No change in total volume
  - 50% increase in residual volume
  - Compromised gas exchange in lower lung regions
  - Reduced compliance of the bony thorax
  - Decreased strength of the respiratory muscles and diaphragm
  - Age-related kyphosis and diminished immune response compromise respiratory function and increase the risk of pneumonia and other respiratory infections.
- Adults 65 years of age and older have a yearly death rate from pneumonia or influenza of 9 per 100,000. When smoking, exposure to air pollutants, or occupational exposure to toxic substances, is present, the rate increases to 217 per 100,000. If two or more risk factors are present, the rate rises to 979 per 100,000 (Miller, 2009).

# Focus Assessment Criteria

## Subjective Data

### Assess History of Symptoms (e.g., Pain, Dyspnea, Cough)

Onset: Precipitated by what? Relieved by what?
Description: Relieved by what?
Effects on other body functions:

- Gastrointestinal: nausea, vomiting, anorexia, constipation
- Genitourinary: impotence, kidney function
- Cardiovascular: angina, tachycardia/bradycardia, fluid retention
- Neurosensory: thought processes, headache
- Musculoskeletal: muscle fatigue, atrophy, use of accessory muscles

Effects on lifestyle

Occupation                              Social/sexual functions

Role functions                          Financial status

Effects on activity/exercise

## Assess for Related Factors

### Presence of Contributing or Causative Factors

Smoking ("pack-years": number of packs per day multiplied by the number of smoking years)

Smoking within the 8 weeks before anesthesia or surgery

Allergy (medication, food, environmental factors—dust, pollen, other)

Trauma, blunt or overt (chest, abdomen, upper airway, head)

Surgery/pain:

- Incision of chest/neck/head/abdomen
- Recent intubation

Asthma/chronic obstructive pulmonary disease (COPD)/sinus problems

Environmental factors:

- Toxic fumes (cleaning agents, smoke)
- Extreme heat or cold
- Daily inspired air at work and in the home (humid, dry, level of pollution, level of pollens)

Infection/inflammation

### For Infant, History of:

| | | |
|---|---|---|
| Placement on stomach to sleep | Prematurity | Low birth weight |
| Cesarean birth | Complicated delivery | Breast-feeding formula |

## Objective Data

## Assess for Defining Characteristics

### Mental Status

### Respiratory Status

*Airway:*

| | | |
|---|---|---|
| Spontaneous nasal | Nasal endotracheal tube | Spontaneous mouth |
| Oral endotracheal tube | Oral airway | Tracheostomy |
| Nasal airway | | |

*Description:*

Spontaneous, labored, or nonlabored

Controlled mechanical ventilation (CMV)

Spontaneous intermittent mechanical ventilations (SIMV)

Rate (per minute)

Rhythm

Depth

Symmetric

Type

| | | |
|---|---|---|
| Splinted/guarded | Kussmaul | Use of accessory muscle |
| Cheyne-Stokes | | |

*Cough:*

Effective/Productive (brings forth sputum and clears lungs)

Ineffective/Nonproductive (does not bring forth mucus or clear lungs)

Triggered by what? Relieved by what?

Needs assistance with coughing

*Sputum:*

| | | | |
|---|---|---|---|
| Color | Character | Amount | Odor |

*Breath sounds (detected by auscultation: compare right upper and lower regions to left upper and lower regions; listen to all four quadrants of the chest)*

**Circulatory Status**

Pulse          Blood pressure     Skin color

For more information on Focus Assessment Criteria, visit http://thepoint.lww.com.

<table>
<tr><td>**NOC**<br>Aspiration Control,<br>Respiratory Status</td><td>➤ **Goal**</td></tr>
</table>

The client will have a respiratory rate within normal limits compared with baseline.

### Indicators:

- Express willingness to be actively involved in managing respiratory symptoms and maximizing respiratory function.
- Relate appropriate interventions to maximize respiratory status (varies depending on health status).
- Have satisfactory pulmonary function, as measured by pulmonary function tests.

<table>
<tr><td>**NIC**<br>Airway<br>Management, Cough<br>Enhancement,<br>Respiratory<br>Monitoring,<br>Positioning</td><td>➤ **General Interventions**</td></tr>
</table>

### Determine Causative Factors

Refer to Related Factors.

### Eliminate or Reduce Causative Factors, If Possible

Encourage ambulation as soon as consistent with the medical plan of care.

- If the client cannot walk, establish a regimen for being out of bed in a chair several times a day (e.g., 1 h after meals and 1 h before bedtime).
- Increase activity gradually. Explain that respiratory function will improve and dyspnea will decrease with practice.

**R:** Lying flat causes the abdominal organs to shift toward the chest, thereby crowding the lungs and making it more difficult to breathe.

For neuromuscular impairment:

- Vary the position of the bed, thereby gradually changing the horizontal and vertical position of the thorax, unless contraindicated.
- Assist the client to reposition, turning frequently from side to side (hourly if possible).
- Encourage deep-breathing and controlled-coughing exercises five times every hour.
- Teach the client to use a blow bottle or incentive spirometer every hour while awake. (With severe neuromuscular impairment, the client may have to be awakened during the night as well.)
- For clients with quadriplegia, teach client and caregivers the "quad cough." (Caregiver places a hand on the client's diaphragm and thrusts upward and inward.)
- For a child, use colored water in a blow bottle; have him or her blow up balloons.
- Ensure optimal hydration status and nutritional intake.

**R:** Exercises and movement promote lung expansion and mobilization of secretions. Incentive spirometry promotes deep breathing by providing a visual indicator of the effectiveness of the breathing effort.
**R:** Adequate hydration and humidity liquefy secretions, enabling easier expectoration and preventing stasis of secretions, which provide a medium for microorganism growth (Halm & Krisko-Hagel, 2008). Hydration also helps decrease blood viscosity, which reduces the risk of clot formation.

For the client with a decreased level of consciousness:

- Position the client from side to side with a set schedule (e.g., left side on even hours, right side on odd hours); do not leave the client lying flat on the back.
- Position the client on the right side after feedings (nasogastric tube feeding, gastrostomy) to prevent regurgitation and aspiration.
- Keep the head of the bed elevated 30 degrees unless contraindicated (Institute for Healthcare Improvement, 2008).
- See also *Risk for Aspiration*.

**R:** Lying flat causes the abdominal organs to shift toward the chest, thereby crowding the lungs and making it more difficult to breathe.

Refer the client to physical therapy and respiratory therapy as indicated.

**R:** Interventions that can enhance pulmonary function include exercise conditioning to improve lung compliance, relaxation and breathing training, chest percussion, postural drainage, and psychosocial rehabilitation.

## Prevent the Complications of Immobility

See *Disuse Syndrome*.

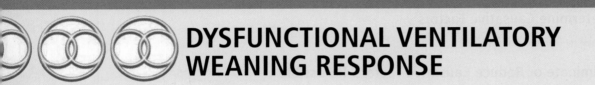

# DYSFUNCTIONAL VENTILATORY WEANING RESPONSE

## DEFINITION

State in which a client cannot adjust to lowered levels of mechanical ventilator support, which interrupts and prolongs the weaning process

## DEFINING CHARACTERISTICS

Dysfunctional ventilatory weaning response (DVWR) is a progressive state, and experienced nurses have identified three levels (Logan & Jenny, 1990): mild, moderate, and severe. The defining characteristics occur in response to weaning.

### Mild

**Major**
Restlessness
Slight increase in respiratory rate from baseline

**Minor**
Expressed feelings of increased oxygen need, breathing discomfort, fatigue, and warmth
Queries about possible machine dysfunction
Increased concentration on breathing

### Moderate

**Major**
Slight increase in blood pressure = 20 mm Hg or less from baseline
Slight increase in heart rate = 20 beats/min or less from baseline
Increase in respiratory rate = 5 breaths/min or less from baseline

**Minor**

| | |
|---|---|
| Hypervigilance to activities | Diaphoresis |
| Inability to respond to coaching | Eye-widening (wide-eyed look) |
| Inability to cooperate | Decreased air entry heard on auscultation |
| Apprehension | Skin color changes: pale, slight cyanosis |
| | Slight respiratory accessory muscle use |

## Severe

### Major
Agitation
Significant deterioration in arterial blood gases from baseline
Increase in blood pressure greater than 20 mm Hg from baseline
Increase in heart rate greater than 20 beats/min from baseline
Rapid, shallow breathing greater than 25 breaths/min

### Minor

| | |
|---|---|
| Cyanosis | Full respiratory accessory muscle use |
| Shallow, gasping breaths | Profuse diaphoresis |
| Paradoxical abdominal breathing | Breathing uncoordinated with the ventilator |
| Adventitious breath sounds | Decreased level of consciousness |

# RELATED FACTORS

## Pathophysiologic

*Related to muscle weakness and fatigue secondary to:*

| | | |
|---|---|---|
| Unstable hemodynamic status | Metabolic/acid–base abnormality | Anemia |
| | | Infection |
| Decreased level of consciousness | Severe disease process | Chronic nutritional deficit |
| | Chronic respiratory disease | Debilitated condition |
| Chronic neuromuscular disability | Multisystem disease | |
| | Fluid/electrolyte imbalance | |

*Related to ineffective airway clearance*

## Treatment-Related

*Related to obstructed airway*
*Related to muscle weakness and fatigue secondary to:*

| | |
|---|---|
| Excess sedation, analgesia | Uncontrolled pain |

*Related to inadequate nutrition (deficit in calories, excess carbohydrates, inadequate fats and protein intake)*
*Related to prolonged ventilator dependence (more than 1 week)*
*Related to previously unsuccessful ventilator weaning attempt(s)*
*Related to too-rapid pacing of the weaning process*

## Situational (Personal, Environmental)

*Related to insufficient knowledge of the weaning process*
*Related to excessive energy demands (self-care activities, diagnostic and treatment procedures, visitors)*
*Related to inadequate social support*
*Related to insecure environment (noisy, upsetting events, busy room)*
*Related to fatigue secondary to interrupted sleep patterns*
*Related to inadequate self-efficacy*
*Related to moderate to high anxiety related to breathing efforts*
*Related to fear of separation from ventilator*
*Related to feelings of powerlessness*
*Related to feelings of hopelessness*

### ■■■■■■ AUTHOR'S NOTE

Dysfunctional Ventilatory Weaning Response (DVWR) is a specific diagnosis within the category of *Risk for Ineffective Respiratory Function. Ineffective Airway Clearance, Ineffective Breathing Patterns*, and *Impaired Gas Exchange* also can be encountered during weaning, either as indicators of lack of weaning readiness or as factors related to the onset of DVWR. DVWR is a separate client state. Its distinctive etiologies and treatments arise from the process of separating the client from the mechanical ventilator.

*(continued)*

■ ■ ■ ■ ■ **AUTHOR'S NOTE** *Continued*

The process of weaning is an art and a science. Because weaning is a collaborative process, the nurse's ability to gain the client's trust and willingness to work is an important determinant of the weaning outcomes, especially with long-term clients. This trust is fostered by the knowledge and self-confidence nurses display and by their ability to deal with clients' specific concerns (Jenny & Logan, 1991).

■ ■ ■ ■ ■ **ERRORS IN DIAGNOSTIC STATEMENTS**

### Dysfunctional Weaning Response related to increased blood pressure, heart rate, respiratory rate, and agitation during weaning

This diagnosis does not indicate the reasons for weaning problems. The related factors are evidence of *Dysfunctional Weaning Response*, not causative and contributing factors. The nurse should write the diagnosis with the related factors if they are known, or "unknown etiology" if not known.

Many of the following assessments and interventions apply to the prevention of moderate and severe responses as well as the treatment phases of managing the diagnosis.

■ ■ ■ ■ ■ **KEY CONCEPTS**

### Generic Considerations

- *Weaning* is the process of assisting clients to breathe spontaneously without mechanical ventilation. Weaning success has been defined as spontaneous breathing for 24 h without ventilatory support, with or without an artificial airway.
- Ventilator weaning is a multidisciplinary effort in which the presence of knowledgeable nurses affects the outcomes positively. Experienced nurses agree that weaning is a collaborative process shared with the client that has both a physical and a psychological aspect. For ventilator-dependent clients, it can be a very stressful experience (Logan & Jenny, 1991). Recent works on clients' perceptions of ventilator weaning describe their concerns, which include physical discomfort, nurse caring behaviors, feelings of altered self, and the clients' physical, emotional, and cognitive work involved in weaning (Jenny & Logan, 1998).
- Ventilator-associated complications may occur with prolonged ventilation. A long period of intubation and mechanical ventilation places clients at risk for postoperative pulmonary complications. Systematic daily assessment of the oropharyngeal cavity is necessary for ventilated clients, especially those who are orally intubated, to detect or prevent lesions and infection (Treloar & Stechmiller, 1995). It is not recommended that normal saline instillation before suctioning be a routine practice (Chulay, 2005; Halm & Krisko-Hagel, 2008).
- Various criteria have been proposed for determining weaning readiness. These criteria are measures of oxygenation, respiratory muscle strength, and the ability to ventilate sufficiently to maintain an adequate arterial carbon dioxide level ($Paco_2$). Gaps exist, however, in our knowledge of client responses to ventilator weaning and in the prediction of outcomes. Goodnough Hanneman (1994) suggests that one reason that weaning predictors do not have adequate predictive power may be that the interrelationship of cardiopulmonary pathophysiologic determinants of outcomes is not reflected by independent predictive criteria (e.g., pulmonary mechanics). The ongoing use of a systematic assessment tool may help tailor the process to the client's current status and prevent a premature weaning trial or a dysfunctional weaning response.
- Outcomes after short-term mechanical ventilation differ from those after long-term ventilation. Psychological outlook, ventilatory drive, respiratory muscle strength and endurance, minute volume requirements, and nutritional status appear to have little bearing on short-term ventilator weaning (Morton et al., 2005).
- The physiologic inspiratory work of breathing includes three components (Porth, 2007):
  - Compliance work to expand the elastic forces of the lung
  - Tissue resistance work to overcome the viscosity of the lung and thoracic cage
  - Airway resistance work to overcome the resistance to the flow of air into and out of the lungs
- Mechanical ventilation increases the work of breathing by decreasing airway diameter and increasing its length, thus increasing resistance. During weaning, the clinician manipulates pressure/volume changes to promote reconditioning of the respiratory muscles without causing excessive fatigue (Morton et al., 2005).
- DVWR can involve respiratory inspiratory muscle fatigue, which can take up to 24 to 48 h for recovery. The fatigue increases dyspnea, which, in turn, creates anxiety, triggering more fatigue and increased breathlessness.

# Focus Assessment Criteria

## Subjective Data

### Assess for Defining Characteristics

Concerns about starting or continuing weaning process
Readiness      Previous experience      Expectations
Possibility of failure
Feelings about comfort, rest, and energy status
Knowledge of weaning process

### Assess for Related Factors

Medication history
Tobacco and alcohol use

## Objective Data

### Assess for Defining Characteristics

Respiratory status: Complete respiratory assessment (see Focus Assessment Criteria in *Risk for Ineffective Respiratory Function*)

| | | |
|---|---|---|
| Level of consciousness | Baseline skin color | Airway clearance |
| Secretions (type and amount) | Adventitious breath sounds | Arterial blood gases |
| Use of accessory muscles | Vital signs | |

### Assess for Related Factors

Respiratory disease, acute and chronic diseases
Mechanical ventilator information:

- Ventilator settings and size of endotracheal or tracheostomy tube
- Ventilation history, including reason for ventilation
- Length of time on the ventilator
- Whether weaning has been attempted before, and if so, with what results

Current hemodynamic, nutritional, infection, and pain status
For more information on Focus Assessment Criteria, visit http://thepoint.lww.com.

---

**NOC**

Anxiety Control, Respiratory Status, Vital Signs Status, Knowledge: Weaning, Energy Conservation

## ➤ Goal

The client will achieve progressive weaning goals.

### Indicators:

- Spontaneous breathing for 24 h without ventilatory support *or*
- Demonstrate a positive attitude toward the next weaning trial: collaborate willingly with the weaning plan, communicate comfort status during the weaning process, attempt to control the breathing pattern, and try to control emotional responses
- Be tired from the work of weaning, but not exhausted

---

**NIC**

Anxiety Reduction, Preparatory Sensory Information, Respiratory Monitoring, Ventilation Assistance, Presence, Endurance

## General Interventions

### If Applicable, Assess Causative Factors for Previous Unsuccessful Weaning Attempts

Refer to Related Factors.

### Determine Readiness for Weaning (Morton et al., 2005)

Respiratory rate less than 35 breaths/min

Oxygen concentration of 40% or less on the ventilator
Negative inspiratory pressure less than –20
Positive expiratory pressure greater than +30
Spontaneous tidal volume greater than 5 mL/kg
Vital capacity greater than 10 to 15 mL/kg
Rested, controlled discomfort
Willingness to try weaning
Absence of fever
Normal hemoglobin levels

**R:** Research has proven these predictors for successful weaning.

## If Readiness for Weaning Is Present, Engage the Client in Establishing the Plan

Explain the weaning process.
Negotiate progressive weaning goals.
Create a visual display of goals that uses symbols to indicate progression (e.g., bar or line graph to indicate increasing time off ventilator).
Explain that these goals will be reexamined daily with the client.
Refer to unit protocols for specific weaning procedures.

**R:** An initial step in the weaning plan is the careful preparation of clients. This includes teaching them about their collaborative weaning role, maximizing their energy resources and physical rest, enhancing their psychological willingness to proceed, and reinforcing their belief that they can perform the work of weaning (Jenny & Logan, 1998). Clients may have difficulty expressing their thoughts, so nurses must use multiple communication methods and persist until an effective method is found.

## Explain the Client's Role in the Weaning Process

From initial intubation, promote the understanding that mechanical ventilation is temporary.
Share nurses' expectations of their collaborative work role when the client is judged ready to wean.
Help the client to understand the importance of communicating comfort status and trying to reach the current weaning goals, and that rest will be allowed throughout the process.

**R:** The strategies can increase psychological readiness.

## Strengthen Feelings of Self-Esteem, Self-Efficacy, and Control

Reinforce self-esteem, confidence, and control through normalizing strategies such as grooming, dressing, mobilizing, and conversing socially about things of interest to the client.
Permit as much control as possible by informing the client of the situation and his or her progress, permitting shared decision-making about details of care, following the client's preferences as far as possible, and improving comfort status.
Increase confidence by praising successful activities, encouraging a positive outlook, and reviewing positive progress to date. Explain that people usually succeed in weaning; reassure the client that you will be with him or her every step of the way.
Demonstrate confidence in the client's ability to wean.
Maintain the client's confidence by adopting a weaning pace that ensures success and minimizes setbacks.*
Explain what you are doing and why, to reduce the client's vigilance and feelings of uncertainty.
Note concerns that hinder comfort and confidence (family members, topics of conversation, room events, previous weaning failures); discuss them openly. Reduce them, if possible.

**R:** Successful weaning is both an art and a science. The art depends on using subjective clinical judgment about the individual situation. The science involves the theories of oxygen exchange, carbon dioxide exchange, and mechanical efficiency (Henneman, 2001). Nurses are a critical factor in imparting a

---

*May require a primary professional's order.

positive outlook, creating a secure environment, enhancing feelings of self-esteem and self-confidence, and helping clients deal with setbacks through their ability to combine the art and science of weaning (Jenny & Logan, 1994).

## Reduce Negative Effects of Anxiety and Fatigue

Monitor status frequently to avoid undue fatigue and anxiety. Use a systematic, comprehensive tool. A pulse oximeter is a noninvasive and unobtrusive way to monitor oxygen saturation levels.
Provide regular periods of rest before fatigue advances:

- Reduce activities.
- Maintain or increase ventilator support and/or oxygen in consultation with a physician.

During a rest period, dim lights, post "do not disturb" signs, and play instrumental music with 60 to 80 beats/min. Allow the client to select type of music (Chan, 1998).
Encourage calmness and breath control by reassuring the client that he or she can and will succeed.
Consider use of alternative therapies such as music, hypnosis, and biofeedback.
If the client is becoming agitated, calm him or her down while remaining at the bedside, and coach him or her to regain breathing control. Monitor oxygen saturation and vital signs closely during this intervention.
If the weaning trial is discontinued, address the client's perceptions of weaning failure. Reassure the client that the trial was good exercise and a useful form of training. Remind the client that the work is good for the respiratory muscles and will improve future performance.

**R:** Successful weaning depends on adequate energy resources, careful use of available energy, and skilled withdrawal of the ventilator support within the limits of the client's ability to tolerate additional breathing work. Altered or depleted energy reserve enhances fatigue. Thus, energy-conservation techniques are crucial to all weaning approaches (Jenny & Logan, 1998; Logan & Jenny, 1990).

## Create a Positive Weaning Environment That Increases Feelings of Security

Provide a room with a quiet atmosphere, low activity, soft music, and no chatter within the client's hearing.

**R:** Music with 60 to 80 beats/min decreases arousability of the CNS and exerts a hypnotic, relaxed state (Chan, 1998).

Delegate the most skilled staff to wean clients who have experienced moderate to severe responses or who are at high risk for doing so.
Remain visible in the room to reinforce feelings of safety.
Reassure the client that help is immediately available, if needed.
Monitor visitors' effects on the client; help visitors understand how they can best assist.
Encourage supportive visitors when possible during the weaning process. Visits from people who upset the client should be postponed.
Ensure that clients are included in discussions that they are likely to overhear.

**R:** Weaning setbacks are common and require client support. During prolonged weaning, the client must be psychologically motivated to wean. Music therapy appears to have a beneficial effect in promoting relaxation in mechanically ventilated clients (Chan, 1998). Feelings of powerlessness, hopelessness, and depression are combated with active decision-making with the client, explanation of sensations experienced, positive feedback, and conveyance of hopefulness, encouragement, and support (Logan & Jenny, 1991).

## Promote Optimal Energy Resources

Assist client to cough and deep-breathe regularly, and use prescribed bronchodilators, humidification, and suctioning to improve air entry.
Ensure that nutritional support falls within current guidelines for ventilated and weaning clients.
Provide sufficient rest periods to prevent undue fatigue.

Use ventilator support at night if necessary to increase sleep time, and try to avoid unnecessary awakening.

Monitor the disease processes to determine the body systems' stability.

**R:** To maintain adequate energy levels, nutritional support is necessary. It should avoid creating the complications of lipogenesis, overfeeding, and excessive carbohydrate loading to prevent excessive levels of carbon dioxide and respiratory acidemia.

## Control Activity Demands

Coordinate necessary activities to promote adequate time for rest or relaxation.

Ensure that all staff follow the individualized care plan.

Coach the client in breath control by regular demonstrations of slow, deep, rhythmic patterns of breathing. Help the client to synchronize breathing with the ventilator.

If the client's concentration starts to create tension and increase anxiety, provide distraction in the form of supportive visitors, radio, television, or conversation.

**R:** As ventilator support is withdrawn, clients have to work harder. Their work of weaning involves controlling their breathing, communicating their comfort status, cooperating with the therapeutic regimen, and trying to control their emotional responses to feelings of fatigue and anxiety (Jenny & Logan, 1991).

## Follow the Institution's Multidiscipline Weaning Protocol

Document the specifics of the plan with a timetable.

Establish predetermined criteria for terminating the weaning process.

Outline each discipline's responsibilities

Review goals and progress at each shift. Document response.

Collaborate if revisions are needed.

**R:** Collaborative weaning plans with clear goals and responsibilities and timetable have decreased ventilator and ICU days.

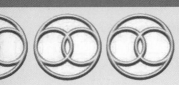

# RISK FOR DYSFUNCTIONAL VENTILATORY WEANING RESPONSE

## DEFINITION

State in which a client is at risk for experiencing an inability to adjust to lowered levels of mechanical ventilator support during the weaning process, related to physical and/or psychological unreadiness to wean

## RISK FACTORS

### Pathophysiologic

*Related to airway obstruction*
*Related to muscle weakness and fatigue secondary to:*

| | | |
|---|---|---|
| Impaired respiratory functioning | Decreased level of consciousness | Unstable hemodynamic status |
| Metabolic abnormalities | Fever | Acid–base abnormalities |
| Dysrhythmia | Anemia | Mental confusion |
| Fluid and/or electrolyte | Severe disease | Infection |
| | | Multisystem disease |

imbalance

## Treatment-Related

*Related to ineffective airway clearance*
*Related to excess sedation, analgesia*
*Related to uncontrolled pain*
*Related to fatigue*
*Related to inadequate nutrition (deficit in calories, excess carbohydrates, inadequate fats and protein intake)*
*Related to prolonged ventilator dependence (more than 1 week)*
*Related to previous unsuccessful ventilator weaning attempt(s)*
*Related to too-rapid pacing of the weaning process*

## Situational (Personal, Environmental)

*Related to muscle weakness and fatigue secondary to:*
Chronic nutritional deficit      Obesity      Ineffective sleep patterns
*Related to knowledge deficit related to the weaning process*
*Related to inadequate self-efficacy related to weaning*
*Related to moderate to high anxiety related to breathing efforts*
*Related to fear of separation from ventilator*
*Related to feelings of powerlessness*
*Related to depressed mood*
*Related to feelings of hopelessness*
*Related to uncontrolled energy demands (self-care activities, diagnostic and treatment procedures, visitors)*
*Related to inadequate social support*
*Related to insecure environment (noisy, upsetting events, busy room)*

■■■■■■ **AUTHOR'S NOTE**

See *Dysfunctional Ventilatory Weaning Response.*

■■■■■■ **ERRORS IN DIAGNOSTIC STATEMENTS**

See *Dysfunctional Ventilatory Weaning Response.*

■■■■■■ **KEY CONCEPTS**

### Generic Considerations

- Clients at high risk for unsuccessful ventilator weaning are those who, for one reason or another, do not meet the traditional criteria for readiness to wean, such as:
  - Respiratory rate less than 25 breaths/min
  - Oxygen concentration of 40% or less on the ventilator
  - Negative inspiratory pressure less than –20
  - Positive expiratory pressure greater than +30
  - Spontaneous tidal volume greater than 5 mL/kg
  - Vital capacity greater than 10 to 15 mL/kg
  - Adequate arterial blood gases for client
  - Rested, controlled discomfort
- Although weaning as soon as possible is important to avoid muscle deconditioning and complications related to prolonged endotracheal intubation and tracheostomy, premature attempts may be counterproductive because of adverse physiologic and psychological effects.

*(continued)*

▪▪▪▪▪▪ **KEY CONCEPTS** *Continued*

- Because weaning is a collaborative process, the nurse's ability to gain the client's trust and willingness to work is an important determinant of outcomes, especially with long-term clients. This trust is fostered by the knowledge and self-confidence nurses display and by their ability to deal with the client's specific concerns (Jenny & Logan, 1991).
- Weaning collaboration involves specific roles for both the nurse and the client. The nurse must know the client, manage his or her energy, and assist with the work of weaning. The client's collaborative work requires a trust relationship, and the belief that he or she will be protected during weaning.
- Respiratory muscles must be stressed to a certain point of fatigue and then allowed to rest. The critical point of fatigue and duration of rest have not been documented in the literature, and this judgment depends on clinical expertise (Slutsky, 1993).
- Dysfunctional ventilatory weaning is usually multifactorial. Marini (1991) notes that, at the bedside, the subjective assessment of the weaning trial by an experienced clinician remains the most reliable predictor of weaning success or failure. Close monitoring of the client's weaning work is needed to prevent serious respiratory fatigue, which can require up to 24 to 48 h of recovery before the client can proceed.
- A dysfunctional weaning response to a weaning trial also can influence the client's motivation and self-efficacy, creating doubt about the ability to wean and weakening the resolve to work (Jenny & Logan, 1991).

## Focus Assessment Criteria

See *Dysfunctional Ventilatory Weaning Response*.

**NOC**
Refer to
*Dysfunctional
Ventilatory Weaning
Response*

## ➤ Goals

The client will:

- Demonstrate a willingness to start weaning.
- Demonstrate a positive attitude about ability to succeed.

### *Indicators:*

- Maintain emotional control.
- Collaborate with planning of the weaning.

**NIC**
Refer to
*Dysfunctional
Ventilatory Weaning
Response*

## ➤ General Interventions

Refer to *Dysfunctional Ventilatory Weaning Response*

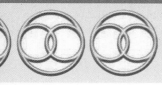

# INEFFECTIVE AIRWAY CLEARANCE

## DEFINITION

State in which a client experiences a threat to respiratory status related to inability to cough effectively

## DEFINING CHARACTERISTICS

### Major (Must Be Present, One or More)

Ineffective or absent cough
Inability to remove airway secretions

### Minor (May Be Present)

Abnormal breath sounds
Abnormal respiratory rate, rhythm, and depth
Related Factors
See *Risk for Ineffective Respiratory Function*.

## ▰▰▰▰▰ KEY CONCEPTS

See *Risk for Ineffective Respiratory Function*.

## Focus Assessment Criteria

See *Risk for Ineffective Respiratory Function*.

**NOC**
Aspiration Control, Respiratory Status

## ➤ Goal

The client will not experience aspiration.

### Indicators:

* Demonstrate effective coughing and increased air exchange.
* Explain rationale for interventions to promote coughing:

**NIC**
Cough Enhancement, Airway Suctioning, Positioning, Energy Management

## ➤ General Interventions

The nursing interventions for the diagnosis *Ineffective Airway Clearance* represent interventions for any client with this nursing diagnosis, regardless of the related factors.

### Assess for Causative or Contributing Factors

Refer to Related Factors.

### Assess and Evaluate

Sputum (color, volume, odor)
Respiratory status before and after coughing exercises (breath sounds, rate, rhythm)

**R:** These assessments can detect abnormal sputum (green, yellow, bloody, and retained secretions).

Provide oral care with a toothbrush every 4 h.

**R:** Oral care with a toothbrush reduces plaque and bacteria. Optimal oral care can improve appetite and promote positive interactions by reducing odor. Reducing bacterial colonization prevents ventilator-associated pneumonia (Munro & Grap, 2004).

## Reduce or Eliminate Barriers to Airway Clearance

### Inability to Maintain Proper Position

Assist with positioning frequently; monitor for *Risk for Aspiration* (see *High Risk for Aspiration*).

### Ineffective Cough

Instruct the client on the proper method of controlled coughing:

• Breathe deeply and slowly while sitting up as high as possible.

**R:** Sitting upright shifts the abdominal organs away from the lungs, enabling greater expansion.

• Use diaphragmatic breathing.

**R:** Diaphragmatic breathing reduces the respiratory rate and increases alveolar ventilation.

• Hold the breath for 3 to 5 s, then slowly exhale as much of this breath as possible through the mouth (lower rib cage and abdomen should sink down).
• Take a second breath, hold, slowly exhale, and cough forcefully from the chest (not from the back of the mouth or throat), using two short, forceful coughs.
• Increase fluid intake if not contraindicated.

**R:** Deep breathing dilates the airways, stimulates surfactant production, and expands the lung tissue surface, thus improving respiratory gas exchange. Coughing loosens secretions and forces them into the bronchus to be expectorated or suctioned. In some clients, "huffing" breathing may be effective and is less painful.

### Pain or Fear of Pain Related to Surgery or Trauma

Assess present analgesic regimen:

• Administer pain medications as needed.
• Coordinate analgesic doses with coughing sessions (e.g., give doses 30 to 60 min before coughing sessions).
• Assess medication's effectiveness: Is the client too lethargic? Is he or she still in pain?
• Note time when the client appears to have the best pain relief with optimal level of alertness and physical performance. This is the time for active breathing and coughing exercises.

Provide emotional support:

• Explain the importance of coughing after pain relief.
• Reassure that suture lines are secure and that splinting by hand or pillow will minimize pain of movement.

Use appropriate comfort measures for the site of pain:

• Splint abdominal or chest incisions with hand, pillow, or both.

For sore throat:

• Provide humidity unless contraindicated.
• Consider warm saline gargle every 2 to 4 h.
• Consider use of an anesthetic lozenge or gargle, especially before coughing sessions.
• Examine the throat for exudate, redness, and swelling; note if it is associated with fever.
• Explain that a sore throat is common after anesthesia and should be a short-term problem.

Maintain good body alignment to prevent muscular pain and strain:

• Acquire and use extra pillows on both sides, especially the affected side, for support.
• Position the client to prevent slouching and cramping positions of the thorax and abdomen; reassess positioning frequently.

Assess understanding of the use of analgesia to enhance breathing and coughing effort:

- Teach during periods of optimal level of consciousness.
- Continually reinforce the rationale for the plan of nursing care. ("I will be back to help you cough when the pain medicine is working and you can be most effective.")

**R:** Pain or fear of pain can inhibit participation in coughing and breathing exercises. Adequate pain relief is essential.

**R:** Coughing exercises are fatiguing and painful. Emotional support provides encouragement.

### Viscous (Thick) Secretions

Maintain adequate hydration (increase fluid intake to 2 to 3 quarts a day if not contraindicated by decreased cardiac output or renal disease).

**R:** Secretions must be sufficiently liquid to enable expulsion.

Maintain adequate humidity of inspired air.

**R:** Thick secretions are difficult to expectorate and can cause mucous plugs, leading to atelectasis.

### Fatigue, Weakness, and Drowsiness

Plan and bargain for rest periods ("Work to cough well now; then I can let you rest.").
Vigorously coach and encourage coughing, using positive reinforcement ("You worked hard; I know it's not easy, but it is important.").
Be sure the coughing session occurs at the peak comfort period after analgesics, but not peak level of sleepiness.
Allow for rest after coughing and before meals.
For lethargy or decreased level of consciousness, stimulate the client to breathe deeply hourly ("Take a deep breath.").

**R:** Coughing exercises are fatiguing and painful. Emotional support provides encouragement.

### For Chronic, Unrelieved Coughing:

Minimize irritants in the inspired air (e.g., dust, allergens).
Provide periods of uninterrupted rest.
Administer prescribed medications—cough suppressant, expectorant—as ordered by the physician/nurse practitioner (withhold food and drink immediately after administration of medications for best results).

**R:** Uncontrolled coughing is tiring and ineffective and may contribute to bronchitis.

## Provide Health Teaching and Referrals, as Indicated

Teach the client and family:

- Hydration requirements
- Mouth care
- Effective coughing techniques
- Signs of infection (change in sputum color, fever)

Refer to Home Health nursing if needed.

**R:** Instructions to continue effective coughing at home are needed to prevent retention of secretions and infection.

**Pediatric Interventions**

Instruct parents on the need for the child to cough, even if it is painful.
Allow an adult and older child to listen to the lungs and describe if clear or if rales are present.
Consult with a respiratory therapist for assistance, if needed.

**R:** Explaining and demonstrating the benefits of coughing can increase parent and child cooperation.

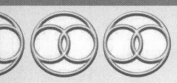

# INEFFECTIVE BREATHING PATTERNS

## DEFINITION

State in which a client experiences an actual or potential loss of adequate ventilation related to an altered breathing pattern

## DEFINING CHARACTERISTICS

### Major (Must Be Present, One or More)

Changes in respiratory rate or pattern (from baseline)
Changes in pulse (rate, rhythm, quality)

### Minor (May Be Present)

Orthopnea                                              Dysrhythmic respirations
Tachypnea, hyperpnea, hyperventilation    Splinted/guarded respirations

## RELATED FACTORS

See *Risk for Ineffective Respiratory Function.*

### ■■■■■ AUTHOR'S NOTE

See *Risk for Ineffective Respiratory Function.*

### ■■■■■ ERRORS IN DIAGNOSTIC STATEMENTS

See *Risk for Ineffective Respiratory Function.*

### ■■■■■ KEY CONCEPTS

#### Generic Considerations

- Hyperventilation is overbreathing with reduced $Pco_2$ and respiratory alkalosis.
- Causes of hyperventilation syndrome are organic (drug effects, CNS lesions), physiologic (response to high altitude, heat, exercise), emotional (anxiety, hysteria, anger, depression), and habitual faulty breathing habits (rapid, shallow breathing) (Porth, 2007).
- Symptoms of hyperventilation syndrome are headache, dyspnea, numbness and tingling, lightheadedness, chest pain, palpitations, and, occasionally, syncope (Porth, 2007).
- Panic can manifest with hyperventilation, and people with panic disorders can hyperventilate.
- All nurses involved in caring for clients with COPD must be skilled at teaching pursed-lip breathing, a critical survival skill that these clients must learn to maintain function. Studies show that pursed-lip breathing decreases respiratory rate, increases tidal volume, decreases arterial $CO_2$, increases arterial oxygen, and improves exercise performance.
- Teach the client to inhale through the nose, not too deeply. Breathe out through the mouth while holding the lips (except for a section in the center) together. Exhalation should be at least twice as long as inhalation and should be a steady stream of air without blowing too hard.

**NOC**
Respiratory Status,
Vital Signs Status,
Anxiety Control

➤ **Goals** _____

*Indicators:*

• Achieve respiratory rate within normal limits, compared with baseline (8 to 24/min).
• Express relief of (or improvement in) feelings of shortness of breath.
• Relate causative factors and ways of preventing or managing them.

**NIC**
Respiratory
Monitoring,
Progressive Muscle
Relaxation, Teaching,
Anxiety Reduction

➤ **General Interventions** _____

## Assess History of Symptoms and Causative Factors

Previous episodes—when, where, circumstances
Causes:

• Organic and physiologic
• Emotional

Faulty breathing habits

## Remove or Control Causative Factors

Explain the cause.
Stay with the client.
If fear or panic has precipitated the episode:

• Remove the cause of the fear, if possible.
• Reassure the client that measures are being taken to ensure safety.
• Distract the client from thinking about the anxious state by having him or her maintain eye contact with you (or perhaps with someone else he or she trusts); say, "Now look at me and breathe slowly with me like this."
• Consider use of a paper bag as means of rebreathing expired air (expired $CO_2$ will be reinspired, thereby slowing respiratory rate).
• See *Fear*.

Reassure the client that he or she can control breathing; tell him or her that you will help.
Teach controlled breathing techniques (e.g., pursed-lip breathing) or consult with a respiratory therapist for training to overcome faulty breathing patterns.

**R:** Interventions focus on slowing the breathing pattern and educating the client to control response.
**R:** Calming a client with shortness of breath by telling him or her that actions are being taken to improve the situation (e.g., "I'm here, and I will get you through this") is an essential intervention to reduce panic and decrease symptoms.

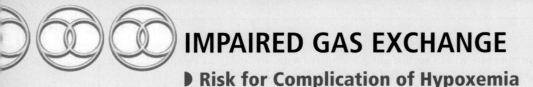

# IMPAIRED GAS EXCHANGE

## ▶ Risk for Complication of Hypoxemia

## DEFINITION

State in which a person experiences an actual or potential decreased passage of gases (oxygen and carbon dioxide) between the alveoli of the lungs and the vascular system

## DEFINING CHARACTERISTICS

### Major (must be present)

Dyspnea on exertion
Minor (may be present)
Tendency to assume three-point position (sitting, one hand on knee and bending forward)
Purse-lip breathing
Lethargy and fatigue
Decreased oxygen content, decreased oxygen saturauion
Cyanosis

## RELATED FACTORS

See related Factors for Inefffective Respiratory Function

### ■■■■■■■ AUTHOR'S NOTE

Respiratory problems that nurses can treat as nursing diagnoses are Ineffective Airway Clearance, Ineffective breathing Patterns, and Risk for Ineffective Respiratory Function. If gas exchange does not improve when these nursing diagnoses are treated, then the problem is a collaborative problem. This should be labeled Risk for Complications of: Hypoxia. In addition the nurse should assess for functional health patterns that decrease oxygenation may affect a sleep, emotional status, fatigue and nutrition and formulated the appropriate nursing diagnoses.

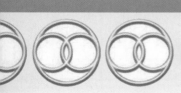

# INEFFECTIVE ROLE PERFORMANCE

## DEFINITION

State in which a client experiences or is at risk of experiencing a disruption in the way he or she perceives his or her role performance

## DEFINING CHARACTERISTICS

### Major (Must Be Present)

Conflict related to role perception or performance

516

## Minor (May Be Present)

Change in self-perception of role

Denial of role

Change in others' perception of role

Change in physical capacity to resume role

Lack of knowledge of role

Change in usual patterns of responsibility

### ■■■■■■ AUTHOR'S NOTE

The nursing diagnosis *Ineffective Role Performance* has a defining characteristic of "conflict related to role perception or performance." All people have multiple roles. Some are prescribed, such as gender and age; some are acquired, such as parent and occupation; and some are transitional, such as elected office or team member.

Various factors affect a client's roles, including developmental stage, societal norms, cultural beliefs, values, life events, illness, and disabilities. When a client has difficulty with role performance, it may be more useful to describe the effect of the difficulty on functioning, rather than to describe the problem as *Ineffective Role Performance*. For example, a client who has experienced a cerebrovascular accident (CVA) may undergo a change from being the primary breadwinner to becoming unemployed. In this situation, the nursing diagnosis *Grieving related to loss of role as financial provider secondary to effects of CVA* would be appropriate. In another example, if a woman could not continue her household responsibilities because of illness and other family members assumed these responsibilities, the situations that may arise would better be described as *Risk for Disturbed Self-Concept related to recent loss of role responsibility secondary to illness and Risk for Impaired Home Maintenance Management related to lack of knowledge of family members*.

A conflict in a family regarding others meeting role obligations or expectations can represent related factors for the diagnosis *Ineffective Family Processes related to conflict regarding expectations of members meeting role obligations*.

Until clinical research defines this diagnosis and the associated nursing interventions, use "ineffective role performance" as a related factor for another nursing diagnosis (e.g., *Anxiety, Grieving,* or *Disturbed Self-Concept*).

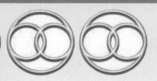

# SELF-CARE DEFICIT SYNDROME

**Self-Care Deficit Syndrome***

Feeding Self-Care Deficit

Bathing Self-Care Deficit

Dressing Self-Care Deficit

Instrumental Self-Care Deficit*

Toileting Self-Care Deficit

## DEFINITION

State in which a client experiences an impaired motor function or cognitive function, causing a decreased ability in performing each of the five self-care activities

## DEFINING CHARACTERISTICS

### Major (One Deficit Must Be Present in Each Activity)

**Self-Feeding Deficits**

Unable to cut food or open packages

Unable to bring food to the mouth

---

*These diagnoses are not currently on the NANDA list but have been included for clarity or usefulness.

**Self-Bathing Deficits (Includes Washing Entire Body, Combing Hair, Brushing Teeth, Attending to Skin and Nail Care, and Applying Makeup)**
Unable or unwilling to wash body or body parts
Unable to obtain a water source
Unable to regulate temperature or water flow
Unable to perceive need for hygienic measures

**Self-Dressing Deficits (Including Donning Regular or Special Clothing, Not Nightclothes)**
Impaired ability to put on or take off clothing
Unable to fasten clothing
Unable to groom self satisfactorily
Unable to obtain or replace articles of clothing

**Self-Toileting Deficits**
Unable or unwilling to get to toilet or commode
Unable or unwilling to carry out proper hygiene
Unable to transfer to and from toilet or commode
Unable to handle clothing to accommodate toileting
Unable to flush toilet or empty commode

**Instrumental Self-Care Deficits**

| | |
|---|---|
| Difficulty using telephone | Difficulty accessing transportation |
| Difficulty laundering, ironing | Difficulty managing money |
| Difficulty preparing meals | Difficulty with medication administration |
| Difficulty shopping | |

# RELATED FACTORS

## Pathophysiologic

*Related to lack of coordination secondary to (specify)*
*Related to spasticity or flaccidity secondary to (specify)*
*Related to muscular weakness secondary to (specify)*
*Related to partial or total paralysis secondary to (specify)*
*Related to atrophy secondary to (specify)*
*Related to muscle contractures secondary to (specify)*
*Related to visual disorders secondary to (specify)*
*Related to nonfunctioning or missing limb(s)*
*Related to regression to an earlier level of development*
*Related to excessive ritualistic behaviors*
*Related to somatoform deficits (specify)*

## Treatment-Related

*Related to external devices (specify: casts, splints, braces, intravenous [IV] equipment)*
*Related to postoperative fatigue and pain*

## Situational (Personal, Environmental)

| | | |
|---|---|---|
| *Related to cognitive deficits* | *Related to fatigue* | *Related to pain* |
| *Related to decreased motivation* | *Related to confusion* | *Related to disabling anxiety* |

## Maturational

**Older Adult**
*Related to decreased visual and motor ability, muscle weakness*

### ▪▪▪▪▪ AUTHOR'S NOTE

Self-care encompasses the activities needed to meet daily needs, commonly known as activities of daily living (ADLs), which are learned over time and become lifelong habits. Self-care activities involve not only what is to be done (hygiene, bathing, dressing, toileting, feeding), but also how much, when, where, with whom, and how (Miller, 2009).

In every client, the threat or reality of a self-care deficit evokes panic. Many people report that they fear loss of independence more than death. A self-care deficit affects the core of self-concept and self-determination. For this reason, the nursing focus for self-care deficit should be not on providing the care measure, but on identifying adaptive techniques to allow the client the maximum degree of participation and independence possible.

The diagnosis *Total Self-Care Deficit* once was used to describe a client's inability to complete feeding, bathing, toileting, dressing, and grooming (Gordon, 1982). The intent of specifying "Total" was to describe a client with deficits in several ADLs. Unfortunately, sometimes its use invites, according to Magnan (1989, personal communication), "preconceived judgments about the state of an individual and the nursing interventions required." The client may be viewed as in a vegetative state, requiring only minimal custodial care. *Total Self-Care Deficit* has been eliminated because its language does not denote potential for growth or rehabilitation.

Currently not on the NANDA list, the diagnosis *Self-Care Deficit Syndrome* has been added here to describe a client with compromised ability in all five self-care activities. For this client, the nurse assesses functioning in each area and identifies the level of participation of which the client is capable. The goal is to maintain current functioning, to increase participation and independence, or both. The syndrome distinction clusters all five self-care deficits together to enable grouping of interventions when indicated, while also permitting specialized interventions for a specific deficit.

The danger of applying a Self-Care Deficit diagnosis lies in the possibility of prematurely labeling a client as unable to participate at any level, eliminating a rehabilitation focus. It is important that the nurse classify the client's functional level to promote independence. (Refer to the functional level classification scale in Focus Assessment Criteria.) Use this scale with the nursing diagnosis (e.g., *Toileting Self-Care Deficit* [2]). Continuous reevaluation also is necessary to identify changes in the client's ability to participate in self-care.

### ▪▪▪▪▪ ERRORS IN DIAGNOSTIC STATEMENTS

1. *Toileting Self-Care Deficit related to insufficient knowledge of ostomy care*
   The diagnosis *Toileting Self-Care Deficit* describes a client who cannot get to, sit on, or rise from the toilet, or perform clothing and hygiene activities related to toileting. Insufficient knowledge of ostomy care does not apply. Depending on the risk factors or signs and symptoms, the diagnosis of *Ineffective Management of Therapeutic Regimen related to insufficient knowledge of ostomy care* would apply.
2. *Dressing Self-Care Deficit related to inability to fasten clothing*
   Inability to fasten clothing represents a sign or symptom of *Dressing Self-Care Deficit*, not a related factor. Using a focus assessment, the nurse needs to determine the contributing factors (e.g., insufficient knowledge of adaptive techniques needed).
3. *Self-Care Deficit Syndrome related to cognitive deficits*
   As a syndrome diagnosis, no related factors are indicated and, in fact, they are not very useful for treatment. Instead, the nurse should write the diagnosis as *Self-Care Deficit Syndrome: Feeding (1), Bathing (4), Dressing (4), Toileting (5), Instrumental (2)*. The number code indicates the present level of functioning needed. The goals or outcome criteria should represent improved or increased functioning.

### ▪▪▪▪▪ KEY CONCEPTS

#### Generic Considerations

- The concept of self-care emphasizes each client's right to maintain individual control over his or her own pattern of living. (This applies to both the ill client and the well client.)
- It is acceptable to be dependent on others to provide basic physiologic and psychological needs for a limited time.
- Regression in ability to perform self-care activities may be a defense mechanism to threatening situations.

*(continued)*

■■■■■■ **KEY CONCEPTS** *Continued*

- Neglect of an extremity refers to the memory loss of the presence of an extremity (e.g., a client who has had a stroke or brain injury resulting in partial paralysis may ignore the arm or leg on the affected side of the body).
- The following key elements promote relearning of self-care tasks:
  - Providing a structured, consistent environment and routine
  - Repeating instructions and tasks
  - Teaching and practicing tasks during periods of least fatigue
  - Maintaining a familiar environment and teacher
  - Using patience, determination, and a positive attitude (by both learner and teacher)
  - Practice, practice, practice
- Lubkin (1995) describes four principles to motivate:
  - Uncover hidden resources.
  - Increase underused abilities.
  - Initiate positive life patterns.
  - Flourish within existing limitations.

## Endurance

- The endurance or ability of the client to maintain a given level of performance is influenced by the ability to use oxygen to produce energy (related to the optimal functioning of the heart and respiratory and circulatory systems) and the functioning of the neurologic and musculoskeletal systems. Thus, clients with alterations in these systems have increased energy demands or decreased ability to produce energy.
- Stress is energy-consuming; the more stressors a client has, the more fatigue he or she experiences. Stressors can be personal, environmental, disease-related, and treatment-related. Examples of possible stressors follow:

| *Personal* | *Environmental* | *Disease-Related* | *Treatment-Related* |
|---|---|---|---|
| Age | Isolation | Pain | Walker |
| Support system | Noise | Anemia | Medications |
| Lifestyle | Unfamiliar setting | Diagnostic studies | |

- Signs and symptoms of decreased oxygen in response to activity (e.g., self-care, mobility) are as follows:
  - Sustained increased heart rate 3 to 5 min after ceasing the activity, or a change in the pulse rhythm
  - Failure of systolic blood pressure reading to increase with activity, or a decrease in value
  - Decrease or excessive increase in respiratory rate and dyspnea
- Weakness, pallor, or cerebral hypoxia (confusion, incoordination)

Refer to Key Concepts under *Activity Intolerance* for additional information.

## Pediatric Considerations

- Infants and young children depend on caregivers for assistance with ADLs.
- Parents/caregivers can facilitate a child's mastery of self-care skills. The desired outcome is that the child participates in his or her care to the maximum of ability (Hockenberry & Wilson, 2009).
- The nurse should assess each child's unique ability to engage in self-care activities to promote control over self and environment.
- Children with cancer with higher self-concept scores performed more self-care practices and received less dependent care from their mothers (Mosher & Moore, 1998).
- When self-care requirements are met by oneself or others, self-concept is lower (Mosher & Moore, 1998).

## Geriatric Considerations

- Age-related changes do not in themselves cause self-care deficits. Older adults do, however, have an increased incidence of chronic diseases that can compromise functional ability (e.g., arthritis, cardiac disorders, visual impairment).
- Older adults with dementia have varying degrees of difficulty with self-care activities depending on memory deficits, ability to follow directions, and judgment (Miller, 2009).
- Sixty-three percent of older nursing home residents cannot perform basic ADLs because of cognitive impairment (Miller, 2009).
- Caregivers frequently promote excess disability and quicker deterioration in older adults because they believe independent behavior is atypical (Miller, 2009).

## Transcultural Considerations

- In some cultures, family members may show their concern for the sick relative by doing as much as possible for him or her (e.g., feeding, bathing). This practice may prevent the client from actively participating in a rehabilitation program (Andrews & Boyle, 2008).
- All cultures have rules, often unspoken, about who touches whom, when, and where (Andrews & Boyle, 2008).

## Focus Assessment Criteria

### Subjective and Objective Data

#### Evaluate Each ADL Using the Following Scale:

0 = Is completely independent
1 = Requires use of assistive device
2 = Needs minimal help
3 = Needs assistance and/or some supervision
4 = Needs total supervision
5 = Needs total assistance or unable to assist

### Assess for Defining Characteristics

#### Self-Feeding Abilities

| | | |
|---|---|---|
| Swallowing | Selecting foods | Chewing |
| Using utensils and cutting food | Seeing | Opening cartons |
| Drinking from cup | | |

#### Self-Bathing Abilities

| | |
|---|---|
| Undressing to bathe | Reaching water source |
| Differentiating water temperatures | Washing body parts |
| Performing oral care | Obtaining equipment (water, soap, towels) |

#### Self-Dressing/Grooming Abilities

| | | |
|---|---|---|
| Putting on or taking off clothing | Fastening clothing | Brushing teeth |
| Selecting appropriate clothing | Cleaning/trimming nails | Plugging in cord |
| Retrieving appropriate clothing | Washing and styling hair | Using deodorant |
| Shaving | | |

#### Self-Toileting Abilities

| | |
|---|---|
| Getting to toilet and undressing | Redressing |
| Performing hygiene (washing hands) | Rising from toilet |
| | Sitting on toilet |
| Can use tampon/sanitary napkin | Cleaning self/flushing toilet |

## Instrumental ADLs

*Telephone:*

| Ability to dial | Ability to talk, hear | Ability to answer |

*Transportation:*

| Ability to drive | Access to transportation |

*Laundry:*

| Availability of washer | Ability to wash, iron | Ability to put away |

*Food procurement and preparation:*

| Ability to cook | Ability to select foods | Ability to shop |

*Medications*

| Ability to remember | Ability to administer |

## Finances

Ability to write checks and pay bills

Ability to handle cash transactions (simple, complex)

## Assess for Related Factors

Ability to remember

Judgment

Ability to follow directions

Ability to identify/express needs

Ability to anticipate needs (food, laundry)

Social supports:

* Support people
* Availability of help with transportation, shopping, money management, laundry, housekeeping, and food preparation
* Community resources

Motivation

Endurance

For more information on Focus Assessment Criteria, visit http://thepoint.lww.com.

---

**NOC**

See Bathing, Feeding, Dressing, Toileting, and/or Instrumental Self-Care Deficit

➤ ## Goal

The client will participate in feeding, dressing, toileting, and bathing activities (specify what the client can perform with assistance and unassisted)

### Indicators:

* Identify preferences in self-care activities (e.g., time, products, location).
* Demonstrate optimal hygiene after assistance with care.

---

**NIC**

See Feeding, Bathing, Dressing, Toileting, and/or Instrumental Self-Care Deficit

➤ ## General Interventions

### Assess for Causative or Contributing Factors

Refer to Related Factors.

*Use the Following Scale to rate the client's ability to perform:*

0 = Is completely independent

1 = Requires use of assistive device

2 = Needs minimal help

3 = Needs assistance and/or some supervision

4 = Needs total supervision

5 = Needs total assistance or unable to assist

**R:** This coding allows for establishing a baseline to evaluate progress from.

## Promote Optimal Participation

Consult with a physical therapist to assess present level of participation and for a plan.

- Determine areas for potentially increased participation in each self-care activity.
- Explore the client's goals and determine what the learner perceives as his or her own needs.
- Compare what the nurse believes are the learner's needs and goals, and then work to establish mutually acceptable goals.
- Allow ample time to complete activities without help. Promote independence, but assist when the client cannot perform an activity.

**R:** Offering choices and including the client in planning care reduces feelings of powerlessness; promotes feelings of freedom, control, and self-worth; and increases the client's willingness to comply with therapeutic regimens. Optimal education promotes self-care.

## Promote Self-Esteem and Self-Determination

Determine preferences for:

| | | |
|---|---|---|
| Schedule | Products | Methods |
| Clothing selection | Hair styling | |

During self-care activities, provide choices and request preferences.

Do not focus on disability.

Offer praise for independent accomplishments.

**R:** Inability to care for oneself produces feelings of dependency and poor self-concept. With increased ability for self-care, self-esteem increases.

## Evaluate the Client's Ability to Participate in Each Self-Care Activity (Feeding, Dressing, Bathing, Toileting)

Reassess ability frequently and revise code as appropriate.

**R:** Coding each self-care ability provides a baseline to evaluate progress.

## Refer to Interventions Under Each Diagnosis—Feeding, Bathing, Dressing, Toileting, and Instrumental Self-Care Deficit—as Indicated

**R:** Enhancing a client's self-care abilities can increase his or her sense of control and independence, promoting overall well-being.

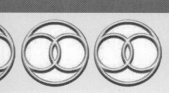

# FEEDING SELF-CARE DEFICIT

## DEFINITION

State in which a client experiences an impaired ability to perform or complete feeding activities for himself or herself

## DEFINING CHARACTERISTICS

Unable to cut food or open food packages
Unable to bring food to mouth

# RELATED FACTORS

See *Self-Care Deficit Syndrome*.

## ▪▪▪▪▪▪ AUTHOR'S NOTE

See *Self-Care Deficit Syndrome*.

## ▪▪▪▪▪▪ ERRORS IN DIAGNOSTIC STATEMENTS

See *Self-Care Deficit Syndrome*.

## ▪▪▪▪▪▪ KEY CONCEPTS

See *Self-Care Deficit Syndrome*.

## Focus Assessment Criteria

See *Self-Care Deficit Syndrome*.

**NOC**

Nutritional Status, Self-Care: Eating, Swallowing Status

## ➤ Goal

The client will demonstrate increased ability to feed self or report that he or she needs assistance.

### Indicators:

- Demonstrate ability to make use of adaptive devices, if indicated.
- Demonstrate increased interest and desire to eat.
- Describe rationale and procedure for treatment.
- Describe causative factors for feeding deficit.

**NIC**

Feeding, Self-Care Assistance: Feeding, Swallowing Therapy, Teaching, Aspiration Precautions

## ➤ General Interventions

### Assess Causative Factors

### Refer to Related Factors

### Use the Following Scale to Rate the Client's Ability to Perform

0 = Is completely independent
1 = Requires use of assistive device
2 = Needs minimal help
3 = Needs assistance and/or some supervision
4 = Needs total supervision
5 = Needs total assistance or unable to assist

**R:** This coding allows for establishing a baseline from which to evaluate progress.

## Provide Opportunities to Relearn or Adapt to Activity

### Common Nursing Interventions for Feeding

Ascertain from the client or family members what foods the client likes or dislikes.
Ensure the client eats meals in the same setting with pleasant surroundings that are not too distracting.
Maintain correct food temperatures (hot foods hot, cold foods cold).
Provide pain relief because pain can affect appetite and ability to feed self.

Provide good oral hygiene before and after meals.

Encourage the client to wear dentures and eyeglasses.

Assist the client to the most normal eating position suited to his or her physical disability (best is sitting in a chair at a table).

Provide social contact during eating.

**R:** These strategies attempt to normalize mealtime to increase participation and intake.

### Specific Interventions for People with Sensory/Perceptual Deficits

Encourage the client to wear prescribed corrective lenses.

Describe the location of utensils and food on the tray or table.

Describe food items to stimulate appetite.

For perceptual deficits, choose different-colored dishes to help distinguish items (e.g., red tray, white plates).

Ascertain usual eating patterns and provide food items according to preference (or arrange food items in clocklike pattern); record on the care plan the arrangement used (e.g., meat, 6 o'clock; potatoes, 9 o'clock; vegetables, 12 o'clock).

Encourage eating of "finger foods" (e.g., bread, bacon, fruit, hot dogs) to promote independence.

Avoid placing food to the blind side of the client with field cut until visually accommodated to surroundings; then encourage him or her to scan the entire visual field.

**R:** Enhancing a client's self-care abilities can increase his or her sense of control and independence, promoting overall well-being.

### Specific Interventions for People with Missing Limbs

Provide an eating environment that is not embarrassing to the client; allow sufficient time for eating.

Provide only the supervision and assistance necessary for relearning or adaptation.

To enhance independence, provide necessary adaptive devices:
- Plate guard to avoid pushing food off the plate
- Suction device under the plate or bowl for stabilization
- Padded handles on utensils for a more secure grip
- Wrist or hand splints with clamp to hold eating utensils
- Special drinking cup
- Rocker knife for cutting

Assist with set-up if needed, opening containers, napkins, condiment packages; cutting meat; and buttering bread.

Arrange food so client has enough space to perform the task of eating.

**R:** Assistive devices can improve self-care abilities

### Specific Interventions for People with Cognitive Deficits

Provide an isolated, quiet atmosphere until the client can attend to eating and is not easily distracted from the task.

Supervise the feeding program until there is no danger of choking or aspiration.

Orient the client to location and purpose of feeding equipment.

Avoid external distractions and unnecessary conversation.

Place the client in the most normal eating position he or she can physically assume.

Encourage the client to attend to the task, but be alert for fatigue, frustration, or agitation.

Provide one food at a time in usual sequence of eating until the client can eat the entire meal in normal sequence.

Encourage the client to be tidy, to eat in small amounts, and to put food in the unaffected side of the mouth if paresis or paralysis is present.

Check for food in cheeks.

Refer to *Impaired Swallowing* for additional interventions.

**R:** Strategies are needed to reduce environmental distractions and to increase attention to the task.

## Initiate Health Teaching and Referrals, as Indicated

Ensure that both client and family understand the reason and purpose of all interventions. Proceed with teaching as needed:

* Maintain safe eating methods.
* Prevent aspiration.
* Use appropriate eating utensils (avoid sharp instruments).
* Test the temperature of hot liquids and wear protective clothing (e.g., paper bib).
* Teach the use of adaptive devices.

**R:** Eating has physiologic, psychological, social, and cultural implications. Increasing one's control over meals promotes overall well-being.

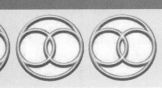

# BATHING SELF-CARE DEFICIT

## DEFINITION

State in which a client experiences an impaired ability to perform or complete bathing/hygiene activities for himself or herself

## DEFINING CHARACTERISTICS

Self-bathing deficits (including washing the entire body, combing hair, brushing teeth, attending to skin and nail care, and applying makeup):

* Unable or unwilling to wash body or body parts
* Unable to obtain a water source
* Unable to regulate temperature or water flow
* Inability to perceive need for hygienic measures

## RELATED FACTORS

See *Self-Care Deficit Syndrome.*

### ■■■■■■ AUTHOR'S NOTE
See *Self-Care Deficit Syndrome.*

### ■■■■■■ ERRORS IN DIAGNOSTIC STATEMENTS
See *Self-Care Deficit Syndrome.*

### ■■■■■■ KEY CONCEPTS
See *Self-Care Deficit Syndrome.*

## Focus Assessment Criteria

See *Self-Care Deficit Syndrome.*

**NOC**
Self-Care: Activities
of Daily Living, Self-
Care: Bathing

## ➤ Goal

The client will perform bathing activity at expected optimal level or report satisfaction with accomplishments despite limitations.

### Indicators:

- Relate a feeling of comfort and satisfaction with body cleanliness.
- Demonstrate the ability to use adaptive devices.
- Describe causative factors of the bathing deficit.

**NIC**
Self-Care Assistance:
Bathing Teaching:
Individual

## ➤ General Interventions

### Assess Causative Factors.

Refer to Related factors

### Use the Following Scale to Rate the Client's Ability to Perform:

0 = Is completely independent
1 = Requires use of assistive device
2 = Needs minimal help
3 = Needs assistance and/or some supervision
4 = Needs total supervision
5 = Needs total assistance or unable to assist

**R:** This coding allows for establishing a baseline from which to evaluate progress.

## Provide Opportunities to Relearn or Adapt to Activity

### General Nursing Interventions for Inability to Bathe

Bathing time and routine should be consistent to encourage optimal independence.
Encourage the client to wear prescribed corrective lenses or hearing aid.
Keep the bathroom temperature warm; ascertain the client's preferred water temperature.
Provide for privacy during bathing routine.
Elicit from the client his or her usual bathing routine.
Keep the environment simple and uncluttered.
Observe skin condition during bathing.
Provide all bathing equipment within easy reach.
Provide for safety in the bathroom (nonslip mats, grab bars).
When the client is physically able, encourage the use of either a tub or shower stall, depending on which he or she uses at home. (The client should practice in the hospital in preparation for going home).
Provide for adaptive equipment as needed:

- Chair or stool in bathtub or shower
- Long-handled sponge to reach back or lower extremities
- Grab bars on bathroom walls where needed to assist in mobility
- Bath board for transferring to tub chair or stool
- Safety treads or nonskid mat on floor of bathroom, tub, and shower
- Washing mitts with pocket for soap
- Adapted toothbrushes
- Shaver holders
- Handheld shower spray

Provide for relief of pain that may affect the client's ability to bathe self.*

**R:** Offering choices and including the client in planning care reduces feelings of powerlessness; promotes feelings of freedom, control, and self-worth; and increases the client's willingness to comply with therapeutic regimens. Assistive devices can improve self-care abilities.

---

*May require a primary care professional's order.

## Specific Interventions for Bathing for People with Visual Deficits

Place bathing equipment in a location most suitable to the client.

Avoid placing bathing equipment to the blind side if the client has a field cut and is not visually accommodated to surroundings.

Keep the call bell within reach if the client is to bathe alone.

Give the client with visual impairment the same degree of privacy and dignity as any other client.

Announce yourself before entering or leaving the bathing area.

Observe the client's ability to locate all bathing utensils.

Observe the client's ability to perform mouth care, hair combing, and shaving.

Provide place for clean clothing within easy reach.

**R:** Inability to perform self-care produces feelings of dependency and poor self-concept. With increased ability for self-care, self-esteem increases (Maher et al., 1998).

## Specific Interventions for Bathing for People with Affected or Missing Limbs

Bathe early in the morning or before bed at night to avoid unnecessary dressing and undressing.

Encourage client to use a mirror during bathing to inspect the skin of paralyzed areas.

Encourage the client with amputation to inspect the remaining foot or stump for good skin integrity.

For limb amputations, bathe the stump twice a day and be sure it is dry before wrapping it or applying the prosthesis.

Provide only the supervision or assistance necessary for relearning the use of extremity or adaptation to the handicap.

For lack of sensation, encourage the use of the affected area in the bathing process. (A client tends to forget the existence of body parts in which there is no sensation.)

**R:** Inability to perform self-care produces feelings of dependency and poor self-concept. With increased ability for self-care, self-esteem increases (Maher et al., 1998).

## Specific Interventions for Bathing for People with Cognitive Deficits

Provide a consistent time for bathing as part of a structured program to help decrease confusion.

Keep instructions simple and avoid distractions; orient the client to the purpose of bathing equipment and put toothpaste on the toothbrush.

If the client cannot bathe the entire body, have him or her bathe one part until he or she does it correctly; give positive reinforcement for success.

Supervise activity until the client can safely perform the task unassisted.

Encourage attention to the task, but be alert for fatigue that may increase confusion.

Apply firm pressure to the skin when bathing; it is less likely to be misinterpreted than a gentle touch.

Use a warm shower or bath to help a confused or agitated client to relax.

**R:** Strategies are needed to reduce environmental distractions and to increase attention to the task.

## Initiate Health Teaching and Referrals, as Indicated

Communicate to staff and family members the client's ability and willingness to learn.

Teach the use of adaptive devices.

Ascertain bathing facilities at home and assist in determining if there is any need for adaptations; refer to occupational therapy or social service for help in obtaining needed home equipment.

Teach the client to use the tub or shower stall, depending on what is used at home.

If the client is paralyzed, instruct the client or family to demonstrate complete skin check on key areas for redness (buttocks, bony prominences).

Teach the family to maintain a safe bathing environment.

**R:** Cleanliness is important for comfort, positive self-esteem, and social interactions.

Inability to care for oneself produces feelings of dependency and poor self-concept. With increased ability for self-care, self-esteem increases.

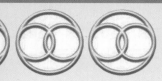

# DRESSING SELF-CARE DEFICIT

## DEFINITION

State in which a client experiences an impaired ability to perform or complete dressing and grooming activities for himself or herself

## DEFINING CHARACTERISTICS

Self-dressing deficits (including donning regular or special clothing, not nightclothes):

- Impaired ability to put on or take off clothing
- Unable to fasten clothing
- Unable to groom self satisfactorily
- Unable to obtain or replace articles of clothing

## RELATED FACTORS

See *Self-Care Deficit Syndrome*.

### ██████ AUTHOR'S NOTE

See *Self-Care Deficit Syndrome*.

### ██████ ERRORS IN DIAGNOSTIC STATEMENTS

See *Self-Care Deficit Syndrome*.

### ██████ KEY CONCEPTS

See *Self-Care Deficit Syndrome*.

## Focus Assessment Criteria

See *Self-Care Deficit Syndrome*.

**NOC**
Self-Care: Activities of Daily Living, Self-Care: Dressing

## ► Goal

The client will demonstrate increased ability to dress self or report the need to have someone else assist him or her to perform the task.

### Indicators:

- Demonstrate ability to use adaptive devices to facilitate independence in dressing.
- Demonstrate increased interest in wearing street clothes.
- Describe causative factors for dressing deficits.
- Relate rationale and procedures for treatments.

**NIC**
Self-Care Assistance: Dressing/Grooming, Teaching: Individual, Dressing

## ► General Interventions

### Assess Causative Factors

Refer to Related Factors.

## Use the Following Scale to Rate the Client's Ability to Perform

> 0 = Is completely independent
> 1 = Requires use of assistive device
> 2 = Needs minimal help
> 3 = Needs assistance and/or some supervision
> 4 = Needs total supervision
> 5 = Needs total assistance or unable to assist

> **R:** This coding allows for establishing a baseline from which to evaluate progress.

## Provide Opportunities to Relearn or Adapt to Activity

### General Nursing Interventions for Self-Dressing

> Encourage the client to wear prescribed corrective lenses or hearing aid.
> Promote independence in dressing through continual and unaided practice.
> Choose loose-fitting clothing with wide sleeves and pant legs and front fasteners.
> Allow sufficient time for dressing and undressing, because the task may be tiring, painful, or difficult.
> Plan for the client to learn and demonstrate one part of an activity before progressing further.
> Lay clothes out in the order in which the client will need them to dress.
> Provide dressing aids as necessary (some commonly used aids include dressing stick, Swedish reacher, zipper pull, buttonhook, long-handled shoehorn, and shoe fasteners adapted with elastic laces, Velcro closures, or flip-back tongues. (All garments with fasteners may be adapted with Velcro closures.)
> Encourage the client to wear ordinary or special clothing rather needed, increase.
> If needed, increase participation in dressing by medicating for pain 30 min before it is time to dress or undress, if indicated.*
> Provide for privacy during dressing routine.
> Provide for safety by ensuring easy access to all clothing and by ascertaining the client's performance level.

> **R:** Inability to care for oneself produces feelings of dependency and poor self-concept. With increased ability for self-care, self-esteem increases. Optimal personal grooming promotes psychological well-being.

### Specific Interventions for Dressing for People with Visual Deficits

> Allow the client to select the most convenient location for clothing and adapt the environment to accomplish the task best (e.g., remove unnecessary barriers).
> Announce yourself before entering or leaving the dressing area.
> If the client has a field cut, avoid placing clothing to the blind side until he or she is visually accommodated to the surroundings; then encourage him or her to turn the head to scan the entire visual field.

> **R:** Strategies used include consistent placement of items needed for dressing.

### Specific Interventions for Dressing for People with Cognitive Deficits (Miller, 2009)

> Keep verbal communication simple:
>
> - Ask yes/no questions.
> - Use one-step requests (e.g., "put your sock on").
> - Praise after each step.
> - Be specific and concise.
> - Call the client by name.
> - Use the same word for the same thing (e.g., "shirt").
> - Dress the bottom half, and then the top half.
>
> Prepare an uncluttered environment:

---

* May require a primary care professional's order.

- Ensure good lighting.
- Make bed; minimize visual clutter.
- Lay clothes face down.
- Place clothes in the order that they will be used.
- Allow the client a choice from only two pieces.
- Place matching clothes together on hangers.
- Remove dirty clothes from the dressing area.

Provide nonverbal cues:

- Hand one clothing item at a time in correct order.
- Place shoes beside the correct foot.
- Use gestures to explain.
- Point or touch the body part to be used.
- If the client cannot complete all the steps, always allow him or her to finish the dressing step, if possible—zipper pants, buckle belt.
- Decrease assistance gradually.

**R:** Strategies are needed to reduce environmental distractions and to increase attention to the task.

## Initiate Health Teaching and Referrals, as Indicated

### Access a Home Health Nurse for an In-Home Evaluation

**R:** An in-home health nurse assessment is critical for self-care activities to be maintained and/or progressed to a higher level.

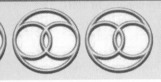

# INSTRUMENTAL SELF-CARE DEFICIT

## DEFINITION

State in which a client experiences an impaired ability to perform certain activities or access certain services essential for managing a household

## DEFINING CHARACTERISTICS

Observed or reported difficulty with one or more of the following:

- Using a telephone
- Accessing transportation
- Laundering and ironing
- Preparing meals
- Shopping (food, clothes)
- Managing money
- Administering medication

## RELATED FACTORS

See *Self-Care Deficit Syndrome*.

## ■■■■■ AUTHOR'S NOTE

*Instrumental Self-Care Deficit* is not currently on the NANDA list but has been added here for clarity and usefulness. This diagnosis describes problems in performing certain activities or accessing certain services needed to live in the community (e.g., phone use, shopping, money management). This diagnosis is important to consider in discharge planning and during home visits by community nurses.

## ■■■■■ ERRORS IN DIAGNOSTIC STATEMENTS

### Instrumental Self-Care Deficit related to possible inability to plan meals and manage laundry

When a nurse suspects that a client or family may have compromised ability to engage in certain activities needed to live in and run a household, the nurse should label the diagnosis *Possible Instrumental Self-Care Deficit* and add related factors representing why he or she suspects the diagnosis (e.g., *related to difficulty remembering routine tasks or related to poor planning skills*). The nurse detecting evidence of memory or judgment difficulties could interpret this as a risk factor for *Risk for Instrumental Self-Care Deficit*.

## ■■■■■ KEY CONCEPTS

### Generic Considerations

- Brody (1985) found that, to live in the community, a client has to perform or have assistance with six ADLs as well as additional activities.
- Instrumental ADLs include housekeeping, preparing and procuring food, shopping, laundering, ability to self-medicate safely, ability to manage money, and access to transportation (Miller, 2009). Instrumental ADLs require more complex tasks than ADLs.
- Maintaining people in the community, rather than in nursing homes, has significant financial benefit. In 1981, 25% of all U.S. health care expenditures for older adults went to nursing homes, but only 5% of older adults were receiving care in these facilities. Medicaid covers about 90% of public spending for nursing home care (Miller, 2009).
- Maintaining people in the community, rather than in nursing homes, also maintains autonomy, strengthens family life, and affirms the value of older adults in our society.

## Focus Assessment Criteria

See *Self-Care Deficit Syndrome*.

**NOC**
Self-Care: Instrumental Activities of Daily Living (IADL)

## ➤ Goal

The client or family will report satisfaction with household management.

### Indicators:

- Demonstrate use of adaptive devices (e.g., telephone, cooking aids).
- Describe a method to ensure adherence to medication schedule.
- Report ability to make calls and answer the telephone.
- Report regular laundering by self or others.
- Report daily intake of at least two nutritious meals.
- Identify transportation options to stores, physician, house of worship, and social activities.
- Demonstrate management of simple money transactions.
- Identify people who will assist with money matters.

**NIC**
Teaching: Individual,
Referral, Family
Involvement
Promotion

> ## General Interventions

### Assess for Causative and Contributing Factors; Refer to Related Factors

#### Use the Following Scale to Rate the Client's Ability to Perform:

0 = Is completely independent
1 = Requires use of assistive device
2 = Needs minimal help
3 = Needs assistance and/or some supervision
4 = Needs total supervision
5 = Needs total assistance or unable to assist

**R:** This coding allows for establishing a baseline to evaluate progress from.

## Assist the Client in Identifing Self-Help Devices

### Grooming/Dressing Aids

See *Impaired Physical Mobility*.

### Kitchen/Eating Aids

Dishes with one side built up
Built-up handles on cutlery (use plastic foam curlers)
Bulldog clip to secure a straw in a glass
Built-up corner of a cutlery board to hold and anchor food or pot (e.g., to butter toast, mash potatoes)
Mounted jar opener
Nonskid material applied under dishes (same strips used to prevent slipping in bathtub)
Two-sided suction holder to hold dishes in place

**R:** A variety of assistive devices are available to be used in the kitchen.

### Communication/Security

Motion-activated lights near walkway/entrance
Nightlight for path to the bathroom
Light next to the bed
Specially adapted telephones (amplified, big buttons)
Specially adapted safety devices (bracelet alarm)

**R:** A variety of assistive devices is available to prevent injury and to call for assistance.

## Promote Self-Care and Safety for the Client with Cognitive Deficit

### Evaluate Activities that Are Achievable

Turn lights on before dark.
Use nightlights.
Keep the environment simple and uncluttered.
Use clocks and calendars as cues.
Mark on calendar (using picture symbols) reminders for shopping, laundry, cleaning, doctor's appointments, and the like.

**R:** Interventions focus on assisting the client and family to maintain safely as much functional independence as possible (Miller, 2009).

### For Laundry, Teach the Client to:

Separate dark and light clothes.
Use pictures to illustrate steps for washing clothes.
Mark cup with line to indicate amount of soap needed.

Minimize ironing.

Use an iron with automatic shutoff mechanism.

**R:** Interventions focus on assisting the client and family to maintain safely as much functional independence as possible (Miller, 2009).

## Evaluate the Client's Ability to Select, Procure, and Prepare Nutritious Food Daily

Prepare a permanent shopping list with cues for essential foods and products.

Teach the client to review the list before shopping, check items needed, and, in the store, check off items selected. (Use a pencil that can be erased to reuse list.)

Teach the client how to shop for single-person meals (refer to *Imbalanced Nutrition* for specific techniques).

If possible, teach the client to use a microwave to reduce the risk of heat-related injuries or accidents.

**R:** Interventions focus on assisting the client and family to maintain as much functional independence as possible (Miller, 2009).

## Offer Hints to Improve Adherence to Medication Schedule

Have someone place medications in a commercial pill holder divided into 7 days.

Take out the exact amount of pills for the day. Divide them in small cups, each labeled with time of day.

If needed, draw a picture of the pills and the quantity on each cup.

Teach the client to transfer the pills from cup to small plastic bag when planning to be away from home.

Tell the client whom to call for instructions if he or she misses a dose.

**R:** Simple strategies can be used to remember the medication schedule and prevent errors.

**R:** Interventions focus on assisting the client and family to maintain as much functional independence as possible (Miller, 2009).

## Initiate Health Teaching and Referrals, as Indicated

Discuss the importance of identifying the need for assistance.

Discuss the possibility of bartering for services (e.g., wash the neighbor's clothes in exchange for shopping help).

Identify a person who can provide immediate help (e.g., neighbor, friend, hotline).

Identify sources for help with laundry, shopping, and money matters.

## Determine Available Sources of Transportation (Neighbors, Relatives, Community Centers)

Church groups or social service agency)

Refer the client to community agencies for assistance (e.g., Department of Social Services, area agency on aging, senior neighbors, public health nursing, Meals on Wheels).

**R:** Community resources, neighbors, and /or religious groups can assist the client when caregivers are unavailable or nonexistent (Miller, 2009).

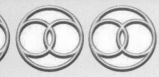

# TOILETING SELF-CARE DEFICIT

## DEFINITION

State in which a client experiences an impaired ability to perform or complete toileting activities for himself or herself

## DEFINING CHARACTERISTICS

Unable or unwilling to get to toilet or commode
Unable or unwilling to carry out proper hygiene
Unable to transfer to and from toilet or commode
Unable to handle clothing to accommodate toileting
Unable to flush toilet or empty commode

## RELATED FACTORS

See *Self-Care Deficit Syndrome*.

■■■■■ **AUTHOR'S NOTE**

See *Self-Care Deficit Syndrome*.

■■■■■ **ERRORS IN DIAGNOSTIC STATEMENTS**

See *Self-Care Deficit Syndrome*.

■■■■■ **KEY CONCEPTS**

See *Self-Care Deficit Syndrome*.

## Focus Assessment Criteria

See *Self-Care Deficit Syndrome*.

**NOC**
Self-Care: Activities of Daily Living, Self-Care: Hygiene, Self-Care: Toileting

## ➤ Goal

The client will demonstrate increased ability to toilet self or report the need to have someone assist him or her to perform the task (specify when assistance is needed).

### Indicators:

• Demonstrate the ability to use adaptive devices to facilitate toileting.
• Describe causative factors for toileting deficit.
• Relate the rationale and procedures for treatment.

**NIC**
Self-Care Assistance: Toileting, Self-Care Assistance: Hygiene, Teaching Individual, Mutual Goal Setting

## ➤ General Interventions

### Assess Causative Factors

Refer to Related Factors.

## Use the Following Scale to Rate the Client's Ability to Perform:

0 = Is completely independent
1 = Requires use of assistive device
2 = Needs minimal help
3 = Needs assistance and/or some supervision
4 = Needs total supervision
5 = Needs total assistance or unable to assist

**R:** This coding allows for establishing a baseline to evaluate progress from.

## Provide Opportunities to Relearn or Adapt to Activity

### Common Nursing Interventions for Toileting Difficulties

Encourage the client to wear prescribed corrective lenses or hearing aid.
Obtain bladder and bowel history from the client or significant other (see *Impaired Bowel Elimination* or *Impaired Urinary Elimination*).
Ascertain the communication system the client uses to express the need to toilet.
Maintain a bladder and bowel record to determine toileting patterns.
Provide adequate fluid intake and a balanced diet to promote adequate urinary output and normal bowel evacuation.
Promote normal elimination by encouraging activity and exercise within the client's capabilities.
Avoid development of "bowel fixation" by less frequent discussion and inquiries about bowel movements.
Be alert to the possibility of falls when toileting the client (be prepared to ease him or her to the floor without injuring either of you).
Achieve independence in toileting by continual and unaided practice.
Allow sufficient time for the task of toileting to avoid fatigue. (Lack of sufficient time to toilet may cause incontinence or constipation.)
Avoid the use of indwelling and condom catheters to expedite bladder continence (if possible).

**R:** The client's maximum involvement in toileting activities can reduce the embarrassment associated with needing assistance with toileting (Maher et al., 1998).
**R:** These strategies provide a structured, consistent environment and routine for achieving client goals.

### Specific Interventions for Toileting for People with Visual Deficits

Keep the call bell easily accessible so the client can quickly obtain help to toilet; answer the call bell promptly to decrease anxiety.
If the bedpan or urinal is necessary for toileting, be sure it is within the client's reach.
Avoid placing toileting equipment to the blind side of a client with field cut. (When he or she is visually accommodated to surroundings, you may suggest he or she search the entire visual field for equipment.)
Announce yourself before entering or leaving the toileting area.
Observe the client's ability to obtain equipment or get to the toilet unassisted.
Provide for a safe and clear pathway to toilet area.

**R:** These strategies provide a structured, consistent environment and routine for achieving client goals.

### Specific Interventions for Toileting for People with Affected or Missing Limbs

Provide only the supervision and assistance necessary for relearning or adapting to the prosthesis.
Encourage the client to look at the affected area or limb and use it during toileting tasks.
Encourage useful transfer techniques taught by occupational or physical therapy. (The nurse becomes familiar with the planned mode of transfer.)
Provide the necessary adaptive devices to enhance independence and safety (commode chairs, spill-proof urinals, fracture bedpans, raised toilet seats, support side rails for toilets).
Provide for a safe and clear pathway to toilet area.

**R:** A variety of assistive devices and techniques are available to prevent injury and promote self-care.

### Specific Interventions for Toileting for People with Cognitive Deficits

Offer toileting reminders every 2 h, after meals, and before bedtime.

When the client can indicate the need to toilet, begin toileting at 2-h intervals, after meals, and before bedtime.

Answer the call bell immediately to avoid frustration and incontinence.

Encourage wearing ordinary clothes. (Many confused people are continent while wearing regular clothing.)

Avoid the use of bedpans and urinals; if physically possible, provide a normal atmosphere of elimination in bathroom. (The toilet used should remain constant to promote familiarity.)

Give verbal cues as to what is expected of the client and positive reinforcement for success.

Work to achieve daytime continence before expecting nighttime continence. (Nighttime incontinence may continue after daytime continence has returned.)

See *Impaired Urinary Elimination* for additional information on incontinence.

**R:** Interventions focus on assisting the client and family to maintain safely as much functional independence as possible (Miller, 2009).

## Initiate Health Teaching and Referrals, as Indicated

## Assess the Understanding and Knowledge of the Client and Significant Others of Foregoing Interventions and Rationales

### Ensure an In-Home Evaluation by a Home Health Nurse

**R:** Community resources, neighbors, and /or religious groups can assist the client in maintaining self-care even when caregivers are unavailable or nonexistent (Miller, 2009).

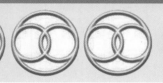

# DISTURBED SELF-CONCEPT

**Disturbed Self-Concept***

Disturbed Body Image
Disturbed Personal Identity
Disturbed Self-Esteem
Chronic Low Self-Esteem
Situational Low Self-Esteem
Risk for Situational Low Self-Esteem

## DEFINITION

State in which a person experiences or is at risk of experiencing a negative state of change about the way he feels, thinks, or views himself. It may include a change in body image, self-esteem, or personal identity (Boyd, 2004).

## DEFINING CHARACTERISTICS

This diagnosis reflects a broad diagnostic category which can be used initially until more specific assessment data can support a more specific nursing diagnosis as Disturbed Body Image or Disturbed Self-Esteem.

---

*This diagnosis is not currently on the NANDA list but has been included for clarity of usefulness.

Some examples of signs and symptoms are:

(Observed or reported)

Verbal or nonverbal negative response to actual or perceived change in structure and/or function (e.g., shame, embarrassment, guilt, revulsion)

Expressions of shame or guilt

Rationalizes away or rejects positive feedback and exaggerates negative feedback about self

Hypersensitivity to slight criticism

Episodic occurrence of negative self-appraisal in response to life events in a person with a previously positive self-evaluation

Verbalization of negative feelings about self (helplessness, uselessness)

## RELATED FACTORS

A disturbed self-concept can occur as a response to a variety of health problems, situations, and conflicts. Some common sources follow.

### Pathophysiologic

*Related to change in appearance, lifestyle, role, response of others secondary to:*

| | | |
|---|---|---|
| Chronic disease | Severe trauma | Loss of body parts |
| Pain | Loss of body functions | |

### Situational (Personal, Environmental)

*Related to feelings of abandonment or failure secondary to:*

Divorce, separation from or death of a significant other

Loss of job or ability to work

*Related to immobility or loss of function*

*Related to unsatisfactory relationships (parental, spousal)*

*Related to sexual preferences (homosexual, lesbian, bisexual, abstinent)*

*Related to teenage pregnancy*

*Related to gender differences in parental child rearing*

*Related to experiences of parental violence*

*Related to change in usual patterns of responsibilities*

### Maturational

**Middle Aged**

Loss of role and responsibilities

**Older Adult**

Loss of role and responsibilities

■ ■ ■ ■ ■ ■  **AUTHOR'S NOTE**

Self-concept reflects self-view, encompassing body image, esteem, role performance, and personal identity. Self-concept develops over a lifetime and is difficult to change. It is influenced by interactions with the environment and others, and by the person's perceptions of how others view him or her.

*Disturbed Self-Concept* represents a broad diagnostic category under which fall more specific nursing diagnoses. Initially, the nurse may not have sufficient clinical data to validate a more specific diagnosis, such as *Chronic Low Self-Esteem* or *Disturbed Body Image*; thus, he or she can use *Disturbed Self-Concept* until data can support a more specific diagnosis.

Self-esteem is one of the four components of self-concept. *Disturbed Self-Esteem* is the general diagnostic category. *Chronic Low Self-Esteem* and *Situational Low Self-Esteem* represent specific types of *Disturbed Self- Esteem* and thus involve more specific interventions. Initially, the nurse may not have sufficient clinical data to validate a more specific diagnosis, such as *Chronic Low Self-Esteem* or *Situational Low Self-Esteem*. Refer to the major defining characteristics under these categories for validation.

*Situational Low Self-Esteem* is an episodic event; repeated occurrence, continuous negative self-appraisals over time, or both can lead to *Chronic Low Self-Esteem* (Willard, 1990, personal communication).

## ERRORS IN DIAGNOSTIC STATEMENTS

1. *Disturbed Self-Concept related to substance abuse*
   Although a relationship exists between negative self-concept and alcohol and/or drug abuse, listing substance abuse as a related factor does not describe the nursing focus. If the person acknowledged a substance abuse problem and expressed a desire for assistance, the diagnosis *Ineffective Coping related to inability to constructively manage stressors without alcohol or drugs* could be appropriate. If the person denied a problem, the diagnosis *Ineffective Denial related to lack of acknowledgment of substance abuse/dependency* would apply—if the nurse will address the denial. A nurse with data that suggest or confirm *Disturbed Self-Concept* should explore contributing factors (e.g., guilt influenced by social stigma). The nurse can use "unknown etiology" until focus assessment identifies contributing factors.

2. *Disturbed Body Image related to mastectomy*
   Mastectomy can produce various responses, including grief, anger, and negative feelings about self. A woman undergoing breast surgery for cancer is at high risk for both *Disturbed Body Image* and *Disturbed Self-Esteem*. Thus, the diagnosis *Risk for Disturbed Self-Concept related to perceived negative effects of changed appearance and diagnosis of cancer* would be most appropriate. A nurse with data to support *Disturbed Self-Concept* should record it as an actual diagnosis with these same related factors and including "as evidenced by" to specify signs and symptoms of or manifestations (e.g., *Disturbed Self-Concept related to perceived negative effects of changed appearance and diagnosis of cancer, as evidenced by reports of negative feelings about "new self" and determination not to let husband see her*).

## KEY CONCEPTS

### Generic Considerations

- Both the client and the nurse have their own personal self-concept. To deal effectively with others, the nurse must be aware of his or her own behavior, feelings, attitudes, and responses.
- Self-concept involves a person's feelings, attitudes, and values and affects his or her reactions to all experiences.
- A person's self-concept evolves from infancy through old age. With aging, new skills and challenges emerge. Successful completion of developmental tasks contributes to a positive self-concept (Boyd, 2005).
- Interactions with others, the sociocultural milieu, and developmental task completion influence self-concept (Boyd, 2005).
- The concept of self includes components of body image, self-esteem, and personal identity (Boyd, 2005).
  - *Body Image:* The sum of the conscious and unconscious attitudes the person has toward his or her body. It includes present and past perceptions.
  - *Self-Esteem:* The individual's personal judgment of his or her own worth obtained by analyzing how well his or her behavior conforms to self-ideals. High self-esteem is rooted in unconditional acceptance of self, despite mistakes, defeats, and failures, as an innately worthy and important being.
  - *Personal Identity:* The organizing principle of the personality that accounts for the unity, continuity, consistency, and uniqueness of the individual. It connotes autonomy and includes self-perceptions of sexuality. Identity formation begins in infancy and proceeds throughout life, but is the major task of adolescence.
- Body image consists of three components: body reality, body ideal, and body presentation (Price, 1990).
  - *Body Reality:* The body as it really exists, constrained by the effects of human genetics and the wear and tear of life in the external environment (as it might be described in a formal physician's examination). It changes both as a result of the aging process and because we use and abuse it. Abrupt changes in body reality are associated with trauma, malignancy, infection, and malnutrition.
  - *Body Ideal:* This is the picture in our heads of how we would like the body to look and to perform. Influences include societal and cultural norms, advertising, and changing attitudes toward fitness and health. Changes in body reality threaten body ideal, but disorders of body ideal (e.g., anorexia nervosa) also may affect the equilibrium directly.
  - *Body Presentation:* Body reality only rarely meets body ideal standards. In the effort to make these two balance, body presentation is used. This is how the body is literally presented to the outside environment: the way we dress, groom, walk, talk, pose limbs, and use props such as walking sticks or hearing aids. Equally, paralysis or loss of limb (body reality) also affects facility in body presentation. Much presentation is for public consumption, laden with symbolic value.

*(continued)*

■ ■■ ■ ■ ■ **KEY CONCEPTS** *Continued*

- Disturbances in the components of self-concept are described as follows:
  - *Body Image:* Viewing oneself differently as a result of actual or perceived changes in body structure or function
  - *Self-Ideal:* A change in self-expectations/striving
  - *Self-Esteem:* Lack of confidence in ability to accomplish that which is desired
  - *Role Performance:* Inability to perform those functions and activities expected of a particular role in a given society
  - *Personal Identity:* Disturbance in perception of self ("Who am I?")

## LOSS OF BODY PART/FUNCTION

- People have a concept of self that includes feelings about self-worth, attractiveness, worth of love, and capabilities. A physical injury assaults one's mental image of one's own body and person. This injury or loss involves the grieving process.
- Facial disfigurement causes the most changes in body image and self-concept.
- Bergamasco et al. (2002) identified two critical incidents in burned persons: noticing the changes in their bodies (e.g., mirror) and noticing that others are aware of their scars.
- Factors that influence successful reimaging are the person's perspective on value of lost function, nature of change, prior life experiences, self-esteem, social support, and others' attitudes, and access to medical technology.
- The grieving process in response to a recent loss of body part or function has been described as (Friedman-Campbell & Hart, 1984):
  - Shock/denial
    - Denies injury or severity of the injury
    - Allows self to think of loss only minimally to protect self
    - Intellectually accepts the loss but denies it emotionally
  - Developing awareness
    - Realizes the effects of the loss on self
    - Experiences acute somatic feelings of loss
    - Displaces anger
    - Is preoccupied with guilt and blaming
    - Mourns the loss and withdraws
    - Shuns change and clings to routines
  - Managing loss of body function
    - Begins to deal with the effects of the loss on self
    - Frees self slowly from the bondage of the loss
    - Readjusts to changed environment
    - Invests in new relationships

## SELF-ESTEEM

- Self-esteem evolves from a comparison between self-concept and self-ideal. The greater the congruency, the higher is the self-esteem.
- Self-esteem derives from the person's own perceptions of competency and efficacy and from appraisals of others. In general, people hold positive self-enhancing beliefs about themselves, the world, and the future. These biased perceptions are considerably more positive than objective evidence indicates.
- As self-esteem declines, so does a person's belief that he or she can exert control over the environment. Likewise, as personal control is perceived to decrease, so does self-esteem. Attributing failure to a lack of ability (internal cause) leads to decreased expectations and motivation.
- In response to a threat to person's self-concept, three cognitive processes protect self-esteem:
  - Searching for meaning in the experience
  - Regaining mastery over the event; exerting personal control
  - Self-enhancement ("How am I managing compared with others?")
- The following behaviors are associated with low self-esteem: rigidity; procrastination; repetitive, unnecessary apologies; minimizing one's abilities; emphasizing deficits; expecting failure; self-destructive behaviors; approval-seeking behavior; inability to accept compliments; disregard for one's own opinions; difficulty in forming close relationships; and inability to say "no" when appropriate (Miller, 2009).

*(continued)*

■■■■■■ **KEY CONCEPTS** *Continued*

• Low self-esteem has been regarded as an important cause of violence; however, the opposite view is theoretically viable. Violence appears often as a result of threatened egotism (that is, highly favorable views of self that some person or circumstance disputes). This is the dark side of high self-esteem.

## Pediatric Considerations

• Self-concept is learned. A child's concept of self, for example, emerges as a result of changes during earlier developmental stages.
• To develop and maintain self-esteem, a child needs to feel worthwhile, different in some way, and superior to and more lovable than any other child (Hockenberry & Wilson, 2009, Hockenberrry et.al 2009).
• Self-esteem increases as a child develops meaningful relationships and masters developmental tasks. Early adolescence is a time of risk to self-esteem as the adolescent strives to define an identity and sense of self within a peer group (Boyd, 2005).
• Present and past perceptions of his or her body, physiologic functioning, developmental maturation, and responses from others influence a child's development of body image. Adolescence is probably the critical period of development for body image formation, as pubertal changes force alteration of the adolescent's body image. The development of a positive body image by age is charted below (Boyd, 2005):

| Age | Developmental Task |
|---|---|
| Birth to 1 year | Learns to tolerate small frustrations<br>Learns to trust |
| 1 to 3 years | Learns to like body<br>Learns mastery of<br>    Motor skills<br>    Language skills<br>    Bowel training |
| 3 to 6 years | Learns initiative<br>Learns sex typing<br>Identifies with parent models<br>Increases skills (motor, language) |
| 6 to 12 years | Develops a sense of industry<br>Has a clear sex role identification<br>Learns peer interaction<br>Develops academic skills |
| Adolescence | Establishes self-identity and sexual role<br>Uses abstract thought<br>Develops personal value system |

• Children learn to see themselves in the way that parents and significant others see them.
• To develop a healthy personality, a child needs a positive and accurate body image, realistic self-ideal, positive self-concept, and high self-esteem.
• Although obese children and adolescents may be at particular risk for developing body image or self-esteem disturbance, lower self-esteem is more likely in children who believe they are responsible for their excess weight, as compared with those who attribute their excess weight to an external cause. Lower self-esteem is also found in those children who believe that their excess weight hinders their social interaction (Pierce & Wardle, 1997).
• Negative self-concepts have been associated with self-destructive health behaviors in children and adolescents, such as overeating, alcoholism, smoking, and drug abuse (Winkelstein, 1989).
• Mastery describes positive coping with stress. Successful coping enhances self-esteem.

## Geriatric Considerations

- According to Miller (2009), self-esteem is "one of the characteristics most highly associated with both depression and happiness" in older adults.
- Self-esteem depends on interactions with others and on others' opinions. In Western societies, a generally negative view of aging can contribute to an older adult's decreased self-esteem.
- Many variables interact to produce a decline in self-esteem in older adults, including negative societal attitudes, decreased social interactions, and decreased power and control over the environment.
- Meisenhelder (1985) reported that the following people exert the most significant influence on self-esteem in older adults: spouse, peers (most important for men), authority figures (most important for women), people they live with, and people in the immediate social, work, and church environments.
- Environmental factors in long-term care facilities that can influence self-esteem of older residents include decor, social roles, choices available, architectural design, space, and privacy (Miller, 2009).
- Older adults with poor health, high degree of disability, and daily pain report the lowest self-esteem (Hunter, Linn, & Harris, 1981–1982).

## Transcultural Considerations

In the Latin culture, the man is the head of the household and has authority over his family. He must provide for and protect his family. Self-image and family image are intertwined. Anything that challenges his ability to provide for his family challenges his very core or self-concept (Andrews & Boyle, 2008).

# Focus Assessment Criteria

*Disturbed Self-Concept* is manifested in a variety of ways. A person may respond with an alteration in another life process (see *Spiritual Distress*, *Fear*, *Ineffective Coping*). The nurse should be aware of this and use the assessment data to ascertain the dimensions affected.

It may be difficult for the nurse to identify the cues and make the inferences necessary to diagnose a self-concept disturbance. Each person reacts differently to loss, pain, disability, and disfigurement. Therefore, the nurse should determine a person's usual reactions to problems and feelings about himself or herself before attempting to diagnose a change.

## Subjective Data
### Assess for Defining Characteristics

**Self Views**
"Describe yourself."
"What do you like most/least about yourself?"
"What do you/others want to change about you?"
"What do you enjoy?"
"Has being ill affected how you see yourself?"

**Identity**
"What personal achievements have given you satisfaction?"
"What are your future plans?"

**Role Responsibilities**
"What do you do for a living? Job responsibilities? Home responsibilities?"
"Are these satisfying?"
If the person has had a role change, how has it affected lifestyle and relationships?

**Somatic Problems**
"Do you feel fearful, anxious, or nervous?"
"Ever feel like you are falling apart? Dizziness? Aches and pains? Shortness of breath? Palpitations? Urinary frequency? Nausea/vomiting? Sleep problems? Fatigue? Loss of sexual interest?"

### Affect and Mood
"How do you feel now?"
"How would you describe your usual mood?"
"What things make you happy/upset?"

### Body Image
"What do you like most/least about your body?"
"What limitations do you think will result?"
"How do you feel about this illness/disability?"
"Has it changed the way you feel about yourself or the way others respond to you?"
Children may be able to draw self-portraits.

## Assess for Related Factors

### *Stress Management*

"How do you manage stress?"
"To whom do you go for help with a problem?"

### *Support System*

"Any problems in current relationships?"
"How does your family feel about your illness?" "Do they understand?"
"Does your family regularly discuss problems?"
"What other supports do you have? Spiritual? Social?"

## Objective Data

### *Assess for Defining Characteristics*

#### General Appearance
Facial expression
Body posture/language (eye contact, head and shoulder flexion, gait/stride)

#### Thought Processes/Content
Orientation
Suspicious
Homicidal/suicidal ideation
Rambling
Sexual preoccupation
Delusions (grandeur, persecution, reference, influence, or bodily sensations)
Difficulty concentrating
Slowed thought processes
Poor memory or may even be missing large portions of personal history
Impaired judgment
Anxiety

#### Behavior
School problems (truancy, low/drop in grades)
Problems on job (lateness, decreased productivity, accident-prone, burnout symptoms)
Social withdrawal
Sexual behavior (increase, decrease, promiscuity)

#### Communication Patterns
With significant others
   Relates well    Dependent
   Hostile       Demanding

#### Nutritional Status
Appetite
Eating patterns
Weight (gain/loss)

**Rest–Sleep Pattern**

Recent change

For more information on Focus Assessment Criteria, visit http://thepoint.lww.com.

**NOC**
Quality of Life,
Depression Level,
Depression Self-
Control Self-Esteem,
Coping

### ➤ Goal

The person will demonstrate healthy adaptation and coping skills.

#### Indicators

- Appraise self and situations realistically without distortions.
- Verbalize and demonstrate increased positive feelings.

**NIC**
Hope Instillation,
Mood Management,
Values Clarification,
Counseling,
Referral, Support
Group, Coping
Enhancement

### ➤ General Interventions

Nursing interventions for the various problems that might be associated with a diagnosis of *Disturbed Self-Concept* are very similar.

### Contact the Client Frequently and Treat Him or Her with Warm, Positive Regard

**R:** Frequent contact by the caregiver indicates acceptance and may facilitate trust. The client may be hesitant to approach the staff because of negative self-concept.

### Encourage the Client to Express Feelings and Thoughts About the Following:

| | | |
|---|---|---|
| Condition | Progress | Prognosis |
| Effects on lifestyle | Support system | Treatment |

**R:** Encouraging the client to share feelings can provide a safe outlet for fears and frustrations and can increase self-awareness.

### Provide Reliable Information and Clarify Any Misconceptions

**R:** Misconceptions can increase anxiety and damage self-concept needlessly.

### Explain the Process of Reimaging (Refer to Key Concepts—Loss of Body Parts or Functions)

Explain that reimaging oneself after a loss of appearance or function is distinct and unique.

Advise that the process takes at least 1 year.

Assist client to examine societal homophobia and its results, so it is not internalized. Link him or her to appropriate groups and organizations.

Provide maternal education and a sound supportive system, which includes alternatives for care of the infant when delivered.

Provide education and refer to support groups that promote empowerment and change of focus to assist in evaluating and raising quality of life.

**R:** The client may tend to focus only on the change in self-image and not on the positive characteristics that contribute to the whole concept of self. The nurse must reinforce these positive aspects and encourage the client to reincorporate them into the new self-concept.

### Help Client to Identify Positive Attributes and Possible New Opportunities

### Assist with Hygiene and Grooming, as Needed

**R:** Participation in self-care and planning can aid positive coping.

### Encourage Visitors

**R:** Frequent visits by support people can help the client feel that he or she is still a worthwhile, acceptable person, which should promote a positive self-concept.

## Help Client Identify Strategies to Increase Independence and to Maintain Role Responsibilities

Prioritizing activities

Using mobility aids and assistive devices, as needed

**R:** Participation in self-care and planning can aid positive coping.

**R:** A strong component of self-concept is the ability to perform functions expected of one's role, thus decreasing dependency and reducing the need for others' involvement.

## Discuss with Client's Support System the Importance of Communicating the Client's Value and Importance to Them

**R:** Communication of the client's values enhances self-esteem and promotes adjustment.

**R:** Optimism enhances social relationships and enables a person to make more effective use of social supports to maintain self-esteem. Supportive friends and family can bolster self-esteem by reinforcing a sense of personal control through suggestions and resources and a sense of confidence (Morse, 1997).

## Initiate Health Teaching, as Indicated

Teach person what community resources are available, if needed (e.g., mental health centers, self-help groups such as Reach for Recovery, Make Today Count).

Refer to specific health teaching issues under *Disturbed Body Image*, *Disturbed Self-Esteem* (*Chronic* and *Situational*).

**R:** Addressing spiritual issues within the counseling process involves an accurate assessment of spiritual functioning and relevant interventions used with discretion and respect for client beliefs.

**R:** Nurses must receive adequate education and keep their knowledge updated. Nurses should receive regular clinical supervision and support to ensure that they can provide therapeutic care for patients with self-concept disturbances.

### Pediatric Interventions

Allow the child to bring his or her own experiences into the situation (e.g., "Some children say that an injection feels like an insect sting; some say they don't feel anything. After we do this, you can tell me how it feels"; Johnson, 1995).

**R:** Allowing the child to describe the experience supports that he or she is unique.

Avoid using "good" or "bad" to describe behavior. Be specific and descriptive (e.g., "You really helped me by holding still. Thank you for helping"; Johnson, 1995).

**R:** It is more helpful to be specific and descriptive when praising a child rather than describing behavior as "good" or "bad."

Connect previous experiences with the present one (e.g., "The x-ray camera will look different from the last time. You will have to hold real still again. The table will move, too"; Johnson, 1995).

**R:** The nurse can provide information that helps the child make sense of the situation by linking the present or future experience to past experience.

Convey optimism with positive self-talk (e.g., "I am so busy today. I wonder if I will get all my work done? I bet I can." or "When you come back from surgery you will need to stay in bed. What would you like to do when you come back?").

**R:** Positive self-talk denotes optimism to the child.

Help the child plan playtime with choices. Encourage crafts that produce an end product.

**R:** Allowing the child choices and productive play can enhance self-concept.

Encourage interactions with peers and supportive adults.

Encourage child to decorate room with crafts and personal items.

**R:** Skill building and positive social relationships increase a child's sense of value and worth

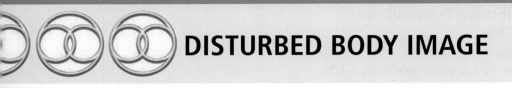

# DISTURBED BODY IMAGE

## DEFINITION

State in which a person experiences or is at risk to experience a disruption in the way he or she perceives one's body

## DEFINING CHARACTERISTICS

### Major (Must Be Present)

Verbal or nonverbal negative response to actual or perceived change in structure and/or function (e.g., shame, embarrassment, guilt, revulsion)

### Minor (May Be Present)

Not looking at body part
Not touching body part
Hiding or overexposing body part
Change in social involvement
Negative feelings about body; feelings of helplessness, hopelessness, powerlessness, vulnerability
Preoccupation with change or loss
Refusal to verify actual change
Depersonalization of part or loss
Self-destructive behaviors (e.g., mutilation, suicide attempts, overeating/undereating)

## RELATED FACTORS

### Pathophysiologic

***Related to changes in appearance secondary to***
Chronic disease     Loss of body part  Loss of body function
Severe trauma       Aging
***Related to unrealistic perceptions of appearance secondary to***
Psychosis   Anorexia nervosa  Bulimia

### Treatment-Related

***Related to changes in appearance secondary to***
Hospitalization      Surgery  Chemotherapy
Radiation

### Situational (Personal, Environmental)

***Related to physical trauma secondary to***
Sexual abuse
Rape (perpetrator known or unknown)
Assault
***Related to effects of (specify) on appearance***
Obesity    Immobility     Pregnancy

## ▪▪▪▪▪ AUTHOR'S NOTE

See *Disturbed Self-Concept.*

■ ■ ■ ■ ■ ■ **ERRORS IN DIAGNOSTIC STATEMENTS**
See *Disturbed Self-Concept*.

**NOC**
Body Image, Child
Development:
(specify age),
Grief Resolution,
Psychosocial
Adjustment: Life
Change, Self-Esteem

## ➤ Goals

The person will implement new coping patterns and verbalize and demonstrate acceptance of appearance (grooming, dress, posture, eating patterns, presentation of self).

### *Indicators*

• Demonstrate a willingness and ability to resume self-care/role responsibilities.
• Initiate new or reestablish contacts with existing support systems.

**NIC**
Self-Esteem
Enhancement,
Counseling,
Presence, Active
Listening, Body
Image Enhancement,
Grief Work
Facilitation, Support
Group, Referral

## ➤ General Interventions

### Establish a Trusting Nurse–Client Relationship

Encourage person to express feelings, especially about the way he or she feels, thinks, or views self.
Acknowledge feelings of hostility, grief, fear, and dependency; teach strategies for coping with emotions.
Explore belief system (e.g., does pain, suffering, loss mean punishment?)
Encourage client to ask questions about health problem, treatment, progress, and prognosis.
Provide reliable information and reinforce information already given.
Clarify any misconceptions about self, care, or caregivers.
Avoid criticism.
Provide privacy and a safe environment.
Use therapeutic touch, with person's consent.
Encourage client to connect with spiritual beliefs and values regarding a higher power.

**R:** Frequent contact by the caregiver indicates acceptance and may facilitate trust. The client may be hesitant to approach the staff because of negative self-concept; the nurse must reach out.

## Promote Social Interaction

Assist client to accept help from others.
Avoid overprotection, but limit the demands made.
Encourage movement.
Prepare significant others for physical and emotional changes.
Support family as they adapt.
Encourage visits from peers and significant others.
Encourage contact (letters, telephone) with peers and family.
Encourage involvement in unit activities.
Provide opportunity to share with people going through similar experiences.
Discuss the importance of communicating the client's value and importance to them with his or her support system.

**R:** Social interactions can reaffirm that the person is acceptable and that previous support system is still intact. Isolation can increase feelings of guilt, fear and embarrassment.

## Provide Specific Interventions in Selected Situations

### *Loss of Body Part or Function*

Assess the meaning of the loss for the person and significant others, as related to visibility of loss, function of loss, and emotional investment.
Explore and clarify misconceptions and myths regarding loss or ability to function with loss.
Expect the person to respond to the loss with denial, shock, anger, and depression.
Be aware of the effect of the responses of others to the loss; encourage sharing of feelings between significant others.

Validate feelings by allowing the person to express his or her feelings and to grieve.

Use role playing to assist with sharing; if person says, "I know my husband will not want to touch me with this colostomy," take the husband's role and discuss her colostomy, then switch roles so she can act out her feelings about her husband's response.

Explore realistic alternatives and provide encouragement.

Explore strengths and resources with person.

Assist with the resolution of a surgically created alteration of body image:

- Replace the lost body part with prosthesis as soon as possible.
- Encourage viewing of site.
- Encourage touching of site.
- Encourage activities that encompass new body image (e.g., shopping for new clothes).

Teach about the health problem and how to manage.

Begin to incorporate person in care of operative site.

Gradually allow person to assume full self-care responsibility, if feasible.

Teach person to monitor own progress (Miller, 2009).

Refer to *Sexual Dysfunction* for additional information, if indicated.

Identifying personal attributes and strengths can help the client focus on the positive characteristics that contribute to the whole concept of self rather than only on the change in body image. The nurse should reinforce these positive aspects and encourage the client to reincorporate them into the new self-concept.

**R:** Identifying personal attributes and strengths can help the client focus on the positive characteristics that contribute to the whole concept of self rather than only on the change in body image. The nurse should reinforce these positive aspects and encourage the client to reincorporate them into the new self-concept.

**R:** Participation in self-care and planning promotes positive coping with the change.

## Changes Associated with Chemotherapy (Camp-Sorrell, 2007)

Discuss the possibility of hair loss, absence of menses, temporary or permanent sterility, decreased estrogen levels, vaginal dryness, and mucositis.

Encourage client to share concerns, fears, and perception of the effects of these changes on life.

Explain where hair loss may occur (head, eyelashes, eyebrows; axillary, pubic, and leg hair).

Explain that hair will grow back after treatment but may change in color and texture.

Encourage client to select and wear a wig before hair loss. Suggest consulting a beautician for tips on how to vary the look (e.g., combs, clips).

Encourage the wearing of scarves or turbans when wig is not on.

Teach client to minimize the amount of hair loss by:

- Cutting hair short
- Avoiding excessive shampooing, using a conditioner twice weekly
- Patting hair dry gently
- Avoiding electric curlers, dryers, and curling irons
- Avoiding pulling hair with bands, clips, or bobby pins
- Avoiding hair spray and hair dye
- Using wide-tooth comb, avoiding vigorous brushing

Refer client to American Cancer Society for information about new or used wigs. Inform the client that the wig is a tax-deductible item.

**R:** Open, honest discussions—expressing that changes will occur but that they are manageable—promote feelings of control. Participation in self-care and planning promotes positive coping with the change.

Discuss the difficulty that others (spouse, friends, coworkers) may have with visible changes.

Encourage client to initiate calls and contacts with others who may be having difficulty.

Encourage client to ask for assistance of friends, relatives. Ask person if the situation were reversed, what he or she would want to do to help a friend.

Allow significant others opportunities to share their feelings and fears.

Assist significant others to identify positive aspects of the client and ways this can be shared.
Provide information about support groups for couples.

**R:** Increased social interaction through involvement in groups enables a person to receive social and intellectual stimulation, which enhances self-esteem.

### Anorexia Nervosa, Bulimia Nervosa

Differentiate between body image distortion and body image dissatisfaction.
Refer individuals for psychiatric counseling.

### Psychoses

Refer to *Confusion* for specific information and interventions.

### Sexual Abuse

Refer to *Disabled Family Coping* for specific information and interventions.

### Sexual Assault

Refer to *Rape Trauma Syndrome* for specific information and interventions.

### Assault

Refer to *Post-Trauma Response* for specific information and interventions.

## Initiate Health Teaching, as Indicated

Teach what community resources are available, if needed (e.g., mental health centers, self-help groups such as Reach for Recovery, Make Today Count).

**R:** Professional counseling is indicated for a client with poor ego strengths and inadequate coping resources.

**R:** Increased social interaction through involvement in groups enables a person to receive social and intellectual stimulation, which enhances self-esteem.

Teach wellness strategies (see *Health-Seeking Behaviors*).

**Pediatric Interventions**

### For Hospitalized Child

Prepare child for hospitalization, if possible, with an explanation and a visit to the hospital to meet personnel and examine the environment.
Provide familiarities/routines of home as much as possible (e.g., favorite toy or blanket, story at bedtime).
Provide nurturance (e.g., hug).

**R:** Attempts to retain the normality of the child's world can help to increase security (Hockenberry & Wilson, 2009).

Provide child with opportunities to share fears, concerns, and anger:
Provide play therapy

- Correct misconceptions (e.g., that the child is being punished; that parents are angry).
- Encourage family to stay with or visit child, despite the child's crying when they leave; teach them to provide accurate information about when they will return to reduce fears of abandonment.
- Allow parents to help with care.
- Ask child to draw a picture of self, and then ask for a verbal description.

**R:** Play therapy puts the child in control by providing opportunities to make choices (Hockenberry & Wilson, 2009).

*(continued)*

**Pediatric Interventions**
*Continued*

Assist child to understand experiences:

- Provide an explanation ahead of time, if possible.
- Explain sensations and discomforts of condition, treatments, and medications.
- Encourage crying.

**R:** Interventions that provide expressive outlets for tension and fear can help maintain the child's integrity (Hockenberry & Wilson, 2009).

### Discuss with Parents How Body Image Develops and What Interactions Contribute to Their Child's Self-Perception

Teach the names and functions of body parts.
Acknowledge changes (e.g., height).
Allow some choices for what to wear.

**R:** Opportunities for choices and success enhance self-esteem and coping.

### For Adolescents

Discuss with parents the adolescent's need to "fit in":

- Do not dismiss concerns too quickly.
- Be flexible and compromise when possible (e.g., clothes are temporary, tattoos are not).
- Negotiate a time period to think about options and alternatives (e.g., 4 to 5 weeks).
- Provide with reasons for denying a request. Elicit adolescent's reasons. Compromise if possible (e.g., parents want curfew at 11:00; adolescent wants 12:00; compromise at 11:30).

Provide opportunities to discuss concerns when parents are not present.
Prepare for impending developmental changes.

**R:** Opportunities for open dialogue, choices and success enhance self-esteem and coping.

**Maternal Interventions**

Encourage the woman to share her concerns.
Attend to each concern, if possible, or refer her to others for assistance.
Discuss the challenges and changes that pregnancy and motherhood bring.
Encourage her to share expectations: her own and those of her significant others.
Assist her to identify sources for love and affection.

**R:** Open, honest discussions—expressing that changes will occur but that they are manageable—promote feelings of control.

Provide anticipatory guidance to both parents-to-be concerning:
- Fatigue and irritability
- Appetite swings
- Gastric disturbances (nausea, constipation)
- Back and leg aches
- Changes in sexual desire and activity (e.g., sexual positions as pregnancy advances)
- Mood swings
- Fear (for self, for unborn baby, of loss of attractiveness, of inadequacy as a parent)

Encourage sharing of concerns between spouses.

**R:** Support can be given more freely and more realistically if others are prepared.

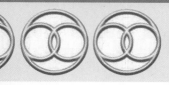

# DISTURBED PERSONAL IDENTITY

## DEFINITION

State in which a person experiences or is at risk of experiencing an inability to distinguish between self and non-self

## DEFINING CHARACTERISTICS*

Appears unaware of or uninterested in others or their activities
Unable to identify parts of the body or body sensations e.g. enuresis
Excessively imitates other's activities or words
Fails to distinguish parent/caregiver as a whole person
Becomes distress with bodily contact with others
Spends long periods of time in self-stimulating behaviors (self-touching, sucking, rocking
Needs ritualistic behaviors and sameness to control anxiety.
Cannot tolerate being separated from parent/caregiver.

## RELATED FACTORS†

### Pathophysiologic

Related to biochemical imbalance
Related to impaired neurologic development or dysfunction

### Maturational

Related to failure to develop attachment behaviors resulting in fixation at autistic phase of development
Related to interrupted or uncompleted separation / individualization process resulting in extreme
  separation anxiety

## ■■■■■ AUTHOR'S NOTE

Disturbed Personal Identity is a very complex diagnosis and should not be used to label autism. It may be more clinically useful in nursing to use Anxiety and/or Impaired Social Interactions for the nursing focus.

---

*Varcarolis, 2006, p. 204.
†Varcarolis, 2006, p. 103.

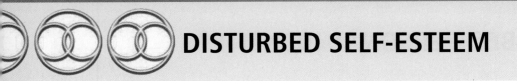

# DISTURBED SELF-ESTEEM

## DEFINITION

State in which a person experiences or is at risk of experiencing negative self-evaluation about self or capabilities

## DEFINING CHARACTERISTICS
## (LEUNER ET AL., 1994; NORRIS & KUNES-CONNELL, 1987)

### Major (Must be Present, One or More)

(Observed or reported)
Self-negating verbalization
Expressions of shame or guilt
Evaluates self as unable to deal with events
Rationalizes away or rejects positive feedback and exaggerates negative feedback about self
Lack of or poor problem-solving ability
Hesitant to try new things or situations
Rationalizes personal failures
Hypersensitivity to slight criticism

### Minor

Lack of assertion
Overly conforming
Indecisiveness
Passive
Seeks approval or reassurance excessively
Lack of culturally appropriate body presentation (posture, eye contact, movements)
Denial of problems obvious to others
Projection of blame or responsibility for problems

## RELATED FACTORS

*Disturbed Self-Esteem* can be either episodic or chronic. Failure to resolve a problem or multiple sequential stresses can result in chronic low self-esteem (CLSE). Those factors that occur over time and are associated with CLSE are indicated by "CLSE" in parentheses.

### Pathophysiologic

*Related to change in appearance secondary to*
Loss of body parts
Loss of body functions
Disfigurement (trauma, surgery, birth defects)
*Related to biochemical /neurophysiologic imbalance*

### Situational (Personal, Environmental)

*Related to unmet dependency needs*
*Related to feelings of abandonment secondary to*
Death of significant other          Separation from significant other
Child abduction/murder
*Related to feelings of failure secondary to*
Loss of job or ability to work          Increase/decrease in weight          Unemployment

| Financial problems | Premenstrual syndrome | Relationship problems |
| Marital discord | Separation | Stepparents |
| In-laws | | |

*Related to assault (personal, or relating to the event of another's assault—e.g., same age, same community)*

*Related to failure in school*

*Related to history of ineffective relationship with parents (CLSE)*

*Related to history of abusive relationships (CLSE)*

*Related to unrealistic expectations of child by parent (CLSE)*

*Related to unrealistic expectations of self (CLSE)*

*Related to unrealistic expectations of parent by child (CLSE)*

*Related to parental rejection (CLSE)*

*Related to inconsistent punishment (CLSE)*

*Related to feelings of helplessness and/or failure secondary to institutionalization*

| Mental health facility | Orphanage | Jail | Halfway house |

*Related to history of numerous failures (CLSE)*

## Maturational

### Infant/Toddler/Preschool
*Related to lack of stimulation or closeness (CLSE)*

*Related to separation from parents/significant others (CLSE)*

*Related to continual negative evaluation by parents*

*Related to inadequate parental support (CLSE)*

*Related to inability to trust significant other (CLSE)*

### School-Aged
Related to failure to achieve grade-level objectives

Related to loss of peer group

Related to repeated negative feedback

### Adolescent
Related to loss of independence and autonomy secondary to (specify)

Related to disruption of peer relationships

Related to scholastic problems

Related to loss of significant others

### Middle-Aged
Related to changes associated with aging

### Older Adult
Related to losses (people, function, financial, retirement)

## ▪▪▪▪▪ AUTHOR'S NOTE
See *Disturbed Self-Concept.*

## ▪▪▪▪▪ ERRORS IN DIAGNOSTIC STATEMENTS
See *Disturbed Self-Concept.*

## ▪▪▪▪▪ KEY CONCEPTS
See *Disturbed Self-Concept.*

## Focus Assessment Criteria

See *Disturbed Self-Concept.*

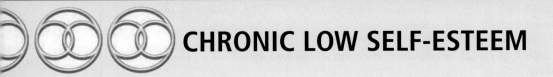

# CHRONIC LOW SELF-ESTEEM

## DEFINITION

State in which a person experiences a long-standing negative self-evaluation about self or capabilities

## DEFINING CHARACTERISTICS
## (LEUNER ET AL., 1994; NORRIS & KUNES-CONNELL, 1987)

### Major (80% to 100%)

**Long-Standing or Chronic**
Self-negating verbalization
Expressions of shame/guilt
Evaluates self as unable to deal with events
Rationalizes away/rejects positive feedback and exaggerates negative feedback about self
Hesitant to try new things/situations
Exaggerating negative feedback

### Minor (50% to 79%)

Frequent lack of success in work or other life events
Overly conforming, dependent on others' opinions
Lack of culturally appropriate body presentation (eye contact, posture, movements)
Nonassertive/passive
Indecisive
Excessively seeks reassurance

## RELATED FACTORS

See *Disturbed Self-Esteem.*

## ■■■■■ AUTHOR'S NOTE

See *Disturbed Self-Concept.*

## ■■■■■ ERRORS IN DIAGNOSTIC STATEMENTS

See *Disturbed Self-Concept.*

**NOC**
Depression Level,
Depression Self-
Control, Anxiety
Level, Quality of Life,
Self-Esteem

## ► Goals

The person will identify positive aspects of self and a realistic appraisal of limitations.

### Indicators

• Modify excessive and unrealistic self-expectations.
• Verbalize acceptance of limitations.
• Verbalize nonjudgmental perceptions of self.
• Cease self-abusive behavior.
• Begin to take verbal and behavioral risks.

<table>
<tr><td>

**NIC**
Hope Instillation,
Anxiety Reduction,
Self-Esteem
Enhancement,
Coping
Enhancement,
Socialization
Enhancement,
Referral

</td></tr>
</table>

# ➤ General Interventions

## Assist the Person to Reduce Present Anxiety Level

Be supportive, nonjudgmental.
Accept silence, but let him or her know you are there.
Orient as necessary.
Clarify distortions; do not use confrontation.
Be aware of your own anxiety and avoid communicating it to the person.
Refer to *Anxiety* for further interventions.

**R:** People with low self-esteem are usually anxious, fearful people. Anxiety levels must be mild or moderate before other interventions can be effective (Mohr, 2007).

## Enhance the Person's Sense of Self

Be attentive.
Respect personal space.
Validate your interpretation of what he or she is saying or experiencing ("Is this what you mean?").
Help him or her to verbalize what he or she is expressing nonverbally.
Assist client to reframe and redefine negative expressions (e.g., not "failure," but "setback").
Use communication that helps to maintain his or her individuality ("I" instead of "we").
Pay attention to person, especially new behavior.
Encourage good physical habits (healthy food and eating patterns, exercise, proper sleep).
Provide encouragement as he or she attempts a task or skill.
Provide realistic positive feedback on accomplishments.
Teach person to validate consensually with others.
Teach and encourage esteem-building exercises (self-affirmations, imagery, mirror work, use of humor, meditation/prayer, relaxation).
Respect need for privacy.
Assist in establishing appropriate personal boundaries.
Provide consistency among staff (Miller, 2009).

**R:** Strategies focus on helping the person reexamine negative feelings about self and identifying positive attributes.

**R:** Strategies focus on helping the person reexamine negative feelings about self and identifying positive attributes.

**R:** Persons with low self-esteem have difficulty asking appropriately for what they need or want. (Varcarolis, 2006)

## Promote Use of Coping Resources

Identify the client's areas of personal strength.

| | | |
|---|---|---|
| Sports, hobbies, crafts | Health, self-care | Work, training, education |
| Imagination, creativity | Writing skills, math | Interpersonal relationships |

Share your observations with the person.
Provide opportunities for person to engage in the activities.

**R:** Client collaboration is necessary for him or her to assume ultimate responsibility for behavior (Stuart & Sundeen, 2002).

## Assist to Identify Cognitive Distortions that Increase Negative Self-Appraisal (Varcarolis, 2006)

Overgeneralization
  Teach to focus on each event as separate
Self-Blame
  Teach to evaluate if she /he is really responsible and why.
Mind-Reading
  Advise to clarify verbally what he/she thinks is happening

Discounting positive responses of others
Teach to respond with only - Thank You

**R:** These cognitive distortions reinforce negative inaccurate perception of self and the world (Varcarlois, 2006)

## Provide Opportunities for Positive Socialization

Encourage visits/contact with peers and significant others (letters, telephone).
Be a role model in one-to-one interactions.
Involve in activities, especially when strengths can be used.
Do not allow person to isolate self (refer to *Social Isolation* for further interventions).
Involve client in supportive group therapy.
Teach social skills as required (refer to *Impaired Social Interaction* for further interventions).
Encourage participation with others sharing similar experiences.

**R:** Opportunities for the person to be successful increases self-esteem (Stuart & Sundeen, 2006).
**R:** Role modeling positive socialization can decrease feelings of isolation and can encourage a more realistic appraisal of self (Varcarolis, 2006).

## Set Limits on Problematic Behavior Such as Aggression, Poor Hygiene, Ruminations, and Suicidal Preoccupation

Refer to *Risk for Suicide* and/or *Risk for Violence* if these are assessed as problems.

## Provide for Development of Social and Vocational Skills

Refer for vocational counseling.
Involve client in volunteer organizations.
Encourage participation in activities with others of same age.
Arrange for continuation of education (e.g., literacy class, vocational training, art/music classes).

**R:** Opportunities for success can increase self-esteem.

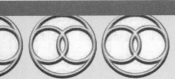

# SITUATIONAL LOW SELF-ESTEEM

## DEFINITION

State in which a person who previously had positive self-esteem experiences negative feelings about self in response to an event (loss, change)

## DEFINING CHARACTERISTICS (LEVNER ET AL., 1994; NORRIS & KUNES-CONNELL, 1987)

### Major (80% to 100%)

Episodic occurrence of negative self-appraisal in response to life events in a person with a previously positive self-evaluation
Verbalization of negative feelings about self (helplessness, uselessness)

### Minor (50% to 79%)

Self-negating verbalizations
Expressions of shame/guilt

Evaluates self as unable to handle situations/events
Difficulty making decisions

# RELATED FACTORS

See *Disturbed Self-Esteem*.

## ■■■■■■ AUTHOR'S NOTE

See *Disturbed Self-Concept*.

## ■■■■■■ ERRORS IN DIAGNOSTIC STATEMENTS

See *Disturbed Self-Concept*.

## ■■■■■■ KEY CONCEPTS

### Generic Considerations

- Qualities of a healthy personality are (Stuart & Sundeen, 2002)
- Positive and accurate body image
- Realistic self-ideal
- Positive self-concept
- High self-esteem
- Satisfying role performance
- Clear sense of identity
- People with healthy personalities can experience a change in their positive self-perception in response to a profound event or a series of negative experiences (Stuart & Sundeen, 2002).
- Responses to a situation that challenges a person's previously positive view of self are feelings of being weak, helpless, or hopeless; fear; vulnerability; and feelings of being fragile, incomplete, worthless, and inadequate (Stuart & Sundeen, 2006).

---

**NOC**

Decision-Making, Grief Resolution, Psychosocial Adjustment: Life Change, Self-Esteem

## ➤ Goals

The person will express a positive outlook for the future and resume previous level of functioning.

### Indicators

- Identify source of threat to self-esteem and work through that issue.
- Identify positive aspects of self.
- Analyze his or her own behavior and its consequences.
- Identify one positive aspect of change.

---

**NIC**

Active Listening, Presence, Counseling, Cognitive Restructuring, Family Support, Support Group, Coping Enhancement

## ➤ General Interventions

### Assist Client to Identify and to Express Feelings

Be empathic, nonjudgmental.
Listen. Do not discourage expressions of anger, crying, and so forth.
Ask what was happening when he or she began feeling this way.
Clarify relationships between life events.

**R:** Self-acceptance can be increased with clarification of feelings and thoughts.

## Assist Client to Identify Positive Self-Evaluations

How has he or she handled other crises?
How does he or she manage anxiety—through exercise, withdrawal, drinking/drugs, talking?

Reinforce adaptive coping mechanisms.

Examine and reinforce positive abilities and traits (e.g., hobbies, skills, school, relationships, appearance, loyalty, industriousness).

Help client accept both positive and negative feelings.

Do not confront defenses.

Communicate confidence in person's ability.

Involve person in mutual goal setting.

Have client write positive true statements about self (for his or her eyes only); have client read the list daily as a part of normal routine.

Reinforce use of esteem-building exercises (self-affirmations, imagery, meditation/prayer, relaxation, use of humor).

## Assist to Identify Cognitive Distortions that Increase Negative Self-Appraisal (Varcarolis, 2006)

Overgeneralization

Teach to focus on each event as separate

Self-Blame

Teach to evaluate if she/he is really responsible and why.

Mind-Reading

Advise to clarify verbally what he/she thinks is happening

Discounting positive responses of others

Teach to respond with only - Thank You

**R:** These cognitive distortions reinforce negative, inaccurate perception of self and the world (Varcarlois, 2006)

## Assess and Mobilize Current Support System

Does he or she live alone? Is he or she employed?

Does he or she have available friends and relatives?

Is religion a support?

Has he or she previously used community resources?

Refer client to vocational rehabilitation for retraining.

Support returning to school for further training.

Assist client to involve local volunteer organizations (senior citizens employment, foster grandparents, local support groups).

Arrange continuation of school studies for students.

**R:** Social support increases resourcefulness, self-esteem, and well-being (Dirsken, 2000).

## Assist Client to Learn New Coping Skills

Practice self-talk (Murray, 2000):
• Write a brief description of the change and its consequence (e.g., My spouse has had an affair. I am betrayed.).
• Write three things that may be useful about this situation.

Communicate that the person can handle the change.

Challenge the person to imagine positive futures and outcomes.

Encourage a trial of new behavior.

Reinforce the belief that the person does have control over the situation.

Obtain a commitment to action.

**R:** Self-talk does not imply that one likes the change; however, it helps one find potential benefits of the change (Murray, 2000).

## Assist Person to Manage Specific Problems

Rape—refer to *Rape-Trauma Syndrome*.
Loss—refer to *Grieving*.

Hospitalization—refer to *Powerlessness* and *Parental Role Conflict*.
Ill family member—refer to *Interrupted Family Processes*.
Change or loss of body part—refer to *Disturbed Body Image*.
Depression—refer to *Ineffective Coping* and *Hopelessness*.
Domestic violence—refer to *Disabled Family Coping*.

### Pediatric Interventions

Provide opportunities for child to be successful and needed.
Personalize the child's environment with pictures, possessions, and crafts he or she made.
Provide structured and unstructured playtime.
Ensure continuation of academic experiences in the hospital and home. Provide uninterrupted time for schoolwork.

**R:** See *Disturbed Self-Concept*.

### Geriatric Interventions

Acknowledge person by name.
Use a tone of voice that you use for your peer group.
Avoid words associated with infants (e.g., "diapers").
Ask about family pictures, personal items, and past experiences.
Avoid attributing disabilities to "old age."
Knock on door of bedrooms and bathrooms.
Allow enough time to accomplish tasks at own pace.

**R:** Because self-esteem depends partially on the responses of others, caregivers must reflect respect for the aged as competent adults (Miller, 2009).

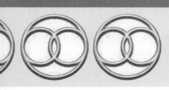

# RISK FOR SITUATIONAL LOW SELF-ESTEEM

## DEFINITION

State in which a person who previously had a positive self-esteem is at risk to experience negative feelings about self in response to an event (loss, change)

## RISK FACTORS

See *Situational Low Self-Esteem*.

### ■■■■■ AUTHOR'S NOTE

See *Situational Low Self-Esteem*.

### ■■■■ ERRORS IN DIAGNOSTIC STATEMENTS

See *Situational Low Self-Esteem*.

■■■■■■ **KEY CONCEPTS**

See *Situational Low Self-Esteem*.

## Goal

The person will continue to express a positive outlook for the future to identify positive aspects of self.

### Indicators

• Identify threats to self-esteem.
• Identify one positive aspect of change.

## General Interventions

See *Situational Low Self-Esteem*.

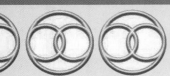

# RISK FOR SELF-HARM

**Risk for Self-Harm\***

Risk for Self-Abuse
Self-Mutilation
Risk for Self-Mutilation
Risk for Suicide

## DEFINITION

State in which a client is at risk for inflicting direct harm on himself or herself. This may include one or more of the following: self-abuse, self-mutilation, suicide.

## DEFINING CHARACTERISTICS

### Major (Must Be Present, One or More)

Expresses desire or intent to harm self
Expresses desire to die or commit suicide
Past history of attempts to harm self

### Minor

**Reported or Observed:**

| | | |
|---|---|---|
| Depression | Hopelessness | Poor self-concept |
| Helplessness | Hallucinations/delusions | Lack of support system |
| Substance abuse | Emotional pain | Poor impulse control |
| Hostility | Agitation | |

## RELATED FACTORS

*Risk for Self-Harm* can occur as a response to a variety of health problems, situations, and conflicts. Some sources are listed next.

———————

\*These diagnoses are not currently on the NANDA list but have been included for clarity of usefulness.

## Pathophysiologic

*Related to feelings of helplessness, loneliness, or hopelessness secondary to:*
Disabilities
Terminal illness
Chronic illness
Chronic pain
Chemical dependency
Substance abuse
New diagnosis of positive human immunodeficiency virus (HIV) status
Mental impairment (organic or traumatic)
Psychiatric disorder

| | | |
|---|---|---|
| Schizophrenia | Personality disorder | Bipolar disorder |
| Adolescent adjustment disorder | Post-trauma syndrome | Somatoform disorders |

## Treatment-Related

*Related to unsatisfactory outcome of treatment (medical, surgical, psychological)*
*Related to prolonged dependence on:*

| | | |
|---|---|---|
| Dialysis | Chemotherapy/radiation | Insulin injections |
| Ventilator | | |

## Situational (Personal, Environmental)

*Related to:*
Incarceration
Depression
Ineffective coping skills
Parental/marital conflict
Substance abuse in family
Child abuse
Real or perceived loss secondary to:

| | | | |
|---|---|---|---|
| Finances/job | Separation/divorce | Status/prestige | Natural disaster |
| Death of significant others | Threat of abandonment | Someone leaving home | |

*Related to wish for revenge on real or perceived injury (body or self-esteem)*

## Maturational

**Adolescent**
*Related to feelings of abandonment*
*Related to peer pressure*
*Related to unrealistic expectations of child by parents*
*Related to depression*
*Related to relocation*
*Related to significant loss*

**Older Adult**
*Related to multiple losses secondary to:*

| | | | |
|---|---|---|---|
| Retirement | Social isolation | Significant loss | Illness |

### ■■■■■ AUTHOR'S NOTE

*Risk for Self-Harm* represents a broad diagnosis that can encompass self-abuse, self-mutilation, and/or risk for suicide. Although initially they may appear the same, the distinction lies in the intent. Self-mutilation and self-abuse are pathologic attempts to relieve stress temporarily, whereas suicide is an attempt to die to relieve stress permanently (Carscadden, 1992, personal communication). *Risk for Self-Harm* also can be a useful early diagnosis when insufficient data are present to differentiate one from the other.

*(continued)*

■■■■■■ **AUTHOR'S NOTE** *Continued*

> *Risk for Suicide* has been in this author's work for over 20 years. *Risk for Suicide* was added to the NANDA list in 2006. Previously, *Risk for Violence to Self* was included under *Risk for Violence*. The term *violence* is defined as a swift and intense force or a rough or injurious physical force. As the reader knows, suicide can be either violent or nonviolent (e.g., overdose of barbiturates). Using the term "violence" in this diagnostic context, unfortunately, can lead to non-detection of a client at risk for suicide because of the perception that the client is not capable of violence.
>
> *Risk for Suicide* clearly denotes a client at high risk for suicide and in need of protection. Treatment of this diagnosis involves validating the risk, contracting with the client, and providing protection. Treatment of the client's underlying depression and hopelessness should be addressed with other applicable nursing diagnoses (e.g., *Ineffective Coping, Hopelessness*).

■■■■■■ **ERRORS IN DIAGNOSTIC STATEMENTS**

### Risk for Suicide related to recent diagnosis of cancer

In this situation, the recent diagnosis of cancer in itself is not a risk factor for suicide. The client must be depressed, severely stressed, and exhibiting suicidal intentions. The nurse must not automatically label a client as suicidal based on a single crisis or severe physical disability. All *Risk for Self-Harm* diagnostic statements should contain both verbal and nonverbal cues to suicidal intent (e.g., *Risk for Suicide related to remarks about life being unbearable and reports of giving belongings away*).

■■■■■■ **KEY CONCEPTS**

### Generic Considerations

- Violence, whether directed toward oneself or others, can elicit strong reactions from people. Nurses, whose profession encompasses caregiving, health promotion, and nurturance, must examine their own attitudes, responses, and behavior toward violence.
- Because much of the practice of self-harm is a "shame-based" problem, the condition is more likely to be underreported rather than overreported. Identification is difficult, because so many who engage in self-harm become extremely adept at hiding the causes of their injuries.
- Self-harm is found in people from all economic and educational backgrounds, and in both men and women. It usually appears in the early teenage years, although it may commence before adolescence. It frequently is associated with long-term effects of physical, psychological, and sexual abuse during childhood.
- Many people who harm themselves are given a psychiatric diagnosis of personality disorder or, more specifically, borderline personality disorder, although other psychiatric diagnoses may be associated with self-harm (see the Pathophysiologic section). An important consideration is that not all people with these diagnoses harm themselves, and not all self-injurers qualify for these diagnoses. Treatment will differ depending on the diagnosis (Carscadden, 1997).
- The client who has delusions or hallucinations (either schizophrenic or drug-induced) presents a different rationale for self-harm. Delusions and hallucinations must be brought under control. Meanwhile, the client's safety is essential. Self-harm also may be prevalent with mentally challenged people, and management in this particular population will differ again, owing to the cognition level of the self-injurer.
- Often repetitive and chronic in nature, self-harm frequently distorts or disrupts the client–therapist relationship and increases the need for and length of hospitalizations. These hospitalizations often exacerbate the problem further. Hospitalization usually increases the client's dependency and decreases his or her accountability.

## Self-Harm

- There are various levels or stages in impending self-harm. The transition from one level to another may be rapid or slowly progressive. The client may or may not be aware of the stages and the transition. Awareness of each stage and its characteristics facilitates intervention. The earlier the stage, the clearer the thinking, the less intense the feelings, and the more control the client has. A client can easily identify stages once he or she learns the defining characteristics (Carscadden, 1993a).

- Although self-harm may create a sense of urgency, imminent disaster, and a strong and immediate sense of responsibility in the listener or observer, one must be careful not to be caught up in this and feel compelled to do something. (This excludes the psychotic and mentally challenged population.) The very act of trying to intervene or prevent the behaviors may increase the likelihood of more serious harm, including completed suicide. The risk increases because (a) the more often intervention takes place, the more likely death by mistake will occur (wrong pills, too many, the expected rescue being thwarted); (b) there may be a need to use increasingly dangerous methods to get the same result; or (c) before long, countertransference hate sets in. In an empathic, yet matter-of-fact manner, the nurse must convey that the client's actions are in his or her hands alone and that no one can be his or her guardian or savior. This is the hardest thing for anyone to say; however, for the self-injurer to survive and mature, he or she must become responsible for his or her own actions. If someone else takes control, the self-injurer will not progress (Carscadden, 1998).
- Families are often the forgotten sufferers in the self-harm syndrome. They are caught in the same shame-based system as the self-injurer, and this often precludes their reaching out for help with the bewilderment, frustration, and helplessness experienced in day-to-day living with the self-injurer. They need assistance in demystifying self-harm, identifying how it has affected them, and examining some coping methods for supporting themselves and the self-injurer on the road to recovery. Educational and support groups as well as family counseling are good ways to begin this process (Carscadden, 1997).

## Suicide

- Suicidal behavior is an attempt to escape from intolerable life stressors that have accumulated over time. It is accompanied by intense feelings of hopelessness, little social support, and insufficient coping skills to manage extreme stressors that are present (Boyd, 2005).
- Lack of healthy coping skills and use of avoidant behaviors such as alcohol and drugs frequently are correlated with suicidal behavior.
- A suicidal crisis happens both to the client and to his or her support system. Suicide may be seen as a viable alternative both by the client and by significant others.
- Depression, low self-esteem, helplessness, and hopelessness are positively related to suicide. The greater the degree of hopelessness, the greater is the risk for suicide. Loss clearly increases the risk of suicide. Cumulative losses increase the risk dramatically.
- People exhibiting poor reality testing, delusions, and poor impulse control are at high risk. Alcohol and drugs tend to lower impulse control.
- Changes in behavior (e.g., giving away possessions) may signal an increase in risk. A client may appear to be better just before an attempt. This may result from feelings of relief after making a decision.
- Demographic factors can help identify people at high risk for suicide:
  - White men over 65 have the highest suicide rate in the United States. Risk increases linearly as the client ages (Boyd, 2005).
  - Adolescents also represent a high-risk group.
  - More women attempt suicide, but men complete suicide more often.
  - Unemployment and frequent job changes are associated with an increased risk.
  - Alcohol is associated with a high risk.
  - The greater the satisfaction with social relationships, the lower the risk will be; thus, divorce, separation, and widowhood increase the risk.
  - Previous attempts place people in a high-risk group because they are likely to repeat.
  - The more resources that are available, the more likely it is that the crisis can be managed effectively. Resources include personal support systems, employment, physical and mental abilities, finances, and housing.
  - Some people use suicide attempts as a way to cope with stress. The more frequent the attempts and the more lethal, the higher the current risk. Suicidal ideation moves from the general to the specific, with more detailed plans representing a higher risk. An event may precipitate an attempt. The difference between a negative life event and one that may lead to a suicide attempt is that with the latter, the client already has engaged in significant suicidal ideation.

- Lethality describes "the probability that a client will successfully complete suicide." It is determined by the "seriousness of the intent and the likelihood that the planned method of death will succeed" (Boyd, 2005, p. 860).
- Nurses should use verbal and nonverbal clues to assess risk, because seriously suicidal people may deny suicidal thoughts.
- Prediction of suicide risk is not an exact science. Some errors that can be made result from:
  - Overreliance on mood as an indicator; not all people who commit suicide are clinically depressed.
  - Reliance on intuition; many people can totally conceal their intention.
  - Failure to assess support system.
  - Countertransference, particularly the failure of the therapist to acknowledge negative feelings that are aroused.
- One in five suicide victims had contact with mental health services or the primary care providers (PCP) within one month of their suicide (Ortiz, 2006).
- Levels of risk can be assessed as low or high. Not all of the following parameters are necessarily present in any one client (Varcarolis, 2006).

*High:*

| | |
|---|---|
| Adolescent or older than 45 years of age | Male |
| Divorced, separated, or widowed | Isolated socially |
| Professional worker | Unemployed or lack of stable job history |
| Chronic or terminal illness | Severe depression |
| Delusions/hallucinations | Severe anxiety |
| Hopelessness/helplessness | Multiple attempts |
| Intoxicated or addicted | With a specific plan |
| Frequent or constant suicidal thoughts | Method is highly lethal |
| Means readily available | |

*Low:*

| | |
|---|---|
| 25 to 45 years of age | Younger than 12 years |
| Married | Blue-collar worker |
| No serious medical problems | No specific plan, or plan with low lethality |
| Female | Socially active |
| Employed | Infrequent substance abuse |
| Fleeting thoughts (if plan is vague) | |

- In an HIV-positive client, the risk for suicide is greatest "shortly after learning of one's infection and at the late stages of AIDS" (Siegel & Meyer, 1999, p. 53).
- The AIDS-related multiple losses that HIV-negative gay men may experience can result in repetitive overwhelming emotions, physical exhaustion, and spiritual demoralization. If coupled with shunning and isolation, despair is increased and chronic (Mallinson, 1999).

## Pediatric Considerations

- The preteen and early adolescent years are often when self-harm begins to manifest itself. Adults must be in tune with changes in behavior and changes in apparel and be highly suspicious of multiple "accidents."
- Suicide is the second leading cause of death during adolescence. A significant trend is the rise among people in the younger age groups.
- Suicide in children (5 to 14 years of age) tends to be more impulsive than in other age groups. Hyperactivity also seems to contribute to the impulsive nature.
- Recognition of depression in adolescents is often difficult because they mask their feelings with bored and angry behavior. Some symptoms include being sad or blue, withdrawal from social activities, trouble concentrating, somatic complaints, changes in sleep or eating patterns, and feelings of guilt or inadequacy.
- Suicidal adolescents rarely have close friends and exhibit poor peer relationships.
- Gay youths are estimated to be two to three times more likely to attempt suicide than their heterosexual peers. As many as 30% of suicides annually are believed to be gay teens.

- Suicide is the leading cause of death among adolescents. A frequent factor is lack of or loss of a meaningful relationship (Hockenberry & Wilson, 2009).
- Suicide attempts among Hispanic adolescent girls were reported to be 19.3%. Significant related factors included family history of suicide attempt, history of sexual or physical abuse, and environmental stress (Giger & Davidhazar, 2009).

## Geriatric Considerations

- White men older than 65 years have twice the rate of suicide of all other age groups. They constitute 18.5% of the population but commit 23% of all suicides (Miller, 2009)
- Retirement, loss of vigor, and loss of a meaningful role negatively affect the self-esteem of older men.
- Older adults tend to complete suicide when they attempt it. The ratio of attempts to completion is 4:1, whereas for younger people it is approximately 200:1 (McIntosh, 1985).
- Alcohol contributes to depression. Depression increases alcohol use. Both are significant risk factors for suicide in older adults.
- Depressed older adults usually talk less about suicide than younger adults but use more violent means and are more often successful (Miller, 2009)
- Suicide potential often is overlooked because of the prevalent view that older adults are generally passive and nonviolent. In addition, complaints about depression and hopelessness may be subtle and thus easily ignored in older adults (Miller, 2009)
- Older adults communicate their intentions less frequently and they use more lethal means (Mellick, Buckwalter, & Stolley, 1992). Families, senior citizen centers, clergy, and physicians are the network that can most readily identify the potential problem.
- Older adults have higher rates of contact with primary care providers within one month of their suicide (Luoma, Martin, & Perason, 2002).

## Transcultural Considerations

- Acceptance of sudden, violent death is difficult for family members in most societies (Andrews & Boyle, 2008).
- Islamic law strictly forbids suicide. Some religions (e.g., Catholicism) do not permit church funerals for suicide victims.
- The Northern Cheyenne Indians believe suicide or any violent death prevents the spirit from entering the spirit world (Andrews & Boyle, 2008).
- Suicide of elderly Eskimos, who could no longer contribute to the sustenance of the tribe, was expected (Giger & Davidhizar, 2009).

# Focus Assessment Criteria

The nurse must be able to differentiate between the diagnoses of *Risk for Suicide* and *Risk for Self-Mutilation* or *Self-Abuse*. Although initially they may appear (in action) or sound (in statements) the same, the distinction lies in the intent. Self-mutilation and self-abuse are pathologic attempts to relieve stress (temporary reprieve), whereas suicide is an attempt to die (to relieve stress permanently). The nurse will be able in the assessment to gather data that enable him or her to distinguish which diagnosis is appropriate for the client. It is prudent to remember that some clients may become so self-harmful that they eventually die, even though they are not intentionally suicidal.

## Subjective Data

### Assess for Risk Factors

**Psychological Status**
*Present concerns:*
- Have you experienced a severe stressor recently?
- How are you feeling?
- Do you want to hurt yourself?
- Can you tell me the reason?
- Do you want to die or just have the pain (thoughts/feelings) go away?

*Assess for Risks of Suicide:*

- Age: Is the client 19 years or younger or 45 years old or older (especially over age 65)?
- Gendr: Is the client a man?
- Emotional State: Is the client depressed? Does the client abuse alcohol?
- Social Supports: Does the client have significant friends, meaningful employment, and spiritual or religious supports?
- Spouse: Is the client widowed, separated, divorced, or single?
- Illness: Does the client have a chronic, debilitating, or severe illness?
- Previous Attempt: Has the client attempted suicide before?
- Method: Is there a specific plan (e.g., pills, wrist slashing, shooting)? Plans for rescue?
- Availability: Is the method accessible? Is access easy or difficult?
- Specificity: How specific is the plan?
- Lethality: How lethal is the method?

*Feelings of:*

| | | |
|---|---|---|
| Hopelessness | Anger/hostility | Helplessness |
| Guilt/shame | Isolation/abandonment | Impulsivity |

*Chemical dependency/substance abuse:*
Assess if the client is suffering from withdrawal or is under the influence. Chemical use lowers cognition ability and raises the level of impulsivity.

*History of psychiatric problems*
Previous history of self-harm:

| | | |
|---|---|---|
| Methods | How recent | Ensures rescue will be made |
| Lethality | Number of times | |

Outpatient follow-up support system

## Medical Status
Acute or chronic illness—how is it affecting life?
Prescribed drugs:

- What is the client using?
- Does he or she take it according to the directions?

## Sources of Stress in Past Environment
Job change/loss
Failure in work/school
Threat of financial loss
Divorce/separation
Death of significant other
Illness/accident
Alcohol/drug use in family
Parental rejection
Dysfunctional family dynamics
Physical, psychological, or sexual abuse
Unrealistic expectations:

- Of child by parent
- Of parent by child
- Of self

Severe trauma

## Sources of Stress in Current Environment
Any of the above (past environment)
Threat of criminal prosecution
Alcohol/drug use by the client
Role change/responsibilities
Any threat to self-concept (real or perceived)

### Assessment of the Client's Awareness of Self-Harm Activities

Acknowledgment or denial—does the client admit self-harm or claim to have "accidents"?
What are the benefits or reasons for self-harm?

- Is communication nonverbal—the client gains someone's attention and coerces others for his needs
- Makes others believe—physical evidence of pain
- Demonstrates the feeling of hopelessness
- Demonstrates outside what the client feels like inside (ugly, scarred, garbage)
- Feels he or she deserves it—bad, ugly, evil, or crazy
- Releases pain and anger—use of self-harm is a safety valve to prevent suicide
- Reestablishes control over one's body
- Verifies there is still life—physical evidence of life in flow of blood
- Is sadomasochistic pleasure
- Is an addiction to near death

Can the client identify specifics in the process?
- Personal triggers
  - Sensory input
  - Situations
  - Particular types of people or places
- Flashbacks or nightmares

Does the client disassociate or "numb out"?
Can the client identify levels or stages before the act of self-harm?
Motivation to cease self-harm:
- Wants to stop and is willing to work toward that end
  - Wants emotional pain to stop; sees self-harm as part of that pain and is considering change
  - Unwilling to give up self-harm behavior

### Support System

Who is relied on during periods of stress?
Are they available?
What is their reaction to the current situation?

| | | |
|---|---|---|
| Denial | Helplessness/frustration | |
| Not receptive to helping | Concern and willingness to help | Anger/guilt |
| Personal and financial resources | | |
| Employment | Housing | Finances |

## Objective Data

### *Assess for Risk Factors*

**General Appearance**

| | | |
|---|---|---|
| Facial expression | Apparel | Posture |

**Behavior During Interview**

| | | |
|---|---|---|
| Agitated | Hostile | Restless |
| Cooperative | Withdrawn | Disassociated |

**Communication Pattern**

| | | |
|---|---|---|
| Hopeless/helpless (subjective) | Allusive | Denial |
| Suicidal expressions | Delusional | Indecisive |
| Hallucinates | Pressured speech | Misinterprets |
| Difficulty concentrating | Supersensitive (subjective) | |

**Nutritional Status**

| | | |
|---|---|---|
| Appetite | Bulimic behavior | Weight (anorectic, obese) |

**Sleep–Rest Pattern**

| | | |
|---|---|---|
| Afraid of dark | Easily awakened | Difficulty falling asleep |
| Sleeps too much | Difficulty staying asleep | Nightmares |

## Physical Manifestations

| | | |
|---|---|---|
| Tremors | Heart palpitations | Agitation |
| Tightness of chest | Hyperalertness | Buzzing in head |
| Shortness of breath | Fists clench | Perspiration |
| Aches and pains: stomach, head, muscles | Change in facial color | |

## Evidence of Self-Harm

*Be highly suspicious if:*

There have been repeated accidents · Client wears long sleeves in hot weather
Client is reluctant to uncover parts of body

*Look for:*

| | | | |
|---|---|---|---|
| Scars | Lumps/bumps | Open cuts | Reddened, irritated areas |
| Sores | Burn marks | Areas that do not heal as expected | Clumps/patches of missing hair |

*Body parts often affected:*

Wrists, arms, legs, feet · Head, face, eyes, neck · Chest, abdomen · Genitals

*Behaviors of self-mutilation:*

| | | | |
|---|---|---|---|
| Cutting | Picking | Slashing | Gouging |
| Stabbing | Head smashing | Scratching | Hitting (e.g., fists against walls) |

Burning (cigarettes, lighters, matches, stove, clothes iron, curling iron)
Use of corrosives (e.g., drain cleaner)

*Behaviors of self-abuse:*

| | | | |
|---|---|---|---|
| Head banging | Slapping | Picking | Scratching |

Nonlethal use of drugs/poison
Anorectic/bulimic behaviors
Swallowing foreign objects (glass, needles, safety pins, straight pins, various hardware [e.g., nails, screws])
Hair pulling
Excessive rubbing
Noncompliance with treatment for serious physical or medical conditions (e.g., diabetes)
For more information on Focus Assessment Criteria, visit http://thepoint.lww.com.

**NOC**
Aggression Self-Control, Impulse Self-Control

## ➤ Goal

The client will choose alternatives that are not harmful.

### *Indicators:*

- Acknowledge self-harm thoughts.
- Admit to use of self-harm behavior if it occurs.
- Be able to identify personal triggers.
- Learn to identify and tolerate uncomfortable feelings.

**NIC**
Presence, Anger Control, Environmental Management: Violence Prevention, Behavior Modification, Security Enhancement, Therapy Group, Coping Enhancement, Impulse Control Training, Crisis Intervention

## ➤ General Interventions

### Establish a Trusting Nurse–Client Relationship

Demonstrate acceptance of the client as a worthwhile person through nonjudgmental statements and behavior.
Ask questions in a caring, concerned manner.
Encourage expression of thoughts and feelings.
Actively listen or provide support by just being there if the client is silent.
Be aware of the client's supersensitivity.
Label the behavior, not the client.
Be honest in your interactions.
Assist the client in recognizing hope and alternatives.
Provide reasons for necessary procedures or interventions.

Maintain the client's dignity throughout your therapeutic relationship.

**R:** Frequent contact by the caregiver indicates acceptance and may facilitate trust. The client may be hesitant to approach the staff because of negative self-concept; the nurse must reach out.

## Validate Reality

### Schizophrenia or Drug-Induced Psychosis

Tell the client, "You are safe."

Use a quiet, calming voice.

Use "talk downs" when the client has taken a hallucinogenic drug. If agitation increases, stop immediately.

Orient the client as required. Point out sensory/environmental misperceptions without belittling his or her fears or indicating disapproval of verbal expressions.

Reassure the client that this will pass.

Watch for signs of increased delusional thinking and/or frightening hallucinations (increased anxiety, agitation, irritability, pacing, hypervigilance).

### Post-Trauma or Dysfunctional

Tell the client, "You are not bad, crazy, or hopeless."

Say you believe the client when he or she tells you personal history; many grew up in denial or minimization.

Let the client know he or she is not the only one.

**R:** The client is acceptable as a person; the behavior is not acceptable.

## Help Reframe Old Thinking/Feeling Patterns (Carscadden, 1993a)

Encourage the belief that change is possible.

Assist the client to identify thought–feeling–behavior concept.

Help the client assess payoffs and drawbacks to self-harm.

Rename words that have a negative connotation (e.g., "setback," not "failure").

Encourage identification of personal triggers.

Assist the client in exploring viable alternatives.

Help the client to examine feelings of ambivalence about recovery.

Encourage the client to become comfortable with and to use feelings.

**R:** Expressing feelings and perception increases the client's self-awareness and helps the nurse plan effective interventions to address his or her needs. Validating the client's perceptions provides reassurance and can decrease anxiety.

## Facilitate the Development of New Behavior

Validate good coping skills already in existence.

Serve as a role model in your own behavior and interactions.

Encourage the use of positive affirmations, meditation and relaxation techniques, and other esteem-building exercises.

Promote the concept of being helpful instead of helpless.

Encourage journaling: keeping a diary of triggers, thoughts, feelings, and alternatives that work or do not work.

Assist the client to develop body awareness as a method of ascertaining triggers and determining levels of impending self-harm.

Assist with role playing to work on situations/relationships.

Promote the development of healthy self-boundaries for the client.

**R:** Expressing feelings and perception increases the client's self-awareness and helps the nurse plan effective interventions to address his or her needs. Validating the client's perceptions provides reassurance and can decrease anxiety.

## Endorse an Environment that Demotes Self-Harm

How much control or influence a professional exerts in this area will depend on the diagnosis, the environmental setting, and the policies of that setting (e.g., a client's home, residential setting, treatment facility, or institution). If mandated by the setting's policies to intervene in self-harm attempts, the following interventions should take place.

### Structure the Client's Time and Activities

Provide a scheduled day that meets the client's need for activity and rest.
Encourage activities with others without competitiveness.
Relieve pent-up tension and purposeless hyperactivity with physical activity (e.g., brisk walk, dance therapy, aerobics).

**R:** It is important not to reward the act of self-harm with reinforcements (negative or positive). Treatment of the injury should be done matter-of-factly, much like removing a splinter, but also provide the client with dignity. Returning to activities/schedules as quickly as possible restores responsibility to the client.

### Reduce Excessive Stimuli

Provide a quiet, serene atmosphere.
Establish firm, consistent limits while giving the client as much control/choice as possible within those boundaries.
Intervene at the earliest stages to assist the client in regaining control, prevent escalation, and allow treatment in the least restrictive manner.
Keep communication simple. Agitated people cannot process complicated communication.
Provide an area where the client can retreat to decrease stimuli (e.g., time-out room, quiet room; clients on hallucinogens need a darkened, quiet room with a nonintrusive observer).
Remove potentially dangerous objects from the environment (if the client is in crisis stage).

**R:** A quiet environment reduces reactivity, enhances calm feelings, and decreases the likelihood of confusion and fear.

### Promote the Use of Alternatives

Stress that there are always alternatives.
Stress that self-harm is a choice, not something uncontrollable.
Allow opportunities for verbal expression of thoughts and feelings (e.g., anger, depression).
Provide acceptable physical outlets (e.g., yelling, pounding pillow, tearing up newspapers, using clay or Play-Doh, taking a brisk walk).
Provide for less physical alternatives (e.g., relaxation tapes, soft music, warm bath, diversional activities).

**R:** Self-destructive behavior can be the result of anger or sadness turned inward.

### Determine Present Level of Impending Self-Harm, If Indicated

**Beginning Stage (Thought Stage)**
Provide soothing touch if permitted by the client (predetermined).
Remind the client that this is an "old tape" and to replace it with new thinking and belief patterns.
Provide nonintrusive, calming alternatives.

**Climbing Stage (Feeling Stage)**
Remind the client to consider alternatives.
Give as much control to the client as possible to support his or her accountability.
Are you in control?     How can I help?     Would you like me to assist?
Provide more intense interventions at this stage.
Encourage the client to turn over any potential items of self-harm.

**Crisis Stage (Behavior Stage)**
Give positive feedback if the client chooses an alternative and does not harm himself or herself.
Ask the client to put down any object of harm if he or she possesses one.
Continue to emphasize there are always alternatives.

Restrain the client only if he or she becomes out of control.

Release the client from restraints as soon as possible to give responsibility back to him or her. "Are you in control now?" "Are you feeling safe?"

Remain calm and caring throughout the crisis period.

Attend to practical issues in a nonpunitive, nonjudgmental manner.

**R:** Control of environment is a basic, but not to be discounted, intervention. A structured schedule provides boundaries and security, enhancing the sense of safety. A quiet environment reduces reactivity, enhances calm feelings, and decreases the likelihood of confusion and fear. Gross motor activity in a protected environment can lessen aggressive drives, whereas rest periods promote opportunities for relaxation, calm the emergency response, and reconnect body/mind/heart.

### Postcrisis Stage

Give positive reinforcements if the client did not harm himself or herself.

Assist the client in problem-solving on how to divert himself before the crisis stage.

Assess the degree of injury/harm if the client did not choose the alternative.

Provide assistance or medical care, as necessary.

Pay as little attention as possible to the act of self-harm and focus on prior stages (e.g., "Can you remember what triggered you?" "What kinds of things were going through your mind?" "What do you think you might have done instead?").

Return the client to normal activities/routine as soon as possible.

**R:** Maladaptive behaviors can be replaced with healthy ones to manage stress and anxiety (Stuart & Sundeen, 2006).

## Initiate Support Systems to Community, When/Where Indicated

### Teach Family

Constructive expression of feelings

How to recognize levels of impending self-harm

How to assist with appropriate interventions

How to deal with self-harm behavior/results

### Supply Phone Number of 24-h Emergency Hotlines

Provide referral to:

| | | |
|---|---|---|
| Individual therapist | Family counseling | Peer support group |
| Leisure/vocational counseling | Halfway houses | Other community resources |

**R:** Many mental health conditions are chronic and require ongoing access to resources for family and client.

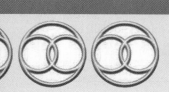

# RISK FOR SELF-ABUSE

## DEFINITION

State in which a person is at risk to perform a deliberate act on the self, without the intent to kill, that may or may not cause harm to the body

## DEFINING CHARACTERISTICS

### Major (Must Be Present, One or More)

Expresses a desire or intent to harm self

Evidence of self-abuse, including:

- Head banging
- Slapping
- Picking
- Scratching
- Nonlethal use of drugs/poison
- Anorectic/bulimic behaviors
- Swallowing foreign objects, (glass, needles, safety pins, straight pins, various hardware [eg, nails, screws])

## RELATED FACTORS

See *Risk for Self-Harm*.

■■■■■■ **AUTHOR'S NOTE**

See *Risk for Self-Harm*.

■■■■■■ **ERRORS IN DIAGNOSTIC STATEMENTS**

See *Risk for Self-Harm*.

■■■■■■ **KEY CONCEPTS**

See *Risk for Self-Harm*.

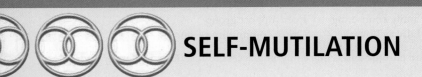

# SELF-MUTILATION

## DEFINITION

State in which a client has performed a deliberate act on the self with the intent to injure, not kill, that produces immediate tissue damage

## DEFINING CHARACTERISTICS

Expresses desire or intent to harm self
Past history of attempts to harm self, including:

| Cutting | Scratching | Slashing |
| Picking | Stabbing | Gouging |

## RELATED FACTORS

See *Risk for Self-Harm*.

■■■■■ **AUTHOR'S NOTE**

See *Risk for Self-Harm*.

■■■■■■ **ERRORS IN DIAGNOSTIC STATEMENTS**
See *Risk for Self-Harm.*

■■■■■■ **KEY CONCEPTS**
See *Risk for Self-Harm.*

## Focus Assessment

See *Risk for Self-Harm.*

## General Interventions

See *Risk for Self-Harm.*

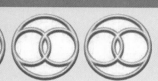

# RISK FOR SELF-MUTILATION

## DEFINITION

State in which a client is at risk to perform a deliberate act on the self with the intent to injure, not kill, that produces immediate tissue damage

## RELATED FACTORS (VARCAROLIS, 2006)

### Pathophysiologic

Related to biochemical/neurophysiologic imbalance secondary to:
Bipolar disorder     Autism     Mentally impaired

### Personal

Related to history of self-injury
Related to history of physical, emotional, or sexual abuse
Related to ineffective coping skills
Related to inability to verbally express feelings

### Maturational

Children/Adolescents
Related to abuse

■■■■■■ **AUTHOR'S NOTE**
See *Risk for Self-Harm.*

■■■■■■ **ERRORS IN DIAGNOSTIC STATEMENTS**
See *Risk for Self-Harm.*

## ■ ■ ■ ■ ■ ■ KEY CONCEPTS

See *Risk for Self-Harm.*

**NOC**

Impulse-Self Control, Self-Mutilation Restraint

### ➤ Goal

The client will identify persons to contact if thoughts of self-harm occur.

### *Indicators*

*Long term (Varcarolis, 2006):*
- State the desire to not harm self.
- Name at least one acceptable alternative to the client's situation.
- Identify at least one goal for the future.

*Short term:*
Make a no-harm contract for the next 24 h and renew it each a day
- Verbalize feelings of anger, loneliness, and hopelessness.
- Identify alternative coping mechanisms.

**NIC**

Active Listening, Coping Enhancement, Impulse Control Training, Behavior Management: Self-Harm, Hope Instillation, Contracting, Surveillance: Safety

### ➤ General Interventions (Varcarolis, 2006)

#### Assess for a History of Self-Mutilation

- Onset, characteristics
- Frequency
- Preceding events

**R:** Interventions can be planned depending upon the assessment data.

#### Explore for Feeling Before the Act of Mutilation and What They Mean (e.g., Gain Control over Others, Attention, Method to Feel Alive, Expression of Guilt or Self-Hate)

**R:** Exploring feeling can help the client gain insight into self-mutilation.

### Establish a Written No Harm Contract with Specific Steps to Initiate When Feeling of Self-Mutilation Occur and Identify Persons to Contact

**R:** Contracts encourage responsibility for healthier behavior and convey confidence in the client.

### Respond to Self-Mutilation Episodes Matter-of-Factly

**R:** A neutral approach decreases blaming and discourages special attention for the episode.

### Provide Treatment for Injuries and What Provoked the Act

**R:** This discussion helps to identify triggers.

### Collaborate on Alternative Behaviors to Self-Mutilation

Avoidance of certain activities that trigger behavior
Discussion of intense feelings with designated person before self-mutilation

**R:** Alternative behaviors provide opportunities to deal with feeling constructively.

### Clearly Establish Limits on Behavior

**R:** "Consistency can establish a sense of security" (Varcarlosis, 2006, p. 262).

### Initiate Referrals as Needed

Connect with community resources (therapist, support groups).

**R:** Therapy will need to be continued with the frequency changing with progress or relapse.

# RISK FOR SUICIDE

## DEFINITION

State in which a client is at risk for killing himself or herself

## DEFINING CHARACTERISTICS

### Major (Must Be Present)

Suicidal behavior (ideation, talk, plan, available means)
Previous suicidal attempts
Suicidal cues (Varcarolis, 2006, p. 483)
Overt ("No one will miss me"," I am better off dead", "I have nothing to live for")
Covert (making out a will, giving valuables away, writing forlorn love notes, acquiring life insurance)

### Minor

Statements of despair, hopelessness, and helplessness

## RELATED FACTORS

See *Risk for Self-Harm.*

## ▣▣▣▣▣ KEY CONCEPTS

See *Risk for Self-Harm.*

## Focus Assessment Criteria

Refer to *Risk for Self-Harm*

**NOC**
Impulse-Self Control,
Suicide Self-Restraint

➤ ## Goal

The client will identify persons to contact if suicidal thoughts occur, and he or she will not commit suicide.

### Indicators

*Long term (Varcarolis, 2006):*
• State the desire to live.
• Name at least one acceptable alternative to his or her situation.
• Identify at least one goal for the future.

*Short term:*
Make a no-suicide contract for the next 24 h and renew it each a day
• Verbalize feelings of anger, loneliness, and hopelessness.
• Identify alternative coping mechanisms.

**NIC**
Active Listening,
Coping
Enhancement,
Suicide Prevention,
Impulse Control
Training, Behavior
Management:
Self-Harm, Hope
Instillation,
Contracting,
Surveillance: Safety

# ➤ General Interventions

## Assist the Client in Reducing His or Her Present Risk for Self-Destruction

### Assess Level of Present Risk (Table II.14):

High          Moderate          Low

### Assess Level of Long-Term Risk:

Lifestyle          Lethality of plan          Usual coping mechanisms
Support available

## Provide a Safe Environment Based on Level of Risk; Notify All Staff that the Client Is at Risk for Self-Harm; Use Both Written and Oral Communication (Varcarolis, 2006)

### Initiate Suicide Precaution for Immediate Management for the High-Risk Client

When the client is being constantly observed, he or she is not to be allowed out of sight, even though privacy is lost. Arm's length is the most appropriate space for a high-risk client.

## TABLE II.14 ASSESSING THE DEGREE OF SUICIDAL RISK

| Behavior or Symptom | Intensity of Risk | | |
|---|---|---|---|
| | Low | Moderate | High |
| Anxiety | Mild | Moderate | High, or panic state |
| Depression | Mild | Moderate | Severe or a sudden change to a happy or peaceful state** |
| Isolation/withdrawal | Some feelings of isolation, no withdrawal | Some feelings of hopelessness, and withdrawal | Hopeless, withdrawn, and self-deprecating, isolation |
| Daily functioning | Effective<br>Good grades in school*<br>Close friends<br>No prior suicide attempt<br>Stable job | Moody<br>Some friends<br>Prior suicidal thoughts | Depressed<br>Poor grades*<br>Few or no close friends<br>Prior suicide attempts<br>Erratic or poor work history |
| Lifestyle | Stable | Moderately stable | Unstable |
| Alcohol/drug use | Infrequently to excess | Frequently to excess | Continual abuse |
| Previous suicide attempts | None or of low lethality (few pills) | One or more (pills, superficial wrist slash) | One or more (entire bottle of pills, gun, hanging) |
| Associated events | None, or an argument | Disciplinary action*<br>Failing grades*<br>Work problems<br>Family illness | Relationship breakup<br>Death of a loved one<br>Loss of job<br>Pregnancy* |
| Purpose of act | None, or not clear | Relief of shame or guilt<br>To punish others<br>To get attention | Wants to die<br>Escape to join deceased<br>Debilitating disease |
| Family's reaction and structure | Supportive<br>Intact family<br>Good coping and mental health<br>No history of suicide | Mixed reaction<br>Divorced/separated<br>Usually copes and understands | Angry and unsupportive<br>Disorganized<br>Rigid/abusive<br>Prior history of suicide in family |
| Suicide plan (method, location, time) | No plan | Frequent thoughts, occasional ideas about a plan | Specific plan |

*Applies only to children and adolescents.
**Added by this author.
Adapted from Hatton, C. L. & McBride, S. (1984). Suicide: Assessment and intervention. Norwalk, CT: Appleton-Century-Crofts; and Jackson, D. B. & Saunders, R. B. (1993). Child health nursing. Philadelphia: J. B. Lippincott.

### Initiate Suicide Observation for Risk Persons

Provide 15 minute visual check of mood, behaviors, and verbatim statements.

**R:** The level of protection of the client will be determined by his or her risk for suicide.

### Ensure the Following:

Restrict glass, nail files, scissors, nail polish remover, mirrors, needles, razors, soda cans, plastic bags, lighters, electric equipment, belts, hangers, knives, tweezers, alcohol, and guns.

Provide meals in a closely supervised area, usually on the unit or in client's room:

- Ensure adequate food and fluid intake.
- Use paper/plastic plates and utensils.
- Check to be sure all items are returned on the tray.

When administering oral medications, check to ensure that all medications are swallowed.

Designate a staff member to provide checks on the client as designated by the institution's policy. Provide relief for the staff member.

Restrict the client to the unit unless specifically ordered by physician. When the client is off unit, provide a staff member to accompany him or her.

Instruct visitors on restricted items (e.g., ensure they do not give the client food in a plastic bag).

The client may use restricted items in the presence of staff, depending on level of risk. Acutely suicidal people Provide a hospital gown to deter the client from leaving the facility. As risk decreases, the client may be allowed own clothing.

Conduct room searches periodically according to institution policy.

Use seclusion and restraint if necessary (refer to *Risk for Violence* for discussion).

Notify the police if the client leaves the facility and is at risk for suicide.

Keep accurate and thorough records of the client's behaviors and all nursing assessments and interventions.

**R:** High-risk suicidal persons should be admitted to a closely supervised environment and should not be allowed access to certain items.

**R:** Although it is impossible to create a completely safe environment, removal of dangerous objects and close observation convey a nonverbal message of concern.

## Emphasize the Following (Varcarolis, 2006, p. 484)

The crisis is temporary.
Unbearable pain can be survived.
Help is available.
You are not alone.

**R:** "These statements give perspective to the person and help offer hope for the future" (Varcarolis, 2006, p. 484).

### Observe for a Sudden Change in Emotions from Sad, Depressed to Elated, Happy, or Peaceful

**R:** A sudden change in emotions can indicate the risk of suicide is very high as the client seeks a way to lose the emotional pain.

### Help Build Self-Esteem and Discourage Isolating Behaviors

Be nonjudgmental and empathic.
Be aware of own reactions to the situation.
Provide genuine praise.
Encourage interactions with others.
Divert attention to the external world (e.g., odd jobs).
Convey a sense that the client is not alone (use group or peer therapy).
Seek out the client for interactions.
Set limits by informing the client of the rules.

Use a firm, consistent approach.

Provide planned daily schedules for people with low impulse control.

**R:** Suicidal individuals are usually ambivalent about the decision. Staff can work with the positive goals to effect a change in attitude and to promote socialization.

### Assist the Client to Identify and Contact Support System

Inform family and significant others.

Enlist support.

Do not provide false reassurance that behavior will not recur.

Point out vague or unclear messages from the client or support system.

Encourage an increase in social activity.

**R:** Caregivers can become immobilized or drained by the acutely suicidal client. Feelings of hopelessness are often communicated to the caregiver.

### Assist the Client in Developing Positive Coping Mechanisms

Encourage appropriate expression of anger and hostility.

Set limits on ruminations about suicide or previous attempts.

Assist the client in recognizing predisposing factors: "What was happening before you started having these thoughts?"

Facilitate examination of life stresses and past coping mechanisms.

Explore alternative behaviors.

Anticipate future stresses and assist in planning alternatives.

Use appropriate behavior modification techniques for noncompliant, resistive people.

Help the client to identify negative thinking patterns and direct the client to practice altering them.

Involve the client in planning the treatment goals and evaluating progress.

Refer to *Anxiety*, *Ineffective Coping*, and *Hopelessness* for further interventions.

**R:** The client's participation in their plan of care can increase their sense of responsibility and control (Schulz & Videbeck, 2002).

### Initiate Health Teaching and Referrals, When Indicated

Provide teaching that prepares the client to deal with life stresses (relaxation, problem-solving skills, how to express feelings constructively).

Refer for peer or group therapy.

Refer for family therapy, especially when a child or adolescent is involved.

Teach the family limit-setting techniques.

Teach the family constructive expression of feelings.

Instruct significant others in how to recognize an increase in risk: change in behavior, verbal or nonverbal communication, withdrawal, or signs of depression.

Supply the phone number of 24-h emergency hotline.

Refer to vocational training if appropriate.

Refer to halfway house or other agencies, as appropriate.

Refer for ongoing psychiatric follow-up.

Refer to senior citizen centers or other agencies to increase leisure activities.

Initiate referral for family intervention after a completed suicide.

**R:** Interventions are based on the type of risk the client presents. Long-term treatment is often more difficult to institute than emergency care in some communities.

**Pediatric Interventions**

Take all suicide threats seriously. Listen carefully.

**R:** All threats or gestures to hurt oneself must be taken seriously regardless of the child's developmental age. Suicide attempts or threats may not represent a true desire to die, but they definitely represent a cry for help.

*(continued)*

**Pediatric Interventions**
*Continued*

Determine whether the child understands the finality of death (e.g., "What does it mean to die?" "Have you ever seen a dead animal on the road? Can it get up and run?").
Engage parents, friends, school personnel, and the client in behavior contracts to "keep safe."

**R:** Parents, friends, and school personnel should be enlisted to help.

Explore feelings and reason for suicidal feelings.

**R:** Suicidal threats and ideation signal a crisis that requires specific care.

Consult with a psychiatric expert regarding the most appropriate environment for treatment.

**R:** Treatment strategies depend on the child's living situation, psychiatric history, and support system available.

Participate in programs in school to teach about the symptoms of depression and signs of suicidal behavior.

**R:** Children who attempt suicide may have marked depression (Varcarolis, 2006).

With adolescents, explore (Mohr, 2007; Hockenberry et al., 2009):
Family problems
Mental status
Strength of support systems
Disruption of friendship or romantic relationship
Seriousness of the attempt
Presence of performance failure (e.g., examination, course)
Recent or upcoming change (change of school, relocation)
Sexual orientation
Convey empathy regarding problems and/or losses.
Be alert for symptoms of a masked depression (e.g., boredom, restlessness, irritability, difficulty concentrating, somatic preoccupation, excessive dependence on or isolation from others, especially adults; Mohr, 2007).

**R:** Certain stressors are especially significant for adolescents, who are developmentally preoccupied with status, peers, and appearances (Varcarolis, 2006).

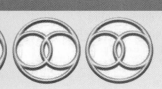

# INEFFECTIVE SELF-HEALTH MANAGEMENT

## DEFINITION

Pattern in which a person experiences or is at risk to experience difficulty integrating into daily living a program for treatment of illness that meets specific health goals.

## DEFINING CHARACTERISTICS

### Major (Must Be Present, One or More)

Verbalized desire to manage the treatment of illness and prevention of complications
Verbalized difficulty with one or more prescribed regimens for treatment of illness and its effects or prevention of complications

## Minor (May Be Present)

Acceleration (expected or unexpected) of illness symptoms
Verbalized to include treatment regimens in daily routines
Verbalized to reduce risk factors for progression of illness and sequelae

# RELATED FACTORS

## Treatment-Related

*Related to:*

| | | |
|---|---|---|
| Complexity of therapeutic regimen | Complexity of health care system | Financial cost of regimen<br>Side effects of therapy |

## Situational (Personal, Environmental)

*Related to:*

| | | |
|---|---|---|
| Previous unsuccessful experiences | Mistrust of health care personnel | Health belief conflicts |
| Questions seriousness of problem | Insufficient knowledge | Questions susceptibility<br>Mistrust of regimen |
| Questions benefits of regimen | | Insufficient confidence |
| | | Decisional conflicts |

Related to insufficient,or unavailable family support.

*Related to barriers to comprehension secondary to:*

Cognitive deficits   Fatigue   Hearing impairments
Motivation  Anxiety  Memory problems

■■■■■■ **AUTHOR'S NOTE**

*Ineffective Self-Help Management* is a very useful diagnosis for nurses in most settings. Individuals and families experiencing various health problems, acute or chronic, usually face treatment programs that require changes in previous functioning or lifestyle. These changes or adaptations can be instrumental in influencing positive outcomes.

This diagnosis describes individuals or families experiencing difficulty achieving positive outcomes. The nurse is the primary professional who, with the client, determines available choices and how to achieve success. The primary nursing interventions are exploring the options available and teaching the client how to implement a treatment plan

When a person faces a complex regimen or has compromised functioning that impedes successful management, the diagnosis *Risk for Ineffective Self-Health Management* would be appropriate. In addition to teaching how to manage the regimen, the nurse also must assist the client to identify the adjustments needed because of a functional deficit.

*Ineffective Self-Health Management* focuses on assisting the person and family to manage the illness and to prevention complications at home. A new Nursing Diagnosis, Risk–Prone Health Behavior, approved in 2006, is different. This diagnosis focuses on habits or lifestyles which are unhealthy and can aggravate an existing condition or contribute to developing a disorder.

■■■■■■ **ERRORS IN DIAGNOSTIC STATEMENTS**

1. *Ineffective Self-Health Management related to a decision not to follow low-salt diet*

    When client makes a decision not to adhere to a therapeutic regimen, the nurse must explore with the client the circumstances surrounding this decision. The diagnosis *Ineffective Self-Health Management related to unknown etiology as evident by not adhering to low-salt diet* is useful. The nurse must collect more data to determine if the client wants to adhere to the diet, or if the client understands the rationale for it. Did the client desire to adhere to the diet but encounter difficulty? Did the client adhere to the diet but experience no positive effects? Nursing intervention strategies would differ with each contributing factor. The following nursing diagnosis is an example of a client who desires to comply but is having difficulty: *Ineffective Self-Health Management related to unplanned meals associated with frequent air travel schedule.*

■■■■■ **KEY CONCEPTS**

## Generic Considerations

- The Stages of Change Model (Transtheoretical Model of Change) can provide interventions to assist people with lifestyle modifications for disease prevention and management. The five stages are *precontemplation*, *contemplation*, *action*, *maintenance*, and *relapse*. People in the precontemplation stage are not considering change because of denial or past failures. People in the contemplation stage are ambivalent about change. Once they decide to make a specific change, they reach the preparation, action, and maintenance stages. The relapse stage is expected (Zimmerman et al., 2000).

- Self-efficacy is a theory that describes a person's evaluation of his or her capacity to manage or to change behaviors to manage stressful situations. Successful management depends on the person believing that the behavior change will improve the situation (outcome expectancy) and that he or she can make the behavior change (self-efficacy expectancy; Bandura, 1982).

- Health education is the teaching–learning process of influencing client and family behavior through changes in knowledge, attitudes, and beliefs and by acquiring psychomotor skills. The goal of client teaching is to help the client assume responsibility for self-care.

- Physical factors that affect learning or the learner include the following (Redman & Thomas, 1996):
    Acute illness
    Fluid and electrolyte imbalance
    Nutritional status
    Illness or treatments that interfere with mental alertness (pain, medications)
    Illness or treatments that interfere with motor abilities (fatigue, equipment)
    Activity tolerance (endurance)

- Personal factors that affect learning or the learner include the following:
    Age Past experiences or knowledge

| | |
|---|---|
| Intelligence | Locus of control |
| Reading ability | Perceived seriousness of condition |
| Level of motivation | Level of anxiety |
| Denial of disease process | Perceived susceptibility to complications |
| Prognosis | Depression |
| Stage of adaptation to illness | Ability to control progression or to cure condition |

- Socioeconomic factors that affect learning include the following:

| | |
|---|---|
| Language | Cultural background |
| Lifestyle | Transportation |
| Support system | Health care facility |
| Financial status | Drugstore |
| Past health care experiences | |

- Factors resulting in ineffective teaching include the following (Redman & Thomas, 1996):
    - Inadequate or no assessment before teaching
    - Assessment data not communicated or not considered when teaching (the most influential assessment factors are psychological status, physical stability, educational level, cultural background, socioeconomic status)
    - Teaching not individualized
    - Information not presented at a level consistent with the client's ability
    - Tendency to talk down to client
    - Use of misunderstood terms
    - Fragmented presentation of information
    - Too much information given, with important information hidden or lost among irrelevant information
    - No repetition of information
    - No feedback given in relation to process (or client is punished for not learning)
    - No evaluation made of client learning

## Geriatric Considerations

- The ability to manage one's therapeutic regimen profoundly influences self-esteem and independence. Using education to increase the self-care capacity of older adults can be an effective way to meet their self-esteem needs (Rakel, 1991; Miller, 2009).
- It is a myth that older adults cannot learn new concepts and skills. Some changes during aging may deter learning, such as decreased visual acuity, decreased hearing, slowing of information processing, decreased attention span, difficulty in unlearning habits, fear of uncertainty or failure, decreased problem solving, and the need for a longer time and more repetition to retain learning (Rakel, 1991; Miller, 2009).

## Transcultural Considerations

- Because the dominant US culture is future oriented, it values a lifestyle that promotes health and prevents disease. This value is challenged when a client or family of another culture is oriented to the present (Andrews & Boyle, 2008).
- Clients with an external locus of control believe that outside factors or forces determine health. This belief challenges the entire concept of health promotion (Andrews & Boyle, 2008).
- Folk remedies are treatments or practices that cultural groups use to stay healthy or to treat illnesses. Spector (1985) questioned students of various cultures to determine health and illness behaviors. Box II.3 illustrates some of her findings.
- Folk remedies are used to treat many illnesses, such as headaches, colds, rashes, coughs, sore throats, constipation, fever, warts, and menstrual cramps. Examples of folk remedies for headaches include lying down and resting in complete darkness (Canadian); boiling a beef bone, breaking up toast in the broth, and drinking (German); applying a cold or hot face cloth to the forehead and resting (Irish); putting a kerchief with ice around the head (Italian); and taking aspirin and hot liquids (Spector, 1985).
- Some folk remedies may be misdiagnosed as abuse. Three folk practices of Southeast Asians leave marks on the body that providers may interpret as signs of violence or abuse. *Cao gio* is rubbing the skin with a coin to produce dark blood or ecchymotic strips; it is done to treat colds and flu-like symptoms. *Bat gio* is skin pinching on the temples to treat headaches or on the neck for sore throat; if petechiae or ecchymoses appear, the treatment is a success. *Poua* is burning the skin with the tip of a dried, weed like grass; it is believed the burning will cause the noxious element that causes the pain to exude (Andrews & Boyle, 2008).

## Focus Assessment Criteria

### Subjective Data

#### *Assess for Defining Characteristics*

**Determine Present Knowledge of**
Illness
Severity     Susceptibility to complications          Prognosis
Ability to cure it or control progression
Treatment/diagnostic studies
Preventive measures

**Does Anything Interfere with Adherence to the Prescribed Health Behavior?**
Learning needs (perceived by client, family)

#### *Assess for Related Factors*

**History of Disease**
Onset
Effects on lifestyle (relationships, work, leisure, finances)
Symptoms

---

### BOX II.3  FOLK REMEDIES TO MAINTAIN HEALTH

Wine: It

Eat wholesome, balanced foods: It, P, S, A, BA, EB, FC, G, I, IC

Dress right for weather: BA, NA, EB, FC, FCC, G, IC

Cleanliness: BA, CC, EC, G, I, IC, N

Daily walks: EB, EC, S

Pray daily: BA, CC

Read: EB

Take baths: EC

Open bedroom windows at night: EC

Enough sleep: FCC, IC

Cod liver oil daily: FC, N, P, S

Exercise: FCC, IC, It

Take aspirin: G

Wear holy medals: IC

Brush teeth: I

Early to bed: It

Hard bread: It

Routine medical examination: S

Medical care when sick: EE, P

Rest: EC, FC, IC, N, P

Spector, R. E. (1985). *Cultural diversity in health and illness* (2nd ed.). Norwalk, CT: Appleton-Century-Crofts.
Code: A, Asian; BA, black African; CC, Canadian Catholic; EE, Eastern Europe, Jewish; EB, English Baptist; EC, English Catholic; FC, French Catholic; FCC, French Canadian Catholics; G, German Catholics; I, Iran Islam; IC, Irish Catholic; It, Italian; N, Norwegian; P, Polish; S, Swedish; NA, Native American.

---

### Stage of Adaptation to Disease

| | | |
|---|---|---|
| Disbelief | Anger | Denial |
| Awareness | Depression | Acceptance |

### Learning Ability (Client, Family)

| | | |
|---|---|---|
| Level of education | Language spoken | Ability to read |
| Language understood | | |

### Cultural Factors

| | | |
|---|---|---|
| Health care beliefs and practices | Values | Lifestyle |
| Traditions | | |

## Objective Data

### *Assess for Related Factors*

#### Ability to Perform Prescribed Procedures

Competency        Accuracy

#### Level of Cognitive and Psychomotor Development

Age              Ability to read and write

#### Presence of Sensory Deficits

| | | |
|---|---|---|
| Vision | Taste (altered or lost) | Hearing |
| Touch | Smell (altered or lost) | |

**Presence of barriers to care at home**

Cost of care        Complexity of treatments        Unavailable /inadequate assistances

For more information on Focus Assessment Criteria, visit http://thepoint.lww.com.

**NOC**

Compliance
Behavior,
Knowledge:
Treatment Regimen/
Procedure,
Participationin
Health Care
Decisions, Treatment
Behavior: Illness or
Injury

## ➤ Goal

The person/family will relate the intent to implement a treatment plan needed or desired for recovery from illness and prevention of recurrence or complications.

### *Indicators*

- Relate less anxiety regarding home management of the condition.
- Describe disease process, causes of and factors contributing to symptoms.
- Demonstrate or describe the treatment regimen for disease or symptom control.

**NIC**

Teaching: Disease
process, Referral,
Family Support,
Health System
Guidance

## ➤ General Interventions

### Identify Causative or Contributing Factors that Impede Effective Management

Refer to Related Factors.

### Identify and Emphasize Strengths

Past coping successes
Their perception of the problem
Their perception of the care needed
Parent–child relationship
Family caregiving abilities

### Consider Cultural Preferences or Practices

What does family do to maintain health?
What does family do to prevent illness?
What home remedies do you or your family use?

### Promote Confidence and Positive Self-Efficacy (Bandura, 1982)

Explore past successful management of problems.
Emphasize past successful coping.
Tell stories of other "successes."
If appropriate, encourage opportunities to witness others successfully coping in a similar situation.
Encourage participation in self-help groups.

**R:** A major determinant of self-efficacy is past successful coping in a similar situation (Bandura, 1982). In contrast, past unsuccessful management of a similar situation is a deterrent.

### Reduce or Eliminate Barriers to Learning

### *Adapt Teaching to Person's Physical and Psychological Status*

Comfort levels
Fatigue levels
Not concurrent with peaks of medications that alter perception or cognition

**R:** Fatigue and pain can negatively affect learning. Barriers to learning will decrease retention and increase frustration.

### *Allow Person to Work Through and Express Intense Emotions Before Beginning to Teach*

## Examine Person's Health Beliefs and Past Experiences Related to Illness; Assess Their Effects on Desire to Learn.

Delay Teaching Until Person is Ready.

**R:** Client motivation is one of the most important variables affecting how much learning takes place.

## Reduce Anxiety

Encourage verbalization.
Listen attentively.
Meet person's expressed needs before giving other information.
Develop trust with frequent, consistent interactions.
Give correct, relevant information.
Give nonthreatening information before delivering more anxiety-producing information.
Explain reason for and intended effect of treatment; emphasize the positive.
Explore with person the effects of a new diagnosis, treatment, or surgery on significant others.
Do not overwhelm person with too much information if anxiety is high or physical condition is unstable.
Allow person to maintain some control over self and routines by involving him or her in care.

**R:** Learning depends on physical and emotional readiness. The client needs to be relatively free of pain and extreme anxiety. High anxiety decreases learning, whereas slight anxiety may increase learning.

## Initiate Teaching Home Care

Determine if the person in inexperienced in the situation.
When providing care explain to person the procedure.
Emphasize important points (safety, infection prevention).
Allow the person to participate if possible.
Present information at a level consistent with the client's ability.
Adjust the explanation according to person's physical abilty.
Use terminology that is commonly known:

- Avoid too much information at the first session
- Repeat important points of information
- Ask client to share what he or she learned and what additional information is desired
- Write down step by step the procedure and what signs of complications should be reported

**R:** An assessment before and during teaching facilitates the meaningfulness, efficacy, and overall success of the teaching–learning process by defining *what* content should be present, *how* the content should be given, *when* the client is ready to learn, and *who* should be included.

## Ensure Family are Included in Teaching Sessions

Explain and discuss:

- Disease process
- Treatment regimen (medications, diet, procedures, exercises, equipment)
- Rationale for regimen
- Expectations (client, family) of regimen
- Side effects of regimen
- Lifestyle changes needed
- Methods to monitor condition
- Follow-up care needed
- Signs/symptoms of complications
- Resources, support available
- Home environment alterations needed

**R:** Research has shown that, when family members are involved in care, client cooperation and positive adjustment to the experience increase (Leske, 1993).

## Initiate Health Teaching and Referral as Indicated

Consult with discharge planner or social services to determine what resouces are needed at home.
Ensure a home health nurse assessment at discharge
Ensure sufficient supplies at discharge

**R:** Complex treatment plans require careful planning and continued nursing involvement after discharge.

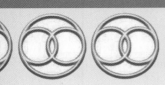

# INEFFECTIVE SEXUALITY PATTERNS

**Ineffective Sexuality Patterns**

Related to Prenatal and Postpartum Changes
Sexual Dysfunction

## DEFINITION

State in which a client expresses concern regarding own sexuality

## DEFINING CHARACTERISTICS

### Major (Must Be Present)

Actual concerns regarding sexual behaviors, sexual health, sexual functioning, or sexual identity.

### Minor (May Be Present)

Expression of concern about sexual behaviors, health, functioning, or sexual identity.
Expression of concern about impact a medical diagnosis or treatment for a medical condition may have on sexual functioning or sexual desirability.

## RELATED FACTORS

Ineffective sexual patterns can occur as a response to various health problems, situations, and conflicts. Some common sources are listed next.

### Pathophysiologic

***Related to biochemical effects on energy and libido secondary to:***
*Endocrine:*
Diabetes mellitus          Hyperthyroidism
Addison's disease          Decreased hormone production
Myxedema                   Acromegaly
*Genitourinary:*
Chronic renal failure
*Neuromuscular and skeletal:*
Arthritis
Amyotrophic lateral sclerosis
Multiple sclerosis
Disturbances of nerve supply to brain, spinal cord, sensory nerves, or autonomic nerves
*Cardiorespiratory:*
Peripheral vascular disorders          Cancer
Myocardial infarction                  Congestive heart failure

Chronic respiratory disorders
***Related to fears associated with (sexually transmitted diseases [STDs]) (specify):***
Human immunodeficiency virus (HIV)/Acquired immunodeficiency syndrome (AIDS)
Human papilloma virus        Herpes        Gonorrhea
Chlamydia        Syphilis
***Related to effects of alcohol on performance***
***Related to decreased vaginal lubrication secondary to (specify)***
***Related to fear of premature ejaculation***
***Related to pain during intercourse***
***Related to fear of pregnancy***
Treatment-Related
***Related to effects of:***
Medications (Table II.15)
Radiation therapy
***Related to altered self-concept from change in appearance (trauma, radical surgery)***

## Situational (Personal, Environmental)

***Related to partner problem (specify):***
Unwilling        Not available        Uninformed
Abusive        Separated, divorced
***Related to no privacy***
***Related to stressors secondary to:***
Job problems        Value conflicts        Financial worries
Relationship conflicts
***Related to misinformation or lack of knowledge***
***Related to fatigue***
***Related to fear of rejection secondary to obesity***
***Related to pain***
***Related to fear of sexual failure***
***Related to fear of pregnancy***
***Related to depression***
***Related to anxiety***
***Related to guilt***
***Related to history of unsatisfactory sexual experiences***

## Maturational

**Adolescent**
***Related to ineffective role models***
***Related to negative sexual teaching***
***Related to absence of sexual teaching***

**Adult**
***Related to adjustment to parenthood***
***Related to effects of menopause on libido and vaginal tissue atrophy***
***Related to values conflict***
***Related to effects of pregnancy on energy levels and body image***
***Related to effects of aging on energy levels and body image***
***Related to unavailable partner***

### ▪▪▪▪▪ AUTHOR'S NOTE

The diagnoses *Ineffective Sexuality Patterns* and *Sexual Dysfunction* are difficult to differentiate. *Ineffective Sexuality Patterns* represents a broad diagnosis, of which sexual dysfunction can be one part. *Sexual Dysfunction* may be used most appropriately by a nurse with advanced preparation in sex therapy. Until *Sexual Dysfunction* is well differentiated from *Ineffective Sexuality Patterns*, most nurses should not use it.

## TABLE II.15  DRUGS THAT AFFECT SEXUALITY

| Drug | Effect on Sexuality |
|---|---|
| Alcohol | In small amounts, may increase libido and decrease sexual inhibitions<br>In large amounts, impairs neural reflexes involved in erection and ejaculation<br>Chronic use causes impotence and sterility in men; decreased desire and orgasmic dysfunction in women |
| Amyl nitrate | Peripheral vasodilator reputed to cause intensified orgasms when inhaled at time of orgasm<br>May cause loss of erection, hypotension, and syncope |
| Antidepressants | Peripheral blockage of nervous innervation to sex organs<br>Significant percentage of impotence and ejaculatory dysfunction in men<br>Decreased libido in both genders |
| Antihistamines | Block parasympathetic innervation of sex organs<br>Sedative effect may decrease desire<br>Decrease in vaginal lubrication |
| Antihypertensives | Libido may be decreased in both genders<br>Some cause impotence and ejaculatory problems in up to 50% of men<br>See specific class of medications. |
| Antispasmodics | Inhibit parasympathetic innervation of sex organs.<br>May cause impotence |
| Chemotherapeutics | Combination therapy may cause azoospermia or oligospermia in men and temporary or permanent menopause in women; fertility may be temporarily or permanently altered; libido may be decreased and body image altered. |
| Cocaine | Short-term use is reported to enhance sexual experience.<br>Chronic use causes loss of desire and sexual dysfunction in both sexes. |
| Hormones | Estrogen suppresses sexual function in men.<br>Testosterone may increase libido in both sexes but causes virilization in women.<br>Chronic use of anabolic steroids causes testicular atrophy, decreased testosterone and decreased sperm production; may cause permanent sterility. |
| Marijuana | May decrease sexual inhibitions.<br>Chronic use may cause decreased libido and impotence. |
| Narcotics | Chronic use causes decreased libido in both sexes.<br>Testosterone levels and amount of semen decreased.<br>Erectile and ejaculatory dysfunction common. |
| Oral contraceptives | Remove fear of pregnancy.<br>May cause decreased libido. |
| Sedatives/ tranquilizers | Initially and in low doses may enhance sexual pleasure due to relaxation and decrease of inhibitions.<br>Long-term use decreases libido and may cause orgasmic dysfunction and impotence. |
| Diuretics | May cause erectile, ejaculatory, and libido problems, especially at higher doses. |
| Anxiolytics | Altered libido in both genders; erectile problems and delayed ejaculation in men. |
| Sildenafil citrate (Viagra) | Enhances erectile ability in men with impaired potency. |

## ERRORS IN DIAGNOSTIC STATEMENTS

1. *Ineffective Sexuality Patterns related to reports of absent libido*
   Report of absent libido represents a symptom of *Ineffective Sexuality Patterns*, not a "related to" statement. If further assessment revealed the client's dissatisfaction with present sexual patterns, the nurse could record the diagnosis *Ineffective Sexuality Patterns related to unknown etiology*, as evidenced by reports of absent libido. The use of "unknown etiology" in this diagnostic statement prompts focus assessments to determine contributing factors (e.g., stress, medication side effects).
2. *Sexual Dysfunction related to impotence secondary to spinal cord injury*
   How would the nurse treat this diagnosis? A nurse planning to explore feelings and to provide information and referrals would not be treating sexual dysfunction. Instead, the nursing focus would be best described in the diagnosis *Anxiety related to effects of spinal cord injury on sexual function and insufficient knowledge of causes and community resources available.*

■■■■■■ **KEY CONCEPTS**

## Generic Considerations

- Sexual health is the integration of somatic, emotional, intellectual, and social aspects of a sexual being in ways that are enriching and that enhance personality, communication, and love.
- Sexual behaviors are the behaviors a client uses to communicate feelings and attitudes about sexuality. They include behaviors used in release of sexual tension, either alone or with another client to attain sexual satisfaction, or for procreation (Wilmoth, 1993).
- All people are sexual beings. Sexuality is an integral part of identity.
- Sexuality encompasses how a client feels about himself or herself and how a client interacts with others.
- Sexual function refers to psychological and physiologic ability to perform in a sexually satisfying manner, with or without a partner, old or young.
- Age, marital and/or relationship status, sexual orientation, personal value system, sexual knowledge, resources (social, economic, geographic), culture, physical health, and emotional health influence sexuality and sexual function (Katzun, 1990; Smith, 1993).
- Research shows that many people with a serious illness experience decreased sexual desire, decreased frequency of sexual activity, and/or decreased satisfaction with sexual function.
- The characteristics of a sexually healthy client are as follows:
  - Positive body image despite the body's packaging
  - Acceptance of sexual and body functions as normal and natural
  - Accurate knowledge about human sexuality and sexual functioning
  - Recognition and acceptance of own sexual feelings
  - Capacity for intimacy in relationships
  - Acceptance of mistakes/imperfections in self and others
  - Prevention of pregnancy when it is not desired
  - Protection of self from STDs
- Sexual expression is not limited to sexual intercourse; it includes closeness and touch, as well as other forms of verbal and nonverbal communication.

## Medications and Sexuality

- Drugs can influence sexual functioning positively and negatively (see Table II.15).
- The client has the right to be educated about all medication side effects, including those affecting sexuality.

## The Nurse's Role in Discussing Sexuality

- The nurse must become educated regarding sexuality and sexual health through the life span. It is important for the nurse to examine his or her own beliefs and feelings concerning sexuality, sexual function, and what is considered sexually normal and abnormal.
- Many nurses have difficulty providing care in the area of sexuality and do not address sexual concerns unless the client asks specific questions. Research indicates, however, that many clients wish nurses and other health care professionals would initiate discussion of sexuality.
- The PLISSIT model (Annon, 1976) is helpful for the nurse generalist providing care in the area of sexuality:
  - **Permission:** Convey to the client and significant other a willingness to discuss sexual thoughts and feelings (e.g., "Some people with your diagnosis have concerns about how it will affect sexual functioning. Is this a concern for you or your partner?").
  - **Limited Information:** Provide the client and significant other with information on the effects certain situations (e.g., pregnancy), conditions (e.g., cancer), and treatments (e.g., medications) can have on sexuality and sexual function.
  - **Specific Suggestions:** Provide specific instructions that can facilitate positive sexual functioning (e.g., changes in coital positions).
  - **Intensive Therapy:** Refer people who need more help to an appropriate health care professional (e.g., sex therapist, surgeon).
- Giving a client "permission" to discuss sexual concerns is by far the most important aspect of nursing care in the area of sexuality. The nurse should give permission by:

*(continued)*

■■■■■ **KEY CONCEPTS** *Continued*

- Including sexuality in the initial health history and addressing questions on sexuality in a manner similar to questions on bowel and bladder function. This helps the client see that nurses view sexuality as a routine part of human health.
- Offering to discuss sexual concerns at appropriate times during the client's hospitalization/visit (Wilmoth, 1994a).
- The nurse should assure the client of the confidentiality of all data on sexuality and obtain permission from the client before making a referral for a sexual problem.

### Contraception and STDs

- Research has shown that the use of mechanical barrier methods (condom, diaphragm, vaginal sponge, cervical cap) and/or chemical barriers containing nonoxynol-9 (foam, jelly, cream) are effective in reducing the transmission of HIV and other STDs.
- Use of the intrauterine device, oral contraceptives, Norplant, Depo-Provera, or sterilization provides *no* protection from STDs. Clients using these methods must be counseled to use a chemical or mechanical barrier method to protect them from disease.

## Pediatric Considerations

- Sex role identification begins in infancy and is determined by adolescence.
  - Infants can identify body parts by the end of the first year.
  - Toddlers learn gender differentiation.
  - Preschoolers frequently engage in masturbation and sex play with peers (e.g., comparing genitals).
  - School-aged children continue to gain awareness about their sex role identity. Although masturbation and sex play are common in the young school-aged child, the older school-aged child becomes involved in purposeful sexual behavior (e.g., hugging, kissing members of the opposite sex (Hockenberry & Wilson, 2009).
  - Adolescents experience altered body image in response to the physical changes of puberty. The key developmental task of adolescence is identity formation, which is influenced by sexual maturation and assuming a sex role (Hockenberry & Wilson, 2009).
- Parents are the primary force in sex education in a child's life. This includes what is not said as well as what is said.
- Formal sex education, presented from a life span approach, is best offered during middle childhood. Topics should include sexual maturation and the process of reproduction.
- STDs continue to be a major cause of morbidity among adolescents and young adults. The highest rates of chlamydial infections in females occur in adolescents (CDC, 2000).
- Risky behavior by adolescents and young adults increases their vulnerability to STDs, pelvic inflammatory disease, infertility, AIDS, and chronic incurable conditions such as hepatitis B or C virus infection, human papilloma virus (HPV) infection, and genital herpes.
- Half of ninth through twelfth graders report having had sexual intercourse (CDC, 2000).
- About 16% of high-school students report having four or more sexual partners (CDC, 2000).
- Only 58% of high-school students reported using a condom. Only 16% reported using birth control (CDC, 2000).

## Maternal Considerations

- Pregnant women have varying degrees of sexual desire during pregnancy.
- Some women are very sexually excitable.
- Some women are not very desirous of sex.
- Libido changes by large degrees during different stages of pregnancy.
- A woman's body image affects her sexuality. (If thinness is an attribute, then many pregnant women are confused about changing size.)
- A woman's attitude toward her body can influence her partner's sexual attraction toward her.
- The postpartum period is a time of self-doubt. For the first 6 weeks, a new mother feels lost, overwhelmed, tired, depressed, ignorant, and isolated. Her self-esteem as well as her sexuality may suffer.

- Polomeno (1999) found the postnatal sexual concerns of men and women (M, men; W, women) to be:
  - Having time for each other (M, W)
  - Sexual intercourse the first time (M, W)
  - Separating oneself from the baby (W)
  - Contraception (M, W)
  - Reactivating the passion, fun, and romance (M, W)
  - To be desired (W)
  - Fatigue and its impact on sexual desire (W)
  - Postpartum depression (M)
  - Balancing intimacy and the baby (W)
  - Time required for healing (W)
  - Fear of pain (M, W)
  - His perception of her and her body (W)

## Geriatric Considerations

- Older adults are psychologically and physically capable of engaging in sexual activity regardless of age-related changes in sexual anatomy and physiology.
- Sexual activity is often beneficial for older adults, reducing anxiety while providing intimacy and improving quality of life.
- Women experience decreased breast tone, thinning and loss of elasticity of the vaginal wall, decreased vaginal lubrication, and shortening of vaginal length from loss of circulating estrogen (Miller, 2009).
- Men experience decreased production of spermatozoa, decreased ejaculatory force, and smaller, less firm testicles. Direct stimulation may be required to achieve an erection; however, the erection may be maintained for a longer time (Miller, 2009).
- The need for intimacy and touch is especially important for older adults, who may be experiencing diminishing meaningful relationships.
- Past sexual function (enjoyment, interest, frequency) serves as a predictor of sexual activity in older adults. To be capable of sexual activity in old age, the client must participate in sexual activity throughout life.
- Adult children and caregivers commonly view sexual activities of older adults as immoral, inappropriate, and negative (Miller, 2009).
- The sexual functioning of older adults is most influenced by myths and misunderstanding. According to Miller (2009), because sex is so closely identified with youthfulness, the stereotype of "sexless seniors" is widely believed.

## Transcultural Considerations

- People of some cultures (e.g., Hispanic, Native American) are very hesitant to discuss sexuality.
- Horn (1993) reports that black women view child-bearing as a validation of their femaleness. White teenage girls approve of prevention of pregnancy; Indian teenage girls value pregnancy (Horn, 1993).
- Some cultures view the postpartum period as a state of impurity. Certain foods and practices are taboo (e.g., intercourse). The woman may be secluded during postpartum bleeding. Some cultures end seclusion with a ritual bath (e.g., Navajo, Hispanic, Orthodox Jewish; Andrews & Boyle, 2008).
- Native American women believe in the importance of monthly menstruation to maintain physical well-being and harmony (Andrews & Boyle, 2008).

# Focus Assessment Criteria

## Guidelines for Taking a Sexual History

Discuss sexuality in a private, relaxed setting to ensure confidentiality.

Do not judge the client by your own beliefs/practices.

Permit the client to refuse to answer.

Clarify your vocabulary; use slang terms if needed to convey meaning.

Assess only those areas pertinent for this client at this time.

Strive to be open, warm, objective, unembarrassed, and reassuring.

Keep in mind that it is more appropriate to assume that the client has had some sexual experience than to assume none.

Several sessions may be necessary to complete the interview.

## Subjective Data

### Determine History

| | |
|---|---|
| Age, sex, marital/relationship status | Communication patterns with significant others |
| Sexual orientation/preference | Quality of relationship with significant other |
| Number of children and siblings | Religious and cultural background |
| Sexual abuse | Job and financial status |
| Depression | Medical and surgical history |
| Medications | Drug and alcohol use (present and past) |

### Assess Concerns and Sexuality Patterns

How has your health problem affected your ability to function as a wife/mother/partner/father/ husband; Wilmoth, 1994a?

How has your health problem affected the way you feel about yourself as a man/woman; Wilmoth, 1994a?

How has your health problem affected your ability to function sexually (Wilmoth, 1994a)?

### Sexual Function

Usual pattern

Present pattern

Satisfaction (client, partner)

Desire (client, partner)

Erection problems for man (attaining, sustaining)

Ejaculation problems for man (premature, retarded, retrograde)

Decreased lubrication for woman

Decreased orgasm for woman

### Sexual Problem

Description

Onset (when, gradual/sudden)

Pattern over time (increased, decreased, unchanged)

Client's concept of cause

Knowledge of problem by others (partner, physician, others)

Expectations

### School-Aged Child

Knowledge:

- "What is the difference between boys and girls?"
- "What do you know about having babies?"
- "Who taught you? At what age?"

Body changes:

- "Is your body changing in any way? How? Why?"
- "How do you feel about these changes?"

Masturbation:

- "Almost everyone touches their body; how do you feel about this?"

### Adolescent

Knowledge and attitudes:

- "What are your parents' attitudes toward sex, nudity, and touching?"
- "How are subjects discussed in your home?"

- "How does pregnancy occur?"
- "What are some methods of birth control?"
- "What do you know about sexually transmitted diseases?"

Body changes:

- "Is your body changing in any way? How? Why?"
- "How do you feel about these changes?"

Sexual activity:

- "Some young people are sexually active and others choose not to be sexually active; what are your beliefs about this?"
- "Are you sexually active? If so, describe the type of birth control and safe sex practices you use."
- "Some teens are attracted to people of their gender; have you experienced these feelings?"(Smith, 1993).

### Senior Citizens

Knowledge:

- "How do you feel when you hear that older adults have little interest in sexuality?"
- "What do you know about sexually transmitted diseases?"

Body changes:

- "How do you feel about the way your body has aged?"
- "What do you do to make yourself feel good about yourself sexually?"

Sexual activity:

- "Do you feel loved, valued by others?"
- "How are your needs for touching and intimacy met?"
- "Have you been able to maintain your sexual activity?"

### Assess for Related Factors

See Related Factors.
For more information on Focus Assessment Criteria, visit http://thepoint.lww.com.

---

**NOC**
Body Image, Self-Esteem, Role Performance, Sexual Identity

## ➤ Goals

The client will resume previous sexual activity or engage in alternative satisfying sexual activity.

### Indicators:

- Identify effects of stressors, loss, or change on sexual functioning.
- Modify behavior to reduce stressors.
- Identify limitations on sexual activity caused by a health problem.
- Identify appropriate modifications in sexual practices in response to these limitations.
- Report satisfying sexual activity.

---

**NIC**
Behavioral Management, Sexual Counseling, Emotional Support, Active Listening, Teaching: Sexuality

## ➤ General Interventions

### Assess for Causative or Contributing Factors (See Related Factors)

### Explore the Client's Patterns of Sexual Functioning

Encourage him or her to share concerns; assume that all clients have had some sexual experience, and convey a willingness to discuss feelings and concerns.

**R:** Many clients are reluctant to discuss sexuality issues. A relaxed approach can encourage the client to share feelings and concerns.

## Discuss the Relationship Between Sexual Functioning and Life Stressors

Clarify the relation between stressors and problem in sexual functioning.

Explore options available for reducing the effects of the stressor on sexual functioning (e.g., increase sleep, increase exercise, modify diet, explore stress reduction methods).

**R:** Explaining that impaired sexual functioning has a physiologic basis can reduce feelings of inadequacy and decreased self-esteem; this actually may help improve sexual function.

## Reaffirm the Need for Frank Discussion Between Sexual Partners

Explain how the client and partner can use role playing to discuss concerns about sex.

**R:** Role playing helps a client gain insight by placing himself or herself in another's position, and allows more spontaneous sharing of fears and concerns.

Reaffirm the need for closeness and expressions of caring through touching, massage, and other means.

Suggest that sexual activity need not always culminate in vaginal intercourse, but that the partner can reach orgasm through noncoital manual or oral stimulation.

**R:** Sexual pleasure and gratification are not limited to intercourse. Other expressions of caring may prove more meaningful.

## With Acute or Chronic Illness

### *Eliminate or Reduce Causative or Contributing Factors, If Possible, and Teach the Importance of Adhering to Medical Regimen Designed to Reduce or Control Disease Symptoms*

### *Provide Limited Information and Specific Suggestions*

Provide appropriate information to client and partner concerning actual limitations on sexual functioning caused by the illness (limited information).

Teach possible modifications in sexual practices to assist in dealing with limitations caused by illness. See Table II.16 for more details.

**R:** Both partners probably have concerns about sexual activity. Repressing these feelings hurts the relationship.

## Facilitate Adaptation to Change in or Loss of Body Part

Assess the stage of adaptation of the client and partner to the loss (denial, depression, anger, resolution; see *Grieving*).

Encourage adherence to the medical regimen to promote maximum recovery.

Encourage the couple to discuss the strengths of their relationship and to assess the influence of the loss on these strengths.

Clarify the relationship between loss or change and the problem in sexual functioning.

**R:** Providing accurate information on the effect of cord injury on sexual functioning can prevent false hope or give real hope, as appropriate.

## Teach Possible Modifications in Sexual Practices to Assist in Dealing with Limitations Caused by Illness (Specific Suggestions)

Refer to Table II.16 for Specific Suggestions

## Provide Referrals as Indicated:

Enterostomal therapist    Physician

Nurse specialist    Sex therapist

**R:** Specialist interventions may be needed.

## TABLE II.16  DISORDERS THAT ALTER SEXUALITY

| Health Problem | Sexual Complication | Nursing Intervention |
|---|---|---|
| Diabetes mellitus | *Men:* Erectile difficulties due to diabetic neuropathies or microangiopathy<br>*Women:* Decreased desire; decreased vaginal lubrication | LI: Encourage proper metabolic control.<br>SS: Eventually may require penile implant; refer to urologist.<br>LI: Encourage proper metabolic control; teach signs and symptoms of vaginitis.<br>SS: Suggest use of water-soluble lubricating jelly. |
| Chronic obstructive pulmonary disease | Activity intolerance due to exertional dyspnea; coughing and expectoration<br><br>Anxiety | LI: Teach controlled breathing; plan intercourse for time of peak effect from medications; avoid sex after large meal or physical exertion, or immediately after awakening; plan for nonhurried, relaxed, low-stress encounters, for losses.<br>SS: Suggest positions that minimize chest pressure (sitting or side-lying); explain that waterbeds also help decrease exertion during sex. |
| Arthritis | Pain, joint stiffness, fatigue<br><br><br><br>Decreased libido from steroid medications | LI: Explain that arthritis has no effect on physiologic aspects of sexual functioning.<br>SS: Suggest that the couple plan intercourse for time of peak medication effects; promote joint relaxation by taking warm bath/shower alone/with partner; perform mild range-of-motion exercises.<br>LI: Teach that decreased desire is a common side effect of medication. |
| Transurethral resection of the prostate (TURP) to treat benign prostatic hypertrophy | Retrograde ejaculation due to damage to internal bladder sphincter | LI: Explain that erection and orgasm will still occur, but ejaculate will be decreased or absent; urine will be cloudy. |
| Cardiovascular disease | Anxiety, fear of performance, fear of chest pain, death, decreased desire, decreased arousal, decision of partner to stop sexual activity | LI: Explain that infarction has no direct effect on physiologic sexual functioning; activity usually is safe 5–8 weeks' postinfarction, based on Index of Sexual Readiness (ability to take brisk walk, climb two flights of stairs without chest pain).<br>Teach to avoid sexual activity after large meal, drinking alcohol, or in room with extremes in temperature. Point out that some medications may cause sexual dysfunction (see Table II-24).<br>SS: Encourage nonsexual touching; suggest positions that conserve energy (side-to-side lying, supine lying position, or sitting in chair with partner on top); explore option of masturbation; assure that oral–genital sex does not place additional strain on heart.<br>Warn to avoid anal sex because anal penetration stimulates vagus nerve and decreases cardiac function. |
| Chronic renal failure (CRF) | Chronic/recurrent uremia can produce state of depression, decreased sexual desire and arousal<br>Untreated CRF causes cessation of ovulation and menses in women and causes atrophy of testicles, decreased spermatogenesis, decreased plasma testosterone, and erectile dysfunction in men. Dialysis may restore ovulation and menses in women and return testosterone levels to normal in men; sexual desire may return to predisease levels with treatment. | LI: Acknowledge that stress of disease and dialysis may cause decreased desire; encourage nonsexual touching without pressure to perform.<br>Reassure that these problems are usually reversible with dialysis. Warn that birth control should be continued because fertility may return. Explain that sexual dysfunction may be a product of emotional stress and the physiologic components of the disease.<br>SS: Explain that measurement of nocturnal penile tumescence can distinguish between organic and psychological causes of sexual dysfunction in men. |
| Total abdominal hysterectomy with bilateral salpingo-oophorectomy | Loss of circulating estrogen<br><br><br><br>Postoperative psychological adjustment or change in sexual identity, grieving, loss of reproductive capacity | LI: Teach signs and symptoms of menopause, use of water-soluble vaginal lubricants.<br>Encourage discussion with physician about estrogen replacement creams. Explain that in most cases intercourse may be resumed after 6-week postoperative visit.<br>Explore the meaning of uterine and ovarian loss to the woman. Assure her that the surgery will not change her ability to respond and function sexually. |

*(continued)*

## TABLE II.16 DISORDERS THAT ALTER SEXUALITY (Continued)

| Health Problem | Sexual Complication | Nursing Intervention |
|---|---|---|
| Enterostomal surgery Anterior–posterior resection | *Women:* Loss of uterus and ovaries; shortening of vagina | LI: See above. |
| | *Men:* Erectile dysfunction, decrease in amount/force of ejaculate or retrograde ejaculation due to interruption of sympathetic and parasympathetic nerve supply | SS: Suggest coital positions that decrease depth of penetration (e.g., side-to-side lying, man on top with legs outside the woman's, woman on top). |
| | *Note:* Amount of rectal tissue removed appears to determine degree of dysfunction. | LI: Explain that erectile dysfunction may be temporary or permanent. Encourage use of touch and other noncoital means of sexual communication. |
| Colostomy/ ileostomy | Alteration in sexual self-concept, body image | LI: Allow person to express feelings about change in body appearance; encourage communication with partner. |
| | Decrease in desire, arousal, and orgasm | LI: Teach that fatigue and decreased desire are common after surgery. Discuss ways to increase sexual attractiveness; suggest wearing sexy lingerie or other clothing to hide appliance. |
| | Anxiety over spillage, odor | Teach to empty bag before sexual activity; encourage to maintain a sense of humor, because accidents will sometimes occur. |
| Spinal cord injury | Erectile dysfunction in men (varies with age and type of surgery) | Encourage alternative ways to express sexuality if intercourse is not possible. |
| | Sexual disability depends on level and type of cord injury: after injury, separation of genital sexual functioning and cerebral eroticism | LI: Discuss sexual options available depending on extent of injury (e.g., a waterbed to amplify pelvic movements). Encourage continued use of contraceptives, as appropriate. |
| | Men with complete upper motor neuron injury may not be able to ejaculate. | SS: Discuss alternate positions (e.g., partner on top). Encourage experimentation with vibrators, massage, and other means of sexual expression. May be a candidate for a penile implant. May have urinary tract infection. Refer to a urologist. |

*Note:* Much information is available on the sexual implications of spinal cord injury. The reader is referred to available literature on this subject.

| Health Problem | Sexual Complication | Nursing Intervention |
|---|---|---|
| Cancer | Sexual implications depend on site of disease and treatment. | LI: Encourage expression of anxiety and fear; encourage grieving for losses. |
| | May feel guilty about desiring touch, need for sexual activity | Assure that sexual expression, even when one has cancer, is natural, and that need for intimacy often increases during this time. |
| | Changes in role function and sexually defined gender roles | Encourage discussion between partners about this; encourage negotiation about role changes, which may be temporary. |
| | Fear of being contagious | Assure person and partner that the disease cannot be transmitted through sexual activity. |
| | Change in body image | Discuss purchase of wig, false eyelashes before hair loss; suggest sexy lingerie, other ways to pamper oneself to increase feelings of sexual desirability and attractiveness. |
| | Fatigue | Explain that severe fatigue may hinder sexual desire and that fatigue does not indicate rejection of partner. Encourage verbal and nonverbal communication between person and partner. |
| Chemotherapy | *Alkylating agents, antimetabolites, and antitumor antibiotics:* Amenorrhea, oligospermia, azoospermia, decreased desire, ovarian dysfunction, erectile dysfunction | LI: Encourage discussion about changes in body appearance/function. |
| | *Vinca alkaloids:* Retrograde ejaculation, erectile dysfunction, decreased desire, ovarian dysfunction, temporary decrease in sexual desire/arousal | Explore option of sperm banking. Urge to continue use of contraceptives. False-positive Pap smear possible. Encourage nonsexual touching; rest; avoidance of alcoholic beverages, narcotics, and sedatives before sexual activity; use of water-soluble lubricants to decrease vaginal irritation; avoidance of oral and anal sex during periods of neutropenia. |
| | Genetic teratogenicity and mutagenicity | Encourage the couple to seek genetic counseling before conception. |
| Radiation therapy | Most side effects are site-dependent; however, side effects such as fatigue, neutropenia, anorexia generally are present in all people. | LI: Teach to plan sexual activity after rest periods and to use positions that require less exertion for the patient. Encourage nonsexual touching and communication. Teach that patient is not radioactive during external treatment. Teach site-specific side effects and impact on sexual functioning. |

LI = limited information; SS = specific suggestion.

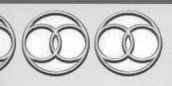

# INEFFECTIVE SEXUALITY PATTERNS

## ▶ Related to Prenatal and Postpartum Changes

**NOC**
Self-Esteem,
Body Image, Role
Performance

➤ **Goal**

The client will express increased satisfaction with sexual patterns.

### Indicators:

- Identify factors that can hinder sexuality.
- Share concerns.

**NIC**
Sexual Counseling,
Anticipatory
Guidance, Teaching:
Sexuality, Body
Image Enhancement,
Support System
Enhancement

➤ **Interventions**

### Assess Sexual Patterns During and After Pregnancy

#### Prenatal

Has the pregnancy made many changes in your life and sexual relationship?
Are there any concerns or worries about your sexual relationship during pregnancy or afterward?
What has your physician said about sex during pregnancy?
How does the pregnancy make you feel? (Ask both partners.)
How do you feel about changes in appearance?
How do you feel about changes in emotions?
How do you feel about one another's experience of the pregnancy?
What are your feelings about sex during pregnancy? Cultural influences?
What have you heard about what you should or should not do sexually during pregnancy?
Have you experienced any physical difficulties with intercourse during pregnancy?
How do you think having a baby will change your life? How do you plan to manage these changes?
How do you feel physically?
What medications do you take?
Have you had any recent changes in your health?

**R:** Preparation of the woman and her partner for the changes associated with pregnancy, labor, delivery, and postpartum can reduce anxiety.

#### Postpartum

Are you still bleeding?
Have you resumed sexual activity?
Are you concerned about conceiving again?
Has breastfeeding altered your sexual relationship?
How has having a baby affected your sexuality?
Is your episiotomy healed and comfortable during intercourse?
Have you experienced a lack of lubrication since delivery?
Do you ever have time alone with your partner?

**R:** Exploring sexual patterns, concerns, and fears can provide opportunities to correct misinformation and to open dialogue between partners.

### Reduce or Eliminate Contributing Factors

#### Body Changes

Provide literature or suggested reading list to establish knowledge about pregnancy and changes.
Refer to community resources.

Refer to early pregnancy classes.
Refer to childbirth preparation classes.
View video about sex during pregnancy.
Suggest alternative sexual positions for later pregnancy to prevent abdominal pressure.

| | |
|---|---|
| Side-lying | Woman on hands and knees |
| Woman kneeling | Woman on top |
| Woman standing | Woman astride man |

Discuss postpartum changes.
Provide literature.
Give reassurance about these changes:

- Episiotomy
- Lochia—how long it will last, how it will change
- Lubrication
- Uterine resolution
- Flabby abdominal musculature
- Breast engorgement
- Breast leakage during lovemaking

Reassure the woman that this state is temporary and will resolve in 2 to 3 months.
Refer her to a postpartum exercise class.

**R:** Pregnancy is a time of stress for both man and woman; to deny physical closeness at a time when both partners are struggling can add to tension and alienation.

**R:** Preparation of the woman and her partner for the changes associated with pregnancy, labor, delivery, and postpartum can reduce anxiety.

## Change in Sex Drive

Reassure the woman that sexual attitudes change throughout pregnancy from feeling very desirous of sex to wanting only to be cuddled.
Support acceptance of whatever pleasuring may be desired. Encourage flexibility and alternative sexual patterns (e.g., oral sex, mutual masturbation, fondling, stroking, massage, vibrators).
Encourage honest communication with her partner concerning desires or changes in interest.

**R:** The woman may worry about her partner's acceptance; the man may be afraid of hurting the woman and needs to know that sexual activity does not harm the fetus.

Fatigue
Acknowledge this as a factor, especially during first trimester and again during the last month.
Fatigue can be a major contributor to postpartum sexual problems.
Encourage the client to make time for her relationship, in sexual as well as other contexts.
Encourage the client to ask for help, hire a sitter, and so forth.
**R:** Helping the couple understand what factors affect libido (e.g., fatigue) can reduce feelings of rejection.

## Emotional Liability

Encourage the woman and/or partner to discuss emotions:

- Postpartum emotional changes can be intense. They can be hormonally influenced but are aggravated by fatigue and loss of identity.
- Conflicting feelings are common. Woman and partner need an opportunity to discuss.
  - Resentment of partner is common; this will certainly affect sexual rapport.
  - Resentment of the infant can create intense guilt and may cause the woman to cling more to the child and reject others. Or she may become depressed and less responsive to infant and partner.
  - Expression and acceptance of feelings are imperative.

Listen—allow time for the client to elaborate on feelings.
Reassure that these feelings are normal.
Recommend reading material.
Refer to other pregnant couples for verification.

Relate your own experiences, if appropriate.

Refer to therapy, if indicated.

**R:** Communication problems are the most common type of marital problems. Couples are encouraged to share their sexual needs and preferences.

### Fear of Damaging Fetus

Reassure that, unless problems exist (preterm labor, previous early loss, bleeding or rupture of membranes), intercourse is allowed until labor begins.

Refer to a physician for reassurance.

Explore misinformation. Use anatomic charts to show protection of the baby in the uterus.

Inform the couple that orgasm causes contractions that are not harmful and will subside.

**R:** Barring complications, a pregnant woman is free to engage in sexual activity with her partner to the extent that it is comfortable and desired.

### Dyspareunia in Pregnancy

Explore what pain is experienced and when.

Suggest alternative positions:

Woman on top    Posterior–vaginal entry    Side-lying

Suggest use of water-soluble lubricant.

Refer to a physician if pain continues.

**R:** Alternative sexual positions can prevent abdominal pressure or deep penetration.

### Dyspareunia Postpartum

Explore what pain is experienced and under what circumstances.

Assess healing of the episiotomy:

- The incision heals on the surface after 1 week.
- Dissolvable stitches can take up to 1 month to resolve; there may be tenderness and swelling until then.
- Nerves can remain sensitive and tender for as long as 6 months.

Suggest varied positions.

Suggest use of water-soluble lubricant (nursing women report reduced vaginal lubrication during the entire nursing experience).

Teach the woman to identify her pelvic floor muscles and strengthen them with exercise:

- "For posterior pelvic floor muscles, imagine you are trying to stop the passage of stool, and tighten your anus muscles without tightening your legs or your abdominal muscles."
- "For anterior pelvic floor muscles, imagine you are trying to stop the passage of urine; tighten the muscles (back and front) for 4 seconds, and then release them; repeat ten times, four times a day" (can be increased to four times an hour if indicated).

Instruct the woman to stop and start the urinary stream several times during voiding.

Refer the woman to a physician, nurse midwife, or nurse practitioner if pain continues.

**R:** Discomfort with sexual activity will decrease libido in women.

### Guilt Over Baby

Encourage discussion; reassure that these feelings are normal; allow time to elaborate.

Expression of these feelings often creates a release and relaxation.

Include partner in discussion. (Both may have similar feelings they have not felt free to express to each other.)

Refer to postpartum support groups.

Refer to psychological or social assistance if pathology is observed.

Encourage the couple to allow themselves to get help in caring for the infant. They need time alone. Suggest they arrange a "date" where they can be alone, with no threat of intrusion of a crying baby. They may then be able to rediscover or renew their intimacy.

**R:** Fathers need to make their own adjustment, both pre-and postnatally. They may feel lost, displaced, or left out. They may have confusing feelings of resentment, especially as the infant suckles the breast (Barclay et al., 1996; Donoran, 1995).

## Fear of Pregnancy

Encourage discussion.

Explore contraceptive choices.

Refer the woman to a nurse practitioner or gynecologist for contraception.

Inform the woman that breastfeeding does not provide effective contraception and that prepregnancy contraceptive devices may no longer fit:

- Warn that, although some oral contraceptives can be used while nursing, they usually significantly reduce milk supply.

**R:** Fear of pregnancy can diminish libido in men and women.

## Techniques to Increase the Couple's Connectiveness (Polomeno, 1999)

Explore fears and anxieties (separately).

Discuss barriers to disclosing fears and anxieties.

Role-play disclosure of fears and anxieties.

Encourage the couple to share the "little things" that represent caring.

**R:** For women, "little things" that represent caring have the same value, whether it is helping with household chores or planning a dinner out. For men, small acts earn small points whereas big gifts earn big points (Gray, 1995).

Instruct on "heart talks." One partner talks for 5 min with no interruption or arguing. The other partner then has a chance to talk. At the end, the couple hugs and says, "I love you" (Polomeno, 1999).

Instruct on "sexual conversation" (Gray, 1995). Useful questions are:

- What do you like about having sex with me?
- Would you like more sex?
- Would you like more or less foreplay?
- Is there a way that you would like me to touch you?

Talk regarding keeping romance alive.

Set aside regular time with each other.

Hold hands.

Send messages that the other partner is appreciated.

**R:** "Romance is important in keeping love, passion, and sex alive in a couple's relationship" (Polomeno, 1999, p 15).

**R:** Romance conveys to a woman that she is important and respected. When a woman appreciates her male partner's efforts, he feels more loved and encouraged to be more romantic (Gray, 1995).

## Initiate Health Teaching and Referrals

Teach couples to abstain from intercourse and seek the advice of their health care provider if any of the following are present (Gilbert & Harmon, 1998):

| | |
|---|---|
| Vaginal bleeding | Premature dilation |
| Multiple pregnancy | Engaged fetal head or lightening |
| Placenta previa | Rupture of membranes |
| History of premature delivery | History of miscarriage |

If any of the above are present, the couple should not engage in *any* sex play. Couples should be instructed to ask *very specific* questions about what is allowed and what is not allowed.

**R:** Intercourse and orgasm are safe for most women, except those with high-risk pregnancies. Semen contains prostaglandin, which may hasten cervical thinning (Gilbert & Harmon, 1998). Orgasm even without intercourse is contraindicated in high-risk pregnancies in most circumstances.

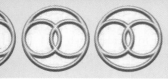

# SEXUAL DYSFUNCTION

## DEFINITION

State in which a client experiences or is at risk of experiencing a change in sexual function that is viewed as unrewarding or inadequate

## DEFINING CHARACTERISTICS

### Major (Must Be Present, One or More)

Verbalization of problem with sexual function
Meets *DSM-IV* criteria for Sexual Dysfunction

### Minor (May Be Present)

Fears future limitations on sexual performance
Misinformed about sexuality
Lacks knowledge about sexuality and sexual function
Value conflicts involving sexual expression (cultural, religious)
Altered relationship with significant other
Dissatisfaction with sex role (perceived or actual)

▪▪▪▪▪▪ **AUTHOR'S NOTE**
See *Ineffective Sexuality Patterns.*

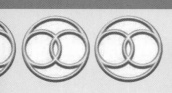

# RISK FOR SHOCK

## ▶ Risk for Complications of Hypovolemia

## DEFINITION

The state in which a client is at risk for inadequate blood flow to the body's tissues which may lead to life-threatening cellular dysfunction

## RISK FACTORS

Hypertension
Hypovolemia
Hypoxemia
Hypoxia
Infection
Sepsis
Systemic inflammatory response syndrome

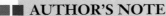

**AUTHOR'S NOTE**

This newly accepted diagnosis by NANDA-I represents several collaborative problems. In order to decide which of the following collaborative problems is appropriate for an individual client, determine what you are monitoring for. Which of the following describes the focus of nursing for this client?

- Risk for Complications of Hypertension
- Risk for Complications of Hypovolemia
- Risk fro Complications of Sepsis
- Risk for Complications of Decrease Cardiac Output
- Risk for Complications of Hypoxemia
- Risk for Complications of Allergic Reaction
- Refer to Section 3 for goals and interventions for each of the above collaborative problems.

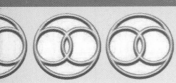

# DISTURBED SLEEP PATTERN

**Disturbed Sleep Pattern**

Insomnia
Sleep Deprivation

## DEFINITION

State in which a client experiences a change in the quantity or quality of one's rest pattern that causes discomfort or interferes with desired lifestyle

## DEFINING CHARACTERISTICS

### Major (Must Be Present)

**Adults**
Difficulty falling or remaining asleep

### Minor (May Be Present)

**Adults**
Fatigue on awakening or during the day          Dozing during the day
Agitation                                       Mood alterations

**Children**
Reluctance to retire
Persists in sleeping with parents
Frequent awakening during the night

## RELATED FACTORS

Many factors can contribute to disturbed sleep patterns. Some common factors follow.

### Pathophysiologic

*Related to frequent awakenings secondary to:*
*Impaired Oxygen Transport*
Angina                    Respiratory disorders          Peripheral arteriosclerosis
Circulatory disorders

*Impaired Elimination; Bowel or Bladder*

| | | |
|---|---|---|
| Diarrhea | Retention | Constipation |
| Dysuria | Incontinence | Frequency |

*Impaired Metabolism*

| | | |
|---|---|---|
| Hyperthyroidism | Hepatic disorders | Gastric ulcers |

## Treatment-Related

***Related to difficulty assuming usual position secondary to (specify)***
***Related to excessive daytime sleeping or hyperactivity secondary to (specify medication)***

| | | |
|---|---|---|
| Tranquilizers | Sedatives | Amphetamines |
| Monoamine oxidase inhibitors | Hypnotics | Barbiturates |
| Antidepressants | Corticosteroids | Antihypertensives |

## Situational (Personal, Environmental)

***Related to excessive hyperactivity secondary to:***

| | | |
|---|---|---|
| Bipolar disorder | Attention-deficit disorder | Panic anxiety |
| Illicit drug use | | |

***Related to excessive daytime sleeping***
***Related to depression***
***Related to inadequate daytime activities***
***Related to pain***
***Related to anxiety response***
***Related to discomforts secondary to pregnancy***
***Related to lifestyle disruptions***

| | | |
|---|---|---|
| Occupational | Emotional | Social |
| Sexual | Financial | |

***Related to environmental changes (specify)***
Hospitalization (noise, disturbing roommate, fear)
Travel
***Related to fears***
***Related to circadian rhythm changes***

## Maturational

**Children**
***Related to fear of dark***
Related to fear
Related to enuresis
Related to inconsistent parenteral responses
Related to inconsistent sleep rituals

**Adult Women**
***Related to hormonal changes (e.g., perimenopausal)***

## ▪▪▪▪▪ AUTHOR'S NOTE

Sleep disturbances can have many causes or contributing factors. Some examples are asthma, tobacco use, stress, marital problems, and traveling. Disturbed Sleep Pattern describes a situation that is probably transient due to a change in the client or environment (e.g., acute pain, travel, hospitalization). Risk for Disturbed Sleep Pattern can use used when a client is at risk due to travel or shift work. Insomnia describes a client with a persistent problem falling asleep or staying asleep as chronic pain and multiple chronic stressors. It may be clinically useful to view sleep problems as a sign or symptom of another nursing diagnosis such as *Stress Overload, Pain, Ineffective Coping, Dysfunctional Family Coping*, or *Risk-Prone Health Behavior*.

# ERRORS IN DIAGNOSTIC STATEMENTS

1. *Insomnia related to apnea*
   This diagnosis requires monitoring and co-management by nurses and physicians; thus, the nurse should write it as the collaborative problem *RC of Sleep Apnea*.
2. *Disturbed Sleep Pattern related to hospitalization*
   This diagnosis does not reflect the treatment needed. The effects of hospitalization on sleep should be specified, such as in *Disturbed Sleep Pattern related to changes in usual sleep environment, unfamiliar noises, and interruptions for assessments*.

# KEY CONCEPTS

## Generic Considerations

- Sleep involves two distinct stages: rapid eye movement (REM) and non-rapid eye movement (NREM). NREM sleep constitutes about 75% of total sleep time; REM sleep accounts for the remaining 25% (Porth, 2006).
- The entire sleep cycle is completed in 70 to 100 min; this cycle repeats itself four or five times during the course of the sleep period.
- Sleep is a restorative and recuperative process that facilitates cellular growth and repair of damaged and aging body tissues. During NREM sleep, metabolic, cardiac, and respiratory rates decrease to basal levels and blood pressure decreases. There is profound muscle relaxation, bone marrow mitotic activity, and accelerated tissue repair and protein synthesis. During REM sleep, the sympathetic nervous system accelerates, with erratic increases in cardiac output and heart and respiratory rate. Perfusion to gray matter doubles, and cognitive and emotional information is stored, filtered, and organized (Boyd, 2005).
- The active phase of the sleep cycle, REM sleep, is characterized by increased irregular vital signs, penile erections, flaccid musculature, and release of adrenal hormones. REM sleep occurs approximately four or five times a night and is essential to a client's sense of well-being. REM sleep is instrumental in facilitating emotional adaptation; a client needs substantially more REM sleep after periods of increased stress or learning (Blissitt, 2001).
- Percentage of time in bed at night actually spent asleep, or *sleep efficiency*, influences perception of the quality of sleep. Studies report that younger people typically report sleep efficiency of 80% to 95%, whereas older people report 67% to 70% (Hayashi & Endo, 1982).
- Sleep deprivation results in impaired cognitive functioning (memory, concentration, judgment) and perception, mental fatigue, reduced emotional control, and increased suspicion, irritability, depression, and disorientation. It also lowers the pain threshold and decreases production of catecholamines, corticosteroids, and hormones (Boyd, 2001; Dines-Kalinowski, 2000).
- The average amount of sleep needed according to age follows:

| Age | Hours of Sleep |
| --- | --- |
| Newborn | 14 to 18 |
| 6 months | 12 to 16 |
| 6 months to 4 years | 12 to 13 |
| 5 to 13 years | 7 to 8.5 |
| 13 to 21 years | 7 to 8.75 |
| Adults younger than 60 | 6 to 9 |
| Adults older than 60 | 7 to 8 |

- Hammer (1991) identified three subcategories of *Disturbed Sleep Pattern*: latency or difficulty falling asleep, interrupted, and early-morning awakening.
- People with depression report early-morning awakenings and inability to return to sleep. People with anxiety complain of insomnia and multiple awakenings (Boyd, 2005).
- Hypnotics contribute to sleep disturbances through the following mechanisms:
  - Requiring increasing dosage as a result of tolerance
  - Depressing central nervous system (CNS) function
  - Producing paradoxic effects (nightmares, agitation)
  - Interfering with REM and deep sleep stages
  - Causing daytime somnolence owing to a very long half-life

*(continued)*

■■■■■■■ **KEY CONCEPTS** *Continued*

• Sleep disturbances are reported by 50% to 100% of peri- and postmenopausal women. These sleep disturbances are caused by hot flashes and sweating caused by hormonal changes (Landis & Moe, 2004).
Sleep disturbances in peri- and postmenopausal women are caused by the re-regulation of neuroendocrine hypothalamic function and changes in the amount and type of sex steroid hormones. These changes affect mood, cognition, stress reactivity, body temperature, and sleep/wake cycles (Landis & Moe, 2004).

## Pediatric Considerations

• Children exhibit wide variations in amount and distribution of sleep (Cureton-Lane & Fontaine, 1997).

| Age | Hours of Sleep |
| --- | --- |
| Newborn | 16 h |
| 12 months | 10 h, 3-h nap |
| 24 months | 11 h, 2-h nap |
| 4 years | 10.5 h |
| 7 years | 10 h |
| 12 years | 9 h |
| 16 years | 8 h |

• Sleep affects a child's growth and development as well as the family unit as a whole.
• As children mature, the number of hours spent in sleep decreases. Moreover, the quality of sleep changes with maturity. Sleep is characterized as being deep and restful 50% of the time in an infant versus 80% of the time in the older child (Hockenberry & Wilson, 2009).

## Maternal Considerations

• The activity of the fetus can interfere with sleep late in pregnancy. Dyspnea can occur if the mother is lying flat (Pillitteri, 2009).
• The effects of maternal rest/sleep deprivation may negatively affect the woman's ability to acquire and sustain her new role (Larkin & Butler, 2000).

## Geriatric Considerations

• Research has found that sleep efficiency declines with advancing age, so more time is needed in bed to achieve restorative sleep. Sleep time decreases with age (e.g., 6 h by 70 years). Stages 3 and 4 and REM sleep decrease with aging (Hammer, 1991).
• Sleep pattern disturbances are the most frequent complaint among older adults (Hammer, 1991).
• Older adults have more difficulty falling asleep, are more easily awakened, and spend more time in the drowsiness stage and less time in the dream stages than do younger people (Miller, 2009).
• Miller (2009) reports that approximately 70% of older adults complain of sleep disturbances, usually involving daytime sleepiness, difficulty falling asleep, and frequent arousals.

# Focus Assessment Criteria

## Subjective Data

### *Assess for Defining Characteristics*

**Sleep Patterns (Present, Past)**
Rate sleep on a scale of 1 to 10 (10 = rested, refreshed)
Usual bedtime and arising time
Difficulty in getting to sleep, staying asleep, or awakening (number)
Naps

### Sleep Requirements

To establish the amount of sleep a client needs, have him or her go to bed and sleep until waking in the morning (without an alarm clock). The client should do this for a few days. Calculate the average of the total sleeping hours, subtracting 20 to 30 min, which is the time most people need to fall asleep.

### History of Symptoms

Complaints of:

| | |
|---|---|
| Sleeplessness | Fear (nightmares, dark, maturational situations) |
| Depression | |
| Anxiety | Irritability |

## Assess for Related Factors

Refer to Related Factors.

## Objective Data

## Assess for Defining Characteristics

*Physical characteristics*
Drawn appearance (pale, dark circles under eyes, puffy eyes)
Yawning
Dozing during the day
Decreased attention span
Irritability
For more information on Focus Assessment Criteria, visit http://thepoint.lww.com.

---

**NOC**

Rest, Sleep, Well-Being, Parenting Performance

## ➤ Goal

The client will report an optimal balance of rest and activity.

### Indicators:

- Describe factors that prevent or inhibit sleep.
- Identify techniques to induce sleep.

---

**NIC**

Energy Management, Sleep Enhancement, Relaxation Therapy, Exercise Promotion, Environmental Management, Parent Education: Childrearing Family

## ➤ General Interventions

Because various factors can disrupt sleep patterns, the nurse should consult the index for specific interventions to reduce certain factors (e.g., pain, anxiety, fear). The following suggests general interventions for promoting sleep and specific interventions for selected clinical situations.

### Identify Causative Contributing Factors

Refer to Related Factors
Explain sleep cycles includes REM, NREM, and wakefulness and sleep requirements.

**R:** Sleep cycle. A client typically goes through four or five complete sleep cycles each night. Awakening during a cycle may cause him or her to feel poorly rested in the morning.

**R:** Although many believe that a client needs 8 h of sleep each night, no scientific evidence supports this belief. Individual sleep requirements vary greatly. In general, a client who can relax and rest easily requires less sleep to feel refreshed. With age, total sleep time usually decreases—especially stage 4 sleep—and stage 1 sleep increases.

### Reduce or Eliminate Environmental Distractions and Sleep Interruptions

Assess with client and family their usual bedtime routine—time, hygiene practices, rituals such as reading—and adhere to it as closely as possible.
Encourage or provide evening care:

- Bathroom or bedpan

- Personal hygiene (mouth care, bath, shower, partial bath)
- Clean linen and bedclothes (freshly made bed, sufficient blankets)

**R:** Sleep is difficult without relaxation, which the unfamiliar hospital environment can hinder.

### Noise

Close the door to the room.
Pull the curtains.
Unplug the telephone.
Use "white noise" (e.g., fan; quiet music; tape of rain, waves).
Eliminate 24-h lighting.
Provide night lights.
Decrease the amount and kind of incoming stimuli (e.g., staff conversations).
Cover blinking lights with tape.
Reduce the volume of alarms and televisions.
Place the client with a compatible roommate, if possible.

### Interruptions

Organize procedures to minimize disturbances during sleep period (e.g., when the client awakens for medication, also administer treatments and obtain vital signs).
Avoid unnecessary procedures during sleep period.
Limit visitors during optimal rest periods (e.g., after meals).
If voiding during the night is disruptive, have the client limit nighttime fluids and void before retiring.

**R:** Researchers have reported that the chief deterrents to sleep in critical care clients were activity, noise, pain, physical condition, nursing procedures, lights, vapor tents, and hypothermia.

## Increase Daytime Activities, as Indicated

Establish with the client a schedule for a daytime program of activity (walking, physical therapy).
Discourage naps longer than 90 min.
Encourage naps in the morning.
Limit the amount and length of daytime sleeping if excessive (i.e., more than 1 h).
Encourage others to communicate with the client and stimulate wakefulness.

**R:** Early-morning naps produce more REM sleep than do afternoon naps. Naps longer than 90 min long decrease the stimulus for longer sleep cycles in which REM sleep is obtained.

## Promote a Sleep Ritual or Routine

- Maintain a consistent daily schedule for waking, sleeping, and resting (weekdays, weekends).
- Arise at the usual time even after not sleeping well; avoid staying in bed when awake.
- Use the bed only for activities associated with sleeping; avoid TV watching.
- If the client is awakened and cannot return to sleep, tell him or her to get out of bed and read in another room for 30 min.
- Take a warm bath.
- Consume a desired bedtime snack (avoid highly seasoned and high-roughage foods) and warm milk
- Use herbs that promote sleep (e.g., lavender, ginseng, chamomile, valerian, rose hips, lemon balm passion flower [Milller, 2009]). Consult with the primary care provider prior to use.
- Avoid alcohol, caffeine, and tobacco at least 4 h before retiring.
- Go to bed with reading material.
- Get a back rub or massage.
- Listen to soft music or a tape-recorded story.
- Practice relaxation/breathing exercises.

**R:** Sleep rituals prepare the mind, body, and spirit for rest and decrease cortical responses.
**R:** Warm milk contains L-tryptophan, which is a sleep inducer.
**R:** Caffeine and nicotine are CNS stimulants that lengthen sleep latency and increase nighttime wakening (Miller, 2009).

**R:** Alcohol induces drowsiness but suppresses REM sleep and increases the number of awakenings (Miller, 2009).

Use pillows for support.

**R:** Pillows can support a painful limb, pregnant or obese abdomen, or the back.

Ensure that the client has at least four or five periods of at least 90 min each of uninterrupted sleep every 24 h.
Document the amount of the client's uninterrupted sleep each shift.

**R:** To feel rested, a client usually must complete an entire sleep cycle (70 to 100 min) four or five times a night.

## Provide Health Teaching and Referrals, as Indicated

Teach an at-home sleep routine (Miller, 2009). See above for specifics.
Teach the importance of regular exercise (walking, running, aerobic dance) for at least 30 min three times a week (if not contraindicated). Avoid exercise in the evening.

**R:** Regular exercise can reduce stress and promote sleep.

Explain risks of hypnotic medications with long-term use.

**R:** There is a risk for development of tolerance and interference with daytime functioning.
Refer a client with a chronic sleep problem to a sleep disorders center.
For peri- and postmenopausal women, explain the following:

* Sedative and hypnotic drugs begin to lose their effectiveness after 1 week of use, requiring increasing dosages and leading to the risk of dependence.
* Warm milk contains L-tryptophan, which is a sleep inducer.
* Caffeine and nicotine are CNS stimulants that lengthen sleep latency and increase nighttime wakening (Miller, 2009).
* Alcohol induces drowsiness but suppresses REM sleep and increases the number of awakenings (Miller, 2009).
* Early-morning naps produce more REM sleep than do afternoon naps. Naps longer than 90 min long decrease the stimulus for longer sleep cycles in which REM sleep is obtained.

**R:** Sleep disturbances during the perimenopausal period are attributed to hot flashes and hormonal fluctuations.

Pediatric
Interventions

### Explain the Sleep Differences of Infants and Toddlers (Murray, Zentner, & Yakimo, 2009, p. 311)

| | |
|---|---|
| 15 months | Shorter morning nap, needs afternoon nap |
| 17 to 24 months | Has trouble falling asleep |
| 18 months | Has a favorite sleep toy, pillow, or blanket |
| 19 months | Tries to climb out of bed |
| 20 months | May awake with nightmares |
| 21 months | Sleeps better, shorter afternoon naps |
| 24 months | Wants to delay bedtime, needs afternoon nap, sleeps less time |
| 2 to 3 years | Can change to bed from crib, needs closely spaced side rails |

**R:** There are age-related sleep requirements and behavior.

Explain night to the child (stars and moon).
Discuss how some people (nurses, factory workers) work at night.
Explain that when night comes for them, day is coming for other people elsewhere in the world.
If a nightmare occurs, encourage the child to talk about it, if possible. Reassure the child that it is a dream, even though it seems very real. Share with the child that you have dreams too.

*(continued)*

**Pediatric Interventions**
*Continued*

**R:** Children need to understand nighttime and be assisted to prepare for it. Preparation for bedtime involves switching the child from activity to bedtime gradually. It is a time for calmness, reassurance, and closeness.

### Stress the Importance of Establishing a Sleep Routine (Murray, Zentner, & Yakimo, 2009, p. 313)

- Set a definite time and bedtime routine. Begin 30 min before bedtime. Try to prevent an overtired, agitated child.
- Establish a bedtime ritual with bath, story-reading, and soft music.
- Ensure that the child has his or her favorite bedtime object/toy, pillow, blanket, etc.
- Quietly talk and hold the child.
- Avoid TV and videos.
- If the child cries, go back in for a few minutes and reassure for less than a minute. Do not pick up the child. If crying continues, return in 5 minutes and repeat the procedure.
- "If extended crying continues, lengthen the time to return to the child to 10 minutes" (p. 313). Eventually the child will fatigue and fall asleep.
- "The child should remain in his or her bed rather than co-sleep for part or all of the night with parents" (p. 313). Occasional exceptions can be made for family crises, trauma, and illness.

**R:** "Bedtime rituals become a precedent for other separations and help the child strengthen a sense of trust and build autonomy" (p. 313). Co-sleeping with parents interferes with parental restorative sleep and promotes the child as in charge.

Provide a night light or a flashlight to give the child control over the dark.
Reassure the child that you will be nearby all night.

**R:** Children can be helped to learn that their beds are safe places. Bedtime is often difficult with sleep problems commonly related to resistance to separation and normal fears.

**Maternal Interventions**

Discuss reasons for sleeping difficulties during pregnancy (e.g., leg cramps, backache, fetal movements).
Teach the client how to position pillows in side-lying position (one between legs, one under abdomen, one under top arm, one under head).

**R:** Interventions that reduce discomfort of enlarging the uterus can promote sleep (Pillitteri, 2009).

Refer to General Interventions for Sleep Promotion Strategies.

**Geriatric Interventions**

### Explain the Age-Related Effects on Sleep
**R:** Older adults have more difficulty falling asleep, are more easily awakened, and spend more time in the drowsiness stage and less time in the dream stages than do younger people (Miller, 2009).

### Explain that Medications (Prescribed, Over-the-Counter) Should Be Avoided Because of Their Risk for Dependence and the Risks of Drowsiness.
If the client needs sleeping pills occasionally, advise him or her to consult primary care provider for a type with a short half-life.

**R:** Over-the-counter sleep aids contain antihistamines which can cause dizziness and risk for falls.

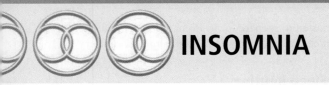

# INSOMNIA

## DEFINITION

The state in which a client reports a persistent pattern of difficulty falling asleep and frequent awakening that disrupts daytime life

## DEFINING CHARACTERISTICS

### Major (Must Be Present)

**Adults**

Report persistent difficulty falling or remaining asleep.

### Minor (May Be Present)

**Adults**

Fatigue on awakening or during the day          Dozing during the day

## RELATED FACTORS

### Pathophysiologic

*Related to frequent awakenings secondary to:*
*Impaired Oxygen Transport:*

| | | |
|---|---|---|
| Angina | Respiratory disorders | Peripheral arteriosclerosis |
| Circulatory disorders | | |

*Impaired Elimination; Bowel or Bladder:*

| | | |
|---|---|---|
| Diarrhea | Retention | Constipation |
| Dysuria | Incontinence | Frequency |

*Impaired Metabolism:*

| | | |
|---|---|---|
| Hyperthyroidism | Hepatic disorders | Gastric ulcers |

### Situational (Personal, Environmental)

*Related to excessive hyperactivity secondary to:*

| | | |
|---|---|---|
| Bipolar disorder | Attention-deficit disorder | Panic anxiety |
| Illicit drug use | | |

*Related to excessive daytime sleeping*
*Related to depression*
*Related to inadequate daytime activities*
*Related to chronic pain*
*Related to anxiety response*
*Related to environmental changes (specify)*
*Related to fears*
*Related to frequent awakenings by children*

**Adult Women**
*Related to hormonal changes (e.g., perimenopausal)*

## General Interventions

Have the client keep a sleep–wake diary for one month to include bedtime, arising time, difficulty getting sleep, number of awakenings (reason), and naps.

**R:** Sleep diaries provide data to improve the validity of assessment.

Review the diary with the client.

**R:** Examining the diary can identify if a sleep problem exists.

Evaluate if there is a physiologic condition or medication that is interfering with sleep. Refer to related factors under Pathophysiologic and Treatment-Related. Refer to the primary care provider for management.

Evaluate if a psychological state is interfering with sleep. Refer to Situation-Related Factors. Refer to Mental Health Professions.

Determine if the lifestyle or life events are interfering with sleep. Refer to other nursing diagnoses if appropriate: *Grieving, Stress Overload, Ineffective Coping,* or *Risk-Prone Health Behavior.*

**R:** Sleep disturbances can have many causes with varied interventions.

**Refer to Disturbed Sleep Pattern for Interventions to Establish a Sleep Ritual or Routine**

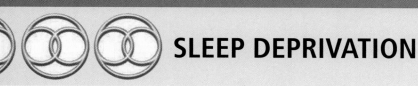

# SLEEP DEPRIVATION

## DEFINITION

State in which a client experiences prolonged periods of time without sustained, natural, periodic states of relative unconsciousness

### ▪▪▪▪▪▪ AUTHOR'S NOTE

This diagnostic label represents a situation in which the client's sleep is insufficient. It is difficult to differentiate this diagnosis from the others. Refer to Disturbed Sleep Pattern for interventions.

## DEFINING CHARACTERISTICS

Refer to *Disturbed Sleep Pattern.*

## RELATED FACTORS

Refer to *Disturbed Sleep Pattern.*

## Goal/Interventions

Refer to *Disturbed Sleep Pattern.*

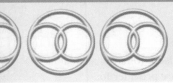

# IMPAIRED SOCIAL INTERACTION

## DEFINITION

State in which a client experiences or is at risk of experiencing negative, insufficient, or unsatisfactory responses from interactions

## DEFINING CHARACTERISTICS

Social isolation is a subjective state. Thus, the nurse must validate all inferences about a client's feelings of aloneness because the causes vary and people show their aloneness in different ways.

### Major (Must be Present, One or More)

Expresses feelings of aloneness or rejection
Desires more contact with people
Reports insecurity in social situations
Describes a lack of meaningful relationships

### Minor (May be Present)

Time passing slowly ("Mondays are so long for me.")
Inability to concentrate and make decisions
Feelings of uselessness
Feelings of rejection
Underactivity (physical or verbal)
Appearing depressed, anxious, or angry
Failure to interact with others nearby
Sad, dull affect
Uncommunicative
Withdrawn
Poor eye contact
Preoccupied with own thoughts and memories

## RELATED FACTORS

Impaired social interactions can result from a variety of situations and health problems related to the inability to establish and maintain rewarding relationships. Some common sources follow.

### Pathophysiologic

*Related to embarrassment, limited physical mobility or energy secondary to:*
Loss of body function          Loss of body part          Terminal illness
*Related to communication barriers secondary to:*
Hearing deficits          Speech impediments          Mental retardation
Chronic mental illness          Visual deficits

### Treatment-Related

*Related to surgical disfigurement*
*Related to therapeutic isolation*

### Situational (Personal, Environmental)

*Related to alienation from others secondary to:*

| Constant complaining | High anxiety | Rumination |
|---|---|---|
| Impulsive behavior | Overt hostility | Delusions |
| Manipulative behaviors | Hallucinations | Mistrust or suspicions |
| Disorganized thinking | Illogical ideas | Dependent behavior |
| Egocentric behavior | Strong unpopular beliefs | Emotional immaturity |
| Depressive behavior | Aggressive responses | |

*Related to language/cultural barriers*
*Related to lack of social skills*
*Related to change in usual social patterns secondary to:*

| Divorce | Relocation | Death |
|---|---|---|

## Maturational

### Child/Adolescent
*Related to inadequate sensory stimulation*
*Related to altered appearance*
*Related to speech impediments*

### Adult
*Related to loss of ability to practice vocation*

### Older Adult
*Related to change in usual social patterns secondary to:*

| Death of spouse | Functional deficits | Retirement |
|---|---|---|

## ■■■■■■ AUTHOR'S NOTE

Social competence refers to a client's ability to interact effectively with others. Interpersonal relationships assist a client through life experiences, both positive and negative. Positive relationships with others require positive self-concept, social skills, social sensitivity, and acceptance of the need for independence. To interact satisfactorily with others, a client must acknowledge and accept his or her limitations and strengths (Maroni, 1989).

A client without positive mental health usually does not have social sensitivity and, thus, is uncomfortable with the interdependence necessary for effective social interactions. A client with poor self-concept may constantly sacrifice his or her needs for those of others or may always put personal needs before the needs of others.

The diagnosis *Impaired Social Interaction* describes a client who exhibits ineffective interactions with others. If extreme and/or prolonged, this problem can lead to a diagnosis of *Social Isolation*. The nursing focus for *Impaired Social Interaction* is increasing the client's sensitivity to the needs of others and teaching reciprocity.

## ■■■■■■ ERRORS IN DIAGNOSTIC STATEMENTS

### Impaired Social Interaction related to verbalized discomfort in social situations

In this diagnosis, the client's report of discomfort represents a diagnostic cue, not a related factor. The nurse performs a focus assessment to determine reasons for the client's discomfort; until he or she knows these reasons, the nurse can record the diagnosis *Impaired Social Interaction related to unknown etiology*.

## ■■■■■■ KEY CONCEPTS

### Generic Considerations
- Blumer described three premises of human conduct and interactions:
  - Life experiences have different meanings for each client. People respond toward situations and others on the basis of these meanings or significance.
  - People learn meanings from social interactions with others.
  - During encounters, people interpret and apply or modify their previous meanings.
- Social competence is a client's ability to interact effectively with his or her environment.

*(continued)*

■ ■ ■ ■ ■ ■ **KEY CONCEPTS** *Continued*

- Effective reality testing, ability to solve problems, and various coping mechanisms are necessary for the client to be socially competent.
- Both the client and the environment contribute to impaired functioning. A client may be able to function in one environment or situation but not in others.
- Adequate social functioning is associated most often with conjugal living and a stable occupation.

## Chronic Mental Illness

- Chronic mental illness is characterized by recurring episodes over a long period. The extent to which role performance is impaired varies. The extent of impairment is related to social inadequacy.
- Disturbed thought processes may interfere with the client's ability to engage in appropriate social or occupational role behavior.
- Dependency is one of the most consistent features presented. It may be seen through multiple readmissions requiring a large amount of clinician's time, resistance to discharge, resistance to any change including medication, and refusal to leave home.
- The origins of impaired social interactions in people with chronic mental illness vary. For some, it is the result of poor reality testing. If a client cannot perceive reality accurately, it is difficult to manage everyday problems. For others, it may be the result of social isolation or the loss of interpersonal skills because of long-term institutionalization.
- The client with chronic mental illness usually has no friends, is socially isolated, and engages in little community activity (Varcarolis, 2006).
- Deinstitutionalization has decreased the number of institutionalized people and the median length of hospital stay, thus changing the character of today's chronically ill population. An emerging group of people 18 to 35 years of age is distinctly different from older institutionalized adults, in that their lives reflect a transient existence and multiple hospital admissions versus stable, long-term residence in a state hospital.
- People with chronic mental illness often lose their jobs, not because of an inability to do tasks but because of deficits in emotional and interpersonal functions. Research in social skills training has shown that skill-building programs improve posthospital adjustment.

## Pediatric Considerations

- A child is significantly affected when a parent is emotionally disturbed. Emotionally disturbed parents may not be able to meet the physical or safety needs of their children.
- Young children depend on their parents to interpret the world for them. Parents with *Impaired Social Interaction*, *Confusion*, or both may not interpret experiences for the child accurately (Varcarolis, 2006).
- Impaired social interaction may result in *Social Isolation*. Also, see the nursing diagnosis *Impaired Parenting*.
- Adolescents with substance abuse problems use the substance to achieve popularity, to reduce stress, or both. Poor personal and social competence is also present (Johnson, 1995).
- Young people with chronic mental illness exhibit problems with impulse control (e.g., suicidal gestures, legal problems, alcohol/drug intoxication), disturbances in affect (e.g., anger, argumentativeness, belligerence), and poor reality testing, especially when under stress. The population varies from system-dependent, poorly motivated people to system-resistant people with low frustration tolerance and refusal to acknowledge problems (Varcarolis, 2006).
- Despite variations, children and adolescents with chronic mental illness share several factors (Varcarolis, 2006).
- Difficulty maintaining stable, supportive relationships—most have transient, unstable relationships with marginally functional people.
- Repeated errors in judgment—they seem unable to learn from their experiences or to transfer knowledge from one situation to another.
- Vulnerability to stress—those experiencing stress are at greater risk for relapse.
- Patterns of social interaction are demanding, hostile, and manipulative, producing negative reactions among caregivers.

## Geriatric Considerations

- Effective social interactions depend on positive self-esteem. No data suggest that older adults have diminished self-esteem compared with younger adults (Miller, 2009).
- In older adults, common threats to self-esteem include devaluation, dependency, functional impairments, and decreased sense of control (Miller, 2009).
- Depression-related affective disturbances of daily life occur in 27% of older adults. Major depression occurs in 2% of community-living older adults and in 12% of older people living in nursing homes (Varcarolis, 2006).
- Depressed older adults lose interest in social activities and do not display positive interactions when they do interact.

# Focus Assessment Criteria

## Subjective Data

### *Assess for Defining Characteristics*

#### Relationships
Does he or she have friends or family?
Does he or she initiate friendships?
Does he or she initiate contact or wait for friends to make contact?
Is he or she satisfied with social interactions?
What is the reason for dissatisfaction with his social network?

#### Coping Skills
*How does the client respond to stress, conflict?*

| | |
|---|---|
| Substance abuse | Substance abuse (drugs, alcohol, food) |
| Aggression (verbal or physical) | Withdrawal |
| Suicidal ideation or gestures | |

#### Legal History (Arrests, Convictions)

### *Assess for Related Factors*

#### Interaction Patterns and Skills
*Job-related*
Job-seeking and interviewing skills:

- Can identify own job-related assets
- Dresses appropriately
- Asks appropriate questions
- Identifies employment sources
- Can complete an application
- Has realistic employment expectations

Employment history:

- Length of employment
- Reasons for leaving (problems with coworkers or supervisors)
- Frequency of job changes

Interactions with coworkers:

- Contacts outside work

*Living arrangements*
Residential patterns:

- Where? Family, group home, boardinghouse, institution?
- How long?
- Frequency of relocation

- Reasons for relocation

Obstacles to community functioning:

| | |
|---|---|
| Poor personal hygiene | Legal problems |
| Expects self-reliance | Unemployed |
| Lacks leisure activities | Unstable, transient residences |
| Inappropriate behavior in public | Social isolation |

*Leisure/recreation*
"What do you do with your free time?"
What interferes with participating in recreational activities?
Preference for client or group activity.

## Objective Data

### Assess for Related Factors

**General Appearance**
Facial expression (e.g., sad, hostile, expressionless)
Dress (e.g., meticulous, disheveled, seductive, eccentric)
Personal hygiene:
Cleanliness
Clothes (appropriateness, condition)
Grooming

**Communication Pattern**
*Content:*

| | | |
|---|---|---|
| Appropriate | Religiosity | Rambling |
| Worthlessness | Suspicious | Delusions |
| Denial of problem | Obsessions | Exaggerated |
| Homicidal or suicidal plans | Sexually preoccupied | |

*Pattern of speech:*

| | | |
|---|---|---|
| Appropriate | Indecisive | Neologisms |
| Circumstantial (cannot get to point) | Blocking (cannot finish idea) | Word salad |
| Jumps from one topic to another | | |

*Rate of speech:*

| | | |
|---|---|---|
| Appropriate | Reduced | Excessive |
| Pressured | | |

**Relationship Skills**
Can listen and respond appropriately
Has conversational skills
Is withdrawn/preoccupied with self
Shows dependency or passivity
Is demanding/pleading
Is hostile
Has barriers to satisfactory relationships

| | | |
|---|---|---|
| Social isolation | Thought disturbances | Severe depression |
| Chronic mental illness | Panic attacks | Preoccupation with illness |

For more information on Focus Assessment Criteria, visit http://thepoint.lww.com.

**NOC**
Family Functioning, Social Interaction Skills, Social Involvement

## ➤ Goal

The client/family will report increased satisfaction in socialization.

### Indicators:

- Identify problematic behavior that deters socialization.
- Substitute constructive behavior for disruptive social behavior (specify).
- Describe strategies to promote effective socialization.

**NIC**
Anticipatory
Guidance, Behavior
Modification, Family
Integrity Promotion,
Counseling, Behavior
Management,
Family Support,
Self-Responsibility
Facilitation

# ➤ General Interventions

## Provide Support to Maintain Basic Social Skills and Reduce Social Isolation (See Risk for Loneliness or Further Interventions)

### Provide an Individual, Supportive Relationship

Assist the client to manage life stresses.

Focus on present and reality.

Help the client to identify how stress precipitates problems.

Support healthy defenses.

Help the client to identify alternative courses of action.

Assist the client to analyze approaches that work best.

**R:** The client needs continual encouragement to test new social skills and to explore new social situations.

## Provide Supportive Group Therapy

Focus on the here and now.

Establish group norms that discourage inappropriate behavior.

Encourage testing of new social behavior.

Use snacks or coffee to decrease anxiety during sessions.

Model certain accepted social behaviors (e.g., respond to a friendly greeting instead of ignoring it).

Foster development of relationships among members through self-disclosure and genuineness.

Use questions and observations to encourage people with limited interaction skills.

Encourage members to validate their perception with others.

Identify strengths among members and ignore selected weaknesses.

Activity groups and drop-in socialization centers can be used for some clients.

**R:** The nurse models appropriate social skills and uses group therapy as other examples of social skills.

Contact the client when he or she fails to attend a scheduled appointment, job interview, and so forth.

Do not wait for the client to initiate participation.

## Hold People Accountable for Their Own Actions

Contact the client when he or she fails to attend a scheduled appointment, job interview, and so forth.

Do not wait for the to initiate participation.

Treat clients as responsible citizens.

Allow decision-making, but outline limits as necessary.

Do not allow clients to use their illness as an excuse for their behavior.

Set consequences and enforce when necessary, including encounters with the law.

Help to see how clients' behaviors or attitudes contribute to their frequent interpersonal conflicts.

**R:** Passivity or lack of motivation is a part of the illness; thus, caregivers should not simply accept it. Caregivers must use an assertive approach in which the treatment is "taken to the client" rather than waiting for him or her to participate (Varcarolis, 2006).

# Provide for Development of Social Skills

Identify the environment in which social interactions are impaired: living, learning, and working.

Provide instruction in the environment where the client is expected to function, when possible (e.g., accompany to a job site, work with the client in his or her own residence).

Develop an individualized social skill program. Examples of some social skills are grooming and personal hygiene, posture, gait, eye contact, beginning a conversation, listening, and ending a conversation. Include modeling, behavior rehearsal, and homework.

Combine verbal instructions with demonstration and practice.

Be firm in setting parameters of appropriate social behaviors, such as punctuality, attendance, managing illnesses with employers, and dress.

Use the group as a method of discussing work-related problems.

Use sheltered workshops and part-time employment depending on level at which success can best be achieved.

Give positive feedback; make sure it is specific and detailed. Focus on no more than three behavioral connections at a time; too-lengthy feedback adds confusion and increases anxiety.

**R:** Effective social skills can be learned with guidance, demonstration, practice, and feedback (Stuart & Sundeen, 2001).

Convey a "can-do" attitude.

Role-play aspects of social interactions (McFarland et al., 1996):

- How to initiate a conversation
- How to continue a conversation
- How to terminate a conversation
- How to refuse a request
- How to ask for something
- How to interview for a job
- How to ask someone to participate in an activity (e.g., going to the movies)

**R:** Role-playing provides an opportunity to rehearse problematic issues and to receive feedback.

**R:** The nurse models appropriate social skills and uses group therapy as other examples of social skills.

## Assist Family and Community Members in Understanding and Providing Support

Provide facts concerning mental illness, treatment, and progress to family members. Gently help family accept the illness.

Validate family members' feelings of frustration in dealing with daily problems.

Provide guidance on overstimulating or understimulating environments.

Allow families to discuss their feelings of guilt and how their behavior affects the client. Refer to a family support group, if available.

Develop an alliance with family.

Arrange for periodic respite care.

**R:** Interventions for the family are very important for successful rehabilitation of a family member with chronic mental illness (Mohr, 2007).

**R:** Both individuals and families are under stress. The client's behaviors that strain the family include excessively demanding behavior, social withdrawal, lack of conversation, and minimal leisure interests. The family also affects the client's ability to survive in the community by either supportive or nonsupportive behaviors.

## Explore Strategies for Handling Difficult Situations (e.g., Disrupted Communications, Altered Thoughts, Alcohol, and Drug Use; Stuart & Sundeen, 2001)

## Refer to Disabled Family Coping or Confusion for Additional Interventions

**R:** Helping the family learn strategies to handle problem behavior provides a sense of control over their lives (Stuart & Sundeen, 2001).

## Initiate Health Teaching and Referrals, as Indicated

Teach the client (McFarland et al., 1996):

- Responsibilities of role as client (making requests clearly known, participating in therapies)
- To outline activities of the day and to focus on accomplishing them
- How to approach others to communicate
- To identify which interactions encourage others to give him or her consideration and respect
- To identify how he or she can participate in formulating family roles and responsibility to comply

- To recognize signs of anxiety and methods to relieve them
- To identify positive behavior and to experience self-satisfaction in selecting constructive choices

Refer to a variety of social agencies; however, one agency should maintain coordination and continuity (e.g., job training, anger management).

Refer for supportive family therapy as indicated.

Refer families to local self-help groups.

Provide numbers for crisis intervention services.

**R:** Passivity or lack of motivation is a part of the illness; thus, caregivers should not simply accept it. Caregivers must use an assertive approach in which the treatment is "taken to the client" rather than waiting for him or her to participate (Varcarolis, 2006).

**R:** Community resources are vital to successful management and support.

**Pediatric Interventions**

### If Impulse Control Is a Problem:

Set firm, responsible limits.

Do not lecture.

State limits simply and back them up.

Maintain routines.

Limit play to one playmate to learn appropriate play skills (e.g., relative, adult, quiet child).

Gradually increase number of playmates.

Provide immediate and constant feedback.

**R:** Failure to control impulses disrupts socialization (e.g., family, peers, school; Johnson, 1995).

### Discuss Selective Parenting Skills

Reward small increments of desired behavior.

Contract appropriate age-related consequences (e.g., time-out, loss of activity [use of car, bicycle]).

Avoid harsh criticism.

Not disagree in front of child.

Establish eye contact before giving instructions and ask child to repeat back what was said.

Teach older child to self-monitor target behaviors and to develop self-reliance.

**R:** Families can be helped to learn effective parenting skills to enhance the child's success (Hockenberry & Wilson, 2009).

### If Antisocial Behavior Is Present, Help to:

Describe behaviors that interfere with socialization.

Role-play alternative responses.

Limit social circle to a manageable size.

Elicit peer feedback for positive and negative behavior.

**R:** Skills that reduce social deficits can increase social acceptance, control, and self-esteem.

### Assist the Adolescent to Decrease Social Deficits

| | |
|---|---|
| Assertiveness | Anger management |
| Problem solving | Refusal skills |
| Stress management | Values clarification |

**R:** Skills that reduce social deficits can increase social acceptance, control, and self-esteem.

**R:** Failure to control impulses disrupts socialization (e.g., family, peers, school; Johnson, 1995).

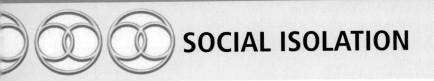

# SOCIAL ISOLATION

## DEFINITION

State in which a client or group experiences or perceives a need or desire for increased involvement with others but is unable to make that contact

## DEFINING CHARACTERISTICS

Social isolation is a subjective state. Thus, the nurse must validate all inferences concerning a client's feelings of aloneness, because the causes vary and people show their aloneness in different ways.

### Major (Must be Present, One or More)

Expressed feelings of aloneness or rejection
Desire for more contact with people
Reports insecurity in social situations
Describes a lack of meaningful relationships

### Minor (May be Present)

Time passing slowly ("Mondays are so long for me.")
Inability to concentrate and make decisions
Feelings of uselessness
Uncommunicative
Feeling of rejection
Withdrawn
Sad, dull affect
Poor eye contact
Preoccupied with own thoughts and memories
Underactivity (physical or verbal)
Appearing depressed, anxious, or angry
Failure to interact with others nearby

## RELATED FACTORS

A state of social isolation can result from a variety of situations and health problems that are related to a loss of established relationships or to a failure to generate these relationships. Some common sources follow.

### Pathophysiologic

*Related to fear of rejection secondary to:*
Obesity
Cancer (disfiguring surgery of head or neck, superstitions of others)
Physical handicaps (paraplegia, amputation, arthritis, hemiplegia)
Emotional handicaps (extreme anxiety, depression, paranoia, phobias)
Incontinence (embarrassment, odor)
Communicable diseases (acquired immunodeficiency syndrome [AIDS], hepatitis)
Psychiatric illness (schizophrenia, bipolar affective disorder, personality disorders)

### Situational (Personal, Environmental)

*Related to death of a significant other*
*Related to divorce*

*Related to disfiguring appearance*

*Related to fear of rejection secondary to:*

| | |
|---|---|
| Obesity | Hospitalization or terminal illness (dying process) |
| Extreme poverty | Unemployment |

*Related to moving to another culture (e.g., unfamiliar language)*

*Related to loss of usual means of transportation*

*Related to history of unsatisfactory relationships secondary to:*

| | | |
|---|---|---|
| Unacceptable social behavior | Drug abuse | Alcohol abuse |
| Delusional thinking | Immature behavior | |

## Maturational

### Child
*Related to protective isolation or a communicable disease*

### Older Adult
*Related to loss of usual social contacts*

### ■■■■■ AUTHOR'S NOTE

In 1994, NANDA added a new diagnosis, *Risk for Loneliness*. Although this diagnosis is only in stage I of a four-stage developmental process, it more accurately adheres to the NANDA definition of "response to." Social isolation is not a response but a cause or contributing factor to loneliness. In addition, a client can experience loneliness even with many people around. This author recommends deleting *Social Isolation* from clinical use and using *Loneliness* or *Risk for Loneliness*.

# CHRONIC SORROW

## DEFINITION

State in which a client experiences, or is at risk to experience, permanent pervasive psychic pain and sadness, variable in intensity, in response to a loved one forever changed by an event or condition and the ongoing loss of normalcy (Teel, 1991)

## DEFINING CHARACTERISTICS

### Major (Must be Present, One or More)

Lifelong episodic sadness to loss of a loved one or loss of normalcy in a loved one who is disabled. Variable intensity

### Minor (May be Present)

| | | | |
|---|---|---|---|
| Anger | Frustration | Fear | Helplessness |

## RELATED FACTORS

### Situational (Personal, Environmental)

*Related to the chronic loss of normalcy secondary to a child's or adult child's condition:*

| | | |
|---|---|---|
| Autism | Severe scoliosis | Chronic psychiatric condition |

Down syndrome      Mental retardation      Spina bifida
Sickle cell disease      Type I diabetes mellitus      Human immunodeficiency virus (HIV)
*Related to lifetime losses associated with infertility*
*Related to ongoing losses associated with a degenerative condition (e.g., multiple sclerosis, Alzheimer's disease)*
*Related to loss of loved one*
*Related to losses associated with caring for a child with fatal illness*

## ■■■■■ AUTHOR'S NOTE

Olchansky identified *Chronic Sorrow* in 1962. Chronic sorrow differs from grieving, which is time-limited and ends in adaptation to the loss. Chronic sorrow varies in intensity but persists as long as the client with the disability or chronic condition lives (Burke et al., 1992). Chronic sorrow also can accompany the loss of a child. It can also occur with an individual who suffers from a chronic disease that regularly impairs his or her ability to live a "normal life" (e.g., paraplegic, AIDS, sickle cell disease).

Chronic sorrow can be described as an "ongoing funeral," because there is no psychological closure or opportunity for resolution (Lindgren et al., 1992; Northington, 2000).

## ■■■■■ ERRORS IN DIAGNOSTIC STATEMENTS

### Chronic Sorrow related to recent death of sister

*Chronic Sorrow* is related to ongoing losses secondary to loss of normalcy. This loss of normalcy can be related to a loved one with a condition that makes a certain relationship impossible. Death of a parent, sibling, or child can affect a client through his or her lifetime. The response to this loss initially can be grieving; however, over time the client may continue to experience pervasive psychic pain. This response can be either *Chronic Sorrow* or *Complicated Grieving*. Careful assessment and discussion can help the nurse differentiate the two.

## ■■■■■ KEY CONCEPTS

- Chronic sorrow is cyclic or recurrent. It is triggered by situations that bring to mind the client's losses, disappointments, or fears (Lindgren et al., 1992).
- Chronic mental illness produces a situation with no predictable end and thus can be a lifelong disruption for the family members.(Eakes, 1995; Mohr, 2007).
- Chronic sorrow is a functional coping response. It is normal, unlike pathologic grief or depression (Burke et al., 1992).
- Response to the death of a loved one could be chronic sorrow. For example, the death of a woman in her 30s could evoke a chronic sorrow response in a surviving sister.
- When a child is disabled, the initial response from the parent will be anxiety, family disorganization, denial, and grief. Then the parent will seek outside help. Unlike grief responses to death, which have some form of closure, parents with *Chronic Sorrow* reexperience the grief response periodically (Kearney & Griffin, 2001).
- When a loved one becomes inaccessible emotionally or cognitively, there are daily reminders of the lost relationship (Teel, 1991). Many situations can trigger recognition of the loss of a hoped-for relationship, such as a school play, school dances, family vacations, dating, and marriages.
- Mallow and Bechtel (1999) found mothers of disabled children responded with chronic sorrow, whereas fathers responded with resignation.
- Parents with children with a developmental disability experience joy and sorrow, hope and no hope, and defiance and despair (Kearney & Griffin, 2001).

# Focus Assessment Criteria

## Subjective Data

### Assess for Defining Characteristics

Perception/Coping

Perception of Child's Abilities, Language Skills, Motor Skills, Social Skills, Friendships, Self-Care Abilities, Past/Recent Illnesses (Melnyk et al., 2001)

Barriers to Coping (Melnyk et al., 2001)

Interfamily relationships

Social support

Financial issues and employment

Changes/stressors in family

For more information on Focus Assessment Criteria, visit http://thepoint.lww.com.

**NOC**
Depression Level, Coping, Mood Equilibrium Acceptance: Health Status

## ➤ Goal

The client will be assisted in anticipating events that can trigger heightened sadness.

### Indicators:

- Express sadness.
- Discuss the losses periodically.

**NIC**
Anticipatory Guidance, Coping Enhancement, Referral, Active Listening, Presence, Resiliency Promotion

## ➤ General Interventions

### Explain Chronic Sorrow

Normal response

Focus on loss of normalcy

Not time-limited

Episodic

Persists throughout life

**R:** Emotions of chronic sorrow occur periodically and are ongoing (Gamino, Hogan, & Sewell, 2002).

## Encourage the Client to Share Feelings Since the Change (e.g., Birth of Child, Accident)

**R:** Families report that open, honest communication is beneficial. They need to know what to expect to help reduce life-span crises (Eakes, 1995).

## Promote Hopefulness (Hockenberry & Wilson, 2009)

- Advise of age-related health promotion needs
- Anticipatory guidance for maturational stages (e.g., puberty)
- Discuss possible age-related self-care responsibilities
- Advise how to negotiate self-care activates between parent and child

**R:** Hopefulness is an internal quality that mobilizes humans into goal-directed action (Hockenberry & Wilson, 2009.)

**R:** Hopefulness can promote increased participation in health-seeking behaviors and an improved sense of well-being and vice versa.

## Prepare the Client for Subsequent Crises Over the Life Span

Gently encourage the client to share lost dreams or hopes.

Assist the client to identify developmental milestones that will exacerbate the loss of normalcy (e.g., school play, sports, prom, dating).

Clarify that feelings will fluctuate (intense, diminished) over the years, but the sorrow will not disappear.

Advise client that these crises may feel like the first response to the "news."

**R:** An empathetic presence that focuses on feelings can reduce feelings of isolation (Eakes et al., 1998).

## Encourage Participation in Support Groups with Others Experiencing Chronic Sorrow and Expression of Grief

Stress the importance of maintaining support systems and friendships.
Share the difficulties of the following (Monsen, 1999):

- Living worried
- Treating the child like other children
- Staying in the struggle

**R:** Parents can learn successful coping mechanisms and prevent social isolation from other parents undergoing a similar experience.

**R:** Monsen (1999) reported that parents of children with spina bifida had a pattern of coping that encompassed living worried, trying to treat the child like other children, and staying strong over the long haul.

## Acknowledge That Parent(s) Is the Child's Expert Caregiver (Melnyk et al., 2001)

Elicit routines from the parents.
Prepare the family for transition to another health care provider (e.g., child to adult providers).
Educate the parents about specific procedures.

**R:** These interventions promote respect and pride (Melnyk et al., 2001).

## Link the Family with Appropriate Services (e.g., Home Health, Respite Counselor)

**R:** Counseling will be needed initially and periodically.

## Refer to **Caregiver Role Strain** for Additional Interventions

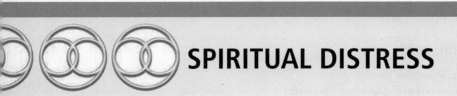

# SPIRITUAL DISTRESS

**Spiritual Distress**

**Related to Conflict Between Religious or Spiritual Beliefs and Prescribed Health Regimen**
**Risk for Spiritual Distress**
**Moral Distress**
**Impaired Religiosity**
**Risk for Impaired Religiosity**

## DEFINITION

State in which a client or group experiences a disturbance in the belief or value system that provides strength, hope, and meaning to life

# DEFINING CHARACTERISTICS

## Major (Must Be Present)

Experiences or expresses a disturbance in spiritual well-being.

## Minor (May Be Present)

Questions meaning of life, death, and suffering
Conveys meaning of life, death, and suffering
Reports no sense of meaning and purpose in life
Lacks enthusiasm for life, feelings of joy, inner peace, or love
Demonstrates discouragement or despair
Feels a sense of spiritual emptiness
Shows emotional detachment from self and others
Experiences alienation from spiritual or religious community
Expresses need to reconcile with self, others, God, or Creator
Exhibits or reports mood changes (frequent crying, depression, apathy, anger)
Presents with sudden interest in spiritual matters (reading spiritual or religious books, watching spiritual or religious programs on television)
Displays sudden changes in spiritual practices (rejection, neglect, doubt, fanatical devotion)
Verbalizes that family, loved ones, peers, or health care providers opposed spiritual beliefs or practices
Questions credibility of religion or spiritual belief system
Requests assistance for a disturbance in spiritual beliefs or religious practice

# RELATED FACTORS

## Pathophysiologic

*Related to challenge in spiritual health or separation from spiritual ties secondary to:*

| | | |
|---|---|---|
| Hospitalization | Pain | Terminal illness |
| Loss of body part or function | Trauma | Debilitating disease |
| Miscarriage, stillbirth | | |

## Treatment-Related

*Related to conflict between (specify prescribed regimen) and beliefs:*

| | | |
|---|---|---|
| Abortion | Isolation | Surgery |
| Amputation | Blood transfusion | Medications |
| Dietary restrictions | Medical procedures | |

## Situational (Personal, Environmental)

*Related to death or illness of significant other*
*Related to embarrassment of expressions of spirituality or religion, such as prayers, meditation, or other rituals*
*Related to barriers to practicing spiritual rituals*

| | |
|---|---|
| Restrictions of intensive care | Lack of privacy |
| Unavailability of special foods/diet | Confinement to bed or room |

*Related to spiritual or religious beliefs opposed by family, peers, health care providers*
*Related to divorce, separation from loved one, or other perceived loss*

■■■■■■ **AUTHOR'S NOTE**

Wellness represents a response to a client's potential for personal growth, involving use of all of a client's resources (social, psychological, cultural, environmental, spiritual, and physiologic). Nurses profess to care for the whole client, but several studies report that they commonly avoid addressing the spiritual dimension of clients, families, and communities (Kendrick & Robinson, 2000).

*(continued)*

■ ■ ■ ■ ■ **AUTHOR'S NOTE** *Continued*

To promote positive spirituality with clients and families, the nurse must possess spiritual self-knowledge. For the nurse, self-evaluation must precede assessment of spiritual concerns, and assessment of spiritual health should be confined to the context of nursing. The nurse can assist people with spiritual concerns or distress by providing resources for spiritual help, by listening nonjudgmentally, and by providing opportunities for meeting spiritual needs (Stoll, 1984; O'Brien, 2003).

Spirituality and religiousness are two different concepts. Burkhart and Solari-Twadell define spirituality as the "ability to experience and integrate meaning and self; others, art, music, literature, nature, or a power greater than oneself" (2001, p. 51). Religiousness is "the ability to exercise participation in the beliefs of a particular denomination of faith community and related rituals" (Burkhart & Solari-Twadell, 2001, p. 51). Although the spiritual dimension of human wholeness is always present, it may or may not exist within the context of religious traditions or practices.

*Impaired Religiousness* was approved by NANDA in 2004. This diagnosis can be used for *Spiritual Distress* when a client has a barrier to practicing his or her religious rituals that the nurse can assist by decreasing or removing. *Impaired Religiosity* would be appropriate.

If a client cannot practice his or her religious rituals, and the nurse cannot alter this situation, *Spiritual Distress* may be more appropriate.

■ ■ ■ ■ ■ **ERRORS IN DIAGNOSTIC STATEMENTS**

### Spiritual Distress related to critical illness and doubts about religious beliefs

Critical illness can challenge a client's spiritual beliefs and evoke feelings of guilt, anger, disappointment, and helplessness. Critical illness, however, does not represent a specific contributing factor or cue to spiritual distress. Until related factors are known, the nurse can record the diagnosis as *Spiritual Distress related to unknown etiology, as evidenced by expressions of doubt about spiritual beliefs*. The nursing focus will be on actively listening to the client's feelings and fears.

■ ■ ■ ■ ■ **KEY CONCEPTS**

### Generic Considerations

- All people have a spiritual dimension, regardless of whether they participate in formal religious practices (Burkhardt, 1994; Carson, 1999). An individual is a spiritual client even when disoriented, confused, emotionally ill, irrational, or cognitively impaired.
- The nurse must consider the client's spiritual nature as part of total care, along with the physical and psychosocial dimensions. Research indicates that most clients feel religion is very important in times of crisis (Kendrick & Robinson, 2000).
- The spiritual may include, but is not limited to religion; spiritual needs include finding, meaning, hope, relatedness, forgiveness or acceptance, or transcendence (Kemp, 2001); creativity and self-expression also may be important to spirituality (Wald & Bailey, 1990). Other descriptions of spirituality include inner strengths, meaning and purpose, and knowing and becoming (O'Brien, 2003; Burkhardt, 1994).
- Health care systems often give spiritual concerns low priority in care planning and delivery. This is less true in hospice organizations, where the spiritual component of care is more likely to be recognized and included (Millison, 1995; O'Brien, 2003).
- Religion influences attitudes and behavior related to right and wrong, family, child-rearing, work, money, politics, and many other functional areas.
- To deal effectively with a client's spiritual needs, the nurse must recognize his or her own beliefs and values, acknowledge that these values may not be applicable to others, and respect the client's beliefs when helping him or her to meet perceived spiritual needs.
- The value of prayers or spiritual rituals to the believer is not affected by whether they can be scientifically "proved" to be beneficial.

*(continued)*

■■■■■■ **KEY CONCEPTS** *Continued*

- Research indicates that many nurses feel inadequately prepared to provide spiritual care, and that fewer than 15% include spirituality in nursing care (Piles, 1990). "Among the reasons that nurses fail to provide spiritual care are the following: (1) They view religious and spiritual needs as a private matter concerning only an individual and his/her Creator; (2) they are uncomfortable about their own religious beliefs or deny having spiritual needs; (3) they lack knowledge about spirituality and the religious beliefs of others; (4) they mistake spiritual needs for psychosocial needs; and (5) they view meeting the spiritual needs of clients as a family or pastoral responsibility not a nursing responsibility" (Andrews & Boyle, 2003, p. 402).

## Pediatric Considerations

- James Fowler's *Stages of Faith Development* (1981) include "Undifferentiated Faith" (infancy) in which the nurse must be concerned with issues of parent–infant bonding as the infant struggles to establish trust, courage, hope, and love.
- In the "Intuitive-Projective Faith" stage (3 to 6 years) (Fowler, 1981), pediatric nurses are encouraged to acknowledge that the child's faith development is influenced by examples, moods, actions, and stories of their faith tradition.
- The "Mythic-Literal" faith stage (7 to 12 years) of development includes the child's internalization of their faith's stories, beliefs, and observances (Fowler, 1981).
- "Synthetic–Conventional" faith (13 to 20 years) stage describes the adolescent's faith development outside of the family context in which faith is included as part of one's identity and outlook (Fowler, 1981). This provides an understanding for the nurse on how the client interacts with family members and external peers.

## Geriatric Considerations

- National Council on Aging defines spiritual well-being as "the affirmation of life in relationship with God, self, community, and environment that nurtures and celebrates wholeness" (http://www.ncoa.org/content.cfm?sectionID 41&detail 393, February 12, 2007).
- There is disagreement among scholars as to whether older adults (over 65 years) become more or less involved in religious or spiritual issues as they age (O'Brien, 2003).
- Older adults tend to view the practice of religion as more important than younger adults.
- While some of the physical and psychosocial deficits of older age may hinder one's religious practices, personal spirituality may deepen (Seymour, 1995).
- Studies of religiosity among older adults demonstrate common religious practices among denominations: prayer, meditation, church membership, participation in religious worship services, study of religious teachings, and spiritual reading (Halstead, 1995).
- For cognitively impaired older adults, traditional prayers learning in one's youth are sometimes remembered and can provide comfort (O'Brien, 2003).
- Factors that contribute to spiritual distress and put older adults at risk include questions concerning life after death as the client ages, separation from formal religious community, and a value–belief system that is continuously challenged by losses and suffering.
- About 75% of all older adults are members of religious organizations. This does not necessarily mean that they attend their formal services and meetings regularly (Miller, 2009).
- James Fowler's *Stages of Faith Development* (1981) for adults include the Conjunctive Faith stage (midlife and beyond) in which the older adult may start to reincorporate earlier religious beliefs and traditions which were previously discarded. Here the nurse acknowledges the individual's more mature spirituality, which aids the patient in finding meaning in his or her illness (O'Brien, 2003).
- A common coping method for older adults, prayer increases feelings of self-worth and hope by reducing sense of aloneness and abandonment. In addition to private prayer and meditation, television and radio often provide adjunct stimuli for spiritual life. Estimates indicate that 60% of viewers of religious television programs are older than 50 years and are primarily women (Bearon & Koenig, 1990).

- Older adults may rely on spiritual life more than most young people because of other limitations in their lives. The spiritual realm allows for satisfying connectedness with others. An older client can counterbalance some of the negative, isolating aspects of aging by identifying with tradition and institutional values. Private religion can help to motivate and provide purpose to life.
- Older adults commonly intertwine their religious beliefs with beliefs about health and illness. The nurse must assess these beliefs appropriately to facilitate the client's understanding of his illness in the context of his religion.

**Transcultural Considerations**

- Religious beliefs, an integral component of culture, may influence a client's explanation of the causes of illness, perception of its severity, and choice of healer. In times of crisis, such as serious illness and impending death, religion may be a source of consolation for the client and family and may influence the course of action believed to be appropriate (Andrews & Boyle, 2008).
- Belonging to a specific cultural group does not imply that the client subscribes to that culture's dominant religion. In addition, even when a client identifies with a particular religion, he or she may not accept all its beliefs or practices (Andrews & Boyle, 2008).
- The nurse's role is not "to judge the religious virtues of individuals but rather to understand" those aspects related to religion that are important to the client and family members (Andrews & Boyle, 2008). Box II.4 was compiled with the intent to assist nurses with this understanding.

## Focus Assessment Criteria

Most spiritual assessment tools reflect a Christian theology, rather than nonreligious spiritual practices. Assessment tools vary on discipline (chaplain, nurse, social worker, physician) and each may identify a particular aspect of spirituality upon which to focus. A comprehensive spiritual assessment should be completed by a professional spiritual care provider, but reassessment of spiritual needs should be performed routinely as the illness experience changes or progresses. A more comprehensive spiritual assessment may only be possible once a trusted nurse–patient relationship has been established. When assessing:

- Use open-ended questions.
- Assess for congruency between affect, behavior, and communication.
- Take note of any objects in the environment that bring the client meaning, such as paintings, religious symbols, photos of nature, or music.
- Initiate assessment by acknowledging that questions may be of a personal or sensitive nature and assess the client's comfort level in answering.
- Note the language of the client's response and adapt questions accordingly.

### Subjective Data

### *Assess for Defining Characteristics*

What is your source of spiritual strength or meaning?
What is your source of peace, comfort, faith, well-being, hope, or worth?
How do you practice your spiritual beliefs?
What practices are important for your spiritual well-being?
Do you have a spiritual leader? If yes, would you like to contact him or her?
How has being ill or hurt affected your spiritual beliefs?
What influence does your faith or beliefs have on how you take care of yourself?
How have your beliefs influenced your behavior during this illness?
What role do your beliefs play in regaining your health?

### *Assess for Related Factors*

How can I help you maintain your spiritual strength (e.g., contact spiritual leader, provide privacy at special times, request reading materials)?

## BOX II.4 OVERVIEW OF RELIGIOUS BELIEFS

### AGNOSTIC

*Beliefs*
It is impossible to know if God exists (specific moral values may guide behavior)

### AMISH

*Illness*
Usually taken care of within family
*Texts*
Bible; Ausbund (16th-century German hymnal)
*Beliefs*
Rejection of all government aid; rejection of modernization
Legally exempt from immunizations

### ARMENIAN

See Eastern Orthodox

### ATHEIST

*Beliefs*
God does not exist (specific moral values may guide behavior)

### BAHA'I

*Illness*
Religion and science are both important
Usual hospital routines and treatments are usually acceptable
*Death*
Burial mandatory; interment near place of death
*Beliefs*
Purpose of religion is to promote harmony and peace
Education very important

### BAPTIST, CHURCHES OF GOD, CHURCHES OF CHRIST, AND PENTECOSTAL (ASSEMBLIES OF GOD, FOURSQUARE CHURCH)

*Illness*
Some practice laying on of hands, divine healing through prayer
May request Communion
Some prohibit medical therapy
May consider illness divine punishment or intrusion of Satan
*Diet*
No alcohol (mandatory for most); no coffee, tea, tobacco, pork, or strangled animals (mandatory for some)
Some fasting
*Birth*
Oppose infant baptism
*Text*
Bible
*Beliefs*
Some practice glossolalia (speaking in tongues)

### BUDDHISM

*Illness*
Considered trial that develops the soul
May wish counseling by priest
May refuse treatment on holy days (1/1, 1/16, 2/15, 3/21, 4/8, 5/21, 6/15, 8/1, 8/23, 12/8, 12/31)
*Diet*
Strict vegetarianism (mandatory for some)
Use of alcohol, tobacco, and drugs discouraged
*Death*
Last-rite chanting by priest
Death leads to rebirth; may wish to remain alert and lucid
*Texts*
Buddha's sermon on the "eightfold path"; the Tripitaka, or "three baskets" of wisdom
*Beliefs*
Cleanliness is of great importance
Suffering is universal

### CHRISTIAN SCIENCE

*Illness*
Caused by errors in thought and mind
May oppose drugs; IV fluid; blood transfusions; psychotherapy; hypnotism; physical examinations; biopsies; eye, ear, and blood pressure screening; and other medical and nursing interventions
Accept only legally required immunizations
May desire support from a Christian Science reader or treatment by a Christian Science nurse or practitioner (a list of these nonmedical practitioners and nurses may be found in the *Christian Science Journal*)
Healing is spiritual renewal
*Death*
Autopsy permitted only in cases of sudden death
*Text*
Bible; *Science and Health With Key to the Scriptures* by Mary Baker Eddy

### CHURCH OF CHRIST

See Baptist

### CHURCH OF GOD

See Baptist

### CONFUCIAN

*Illness*
The body was given by one's parents and should therefore be well cared for
May be strongly motivated to maintain or regain wellness
*Beliefs*
Respect for family and older people very important

### CULTS (VARIETY OF GROUPS, USUALLY WITH LIVING LEADER)

*Illness*
Most practice faith healing

## BOX II.4 OVERVIEW OF RELIGIOUS BELIEFS (Continued)

May reject modern medicine and condemn health personnel as enemies

Therapeutic compliance and follow-up are usually poor

Illness may represent wrong thinking or inhabitation by Satan

*Beliefs*

Expansion of cult through conversions important

May depend on cult environment for definition of reality

### EASTERN ORTHODOX (GREEK ORTHODOX, RUSSIAN ORTHODOX, ARMENIAN)

*Illness*

May desire Holy Communion, laying on of hands, anointing, or sacrament of Holy Unction

Most oppose euthanasia and favor every effort to preserve life

Russian Orthodox men should be shaved only if necessary for surgery

*Diet*

May fast Wednesdays, Fridays, during Lent, before Christmas, or for 6 hours before Communion (seriously ill are exempted)

May avoid meat, dairy products, and olive oil during fast (seriously ill are exempted)

*Birth*

Baptism 8–40 days after birth, usually by immersion (mandatory for some)

May be followed immediately by confirmation

Greek Orthodox only: If death of infant is imminent, nurse should baptize infant by touching the forehead with a small amount of water three times

*Death*

Last rites and administration of Holy Communion (mandatory for some)

May oppose autopsy, embalming, and cremation

*Texts*

Bible; prayer book

*Religious Articles*

Icons (pictures of Jesus, Mary, saints) are very important

Holy water and lighted candles

Russian Orthodox wears cross necklace that should be removed only if necessary

*Other*

Greek Orthodox opposes abortion

Confession at least yearly (mandatory for some)

Holy Communion four times yearly: Christmas, Easter, 6/30, and 8/15 (mandatory for some)

*Dates of holy days may differ from Western Christian calendar*

### EPISCOPAL

*Illness*

May believe in spiritual healing; may desire confession and Communion

*Diet*

May abstain from meat on Fridays; may fast during Lent or before Communion

*Birth*

Infant baptism is mandatory (nurse may baptize infant when death is imminent by pouring water on forehead and saying, "I baptize you in the name of the Father, the Son, and the Holy Spirit")

*Death*

Last rites optional

*Texts*

Bible; prayer book

### FRIENDS (QUAKER)

No minister or priests; direct, individual, inner experience of God is vital

*Diet*

Most avoid alcohol and drugs and favor practice of moderation

*Death*

Many do not believe in afterlife

*Beliefs*

Pacifism important; many are conscientious objectors to war

### GREEK ORTHODOX

See Eastern Orthodox

### HINDUISM

*Illness*

May minimize illness and emphasize its temporary nature

Viewed as result of karma (actions/fate) of previous life

Caused by body and spirit not being in harmony or by tension in interpersonal relationships

Belief in healing responses triggered by treatment

Strong belief in alternative healing practices (e.g., herbal treatments, faith healing)

*Diet*

Various doctrines, many vegetarian; many abstain from alcohol (mandatory for some); beef and pork are forbidden; prefer fresh, cooked foods

*Death*

Believe in immortality of the soul

Seen as rebirth; may wish to be alert; chant prayer

Priest may tie sacred thread around neck or wrist, or body—do not remove

Water is poured into mouth, and family washes body

Cremation preferred—must be soon after death

*Beliefs*

Physical, mental, and spiritual discipline, and purification of body and soul emphasized

Believe in the world as a manifestation of Brahman, one divine being pervading all things

*Texts*

| | |
|---|---|
| Vedas | Ramayana |
| Upanishads | Mahabharata |
| Bhagavad-Gita | Puranas |

*Worship*

Daily prayers, usually in home; quiet meditation

## BOX II.4 OVERVIEW OF RELIGIOUS BELIEFS (Continued)

Rituals may include use of water, fire, lights, sounds, natural objects, special postures, and gestures

### JEHOVAH'S WITNESS

*Illness*

Oppose blood transfusions and organ transplantation (mandatory)

May oppose other medical treatments and all modern science

Oppose faith healing; oppose abortion

*Diet*

Refuses foods to which blood has been added; may eat meats that have been drained

*Text*

Bible

### JUDAISM

*Illness*

Medical care emphasized

Rabbinical consultation necessary for donation and transplantation of organs

May oppose surgical procedures on the Sabbath (sundown Friday to sundown Saturday); seriously ill are exempted

May prefer burial of removed organs or body tissues

May oppose shaving

May wear skull cap and socks continuously, believing head and feet should be covered

*Diet*

Fasting for 24 hours on holy days of Yom Kippur (in September or October) and Tishah-b'Ab (in August)

Matzo replaces leavened bread during Passover week (in March or April)

May observe strict Kosher dietary laws (mandatory for some) that prohibit pork, shellfish, and the eating of meat and dairy products at same meal or with same dishes (milk products, served first, can be followed by meat in a few minutes; reverse is not Kosher); seriously ill are exempted

*Birth*

Ritual circumcision 8 days after birth (mandatory for some); fetuses are buried

*Death*

Ritual burial; society members wash body

Burial as soon as possible

May oppose cremation

Many oppose autopsy and donation of body to science

Most do not believe in afterlife

Generally oppose prolongation of life after irreversible brain damage

*Texts*

Torah (first five books of Old Testament)

Talmud

Prayer book

*Religious Articles*

Menorah (seven-branched candlestick)

Yarmulke (skull cap, may be worn continuously)

Tallith (prayer shawl worn for morning prayers)

Tefillin, or phylacteries (leather boxes on straps containing scripture passages)

Star of David (may be worn around neck)

*Beliefs*

Observation of the Sabbath (Friday evening to Saturday evening) may require not writing, traveling, using electrical appliances, or receiving treatment

### KRISHNA

*Diet*

Vegetarian diet; no garlic or onions

No drugs, alcohol; herbal tea only

*Death*

Cremation mandatory

*Texts*

Vedas

Srimad-Bhagavatam

*Beliefs*

Continual practice of mantra (chant)

Belief in reincarnation

### LUTHERAN, METHODIST, PRESBYTERIAN

*Illness*

May request Communion, anointing and blessing, or visitation by minister or elder

Generally encourages use of medical science

*Birth*

Baptism by sprinkling or immersion of infants, children, or adults

*Death*

Optional last rites or scripture reading

*Texts*

Bible; prayer book

### MENNONITE

*Illness*

Opposes laying on of hands; may oppose shock treatment and drugs

*Texts*

Bible; 18 articles of the Dondecht Confession of Faith

*Beliefs*

Shun modernization; no participation in government, pensions, or health plans

### METHODIST

See Lutheran

### MORMON (CHURCH OF JESUS CHRIST OF LATTER-DAY SAINTS)

*Illness*

May come through partaking of harmful substances such as alcohol, tobacco, drugs, and so forth

May be seen as a necessary part of the plan of salvation

May desire Sacrament of the Lord's Supper to be administered by a Church Priesthood holder

Divine healing through laying on of hands

Church may provide financial support during illness

## BOX II.4 OVERVIEW OF RELIGIOUS BELIEFS (Continued)

*Diet*
 Prohibits alcohol, tobacco, and hot drinks (tea and coffee); sparing use of meats
*Birth*
 No infant baptism; infants are born innocent
*Death*
 Cremation is opposed
*Texts*
 Bible; Book of Mormon
*Religious Articles*
 Special undergarment may be worn by both men and women and should not be removed except during serious illness, childbirth, emergencies, and so forth
*Beliefs*
 Abortion is opposed
 Vicarious baptism for deceased who were not baptized in life

### MUSLIM (ISLAMIC, MOSLEM) AND BLACK MUSLIM

*Illness*
 Opposes faith healing; favors every effort to prolong life
 May be noncompliant because of fatalistic view (illness is God's will)
 Group prayer may be helpful—no priests
*Diet*
 Pork prohibited
 May oppose alcohol and traditional black American foods (corn bread, collard greens)
 Fasts sunrise to sunset during Ramadan (9th month of Muslim year—falls different time each year on Western calendar); seriously ill are exempted
*Birth*
 Circumcision practiced with accompanying ceremony
 Aborted fetus after 30 days is treated as human being
*Death*
 Confession of sins before death, with family present if possible; may wish to face toward Mecca
 Family follows specific procedure for washing and preparing body, which is then turned to face Mecca
 May oppose autopsy and organ transplantation
 Funeral usually within 24 hours after death
*Texts*
 Koran (scriptures); Hadith (traditions)
 Prayer
 Five times daily—on rising, midday, afternoon, early evening, and before bed—facing Mecca and kneeling on prayer rug
 Ritual washing after prayer
*Beliefs*
 All activities (including sleep) restricted to what is necessary for health
 Personal cleanliness very important
 All Muslims: gambling and idol worship prohibited

### PENTECOSTAL

See Baptist

### PRESBYTERIAN

See Lutheran

### QUAKERS

See Friends

### ROMAN CATHOLIC

*Illness*
 Allowed by God because of man's sins, but not considered personal punishment
 May desire confession (penance) and Communion
 Anointing of sick for all seriously ill patients (some patients may equate this with "Last Rites" and assume they are dying)
 Donation and transplantation of organs permitted
 Burial of amputated limbs (mandatory for some)
*Diet*
 Fasting or abstaining from meat mandatory on Ash Wednesday and Good Friday (seriously ill are exempted); optional during Lent and on Fridays
 Fasts from solid food for 1 h and abstains from alcohol for 3 h before receiving Communion (mandatory; seriously ill are exempted)
*Birth*
 Baptism of infants and aborted fetuses mandatory (nurse may baptize in case of imminent death by sprinkling water on the forehead and saying, "I baptize you in the name of the Father, of the Son, and of the Holy Ghost")
*Death*
 Anointing of sick (mandatory)
 Extraordinary artificial means of sustaining life are unnecessary
*Texts*
 Bible; prayer book
*Religious Articles*
 Rosary, crucifix, saints' medals, statues, holy water, lighted candles
*Other*
 Attendance at mass required (seriously ill are exempted) on Sundays or late Saturday and on holy days (1/1, 8/15, 11/1, 12/8, 12/25, and 40 days after Easter)
 Sacrament of Penance at least yearly (mandatory); opposes abortion

### RUSSIAN ORTHODOX

See Eastern Orthodox

### SEVENTH-DAY ADVENTIST (ADVENT CHRISTIAN CHURCH)

*Illness*
 May desire baptism or Communion
 Some believe in divine healing
 May oppose hypnosis
 May refuse treatment on the Sabbath (sundown Friday to sundown Saturday)
 Healthful diet and lifestyle are stressed

**BOX II.4  OVERVIEW OF RELIGIOUS BELIEFS (Continued)**

*Diet*
No alcohol, coffee, tea, narcotics, or stimulants
  (mandatory)
Some abstain from pork, other meat, and shellfish
*Birth*
Opposes infant baptism
*Text*
Bible, especially Ten Commandments and Old Testament

**SHINTO**

*Illness*
May believe in prayer healing
Great concern for personal cleanliness
Physical health may be valued because of emphasis on joy
and beauty of life
Family extremely important in giving care and providing
emotional support
*Beliefs*
Worships ancestors, ancient heroes, and nature
Traditions emphasized; aesthetically pleasing area for wor-
ship important

**SIKHISM**

*Diet*
Frequently vegetarian; may exclude eggs and fish
*Religious Articles*
Men may wear uncut hair, a wooden comb, an iron wrist
band, a short sword, and short trousers. These symbols
should not be disturbed.
*Death*
Cremation mandatory, usually within 24 hours after death

*Text*
Guru Grant Sahab

**TAOIST**

*Illness*
Illness is seen as part of the health/illness dualism
May be resigned to and accepting of illness
May consider medical treatment as interference
*Death*
Seen as natural part of life; body is kept in house for 49 days
Mourning follows specific ritual patterns
*Text*
*Tao-te-ching* by Lao-tzu
*Beliefs*
Aesthetically pleasing area for meditation important

**UNITARIAN UNIVERSALIST**

*Illness*
Reason, knowledge, and individual responsibility are empha-
sized, so may prefer not to see clergy
*Birth*
Most do not practice infant baptism
*Death*
Prefer cremation

**ZEN**

Meditation using lotus position (many hours and years
  are spent in meditation and contemplation): goal is to
  discover simplicity
*Illness*
May wish consultation with Zen master

## Objective Data

### Assess for Defining Characteristics

**Current Practices**
Any religious or spiritual articles (clothing, medals, texts)
Visits from spiritual leader
Visits to place of worship or meditation
Requests for spiritual counseling or assistance

**Response to Interview on Spiritual Needs**
Grief    Doubt    Anxiety    Anger

**Participation in Spiritual Practices**
Rejection or neglect of previous practices
Increased interest in spiritual matters
For more information on Focus Assessment Criteria, visit http://thepoint.lww.com.

**NOC**
Hope, Spiritual
Well-Being

➤ **Goal**

The client will find meaning and purpose in life, including and during illness.

*Indicators:*

- The client expresses his or her feelings related to beliefs and spirituality.
- The client describes his or her spiritual belief system as it relates to illness.
- The client finds meaning and comfort in religious or spiritual practice.

**NIC**
Spiritual Growth
Facilitation, Hope
Instillation, Active
Listening, Presence,
Emotional Support,
Spiritual Support

> ## General Interventions _____

### Assess for Causative and Contributing Factors

Failure of spiritual beliefs to provide an explanation or comfort during a crisis of illness/suffering/
   impending death
Doubting quality or strength of own faith to deal with current crisis
Anger toward God or spiritual beliefs for allowing or causing illness/suffering/death

**R:** The client may view anger at God and a religious leader as "forbidden" and may be reluctant to
   initiate discussions of spiritual conflicts.

### Eliminate or Reduce Causative and Contributing Factors, If Possible

#### *Feeling Threatened and Vulnerable Because of Symptoms or Possible Death*

Inform clients and families about the importance of finding meaning in illness.
Suggest using prayer, imagery, and meditation to view selves as survivors rather than victims.

**R:** According to Stoll (1984, p. 347), "Prayer, private or with a significant other, is overwhelmingly
   reported as the most meaningful spiritual coping strategy and religious practice."
**R:** The nature of the spiritual care a client receives may directly affect the speed and quality of recovery,
   or the quality of the dying experience.
**R:** The nurse should function as an advocate in recognizing and respecting the client's spiritual needs,
   which other health professionals may sometimes overlook or ignore.

#### *Failure of Spiritual Beliefs to Provide Explanation or Comfort During Crisis of Illness/Suffering/Impending Death*

Communicate your concern seriously by being available to listen to feelings, questions, and so forth.
Give "permission" to discuss spiritual matters with the nurse by bringing up the subject of spiritual
   welfare, if necessary.
Use questions about past beliefs and spiritual experiences to assist the client in putting this life event into
   wider perspective.
Assist the client in beginning the problem-solving process and moving toward new spiritual
   understandings, if necessary.
Offer to contact the usual or a new spiritual leader.
Offer to pray/meditate/read with the client if you are comfortable with this, or arrange for another
   member of the health care team if more appropriate.
Provide uninterrupted quiet time for prayer/reading/meditation on spiritual concerns.

**R:** Spirituality influences attitudes and behavior related to right and wrong, family, child-rearing, work,
   money, politics, and many other functional areas.
**R:** According to Stoll (1984, p. 347), "Prayer, private or with a significant other, is overwhelmingly
   reported as the most meaningful spiritual coping strategy and religious practice."
**R:** The nature of the spiritual care a client receives may directly affect the speed and quality of recovery,
   or the quality of the dying experience.
**R:** The physical environment often influences spirituality, so nurses should provide appropriate settings
   whenever possible, considering such aspects as quiet, nature, music, art, and the like.

#### *Doubting Quality of Own Faith to Deal with Current Illness/Suffering/Death*

Be available and willing to listen when client expresses self-doubt, guilt, or other negative feelings.

Silence, touch, or both may be useful in communicating the nurse's presence and support during times of doubt or despair.

Suggest the process of "life review" to identify past sources of strength or spiritual support.

Suggest guided imagery or meditation to reinforce faith/beliefs.

Offer to contact usual or new spiritual leader.

**R:** The physical environment often influences spirituality, so nurses should provide appropriate settings whenever possible, considering such aspects as quiet, nature, music, art, and the like.

**R:** Research shows that people with higher levels of spiritual well-being tend to experience lower levels of anxiety. For many people, spiritual activities provide a direct coping action (Sodestrom & Martinson, 1987) and may improve adaptation to illness (Carson & Green, 1992).

**R:** The nurse should function as an advocate in recognizing and respecting the client's spiritual needs, which other health professionals may sometimes overlook or ignore.

## Anger Toward God or Spiritual Beliefs for Allowing or Causing Illness/Suffering/Death

Express to the client that anger toward God is a common reaction to illness/suffering/death.

Help the client recognize and discuss feelings of anger.

Allow client to problem-solve to find ways to express and relieve anger.

Offer to contact the usual spiritual leader.

Offer to contact another spiritual support person (e.g., pastoral care, hospital chaplain) if the client cannot share feelings with the usual spiritual leader.

**R:** The client may view anger at God and a religious leader as "forbidden" and may be reluctant to initiate discussions of spiritual conflicts.

**R:** The nurse should function as an advocate in recognizing and respecting the client's spiritual needs, which other health professionals may sometimes overlook or ignore.

**R:** Hinton (1999) found that a client's acceptance of impending death was related to the inevitability of death, faith and spiritual values, completing life, belief's diminishing rewards, and sharing.

## Engage in Spiritual Listening (Cameron, 1998)

Avoid lecturing, criticizing, and giving advice.

Avoid using religious dogma as responses.

Use nondirective communication techniques.

Help clients to determine what is right for them.

**Pediatric Interventions**

Encourage children to maintain bedtime or before-meal prayer rituals.

If compatible with the child's religious beliefs:

- Share religious picture book and other religious articles.
- Consult with the family for appropriate books or objects (e.g., medals, statues).
- Explore the child's feelings regarding illness as punishment for wrongdoing (Hockenberry & Wilson, 2009).

**R:** Continuance of usual activities can help the child cope with threatening situations (Hockenberry & Wilson, 2009).

**R:** Because U.S. society has a Judeo-Christian orientation, the nurse must be sensitive to other religious backgrounds (e.g., Buddhist, Hindu, Islamic).

**R:** Often, children view illness or injury as punishment for real or imagined wrongdoing (Hockenberry & Wilson, 2009).

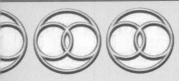

# SPIRITUAL DISTRESS

▶ **Related to Conflict Between Religious or Spiritual Beliefs and Prescribed Health Regimen**

**NOC**
Refer to *Spiritual Distress*

➤ **Goal**_____

The client will find meaning and purpose in life, including the illness experience.

### *Indicators:*

- Express decreased feelings of guilt and fear.
- Relate that he or she is supported in decisions about his or her health regimen.
- State that conflict has been eliminated or reduced.

**NIC**
Refer to *Spiritual Distress*

➤ **General Interventions** _____

### Assess for Causative and Contributing Factors (See Box II.4)

Lack of information about or understanding of spiritual restrictions
Lack of information about or understanding of health regimen
Informed, true conflict
Parental conflict concerning treatment of their child
Lack of time for deliberation before emergency treatment or surgery

**R:** The nurse's role is as an advocate for the family.
**R:** Interventions focus on providing information about all alternatives and the consequences of each option.
**R:** The nurse should be the link between the family and other members of the health care team.
**R:** Court orders to save a child's life remove the parent's right to refuse (Hockenberry & Wilson, 2009).

## Eliminate or Reduce Causative and Contributing Factors, If Possible

### *Lack of Information About Spiritual Restrictions*

Have the spiritual leader discuss restrictions and exemptions as they apply to those who are seriously ill or hospitalized.
Provide reading materials on religious and spiritual restrictions and exemptions.
Encourage the client to seek information from and discuss restrictions with others in the spiritual group.
Chart the results of these discussions.

**R:** The nurse's role is as an advocate for the family.
**R:** Interventions focus on providing information about all alternatives and the consequences of each option.
**R:** The nurse should be the link between the family and other members of the health care team.

### *Lack of Information About Health Regimen*

Provide accurate information about health regimen, treatments, and medications.
Explain the nature and purpose of therapy.
Discuss possible outcomes without therapy; be factual and honest, but do not attempt to frighten or force the client to accept treatment.

**R:** The nurse's role is as an advocate for the family.
**R:** Interventions focus on providing information about all alternatives and the consequences of each option.

### Informed, True Conflict

Encourage the client and physician to consider alternative methods of therapy* (e.g., use of Christian Science nurses and practitioners; special surgeons and techniques for surgery without blood transfusions).

Support the client making an informed decision—even if the decision conflicts with nurse's own values.

Nurse can consult own spiritual leader.

Change assignment so a nurse with compatible beliefs can care for the client.

Arrange for discussions among health care team to share feelings.

**R:** The nurse's role is as an advocate for the family.

**R:** Interventions focus on providing information about all alternatives and the consequences of each option.

## Parental Conflict Over Treatment of the Child

If parents refuse treatment of the child, follow the interventions under informed conflict above.

If parents still refuse treatment, the physician or hospital administrator may obtain a court order appointing a temporary guardian to consent to treatment.

Call the spiritual leader to support the parents (and possibly the child).

Encourage expression of negative feelings.

**R:** The nurse's role is as an advocate for the family.

**R:** Interventions focus on providing information about all alternatives and the consequences of each option.

**R:** The nurse should be the link between the family and other members of the health care team.

**R:** Court orders to save a child's life remove the parent's right to refuse (Hockenberry & Wilson, 2009).

### Emergency Treatment

Consult the family if possible.

Delay treatment, if possible, until spiritual needs have been met (e.g., receiving last rites before surgery)*; send the spiritual leader to the treatment room or operating room, if necessary.

Anticipate reaction and provide support when the client chooses or is forced to accept spiritually unacceptable therapy:

- Depression, withdrawal, anger, and fear
- Loss of will to live
- Reduced speed and quality of recovery

**R:** The nurse's role is as an advocate for the family.

**R:** Interventions focus on providing information about all alternatives and the consequences of each option.

———————

*May require a primary care professional's order.

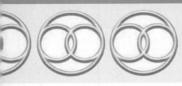

# RISK FOR SPIRITUAL DISTRESS

## DEFINITION

State in which a client or group is at risk of experiencing a disturbance in their belief or value system that provides strength, hope, meaning, and purpose to life

## RISK FACTORS

See *Spiritual Distress*.

### ■■■■■ AUTHOR'S NOTE

See *Spiritual Distress*.

### ■■■■■ ERRORS IN DIAGNOSTIC STATEMENTS

See *Spiritual Distress*.

### ■■■■■ KEY CONCEPTS

See *Spiritual Distress*.

**NOC**
Refer to *Spiritual Distress*

## ➤ Goal

The client will find meaning and purpose in life, including during illness.

### Indicators:

- Practice spiritual rituals.
- Express comfort with beliefs.

**NIC**
Refer to *Spiritual Distress*

## ➤ General Interventions

See *Spiritual Distress*.

---

# MORAL DISTRESS

## DEFINITION

The state in which a person experiences psychological disequilibrium, physical discomforts, anxiety, and/or anguish that results when a person makes a moral decision but does not follow through with the moral behavior

■■■■■■ **AUTHOR'S NOTE**
This newly accepted NANDA I nursing diagnosis has application in all settings where nurses practice. The literature to support this diagnosis when submitted was focused primarily on moral distress in nursing.

If moral distress occurs in a client or family, this author suggests a referral to a professional expert in this area, for example, a counselor, therapist, or nurse spiritual advisor.

This author will present *Moral Distress* as a Department of Nursing—Standard of Practice. This standard addresses prevention of moral distress with specific individual nurse, unit, and department interventions. Strategies for addressing moral distress for individual nurses, on units, in the department of nursing, and in the institution will be presented.

## DEFINING CHARACTERISTICS

### Major

Expresses anguish over difficulty acting on one's moral choice

### Minor

Feelings of:

- Powerlessness
- Anxiety
- Guilt
- Fear
- Frustration
- Anger
- Avoidance

## RELATED FACTORS

The following factors do not cause moral distress in every nurse. If the nurse does not support terminating ventilators on anyone, then she or he would not have moral distress if a terminally ill client was on a ventilator. Moral distress results from a nurse not acting on his or her own moral beliefs and then suffering because of the inaction.

### Situational (Personal, Environmental)

#### End-of-Life Decisions

*Related to providing treatments that were perceived as futile for hopelessly ill person, (e.g., blood transfusions, chemotherapy, organ transplants, mechanical ventilation)*
*Related to conflicting attitudes toward advanced directives*
*Related to participation of life-saving actions when they only prolong dying*

#### Treatment Decisions

*Related to the client's/family's refusal of treatments deemed appropriate by the health care team*
*Related to inability for the family to make the decision to stop ventilator treatment on hopelessly ill person*
*Related to a family's wishes to continue life support even though it is not in the best interest of the client*
*Related to performing a procedure that increases the person's suffering*
*Related to providing care that does not relieve the person's suffering*
*Related to conflicts between wanting to disclose poor medical practice and wanting to maintain trust in the physician*

#### Professional Conflicts

*Related to insufficient resources for care (e.g., time, staff)*
*Related to failure to be included in the decision-making process*
*Related to more emphasis on technical skills and tasks than relationships and caring*

**Cultural Conflicts**
*Related to decisions made for women by male family members*
*Related to cultural conflicts with the American health care system*

## ▪▪▪▪▪▪ KEY CONCEPTS

The following key concepts relate to moral distress in nursing:

- Gutierrez reported "nurses moral judgment and perceptions of appropriate moral actions linked to strong moral values to ease suffering (nonmaleficence), respect client wishes (autonomy), maintain truthfulness (veracity), and distribute scarce health care resources appropriately (justice)" (2005, p.236).
- The intrinsic purpose of a person and a living creature is supernaturally designed (Hanna, 2004). Humans can determine outcomes for others, but "when human beings attempt to manipulate or destroy the 'end' for which someone or something exists," this "manipulation or destruction is immoral and against the true nature of the existence of the person or thing" (Hanna, 2004, pp. 75–76).
- Nurses are in a unique position to advocate for the client and family and assist in decision-making because they are closely integrated with them during caregiving and because they do not benefit financially from treatment decisions that are offered.
- Nurses experience conflicts when attempting to balance authority and responsibility (Corley et al., 2001). Often nurses have more responsibility than authority. Nurses have to respond to dual authorities—physicians who write orders for patients and administrators who employ them.
- Wilkinson (1988) reported that "nurses viewed physicians as punitive and peers and nursing administration as nonsupportive in moral situations" (p. 21).
- Kramer (1974) found that new graduates reported psychological disequilibrium, discomfort, and distress when they found that the values they learned in school were difficult, if not impossible, to apply to the real world.
- Coping behaviors of nurses with moral distress are conscious and unconscious (Wilkinson, 1987–1988).

Unconscious behaviors focus on:

- The immoral actions of others rather than their own
- The powerful constraints preventing their moral actions
- That their care of the client was not negatively affected

Conscious behaviors were:

- Avoidance of the client
- Leaving the unit, the institution, or nursing altogether
- Constraints to follow one's moral actions were identified as external and internal (Wilkinson, 1987–1988):
  - External
    - Physicians
    - Fear of lawsuits
    - Unsupportive nursing administrators, agency administration policies
  - Internal
    - Fear of losing their jobs
    - Self-doubts
    - Futility of past actions
    - Socialization to follow orders
    - Lack of courage
- In the U.S. less than 1 in 5 deaths involves hospitalization with the use of the intensive care unit (Angus et al., 2004). The distinction between critical illness and terminal illness is not clear (Elpern, Covert, & Kleinpell, 2005). Dying while receiving aggressive interventions to extend life produces confusion, conflicts, and distress in caregivers, clients, and families (Elpern et al., 2005).
- In 2001, Corley and coworkers reported that 15% of the nurses studied related that they have left a job because of moral distress. In 2005, the same investigators reported the percentage to be over 25.5%.
- Research identified three categories that contained sources of moral distress in nursing—individual responsibility, not in the patient's best interest, and deception (Corley et al., 2001).

*(continued)*

■■■■■■ **KEY CONCEPTS** *Continued*

- Elpern, Covert, and Klienpell (2005), using the Moral Distress Scale, reported the following factors with the highest levels of moral distress to be related to (Corley et al., 2001):
  - Continue to participate in care for the hopelessly ill client who is being sustained on a ventilator, when no one will make a decision to "pull the plug."
  - Follow a family's wishes to continue life support even though it is not the best interest of the client.
  - Initiate extensive life-saving actions when I think it only prolongs death.
  - Follow the family's wishes for the client's care when I do not agree with them but do so because the hospital administration fears a lawsuit.
  - Carry out the physician's orders for unnecessary tests and treatments for terminally ill patients.
  - Provide care that does not relieve the client's suffering because the physician fears increasing doses of pain medication will cause death (Elpern et al., 2005, p. 526).
- In 2005, Corley and colleagues reported that unsafe staffing was the highest source of moral distress.

## Focus Assessment Criteria

### Subjective Data

#### *Assess for Psychological Disequilibrium Associated with a Situation or Situations Identified Under Related Factors*

> Powerlessness
> Anger
> Frustrations
> Guilt
> Frustration
> Avoidance

#### *Assess for Related Factors*

> Refer to Related Factors.

**NOC**
Suffering Level,
Social Support,
Hope, Fear Control

## ➤ Goal

The nurse will relate strategies to prevent or reduce moral distress.

### *Indicators:*

Identify source (s) of moral distress.
Share their distress with a colleague.
Identify two strategies to enhance decision-making with clients and family.
Identify two strategies to enhance discussion of the situation with the physician.
Identify institutional strategies to decrease moral distress in nurses.

**NIC**
Refer to *Spiritual Distress*

## ➤ Interventions

### Explore Moral Work and Action

Educate yourself about moral distress. Refer to articles on the reference list.
Share your stories of moral distress. Elicit stories from coworkers.
Read stories of moral action. Refer to Gordon's *Life Support: Three Nurses on the Front Lines* and Kritek's *Reflections on Healing: A Central Construct* (see the reference list).

**R:** Stories can help nurses identify strengths, insights, shared distress, and options for moral actions (Tiedje, 2000). Nurses responded positively when they were asked to discuss their feelings regarding moral issues (Elpern et al., 2005).

## Investigate How Clinical Situations that Are Morally Problematic Are Managed in the Institution; If an Ethics Committee Exists, Determine Its Mission and Procedures

> **R:** Organizational practices that support open discussions of patient care issues and problems with ethical and moral implications contribute to perceptions of an ethical climate for clinicians.

## Do Not Try to Avoid Moral Distress

> **R:** Responding to moral distress is viewed as negative (Hanna, 2004). It can also be viewed "as a life challenge that develops moral character for those who manage it well" (Hanna, 2004, p. 77).

## Initiate Dialogue with the Client, If Possible, and Family

> Explore what the perception of the situation is.
> Pose questions, for example, "What options do you have in this situation?"
> Elicit feelings about the present situation.

## Gently Explore Client/Family End-of-Life Decisions

> **R:** Direct but gentle inquiries and discussions can assist the client/family to examine the situation clearly and the implications of treatment options and decisions.

## If Indicated, Explain "No Code" Status and Explain the Focus of Palliative Care that Replaces Aggressive Care

> **R:** Often families think that "no code" status means no care. Palliative care focuses on comfort during the dying process.

## Dialogue With Unit Colleagues About the Situation that Causes You Moral Distress

> **R:** Elpern et al. (2005) found that nurses were relieved that their personal distress was shared and that they were not unique in their feelings.

## Enlist a Colleague as a Coach or Engage as a Coach for a Coworker

> **R:** A coach is a client who can listen, guide, and provide feedback through the process (Tiedje, 2000).

## Start with an Approach to Address an Unsatisfactory Moral Clinical Situation that Has a Low Risk; Evaluate the Risks Before Taking Action; Be Realistic

> **R:** Moral action takes courage. Risk-taking is a skill that can be learned.

## Engage in Open Communication with Other Involved Colleagues. Start Your Conversation with Your Concern, for Example, "I Am Not Comfortable with. . . . , The Family Is Asking/Questioning/ Feeling . . . , Mr. X Is Asking/Questioning/Feeling. . . ."

> **R:** Each professional has rights and duties, and conflict may be able to be resolved through open communication and sharing of feelings and values (Caswell & Cryer, 1995). Nonthreatening language can reduce embarrassment and blaming.

## Dialogue with Other Professionals: Chaplains, Manager, Social Worker, or Ethics Committee

> **R:** Nurses can be assisted in moral work with support from others in the organization.

Incorporate Health Promotion and Stress Reduction in Your Lifestyle; Advocate for End-of-Life Decision Dialogues in All Families; Refer to *Stress Overload* and *Altered Health Maintenance*

**R:** Healthy lifestyles can reduce stress and increase energy levels for moral work.

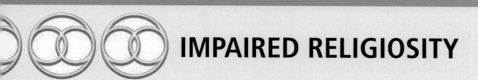

# IMPAIRED RELIGIOSITY

## DEFINITION

State in which a client or group has an impaired ability to exercise reliance on beliefs of a particular denomination or faith community and to participate in related rituals

▪▪▪▪▪▪ **AUTHOR'S NOTE**
Refer to *Spiritual Distress*.

## DEFINING CHARACTERISTICS

Individuals experience distress because of difficulty in adhering to prescribed religious rituals, for example:

Religious ceremonies
Dietary regulations
Certain clothing
Prayer
Request to worship
Holiday observances
Separation from faith community
Emotional distress regarding religious beliefs and/or religious social network
Need to reconnect with previous belief patterns and customs
Questions religious belief patterns and customs

## RELATED FACTORS

### Pathophysiologic

*Related to sickness/illness*
*Related to suffering*
*Related to pain*

### Situational

*Related to personal crisis related to activity*
*Related to fear of death*
*Related to embarrassment at practicing spiritual rituals*
*Related to barriers to practicing spiritual rituals*
Intensive care restrictions
Confinement to bed or the room
Lack of privacy

Lack of availability of special foods/diets

Hospitalization

***Related to crisis within the faith community which causes distress in the believer***

## KEY CONCEPTS

Refer to *Spiritual Distress*.

- To assist people in spiritual distress, the nurse must know certain beliefs and practices of various spiritual groups. Box II.4 provides information on the beliefs and practices that relate most directly to health and illness. It is intended as a reference only. Major religions, denominations, and spiritual groups are arranged alphabetically. Denominations with similar practices and restrictions are grouped together. Not every member of each religion adheres to all practices and beliefs set forth. It is important to verify with the client their unique practices and traditions when asking questions about religious preference. No attempt is made to discuss the broad beliefs and philosophies of the selected groups; see References/Bibliography for texts supplying such in-depth information.

## Focus Assessment Criteria

Refer to *Spiritual Distress*.

**NOC**
Spiritual Well-Being

## ➤ Goal

The client will express satisfaction with ability to practice or exercise beliefs and practices.

### *Indicators:*

- Continue spiritual practices not detrimental to health.
- Express decreasing feelings of guilt and anxiety.

**NIC**
Spiritual Support

## ➤ General Interventions

### Explore Whether the Client Desires to Engage in an Allowable Religious or Spiritual Practice or Ritual; If So, Provide Opportunities To Do So

**R:** For a client who places a high value on prayer or other spiritual practices, these practices can provide meaning and purpose and can be a source of comfort and strength (Carson, 1999).

**R:** Privacy and quiet provide an environment that enables reflection and contemplation.

**R:** These measures can help the client maintain spiritual ties and practice important rituals.

### Express Your Understanding and Acceptance of the Importance of the Client's Religious or Spiritual Beliefs and Practices

**R:** Conveying a nonjudgmental attitude may help reduce the client's uneasiness about expressing his beliefs and practices.

**R:** The nurse—even one who does not subscribe to the same religious beliefs or values of the client—can still help him meet his spiritual needs.

### Assess for Causative and Contributing Factors

Hospital or nursing home environment

Limitations related to disease process or treatment regimen (e.g., cannot kneel to pray owing to traction; prescribed diet differs from usual religious diet)

Fear of imposing on or antagonizing medical and nursing staff with requests for spiritual rituals

Embarrassment over spiritual beliefs or customs (especially common in adolescents)

Separation from articles, texts, or environment of spiritual significance

Lack of transportation to spiritual place or service

Spiritual leader unavailable because of emergency or lack of time

**R:** Privacy and quiet provide an environment that enables reflection and contemplation.

**R:** The nurse—even one who does not subscribe to the same religious beliefs or values of the client—can still help him meet his spiritual needs.

**R:** These measures can help the client maintain spiritual ties and practice important rituals.

## Eliminate or Reduce Causative and Contributing Factors, If Possible

### Limitations Imposed by the Hospital or Nursing Home Environment

Provide privacy and quiet as needed for daily prayer, visit of spiritual leader, and spiritual reading and contemplation:

• Pull the curtains or close the door.
• Turn off the television and radio.
• Ask the desk to hold calls, if possible.
• Note the spiritual interventions on Kardex and include in the care plan.

Contact the spiritual leader to clarify practices and perform religious rites or services, if desired:

• Communicate with the spiritual leader concerning the client's condition.
• Address Roman Catholic, Orthodox, and Episcopal priests as "Father," other Christian ministers as "Pastor," and Jewish rabbis as "Rabbi."
• Prevent interruption during the visit, if possible.
• Offer to provide a table or stand covered with a clean white cloth.

Inform the client about religious services and materials available within the institution.

**R:** Conveying a nonjudgmental attitude may help reduce the client's uneasiness about expressing his beliefs and practices.

**R:** Privacy and quiet provide an environment that enables reflection and contemplation.

**R:** The nurse—even one who does not subscribe to the same religious beliefs or values of the client—can still help him or her meet his or her spiritual needs.

### Limitations Related to Disease Process or Treatment Regimen

Encourage spiritual rituals not detrimental to health (see Box II.4):

• Assist clients with physical limitations in prayer and spiritual observances (e.g., help to hold rosary; help to kneeling position, if appropriate).
• Assist in habits of personal cleanliness.
• Avoid shaving if beard is of spiritual significance.
• Allow the client to wear religious clothing or jewelry whenever possible.
• Make special arrangements for burial of respected limbs or body organs.
• Allow the family or spiritual leader to perform ritual care of the body.
• Make arrangements as needed for other important spiritual rituals (e.g., circumcisions).

Maintain diet with spiritual restrictions when not detrimental to health (see Box II.4):

• Consult with a dietitian.
• Allow fasting for short periods, if possible.*
• Change the therapeutic diet as necessary.*
• Have family or friends bring in special food, if possible.
• Have members of the spiritual group supply meals to the client at home.
• Be as flexible as possible in serving methods, times of meals, and so forth.

**R:** For a client who places a high value on prayer or other spiritual practices, these practices can provide meaning and purpose and can be a source of comfort and strength (Carson, 1999).

**R:** The nurse—even one who does not subscribe to the same religious beliefs or values of the client—can still help the client meet his spiritual needs.

**R:** These measures can help the client maintain spiritual ties and practice important rituals.

**R:** Many religions prohibit certain behaviors; complying with restrictions may be an important part of the client's worship.

---

*May require a primary care professional's order.

### Fear of Imposing or Embarrassment

Communicate acceptance of various spiritual beliefs and practices.

Convey a nonjudgmental, respectful attitude.

Acknowledge the importance of spiritual needs.

Express the willingness of the health care team to help in meeting spiritual needs.

Provide privacy and ensure confidentiality.

**R:** Conveying a nonjudgmental attitude may help reduce the client's uneasiness about expressing his beliefs and practices.

**R:** The nurse—even one who does not subscribe to the same religious beliefs or values of the client—can still help the client meet his spiritual needs.

### Separation from Articles, Texts, or Environment of Spiritual Significance

Question the client about missing religious or spiritual articles or reading material (see Box II.4).

Obtain missing items from the clergy in the hospital, spiritual leader, family, or members of the spiritual group.

Treat these articles and books with respect.

Allow the client to keep spiritual articles and books within reach as much as possible, or where they can be easily seen.

Protect from loss or damage (e.g., a medal pinned to a gown can be lost in the laundry).

Recognize that articles without overt religious meaning may have spiritual significance for the client (e.g., wedding band).

Use spiritual texts in large print, in Braille, or on tape when appropriate and available.

Provide an opportunity for the client to pray with others or be read to by members of his or her own religious group or a member of the health care team who feels comfortable with these activities.

**R:** For a client who places a high value on prayer or other spiritual customs, these practices can provide meaning and purpose and can be a source of comfort and strength (Carson, 1999).

**R:** Privacy and quiet provide an environment that enables reflection and contemplation.

**R:** These measures can help the client maintain spiritual ties and practice important rituals.

### Lack of Transportation

Take the client to the chapel or quiet environment on hospital grounds.

Arrange transportation to the church or synagogue for the client in home.

Provide access to spiritual programming on radio and television when appropriate.

**R:** Privacy and quiet provide an environment that enables reflection and contemplation.

**R:** The nurse—even one who does not subscribe to the same religious beliefs or values of the client— can still help the client meet his spiritual needs.

### Spiritual Leader Unavailable Because of Emergency or Lack of Time

Baptize the critically ill newborn of Greek Orthodox, Episcopal, or Roman Catholic parents (see Box II.4).

Perform other mandatory spiritual rituals, if possible.

Offer a visit from the hospital spiritual care professional.

**R:** For a client who places a high value on prayer or other spiritual customs, these practices can provide meaning and purpose and can be a source of comfort and strength (Carson, 1999).

**R:** The nurse—even one who does not subscribe to the same religious beliefs or values of the client—can still help the client meet his spiritual needs.

**R:** These measures can help the client maintain spiritual ties and practice important rituals.

## Suggested Readings

1. Jews and Seventh-Day Adventists would find Psalms 23, 34, 42, 63, 71, 103, 121, and 127 appropriate.
2. Christians would also appreciate I Corinthians 13, Matthew 5:3–11, Romans 12, and the Lord's Prayer.

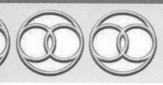

# RISK FOR IMPAIRED RELIGIOSITY

## DEFINITION

The state in which a client is at risk for impaired ability to exercise reliance on beliefs of a particular denomination or faith community and to participate in related rituals

## RELATED FACTORS

Refer to *Impaired Religiosity*.

**NOC**
Spiritual Well-Being

## ➤ Goal

The client will express continued satisfaction with religious activities.

### *Indicators:*

• Continue to practice religious rituals.
• Described increased comfort after assessment.

**NIC**
Spiritual Support

## ➤ General Interventions

Refer to *Impaired Religiosity* for interventions.

---

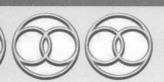

# STRESS OVERLOAD

## DEFINITION

State in which an individual or group experience overwhelming, excessive amounts and types of demands that require action

## DEFINING CHARACTERISTICS

### Physiologic

| | | |
|---|---|---|
| Headaches | Indigestion | Sleep difficulties |
| Restlessness | Fatigue | |

### Emotional

| | | |
|---|---|---|
| Crying | Anger | Edginess |
| Impatience | Nervousness | Easily upset |
| Overwhelmed | Feeling sick | |

### Cognitive

| | | |
|---|---|---|
| Memory loss | Constant worry | Forgetfulness |
| Loss of humor | Difficulty making decisions | Trouble thinking clearly |

## Behavioral

| | | | |
|---|---|---|---|
| Isolation | Intolerance | Lack of intimacy | Compulsive eating |
| Excessive smoking | Resentment | | |

## RELATED FACTORS

The related factors for *Stress Overload* for one person can be multiple coexisting stressors that can be pathophysiologic, maturational, treatment related, situational, environmental, and/or personal.

## Pathophysiologic

Related to coping with:

- Acute illness (myocardial infarction, fractured hip)
- Chronic illness (arthritis, depression, COPD)
- Terminal illness
- New diagnosis (cancer, genital herpes, HIV, multiple sclerosis, diabetes mellitus)
- Disfiguring condition

## Situational (Personal, Environmental)

Related to actual or anticipated loss of a significant other secondary to:

| | |
|---|---|
| Death, dying | Moving |
| Divorce | Military duty |

Related to coping with:

| | | |
|---|---|---|
| Dying | War | Assault |

Related to actual or perceived change in socioeconomic status secondary to:

| | |
|---|---|
| Unemployment | New job |
| Promotion | Illness |
| Destruction of personal property | |

Related to coping with:

| | |
|---|---|
| Family violence | New family member |
| Substance abuse | Relationship problems |

## Maturation

Related to coping with:

| | |
|---|---|
| Retirement | Financial changes |
| Loss of residence | Functional losses |

■■■■■■ **AUTHOR'S NOTE**

This diagnosis represents a person in an overwhelming situation influenced by multiple varied stressors. If stress overload is not reduced, the person will deteriorate and is in danger of injury and illness.

■■■■■■ **KEY CONCEPTS**

Refer to *Anxiety* and *Ineffective Coping* for specific information on anxiety and ineffective coping.

- Stress is always present in all persons. Stress is the physical, psychological, social, or spiritual effect of life's pressures and events (Edelman & Mandle, 2006).
- Stress is an interactive process in response to the loss or threat of loss of homeostasis or well-being (Cahill, 2002).
- Stress is a psychological, emotional state experienced by an individual in response to a specific stressor or demand that results in harm, either temporary or permanent, to the person (Ridner, 2004, p. 539).
- Excessive stress requires recognition, perception and adaptation (Cadhill, 2001).

*(continued)*

■■■■■■ **KEY CONCEPTS** *Continued*

- A chronic state of stress or repeated episodes of psychological stress (depression, anger, hostility, anxiety) can lead to cardiovascular disease, arteriosclerosis, headaches, and gastrointestinal disorders (Edelman & Mandle, 2006).
- In response to stress, individuals initiate or increase unhealthy behaviors such as overeating, sedentary lifestyle, excessive use of drugs or alcohol, smoking, and social isolation (USDHHS, 2000).

## Focus Assessment

### Subjective/Objective

### Ask Person to Rate His or Her Usual Level of Stress

0 = little     10 = overwhelming

### Ask Person to Describe How His or Her Stress is Affecting the Ability to Function

Work
Sleep
Relationships

### Assess for Feelings of:

| | |
|---|---|
| Anger | Unhappiness |
| Impatience | Edginess |
| Despair | Boredom |
| Apathy | Easily upset |
| Lack of intimacy | Intolerance |

### Assess for Cognitive Symptoms.

| | |
|---|---|
| Forgetfulness | Constant worry |
| Memory loss | Thoughts of abandonment |
| Difficulty making decisions | Loss of sense of humor |

### Assess for Overuse of

| | |
|---|---|
| Sleep | Tobacco |
| Alcohol | Food |
| Drugs (prescription, street) | |

**NOC**
Well–Being: Health Beliefs; Anxiety Reduction; Coping; Knowledge: Health Promotion; Knowledge: Health Resources

## Goal

The person will verbalize intent to change two behaviors to decrease or manage stressors.

### Indicators

- Identify stressors that can be controlled and those that can not.
- Identify one successful behavior change to increase stress management.
- Identify one behavior to reduce or eliminate, to increase successful stress management.

**NIC**
Assist the Person to Appraise Their Present Stressors and Categorize Them as: Extrinsic (No Control); Intrinsic (Some Control)

## Interventions

### Assist Them to Recognize Their Thoughts, Feelings, Actions and Physiologic Responses.

**R:** Self-awareness can help the person reframe and reinterpret their experiences (Edelman & Mandle, 2006).

## Teach the Person How to Break the Cycle of Their Stress in a Traffic Jam and that There Are Increases in Heart Rate, Respirations, and Strong Feelings of Anger (Edelman & Mandle, 2006).

Purposefully distract yourself by thinking of something pleasant.

Engage in a diversional activity.

Initiate relaxation breaking: inhale through nose, taking 4 seconds.

Refer to resources to learn relaxation techniques such as audiotapes, printed material, yoga.

**R:** Faced with overwhelming multiple stressors, the person can be assisted to differentiate which stressors can be modified or eliminated (Edelman & Mandel, 2006).

## Ask the Person to List One or Two Changes They Would Like to Make in the Next Week.

Diet (eat one vegetable a day)

Exercise (walk one to two blocks each day)

**R:** In a person who is already overwhelmed, small changes in lifestyle may have a higher chance for success and will increase confidence (Bodenheimer, MacGregor, & Shariffi, 2005).

## If Sleep Disturbances Are Present, Refer to Insomnia.

Ask what activity brings them feelings of peace, joy and happiness. Ask them to incorporate one of these activities each week.

**R:** Persons overwhelmed usually deny themselves such activities. Leisure can break the stress cycle (Wells-Federman, 2000).

## If Spiritual Needs Are Identified as Deficient, Refer to Spiritual Distress.

Ask what is important, and if change is needed to include in life.

**R:** Values clarification assists the overwhelmed person to identify what is meaningful and valued and if it is present in their actual living habits (Edelman & Mandle, 2006).

## Assist the Person to Set Realistic Goals to Achieve a More Balanced Health-Promoting Lifestyle (Wells-Federman, 2000).

What is most important?

What aspects of your life would you like to change most?

What is the first step?

When?

**R:** Setting realistic goals with increase confidence and success (Bodenheimer, MacGregor, & Shariffi, 2005).

## Initiate Health Teaching and Referrals as Necessary.

If person is engaged in substance or alcohol abuse, refer for drug and alcohol abuse.

If person has severe depression or anxiety, refer for professional counseling.

If family functioning is disabled, refer for family counseling.

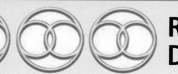

# RISK FOR SUDDEN INFANT DEATH SYNDROME

## DEFINITION

State in which an infant younger than 1 year old is at risk to experience sudden death, unexpected by history and unexplained by postmortem examination

## RISK FACTORS

No single risk factor. Several risk factors combined may be contributory (refer to Related Factors).

## RELATED FACTORS (MCMILLAN ET AL., 1999)

### Pathophysiologic

***Related to increased vulnerability secondary to:***

| | | |
|---|---|---|
| Cyanosis | Hypothermia | Fever |
| Poor feeding | Irritability | Respiratory distress |
| Tachycardia | Tachypnea | Low birth weight* |
| Small for gestational age* | Prematurity* | Low Apgar score (less than 7) |

History of diarrhea, vomiting, or listlessness 2 weeks before death

***Related to increased vulnerability secondary to prenatal maternal:***

| | | |
|---|---|---|
| Anemia* | Urinary tract infection | Poor weight gain |

Sexually transmitted infections
Situational (Personal, Environmental)

***Related to increased vulnerability secondary to maternal:***

| | | |
|---|---|---|
| Cigarette smoking* | Drug use during pregnancy | Lack of breastfeeding* |
| Inadequate prenatal care* | Low educational levels* | Single mother* |
| Multiparity with first | Young maternal age (less than 20)* | Young maternal age pregnancy* |

***Related to increased vulnerability secondary to:***

| | | |
|---|---|---|
| Crowded living conditions* | Sleeping on stomach* | Poor family financial status |
| Cold environment | Low socioeconomic status | |

***Related to increased vulnerability secondary to:***

| | | |
|---|---|---|
| Male gender* | Native Americans* | Multiple births |
| African Descent* | Previous sudden infant death syndrome (SIDS) death in family | |

## ■■■■■ ERRORS IN DIAGNOSTIC STATEMENTS

### Risk for Sudden Infant Death Syndrome related to low-income parents

Although poor living conditions have been linked to SIDS, the wording of this diagnosis is problematic. The following diagnosis would be more clinically useful: *Risk for Sudden Infant Death Syndrome related to insufficient knowledge of caregivers in causes and prevention of SIDS.*

## ■■■■■ KEY CONCEPTS

- SIDS is the leading single cause of death between 7 and 365 days of age (Hockenberry & Wilson, 2009).
- Incidence of SIDS has decreased approximately 40% since the American Academy of Pediatrics (AAP) advised sleeping position on the back for infants in 1996 (AAP, 2000).
- Although etiology is not known, autopsies show consistent pathologic findings as pulmonary edema and intrathoracic hemorrhages.
- There is no evidence that apnea monitors prevent SIDS (Sherratt, 1999).

*Widely accepted; general agreement among investigators.

## Focus Assessment Criteria

Refer to Related Factors.

NOC
Knowledge:
Maternal–Child
Health, Risk Control:
Tobacco Use, Risk
Control, Knowledge:
Infant Safety

## ➤ Goals

The caregiver will reduce or eliminate risk factors that are modifiable.

### *Indicators:*

- Position the infant on the back or side-lying.
- Eliminate smoking in the home, near the infant, and during pregnancy.
- Participate in prenatal and newborn medical care.
- Improve maternal health (e.g., treat anemia, promote optimal nutrition).
- Enroll in drug and alcohol programs, if indicated.

NIC
Teaching: Infant
Safety, Risk
Identification

## ➤ General Interventions

### Explain SIDS to Caregivers and Identify Risk Factors Present

**R:** The primary focus of nursing with parents caring for an infant at risk for SIDS is emotional support.

## Reduce or Eliminate Risk Factors That Can Be Modified

## Determine If Home Cardiorespiratory Monitoring Is Indicated; Consult With Pediatrician or Neonatal/Pediatric Nurse Practitioner (Hockenberry & Wilson, 2009)

Teach parents to focus on the infant when the alarm sounds, not on the machine.
Teach parents to assess:

- Infant's color (pink?)
- Infant's breathing

**R:** To help the family cope with the numerous procedures they must learn, adequate preparation before discharge is critical.

## Teach Environmental Practices to Reduce SIDS

Position infant on the back.
Avoid overheating the infant during sleep.
Avoid soft bedding (e.g., mattresses).
Avoid pillows.
Avoid sleeping with the infant (Anderson, 2000).
Avoid tobacco smoke.

**R:** Sleeping on the abdomen has been linked to SIDS (Hockenberry & Wilson, 2009).
**R:** Maternal smoking during pregnancy and exposure to smoke after birth has been associated with SIDS (American Academy of Pediatrics, 2000).

## Initiate Health Teaching and Referrals as Indicated

Provide instructions on use of the home monitor and CPR if appropriate.
Refer the client to drug and alcohol treatment programs as indicated.
Discuss strategies to stop smoking (refer to index—*smoking*).
Provide emergency numbers as indicated.
Refer to social agencies as indicated.

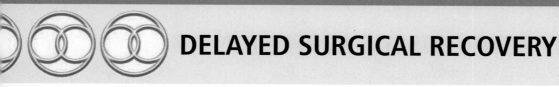

# DELAYED SURGICAL RECOVERY

## DEFINITION (NANDA)

Extension of the number of postoperative days required to initiate and perform self-care activities

■■■■■ **AUTHOR'S NOTE**

This recently accepted diagnosis represents a client who has not achieved recovery from a surgical procedure within the expected time. Based on the defining characteristics from NANDA, some confusion exists regarding the difference between defining characteristics (signs and symptoms) and related factors. A possible use of this diagnosis is as a Risk diagnosis. Persons who are high risk for *Delayed Surgical Recovery*, for example, the obese, those with diabetes mellitus, or cancer, could by identified. Interventions to prevent this state could be implemented. The diagnosis has not been developed sufficiently for clinical use. This author recommends using other nursing diagnoses, such as *Self-Care Deficit*, *Acute Pain*, or *Imbalanced Nutrition*.

## DEFINING CHARACTERISTICS (NANDA)

Postpones resumption of activities (home, work)
Requires help to complete self-care
Loss of appetite with or without nausea
Fatigue

Perceives that more time is needed to recover
Evidence of interrupted healing of surgical area
Difficulty moving about
Venous obstruction/pooling

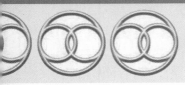

# INEFFECTIVE TISSUE PERFUSION

**Ineffective Tissue Perfusion**

Risk for Decreased Cardiac Tissue Perfusion
Risk for Ineffective Cerebral Tissue Perfusion
Risk for Ineffective Gastrointestinal Tissue Perfusion
Peripheral Tissue Perfusion, Ineffective
Renal Perfusion, Risk for Ineffective

## DEFINITION (NANDA)

Decrease in oxygen resulting in failure to nourish tissues at capillary level

### ■■■■■ AUTHOR'S NOTE

The use of any *Ineffective Tissue Perfusion* diagnosis other than *Peripheral* merely provides new labels for medical diagnoses, labels that do not describe the nursing focus or accountability.

NANDA approved the diagnosis *Ineffective Tissue Perfusion* in 1980. It does not conform to the NANDA definition approved in 1990 (refer to Chapter 2). When using these diagnoses, nurses cannot be accountable for prescribing the interventions for outcome achievement. Instead of using *Ineffective Tissue Perfusion*, the nurse should focus on the nursing diagnoses and collaborative problems applicable because of altered renal, cardiac, cerebral, pulmonary, or gastrointestinal (GI) tissue perfusion. Refer to Section 3 for specific collaborative problems for example: RC of Increased Intracranial Pressure, RC of GI Bleeding

*Ineffective Peripheral Tissue Perfusion* can be a clinically useful nursing diagnosis if used to describe chronic arterial or venous insufficiency or potential thrombophlebitis. (In contrast, acute embolism and thrombophlebitis represent collaborative problems.) A nurse focusing on preventing thrombophlebitis in a postoperative client would write the diagnosis *Risk for Ineffective Peripheral Tissue Perfusion related to postoperative immobility and dehydration*.

### ■■■■■ ERRORS IN DIAGNOSTIC STATEMENTS

1. *Ineffective GI Tissue Perfusion related to esophageal bleeding varices*
   Because this diagnosis actually represents a situation that nurses monitor and manage with nursing and medical interventions, the diagnosis should be rewritten as the collaborative problem *RC of Esophageal bleeding varices*.
2. *Ineffective Cerebral Tissue Perfusion related to cerebral edema secondary to intracranial infections*
   This diagnosis represents merely a new label for encephalitis, meningitis, or abscess. Instead, the nurse should specify collaborative problems to clearly describe and designate the nursing accountability: *RC of Increased intracranial pressure* and *RC of Septicemia*. In addition, certain nursing diagnoses may be indicated (e.g., *Risk for Infection Transmission, Impaired Comfort*).
3. *Ineffective Peripheral Tissue Perfusion related to deep vein thrombosis*
   Deep vein thrombosis is a medical diagnosis that evokes responses for which nurses are accountable: monitoring for and managing, with physician- and nurse-prescribed interventions, physiologic complications (e.g., embolism, venous ulcers). This situation would be represented by collaborative problems such as *RC of Embolism*. In addition, the nurse would intervene independently to prevent complications of immobility and teach how to prevent recurrence, applying nursing diagnoses such as *Disuse Syndrome* and *Risk for Ineffective Health Maintenance related to insufficient knowledge of risk factors*.

# RISK FOR DECREASED CARDIAC TISSUE PERFUSION

## DEFINITION (NANDA)

At risk for a decrease in cardiac tissue perfusion.

## RISK FACTORS (NANDA)

Birth Control Pills (medication side effect of combination pills)*
Cardiac Surgery (treatment)
Cardiac Tamponade (clinical emergency)
Coronary artery spasm (clinical emergency)
Diabetes mellitus (medical diagnosis with multiple complications with associated modifiable risk lifestyles)
Drug abuse (clinical situations with multiple complications)
Elevated C-reactive protein (positive laboratory test)
Family history of coronary artery disease (factor with associated modifiable risk lifestyles)
Hyperlipidemia (medical diagnosis with associated modifiable risk lifestyles)
Hypertension (medical diagnosis with multiple complications with associated modifiable risk lifestyles)
Hypoxemia (complication)
Hypovolemia (complication)
Hypoxia (complication)
Lack of knowledge of modifiable risk factors (e.g. smoking, sedentary lifestyle, obesity)
(These relate to nursing diagnoses of Risk Prone Health Behavior and/or Ineffective Self-Health Management)

## ■■■■■■ ▶ AUTHOR'S NOTE

This new NANDA-I nursing diagnosis represents a collection of risk factors that have very different clinical implications. Some have a collection of physiological complications that are related to the situation and can be labeled as Risk for Complications of Cardiac Surgery, RC of Acute Coronary Syndrome, RC of Diabetes Mellitus. Some are single complications as RC of Hypovolemia and RC of Hypoxia

For example, Risk for Complications of Cocaine Abuse would describe monitoring and management of complications as cardiac/vascular shock, seizures, coma, respiratory insufficiency, stroke and hyperpyrexia. These are different for Risk for Complications of Alcohol Abuse would describe the monitoring and management of complications of delirium tremors, seizures, autonomic hyperactivity, hypovolemia, hypoglycemia. alcohol hallucinosis and cardio/vascular shock.

Some are medical emergencies as cardiac tamponade, coronary artery spasm or occlusion, which have protocols for medical interventions.

Birth control pills can have a side effects of nausea, breast discomforts, elevated blood pressure and adverse events as cardio-vascular or cerebral thrombus, using a nursing diagnosis as Risk for Decreased Cardiac Perfusion to describe one adverse event is not clinically usefully. If a diagnosis is needed for this clinical situation, use Risk for Complications of Medication Therapy Adverse Effects, specifically Risk for Complications of Oral Combination Contraception Therapy.

---

*Text in parentheses has been added by author.

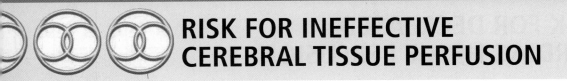

# RISK FOR INEFFECTIVE CEREBRAL TISSUE PERFUSION

## DEFINITION

The state in which an individual is at risk for a decrease in cerebral tissue circulation

## RISK FACTORS

Abnormal partial thromboplastin time
Akinetic left ventricular segment
Arterial dissection
Atrial myxoma
Carotid stenosis
Coagulopathies (e,g, sickle cell anemia)
Disseminated intravascular coagulation
Head trauma
Hypertension
Left Atrial appendage thrombosis
Mitral stenosis
Recent Myocardial infarction
Substance abuse
Treatment-related side effects
    (cardiopulmonary bypass, medications)

Abnormal Prothrombin time
Aortic atherosclerosis
Atrial fibrillation
Brain Tumor
Cerebral aneurysm
Dilated Cardiomyopathy
Embolism
Hypercholesterolemia
Endocardiitis
Mechanical prosthetic valve
Neoplasm of the brain
Sick sinus syndrome
Thrombolytic Therapy

■■■■■■ **AUTHOR'S NOTE**

This newly Accepted NANDA-I nursing diagnosis represents a collection of risk factors that have very different clinical implications. Some are physiological complications that are related to a medical diagnosis or treatment and can be labeled as Risk for Complications of Head Trauma, RC of Brain Tumor, or RC of Thrombolytic Therapy. These clinical situations have both nursing diagnoses and collaborative problems that require interventions.

   For example Risk for Complications of Cranial Surgery would have the following collaborative problems:

* RC of Increase Intracranial Pressure
* RC of Hemorrhage, Hypovolemia/shock,
* RC of Thromboembolism
* RC of Cranial nerve dysfunction
* RC of Cardiac Dysrhythmias
* RC of Seizures
* RC of Sensory/Motor Alterations

Nursing diagnoses associated with this clinical situation:*
Anxiety to impending surgery and fear of outcomes
Acute Pain related to compression /displacement of brain tissue and increased intracranial pressure
Risk for Ineffective Self Heath Management Related to Insufficient Knowledge of wound care signs and symptoms of complications, restrictions ands follow-up care.

---

*For more specific care plans with nursing interventions/rationales and outcomes for clinical situations (Medical Diagnoses e.g. Acute Coronary Syndrome, Hypertension, Stroke, Surgical Procedures e.g. Coronary Bypass Surgery, Therapies Treatments e.g. Anticoagulant Therapy, Pacemaker Insertion and 70 other situations refer to Carpenito-Moyet, L.J. (2009). *Nursing Care Plans and Documentation* (5th ed.). Philadelphia: Lippincott, Williams & Wilkins.

## Interventions/Goals

Refer to section 3 for specific collaborative problems under Risk for Complications of Neurologic Dysfunction

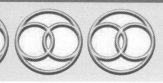

# RISK FOR INEFFECTIVE GASTROINTESTINAL TISSUE PERFUSION

## DEFINITION (NANDA)

At risk for decrease in gastrointestinal circulation

## RISK FACTORS (NANDA)

Abdominal aortic aneurysm
Abnormal partial thromboplastin time
Acute Gastrointestinal bleed
Age greater than 60 years
Coagulopathies (e.g. sickle cell anemia)
Disseminated intravascular coagulation
Gastric Paresis (e.g. diabetes mellitus) gastric ulcer, ischemic colitis, ischemic pancreatitis)
Hemodynamic instability
Myocardial infarction
Treatment-related side effects (e.g., cardiopulmonary bypass, medications, anesthesia, gastric surgery)

Abdominal compartment Syndrome
Abnormal Prothrombin time
Acute gastrointestinal hemorrhage
Anemia
Diabetes Mellitus
Female gender
Gastrointestinal disease (e.g. duodenal or
Liver Dysfunction
Poor left ventricular performance
Stroke
Renal failure
Vascular Disease (e.g., peripheral vascular disease, aortoiliac occlusive disease)

### ■■■■■ AUTHOR'S NOTE

This diagnosis is too general for clinical use because it represents a variety of physiological complications related to GI perfusion. These complications are collaborative problems and should be separated to more specific complications as:

* RC of GI Bleeding
* RC of Paralytic Ileus
* RC of Hypovolemia/Shock

## Interventions/Goals

Refer to Section 3 for interventions/rationale and goals for Risk for Complications of GI Bleeding or Paralytic Ileus or Hypovolemia/Shock.

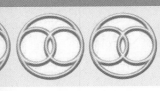

# INEFFECTIVE PERIPHERAL TISSUE PERFUSION

## DEFINITION

State in which a person experiences or is at risk of experiencing a decrease in nutrition and respiration at the peripheral cellular level because of a decrease in capillary blood supply

## DEFINING CHARACTERISTICS

### Major (Must Be Present, One or More)

Presence of one of the following types (see Key Concepts for definitions):

| | |
|---|---|
| Claudication (arterial) | Aching pain (arterial or venous) |
| Rest pain (arterial) | Diminished or absent arterial pulses (arterial) |
| Skin color changes | Pallor (arterial) |
| Reactive hyperemia (arterial) | Cyanosis (venous) |
| Skin temperature changes | Cooler (arterial) |
| Warmer (venous) | Decreased blood pressure (arterial) |
| Capillary refill longer than 3 s (arterial) | |

### Minor (May Be Present)

| | |
|---|---|
| Edema (venous) | Change in sensory function (arterial) |
| Change in motor function (arterial) | Trophic tissue changes (arterial) |
| Hard, thick nails | |
| Loss of hair | |
| Nonhealing wound | |

## RELATED FACTORS

### Pathophysiologic

*Related to compromised blood flow secondary to:*

Vascular disorders

| | | |
|---|---|---|
| Arteriosclerosis | Leriche's syndrome | Venous hypertension |
| Raynaud's disease/syndrome | Aneurysm | Varicosities |
| Arterial thrombosis | Buerger's disease | Deep vein thrombosis |
| Sickle cell crisis | Collagen vascular disease | Cirrhosis |
| Rheumatoid arthritis | Alcoholism | |

Diabetes mellitus
Hypotension
Blood dyscrasias
Renal failure
Cancer/tumor

### Treatment-Related

*Related to immobilization*
*Related to presence of invasive lines*
*Related to pressure sites/constriction (elastic compression bandages, stockings, restraints)*
*Related to blood vessel trauma or compression*

### Situational (Personal, Environmental)

*Related to pressure of enlarging uterus on pelvic vessels*

*Related to pressure of enlarged abdomen on pelvic vessels*

*Related to vasoconstricting effects of tobacco*

*Related to decreased circulating volume secondary to dehydration*

*Related to dependent venous pooling*

*Related to hypothermia*

*Related to pressure of muscle mass secondary to weight lifting*

## ▪▪▪▪▪▪ AUTHOR'S NOTE

See *Ineffective Peripheral Tissue Perfusion.*

## ▪▪▪▪▪▪ ERRORS IN DIAGNOSTIC STATEMENTS

See *Ineffective Peripheral Tissue Perfusion.*

## ▪▪▪▪▪▪ KEY CONCEPTS

### Generic Considerations

- Adequate cellular oxygenation depends on the following processes (Porth, 2007):
  - The ability of the lungs to exchange air adequately ($O_2$–$CO_2$)
  - The ability of the pulmonary alveoli to diffuse oxygen and carbon dioxide across the cell membrane to the blood
  - The ability of the red blood cells (hemoglobin) to carry oxygen
  - The ability of the heart to pump with enough force to deliver the blood to the microcirculation
  - The ability of intact blood vessels to deliver blood to the microcirculation
- Hypoxemia (decreased oxygen content of the blood) results in cellular hypoxia, which causes cellular swelling and contributes to tissue injury.
- *Arterial* blood flow is enhanced by a *dependent* position and inhibited by an *elevated* position. (Gravity pulls blood downward, away from the heart.)
- When an alteration in peripheral tissue perfusion exists, the nurse must consider its nature. The two major components of the peripheral vascular system are the arterial and the venous systems. Signs, symptoms, etiology, and nursing interventions are different for problems in each of these two systems and therefore are addressed separately.
- Changes in arterial walls increase the incidence of stroke and coronary artery disease (Porth, 2006).
- High levels of circulating lipids increase the risk of coronary heart disease, peripheral vascular disease, and stroke (Porth, 2007).

 **Geriatric Considerations**

- Age-related vascular changes include stiffened blood vessels, which cause increased peripheral resistance, impaired baroreceptor functioning, and diminished ability to increase organ blood flow (Miller, 2009). These age-related changes cause the veins to become more dilated and less elastic. Valves of the large leg veins become less efficient. Age-related reductions in muscle mass and inactivity further reduce peripheral circulation (Miller, 2009).
- Physical deconditioning or lack of exercise accentuates the functional consequences of age-related cardiovascular changes. Contributing factors to deconditioning include acute illness, mobility limitations, cardiac disease, depression, and lack of motivation (Miller, 2009).

## Focus Assessment Criteria

See Tables II.17 and II.18.

### TABLE II.17 ARTERIAL INSUFFICIENCY VS VENOUS INSUFFICIENCY: A COMPARISON OF SUBJECTIVE DATA

| Symptom | Arterial Insufficiency | Venous Insufficiency |
|---|---|---|
| **Pain** | | |
| Location | Feet, muscles of legs, toes | Ankles, lower legs |
| Quality | Burning, shocking, prickling, throbbing, cramping, sharp | Aching, tightness |
| Quantity | Increase in severity with increased muscle activity or elevation | Varies with fluid intake, use of support hose, and decreased muscle activity |
| Chronology | Brought on predictably by exercise | Greater in evening than in morning |
| Setting | Use of affected muscle groups | Increases during course of day with prolonged standing or sitting |
| Aggravating factors | Exercise<br>Extremity elevation | Immobility<br>Extremity dependence |
| Alleviating factors | Cessation of exercise<br>Extremity dependence | Extremity elevation<br>Compression stockings or Ace wraps |
| **Paresthesia** | Numbness, tingling, burning, decreased touch sensation | No change unless arterial system or nerves are affected |

### TABLE II.18 ARTERIAL INSUFFICIENCY VS VENOUS INSUFFICIENCY: A COMPARISON OF OBJECTIVE DATA

| Sign | Arterial Insufficiency | Venous Insufficiency |
|---|---|---|
| Temperature | Cool skin | Warm skin |
| Color | Pale on elevation, dependent rubor (reactive hyperemia) | Flushed, cyanotic<br>Typical brown discoloration around ankles |
| Capillary filling | greater than 3 seconds | Nonapplicable |
| Pulses | Absent or weak | Present unless there is concomitant arterial disease, or edema may obscure them |
| Movement | Decreased motor ability with nerve and muscle ischemia | Motor ability unchanged unless edema is severe enough to restrict joint mobility |
| Ulceration | Occurs on foot at site of trauma or at tips of toes (most distal to be perfused)<br>Ulcers are deep with well-defined margins<br>Surrounding tissue is shiny and taut with thin skin | Occurs around ankle (area of greatest pressure from chronic venous stasis due to valvular incompetence)<br>Ulcers shallow with irregular edges<br>Surrounding tissue edematous with engorged veins |

## Subjective Data

### Assess for Defining Characteristics.

Pain (associated with, time of day)          Pallor, cyanosis, paresthesias
Temperature change                           Change in motor function

### Assess for Related Factors.

**Medical History**
See Related Factors.

**Risk Factors**
Smoking (never, quit, years)
Immobility
History of phlebitis
Sedentary lifestyle

Family history of heart disease, vascular disease, stroke, kidney disease, or diabetes mellitus
Stress

**Medications**
Type     Side effects     Dosage

## Objective Data

### *Assess for Defining Characteristics.*

Skin
Temperature (cool, warm)
Color (pale, dependent rubor, flushed, cyanotic, brown discolorations)
Ulcerations (size, location, description of surrounding tissue)
Bilateral pulses (radial, femoral popliteal, posterior tibial, dorsalis pedis)

| | |
|---|---|
| Rate, rhythm | Weak |
| Volume | Normal, easily palpable |
| Absent, nonpalpable | Aneurysmal |

Paresthesia (numbness, tingling, burning)
Edema (location, pitting)
Capillary refill (normal less than 3 seconds)
Motor ability (normal, compromised)
For more information on Focus Assessment Criteria, visit http://thepoint.lww.com.

**NOC** ➤

Sensory Functions;
Cutaneous, Tissue
Integrity, Tissue
perfusion: Peripheral

## Goal

The individual will report a decrease in pain.

### *Indicators:*

• Define peripheral vascular problem in own words.
• Identify factors that improve peripheral circulation.
• Identify necessary lifestyle changes.
• Identify medical regimen, diet, medications, activities that promote vasodilation.
• Identify factors that inhibit peripheral circulation.
• State when to contact physician or health care professional.

**NIC** ➤

Peripheral Sensation
management,
Circulatory Care:
Venous Insufficiency,
Circulatory Care:
Arterial Insufficiency,
Positioning, Exercise
Promotion

## General Interventions

### Assess Causative and Contributing Factors.

Underlying disease     Inhibited arterial blood flow
Inhibited venous blood flow     Fluid volume excess or deficit
Hypothermia or vasoconstriction          Activities related to symptom/sign onset

### Promote Factors that Improve Arterial Blood Flow.

Keep extremity in a dependent position.

**R:** *Arterial* blood flow is enhanced by a *dependent* position and inhibited by an *elevated* position (gravity pulls blood downward, away from the heart).

Keep extremity warm (do not use heating pad or hot water bottle,

**R:** Peripheral vascular disease will reduce sensitivity. The person will not be able to determine if the temperature is hot enough to damage tissue; the use of external heat also may increase the metabolic demands of the tissue beyond its capacity.

Reduce risk for trauma:

• Change positions at least every hour.
• Avoid leg crossing.

- Reduce external pressure points (inspect shoes daily for rough lining).
- Avoid sheepskin heel protectors (they increase heel pressure and pressure across dorsum of foot).
- Encourage range-of-motion exercises.
- Discuss smoking cessation (see *Ineffective Health Maintenance Related to Tobacco Use*).

**R:** Cellular nutrition and function depend on adequate blood flow through the microcirculation

**R:** Tight garments and certain leg positions constrict leg vessels, further reducing circulation.

## Promote Factors that Improve Venous Blood Flow.

Elevate extremity above the level of the heart (may be contraindicated if severe cardiac or respiratory disease is present).

**R:** *Venous* blood flow is enhanced by an *elevated* position and inhibited by a *dependent* position. (Gravity pulls blood downward, away from the heart.)

Avoid standing or sitting with legs dependent for long periods.

Consider the use of elastic compression stockings.

**R:** Compression stockings increase venous return and the rate of venous flow and decrease venous pooling

Teach to:

- Avoid pillows behind the knees or Gatch bed, which is elevated at the knees.
- Avoid leg crossing.
- Change positions, move extremities, or wiggle fingers and toes every hour.
- Avoid garters and tight elastic stockings above the knees.
- Measure baseline circumference of calves and thighs if person is at risk for deep venous thrombosis, or if it is suspected.

**R:** Reduce or remove external venous compression that impedes venous flow.

## Plan a Daily Walking Program.

Refer to *Sedentary Lifestyle* for specific interventions

## *Initiate Health Teaching, as Indicated.*

**Teach Client to**

Avoid long car or plane rides (get up and walk around at least every hour).

Keep dry skin lubricated (cracked skin eliminates the physical barrier to infection).

Wear warm clothing during cold weather.

Wear cotton or wool socks.

Use gloves or mittens if hands are exposed to cold (including home freezers).

Avoid dehydration in warm weather.

**R:** These measures can increase circulation and prevent injuries

Give special attention to feet and toes:

- Wash feet and dry well daily.
- Do not soak feet.
- Avoid harsh soaps or chemicals (including iodine) on feet.
- Keep nails trimmed and filed smooth.

Inspect feet and legs daily for injuries and pressure points.

Wear clean socks.

Wear shoes that offer support and fit comfortably.

Inspect the inside of shoes daily for rough lining.

**R:** Daily foot care can reduce tissue damage and help prevent or detect early further reducing circulation.

**Explain the Relation of Certain Risk Factors to the Development of Atherosclerosis.**

*Smoking*

Vasoconstriction        Elevated blood pressure
Decreased oxygenation of the blood        Increased lipidemia
Increased platelet aggregation

**R:** The effects of nicotine on the cardiovascular system contribute to coronary artery disease, stroke, hypertension, and peripheral vascular disease (Porth, 2006).

*Hypertension/Hyperlipidemia*

**R:** Constant increased pressure causes damage to the vessel lining, which promotes plaque formation and narrowing. *Hyperlipidemia* promotes atherosclerosis

*Sedentary lifestyle*

**R:** Inactivity decreases muscle tone and strength and decreases circulation

*Excess weight (greater than 10% of ideal)*

**R:** Obesity increases peripheral resistance and venous pooling, excess weight increases cardiac workload, causing hypertension (Porth, 2006).

Refer to community resources for lifestyle changes.

**R:** Community resources can assist the client with weight loss, smoking cessation, diet, and exercise programs.

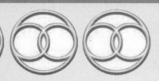

# RISK FOR PERIPHERAL NEUROVASCULAR DYSFUNCTION

## ▶ Risk for Complications of Compartment Syndrome

## DEFINITION

State in which a person is at risk of experiencing a disruption in circulation, sensation, or motion of an extremity

## RISK FACTORS

### Pathophysiologic

*Related to increased volume of (specify extremity) secondary to:*

| | | |
|---|---|---|
| Bleeding (e.g., trauma, fractures) | Arterial obstruction | Coagulation disorder |
| | Venous obstruction/pooling | |

*Related to increased capillary filtration secondary to:*

| | | |
|---|---|---|
| Allergic response (e.g., insect bites) | Frostbite | Hypothermia |
| | Trauma | Nephrotic syndrome |
| Severe burns (thermal, electrical) | Venomous bites (e.g., snake) | |

*Related to restrictive envelope secondary to Circumferential burns*

### Treatment-Related

*Related to increased capillary filtration secondary to:*

Total knee replacement        Total hip replacement

*Related to restrictive envelope secondary to:*

| | | |
|---|---|---|
| Tourniquet | Antishock trousers | Circumferential dressings |
| Ace wraps | Excessive traction | Cast |
| Brace | Air splints | Premature or tight closure of fascial defects |
| Restraints | | |

## ◼◼◼◼◼◼ AUTHOR'S NOTE

This diagnosis represents a situation that nurses can prevent complications by identifying who is at risk and implementing measures to reduce or eliminate causative or contributing factors. *Risk for Peripheral Neurovascular Dysfunction* can change to compartment syndrome. *RC of Compartment Syndrome* is inadequate tissue perfusion in a muscle, usually an arm or leg, caused by edema, which obstructs venous and arterial flow and compresses nerves. The nursing focus for compartment syndrome is diagnosing early signs and symptoms and notifying the physician. The medical interventions required to abate the problem are surgical, such as evacuation of hematoma, repair of damaged vessels, or fasciotomy. Refer to *RC of Compartment Syndrome in Section 3 for specific interventions for either diagnosis.* Students should consult with their faculty for direction to use either *Risk for Peripheral Vascular Dysfunction* or *RC of Compartment Syndrome.*

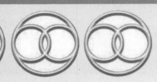

# RISK FOR INEFFECTIVE RENAL PERFUSION

## DEFINITION (NANDA)

At risk for a decrease in blood circulation to the kidney that may compromise health

## RISK FACTORS (NANDA)

| | | |
|---|---|---|
| Abdominal compartment syndrome | Advance age | Bilateral cortical necrosis |
| Burns | Cardiac surgery | Cardiopulmonary bypass |
| Diabetes mellitus | Exposure to toxins | Female glomerulonephritis |
| Hyperlipidemia | Hypertension | Hypovolemia |
| Hypoxemia | Hypoxia | Infection |
| Malignancy | Malignant Hypertension | Metabolic acidosis |
| Multitrauma | Polynephritis | Renal artery stenosis |
| Renal disease (polycystic kidney) | Smoking | |

Systemic inflammatory response syndrome
Treatment-related side effects (e.g. medications)
Vascular embolism vasculitis

## ◼◼◼◼◼◼ AUTHOR'S NOTE

This NANDA-I diagnosis represents a potential complication which is a collaborative problem, Risk for Complications of Renal Insufficiency

If the situation is a medical diagnosis of Acute Kidney Failure or Chronic Renal Disease, Using, Risk for Complications of Acute Kidney Failure would include the following collaborative problems:*

*(continued)*

---

*For a more specific care plans with nursing interventions /rationales and outcomes for clinical situations (medical diagnoses e.g. Chronic Renal Disease, Acute Kidney Failure, surgical procedures, e.g. Nephrectomy, Treatments/procedures e.g. Hemodialysis, Peritoneal Dialysis and 70 other clinical situations, refer to Carpenito-Moyet, L.J. (2009). *Nursing Care Plans and Documentation* (5th ed.). Philadelphia: Lippincott, Williams & Wilkins.

■■■■■■ **AUTHOR'S NOTE** *Continued*

- RC of Fluid Overload
- RC of Metabolic Acidosis
- RC of Acute Albuminemia
- RC of Hypertension
- RC of Pulmonary Edema
- RC of Dysrhythmias
- RC of Gastrointestinal bleeding

Nursing diagnoses associated with this clinical situation:

- Risk for Infection related to invasive procedures
- Imbalanced Nutrition: Less that Body Requirements related to anorexia, nausea, vomiting, loss of taste, loss of smell, stomatitis and dietary restrictions
- Risk for Impaired Tissue Integrity related to retention of metabolic wastes, increased capillary fragility and platelet dysfunction.

## Interventions/Goals

Refer to section 3 for interventions/goal for Risk for Complications of Renal insufficiency
Refer to Section 2 for interventions and goals for specific related nursing diagnoses.

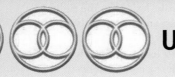

# UNILATERAL NEGLECT

## DEFINITION

State in which a client is unable to attend to or "ignores" the hemiplegic side of the body and/or, on the affected side, objects, persons, or sounds in the environment

## DEFINING CHARACTERISTICS

### Major (Must Be Present, One or More)

Neglect of involved body parts and/or extrapersonal space (hemispatial neglect), and/or
Denial of the existence of the affected limb or side of body (anosognosia)

### Minor (May Be Present)

Difficulty with spatial–perceptual tasks
Hemiplegia (usually of the left side)

## RELATED FACTORS

### Pathophysiologic

Related to the impaired perceptual abilities secondary to:
Cerebrovascular accident    Brain injury/trauma
Cerebral aneurysms    Cerebral tumors

■■■■■■ **AUTHOR'S NOTE**

*Unilateral Neglect* represents a disturbance in the reciprocal loop that occurs most often in the right hemisphere of the brain. This diagnosis also could be viewed as a syndrome diagnosis, *Unilateral Neglect Syndrome*. As mentioned in Chapter 3, syndrome diagnoses encompass a cluster of nursing diagnoses related to the situation. The nursing interventions for *Unilateral Neglect Syndrome* would focus on *Self-Care Deficit*, *Anxiety*, and *Risk for Injury*.

■■■■■■ **ERRORS IN DIAGNOSTIC STATEMENTS**

### Unilateral Neglect related to lack of grooming and hygiene for right side of face, head, and right arm

Lack of grooming on one side of the body can be an indicator of *Unilateral Neglect* if neurologic disease or damage is present; it is not a related factor. When writing the diagnostic statement, the nurse should ask, "How does the nurse treat unilateral neglect?" Because the nursing focus is on teaching adaptive techniques, phrasing the diagnosis *Unilateral Neglect related to lack of knowledge of adaptive techniques* would be appropriate. If *Unilateral Neglect* were viewed as a syndrome diagnosis, the appropriate diagnostic statement would be *Unilateral Neglect Syndrome*. No "related to" is needed with a syndrome diagnosis because the label includes the etiology. The interventions would have the same focus, reducing neglect by using adaptive techniques.

■■■■■■ **KEY CONCEPTS**

### Generic Considerations

- Unilateral neglect is also called hemi-inattention, unilateral asomatognosia (unilateral spatial agnosia, Anton-Babinski syndrome), anosognosia, and atopognosia.
- The most common cause of unilateral neglect is right hemispheric brain damage; primarily, lesions in the right parietal lobe cause this defect. Lesions of the frontal lobe, inferior parietal lobe, thalamus, and striatum also can cause unilateral neglect (Lin, 1996; Katz et al., 2000).
- The right parietal lobe attends to stimuli presented to both the right and left sides; with a lesion of the left parietal lobe, the right parietal lobe could continue attending to the ipsilateral (same side) or contralateral (right-sided) stimuli. Because the left parietal lobe cannot attend to ipsilateral stimuli as well as the right parietal lobe can, however, lesions of the right parietal lobe are more likely to induce a profound contralateral sensory inattention than lesions of the left parietal lobe (Porth, 2007).
- Unilateral neglect is characterized by an unawareness or denial of the affected half of the body, often extending to the extrapersonal space. It can improve after a stroke. Complete recovery did occur in 13% of studied subjects.
- Homonymous hemianopsia (loss of vision on the contralateral side) usually occurs with unilateral neglect. Unilateral neglect and hemianopsia are two separate phenomena, and either can be present without the other. When they occur together, the client has more difficulty compensating for the loss (Porth, 2006).
- Anosognosia (ignorance of paralysis) and dressing apraxia may occur in lesions of either hemisphere but have been observed more frequently in lesions of the nondominant hemisphere.
- The client with a parietal lobe injury demonstrates problems with body schema, spatial judgment, and sensory interpretation.
- In addition, the client with this type of brain injury may exhibit some or all of the following characteristics that complicate the neglect syndrome:
  - Impulsiveness
  - Short attention span
  - Lack of insight into the extent of the disability
  - Diminished learning skills
  - Inability to recognize faces
  - Decrease in concrete thinking
  - Confusion

*(continued)*

■■■■■■ **KEY CONCEPTS** *Continued*

- Prognosis for recovery from many of the behavioral abnormalities associated with right hemisphere stroke is more favorable after hemorrhage as opposed to after infarction (Lin, 1996).
- Early recognition of the existence and extent of these syndromes allows more accurate planning of goals.

### Pediatric Considerations

Children at greatest risk for development of unilateral neglect are those with acquired hemiplegia (e.g., from stroke). Strokes may occur in children with congenital heart disease, sickle cell anemia, meningitis, or head trauma.

### Geriatric Considerations

Most people who experience unilateral neglect are older adults, simply because the incidence of stroke is greatest in this population.

## Focus Assessment Criteria

### Subjective and Objective Data

#### *Assess for Defining Characteristics*

**Client's Perception of the Problem**

**Effects on Activities of Daily Living (ADLs)**
Bathing, grooming, and hygiene—does the client:

Wash the affected side of the body?                 Put dentures in straight?
Shave both sides of the face?                       Comb only part of the hair?
Brush all his or her teeth?                         Apply makeup to both sides of face?
Put eyeglasses on straight?

Feeding—does the client:
Pocket food on the affected side of the mouth?
Eat only half of his or her food (i.e., eat only food on the unaffected side of the plate/tray)?

Dressing—does the client:
Dress the affected limbs?

Mobility/positioning:
When sitting in a wheelchair, does the client lean or tilt toward the unaffected side?
Does the affected arm dangle off the lapboard?
Are the head and eyes turned toward the unaffected side?
When propelling the wheelchair or when ambulating, does the client bump or run into objects on the affected side?

Safety—does the client:
Attempt to walk or transfer out of the chair or bed when unable to ambulate?
Have sensation in the affected limbs?
Frequently injure the affected arm or hand (cuts, bumps, bruises)?
Feel pain when injured?
Realize when injury occurs?
Scan the entire visual field?
Turn the head to the affected side to compensate?
Respond to stimuli presented from the affected side?
Does the affected arm dangle at the side and get caught in the wheelchair spokes, side rails, doorways, and so forth?

For more information on Focus Assessment Criteria, visit http://thepoint.lww.com.

**NOC**
Body Image, Self-
Care Assistance

## ► Goal

The client will demonstrate an ability to scan the visual field to compensate for loss of function/sensation in affected limbs.

### Indicators:

- Identify safety hazards in the environment.
- Describe the deficit and the rationale for treatment.

**NIC**
Unilateral Neglect
Management, Self-
Care Assistance

## ► General Interventions

### Consult With a Neuropsychologist, Physical Therapist, Occupational Therapist, and a Nurse Rehabilitation Specialist to Create a Multidisciplinary Plan with and for the Client

**R:** Treatment for unilateral neglect must be multidisciplinary.

## Assist the Client to Recognize the Perceptual Deficit

Initially adapt the environment to the deficit:

- Position the client, call light, bedside stand, television, telephone, and personal items on the unaffected side.
- Position the bed with the unaffected side toward the door.
- Approach and speak to the client from the unaffected side.
- If you must approach the client from the affected side, announce your presence as soon as you enter the room to avoid startling the client.
- When working with the client's affected extremity, position the unaffected side near a wall to minimize distractions.

Gradually change the client's environment as you teach him or her to compensate and to learn to recognize the forgotten field; move furniture and personal items out of the visual field.

Provide a simplified, well-lit, uncluttered environment:

- Provide a moment between activities.
- Provide concrete cues: "You are on your side facing the wall."

Provide a full-length mirror to help with vertical orientation and to diminish the distortion of the vertical and horizontal plane, which manifests itself in the client leaning toward the affected side.

Use verbal instructions rather than mere demonstrations. Keep instructions simple.

For a client in a wheelchair, obtain a lapboard (preferably Plexiglas); position the affected arm on the lapboard with the fingertips at midline. Encourage the client to look for the arm on the board.

For an ambulatory client, obtain an arm sling to prevent the arm from dangling and causing shoulder subluxation.

When the client is in bed, elevate the affected arm on a pillow to prevent dependent edema.

Constantly cue to the environment.

Encourage the client to wear a watch, favorite ring, or bracelet on affected arm to draw attention to it.

**R:** Strategies are provided to stimulate the individual to focus on the affected side.

## Assist the Client with Adaptations Needed for Self-Care and Other ADLs

### Encourage the Client to Wear Prescribed Corrective Lenses or Hearing Aids

### For Bathing, Dressing, and Toileting:

Instruct the client to attend to the affected extremity side first when performing ADLs.

Instruct the client always to look for the affected extremity when performing ADLs, to know where it is at all times.

Teach the client to dress and groom in front of a mirror.

Suggest using color-coded markers sewn or placed inside shoes or clothes to help distinguish right from left.

Encourage the client to integrate affected extremity during bathing and to feel extremity by rubbing and massaging it.

Use adaptive equipment as appropriate.

Refer to *Self-Care Deficit* for additional interventions.

### For Feeding:

Set up meals with a minimum of dishes, food, and utensils.

Instruct the client to eat in small amounts and place food on unaffected side of mouth.

Instruct the client to use the tongue to sweep out "pockets" of food from the affected side after every bite.

After meals/medications, check oral cavity for pocketed food/medication.

Provide oral care t.i.d. and PRN.

Initially place food in the client's visual field; gradually move the food out of the field and teach the client to scan entire visual field.

Use adaptive feeding equipment as appropriate.

Refer to *Self-Care Deficit: Feeding* for additional interventions.

Refer to *Imbalanced Nutrition: Less than Body Requirements related to swallowing difficulties* if the client has difficulty chewing and swallowing food.

**R:** Adapting the environment minimizes sensory deprivation. Initially, however, attempts should be made to have the client attend to both sides.

**R:** Reminders can help the client adapt to the environment.

## Teach Measures to Prevent Injury

Ensure a clutter-free, well-lighted environment.

## Retrain the Client to Scan Entire Environment

Instruct the client to turn the head past midline to view the scene on the affected side.

Perform activities that require turning the head.

Remind the client to scan when ambulating or propelling a wheelchair.

**R:** Scanning can help prevent injury and increase awareness of entire space.

## Use Tactile Sensation to Reintroduce Affected Arm/Extremity to the Client

Have the client stroke the involved side with the uninvolved hand and watch the arm or leg while stroking it.

Rub different-textured materials to stimulate sensations (hot, cold, rough, soft).

**R:** Cognitive impairments if present can compromise judgment and increase the risk of injury (Katz et al., 2000).

## Instruct the Client to Keep the Affected Arm and/or Leg in View

Position the arm on the lapboard. (Plexiglas lapboards allow the client to view the affected leg, thereby helping to integrate the leg into the body schema.)

Provide an arm sling for an ambulatory client.

Instruct the client to take extra care around sources of heat or cold and moving machinery or parts to protect the affected side from injury.

R: Decreased sensation or motor function increases the vulnerability to injury.

## Initiate Health Teaching and Referrals

Ensure that both the client and family understand the cause of unilateral neglect and the purpose of and rationale for all interventions.

Proceed with teaching as needed.

Explain unilateral neglect.

Instruct the family on how to facilitate the client's relearning techniques (e.g., cueing, scanning visual field).

Teach use of adaptive equipment, if appropriate.

Teach principles of maintaining a safe environment.

**R:** Strategies to improve unilateral neglect and to prevent injury must be ongoing at home.

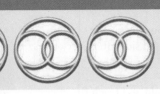

# IMPAIRED URINARY ELIMINATION

**Impaired Urinary Elimination**

Maturational Enuresis*
Functional Incontinence
Reflex Incontinence
Stress Incontinence
Continuous Incontinence
Urge Incontinence
Overflow Incontinence

## DEFINITION

State in which a person experiences or is at risk of experiencing urinary elimination dysfunction

## DEFINING CHARACTERISTICS

### Major (Must Be Present, One or More)

*Reports or experiences a urinary elimination problem, such as:*

| | | |
|---|---|---|
| Urgency | Dribbling | Frequency |
| Bladder distention | Hesitancy | Large residual urine volumes |
| Nocturia | Incontinence | Enuresis |

## RELATED FACTORS

### Pathophysiologic

*Related to incompetent bladder outlet secondary to congenital urinary tract anomalies*

*Related to decreased bladder capacity or irritation to bladder secondary to:*

| | | |
|---|---|---|
| Infection | Glucosuria | Trauma |
| Carcinoma | Urethritis | |

*Related to diminished bladder cues or impaired ability to recognize bladder cues secondary to:*

| | | |
|---|---|---|
| Cord injury/tumor/infection | Diabetic neuropathy | Brain injury/tumor/infection |
| Alcoholic neuropathy | Cerebrovascular accident | Tabes dorsalis |
| Demyelinating diseases | Parkinsonism | Multiple sclerosis |
| Alpha adrenergic agents | | |

### Treatment-Related

*Related to effects of surgery on bladder sphincter secondary to:*

Postprostatectomy    Extensive pelvic dissection

*Related to diagnostic instrumentation*

---

* This diagnosis is not currently on the NANDA list but has been included for clarity or usefulness.

*Related to decreased muscle tone secondary to:*
General or Spinal Anesthesia
Drug Therapy (iatrogenic)

| | | |
|---|---|---|
| Antihistamines | Immunosuppressant therapy | Epinephrine |
| Diuretics | Anticholinergics | Tranquilizers |
| Sedatives | Muscle relaxants | Post-indwelling catheters |

## Situational (Personal, Environmental)

*Related to weak pelvic floor muscles secondary to:*

| | | |
|---|---|---|
| Obesity | Childbirth | Aging |
| Recent substantial weight loss | | |

*Related to inability to communicate needs*

*Related to bladder outlet obstruction secondary to fecal impaction/chronic constipation*

*Related to decreased bladder muscle tone secondary to dehydration*

*Related to decreased attention to bladder cues secondary to:*
Depression
Delirium
Intentional suppression (self-induced deconditioning)
Confusion

*Related to environmental barriers to bathroom secondary to:*

| | | |
|---|---|---|
| Distant toilets | Poor lighting | Unfamiliar surroundings |
| Bed too high | Siderails | |

*Related to inability to access bathroom on time secondary to:*
Caffeine/alcohol use
Impaired mobility

## Maturational

**Child**
*Related to small bladder capacity*
*Related to lack of motivation*

## ■■■■■■ AUTHOR'S NOTE

*Impaired Urinary Elimination* probably is too broad a diagnosis for effective clinical use. For this reason, the nurse should use a more specific diagnosis, such as *Stress Incontinence*, whenever possible. When the etiologic or contributing factors for incontinence have not been identified, the nurse could write a temporary diagnosis of *Impaired Urinary Elimination related to unknown etiology, as evidenced by incontinence*.

The nurse performs a focus assessment to determine whether the incontinence is transient, in response to an acute condition (e.g., infection, medication side effects), or established in response to various chronic neural or genitourinary conditions (Miller, 2009). In addition, the nurse should differentiate the type of incontinence: functional, reflex, stress, urge, or total. The nurse should not use the diagnosis *Continuous Incontinence* unless all other types of incontinence have been ruled out.

## ■■■■■■ ERRORS IN DIAGNOSTIC STATEMENTS

1. *Impaired Urinary Elimination related to surgical diversion*
This diagnosis represents a new label for urostomy and does not focus on the nursing accountability. The nurse should assess a person with a urostomy for its effect on functional patterns and physiologic functioning. For this person, the collaborative problems Risk for Complications of Stomal Obstruction and Risk for Complications of Internal Urine Leakage, as well as nursing diagnoses such as Risk for Disturbed Body Image and Risk for Impaired Health Maintenance, could apply.

*(continued)*

## ■■■■■■ ERRORS IN DIAGNOSTIC STATEMENTS *Continued*

2. *Impaired Urinary Elimination related to renal failure*

This nursing diagnosis renames renal failure and is inappropriate. For this reason, the diagnosis *Excess Fluid Volume related to acute renal failure* also would be incorrect. Renal failure causes or contributes to various actual or potential nursing diagnoses, such as *Risk for Infection* and Risk for Imbalanced Nutrition, and collaborative problems, such as *Risk for Complications of Fluid/Electrolyte Imbalances* and *Risk for Complications of Metabolic Acidosis*.

3. *Continuous Incontinence related to effects of aging*

The physiologic effects of aging on the urinary tract system can influence functioning negatively when other risk factors (e.g., mobility problems, dehydration, side effects of medications, decreased awareness of bladder cues) also are present. This nursing diagnosis projects a biased view of anticipated incontinence in an older adult, with associated use of indwelling catheters, incontinence briefs, and/or bed pads. When this equipment is used, the nurse is not treating incontinence, but rather managing urine. The use of such equipment is a short-term solution. For these situations, *Risk for Infection* and *Risk for Impaired Skin Integrity* would apply. When an older adult has an incontinent episode, the nurse should proceed cautiously before applying the nursing diagnosis label of "incontinence." If factors exist that increase the likelihood of recurrence and the client is motivated, the diagnosis *Risk for Functional/Urge Incontinence related to* (specify—e.g., dehydration, mobility difficulties, decreased bladder capacity) could apply. This diagnosis would focus nursing interventions on preventing incontinence, rather than expecting it as inevitable. For an older person with the combination of functional and urge incontinence, the nurse would focus on assisting him or her to increase bladder capacity and to reduce barriers to bathrooms, using the diagnosis *Functional/Urge Incontinence related to age-related effects on bladder capacity, self-induced fluid limitations, and unstable gait*.

## ■■■■■ KEY CONCEPTS

### Generic Considerations

- The three components of the lower urinary tract that assist to maintain continence are as follows (Porth, 2007):
  - Detrusor muscle in the bladder wall, which allows bladder expansion to increase with volume of urine
  - Internal sphincter or proximal urethra, which, when contracted, prevents urine leakage
  - External sphincter, which by voluntary control provides added support during stressed situations (e.g., over-distended bladder)
- Innervation of the bladder arises from the spinal cord at the levels of S2–S4. The bladder is under parasympathetic control. The cortex, midbrain, and medulla influence voluntary control over urination (Sampselle & DeLancey, 1998).
- The female urethra is 3 to 5 cm long. The male urethra is approximately 20 cm long. The urethra primarily maintains continence, but the cerebral cortex is the principal area for suppression of the desire to micturate.
- Capacity of the normal bladder (without experiencing discomfort) is 250 to 400 mL. The desire to void occurs when 150 to 250 mL of urine is in the bladder.
- The sitting position for the female and the standing position for the male allow optimal relaxation of the external urinary sphincter and perineal muscles.
- Bladder tissue tone can be lost if the bladder is distended to 1000 mL (atonic bladder) or continuously drained (Foley catheter).
- Mechanisms to stimulate the voiding reflex or Credé's method may be ineffective if the bladder capacity is less than 200 mL.
- Alcohol, coffee, and tea have a natural diuretic effect and are bladder irritants.
- Injury to the spinal cord above S2–S4 produces a spastic or reflex bladder tone. Injury to the spinal cord below S2–S4 produces a flaccid or atonic bladder.
- Lesions affecting inhibitory centers in the brain or the pathways transmitting inhibitory impulses to the bladder result in an uninhibited bladder.

### INFECTION

- Stasis or pooling of urine contributes to bacterial growth. Bacteria can travel up the ureters to the kidney (ascending infection).
- Recurrent bladder infections cause fibrotic changes in the bladder wall, with a resultant decrease in bladder capacity.

*(continued)*

■■■■■■ **KEY CONCEPTS** *Continued*

- Urinary stasis, infections, alkaline urine, and decreased urine volume contribute to the formation of urinary tract calculi.

### INCONTINENCE

- Incontinence is transient in as many as 50% of people presenting with the problem. of the remaining group, about 66% can be cured or markedly improved with treatment (Resnick & Yalla, 1985). There are many effective corrective measures for the management of urinary tract disease in older adults, and a positive approach should be taken to minimize the incidence of urinary incontinence

- It is important to determine the natural history of the incontinent pattern. A new onset of incontinence is likely to be the result of a precipitating factor outside the urinary tract (e.g., medications, acute illness, inaccessible toilets, impaired mobility that prevents getting to the toilet on time), which usually can be easily corrected. Incontinence can be either transient (reversible) or established (controllable).

- Causes of transient incontinence include acute confusion, urinary tract infection, atrophic vaginitis, side effects of medications, metabolic imbalance, impaction, mobility problems, urosepsis, depression, and pressure sores.

- Controllable incontinence cannot be cured, but urine removal can be planned

- Certain medications are associated with incontinence. Narcotics and sedatives diminish awareness of bladder cues. Adrenergic agents cause retention by increasing bladder outlet resistance. Anticholinergics (antidepressants, some antiparkinsonian medications, antispasmodics, antihistamines, antiarrhythmics, opiates) cause chronic retention with overflow. Diuretics rapidly increase urine volume and can cause incontinence if voiding cannot be delayed (Miller, 2009).

- People with diabetes mellitus, which can contribute to increased residual urine, frequency, and urgency, may have decreased awareness of bladder fullness.

- Social isolation of people with incontinence can be self-imposed because of fear and embarrassment, or imposed by others because of odor and aesthetics.

- Depression can prevent the person from recognizing or responding to bladder cues and, thus, contributes to incontinence.

- Urinary incontinence affects people of all ages, but most commonly the elderly. Urinary incontinence remains under diagnosed and under reported primarily due to embarrassment (Smeltzer, Bare, Hinkle & Cheever, 2008).

### INTERMITTENT CATHETERIZATION

- This method maintains the tonicity of the bladder muscle, prevents overdistention, and provides for complete emptying of the bladder.

- The initial removal of more than 500 mL of urine from a chronically distended bladder can cause severe hemorrhage, which results when bladder veins, previously compressed by the distended bladder, rapidly dilate and rupture when bladder pressure is abruptly released. (After the initial release of 500 mL of urine, alternate the release of 100 mL of urine with 15-min catheter clamps.)

- The accumulation of more than 500 to 700 mL of urine in a bladder should not be permitted.

- In clients with spinal injuries at the T4 level or above, it is necessary to empty the bladder completely regardless of high volumes (>500 mL) owing to the risk of autonomic dysreflexia. Interruption of the sympathetic nervous system causes the veins not to dilate rapidly.

### CONTINUOUS INCONTINENCE

A cognitively impaired person with continuous incontinence requires caregiver-directed treatment. In institutional settings, indwelling and external catheters or disposal or washable incontinence briefs or pads are beneficial to the caregivers, but detrimental to the incontinent person. Aids and equipment should be considered only after other means have been attempted. In the home setting, the caregiver's needs may take precedence over the cognitively impaired person's. Urinary incontinence is cited as the major reason for seeking institutional care for people living at home (Miller, 2009).

 **Geriatric Considerations**

- Urinary incontinence affects 12% to 49% of older women and 7% to 22% of older men living in the community. Its prevalence increases to about 40% in hospitalized clients and 50% in institutionalized clients (Steeman & Defever, 1998). One of the major problems of incontinence in older adults is that it may be overlooked and not adequately evaluated by professionals; as a result, appropriate treatment is denied. Older clients may not admit to the problem because of attitudes about the inevitability of such complications.

- Age-related physiologic changes result in decreased bladder capacity, incomplete emptying, contractions during filling, and increased residual urine (Miller, 2009).
- Another aspect to consider is loss of dignity. This may be especially evident in patients who need special assistance such as with the use of a bedpan (Wilkinson & Van Leuven, 2007).
- Older adults can comfortably store 250 to 300 mL of urine, compared with a storage capacity of 350 to 400 mL in younger adults.
- The sensation to void is delayed in older adults, which shortens the interval between the initial perception of the urge and the actual need to void, resulting in urgency (Miller, 2009). Any factor that interferes with the older adult's perception to void (e.g., medications, depression, limited fluid intake, neurologic impairments) or delays his or her ability to reach the toilet can cause incontinence.
- Other physiologic components of aging that contribute to incontinence are the diminished ability of kidneys to concentrate urine, decreasing muscle tone of the pelvic floor muscles, and the inability to postpone urination.
- Frequent voiding out of habit or limiting fluids may contribute to urgency by impairing the neurologic mechanisms that signal the need to void, because the bladder is rarely fully expanded.
- The diminished vision, impaired mobility, and decreased energy level that may accompany aging mean that increased time is needed to locate the toilet, which also requires the person to be able to delay urination.
- Older adults experience urgency owing to the bladder's limited capacity and their decreased ability to inhibit bladder contractions.

## Focus Assessment Criteria

### Subjective Data

### *Assess for Defining Characteristics.*

"Do you have a problem with controlling your urine (or going to the bathroom)?"

*History of symptoms*

| | | |
|---|---|---|
| Lack of control | Pain or discomfort | Dribbling |
| Burning | Hesitancy | Change in voiding pattern |
| Urgency | Retention | Frequency |

*Onset and duration*
*Restrictions on lifestyle*

| | | |
|---|---|---|
| Social | Sexual | Occupational |
| Role responsibilities | | |

### Adult Incontinence
*History of continence*

| | |
|---|---|
| Is degree of continence acceptable | History of "weak" bladder |
| | Family history of incontinence |
| Age of attainment of continence | Previous history of enuresis |

*Onset and duration (day, night, just certain times)*
*Factors that increase incidence*

| | | |
|---|---|---|
| Delay in getting to bathroom | Coughing | Laughing |
| When excited | Standing | Leaving bathroom |
| Turning in bed | Running | |

*Perception of need to void*

| | | |
|---|---|---|
| Present | Absent | Diminished |

*Ability to delay urination after urge*

| | |
|---|---|
| Present (how long?) | Absent |

*Sensations before or during micturition*

| | | |
|---|---|---|
| Difficulty starting stream | Need to force urine out | Difficulty stopping stream |
| Lack of sensation to void | Painful straining (tenesmus) | |

*Relief after voiding*
Complete
Continued desire to void after emptying bladder
*Use of catheters, incontinence briefs, bed pads*

### Childhood Enuresis
Onset and pattern (day, night)
Toilet-training history
Family history of bed-wetting
Response of others to child (parents, siblings, peers)

## Assess for Related Factors.

### Physiologic Risk Factors
Fluid intake pattern (type and amount, especially before bedtime)
Dehydration (self-imposed, overuse of diuretics, caffeine, alcohol)
Prostatic hypertrophy
Bladder, vaginal infections
Chronic illnesses (e.g., diabetes, alcoholism, Parkinson's disease, Alzheimer's disease, multiple sclerosis, cerebrovascular accident, vitamin $B_{12}$ deficiency)
Metabolic disturbances (e.g., hypokalemia, hypercalcemia)
Fecal impaction/severe constipation
Certain medications (diuretics, anticholinergics, antihistamines, sedatives, acetaminophen, amitriptylane, aspirin, barbiturates, chlorpropamide, clofibrate, fluphenazine, haloperidol, narcotics)
Multiple or difficult deliveries
Pelvic, bladder, or uterine surgery, disorders

### Environmental Barriers
Location of bathroom within 40 feet
Stairs, narrow doorways
Dim lighting
Ability to locate bathroom in social settings

## Objective Data

## Assess for Defining Characteristics.

### Urination Stream

| | | |
|---|---|---|
| Slow | Sprays | Small |
| Starts and stops | Drops | Slow or hard to start |
| Dribble | | |

### Urine
Color, odor, appearance, specific gravity
Negative or positive for

| | | |
|---|---|---|
| Glucose | Bacteria | Protein |
| Red blood cells | Ketone | |

## Assess for Related Factors.

### Voiding and Fluid Intake Patterns
Record for 2 to 4 days to establish a baseline.
What is daily fluid intake?
When does incontinence occur?

### Muscle Tone
Abdomen firm, or soft and pendulous?
History of recent significant weight loss or gain?

### Reflexes
Presence or absence of cauda equina reflexes
Anal
Bulbocavernosus

**Bladder**

Distention (palpable)

Can it be emptied by external stimuli? (Credé's method, gentle suprapubic tapping, or warm water over the perineum, Valsalva maneuver, pulling of pubic hair, anal stretch)

Capacity (at least 400 to 500 mL)

Residual urine

None

Present (in what amount?)

**Functional Ability**

Get in/out of chair            Walk alone to bathroom            Maintain balance

Manipulate clothing

**Cognitive Ability**

Asks to go to bathroom         Initiates toileting               Aware of incontinence

Expects to be incontinent         with reminders

**Assess for Any**

Constipation                   Depression                        Fecal impaction

Mobility disorders             Dehydration                       Sensory disorders

For more information on Focus Assessment Criteria, visit http://thepoint.lww.com.

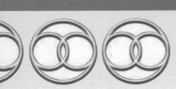

# MATURATIONAL ENURESIS

## DEFINITION

State in which a child experiences involuntary voiding during sleep that is not pathophysiologic in origin

## DEFINING CHARACTERISTICS

### Major (Must Be Present)

Reports or demonstrates episodes of involuntary voiding during sleep

## RELATED FACTORS

### Situational (Personal, Environmental)

Related to stressors (school, siblings)

Related to inattention to bladder cues

Related to unfamiliar surroundings

### Maturational

#### Child

Related to small bladder capacity

Related to lack of motivation

Related to attention-seeking behavior

## ■■■■■ AUTHOR'S NOTE

Enuresis can result from physiologic or maturational factors. Certain etiologies, such as strictures, urinary tract infection, constipation, nocturnal epilepsy, and diabetes, should be ruled out when enuresis is present. These situations do not represent nursing diagnoses.

When enuresis results from small bladder capacity, failure to perceive cues because of deep sleep, or inattention to bladder cues, or is associated with a maturational issue (e.g., new sibling, school pressures), the nursing diagnosis *Maturational Enuresis* is appropriate. Psychological problems usually are not the cause of enuresis but may result from lack of understanding or insensitivity to the problem. Interventions that punish or shame the child must be avoided.

## ■■■■■ ERRORS IN DIAGNOSTIC STATEMENTS

### Maturational Enuresis related to stressors and conflicts

Rather than focus on etiology for maturational enuresis, the nurse should focus on teaching the child and parents management strategies. The nurse also should encourage parents to share their concerns and direct them away from punishing behaviors. Given this nursing focus, the nurse could restate the diagnosis as *Maturational Enuresis related to unknown etiology, as evidenced by reported episodes of bed-wetting.*

## ■■■■■ KEY CONCEPTS

- The newborn may void up to 20 times per day because of small bladder capacity. As the child grows, bladder capacity increases and frequency of urination decreases (Hockenberry et al., 2009).
- Most children by 4 or 5 years of age have complete neuromuscular control of urination (Kelleher, 1997).
- Enuresis is defined as urinary incontinence at any age when urinary control would be expected.
- The etiology of enuresis is complex and not well understood. The following factors have been implicated:
  - Developmental/maturational delay (e.g., small functional bladder capacity, deep sleep, mental retardation)
  - Organic factors (e.g., infection, sickle cell anemia, diabetes, neuromuscular disorders)
  - Psychological/emotional factors (e.g., stressors such as birth of sibling, hospitalization, divorce of parents; Kelleher, 1997)
- Children at risk for overflow retention include those who (Hockenberry et al., 2009).
- Have congenital anomalies of the urinary tract
- Are neurologically impaired
- Have undergone surgery
- Enuresis is primarily a maturational problem and usually ceases between 6 and 8 years of age. It is more common in boys. By adolescence, 99% become continent (Kelleher, 1997).
- There is a high frequency of bed-wetting in children whose parents or other near relatives were bed-wetters (Kelleher, 1997).
- High anxiety can impede the child's ability to master the skills necessary for the maintenance of continence (Morison, 1998).
- Most children with nocturnal enuresis have neither a psychiatric nor an organic illness (Kelleher, 1997).

# Focus Assessment Criteria

## Subjective Data

### *Assess for Defining Characteristics.*

> Onset
> Pattern (day, night)
> Number of episodes in month

### *Assess for Related Factors.*

> Toilet-training history

Family history of bed-wetting
Response of others (parents, peers, siblings)
Recent change or stressor
    School           Relocation     Peers
    Family problems    New sibling
Inattention to bladder cues
Sexual abuse

For more information on Focus Assessment Criteria, visit http://thepoint.lww.com.

---

**NOC**

Urinary Continence, Knowledge: Enuresis, Family Functioning

## ➤ Goal

The child will remain dry during the sleep cycle.

### *Indicator:*

The child and family will be able to list factors that decrease enuresis.

---

**NIC**

Urinary Incontinence Care: Enuresis, Urinary Habit Training, Anticipatory Guidance, Family Support

## ➤ General Interventions

### Ascertain that Physiologic Causes of Enuresis Have Been Ruled Out.

Examples include infections, meatal stenosis, fistulas, pinworms, epispadias, ectopic ureter, and minor neurologic dysfunction (hyperactivity, cognitive delay).

### Determine Contributing Factors.

Refer to Related Factors.

## Promote a Positive Parent–Child Relationship.

Explain to the parents and the child the physiologic development of bladder control.

**R:** This can help to relieve feelings of guilt or blame (Ball & Bindler, 2008).

Explain to parents that disapproval (shaming, punishing) is useless in stopping enuresis but can make child shy, ashamed, and afraid.

**R:** Anger, punishment, and rejection by parents and peers contribute to feelings of shame, embarrassment, and low self-esteem (Carpenter, 1999).

Offer reassurance to child that other children wet the bed at night and that he or she is not bad or sinful. Explain that there is a high rate of remission.

**R:** Explaining that enuresis is developmental reduces blaming of child and parental frustration (Morison, 1998). Self-concept improves in children treated for enuresis compared with those not treated (Longstaffe et al., 2000).

## Reduce Contributing Factors, If Possible.

### *Small Bladder Capacity*

After child drinks fluids, encourage him or her to postpone voiding to help stretch the bladder.

### *Sound Sleeper*

Have child void before retiring.
Restrict fluids at bedtime.
If child is awakened later (about 11 PM) to void, attempt to awaken child fully for positive reinforcement.

### *Too Busy to Sense a Full Bladder (If Daytime Wetting Occurs)*

Teach child awareness of sensations that occur when it is time to void.

Teach child the ability to control urination (have him or her start and stop the stream; have him or her "hold" the urine during the day, even if for only a short time).

Have child keep a record of how he or she is doing; emphasize dry days or nights (e.g., stars on a calendar).

If child wets, have him or her explain or write down (if feasible) why he or she thinks it happened.

**R:** These strategies engage the child in the treatment plan and increase awareness that the problem can be controlled

With school age children assess if the child is using the bathroom at school. Do they get sufficient bathroom breaks? Can a reminder device be used (vibrating watch)

**R:** Arrangements may need to be made with the teacher for extra bathroom time (Ball & Bindler, 2008). The use of devices, such as a vibrating watch, may help remind the child when it is time to use the bathroom (Ball & Bindler, 2008).

## Initiate Health Teaching and Referrals, as Indicated.

For children with enuresis:

Teach child and parents the facts about enuresis.

Teach family techniques to control the adverse effects of enuresis (e.g., plastic mattress covers, use of sleeping bag [machine-washable] when staying overnight away from home).

Explain that the child cannot control bed-wetting but that bed-wetting can be controlled with intervention (Morison, 1998).

Children who believe that they can be helped have the best chance of success (Morison, 1998).

Without implying punishment involve the child in bed changing for nocturnal enuresis (Ball & Bindler, 2008).

**R:** Interventions for nocturnal enuresis must focus on reducing social and emotional stigma (Macaulay, 2004).

Seek opportunities to teach the public about enuresis and incontinence (e.g., school and parent organizations, self-help groups).

Explain how the nocturnal enuresis alarm works.

**R:** The use of an alarm intervention reduces nighttime bed-wetting in the majority of children both during and after treatment (Macaulay et al., 2004).

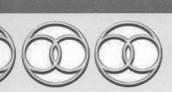

# FUNCTIONAL INCONTINENCE

## DEFINITION

State in which a person experiences incontinence because of a difficulty or inability to reach the toilet in time

## DEFINING CHARACTERISTICS

### Major (Must Be Present)

Incontinence before or during an attempt to reach the toilet

# RELATED FACTORS

## Pathophysiologic

*Related to diminished bladder cues and impaired ability to recognize bladder cues secondary to:*

| | | |
|---|---|---|
| Brain injury/tumor/infection | Alcoholic neuropathy | Cerebrovascular accident |
| Parkinsonism | Demyelinating diseases | Progressive dementia |
| Multiple sclerosis | | |

## Treatment-Related

*Related to decreased bladder tone secondary to:*

| | | |
|---|---|---|
| Antihistamines | Immunosuppressant therapy | Epinephrine |
| Diuretics | Anticholinergics | Tranquilizers |
| Sedatives | Muscle relaxants | |

## Situational (Personal, Environmental)

*Related to impaired mobility*
*Related to decreased attention to bladder cues*
Depression
Intentional suppression (self-induced deconditioning)
Confusion
*Related to environmental barriers to bathroom*

| | | |
|---|---|---|
| Distant toilets | Bed too high | Poor lighting |
| Siderails | Unfamiliar surroundings | |

## Maturational

**Older Adult**
*Related to motor and sensory losses*

## ◼◼◼◼◼ KEY CONCEPTS

- Functional incontinence is the inability or unwillingness of the person with a normal bladder and sphincter to reach the toilet in time.
- Functional incontinence may be caused by conditions affecting physical and emotional ability to manage the act of urination.
- Underlying psychological problems can be a functional etiology of incontinence.
- Approximately 45% of all nursing home residents are incontinent. Of those with bladder incontinence, 82% have limited mobility.

# Focus Assessment Criteria

See *Impaired Urinary Elimination*.

**NOC**
Tissue Integrity,
Urinary Continence,
Urinary Elimination

## ➤ Goal

The person will report no or decreased episodes of incontinence.

### Indicators:

- Remove or minimize environmental barriers at home.
- Use proper adaptive equipment to assist with voiding, transfers, and dressing.
- Describe causative factors for incontinence.

# ➤ General Interventions

## Assess Causative or Contributing Factors.

### Obstacles to Toilet

Poor lighting, slippery floor, misplaced furniture and rugs, inadequate footwear, toilet too far, bed too
   high, side rails up
Inadequate toilet (too small for walkers, wheelchair, seat too low/high, no grab bars)
Inadequate signal system for requesting help
Lack of privacy

## Sensory/Cognitive Deficits

Visual deficits (blindness, field cuts, poor depth perception)
Cognitive deficits as a result of aging, trauma, stroke, tumor, infection

## Motor/Mobility Deficits

Limited upper and/or lower extremity movement/strength (inability to remove clothing)
Barriers to ambulation (e.g., vertigo, fatigue, altered gait, hypertension)

**R:** Barriers can delay access to the toilet and cause incontinence if the client cannot delay urination.
   A few seconds' delay in reaching the bathroom can make the difference between continence and
   incontinence.

## Reduce or Eliminate Contributing Factors, If Possible.

### Environmental Barriers

Assess path to bathroom for obstacles, lighting, and distance.
Assess adequacy of toilet height and need for grab bars.
Assess adequacy of room size.
Provide a commode between bathroom and bed, if necessary.

## Sensory/Cognitive Deficits

*For a person with diminished vision:*
Ensure adequate lighting.
Encourage person to wear prescribed corrective lens.
Provide clear, safe pathway to bathroom.
Keep call bell easily accessible.
If bedpan or urinal is used, make sure it is within easy reach in the same location at all times.
Assess person for safety in bathroom.
Assess person's ability to provide self-hygiene.
*For a person with cognitive deficits:*
Offer toileting reminders every 2 h, after meals, and before bedtime.
Establish appropriate means to communicate need to void.
Answer call bell immediately.
Encourage wearing of ordinary clothes.
Provide a normal environment for elimination (use bathroom, if possible).
Allow for privacy while maintaining safety.
Allow sufficient time for task.
Reorient client to where he or she is and what task he or she is doing.
Be consistent in your approach to person.
Give simple step-by-step instructions; use verbal and nonverbal cues.
Give positive reinforcement for success.
Assess person for safety in bathroom.
Assess need for adaptive devices on clothing to make dressing and undressing easier.
Assess person's ability to provide self-hygiene.

**R:** A client with a cognitive deficit needs constant verbal cues and reminders to establish a routine and
   reduce incontinence

## Provide for Factors that Promote Continence.

### *Maintain Optimal Hydration.*

> Increase fluid intake to 2000 to 3000 mL/day, unless contraindicated.
> Teach older adults not to depend on thirst sensations but to drink liquids even when not thirsty.
> Space fluids every 2 h.
> Decrease fluid intake after 7 PM; provide only minimal fluids during the night.
>
> **R:** Dehydration can prevent the sensation of a full bladder and can contribute to loss of bladder tone. Spacing fluids helps promote regular bladder filling and emptying.
> **R:** Dilute urine helps prevent infection and bladder irritation.
>
> Reduce intake of coffee, tea, cola, alcohol, and grapefruit juice because of their diuretic effect.
>
> **R:** Coffee, tea, colas, and grapefruit juice act as diuretics, which can cause urgency.
>
> Avoid large amounts of tomato and orange juice.
>
> **R:** These beverages make the urine alkaline which promotes infection.
>
> Avoid bladder irritants such as alcohol, caffeine and aspartame (Smeltzer, Bare, Hinkle, & Cheever, 2008). Encourage cranberry juice.\
>
> **R:** Acidic urine deters the growth of most bacteria implicated in cystitis.
>
> Monitor salt intake.
>
> **R:** High salt diets decrease urine production and cause water retention (Wilkinson & Van Leuven, 2007).

### *Maintain Adequate Nutrition to Ensure Bowel Elimination at Least Once Every 3 Days.*

> Promote Micturition.

### *Promote Personal Integrity and Provide Motivation to Increase Bladder Control.*

> Encourage person to share feelings about incontinence and determine its effect on his or her social patterns.
> Convey that incontinence can be cured or at least controlled to maintain dignity.
> Use protective pads or garments only after conscientious reconditioning efforts have been completely unsuccessful after 6 weeks.
> Work to achieve daytime continence before expecting nighttime continence:
>> Encourage socialization.
>> Discourage the use of bedpans.
>> Encourage and assist person to groom self.
>> If hospitalized, provide opportunities to eat meals outside bedroom (day room, lounge).
>> If fear or embarrassment is preventing socialization, instruct person to use sanitary pads or briefs temporarily until control is established.
>> Change clothes as soon as possible when wet to avoid indirectly sanctioning wetness.
>> Advise the oral use of chlorophyll tablets to deodorize urine and feces.
>> See *Social Isolation* and *Ineffective Coping* for additional interventions, if indicated.
>
> **R:** Wearing normal clothing or nightwear helps simulate the home environment, where incontinence may not occur. A hospital gown may reinforce incontinence. Use of bathroom rather than bedpans simulate the home environment

### *Promote Skin Integrity.*

> Identify clients at risk for development of pressure ulcers.
> Avoid harsh soaps and alcohol products.
> Keep moisture away from the skin.
> See *Risk for Impaired Skin Integrity* for additional information.

**R:** Ammonia from urine makes the skin more alkaline and more vulnerable to irritants (Scardillo et al., 1999).

## Teach Prevention of Urinary Tract Infections.

Encourage regular, complete emptying of the bladder.

Ensure adequate fluid intake.

Keep urine acidic; avoid citrus juices, dark colas, coffee, tea and alcohol which act as irritants (Smeltzer, Bare, Hinkle, & Cheever, 2008)

Monitor urine pH.

Teach client to recognize abnormal changes in urine properties.

Increased mucus and sediment

Blood in urine (hematuria)

Change in color (from normal straw-colored) or odor

Teach client to monitor for signs and symptoms of infection:

Elevated temperature, chills, and shaking

Changes in urine properties

Suprapubic pain

Painful urination

Urgency

Frequent small voids or frequent small incontinences

Increased spasticity in spinal cord-injured individuals

Increased urine pH

Nausea/vomiting

Lower back and/or flank pain

**R:** Bacteria multiply rapidly in stagnant urine retained in the bladder. Moreover, overdistention hinders blood flow to the bladder wall, increasing the susceptibility to infection from bacterial growth. Regular, complete bladder emptying greatly reduces the risk of infection.

## Explain Age-Related Effects on Bladder Function and that Urgency and Nocturia Do Not Necessarily Lead to Incontinence.

### *Initiate Health Teaching Referral, When Indicated.*

Refer to visiting nurse (occupational therapy department) for assessment of bathroom facilities at home.

**Geriatric Interventions**

Emphasize that incontinence is not an inevitable age-related event.

**R:** Explaining the cause can motivate the person to participate

Explain not to restrict fluid intake for fear of incontinence.

**R:** Dehydration can cause incontinence by eliminating the sensation of a full bladder (the signal to urinate) and also by reducing the person's alertness to the sensation.

Explain not to rely on thirst as a signal to drink fluids.

**R:** The older adult has an age-related decrease in thirst (Miller, 2009).

Teach the need to have easy access to bathroom at night. If needed, consider commode chair or urinal.

**R:** This is to prevent falls.

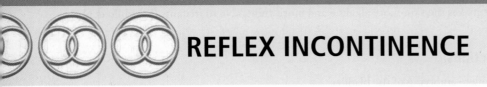

# REFLEX INCONTINENCE

## DEFINITION

State in which a person experiences predictable involuntary loss of urine with no sensation of urge, voiding, or bladder fullness

## DEFINING CHARACTERISTICS

### Major (Must Be Present)

Uninhibited bladder contractions
Involuntary reflexes producing spontaneous voiding
Partial or complete loss of sensation of bladder fullness or urge to void

## RELATED FACTORS

### Pathophysiologic

*Related to impaired conduction of impulses above the reflex arc level secondary to:*
Cord injury/tumor/infection

### ■■■■■■ KEY CONCEPTS

- A lesion above the sacral cord segments (above T12) involving both motor and sensory tracts of the spinal cord results in a reflex bladder. Other common names for this type of bladder dysfunction are spastic, supraspinal, hypertonic, automatic, and upper motor neuron bladder.
- A lesion that does not completely transect the spinal cord can produce variable findings.
- Control from higher cerebral centers is removed in the reflex neurogenic bladder. Therefore, the person cannot start or stop micturition in a voluntary manner.
- The simple spinal reflex arc takes over the control of micturition.
- A positive bulbocavernosus reflex suggests that the voiding reflex (spinal reflex arc) is intact.
- If the opening of the urinary sphincter and the relaxation of the striated muscle surrounding the urinary sphincter are uncoordinated, there is a potential for large residual urine volumes after triggered voiding.
- Autonomic dysreflexia is an abnormal hyperactive reflex activity that occurs only in people with spinal cord injury with a lesion above T8. Most often, these clients have an upper motor neuron bladder (reflex incontinence). This is a life-threatening situation in which the blood pressure rises to lethal levels. Autonomic hyperreflexia is most often caused by stimuli resulting from an overstretched bladder or bowel.

## Focus Assessment Criteria

See *Impaired Urinary Elimination*.

**NOC**
See *Functional Incontinence*

## ➤ Goal

The person will report a state of dryness that is personally satisfactory.

### Indicators:

- Have a residual urine volume of less than 50 mL.
- Use triggering mechanisms to initiate reflex voiding.

684

**NIC**
See also *Functional Incontinence*, Pelvic Muscle Exercise, Weight Management

➤ **General Interventions**

**Assess for Causative and Contributing Conditions.**

Refer to related factors.

**Explain Rationale for Treatments.**

**Develop a Bladder Retraining or Reconditioning Program (See Interventions Under *Continuous Incontinence*).**

**Teach Techniques to Stimulate Reflex Voiding.**

Cutaneous triggering mechanisms
Repeated deep, sharp suprapubic tapping (most effective)
Instruct to:
　Place self in a half-sitting position.
　Tap directly at bladder wall at a rate of seven or eight times for 5 s (35 to 40 single blows).
　Use only one hand.
　Shift site of stimulation over bladder to find most successful site.
　Continue stimulation until a good stream starts.
　Wait approximately 1 min; repeat stimulation until bladder is empty.
　One or two series of stimulations without response signifies that nothing more will be expelled.
If the preceding measures are ineffective, instruct client to perform each of the following for 2 to 3 min, waiting 1 min between attempts.
　Stroking glans penis
　Lightly punching abdomen above inguinal ligaments
　Stroking inner thigh
Encourage person to void or trigger at least every 3 h.
Indicate on intake and output sheet which mechanism was used to induce voiding.
People with abdominal muscle control should use the Valsalva maneuver during triggered voiding.
Teach person that if he or she increases fluid intake, he or she also needs to increase the frequency of triggering to prevent overdistention.
Schedule intermittent catheterization program (see *Continuous Incontinence*).

**R:** Stimulating the reflex arc replaces the internal sphincter of the bladder, allowing urination. Stimulating the bladder wall or cutaneous sites (e.g., suprapubic, pubic) can trigger the reflex arc.
**R:** Preferred cutaneous triggering methods are light, rapid suprapubic tapping, light pulling of pubic hairs, massage of the abdomen, and digital rectal stimulation.
**R:** Use of Credé's maneuver should be avoided with a reflex bladder because the urethra may be damaged or vesicoureteral reflux may occur if the external sphincter is contracted.
**R:** Contraction of abdominal muscles compresses the bladder to empty it.

**Initiate Health Teaching, as Indicated.**

**Arrange an At-Home Assessment by a Home Health Nurse.**

Teach bladder-reconditioning program (see *Continuous Incontinence*).
Teach intermittent catheterization (see *Continuous Incontinence*).
Teach prevention of urinary tract infections (see *Continuous Incontinence*).

**R:** Strategies to control urination must be continued at home

If at high risk for dysreflexia, see *Dysreflexia*.

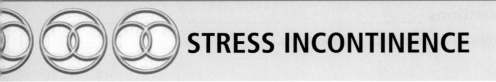

# STRESS INCONTINENCE

## DEFINITION

State in which a person experiences an immediate involuntary loss of urine with an increase in intraabdominal pressure

## DEFINING CHARACTERISTICS

### Major (Must Be Present)

The person reports loss of urine (usually <50 mL) occurring with increased abdominal pressure from standing, sneezing, coughing, running, or lifting heavy objects.

## RELATED FACTORS

### Pathophysiologic

*Related to incompetent bladder outlet secondary to congenital urinary tract anomalies*
*Related to degenerative changes in pelvic muscles and structural supports secondary to estrogen deficiency*

### Situational (Personal, Environmental)

*Related to high intraabdominal pressure and weak pelvic muscles secondary to:*
Obesity          Sex          Pregnancy
Poor personal hygiene     Smoking
*Related to weak pelvic muscles and structural supports secondary to:*
Recent substantial weight loss  Childbirth

### Maturational

**Older Adult**
*Related to loss of muscle tone*

### ■ ■ ■ ■ ■ ■ KEY CONCEPTS

#### Generic Considerations

- Urinary continence is maintained by the junction of the bladder and the urethra, support from the perineal floor, and the muscle around the urethra.
- Stress incontinence is the leakage of small amounts of urine when the urethral outlet cannot control passage of urine in the presence of increased intraabdominal pressure.
- Menopausal decrease in elasticity usually worsens stress incontinence.
- A trial of vaginal estrogen cream in the postmenopausal woman who exhibits a pale, atrophic vaginal vault may help to reduce the incidence of incontinence.
- A stress test is used to help diagnose stress incontinence. It involves observation of the urethral meatus of a client with a full bladder in the standing position while she coughs or strains. Short spurts of urine escaping simultaneously with cough or strain suggest a probable diagnosis of stress incontinence.
- The client with pure stress incontinence has a normal cystometrogram.
- The degrees of stress incontinence are as follows:
  - Grade 1—Urine is lost with sudden increase in abdominal pressure, but never at night.
  - Grade 2—Lesser degrees of physical stress, such as walking, standing erect from a sitting position, or sitting up in bed, produce incontinence.
  - Grade 3—There is continuous incontinence, and urine is lost without any relation to physical activity or to position.

**Maternal Considerations**

Pressure of the uterus can cause stress incontinence, which can be misinterpreted as amniotic fluid.

## Focus Assessment Criteria

See *Impaired Urinary Elimination*.

**NOC**
See *Functional Incontinence*

## ➤ Goal

The person will report a reduction or elimination of stress incontinence.

### Indicator:

Be able to explain the cause of incontinence and rationale for treatments.

**NIC**
See also *Functional Incontinence*, Pelvic Muscle Exercise, Weight Management

## ➤ General Interventions

### Determine Contributing Factors.

### Explain the Effect of Incompetent Floor Muscles on Continence (See Key Concepts).

### Teach Pelvic Muscle Exercises (Dougherty, 1998).

### *Teach How to Self-Assess Whether Exercises Are Being Done Correctly.*

Stand with one foot elevated on a stool, insert finger in vagina, and feel the strength of the contraction. Evaluate the strength of the contraction on a scale of 0 to 5 (Sampselle & DeLancey, 1998):
0 = No palpable contraction
1 = Very weak, barely felt
2 = Weak but clearly felt
3 = Good but not maintained when moderate finger pressure is applied
4 = Good but not maintained when intense finger pressure is applied
5 = Maximum strength with strong resistance
Use a mirror to observe whether the clitoris has downward movement and the anus tightens with contraction.
Consult an incontinence specialist for use of vaginal weights for pelvic floor strengthening.

### *Provide Instructions for Pelvic Muscle Exercises.*

Teach the patient ways to strengthen the pelvic floor muscle.
Tightening muscles as if you were trying to stop urination; this includes tightening the rectal muscles (Wilkinson & Van Leuven, 2007).
Hold the contractions for 5-10 seconds and release. Relax between contractions taking care to keep contraction and relaxation times equal. If you contract for 10 seconds, relax for 10 seconds before next contraction (Wilkinson & Van Leuven, 2007).
Perform 40 to 60 contractions divided in 2-4 sessions each time. These should be spread out through the day and incorporate different positions; sitting, standing and lying (Wilkinson & Van Leuven, 2007).
A good way to remember to do your exercises is to incorporate them into your daily routine. Such as stopping at a traffic light or washing dishes (Wilkinson & Van Leuven, 2007).
Use the urine stop test to measure the effectiveness of a contraction by the time it takes to stop voiding. Advise not to perform the urine stop test more than once a day.

**R:** In stress incontinence, childbirth, trauma, menopausal atrophy, or obesity have weakened or stretched the pelvic floor muscles (pubococcygeus) and levator ani muscles.

**R:** Pelvic floor muscle rehabilitation is an important treatment for strengthening perineal muscles. It is not uncommon to see improvement rates of 48-80% with these exercises. Approximately 6-12 month of treatment may be required before improvement is seen (Wilkinson & Van Leuven, 2007).

## Initiate Health Teaching for People Who Continue to Remain Incontinent After Attempts at Bladder Reconditioning or Muscle Retraining.

Promote personal integrity (see *Continuous Incontinence*).
Promote skin integrity (see *Continuous Incontinence*).
Schedule intermittent catheterization program, if appropriate (see *Continuous Incontinence*).

**Maternal Interventions**

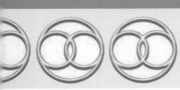

For increased abdominal pressure during pregnancy:
    Teach client to avoid prolonged standing.
    Teach client the benefit of frequent voiding, at least every 2 h.
    Teach pelvic muscle exercises after delivery.

**R:** Pressure of the uterus on the bladder can cause involuntary loss of urine.

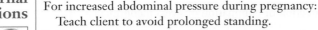

# CONTINUOUS INCONTINENCE

## DEFINITION

State in which a person experiences continuous, unpredictable loss of urine without distention or awareness of bladder fullness

## DEFINING CHARACTERISTICS

### Major (Must Be Present, One or More)

Constant flow of urine without distention
Nocturia more than two times during sleep
Incontinence refractory to other treatments

### Minor (May Be Present)

Unaware of bladder cues to void
Unaware of incontinence

## RELATED FACTORS

Refer to *Impaired Urinary Elimination*.

## KEY CONCEPTS

See *Impaired Urinary Elimination*.

## Focus Assessment Criteria

See *Impaired Urinary Elimination*.

**NOC**
See *Functional Incontinence*

## ➤ Goal

The person will be continent (specify during day, night, 24 h).

### Indicators:

- Identify the cause of incontinence and rationale for treatments.
- Identify daily goal for fluid intake.

**NIC**
See also *Functional Incontinence*, Environmental Management, Urinary Catheterization, Teaching: Procedure/Treatment, Tube Care: Urinary, Urinary Bladder Training

## ➤ General Interventions

### Develop a Bladder Retraining or Reconditioning Program, Which Should Include Communication, Assessment of Voiding Pattern, Scheduled Fluid Intake, and Scheduled Voiding Times.

*Promote Communication Among All Staff Members and Among Individual, Family, and Staff.*

Provide all staff with sufficient knowledge concerning the program planned.
Assess staff's response to program.

### Assess the Person's Potential for Participation in a Bladder-Retraining Program.

Cognition
Desire to change behavior
Ability to cooperate
Willingness to participate

**R:** Continence training programs are either self-directed or caregiver-directed. Self-directed programs of bladder training, retraining, and exercises are for motivated, cognitively intact clients. Caregiver-directed programs of scheduled toileting or habit training are appropriate for motivated caregivers of clients with cognitive impairment (Miller, 2009).

### Provide Rationale for Plan and Acquire Client's Informed Consent.

### Encourage Person to Continue Program by Providing Accurate Information Concerning Reasons for Success or Failure.

### Assess Voiding Pattern.

Monitor and record:
  Intake and output
  Time and amount of fluid intake
  Type of fluid
  Amount of incontinence; measure if possible or estimate amount as small, moderate, or large
  Amount of void, whether it was voluntary or involuntary
  Presence of sensation of need to void
  Amount of retention (amount of urine left in the bladder after an unsuccessful attempt at manual triggering or voiding)
  Amount of residual (amount of urine left in the bladder after either a voluntary or manual triggered voiding; also called a postvoid residual)
Amount of triggered urine (urine expelled after manual triggering [e.g.; tapping, Credé's method])
Identify certain activities that precede voiding (e.g., restlessness, yelling, exercise).
Record in appropriate column.

### Schedule Fluid Intake and Voiding Times.

Provide fluid intake of 2000 mL each day unless contraindicated.
Discourage fluids after 7 PM.

Initially, bladder emptying is done at least every 2 h and at least twice during the night; goal is 2- to 4-h intervals.

If the person is incontinent before scheduled voids, shorten the time between voids.

If the person has a postvoid residual greater than 100 to 150 mL, schedule intermittent catheterization.

### *Reduce Incontinence-Related Irritant Dermatitis (Scardillo et al., 1999).*

Decrease the alkalizing effect of urine on the skin:
  Use a no-rinse perineal cleanser.
  Avoid fragrances, alcohol, and alkaline agents (found in many commercial soaps).
  Apply moisturizer immediately after bathing, when pores are open.
  Select a moisturizer that is occlusive (white petroleum, lanolin, emollients).
Decrease injury with washing:
  Do not try to remove all of the ointment with cleansing.
  Gently wash skin, using very little soap.
  Dry skin very gently by patting, not rubbing.
  Use a moisture-barrier product (e.g., Curity Moisture Barrier Cream; No Sting Barrier Film).

**R:** The essential components of any continence training program (self-directed or caregiver-directed) include motivation, assessment of voiding and incontinence patterns, a regular fluid intake of 2000 to 3000 mL/day, timed voiding of 2- to 4-h intervals in an appropriate place, and ongoing assessment (Miller, 2009).

**R:** Intermittent catheterization, when performed in a health care facility, should follow aseptic technique, because the organisms present in such a facility are more virulent and resistant to drugs than organisms found outside. People at home can practice clean technique because of the lack of virulent organisms in the home environment.

**R:** Dehydration can cause incontinence by eliminating the sensation of a full bladder (the signal to urinate) and also by reducing the person's alertness to the sensation.

### *Schedule Intermittent Catheterization Program (ICP), if Indicated.*

Monitor intake and output.
Fluid intake should be at least 2000 mL/day.
Use sterile catheterization technique in the hospital, clean technique at home.
Desired catheter volumes are less than 500 mL.
Increase or decrease the interval between catheterizations to obtain the desired catheter volumes.
Usual catheterization times are every 4 to 6 h.
Urine volumes may increase at night; thus, it may be necessary to catheterize more frequently at night.
Encourage the client to attempt to void before scheduled catheterization time.
Initially obtain postvoid residuals at least every 6 h.
Terminate ICP when the bladder is consistently emptied voluntarily or by triggering with less than 50 mL residual urine after each void.

**R:** Intermittent self-catheterization, periodic drainage of urine through the use of a catheter in the bladder, is indicated when a neurologic impairment alters bladder emptying.

**R:** Intermittent catheterization, when performed in a health care facility, should follow aseptic technique, because the organisms present in such a facility are more virulent and resistant to drugs than organisms in the home environment.

## Teach ICP to Person and Family for Long-Term Management of Bladder (See Key Concepts).

Explain the reasons for the catheterization program.
Explain the relation of fluid intake and the frequency of catheterization.
Explain the importance of emptying the bladder at the prescribed time, regardless of circumstances, because of the hazards of an overdistended bladder (e.g., circulation contributes to infection, and stasis of urine contributes to bacterial growth).

**R:** Intermittent catheterization provides a decrease in morbidity associated with long-term use of indwelling catheters, increased independence, a more positive self-concept, and more normal sexual relations.

**R:** An over distended bladder reduces blood flow to the bladder wall, making it more susceptible to infection from bacterial growth.

## Teach the Client About the Bladder Reconditioning Program.

Explain rationale and treatments (see Key Concepts).

Explain the schedule of fluid intake, voiding attempts, manual triggering, and catheterization to control incontinence.

Teach person and family the importance of positive reinforcement and adherence to program for best results.

Refer to community nurses for assistance in bladder reconditioning if indicated.

**R:** The essential components of any continence training program (self-directed or caregiver-directed) include motivation, assessment of voiding and incontinence patterns, a regular fluid intake of 2,000 to 3,000 mL/day, time voiding of 2- to 4-h intervals in an appropriate place, and ongoing assessment (Miller, 2009).

## Initiate Health Teaching.

If appropriate, teach intermittent catheterization.

Instruct in prevention of urinary tract infection.

For people living in the community, initiate a referral to the visiting nurse for follow-up and/or regular indwelling catheter changes.

**R:** Long-term catheterization requires use of community nurses.

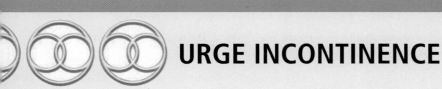

# URGE INCONTINENCE

## DEFINITION

State in which a person experiences an involuntary loss of urine associated with a strong, sudden desire to void

## DEFINING CHARACTERISTICS

### Major (Must Be Present)

Urgency followed by incontinence

## RELATED FACTORS

### Pathophysiologic

*Related to decreased bladder capacity secondary to:*

| | | |
|---|---|---|
| Infection | Cerebrovascular accident | Trauma |
| Demyelinating diseases | Urethritis | Diabetic neuropathy |
| Neurogenic disorders or injury/tumor/infection injury | Alcoholic neuropathy | Brain |
| Parkinsonism | | |

## Treatment-Related

> ***Related to decreased bladder capacity secondary to:***
> Abdominal surgery        Post-indwelling catheters

## Situational (Personal, Environmental)

> ***Related to irritation of bladder stretch receptors secondary to:***
> Alcohol      Caffeine      Excess fluid intake
> ***Related to decreased bladder capacity secondary to frequent voiding***

## Maturational

> Child
> ***Related to small bladder capacity***
>
> Older Adult
> ***Related to decreased bladder capacity***

■■■■■■■ **KEY CONCEPTS**

- Urge incontinence is an involuntary loss of urine associated with a strong desire to void. It is characterized by loss of large volumes of urine and may be triggered by emotional factors, body position changes, or the sight and sound of running water. This type of incontinence is commonly called bladder detrusor instability or vesical instability.
- Detrusor instability is characterized by uninhibited detrusor contractions sufficient to cause urinary incontinence. Common causes include central nervous system disease, hyperexcitability of the afferent pathways, and deconditioned voiding reflexes.
- A person with an uninhibited neurogenic bladder has damage to the cerebral cortex (e.g., cerebrovascular accident, Parkinson's disease, brain injury/tumor) affecting the ability to inhibit urination. Sensation of bladder fullness is also limited; this is manifested by urgency. There is little time between the sensation to void and the uninhibited contraction.
- Warning time is the time a person can delay urination after feeling the urge to void. Diminished warning time can cause incontinence if the person cannot reach a toilet in time.

## Focus Assessment Criteria

See *Impaired Urinary Elimination*.

**NOC**
Refer to *Functional Incontinence*

### ➤ Goal

The person will report no or decreased episodes of incontinence (specify).

### *Indicators:*

- Explain causes of incontinence.
- Describe bladder irritants.

**NIC**
Refer to *Functional Incontinence*

### ➤ General Interventions

### Assess for Causative or Contributing Factors.

Refer to Related Factors.

### Assess Pattern of Voiding/ Incontinence and Fluid Intake.

Maintain optimal hydration (see *Continuous Incontinence*).
Assess voiding pattern (see *Continuous Incontinence*).

# Reduce or Eliminate Causative and Contributing Factors, When Possible.

## *Bladder Irritants*

Infection/inflammation:
Refer to physician for diagnosis and treatment.
Initiate bladder reconditioning program (see *Continuous Incontinence*).
Explain the relation between incontinence and intake of alcohol, caffeine, and colas (irritants).
Explain the risk of insufficient fluid intake and its relation to infection and concentrated urine.

**R:** Optimal hydration is needed to prevent urinary tract infection and renal calculi.

## *Diminished Bladder Capacity*

Determine time between urge to void and need to void (record how long person can delay urination).
For a person with difficulty prolonging waiting time, communicate to personnel the need to respond rapidly to his request for assistance for toileting (note on care plan).
Teach client to increase waiting time by increasing bladder capacity:
Determine volume of each void.
Ask person to "hold off" urinating as long as possible.
Give positive reinforcement.
Discourage frequent voiding that is the result of habit, not need.
Develop bladder reconditioning program (see *Continuous Incontinence*).

**R:** Deconditioning of the voiding reflex can result in incontinence through self-induced or iatrogenic causes. Frequent toileting (more than every 2 h) causes chronic low-volume voiding, which reduces bladder capacity and increases detrusor tone and bladder wall thickness, which, in turn, potentiate incontinent episodes.

## *Overdistended Bladder*

Explain that diuretics are given to help reduce the water in the body; they work by acting on the kidneys to increase the flow of urine.
Explain that in diabetes mellitus, insulin deficiency causes high levels of blood sugar. The high level of blood glucose pulls fluid from body tissues, causing osmotic diuresis and increased urination (polyuria).
Explain that because of the increased urine flow, regular voiding is needed to prevent overdistention of the bladder.
Assess voiding pattern (see *Continuous Incontinence*).
Check postvoid residual; if greater than 100 mL, include intermittent catheterization in bladder reconditioning program.
Initiate bladder reconditioning program (see *Continuous Incontinence*).

**R:** Overdistention results in loss of bladder sensation which causes incontinence episodes.

## *Uninhibited Bladder Contractions*

Assess voiding pattern (see *Continuous Incontinence*).
Establish method to communicate urge to void (document on care plan).
Communicate to personnel the need to respond rapidly to a request to void.
Establish a planned-voiding pattern:
Provide an opportunity to void on awakening; after meals, physical exercise, bathing, and drinking coffee or tea; and before going to sleep.
Begin by offering bedpan, commode, or toilet every half hour initially, and gradually lengthen the time to at least every 2 h.
If person has incontinent episode, reduce the time between scheduled voidings.
Document behavior/activity that occurs with void or incontinence (see *Continuous Incontinence*).
Encourage person to try to "hold" urine until voiding time, if possible.
Consult primary care professional for pharmacological interventions.
Refer to *Continuous Incontinence* for additional information on developing a bladder reconditioning program.

**R:** The essential components of any continence training program (self-directed or caregiver directed) include motivation, assessment of voiding and incontinent patterns, a regular fluid intake of 2000 to

3,000 mL/day, timed voiding of 2 to 4 h intervals in an appropriate place, and ongoing assessment (Miller, 2009).

**Initiate Health Teaching.**

Instruct person on prevention of urinary tract infections (see *Functional Incontinence*).

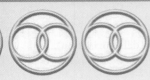

# OVERFLOW INCONTINENCE*

## DEFINITION

State in which a person experiences involuntary loss of urine associated with overdistention of the bladder.

## DEFINING CHARACTERISTICS

### Major (Must Be Present, One or More)

Bladder distention (not related to acute reversible etiology) or
Bladder distention with small, frequent voids or dribbling (overflow incontinence)
100 mL or more residual urine
High post void residual volume observed or reports involuntary leakage of small volumes of urine
Nocturia

## RELATED FACTORS

### Pathophysiologic

*Related to sphincter blockage secondary to:*

| | | |
|---|---|---|
| Strictures | Ureterocele | Bladder neck contractures |
| Prostatic enlargement | Perineal swelling | |

*Related to impaired afferent pathways or inadequacy secondary to:*

| | | |
|---|---|---|
| Cord injury/tumor/infection | Brain injury/tumor/infection | Cerebrovascular accident |
| Demyelinating diseases | Multiple sclerosis | Diabetic neuropathy |
| Alcoholic neuropathy | Tabes dorsalis | |

### Treatment-Related.

*Related to bladder outlet obstruction or impaired afferent pathways secondary to drug therapy (iatrogenic)*

| | | |
|---|---|---|
| Antihistamines | Theophylline | Epinephrine |
| Isoproterenol | Anticholinergics | |

### Situational (Personal, Environmental)

*Related to bladder outlet obstruction secondary to fecal impaction*
*Related to detrusor inadequacy secondary to:*

| | |
|---|---|
| Deconditioned voiding | Association with stress or discomfort |

---

*Previously *Urinary Retention*.

## ■■■■■ KEY CONCEPTS

- Three entities can cause overflow incontinence: bladder outlet obstruction, detrusor inadequacy, and impaired afferent pathways.
- Detrusor inadequacy is characterized by the pressure of uninhibited detrusor contractions sufficient to cause urinary incontinence. One cause of detrusor inadequacy is deconditioned voiding reflexes characterized by anxiety or discomfort associated with voiding. Another cause is central nervous system diseases.
- Impaired afferent pathways occur when both the sensory and motor branches of the simple reflex arc are damaged. Therefore, there are no sensations to tell the person the bladder is full or no motor impulses for emptying the bladder. Thus, the person develops a neurogenic bladder (autonomous). With this type of neurogenic bladder, the person is likely to dribble urine when pressure in the bladder rises because of the bladder filling beyond its normal capacity or because of coughing, straining, or exercising.

## Focus Assessment Criteria

See *Impaired Urinary Elimination*.

**NOC**
See *Functional Incontinence*

## ➤ Goal

The person will achieve a state of dryness that is personally satisfactory.

### Indicators:

- Empty the bladder using Créde's or Valsalva maneuver with a residual urine of less than 50 mL if indicated.
- Void voluntarily.

**NIC**
See also *Functional Incontinence,* Overflow retention Care, Urinary Bladder Training

## ➤ General Interventions

Refer to Related Factors

### Explain Rationale for Treatment.

### Develop a Bladder Retraining or Reconditioning Program (See **Continuous Incontinence**).

Instruct on methods to empty bladder.

### Assist to a Sitting Position.

Teach abdominal strain and Valsalva maneuver; instruct person to:

- Lean forward on thighs.
- Contract abdominal muscles, if possible, and strain or "bear down"; hold breath while straining (Valsalva maneuver).
- Hold strain or breath until urine flow stops; wait 1 min, and strain again as long as possible.
- Continue until no more urine is expelled.

**R:** Valsalva maneuver contracts the abdominal muscles, which manually compresses the bladder.
Teach Credé's maneuver; instruct person to:
Place hands flat (or place fist) just below umbilical area.
Place one hand on top of the other.
Press firmly down and in toward the pelvic arch.
Repeat six or seven times until no more urine can be expelled.
Wait a few minutes and repeat to ensure complete emptying.

**R:** In many clients, Credé's maneuver can help empty the bladder. This maneuver is inappropriate, however, if the urinary sphincters are chronically contracted. In this case, pressing the bladder can force urine up the ureters as well as through the urethra. Reflux of urine into the renal pelvis may result in renal infection.

*Indicate on the Intake and Output Record Which Technique Was Used to Induce Voiding.*

*Obtain Postvoid Residuals After Attempts at Emptying Bladder; If Residual Urine Volumes Are Greater Than 100 mL, Schedule Intermittent Catheterization Program (See Continuous Incontinence).*

**R:** Clean intermittent self-catheterization (CISC) prevents overdistention, helps maintain detrusor muscle tone, and ensures complete bladder emptying. CISC may be used initially to determine residual urine after Credé's maneuver or tapping. As residual urine decreases, catheterization may be tapered. CISC may recondition the voiding reflex in some clients.

### Initiate Health Teaching.

Teach bladder reconditioning program (see *Continuous Incontinence*).
Teach intermittent catheterization (see *Continuous Incontinence*).
Instruct person on prevention of urinary tract infections (see *Continuous Incontinence*).
**R:** If bladder emptying techniques are unsuccessful, other methods of managing incontinence are necessary.

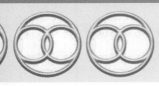

# RISK FOR VASCULAR TRAUMA

**Risk for Vascular Trauma Related to Infusion of Vesicant Medications.**

## DEFINITION

The state in which an individual is at risk for damage to a vein and its surrounding tissues related to the presence of a catheter and/or infused solutions.

## RISK FACTORS

### Treatment-Related

Catheter type*

Impaired ability to visualize the insertion site

Infusion rate*

Length of insertion time

Catheter width*

Inadequate catheter fixation*

Insertions site*

Nature of solution (e.g,. concentration. chemical irritant, temperature, pH)

▚▪▪▪▪▪■ **AUTHOR'S NOTE**

This new NANDA-I diagnosis represents a risk for all persons with intravenous catheters. Procedure manuals on the clinical unit should contain the correct placement, fixation and monitoring of all intravenous sites. Nurses needing these guidelines should refer to the procedure manual. There is no need for practicing nurses to have this diagnosis on the care plan. Students should refer to their fundamentals of nursing text for specific techniques to start, secure, and monitor intravenous therapy. Consult with your faculty to determine if this should be written on your assigned client's care plan.

*(continued)*

_____

*May indicate poor clinical practice.

■■■■■■■ **AUTHOR'S NOTE** *Continued*

Clinically, certain intravenous medications (e.g., chemotherapy, vesicant medications) are extremely toxic and therefore require specific interventions to prevent occurrence and tissue necrosis. Interventions and goals for preventing and responding to extravasation of the intravenous vesicant medications will be outlined for this diagnosis. These interventions are usually also found in a procedure manual.

■■■■■■■ **ERRORS IN DIAGNOSTIC STATEMENTS**

**Risk for Vascular Trauma related to inadequate catheter fixation**

This diagnostic statement contains a related factor that is legally problematic. If the catheter was inadequately secured, then this should be corrected. This is not a nursing diagnosis issue. It is a clinician problem that needs to be addressed and corrected.

Review the preceding Risk Factors; this author has placed an asterisk (*) next to all those listed that may indicate poor clinical practice. These situations should not be listed as related factors for this diagnosis but instead require immediate correction.

■■■■■■■ **KEY CONCEPTS**

- Administration of prescribed intravenous antineoplastic agents requires the nurse to review and know dosage (ranges), solution restrictions when dosage reductions are indicated, administration precautions (time, storage), side effects, and adverse effects.
- Intravenous drugs are categorized as an irritant, nonirritant, or vesicant.
- A local reaction to chemotherapy (e.g., doxorubicin) is a venous flare. It is characterized by a localized erythema, venous streaking, and pruritus along the injected vein. There is no pain or edema and there is a blood return.
- Another local reaction is from an agent carmustine (irritant) that causes pain, venous irritation, and chemical phlebitis. These agents do not cause ulceration if infiltrated.
- A vesicant is a drug that infiltrated (extravasation) causes pain, ulceration, necrosis, and sloughing of damaged tissue. Prolonged extravasation can cause loss of joint or tendon mobility, vascularity, or tendon function.
- Vesicants can be non-antineoplastic drugs (e.g., Levophed, Dilantin). Many antineoplastic drugs are vesicants.
- The physical and emotional impact of an extensive extravasation injury may prompt legal action.
- The best defenses against claims of negligence related to extravasation are the following:
  - To prevent them if possible
  - To detect them quickly
  - To intervene promptly
- Persons receiving vesicants intravenously need close monitoring and should be instructed of the signs and symptoms to report.

## Focus Assessment

### Assess the Insertion Site Prior to Infusion for:

- Leaks
- Redness
- Edema
- Blood return

### Assess the Site During Infusion for:

- Redness
- Swelling (bled at injection site)
- Blood return

**Ask the Client If There Is Any Burning or Pain at the Injection Site**

**Advise the Client to Report Any Sensations
That Occur at the Site During Infusion**

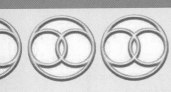

# RISK FOR VASCULAR TRAUMA

## ▶ Related to Infusion of Vesicant Medications

**NOC**
Knowledge
Treatment
Procedure, Risk
Control

### ➤ Goals

The client will report or be monitored for early signs/symptoms of extravasation.

*Indicators:*

- Swelling
- Stinging, burning, or pain at the injection site
- Redness
- Lack of blood return

**NIC**
Intravenous
Insertion, Medication
Administration:
Intravenous,
Surveillance,
Teaching: Procedure/
Treatment, Venous
Access Device (VAD)
Maintenance,
Chemotherapy
Management

### ➤ Interventions

**Prior to Administration of a Prescribed Vesicant
Medication, Review the Agency Protocol, Physician
Order, and Information About the Medication**

**R:** The institutional policy is written to help prevent extravasation and to direct management if it occurs.

**If Inexperienced in This Procedure,
Consult an Experienced Nurse**

**R:** Serious injury from extravasation can be prevented.

**Identify Clients at Increased Risk for Extravasation (Elderly, Debilitated,
Confused, Unable to Communicate, Diabetics, Fragile Veins, General
Vascular Disease) and Monitor Them Continuously During Infusion.**

**R:** Clients who cannot identify and communicate stinging, burning, or pain at the injection site cannot be relied on for early detection of extravasation (Hayden & Goodman, 2005).

**Avoid Infusing Vesicant Drugs:**

- Over joints, bony prominences, tendons, neurovascular bundles, or the antecubital fossa
- When venous or lymphatic circulation is poor
- At sites that have been previously irritated

**R:** These precautions can prevent movement of the catheter and extravasation.

**Never Give Vesicants Intramuscularly or Subcutaneously**

**The Drug Is Toxic to Tissues**

## Prior to Infusion

- Check for blood return gently
- Check all needle or catheter site for leaks, evidence of swelling, or venous thrombosis

**R:** Displacement, damage, or a blockage can be detected before infusion.

## Use the Correct Equipment (IV, Port, Huber-Point Needle) Slowly, in a Steady, Even Flow to Infuse Solution; Check for Blood Return According to Policy

**R:** Early identification of extravasation can prevent serious tissue damage.

## Assess the Client Every _____ per Institution's Policy for:

- Swelling
- Stinging, burning, or pain at the injection site
- Redness
- Lack of blood return

**R:** Extravasation can occur with or without symptoms and signs.

## If the Above Signs or Symptoms Occur, Stop Infusion and Contact an Experienced Nurse, Physician, or Nurse Practitioner Immediately

**R:** The situation requires a rapid diagnosis and actions.

## If Extravasation Occurs, Follow Institutional Policy for Discontinuation, Antidote Administration, Diluents, Site Care, Ice Applications, and Elevation of the Extremity

**R:** The institutional policy and extravasation kit should be available for use.

## Document the Extravasation Event Including Subjective Complaints and Objective Observations with Times and Actions Taken

**R:** The best defense against claims of negligence related to extravasation injuries is to prevent them to the extent possible, to detect them quickly, and to intervene properly.

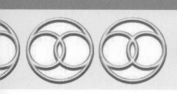

# RISK FOR OTHER-DIRECTED VIOLENCE

## DEFINITION

State in which a client has been, or is at risk to be, assaultive toward others or the environment

## RISK FACTORS

### Major (Must Be Present)

Presence of risk factors (see Related Factors).

# RELATED FACTORS

## Pathophysiologic

*Related to history of aggressive acts and perception of environment as threatening secondary to:*
or
*Related to history of aggressive acts and delusional thinking secondary to:*
or
*Related to history of aggressive acts and manic excitement secondary to:*
or
*Related to history of aggressive acts and inability to verbalize feelings secondary to:*
or
*Related to history of aggressive acts and psychic overload secondary to:*
Temporal lobe epilepsy
Head injury
Progressive central nervous system deterioration (brain tumor)
Hormonal imbalance
Viral encephalopathy
Mental retardation
Minimal brain dysfunction
*Related to toxic response to alcohol or drugs*
*Related to organic brain syndrome*

## Treatment-Related

*Related to toxic reaction to medication*

## Situational (Personal, Environmental)

*Related to history of overt aggressive acts*
*Related to increase in stressors within a short period*
*Related to acute agitation*
*Related to suspiciousness*
*Related to persecutory delusions*
*Related to verbal threats of physical assault*
*Related to low frustration tolerance*
*Related to poor impulse control*
*Related to fear of the unknown*
*Related to response to catastrophic event*
*Related to response to dysfunctional family throughout developmental stages*
*Related to dysfunctional communication patterns*
*Related to drug or alcohol abuse*

■■■■■■ **AUTHOR'S NOTE**

The diagnosis *Risk for Other-Directed Violence* describes a client who has been assaultive or, because of certain factors (e.g., toxic response to alcohol or drugs, hallucinations or delusions, brain dysfunction), is at high risk for assaulting others. In such a situation, the nursing focus is on decreasing violent episodes and protecting the client and others.

The nurse should not use this diagnosis to address underlying problems such as anxiety or poor self-esteem, but instead should refer to the diagnoses *Anxiety*, *Ineffective Coping*, or both to focus on the sources of the violence (spouse, child, older adult). When domestic violence is present or suspected, the nurse should explore the diagnosis *Disabled Family Coping*. A client at risk for suicide would warrant the diagnosis *Risk for Suicide*.

■■■■■ **ERRORS IN DIAGNOSTIC STATEMENTS**

1. *Risk for Other-Directed Violence related to reports of abuse by wife*
   "Reports of abuse by a spouse" represents family dysfunction, which *Risk for Violence* does not cover. Spouse abuse is a complex situation necessitating individual and family therapy. The nursing diagnoses *Disabled Family Coping* and *Ineffective Coping* for the abuser and the victim would be more clinically useful.
2. *Risk for Other-Directed Violence related to poor management or agitation by staff*
   This diagnostic statement is legally problematic and does not offer constructive strategies. When staff management of an agitated client is inappropriate, the nurse must treat this as a staff management problem, not a client problem. If staff members increased the client's agitation because of lack of knowledge, the nurse must outline specific do's and don'ts in the nursing care plan. In addition, an in-service program on identifying precursors to violence and agitation reduction strategies should be held for staff. For the client, the nurse could rewrite the diagnosis as *Risk for Other-Directed Violence related to mental dysfunction and persecutory delusions*.

■■■■■ **KEY CONCEPTS**

### Generic Considerations

- A central theme in violent people is helplessness. Assaultive behavior is a defense against passivity and helplessness.
- Aggressive behavior is a defense against anxiety. This coping mechanism is reinforced because it reduces anxiety by increasing the client's sense of power and control. (Refer to Key Concepts, *Anxiety*, for further discussion of anger.) Interventions that encourage "acting out of anger" reinforce assaultiveness and, thus, are to be avoided.
- Violence is usually preceded by a predictable sequence of events (e.g., a stressor or a series of stressors).
- When brain dysfunction is a prime or contributing factor to violent behavior, social and environmental variables still should be evaluated. Organic impairment may interfere with a client's ability to handle certain stresses. Exposure to or ingestion of toxic chemicals, such as lead and pesticides, can alter a client's normal behavior. Examples of violent behavior in brain dysfunction are biting, scratching, temper outbursts, and mood lability.
- Fear and anxiety can distort perceptions of the environment. Suspicious, delusional people often misinterpret stimuli. Alcohol and drugs also impair judgment and decrease internal controls over behavior.
- People who had a history of emotional deprivation in childhood are particularly vulnerable to attacks on their self-esteem.
- Although the client may identify the person with whom he or she is angry, this may not be the real object of aggression. People often cannot allow themselves to express anger toward a person on whom they are dependent.
- Staff members frequently respond to violent clients with actual fear or overreactions. This can lead to punitive sanctions such as heavier medication, seclusion, or attempts to cope by avoidance and withdrawal from the client. Staff must identify their own reactions to violent individuals so they can manage the situation more effectively. Staff should trust an intuition that the client is potentially violent (Farrell et al., 1998).
- In studies of clients' perception of seclusion, sense of powerlessness seemed to be the worst feeling, followed by fear, humiliation, loneliness, and shame (Norris & Kennedy, 1992).
- Physical aggression in long-term care, such as swearing, biting, kicking, spitting, and grabbing, may be in response to a loss of control over life. The more importance the client attaches to freedom and choice, the more forcefully he or she is likely to respond.

 **Pediatric Considerations**

- In 1994, there were 24,547 victims of violence in the United States; more than one third were younger than 25 years of age. Between 1985 and 1994, homicide rates for males 15 to 19 years of age increased 166% (Dowd, 1998).
- From 1985–1994, the percentage of gun-related homicides rose from 67% to 87% in people 15 to 24 years of age (Dowd, 1998).
- Homicide is the leading cause of death for African-American and Hispanic males 15 to 24 years of age (Dowd, 1998).
- Violent shaking of children, especially those younger than 6 months, can cause fatal intracranial trauma without signs of external head injury (Hockenberry & Wilson, 2009).

- The homicide rate in the United States is 4.3 times higher in children 0 to 4 years of age and 5.8 times higher in children 5 to 14 years of age than in 25 industrialized countries.
- Children who are exposed to community violence experience more depression, anxiety, fear, and aggressive acting-out behaviors than children not exposed (Veenema, 2006).
- During 2001 in the United States, 903,000 children experienced or were at risk for child abuse. Physical abuse of children often results from unreasonable severe corporal punishment or unjustifiable punishment (e.g., hitting an infant for crying) (Varcarolis, 2006).

## Focus Assessment Criteria

(Refer also to Focus Assessment Criteria for *Ineffective Coping, Disabled Family Coping, Confusion,* and *Anxiety*).

### Subjective Data

### *Assess for Risk Factors.*

**Medical History**

| | |
|---|---|
| Hormonal imbalance | Head injury |
| Brain disease | Drug abuse (amphetamines, phencyclidine hydrochloride, marijuana, alcohol, cocaine) |

**Psychiatric History**

| | |
|---|---|
| Previous hospitalizations | Outpatient therapy |

**History of Emotional Difficulties in Client, Family, or Both**

| | |
|---|---|
| Mental retardation | Parental brutality |
| Cruelty to animals | Pyromania |

**Interaction Patterns (Note Changes)**

| | |
|---|---|
| Family | Coworkers |
| Friends | Others |

**Coping Patterns (Past and Present)**

**Sources of Stress in Current Environment**

**Work/School History**

| | |
|---|---|
| How does client function under stress? | Fights in school |
| | Stable employment |
| Level of education attained | Frequency of job changes |
| Learning disabilities | Periods of unemployment |

**Legal History**
Arrests and convictions for violent crimes
Juvenile offenses for violent behavior

**History of Violence**
Assess recency, severity, and frequency:

- "What is the most violent thing you have ever done?"
- "What is the closest you have ever come to striking someone?"
- "In what kinds of situations have you hit someone or destroyed property?"
- "When was the last time this happened?"
- "How often does this occur?"
- "Were you using drugs or alcohol during these episodes?"

**Present Thoughts About Violence**
Identify possible victim and weapon:

- "How do you feel after an incident?"
- "Are you currently having thoughts about harming someone?"

- "Is there anyone in particular you think about harming?" (Identify the victim and the client's access to the victim.)
- "Do you have a specific plan for how you might accomplish this?" (Identify the plan, type of weapon, and availability of weapon.)

### Thought Content
Helplessness
Suspiciousness or hostility
Perceived intention (e.g., "He meant to hit me" in response to a slight bump)
Fear of loss of control
Persecutory delusions
Disorientation

### Child–Adolescent
*Conflict management—impulse control*
How does the child respond to conflict?
History of fights
History of being a victim of bullying

*Relationships*
Has he or she experienced pushing, hitting, being afraid, being hurt, or being forced to have sexual contact?

*Safety*
"Do you feel safe?"
"Are you afraid of someone you know?"
"Have you talked with an adult about this situation?"
If abuse is suspected, refer to *Disabled Family Coping*.

## Objective Data

## *Assess for Risk Factors*

### Body Language
Posture (relaxed, rigid)
Hands (relaxed, rigid, clenched)
Facial expression (calm, annoyed, tense)

### Motor Activity
| | | |
|---|---|---|
| Within normal limits | Pacing | Immobile |
| Agitation | Increased | |

### Affect
| | | |
|---|---|---|
| Within normal limits | Flat | Labile |
| Inappropriate | Controlled | |

For more information on Focus Assessment Criteria, visit http://thepoint.lww.com.

**NOC**
Abuse Cessation, Abusive Behavior Self-Restraint, Aggression Self-Control, Impulse Self-Control

## ➤ Goal

The client will have fewer violent responses or none.

### *Indicators (Varcarolis, 2006):*

- Seeks assistance when emotions are escalating
- Refrains from threatening, loud language toward others
- Responds to external controls when at high risk for loss of control
- Explain rationales for interventions.

**NIC**
Abuse Protection Support, Anger Control Assistance, Environmental Management: Violence Prevention, Impulse Control Training, Crisis Intervention, Seclusion, Physical Restraint

➤ **General Interventions**

The nursing interventions for *Risk for Other-Directed Violence* apply to any client who is potentially violent, regardless of related factors.

## Promote Interactions that Increase the Client's Sense of Trust

Acknowledge the client's feelings (e.g., "You are having a rough time"):

*   Be genuine and empathetic.
*   Tell the client that you will help him or her to control behavior and not do anything destructive.
*   Be direct and frank ("I can see you are angry").
*   Be consistent and firm.

Set limits when the client poses a risk to others. Refer to *Anxiety* for further interventions on limit-setting. Offer choices and options. At times, it is necessary to give in to some demands to avoid a power struggle.

**R:** Setting limits clarifies rules, guidelines, and standards of acceptable behavior and establishes the consequences of violating the rules.

Encourage the client to express anger and hostility verbally instead of "acting out."
Encourage walking or exercise as activities that may diffuse aggression.

**R:** Physical activity can help reduce muscle tension (Alvarey, 1998).

Maintain client's personal space:

*   Do not touch the client.
*   Avoid feelings of physical entrapment of individual or staff.

Be aware of your own feelings and reactions:

*   Do not take verbal abuse personally.
*   Remain calm if you are becoming upset; leave the situation to others, if possible.
*   After a threatening situation, discuss your feelings with other staff.

**R:** Staff activities may be counterproductive to managing aggressive behavior. Recognition and replacement of attitudes such as "I must be calm and relaxed at all times" with "No matter how anxious I feel, I will keep thinking and decide on the best approach" often prevent escalation of aggression.

Observe for cues to increasing anger (Boyd, 2005):

*   Reports of numbness, nausea, and vertigo
*   Choking sensation, chills, and prickly sensations
*   Increased muscle tone, clenched fists, set jaw, and eyebrows lower and drawn together
*   Lips pressed together to form a thin line
*   Flushing or paleness
*   "Goose bumps"
*   Twitching
*   Sweating

**R:** Violence can have a pattern. Early detection can prevent escalation (Varcarolis, 2006).

## Initiate Immediate Management of the High-Risk Client

Allow the client with acute agitation space that is five times greater than that for a client who is in control. Do not touch the client unless you have a trusting relationship.
Avoid physical entrapment of individual or staff.
Convey empathy by acknowledging the client's feelings. Let the client know you will not let him or her lose control. Remind the client of previous successes at self-control.
Do not approach a violent client alone. Often, the presence of three or four staff members is enough to reassure the client that you will not let him or her lose control. Use a positive tone; do not demand or cajole.

**R:** Always place staff safety first. The presence of four or five staff members reassures the client that you will not let him or her lose control. The focus is respect, concern, and safety.

**R:** Assaultive behavior tends to occur when conditions are crowded, are without structure, and involve staff-"demanded" activity (Farrell et al., 1998).

Give the client control by offering alternatives (e.g., walking, talking).
Set limits on actions, not feelings. Use concise, easily understood statements.

**R:** Minimization of anger and ineffective coping are the most frequent factors contributing to escalation of violence (Varcolis, 2006).

Maintain eye contact, but do not stare. Stand at a friendly angle (45 degrees); keep an open posture if the client is standing, and sit when the client sits.

**R:** Maintain the same physical level (e.g., both people either sitting or standing prevents feelings of intimidation). The least aggressive stance is at a 45-degree angle to the person, rather than face to face.

Do not make promises you cannot keep.
Avoid using "always" and "never."

**R:** Although people may verbalize hostile threats and take a defensive stance, most fear losing control and want assistance to maintain their control (Alvarey, 1998).

When interpersonal and pharmacologic interventions fail to control the angry, aggressive client, physical interventions (restraints, seclusion) are the final resort. Always follow hospital protocols (Varocolis, 2006).

**R:** Hospital protocols should be clear regarding how, when, and for what time period a client can be restrained or secluded and the associated nursing care needed (Varicolis, 2006).

## Establish an Environment that Reduces Agitation (Farrell et al., 1998)

Decrease noise level.
Give short, concise explanations.
Control the number of persons present at one time.
Provide asingle or semiprivate room.
Allow the client to arrange personal possessions.
Be aware that darkness can increase disorientation and enhance suspiciousness.
Decrease situations in which the client is frustrated.
Provide music if the client is receptive.

**R:** The client is in an agitated/mentally compromised state. Environmental stimuli unnecessarily increase this state and can increase aggression.

## Assist the Client to Maintain Control over His or Her Behavior

Establish the expectation that he or she can control behavior, and continue to reinforce the expectation. Explain exactly which behavior is inappropriate and why.
Give three options: two offer a choice, whereas the third is the consequence of violent behavior.
Allow time for the client to make a choice.
Provide positive feedback when the client is able to exercise restraint.
Enforce consequences when indicated.
Reassure the client that you will provide control if he or she cannot ("I am concerned about you. I will get [more staff, medications] to keep you from doing anything impulsive.").
Set firm, clear limits when a client presents a danger to self or others ("Put the chair down.").
Call the client by name in a calm, quiet, respectful manner.
Avoid threats; refer to yourself, not policies, rules, or supervisors.
Allow appropriate verbal expressions of anger. Give positive feedback.
Set limits on verbal abuse. Do not take insults personally. Support others (clients, staff) who may be targets of abuse.
Do not give attention to the client who is being verbally abusive. Tell the client what you are doing and why.

Assist with external controls, as necessary:

- Maintain observation every 15 to 30 min.
- Remove items that the client could use as weapons (e.g., glass, sharp objects).
- Assess the client's ability to tolerate off-unit procedures.
- If the client is acutely agitated, be cautious with items such as hot coffee.

**R:** Crisis management techniques can help prevent escalation of aggression and help the client achieve self-control. The least restrictive safe and effective measure should be used (Alvarey, 1998).

**R:** The nurse and the client collaborate to find solutions and alternatives to aggression (Boyd, 2005).

## Plan for Unpredictable Violence

Monitor for cues to potential aggression (Alvarey, 1998).

### *Verbal*

| | | |
|---|---|---|
| Morose silence | Loud, demanding remarks | Illogical responses |
| Negative response to requests | Demeaning remarks | Overt hostility |
| Threats | Sarcasm | Mistrust |

### *Nonverbal Facial Expression*

| | | |
|---|---|---|
| Tense jaw | Staring | Clenched teeth |
| Dilated pupils | Lip biting | Pulsing carotid |

### *Nonverbal Body Language*

| | | |
|---|---|---|
| Hand twisting objects | Stony withdrawal | Aggression toward |
| Confrontational stance | Fist clenching, unclenching (slamming doors) | |
| Pounding, kicking | Pacing | |

Ensure availability of staff before potential violent behavior (never try to assist the client alone when physical restraint is necessary).

Determine who will be in charge of directing personnel to intervene in violent behavior if it occurs.

Ensure protection for self (door nearby for withdrawal, pillow to protect face).

**R:** Crisis management techniques can help prevent escalation of aggression and help the client achieve self-control. The least-restrictive safe and effective measure should be used (Alvarey, 1998).

## Use Seclusion and/or Restraint, If Indicated

Remove client from situation if environment is contributing to aggressive behavior, using the least amount of control needed (e.g., ask others to leave, and take client to quiet room).

Reinforce that you are going to help the client control himself or herself.

Repeatedly tell the client what is going to happen before external control begins.

Ensure that sufficient personnel (5) are present.

Protect client from injuring self or others through use of restraints or seclusion.*

When using seclusion, institutional policy provides specifics; the following are general:

- Observe the client at least every 15 min.
- Search the client before secluding to remove harmful objects.
- Check seclusion room to see that safety is maintained.
- Offer fluids and food periodically (in nonbreakable containers).
- When approaching a client to be secluded, have sufficient staff present.
- Explain concisely what is going to happen ("You will be placed in a room by yourself until you can better control your behavior"); give the client a chance to cooperate.
- Assist with toileting and personal hygiene (assess the client's ability to be out of seclusion; a urinal or commode may need to be used).
- If the client is taken out of seclusion, someone must be present continually.

---

* May require a primary care professional's order.

- Maintain verbal interaction during seclusion (provides information necessary to assess the client's degree of control).
- When the client is allowed out of seclusion, a staff member needs to be in constant attendance to determine whether the client can handle additional stimulation.

When using restraint, institutional policy provides specifics. The following are general measures:

- A client in a four-point or two-point restraint must be in seclusion or with one-on-one nursing care for protection. Seclusion guidelines should be followed.
- Restraints must be loosened every hour (one limb at a time).
- Waist restraints must allow enough arm movement to enable eating/smoking and self-protection against falling.
- Restraints should be padded.
- Restraints never should be attached to side rails, but rather to the bed frame.

Provide an opportunity to clarify the rationale for seclusion and to discuss the client's reactions after the seclusion period is over.

**R:** Seclusion and restraint are options for a client exhibiting serious, persistent aggression. The nurse must protect the client's safety at all times. Use of the least restrictive measures allows the client the most opportunity to regain self-control (Farrell et al., 1998).

### Convene a Group Discussion After a Violent Episode on an Inpatient Unit

Include all those who witnessed the episode (client, staff).
Include client(s) exhibiting the violent behavior, if possible.
Discuss what happened, the consequences, and the feelings of the community.

**R:** After a violent act, leading a group discussion of the event, outcome, and feelings can decrease anxiety, increase understanding of violence, and address preventable problems that occurred.

### Assist the Client in Developing Alternative Coping Strategies When the Crisis Has Passed and Learning Can Occur

Explore what precipitates the client's loss of control ("What was happening before you began to feel like hitting her?").
Assist the client to recall the physical symptoms associated with anger.
Help the client to evaluate where in the chain of events change was possible:

- Use role playing to practice communication techniques.
- Discuss how issues of control interfere with communication.
- Help the client recognize negative thinking patterns associated with low self-esteem.

Help the client to practice negotiation skills with significant others and people in authority.
Encourage increased recreational activities.
Use group therapy to decrease sense of aloneness and increase communication skills.
Instruct or refer for assertiveness training.
Instruct or refer for negotiation skills development.

**R:** Postcrisis discussions can help to foster new and more effective approaches to management of aggressive persons (Varcolis, 2006).

**Pediatric Interventions**

Discuss with parents the methods of disciplining the child. Refer to *Disabled Family Coping* for more information on child abuse if indicated.
Discuss the risks of firearms in the home. Explore the storage of firearms and protective devices (e.g., lockboxes, trigger locks).

*(continued)*

**Pediatric Interventions**
*Continued*

Explore various sources of media violence (e.g., television, video games, music, movies).
Explain strategies to prevent adverse effects of media violence (Willis & Strasburger, 1998):

* Watch television and videos with children.
* If possible, avoid programs that emphasize violence.
* Creatively illustrate when violent acts are punished.
* Explore alternatives to violence (e.g., "What could the man have done besides shooting?")
* When selecting programs, consider:
  * Are good characters violent?
  * Is the violence justified?
  * Are there negative consequences of violence?

Consider the child's age when selecting television programs and movies.

**R:** Discussions that correlate with the actual viewing of violent behavior are more meaningful (Davies & Flannery, 1998).

Engage the child and peers in a nonthreatening manner to discuss age-related violence (e.g., hitting, bullying, throwing objects, date rape).

**R:** Violence is a learned behavior. If it is learned, then prosocial behavior can also be taught as an alternative (Davies & Flannery, 1998).

Role-play high-risk situations, such as:

* Finding a gun in a friend's house
* Bullying a victim
* Refusing sexual advances

**R:** Parents can model appropriate problem-solving strategies. Environments (families, schools, communities) that provide caring and support have high expectations, and provide opportunities for children to participate in discussions that can increase children's hardiness and invulnerability to violence (Edari & McManus, 1998).

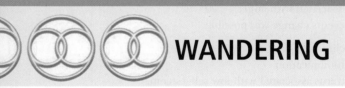

# WANDERING

## DEFINITION

State in which a client with dementia has meandering, aimless, or repetitive locomotion that exposes the client to harm

## DEFINING CHARACTERISTICS

Wandering is frequently incongruent with boundaries, limits, or obstacles.
The client with dementia who acts in the following ways (Algase, 1999):

* Ambulates in an aimless, endless manner
* Has repetitive locomotion in a circular pattern
* Paces repeatedly
* Exceeds or transgresses environmental limits into hazardous or unauthorized locations
* Has spatial disorientation or navigational deficits
* Cannot find what he or she is seeking

## RELATED FACTORS

### Pathophysiologic

*Related to impaired cerebral function secondary to:\**

Cerebrovascular accident          Mental retardation          Alzheimer's dementia or other dementia

*Related to physiologic urge (e.g., hunger, thirst, pain, urination, constipation)*

Situational (Personal, Environmental)

*Related to increased frustration, anxiety, boredom, depression, or agitation*

*Related to over/understimulating environment*

*Related to separation from familiar people and places*

### Maturational

Older Adult

*Related to faulty judgments secondary to motor and sensory deficits, medications*

■■■■■■ **AUTHOR'S NOTE**

This approved NANDA diagnosis is more useful than *Risk for Injury*, which was previously used. *Risk for Injury* focuses on strategies to protect a client from injury. *Wandering* directs interventions to protect the client from injury in addition to addressing the reasons for the wandering behavior, if possible.

■■■■■■ **ERRORS IN DIAGNOSTIC STATEMENTS**

**Wandering related to repetitive episodes of "being lost" in neighborhood**

This diagnosis as written does not have related factors. These related factors are signs of *Wandering*. If the contributing factors to *Wandering* are not known, the nurse can write the diagnosis as *Wandering related to unknown etiology, as evidenced by repetitive episodes of "being lost" in the neighborhood.*

■■■■■■ **KEY CONCEPTS**

- Up to 39% of cognitively impaired nursing home residents and up to 79% of community-residing patients wander (Nelson, 2004).
- Wandering behavior is thought to result from frontal and parietal lobe damage that causes cognitive problems (Maier-Lorentz, 2000). Severity and duration of the dementia correlate with the wandering (Algase, 1999).
- It is uncertain why people wander. Some possible causes are as follows (Brown et al., 1999):
  - Feeling lost
  - Searching for something/someone
  - Overstimulation
  - Anxiety
  - Boredom
  - Needing exercise
- Negative consequences of wandering for patients include elopement, falls, other injuries, and even death (Nelson, 2004).

## Focus Assessment Criteria

### Subjective Data

### *Assess for Related Factors*

Emotional coping patterns
See *Ineffective Coping*.

---

*This related factor must be present. Other related factors also can be present concurrently.

## Objective Data

### *Assess for Defining Characteristics*

Reported episodes of:

Trespassing    Persistent locomotion

Getting lost    Following caregiver    Hyperactivity

Pacing

Locomotion with no apparent destination

For more information on Focus Assessment Criteria, visit http://thepoint.lww.com.

---

**NOC**

Risk Control, Elopement Propensity Risk, Safe Wandering, Family Functioning

## ➤ Goals

The client will not elope or get lost.

### *Indicators for Client/Family:*

• Ambulate safely.
• Caretakers will identify factors that contribute to wandering behaviors.
• Caretakers will anticipate wandering behaviors.

---

**NIC**

Surveillance: Safety, Environmental Management: Safety, Referral, Risk Identification, Security Enhancement

## ➤ General Interventions

### Assess for Contributing Factors

Anxiety

Confusion

Frustration

Boredom

Agitation

Separation from familiar people and places

Faulty judgments

Physiologic urge (hunger, thirst, pain, urination, constipation)

## Reduce or Eliminate Contributing Factors, If Possible

### *Anxiety/Agitation*

Refer to *Anxiety* for interventions.

### *Unfamiliar Environment*

Select a familiar picture to exhibit on the client's door.

Redirect the client if he or she is lost.

Provide a safe route for walking.

Encourage activities that involve exercise (e.g., sweeping, raking).

Create nature scenes in the hallways (Cohen-Mansfield, 1998).

Mark exit door with big signs.

Place horizontal stripes on the exit door or use a cloth panel across the width of the door.

**R:** Safe paths within or on the outside of a unit can provide a release for the need to wander (Logsdon et al., 1998).

**R:** When an environment is enhanced with murals, pictures, and so forth, people with dementia trespass and exit less (Cohen-Mansfield, 1998).

### *Physiologic Urges*

Anticipate need for toileting with a schedule.

Schedule times for fluids and food.

Evaluate for any pain.

**R:** Physiologic needs (e.g., elimination, hunger, thirst) can precipitate wandering.

## Promote a Safe Environment

Install locks on doors and windows.

Install electronic devices with buzzers on doors and property boundaries.

Use pressure-sensitive alarms (doormats, bed sensor, chair sensor).

Provide regular opportunities for the client to walk with a companion or in a safe area.

**R:** Modifying the environment rather than using restraints can decrease stress and agitation (Logsdon et al., 1998).

**R:** People with cognitive impairments need external controls for protection.

## Notify Others (Neighbors, Police, Others in Residence, Staff, Community Resources) About the Client's Wandering Behaviors

Explain the use of electronic devices.

Instruct others to notify the provider if they see the client wandering.

Supply others with a recent photograph and current identification information (age, height, weight, hair color, description of clothes, identifying characteristics) of the client.

Contact the local Alzheimer's Association for safety programs.

**R:** Community residents, personnel, and police need to be alerted to the risk of wandering and injury.

# Part Two
# FAMILY/HOME NURSING DIAGNOSES

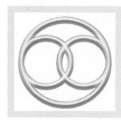

This section focuses on Family and Home Nursing Diagnoses. These diagnoses can be utilized in any setting, for example, a hospital or a home. Community Wellness and Health Maintenance diagnoses related to the family can be found in Part Four. Key concepts related to the family will be relevant to all types of Family and Home Nursing Diagnoses.

## ■■■■■■ KEY CONCEPTS

### Generic Considerations
- Each family has a personality to which each member contributes.
- The family unit may be viewed as a system with:
  - Interdependence among members
  - Interactional patterns that provide structure and support for members
  - Boundaries between the family and the environment and between members, with varying degrees of permeability
- Families change with time. They must accomplish specific tasks that originate from the needs of their members. Table II.19 illustrates the task of the family.
- Each family member influences the entire family unit. Thus, the health of an individual influences the health of the family. Family equilibrium depends on a balance of roles in the family and reciprocation (Clemen-Stone et al., 2002; Duvall, 1977).

*(continued)*

■ ■ ■ ■ ■ ■ **KEY CONCEPTS** *Continued*

- *Stress* is defined as the body's response to any demand made on it. Stress has the potential to become a crisis when the person or family cannot cope constructively. A *crisis* is when a person's usual problem-solving methods are inadequate to resolve a situation.
- "Crisis resolution can be an adaptive process, in which growth and impaired health occur, or it can be maladaptive, resulting in abuse,* illness or even death" (Allender & Spradley, 2006, p. 558).
- The family responding to the crisis returns to pre-crisis functioning, develops improved functioning (adaptation), or develops destructive functioning (maladaptation).
- Constructive or functional coping mechanisms of families facing a stress crisis are as follows (Clemen-Stone et al., 2002):
  - Greater reliance on one another
  - Maintenance of a sense of humor
  - Increased sharing of feeling and thoughts
  - Promotion of each member's individuality
  - Accurate appraisal of the meaning of the problem
  - Search for knowledge and resources about the problem
  - Use of support systems
- Destructive or dysfunctional coping mechanism of families facing a crisis are as follows (Smith-DiJulio, 1998, Carson & Smith-DiJulio, 2006):
  - Denial of the problem
  - Exploitation of one or more members (threats, violence, neglect, scapegoating)
  - Separation (hospitalization, institutionalization, divorce, abandonment)
  - Authoritarianism (no negotiation)
  - Preoccupation of family or members (who lack affection) with appearing close
- Parenthood is a crisis. Some common problems include the following:
  - Increased arguments in adults
  - Fatigue resulting from schedule
  - Disrupted social life
  - Disrupted sex life
  - Multiple losses—actual or perceived (e.g., independence, career, appearance, attention)
- Characteristics of families prone to crisis include the following (Fife, 1985; Smith-DiJulio, 1998; Carson & Smith-DiJulio, 2006):
  - Apathy (resignation to state in life)
  - Poor self-concept
  - Low income
  - Inability to manage money
  - Unrealistic preferences (materialistic)
  - Lack of skills and education
  - Unstable work history
  - Frequent relocations
  - History of repeated inadequate problem solving
  - Lack of adequate role models
  - Lack of participation in religious or community activities
  - Environmental isolation (no telephone, inadequate public transportation)
- A time lag exists between identifying symptoms and help-seeking behavior, which may vary among families, depending on previous experience with the health care system, cultural interpretations of health and illness, and financial concerns.
- Successful outcomes of family efforts to achieve new adaptation after a crisis depend on the following (Nugent, Hughes, Ball & Davis, 1992):
- Cohesiveness in response to past stressors
- Interaction with others in support group
- Belief that family can handle the crisis

———————————

\* Added by this author.

### TABLE II.19 STAGE-CRITICAL FAMILY DEVELOPMENTAL TASKS THROUGH THE FAMILY LIFE CYCLE

| Stage of the Family Life Cycle | Positions in the Family | Stage-Critical Family Developmental Tasks |
|---|---|---|
| 1. Married couple | Wife<br>Husband | Establishing a mutually satisfying marriage<br>Adjusting to pregnancy and the promise of parenthood<br>Fitting into the kin network |
| 2. Child-bearing | Wife–mother<br>Husband–father<br>Infant daughter or son or both | Having, adjusting to, and encouraging the development of infants<br>Establishing a satisfying home for both parents and infant(s) |
| 3. Preschool-aged | Wife–mother<br>Husband–father<br>Daughter–sister<br>Son–brother | Adapting to the critical needs and interests of preschool children in stimulating, growth-promoting ways<br>Coping with energy depletion and lack of privacy as parents |
| 4. School-aged | Wife–mother<br>Husband–father<br>Daughter–sister<br>Son–brother | Fitting into the community of school-aged families in constructive ways<br>Encouraging children's educational achievement |
| 5. Teenage | Wife–mother<br>Husband–father<br>Daughter–sister<br>Son–brother | Balancing freedom with responsibility as teenagers mature and emancipate themselves<br>Establishing postparental interests and careers as growing parents |
| 6. Launching center | Wife–mother–grandmother<br>Husband–father–grandfather<br>Daughter–sister–aunt<br>Son–brother–uncle | Releasing young adults into work, military service, college, marriage, etc. with appropriate rituals and assistance<br>Maintaining a supportive home base |
| 7. Middle-aged parents | Wife–mother–grandmother<br>Husband–father–grandfather | Rebuilding the marriage relationship<br>Maintaining kin ties with older and younger generations |
| 8. Aging family members | Widow–widower<br>Wife–mother–grandmother<br>Husband–father–grandfather | Coping with bereavement and living alone<br>Closing the family home or adapting it to aging<br>Adjusting to retirement |

Duvall, E. M. (1977). *Marriage and family development* (5th ed.). Philadelphia: J. B. Lippincott, reproduced with permission.

## Transcultural Considerations

- The dominant US culture values two goals for families: (1) encouragement and nurturance of each individual and (2) cultivation of healthy, autonomous children. Marital partners are expected to be supportive and share a sense of meaning. Each partner has the freedom for personality development. Children are encouraged to develop their own identity and life directions (Giger & Davidhizar, 2009).
- The family was found to be the principal source of support during illness in seven minority groups (Giger & Davidhizar, 2009).
- In Latin families, the needs of the family are more important than those of the individual. The father is provider, head of the household, and decision maker (Andrews & Boyle, 2008).
- Arab-American families are supposed to be supportive. A family is often criticized as a failure if a member is sent to the hospital for psychiatric care. Arab-American families may appear overindulgent and interfering to compensate for criticism (Giger & Davidhizar, 2009).
- Japanese Americans identify themselves by the generation in which they are born. First- and second-generation Japanese Americans see the family as one of the most important factors in their lives. They manage problems within the family structure. The father and other male members are in the top position. Achievement or failure of one member reflects on the entire family. Caring for elderly parents, usually by the oldest son or unmarried child, is expected. Adult children freely provide their parents with goods, money, and assistance (Andrews & Boyle, 2008; Hashizume & Takano, 1983).
- The nuclear family and the greater Jewish community are the center of Jewish culture. Families are close knit and child oriented. The commandments dictate expected behavior toward parents and within the community (Giger & Davidhizar, 2009).

- For the Vietnamese, family has been the chief source of cohesion and continuity for hundreds of years. Immediate family includes parents, unmarried children, and sometimes the husband's parents and sons with their wives and children. Individual behavior reflects on the whole family. A member is expected to give up personal wishes or ambitions if they disrupt family harmony. Family loyalty is "filial piety," which commands children to obey and honor their parents even after death (Giger & Davidhizar, 2009).

## Families in Crisis

- Abuse is "willful infliction of physical injury or mental anguish and the deprivation by the caregiver of essential services" (Verwoerdt, 1976, as cited in Smith-DiJulio & Holzapfel, 1998) and nurturing. Patterns of family maltreatment can take many forms, including physical abuse, endangerment, sexual abuse, emotional abuse, neglect, and economic abuse (Smith-DiJulio & Holzapfel, 1998; Carson & Smith-DiJulio, 2006).

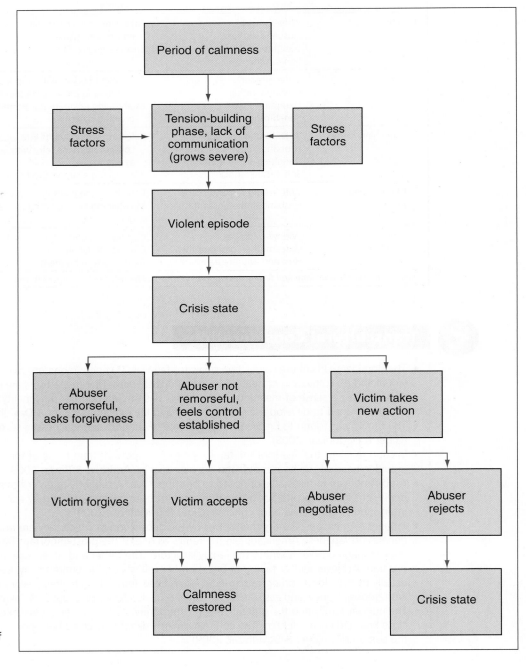

**FIGURE II.3** Escalation of violence.

- "Battering is a discordant, disrespectful and violent behavior exercised by people to attack or injure another person physically, psychologically and sexually" (Willis & Porche, 2004, p. 271).
- It is a criminal activity; no matter the reason, battering is an unacceptable response. Never ask a victim of battering why he or she stays; instead, focus on the criminal behavior and protection for the victim.
- Violence and abuse are choices batterers make.
- People involved in family violence have higher levels of depression, suicidal feelings, self-contempt, inability to trust, and inability to develop intimate relationships in later life (Smith-DiJulio & Holzapfel, 1998; Carson & Smith-DiJulio, 2006).
- Children who witness abuse in their homes after 5 or 6 years of age begin to identify with the aggressor and lose respect for the victim (Smith-DiJulio & Holzapfel, 1998; Carson & Smith-DiJulio, 2006).
- The following are characteristics of abusive families:
  - Poor differentiation of individuals within the family
  - Lack of autonomy
  - Insulation from the influence of others; social isolation
  - Desperate competition for affection and nurturance among members
  - Feelings of helplessness and hopelessness
  - Abuse/violence learned as a way to reduce tension
  - Low tolerance for frustration; poor impulse control
  - Closeness and caring confused with abuse/violence
  - Communication patterns characterized by mixed and double messages
  - High level of conflict surrounding family tasks
  - Nonexistent parental coalition
- The role of the victim is a critical factor in child and spouse abuse. It is socially learned and characterized by helplessness. This occurs when victims learn over time that they cannot control their lives.
- Guilt reactions are common among victims; they frequently feel responsible for the incident. This helps to protect them against feelings of powerlessness.

## Spouse Abuse

- "Domestic violence is a behavior that is chosen by a batterer in order to exercise power and control over another person. The batterer, and only the batterer, decides to use abusive and violent behavior. A battered partner cannot make the abuser stop being violent and/or abusive, as the batterer chooses to use this behavior as a form of control. A battered partner does not ask for, invite or provoke the abuser to be violent. The batterer does not become violent because of the use or abuse of alcohol and/or drugs" (AWARE, 1994, p. 1).
- The sociologic-cultural factors linked to battering are gender and power dynamics, criminal deviance, structural and institutional hierarchies of male dominance, patriarchy, entitlement, family structure, aggressive behaviors, stereotypical views of women, and the intergenerational transmission of violence as a learned behavior (Willis & Porche, 2004).
- Spouse abuse in the form of beatings occurs in 1% of all families. Some form of violence disrupts 50% of U.S. families. About 2% to 4% of all women presenting at the emergency room or primary care setting are battered (Agency for Healthcare Research and Quality, 2002). Three out of every 100 males severely batter their intimate partners within a 1-year period (CDC, 2003). Fifteen percent of all homicides are spouse killings; 50% of the victims are women. Women usually kill their husbands with guns and knives, whereas husbands usually beat wives to death (Chescheir, 1996).
- The battered wife syndrome has three major concepts: cycle of violence (Fig. II.3), learned helplessness, and anticipatory fear (Blair, 1986).
- Learned helplessness can result from childhood experiences, witnessing or receiving abuse, or the outcome of the battering relationship (Blair, 1986).
- Victims of abuse are "brainwashed by terror." They use denial and rationalization when they remain in the battering relationship (Blair, 1986).
- Battered women rarely report incidents to health care providers; rather, they seek assistance for psychosomatic conditions (chest pain, choking sensations, abdominal pain, fatigue, gastrointestinal disorders, and pelvic pain) or with injuries with inappropriate explanations (Greany, 1984). Victims seldom report abuse because of (Blair, 1986):
  - Feelings of guilt and shame
  - Fear of social stigmatization

- Fear of the abuser
- View of violence as normal
- Lack of alternative resources
- Violent episodes
  - Escalate in frequency and severity over time
  - Require less and less provocation to trigger them
  - Include verbal as well as physical abuse
  - Are made more brutal by alcohol use
- Carlson-Catalano (1998) found that of the battered women in her study, all reported they left to protect another loved one (child or pet). None of the women reported that she left because of her own safety or discomfort.
- Women who attempt to defend themselves during the tension-building phase often succeed in preventing the beating, whereas women who attempt to defend themselves during the assault phase often sustain a more brutal beating.
- The abuser's ability to control his spouse directly increases his feelings of autonomy and esteem. Therefore, the fear of loss (and loss of control) of his spouse directly influences his feelings about himself.
- Factors contributing to a battered woman's remaining in the relationship follow:
  - Belief that children need a two-parent family
  - Lack of financial support
  - Lack of a place to go
  - Belief that the abuse will stop
  - Fear for her life or her children's lives
  - Fear of unknown future
- Personal characteristics of the abuser include the following (Else et al., 1993; Smith-DiJulio & Holzapfel, 1998):
  - History of a family devoid of love, affection, and security
  - Unfulfilled, overwhelming need for love and security
  - Unrealistic expectations about others (usually spouse or child) as being able to fill void from childhood, resulting in feelings of rejection, anger, and abuse
  - Blaming of outside factors for everything that goes wrong; blaming of wife for causing him to get angry
  - Denial of the violence or minimizing its severity
  - Impulsiveness
  - Excessive dependence on and jealousy of spouse (usually the only significant relationship he has)
  - Fear of losing her, which can contribute to suicide, homicide, depression, or anger
  - Belief in male supremacy
- Personal characteristics of the battered woman include the following:
  - Low self-esteem, defining of self in terms of partner
  - Unrealistic hopes for change
  - Belief that she has incited her husband to beat her and is to blame
  - Raised in a family that restricted emotional expression (e.g., anger, hugging)
  - Subscribing to the feminine sex-role stereotype
  - History of marrying to escape restrictive, confining family
  - Extreme resourcefulness and self-sufficiency to survive
  - Usually not abused as a child and did not witness abuse
  - View of herself as a victim with no option but to appease her spouse
  - Gradually increased social isolation
  - Belief that partner "can't help it"
- The likelihood of a woman seeking and using assistance for abuse increases if (Sammons, 1981):
  - She has been in the relationship less than 5 years.
  - She is employed.
  - She has friends or relatives who live nearby (within a few miles).
  - She has discussed the abuse with others.
  - The abuse is frequent (daily, weekly), severe (requires medical treatment/hospitalization), or increasing in frequency.

## Pediatric Considerations

- About 3 million cases of suspected child abuse and neglect were reported in 1994, with 2022 deaths (National Center on Child Abuse and Neglect, 1995). Westat, Inc., conducted a federally funded study in 1986 and estimated that the professionals surveyed failed to report almost 40% of sexually abused children, 30% of fatal or serious physical abuse cases, almost 50% of moderate physical abuse cases, and 70% of neglect cases. At the same time, an equally serious problem is a high number of "unfounded" (not indicated) reports of child maltreatment (Besharov, 1990).
- The discrepancy between the reported cases of child abuse and neglect and the estimated number is related to differences in laws defining abuse/neglect, professionals' failure to recognize the signs, ignorance of the law, fear of court involvement, and lack of faith in child protective services. Professionals report only about one third of cases they recognize (Wissow, 1994).
- The nurse may come in contact with an abused child in an emergency room, school, or physician's office or in her personal life (Kauffman, Neill & Thomas, 1986).
- "Child neglect is defined as the failure of the child's parents or caretaker to provide the child with the basic necessities of life, when financially able to do so or when offered reasonable means to do so" (Cowen, 1999, p. 401). Basic necessities are shelter, nutrition, health care, supervision, education, affection, and protection (Cowen, 1999).
- Family interactions in neglectful families are "more chaotic, less able to resolve conflict, less cohesive, less verbally expressive and less warm and empathetic" (Cowen, 1999, p. 409).
- In one study, 85% of cases of neglected children had a parent who was indifferent, intolerant, or overanxious (Browne, 1989).
- Child abuse is a symptom of a family in crisis or a family dysfunction. The crisis can be illness, financial difficulties, or any recent change in the family unit (e.g., new members, loss of a member, relocation) (Cowen, 1999; Kauffman et al., 1986).
- Separation of the infant from its parents, as in the case of prematurity, can reduce the attachment and nurturing behaviors of the mother toward her child. A disproportionate number of abused children were premature or ill at birth (Kauffman et al., 1986).
- Children usually are abused by someone they know: parent, babysitter, relative, or friend of the family.
- Factors that contribute to child abuse include the following (Hockenberry & Wilson, 2009):
  - Lack or unavailability of extended family
  - Economic conditions (e.g., inflation, unemployment)
  - Lack of role model as a child
  - High-risk children (e.g., unwanted, undesired sex or appearance, physically or mentally handicapped, hyperactive, terminally ill)
  - High-risk parents (e.g., single, adolescent, emotionally disturbed, alcoholic, drug addicted, physically ill)
- Characteristic personal patterns of abusers include the following (Kauffman et al., 1986):
  - No dominant ethnic or socioeconomic characteristics
  - History of abuse by and lack of warmth and affection from parents
  - Social isolation (few friends or outlets for tensions)
  - Marked lack of self-esteem, with low tolerance for criticism
  - Emotional immaturity and dependency
  - Distrust of others
  - Inability to admit the need for help
  - Unrealistic expectations for/of child
  - Desire for the child to give them pleasure
- The non-abusing parent, who is usually passive and compliant in the abuse, must be included in the treatment plan (Kauffman et al., 1986).
- The effects of abuse on the parent include termination of parental rights, angry reactions from professionals, court proceedings and court-ordered treatment, reactions of family members and community, and financial obligations (from medical and legal expenses).

## Maternal Considerations

- Studies have shown that 15% to 25% of women are battered during pregnancy.
- Low birth weight correlates with trauma to the fetus and battering.

## Geriatric Considerations

- Elder mistreatment is defined as maltreatment, intentional or unintentional, resulting from actions or inactions of others, within the context of a relationship. Types include physical and psychological mistreatment, neglect, misuse of finances, and violation of personal rights (Miller, 2009). Older adults are increasingly vulnerable to mistreatment as they become economically, physically, socially, and emotionally more dependent and the resources of caretakers are limited.
- It is estimated that over 2 million elders are abused or mistreated each year (American Psychological Association, 2003). Theories of causation include intrafamily violence, learned behavior (cycle of family violence), psychopathology of the abuser, dependency of the elder, dependency of the caregiver, lack of social support, caregiver burden, and poor health of the elder or caregiver, and substance abuse.
- According to Miller (2009), mandatory reporting laws do not require reporters to know that abuse or neglect has occurred, but merely to report it if they suspect it.

## Transcultural Considerations

- Domestic violence is cross-cultural. It exists in every culture and is a sign of individual and family dysfunction.
- Traditional Native American life did not include spouse or child abuse. Unfortunately, domestic violence has evolved and is frequently alcohol-related.

# Children with Special Needs

- Parental tasks for successful adaptation to children with special needs are:
  - Realistically perceive infant's condition and caregiver's needs.
  - Adapt to hospital environment.
  - Assume primary caregiver role.
  - Progress to total responsibility for care at discharge.
- Parenting behaviors are learned through role modeling, role rehearsal, and reference group interaction. External factors, both developmental (birth of a child) and situation (illness and/or hospitalization of a child), require the acquisition of new behaviors or the modification of existing behaviors. Difficulty in mastering the behaviors required for the role transition leads to role strain. Uncertainty about what behaviors the new role requires leads to lack of role clarity. Incompatibility between the new role expectation and already existing expectations leads to role conflict.
- Parents experiencing their child's illness in an acute or a chronic situation face the challenge of role transition to continue effective parenting on either a temporary or permanent basis. The parent must give up the role of parenting a well child and acquire the role of parenting a sick child.
- Role conflicts can develop easily when a child receives home care from a parent or a combination of parents and health care professionals. Role diffusion caused by the intrusion of treatments, providers, or both into the home is a source of stress for the entire family and requires careful role negotiation (Melnyk et al., 2001).
- Unhealthy outcomes resulting from maladaptation to family crisis are as follows:
  - Disturbed parent–child relationship
  - Failure to thrive
  - Vulnerable child syndrome
  - Disturbed marital and family equilibrium
  - Child abuse or neglect
- Clements, Copeland, and Loftus (1990) report in a study of 30 families with chronically ill children that parenting is more difficult at certain critical times: initial diagnosis; increase in physical symptoms; relocation of the child, such as rehospitalization; developmental changes for the child, such as entrance into school; and the physical or emotional absence of one parent (e.g., illness, pregnancy).
- Caring for a child with special needs places high demands on parents' energy, time, and financial resources.
- Fathers of children with special needs are challenged with a situation that they could not protect their family from or control. They have more difficulty adjusting to a son with special needs because of the loss of future joint recreation.

- In a study of 45 mothers of acutely ill children, Schepp (1991) found that predictability of events and anxiety influenced the mother's coping effort. Mothers who knew what to expect were less anxious.
- Strong families appreciate and encourage all members. There is a commitment toward each member and the family unit. There is a clear set of family rules, values, and beliefs.
- Families acquire children through birth, adoption, and remarriage. Sometimes grandparents assume the parenting role for grandchildren because of the loss of parents, substance abuse, or a history of ineffective parenting (Clemen-Stone et al., 2002).
- Although many parents anticipate the birth of their child with pleasure, most are unprepared for the accompanying changes. After a child is born, parental self-concepts develop. For a woman, her role as parent often overshadows her role as wife and individual. For a man, parenthood strengthens his role as husband and worker. Parenting often becomes a dominant role for women and a secondary role for men (Clemen-Stone et al., 2002).
- Situations that contribute to abuse are often related to ineffective individual or family coping. (See *Disabled Family Coping, as evidenced by child abuse*.)

## Alcoholism in Family

- Alcoholism is a family disease. There are approximately 13 million alcoholics in the US; at least 4 million others are affected intimately (APA, 2000b).
- Alcoholism and its denial dominate alcoholic families. When alcohol is the center of the family, developmental tasks are thwarted or ignored. "To keep the family unit intact, each member must change his or her cognitive perceptions to fit into the family's scheme of enabling the drinking to continue, while at the same time denying that it is a problem" (Starling & Martin, 1990, p. 16).
- Alcoholics initially use denial about alcohol to relieve stress. After dependence sets in, they use denial to conceal from the self and others how important alcohol is to functioning (Smith-DiJulio, 1998).
- As destructive interactions continue, family members and the alcoholic move away from each other. The alcoholic turns to liquor, while the family finds other means of escape (Collins, Leonard, & Searles, 1990).
- "Meaningful sobriety is characterized by more than just the abstinence of the alcoholic person. It necessitates an ongoing growth process for all family members to work together toward the goal of a well-functioning family" (Grisham & Estes, 1982, p. 257).
- Wegscheider (1981) described six roles typical in families affected by alcoholism:
- Alcoholic
- Chief enabler—often the spouse; super-responsible, takes on alcoholic duties
- Family hero—high achiever to provide family with some pride to cover up failures
- Scapegoat—defiant, angry, diverts family focus from alcoholism
- Lost child—helpless, powerless
- Mascot—clowning, joking; a form of tension relief to mask underlying terrors
- Wing (1991, 1994) describes a four-stage theory of alcoholism, recovery, and goal setting:
  - Stage I: Denial—alcoholics are coerced into treatment; their goals are to avoid punishment, with no sincere desire to stop drinking.
  - Stage II: Dependence—alcoholics admit that they have a drinking problem and seek treatment to maintain job or a relationship.
  - Stage III: Behavior change—alcoholics attempt to replace unhealthy behaviors with health behaviors.
  - Stage IV: Life planning—alcoholics integrate family, career, and educational goals with sobriety.
- Men entering treatment services perceive alcohol as the cause of their problems. Women reported that they drank because of their problems (Kellet et al., 2000).

### Pediatric Considerations

Children learn definitions of love, intimacy, and trust in their families of origin. The environment in the alcoholic family is chaotic and unpredictable. Roles are unclear. Sometimes, children become the parents and the alcoholic member becomes an outsider in the family.

- Children report being more disturbed by parents arguing rather than one parent's drinking. Children can respond in varied ways (e.g., peacemaker, aggression at school).
- Behavioral problems in children need to be assessed in the context of their purpose for the family.
- Children of alcoholics are accustomed to extra and inappropriate responsibilities (Smith-DiJulio, 1998).

## Transcultural Considerations

- Alcoholism is the number one health problem in the African-American community, reducing longevity with high incidences of acute and chronic alcohol-related diseases. Unemployment has been identified as the primary factor. Treatment programs must be accessible within the community or by public transportation. Black churches serve as a dual role as a site for therapy meetings and as a referral service (Giger & Davidhizar, 2009).
- Alcohol consumption is a way to celebrate life for Mexican Americans. Alcohol contributes to increased incidents and violence. Family pride protects the alcoholic male as long as he provides for the family (Giger & Davidhizar, 2009).
- Alcoholism is found among Native Americans in very high percentages. It is responsible for violence, suicides, and fetal alcohol syndrome. Studies have shown an increased sensitivity to alcohol in this group (Giger & Davidhizar, 2009).

## Parenting

- In the past, because of living in extended families, young children observed and assisted frequently in the birth and care of infants. Today in the United States, because of social mobility and the more isolated nuclear family lifestyle, young men and women often approach parenthood with only a vague recollection of their own childhood, little knowledge of the birthing process, and limited, if any, experience in infant and child care.

## Parent-Infant Bonding

- Bonding cannot be determined "by particular behaviors, but from patterns of behavior" (Goulet et al., 1998, p. 1072). Parent-infant bonding is interactional. Attachment requires proximity, reciprocity, and commitment (Goulet et al., 1998).

- "Children who are cared for in a relatively consistent and predictable way develop confidence in their ability to have a positive influence on their environment and are more likely to express their need for love and security" (Goulet et al., 1998, p. 1078).

- The mother-child relationship begins before conception: planning, confirming, and accepting the pregnancy; feeling fetal movement, accepting the fetus as an individual; giving birth; hearing and seeing the baby; touching and holding the baby; and caring for the baby.

- Participation of the father in caregiving activities has increased in the United States. Fathers who choose a traditional role (allowing the mother to be totally responsible for caretaking activities) must be accessed in their sociocultural context.

- Mercer and Ferketich (1990) studied parental attachment of 121 high-risk women, 61 partners of high-risk women, 182 low-risk women, and 117 partners of low-risk women. They found that the major predictor of parental attachment for all four groups was parental competence.

## Focus Assessment Criteria

### General

Family composition (who resides in home)
Family strengths
Rules/discipline
Financial status
Participation in community activities
Presence of extended family

### Assess:

### *Communication Patterns*

Express open feelings only     Straight messages     No manipulation

## Emotional/Supportive Pattern

*Constructive*

| | | |
|---|---|---|
| Appraise problem accurately | Rely on one another | Show optimism |
| Seek knowledge and resources | Share feelings, thoughts | Deal with problems |
| Use support systems | | |

*Destructive*

| | | |
|---|---|---|
| Deny problems | Use abandonment | Show authoritarianism |
| Exploit members (threats, violence, neglect, scapegoating) | Show apathy | |

# Assess for Recent Changes.

## Addition of New Family Member

Birth    Adoption
Marriage    Elderly relative

## Loss of Family Member

Relocation    Illness        Death

## Change in Family Roles

Financial crisis
Disaster
Conflicts
Family member with a coping problem
Relocation history

## Child Illness or Hospitalization

*History of illness*
Acute or chronic    Resulting from an accident    Congenital or acquired
When diagnosis first made
*Parent's knowledge/experiences*
Experience with own hospitalizations
Experiences with previous hospitalizations of this child or other children
Involvement with medical/nursing care in the home
Communication style and level
Knowledge of child development and understanding of effect of hospitalization on child
Understanding of need for this hospitalization
Desired outcomes from current hospitalization
Involvement in case management for child, if any

## Plans for Dealing with This Hospitalization

Visiting plans and travel arrangements
Desired involvement in care
Plans for acquiring information about child
Plans for self-care
Plans for payment of medical and hospital bills
Plans for meeting other roles while child is hospitalized (e.g., working, care of home and other children)
Other emergent family situations that will affect time and energy needed fro parenting the ill child.

# Assess:

## Parent-Child Interaction (observe each parent/caretaker)

Involvement in caretaking
Comforting of child (touching, holding)
Discipline of child (reasons, methods)

Interpreting hospitalization/illness-related events to child
Support of child's development (play activities, developmental toys)

## Parental Behavior (prenatal, post-delivery)

### Prenatal
Verbalize anticipation
Decide about feeding (breast, bottle)
Seek prenatal care
Follow the regimen
Select a name
Plan layette

### Intrapartum
Participate in decision and birthing process
Verbalize positive feelings
Attempt to see infant as soon as delivered
Respond positively (happy) or negatively (sad, apathetic, disappointed, angry, ambivalent)
Hold and talk to infant
Use baby's name
Talk to baby's father or mother

### Postpartum
Verbalize positive feelings
Seek proximity by holding infant closely; touch and hug
Smile and gaze at infant; seek eye-to-eye contact
Seek family resemblance (e.g., "has my eyes," "sleeps like his father")
Refer to infant by name and sex
Express interest in learning infant care
Perform nurturing behavior (i.e., feeding, changing)

## Assess for Domestic Violence.

Have you ever been emotionally or physically abused by your partner or someone important to you?
In the last year, have you been hit, slapped, kicked, or otherwise physically hurt by someone?
Are you or have you ever been pregnant? If yes, have you been hit, slapped, kicked, or otherwise physically hurt by someone? If yes, by whom? How many times?
Within the last year, has anyone forced you to have sexual activities? If yes, who? Number of times?
Are you afraid of your partner or anyone else you listed above?
Has your partner:

Tried to choke you?
Threatened you with a weapon?
Threatened to try suicide?
Been violent to your children?
Been violent outside the home?
Threatened to kill you?

Does your partner:

Drink to excess?
Use drugs?
Try to control your daily activities?
Have a gun?
Control all the money?
Destroy possessions?
Try to control who your friends are?
Exhibit violent jealousy?

## Assess for Child Abuse Suspicion.

Trauma (fractures, lacerations, bruises, welts, burns, dislocations)
Unexplained or unwitnessed injuries
Nature and extent of injury not consistent with explanation
Injuries in various stages of healing
Injuries to face
Abdominal injuries
Multiple bruises (trunk, buttocks, wrists, ankles, ears, neck, around mouth)
Fractures (rib, metaphyseal, scapular, distal clavicle, all humerus fractures [except supracondylar] in children younger than 3 years, vertebral fractures or subluxations, midshaft ulnar fractures, bilateral fractures)

Bruises of varied colors:

Red, black, or blue Immediate to 5 days

Green        5 to 7 days

Yellow       7 to 10 days

Brown        10 to 14 days

Physical indicators of sexual abuse

| | |
|---|---|
| Vaginal or penile discharges | Venereal diseases |
| Genital or anal injuries or swelling | Pain or itching in genital area |
| | Difficulty walking |
| Pain while urinating | |

Behavioral indicators

| | |
|---|---|
| Wary of adult contact | Afraid to go home |
| Fearful of parents | High pain threshold |
| Excessive effort to please | Excessive seeking of affection |

Indicators of neglect (subjective, objective) (Cowen, 1999; Heindl, 1979)

| | |
|---|---|
| Hunger | Abandonment |
| Inappropriate dress for weather | Poor growth patterns |
| | Delinquency |
| Consistent lack of supervision | Assumes adult responsibilities |
| | Constant fatigue or listlessness |
| Unattended medical or dental needs | |

How soon was medical care sought? Immediately after injury? Day or more later?

Is medical care sought at the same place or are different places used? Why?

Caregiver–sibling interaction

| | |
|---|---|
| Is child afraid of adult? | Are they interacting with each other? |
| Is adult concerned? | Does child report problem with sibling? |
| What happens during fights? | |

## Assess for Caregiver Risk Factors (Cowen, 1999).

| | |
|---|---|
| Poor coping skills | Psychological problems |
| Substance abuse | Poor impulse control |
| Depression | Limited household management skills |
| Limited finances | Inadequate support system |

## Assess for Alcohol Abuse.

### Denial of Problem

### Responses of Family Members

| | | |
|---|---|---|
| Alcohol use influences decisions | Afraid | Worried |
| | Embarrassed | Effects on each member |
| Overall feelings | Behavior problems (children) | Guilt feelings |

### Characteristics of Alcoholic Person

| | | |
|---|---|---|
| Friends drink heavily | Justifies alcohol use | Promises to quit or reduce |
| Is verbally/physically abusive | Drives under influence | Fails to remember events |
| Avoids conversations about alcohol | Has periods of remorse | |

### Family/Social Functions

| | | |
|---|---|---|
| Unsatisfactory, tense | Always include alcohol | Financial, legal problems |

Negative comments of others on drinking behavior

Link symbols with lines that indicate:

| | | |
|---|---|---|
| Marriage | Separation | Divorce |
| Living together | | |

Indicate death with × in symbol or miscarriage with Δ or abortion with ×.

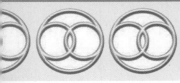

# COMPROMISED FAMILY COPING

## DEFINITION (NANDA)

Usually supportive primary person (family member or close friend) is providing insufficient, ineffective, or compromised support, comfort, assistance, or encouragement that may be needed by the client to manage or master adaptive tasks related to his or her health challenge

## DEFINING CHARACTERISTICS (NANDA)

### Subjective Data

Client expresses or confirms a concern or complaint about significant other's response to his or her health problem.

Significant person describes preoccupation with personal reactions (e.g., fear, anticipatory grief, guilt, anxiety) to client's illness, disability, or to other situational or developmental crises.

Significant person describes or confirms an inadequate understanding or knowledge base, which interferes with effective assistive or supportive behaviors.

### Objective Data

Significant person attempts assistive or supportive behaviors with less than satisfactory results.

Significant person withdraws or enters into limited or temporary personal communication with the client at time of need.

Significant person displays protective behavior disproportionate (too little or too much) to the client's abilities or need for autonomy.

## RELATED FACTORS

See *Interrupted Family Processes*.

■■■■■■ **AUTHOR'S NOTE**

This nursing diagnosis describes situations similar to the diagnosis *Interrupted Family Processes* or *Risk for Interrupted Family Processes*. Until clinical research differentiates this diagnosis from the aforementioned diagnosis, use *Interrupted Family Processes*.

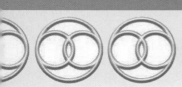

# DISABLED FAMILY COPING

**Disabled Family Coping**

Related to (Specify), as Evidenced by Partner Violence
Related to (Specify), as Evidenced by Child Abuse/Neglect

**High Risk for Disabled Family Coping**

Related to Multiple Stressors Associated with Elder Care

# DEFINITION

The state in which a family demonstrates, or is at risk to demonstrate, destructive behavior in response to an inability to manage internal or external stressors due to inadequate resources (physical, psychological, cognitive)

# DEFINING CHARACTERISTICS

## Major (One Must Be Present)

Abusive or neglectful care of individual(s)
Decisions/actions that is detrimental to family well-being
Abusive or neglectful relationships with other family members

## Minor (May Be Present)

Distortion of reality regarding the health problem
Rejection
Agitation
Aggression
Impaired restructuring of a family unit
Intolerance
Abandonment
Depression
Hostility

# RELATED FACTORS

## Biopathophysiologic

*Related to impaired ability to fulfill role responsibilities secondary to:*
*Any acute or chronic illness*

## Situational (Cliental, Environmental)

*Related to impaired ability to constructively manage stressors secondary to:*
Substance abuse
Alcoholism
Negative role modeling
History of ineffective relationship with own parents
History of abusive relationship with parents
*Related to unrealistic expectations of child by parent*
*Related to unrealistic expectations of parent by child*
*Related to unmet psychosocial needs of child by parent*
*Related to unmet psychosocial needs of parent by child*

■■■■■■ **AUTHOR'S NOTE**

*Disabled Family Coping* describes a family with a history of overt or covert destructive behavior or responses to stressors. This diagnosis necessitates long-term care from a nurse therapist with advanced specialization in family systems and abuse.

The use of this diagnosis in this book focuses on nursing interventions appropriate for a nurse generalist in a short-term relationship (e.g., emergency unit, nonpsychiatric in-house unit) and for any nurse in the position to prevent *Disabled Family Coping* through teaching, counseling, or referrals.

■ ■ ■ ■ ■ ■ **ERRORS IN DIAGNOSTIC STATEMENTS**

**Disabled Family Coping related to reports of beatings by alcoholic husband**

This diagnostic statement is formulated incorrectly and legally inadvisable for a nurse to write. Reported beating by a husband with alcoholism is not the contributing factor, but rather a diagnostic cue. This diagnosis should be written as *Disabled Family Coping related to unknown etiology, as evidenced by wife reporting*, "My husband is an alcoholic and beats me frequently." The quoted statement represents the data as reported by the wife, rather than the nurse's judgment.

---

**NOC**

Caregiver Emotional Health, Caregiver Stressors, Family Coping, Family Normalization

## ➤ Goals

Each family member will set short-term and long-term goals for change.

### Indicators

- Appraise unhealthy coping behaviors for family members.
- Relate expectations for self and family.
- Relate community resources available.

---

**NIC**

Caregiver Support, Referral, Emotional Support, Family Therapy, Family Involvement Promotion

## ➤ General Interventions

### Assist Members to Appraise Family Behaviors.

### Discuss the Effects of Behaviors on Individuals and Family Unit.

Emotions      Roles
Support       Performance

**R:** Families with a dysfunctional member (e.g., an alcoholic) are assisted to see that the entire family is dysfunctional, not just the individual.

### Assist Family to Set Short-Term and Long-Term Goals.

**R:** Short-term goals focus on stabilizing the family as much as possible. Long-term goals focus on changes needed in functioning and establishing patterns to foster lasting changes

### Promote Family Stabilization.

Ask each family member to identify one activity he or she would like to add to their family.
Identify stressors that can be reduced or eliminated. Ask each family member to identify one behavior he or she could control.
Begin to help members to work through resentments of the past.

**R:** Each family member is provided an opportunity to share feelings about the present and past (Smith-DiJulio & Holzapfel, 2006). Interventions focus on helping the family renegotiate roles and patterns of interactive and functioning.

### Improve Family Cohesiveness.

Determine family recreational activities that include all members and are enjoyable.
**R:** Family recreational activities foster family cohesion with positive experiences.

### Initiate Referrals as Needed.

Support groups      Family therapy    Economic Support
**R:** Dysfunctional families have a history of isolation. Interventions focus on increasing their socialization and use of community resources.

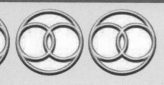

# DISABLED FAMILY COPING

## ▶ Related to (Specify), as Evidenced by Partner Violence

Domestic abuse is defined as any action by an individual intended to harm another client (physical, emotional, financial, social, and sexual) in a shared household.

**NOC**
Family Coping, Family Normalization, Family Functioning, Abuse Protection, Abuse Cessation

## ► Goal

The client will seek assistance for abusive behaviors.

### Indicators

- Discuss the physical assaults and fears
- Identify characteristics of abusers
Describe a safety plan
- Seek assistance for abusive behavior; legally and emotionally.
- Relate community resources available when help is desired.

**NIC**
Caregiver Support, Emotional Support, Referral, Counseling, Decision-Making Support, Support Group, Anger Control Assistance, Abuse Protection Support: Domestic Partner, Conflict Mediation

## ► Interventions

Interventions to address the complexity and magnitude of the problems inherent in domestic violence usually are beyond the scope of a nurse generalist. Those provided here are to assist the nurse who has a short-term interaction with a client.

### Develop Rapport.

Interview in private. Be empathic.
Don't assume you know what the client needs.
Ask, "How can I help you?"
Avoid displaying shock or surprise at the details.
If contact is made by telephone, find out how to get in touch with the victim.

**R:** The victim is tense and afraid, feels helpless, accepts blame, and is hoping for change in the partner (Carlson & Smith-DiJulio, 2006).

## Evaluate Potential Danger to Victim and Others.

### Assess Actual Physical Abuse:

Current and past physical/sexual abuse
When did it happen last?
Are you hurt now?

Are the children hurt?
Assess danger to children

### Assess Support System:

Does she have a safe place to go?
Does she want police called?
Does she need an ambulance?

### Assess Drug and Alcohol Use:

Is victim using drugs/alcohol?
Is abuser using drugs/alcohol?

**R:** Nursing interventions should focus on level of danger, safety and protection. Consequences of rash decisions can be fatal.

## Assess for Factors that Inhibit Victims from Seeking Aid.

### Cliental Beliefs

Fear for safety of self or children     Fear of embarrassment
Low self-esteem                         Guilt (punishment justified)
Myths ("It is normal" or "It will stop")

**R:** The nurse must openly dispel myths that offer explanations and tolerance for battering and wrongly give an illusion of control and rationality (Carson & Smith-DiJulio, 2006).

### Lack of Knowledge of

The severity of the problem     Community resources
Legal rights

**R:** When stressed, individuals solve problems poorly and do not seek outside assistance.

### Lack of Financial Independence or Support System

**R:** Compromised finances or access to alternative housing may be the primary deterrent to seeking help.

## Gently Discuss the Effects of Violence on Children.

- Elicit the client's impression of effects on children
- Greater life-long risks for behavioral and emotional problems
- After age 5-6 children lose respect for the victim and identify with the aggressor

**R:** Family violence is common in histories of juvenile criminals, runaways, violent criminals, prostitutes and those who in turn are violent to others." (Carson & Smith-DiJulio, 2006, p. 507).

## Encourage Decision Making.

Provide an opportunity to validate abuse and talk about feelings; if the acutely injured client is accompanied by a spouse/caregiver who is persistent about staying, make an attempt to see the client alone (e.g., tell her you need a urine specimen and accompany her to the bathroom).
Be direct and nonjudgmental:

- How do you handle stress?
- How does your partner or caregiver handle stress?
- How do you and your partner argue?
- Are you afraid of him?
- Have you ever been hit, pushed, or injured by your partner?

Provide options but allow client to make a decision at her own pace.
Encourage a realistic appraisal of the situation; dispel guilt and myths:

- Violence is not normal for most families.
- Violence may stop, but it usually becomes increasingly worse.
- The victim is not responsible for the violence.

**R:** Nurses must be cautious not to pressure the victim into a premature decision. Victims of abuse are "brainwashed by terror." They use denial and rationalization when they remain in the abusive relationship (Blair, 1986).

## Establish a Safety and/or Escape Plan (Refer to Abuse Specialists/Hotlines).

- Provisions for child safety, pets, designated care giver (provide school/day care with written instructions with permission for other designated adult(s) to pick up child)
- Access to important phone numbers (written) address book
- Destination if leaving
- Extra money, car keys, clothes
- Children's favorite toys, blanket
- Sentimental pictures jewelry
- Important items to take:

Identification, social security cards, birth certificates, credit cards, divorce papers, insurance cards, mortgage or rental papers

- Enlist help of co-workers, family, neighbors, school clientele
- If staying in home increase safety measures e.g. new locks, security systems
- Alert neighbors to call police if they hear or see the problem individual

**R:** A safety plan is a specific plan for a fast escape if the victim identifies "now is the time to leave."

## Assess for Risk Factors Associated with Murder and Suicide.

| | |
|---|---|
| Increased frequency or severity of violence | Violence outside home |
| | Use of weapon or threat with weapon |
| Choking | Gun in house |
| Forced sex | Alcohol/drug abuse |
| Alcohol abuse | Extreme jealousy |
| Death threats | Control of most or all of client's activities |
| Violence toward children | Suicide threat or attempt |

**R:** Fifteen hundred women die every year from domestic violence (Agency for Healthcare Research and Quality, 2002).

## Provide Legal and Referral Information.

Discreetly inform of community agencies available to victim and abuser (emergency and long-term).

| | |
|---|---|
| Hotlines | Legal services |
| Shelters | Counseling agencies |

Mandatory reporting
Discuss the availability of the social service department for assistance.
Consult with legal resources in the community and familiarize the victim with state laws regarding:
Abuse

| | |
|---|---|
| Eviction of abuser | Counseling |
| Temporary support | Protection orders |
| Criminal law | Types of police interventions |

Document Findings and Dialogue (Carlson & Smith-DiJulio, 2006).

**R:** Some states and cities have laws that allow the police to press charges against the abuser when physical evidence of battering exist,. This reduces the pressure for the victim filing charges

Refer for individual, group, or couples counseling.
Explore strategies to reduce stress and more constructively manage stressors (e.g., relaxation exercises, walking, and assertiveness training).

**R:** Battering interventions must take place in the context of a coordinated community and criminal justice response to battering.

## Initiate Health Teaching if Indicated.

Teach the community (e.g., parent–school organizations, women's clubs, and programs for schoolchildren) about the problem of spouse/elder abuse.
Instruct caregivers in how properly to manage an elderly client at home (e.g., transferring to chair, modified appliances, how to maintain orientation).
Refer for financial assistance and transportation arrangements.
Refer for assertiveness training.
Inform family of senior citizen centers or day care programs.
Refer the abuser to the appropriate community service (only refer men who have asked for assistance or admitted their abuse, because revealing the wife's confidential disclosure may trigger more abuse).
To secure additional information, contact National Clearinghouse on Domestic Violence www.ncodv.org.

**R:** Information and referrals are provided to encourage decision making. When stressed individuals have difficulty accessing outside support (Carlson & Smith-DiJulio, 2006).

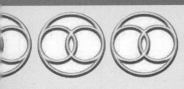

# DISABLED FAMILY COPING

## ▶ Related to (Specify), as Evidenced by Child Abuse/Neglect

Child abuse is an action or inaction that brings injury to a child, including physical and psychological injury, neglect, and sexual abuse.

**NOC**

Family Coping, Family Normalization, Family Functioning, Abuse Protection, Abuse Cessation

## ➤ Goal

The child will be free from injury or neglect.

### Indicators

Receive comfort from another caretaker.
The parent will receive assistance for abusive behavior.
Acknowledge abusive behaviors.

**NIC**

Caregiver Support, Emotional Support, Counseling, Decision-Making Support, Support Group, Anger Control Assistance, Abuse Protection Support: Child, Conflict Mediation, Referral

## ➤ General Interventions

### Identify Families at Risk for Child Abuse.

- Poor differentiation of individual within the family
- Lack of autonomy
- Insulation from the influence of others; social isolation
- Desperate competition for affection and nurturance among members
- Feelings of helplessness and hopelessness
- Abuse/Violence learned as a way to reduce tension
- Low tolerance for frustration; poor impulse control
- Closeness and caring confused with abuse and violence
- Mixed and double message communication patterns
- High level of conflict surrounding family tasks
- Nonexistent parental coalition

### Intervene with Families at Risk.

Establish a relationship with parents that encourages them to share difficulties ("Being a parent is sure difficult [frustrating] work, isn't it?").

Provide parents with access to information about parenting and child development (see *Delayed Growth and Development*).

Provide anticipatory guidance relative to growth and development (e.g., the need to cry in early months; toilet training).

Stress the importance of support systems (e.g., encourage parents to exchange experiences with other parents).

Encourage parents to allow time for their own needs (e.g., exercise three times a week).

Discuss with parents how they respond to parental frustrations (share feelings with other parents) and instruct them not to discipline children when very angry.

Explore other methods of discipline aside from physical punishment.

Refer parents to expert help.

Inform parents of community services (telephone hotlines, clergy).

**R:** Successful interactions with abusing parents must be provided in the context of acceptance and approval to compensate for their low self-esteem and fear of rejection (Wissow, 1994).

**R:** Programs that teach parents to interpret and understand their children's behaviors and to give appropriate responses can reduce child maltreatment.

## Identify Suspected Cases of Child Abuse.

Assess for and evaluate:
Evidence of maltreatment (refer to Focus Assessment Criteria)
History of incident or injury

* Conflicting stories
* Story improbable for child's age
* Story not consistent with injury

Parental behaviors

* Seeks care for a minor complaint (e.g., cold) when other injuries are visible
* Shows exaggerated or no emotional response to the injury
* Is unavailable for questioning
* Fails to show empathy for child
* Expresses anger or criticism of child for being injured
* Demands to take child home if pressured for answers

Child behaviors

* Does not expect to be comforted
* Adjusts inappropriately to hospitalization
* Defends parents
* Blames self for inciting parents to rage

**R:** Identification of child abuse depends on recognizing the physical signs, specific parent behavior, specific child behavior, inconsistencies in injury history, and contributing factors (e.g., familial, environmental) (Boyd, 2005; Kauffman et al., 1986).

**R:** The first priority of care for the abused child is preventing further injury (Hockenberry and Wilson, 2009).

## Report Suspected Cases of Child Abuse.

Know your state's child abuse laws and procedures for reporting child abuse (e.g., Bureau of Child Welfare, Department of Social Services, and Child Protective Services).
Maintain an objective record (Cowen, 1999):

* Health history, including accidental or environmental injuries
* Detailed description of physical examination (nutritional status, hygiene, growth and development, cognitive and functional status)
* Environmental assessment of home (if in community)
* Description of injuries
* Verbal conversations with parents and child in quotes
* Description of behaviors, not interpretation (e.g., avoid "angry father," instead, "Father screamed at child, 'If you weren't so bad this wouldn't have happened.'")
* Description of parent–child interactions (e.g., shies away from mother's touch)

**R:** The nurse should consult the legislation mandating the reporting of child abuse for the specifics of legal definition, penalties for failure to report, reporting procedure, and legal immunity for reporting (Kauffman et al., 1986).

**R:** The first priority of care for the abused child is preventing further injury (Hockenberry & Wilson, 2009).

## Promote a Therapeutic Environment.

### *Provide the Child with Acceptance and Affection.*

Show child attention without reinforcing inappropriate behavior.
Use play therapy to allow child self-expression.
Provide consistent caregivers and reasonable limits on behavior; avoid pity.
Avoid asking too many questions and criticizing parent's actions.

Ensure that play and educational needs are met.

Explain in detail all routines and procedures in age-appropriate language.

**R:** These strategies can reduce the child's stress and role model appropriate behavior for the parent(s).

### Assist Child with Grieving If Foster Home Placement Is Necessary.

Acknowledge that child will not want to leave parents despite severity of abuse.

Allow opportunities for child to express feelings.

Explain reasons for not allowing child to return home; dispel belief it is a punishment.

Encourage foster parents to visit child in hospital.

**R:** Children are attached to their parents despite the abuse (Hockenberry & Wilson, 2009).

### Provide Interventions that Promote Parent's Self-Esteem and Sense of Trust.

Tell them it was good that they brought the child to the hospital.

Welcome parents to the unit and orient them to activities.

Promote their confidence by presenting a warm, helpful attitude and acknowledging any competent parenting activities.

Provide opportunities for parents to participate in child's care (e.g., feeding, bathing).

**R:** Strong negative feelings can interfere with the nurse's judgment and effectiveness and alienate the family (Carlson & Smith-DiJulio, 2006).

## Promote Comfort and Reduce Fear for Child (Carlson & Smith-DiJulio, 2006).

Do not display anger, horror, or shock.

Do not blame abuser.

Reassure child that he or she was not "bad" or at fault.

Do not pressure child to give answers.

Do not force child to undress.

**R:** Children, being egocentric, assume they are responsible for the maltreatment.

## Initiate Health Teaching and Referrals, As Indicated.

### Provide Anticipatory Guidance for Families at Risk.

Assist individuals to recognize stress and to practice management techniques (e.g., plan for time alone away from child).

Discuss the need for realistic expectations of the child's capabilities.

Teach about child development and constructive methods for handling developmental problems (enuresis, toilet training, temper tantrums); refer to Bibliography.

Discuss methods of discipline other than physical (e.g., deprive the child of favorite pastime: "May not ride your bike for a whole day"; "May not play your stereo").

Emphasize rewarding positive behavior.

**R:** Unrealistic expectations for the age of the child and severe punishment techniques increase episodes of violence.

### Disseminate Information to the Community About Child Abuse (e.g., Parent–School Organizations, Radio, Television, Newspaper).

Discuss with parents and parents-to-be the problems of parenting.

Teach those who are at risk of being future abusers.

Discuss constructive stress management.

Teach the signs and symptoms of abuse and the method for reporting.

Focus on abuse as a problem resulting from child-rearing difficulties, not parental deficiencies.

Relay your understanding of stresses, but do not condone abuse.

Focus on the parent's needs; avoid an authoritative approach.

Take opportunities to demonstrate constructive methods for working with children (give the child choices; listen carefully to the child).

Consider developing parenting classes for parents (preventive, corrective) to increase their skills as nurturers and teachers. Weekly topic examples:

| | |
|---|---|
| What is parenting? | Child development and play |
| Discipline and toilet training | Play and nutrition |
| Discipline and common problems | Expectations vs. realities |
| Safety and health | Parental needs |

**R:** Primary prevention (public awareness, community education, parenting classes, nutrition programs) is directed at the general population. Secondary prevention is directed at high-risk groups. Home-based and center-based programs have had positive outcomes (e.g., home visitation programs, substance abuse/mental health referrals, crisis intervention) (Cowan, 1999).

Refer at risk families to a home health nursing agency to assess

- Interaction of family members
- Type of physical contact, eg. comforting, detached, angry
- Parenteral attitudes /conflicts about parenting
- Parenteral history of abuse
- Environmental conditions(sleep areas, play areas, home management)
- Financial status
- Need for immediate services (economic, child care, counseling, protection services)

**R:** The best environment to assess an family functioning is in their home

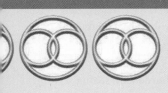

# DISABLED FAMILY COPING

## ▶ Related to Multiple Stressors Associated with Elder Care

**NOC**
Family Coping, Family Normalization, Family Functioning, Abuse Protection, Abuse Cessation

### ➤ Goal

The caregiver will acknowledge the need for assistance with abusive behavior.

### *Indicators*

- Discuss the stressors of elder care.
- Relate strategies to reduce stressors.
- Identify community resources available.

The older adult will be free of abusive behavior.

- Describe methods to increase socialization beyond caregiver.
- Identify resources available for assistance.

**NIC**
Caregiver Support, Emotional Support, Counseling, Support Group, Decision-Making Support, Anger Control Assistance, Abuse Protection Support: Elder, Conflict Mediation, Referral

### ➤ Interventions

### Identify Individuals (Caregiver, Older Adult) at High Risk for Abuse or Neglect.

**Caregiver**
Social isolation
Dependency on elder (financial, emotional); co-residency
Health problems (physical, mental)
Substance abuse

Poor relationship history with elder
Financial problems
Transgenerational violence
Relationship problems

**Older Adult**
Dependent on others for activities of daily living
Isolation
Financial insecurity
Impaired cognitive functioning
Depressive clientality
History of abuse to caregiver
Incontinence

**R:** Perpetrator who initiates violence or neglect considers their own needs to be more important than anyone else. An elder who is dependent for activities of daily living is most vulnerable (Carlson & Smith-DiJulio, 2006).

## Assist Caregivers to Reduce Stressors.

Establish a relationship with caregivers that encourages them to share difficulties.
Encourage them to share experiences with others in same situation.
Evaluate caregiver's ability to provide long-term in-home care.
Explore sources of help (e.g., housekeeping, home-delivered meals, day care, respite care, transportation assistance).
Encourage caregiver to discuss sharing responsibilities with other family members.
Discuss alternative sources of care (e.g., nursing home, senior housing).
Discuss how caregiver can allow time for cliental needs.
Discuss community resources available for help (e.g., crisis hotline, social service, voluntary emergency caregivers).
Refer also to *Caregiver Role Strain*.

**R:** Steinmetz (1988) reported that caregivers' perceptions of stress and feelings of burden are strong predictors of elder abuse.

**R:** Interventions focus on assisting caregivers to reduce stress and select constructive coping responses (Miller, 2009).

## Assist Older Adults to Reduce Risks of Abuse.

Encourage contact with old friends and neighbors if living with relative.
Plan a weekly contact in client with friend, neighbor.
Encourage client to participate in community activities as much as possible.
Encourage client to have his or her own telephone.
Assist client to acquire legal advice.

**R:** Strategies to reduce isolation can protect the client from undetected abuse. Legal advice may be needed to protect accents.

Ensure client is not accepting cliental care in exchange for transfer of assets or property without legal advice.
Ensure client is not living with someone who has a history of violence or substance abuse.

**R:** Strategies for high-risk elders include access and assessment, intervention, follow-up, and prevention.

## Identify Suspected Cases of Elder Abuse (Fulmer & Paveza, 1998).

Signs include the following:

• Failure to adhere to therapeutic regimens, which can pose threats to life (e.g., insulin administration, ulcerated conditions)
• Evidence of malnutrition, dehydration, elimination problems
• Bruises, swelling, lacerations, burns, bites

- Pressure ulcers
- Caregiver not allowing nurse to be alone with elder

Consult with home health nurse to plan a home visit for assessment of signs of abuse or neglect (Smith-DiJulio & Holzapfel, 1998):

- House in poor repair
- Inadequate heat, lighting, furniture, or cooking utensils
- Unpleasant odors
- Inaccessible food
- Old food
- Older adult lying on soiled materials (e.g., urine, food)
- Medication not being taken
- Garbage

**R:** Abused elders usually do not report abuse because of fear of reprisal or abandonment. Rather, elder abuse must be detected.

## Report Suspected Cases.

Consult with supervisor for procedures for reporting suspected cases of abuse.
Maintain an objective record, including:

| | |
|---|---|
| Description of injuries | Conversations with elder and caregivers |
| Description of behaviors | Nutritional, hydration status |

Consider the elder's right to choose to live at risk of harm, providing he or she is capable of making that choice.
Do not initiate an action that could increase the elder's risk of harm or antagonize the abuser.
Respect the elder's right to secrecy and the right for self-determination.

**R:** Each state has specific guideline for reporting suspected cases of elder abuse.

## Initiate Health Teaching and Referrals, as Indicated.

Refer high-risk families to a home health nursing agency to assess (Carson & Smith-DiJulio,2006)

- Environmental Conditions
  inadequate heat, lighting,
  presence of garbage, old food in kitchen, unpleasant odors
  blocked stairways, locks on refrigerator
- Caretaker
  Attitudes conflicts, anger, depression
  Interaction with elder
  Insufficient finances
  Alcohol/drug abuse
- Elder condition
  Unclean, unclean clothes and linens
  Medications not taken properly
  Lack of assistive devices
  Inadequate follow-ups with primary provider
- Need for immediate services (economic, day care, respite, protection services, counseling)

Refer elder for counseling to explore choices.
Explore support services (e.g., respite, home health aide, homemaker services).
Disseminate information to community regarding prevention:

- Publicize support services.
- Seek to assist caregiving families (e.g., companions, respite care, day care centers).
- Seek to establish weekly contact with dependent elderly.
- Attempt to reduce isolation of caregivers and elders.
- Develop procedures for investigation, public education.

**R:** Educational programs serve to advocate for elders and to raise the consciousness of the community.

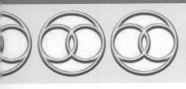

# READINESS FOR ENHANCED FAMILY COPING

## DEFINITION (NANDA)

Effective managing of adaptive tasks by family member involved with the client's health challenge, who now is exhibiting desire and readiness for enhanced health and growth in regard to self and in relation to the client

## DEFINING CHARACTERISTICS (NANDA)

Family member attempting to describe growth impact of crisis on his or her own values, priorities, goals, or relationships

Family member moving in direction of health-promoting and enriching lifestyle that supports and monitors maturational processes, audits and negotiates treatment programs, and generally chooses experiences that optimize wellness

Individual expressing interest in making contact on a one-to-one basis or on a mutual-aid group basis with another client who has experienced a similar situation

## RELATED FACTORS

See *Health-Seeking Behaviors* and *Interrupted Family Processes*.

### ■■■■■ AUTHOR'S NOTE

This nursing diagnosis describes components found in *Interrupted Family Processes* and *Health-Seeking Behaviors*. Until clinical research differentiates the category from the aforementioned categories, use *Interrupted Family Processes* or *Health-Seeking Behaviors*, depending on the data presented.

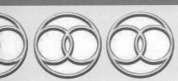

# CONTAMINATION: FAMILY

## DEFINITION

Exposure to environmental contaminants in doses sufficient to cause adverse health effects

## DEFINING CHARACTERISTICS

See Defining Characteristics for *Contamination: Individual and Community*

## RELATED FACTORS

See Related Factors for *Contamination: Individual and Community*

### ■■■■■ KEY CONCEPTS

See Key Concepts for *Contamination: Individual and Community*

## Focus Assessment Criteria

### Assess for Defining Characteristics.

See Defining Characteristics for *Contamination: Individual and Community*

**NOC**
See Contamination: Indiviudal and Community for Possible NOC Outcomes

➤ **Goal**

Family adverse health effects of contamination will be minimized.

**NIC**
See Contamination: Indiviudal and Community for Possible NOC Outcomes. See Also Appropriate NIC Interventions Based on Family's Defining Characteristics

➤ **Interventions**

See *Contamination: Individual and Community* for possible interventions

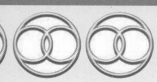

# RISK FOR CONTAMINATION: FAMILY

## DEFINITION

Accentuated Risk of Exposure to Environmental Contaminants in Doses Sufficient to Cause Adverse Health Effects

## RISK FACTORS

See Related Factors under *Contamination: Individual*

## KEY CONCEPTS

See Key Concepts under *Contamination: Individual*

## Focus Assessment Criteria

### Assess for Risk Factors.

Refer to Related Factors under *Contamination: Individual*

**NOC**
See *Risk for Contamination (Individual)* for Possible NOC Outcomes

➤ **Goal**

Family will remain free of adverse effects of contamination.

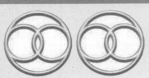

## ➤ Interventions

See *Risk for Contamination: Individual* for Interventions

# INTERRUPTED FAMILY PROCESSES

## DEFINITION

State in which a usually supportive family experiences, or is at risk to experience, a stressor that challenges its previously effective functioning

## DEFINING CHARACTERISTICS

### Major (Must Be Present)

Family system cannot or does not:
Adapt constructively to crisis
Communicate openly and effectively between family members

### Minor (May Be Present)

Family system cannot or does not:
Meet physical needs of all its members
Meet emotional needs of all its members
Meet spiritual needs of all its members
Express or accept a wide range of feelings
Seek or accept help appropriately

## RELATED FACTORS

Any factor can contribute to *Interrupted Family Processes*. Common factors are listed below.

### Treatment-Related

*Related to:*
Disruption of family routines because of time-consuming treatments (e.g., home dialysis)
Physical changes because of treatments of ill family member
Emotional changes in all family members because of treatments of ill family member
Financial burden of treatments for ill family member
Hospitalization of ill family member

### Situational (Personal, Environmental)

*Related to loss of family member*

| | | |
|---|---|---|
| Death | Incarceration | Going away to school |
| Desertion | Separation | Hospitalization |
| Divorce | | |

*Related to addition of new family member*

| | | |
|---|---|---|
| Birth | Marriage | Adoption |

Elderly relative
***Related to losses associated with:***
Poverty                             Economic crisis          Change in family roles
Birth of child with defect          Relocation                  (e.g., retirement)
Disaster
***Related to conflict (moral, goal, cultural)***
***Related to breach of trust between members***
***Related to social deviance by family member (e.g., crime)***

## ■■■■■■ AUTHOR'S NOTE

*Interrupted Family Processes* describes a family that reports usual constructive function but is experiencing an alteration from a current stress-related challenge. The family is viewed as a system, with interdependence among members. Thus, life challenges for individual members also challenge the family system. Certain situations may negatively influence family functioning; examples include illness, an older relative moving in, relocation, separation, and divorce. *Risk for Interrupted Family Processes* can represent such a situation.

   *Interrupted Family Processes* differs from *Caregiver Role Strain*. Certain situations require one or more family members to assume a caregiver role for a relative. Caregiver role responsibilities can vary from ensuring an older parent has three balanced meals daily to providing for all hygiene and self-care activities for an adult or child. *Caregiver Role Strain* describes the mental and physical burden that the caregiver role places on individuals, which influences all their concurrent relationships and role responsibilities. It focuses specifically on the individual or individuals with multiple direct caregiver responsibilities.

## ■■■■■■ ERRORS IN DIAGNOSTIC STATEMENTS

### Interrupted Family Processes Related to Family Not Discussing the Situation

A family's failure to discuss a situation does not represent a related factor, but a possible validation of the problem. If a failure to support one another represents a response to a stressor affecting the family system, *Interrupted Family Processes related to (specify stressor), as evidenced by report of family not discussing the situation* may be appropriate.

---

| NOC |
| --- |
| Family Coping, Family Environment: Internal, Family Normalization, Parenting |

## ➤ Goal

The family will maintain functional system of mutual support for one another.

### Indicators

- Frequently verbalize feelings to professional nurse and one another.
- Identify appropriate external resources available.

| NIC |
| --- |
| Family Involvement Promotion, Coping Enhancement, Family Integrity Promotion, Family Therapy, Counseling, Referral |

## ➤ General Interventions

### Assess Causative and Contributing Factors.

#### Illness-Related Factors

Sudden, unexpected nature of illness
Burdensome, chronic problems
Potentially disabling nature of illness
Symptoms creating disfiguring change in physical appearance
Social stigma associated with illness
Financial burden

### Factors Related to Behavior of Ill Family Member

Refuses to cooperate with necessary interventions
Engages in socially deviant behavior associated with illness: suicide attempts, violence, substance abuse
Isolates self from family
Acts out or is verbally abusive to health professionals and family members

### *Factors Related to the Overall Family Functioning*

Unresolved guilt, blame, hostility, jealousy
Inability to solve problems
Ineffective communication patterns among members
Changes in role expectations and resulting tension
Unclear role boundaries

### *Factors Related to Illness in Family (see also Caregiver Role Strain)*

### *Factors Related to the Community*

Lack of support from spiritual resources (philosophical, religious, or both)
Lack of relevant health education resources
Lack of supportive friends
Lack of adequate community health care resources (e.g., long-term follow up, hospice, respite)

**R:** Common sources of family stress are as follows (Carlson & Smith-DiJulio, 2006):

- External sources of stress (e.g., job or school related) one member is experiencing
- External sources of stress (e.g., finances, relocation) influencing the family unit
- Developmental stressors (e.g., childbearing, new baby, childrearing, adolescence, arrival of older grandparent, marriage of single parents, loss of spouse)
- Situational stressors (e.g., illness, hospitalization, separation, caregiving responsibilities)

## Promote Cohesiveness.

Approach the family with warmth, respect, and support.
Avoid vague and confusing advice and clichés, such as, "Take it easy; everything will be OK."
Keep family members abreast of changes in ill member's condition when appropriate.
Avoid discussing what caused the problem or blaming.
Facilitate communication.
Encourage verbalization of guilt, anger, blame, and hostility and subsequent recognition of own feelings in family members.

**R:** No family is 100% functional; however, healthy families are concerned with each other's needs and encourage expression of feelings (Varcarolis, Carson, & Shoemaker, 2006).

## Assist Family to Appraise the Situation.

What is at stake? Encourage family to have a realistic perspective by providing accurate information and answers to questions. Ensure all family members have input.
What are the choices? Assist family to reorganize roles at home and set priorities to maintain family integrity and reduce stress.
Initiate discussions regarding stressors of home care (physical, emotional, environmental, and financial).
"Family oriented approaches that include helping a family gain insight and make behavioral changes are most successful" (Varcarolis, Carson, & Shoemaker, 2006, p. 746).

## Promote Clear Boundaries between Individuals in Family.

- Ensure that all family members share their concerns
- Elicit the responsibilities of each member
- Acknowledge the differences

**R:** A client's emotional, social and physical functioning is directly related to how clear his/her role is differentiated in the family (Varcarolis, Carson, & Shoemaker, 2006).

## Initiate Health Teaching and Referrals, as Necessary.

Include family members in group education sessions.
Refer families to lay support and self-help groups:
Al-Anon                    Lupus Foundation of America

| Syn-Anon | Arthritis Foundation |
|---|---|
| Alcoholics Anonymous | National Multiple Sclerosis Society |
| Sharing and Caring | American Cancer Society |
| (American Hospital | American Heart Association |
| Association) | American Diabetes Association |
| Ostomy Association | American Lung Association |
| Reach for Recovery | Alzheimer's Disease and Related Disorders Association |

Facilitate family involvement with social supports.

Assist family members to identify reliable friends (e.g., clergy, significant others); encourage seeking help (emotional, technical) when appropriate.

Enlist help of other professionals (social work, therapist, psychiatrist, school nurse).

**R:** Families in stress will need extra encouragement to participate in self-help or other community agencies (Murray, Zenter, & Yakimo, 2009).

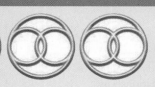

# DYSFUNCTIONAL FAMILY PROCESSES

## ▶ Related to Effects of Alcohol Abuse

## DEFINITION

State in which the psychosocial, spiritual, economic, and physiologic functions of the family members and system are chronically disorganized because of the effects of alcohol abuse

## DEFINING CHARACTERISTICS (LINDEMAN, HOKANSON, & BARTEK, 1994)

### Major (80% to 100%)

**Behaviors**

| | | |
|---|---|---|
| Inappropriate expression of anger | Inadequate understanding or knowledge of alcoholism | Manipulation |
| Dependency | Loss of control of drinking | Denial of problems |
| Impaired communication | Alcohol abuse | Refusal to get help |
| Enabling behaviors | Blaming | Rationalization |
| Inability to meet emotional needs | Broken promises | Ineffective problem solving |
| | | Criticizing |

**Feelings**

| | | |
|---|---|---|
| Hopelessness | Anger | Guilt |
| Powerlessness | Emotional isolation | Worthlessness |
| Vulnerability | Suppressed rage | Repressed emotions |
| Anxiety | Shame | Mistrust |
| Loneliness | Responsible for alcoholic's behavior | Embarrassment |

**Roles and Relationships**

| | | |
|---|---|---|
| Deteriorated family relationships | Inconsistent parenting | Disturbed family dynamics |
| Closed communication systems | Family denial | Marital problems |
| Ineffective spouse communication | Intimacy dysfunction | Disruption of family roles |

## Minor (70% to 79%)

### Behaviors

| | | |
|---|---|---|
| Cannot express or accept wide range of feelings | Inability to get or receive help appropriately | Orientation toward tension relief rather than goal achievement |
| Ineffective decision making | Contradictory, paradoxical communication | Family's special occasions are alcohol centered |
| Failure to deal with conflict | Escalating conflict | Isolation |
| Harsh self-judgment | Failure to send clear messages | Difficulty having fun |
| Lying | Disturbances in concentration | Chaos |
| Immaturity | Substance abuse other than alcohol | Difficulty with life cycle transitions |
| Inability to adapt to change | Stress-related physical illnesses | Failure to accomplish current or past developmental tasks |
| Power struggles | Disturbances in academic performance in children | |
| Verbal abuse of spouse or parent | | |
| Lack of reliability | | |

### Feelings

| | | |
|---|---|---|
| Being different from other people | Lack of identity | Unresolved grief |
| Feelings misunderstood | Loss | Depression |
| Fear | Hostility | Abandonment |
| Moodiness | Confused love and pity | Emotional control by others |
| Dissatisfaction | Confusion | Failure |
| | Being unloved | Self-blaming |

### Roles and Relationships

| | |
|---|---|
| Triangulating family relationship | Inability to meet spiritual needs of members |
| Reduced ability to relate to one another for mutual growth and maturation | Lack of skills necessary for relationships |
| Disrupted family rituals or no family rituals | Lack of cohesiveness |
| Does not demonstrate respect for individuality of its members | Inability to meet security needs of members |
| Low perception of parental support | Decreased sexual communication and individuality of its members |
| Neglected obligations | Pattern of rejection |

## RELATED FACTORS

Because the cause of this diagnosis is alcohol abuse by a family member, no related factors are needed.

### ■■■■■■ AUTHOR'S NOTE

Alcoholism is a family disease. This nursing diagnosis represents the consequences of the disturbed family dynamics related to alcohol abuse by a family member. The NANDA definition of *Interrupted Family Processes* is "the state in which a family that normally functions effectively experiences a dysfunction" (NANDA, 1992, p. 41).

The alcoholic family does not have a history of effective functioning. *Disabled Family Coping* would be more descriptive of the alcoholic family. The diagnosis could be stated as *Ineffective Family Coping*. Further assessment will determine the physical, psychological, spiritual, financial, and developmental effects of alcoholism on the family unit. If clinical research validates that alcoholism affects all these dimensions in all or most families, the diagnosis *Alcoholic Family Syndrome* may prove very useful.

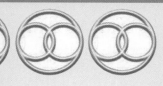

# DYSFUNCTIONAL FAMILY PROCESSES

## ▶ Related to Effects of Alcohol Abuse

**NOC**
Family Coping,
Family Functioning,
Substance Addiction
Consequences

## ➤ Goals

The family will acknowledge the alcoholism in the family.
The family will set short- and long-term goals.

### *Indicators*

- Relate the effects of alcoholism on the family unit and individuals.
- Identify destructive response patterns.
- Describe resources available for individual and family therapy.

**NIC**
Coping
Enhancements,
Referral,
Family Process
Maintenance,
Substance Use
Treatment, Family
Integrity Promotion,
Limit Setting,
Support Group

## ➤ General Interventions

### Establish a Trusting Relationship.

Be consistent; keep promises.
Be accepting and noncritical.
Do not pass judgment on what is revealed.
Focus on family member responses.

**R:** Alcoholism involves shame and stigma which promotes secrets and silence

### Allow Family Members as Individuals and a Group to Share Pent-Up Feelings.

Validate feelings as normal.
Correct inaccurate beliefs.

**R:** Alcoholism disturbs family communication. Sharing feelings is uncommon because of a history of disappointment. Diminished sharing and silence can maintain disturbed families for long periods. Communication focuses mainly on family members trying to control the other client's drinking behavior (Grisham & Estes, 1982).

### Emphasize that Family Members Are Not Responsible for the Client's Drinking (Starling & Martin, 1990; Carlson, Smith, & Julio, 2006).

Explain that emotional difficulties are relationship based rather than "psychiatric."
Instruct that their feelings and experiences are associated frequently with family alcoholism.

**R:** "The potential value of reaching the alcoholic client by first assisting family members should not be underestimated" (Grisham & Estes, 1982, p. 257). The family and health care professional must accept that no certain outcome can be promised for the alcoholic, even when the family gets help.

### Explore the Family's Beliefs About Situation and Goals.

Discuss characteristics of alcoholism; review a screening test (e.g., MAST, CAGE) that outlines characteristics of alcoholism.
Discuss causes and correct misinformation.
Assist to establish short- and long-term goals.

**R:** Wing (1994) proposes that relapses occur for different reasons in each stage. In stage I, relapse accompanies removal of the threat of punishment. Relapse in stage II occurs when the object of dependence (e.g., marriage, job) is secured or lost. Relapses in stages III and IV are less frequent and triggered by unexpected, stressful events. Nursing interactions for people in stages I and II focus on confronting denial and helping them become more internally focused. People in stages III and IV need assistance to learn how to cope with unexpected, stressful events (Wing, 1994).

**743**

## Assist the Family to Gain Insight into Behavior. Discuss Ineffective Methods Families Use.

| | |
|---|---|
| Hiding alcohol or car keys | Anger, silence, threats, crying |
| Making excuses for work, family, or friends | Bailing the client out of jail |
| Does not stop drinking | |
| Increases family anger | |
| Removes the responsibility for drinking from the client | |
| Prevents the client from suffering the consequences of his or her drinking behavior | |

**R:** Interventions focus on assisting the family to change their ineffective communication and response patterns (Carson & Smith-DiJulio, 2006).

## Emphasize that Helping the Alcoholic Means First Helping Themselves.

Focus on changing their response.

Allow the client to be responsible for his or her drinking behavior.

Describe activities that will improve their lives, as individuals and a family.

Initiate one stress management technique (e.g., aerobic exercise, assertiveness course, meditation).

Plan time as a family together outside the home (e.g., museum, zoos, and picnic). If the alcoholic is included, he or she must contract not to drink during the activity and agree on a consequence if he or she does.

**R:** Family members use denial to avoid admitting the problem and dealing with their contribution to it, and in the hope that the problem will disappear if not disclosed (Collins et al., 1990).

## Discuss with Family that Recovery Will Dramatically Change Usual Family Dynamics.

The alcoholic is removed from the center of attention.

All family roles will be challenged.

Family members will have to focus on themselves instead of the alcoholic client.

Family members will have to assume responsibility for their behavior, rather than blaming others.

Behavioral problems of children serve a purpose for the family.

**R:** Ending the drinking behavior threatens the family integrity because the family functioning is centered around the alcoholism (Carlson & Smith-DiJulio, 2006).

## Discuss Possibility of and Contributing Factors to Relapse.

**R:** Wing (1994) proposes that relapses occur for different reasons in each stage. In stage I, relapse accompanies removal of the threat of punishment. Relapse in stage II occurs when the object of dependence (e.g., marriage, job) is secured or lost. Relapses in stages III and IV are less frequent and triggered by unexpected, stressful events. Nursing interactions for people in stages I and II focus on confronting denial and helping them become more internally focused. People in stages III and IV need assistance to learn how to cope with unexpected, stressful events (Wing, 1994).

## If Additional Family or Individual Nursing Diagnoses Exist, Refer to Specific Diagnosis (e.g., Child Abuse, Domestic Violence).

## Initiate Health Teaching Regarding Community Resources and Referrals as Indicated.

| | | |
|---|---|---|
| Al-Anon | Alcoholics Anonymous | Family therapy |
| Individual therapy | Self-help groups | |

**R:** The family is the unit of treatment when one member is an alcoholic. Referrals are needed for long-term therapy.

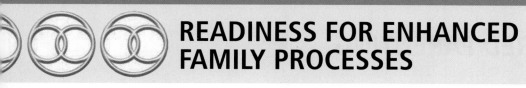

# READINESS FOR ENHANCED FAMILY PROCESSES

## DEFINITION (NANDA)

A pattern of family functioning that is sufficient to support the well-being of family members and can be strengthened

## DEFINING CHARACTERISTICS (NANDA)

- Expresses willingness to enhance family dynamics
- Family functioning meets physical, social, and psychological needs of family members
- Activities support the safety and growth of family members
- Communication is adequate
- Relationships are generally positive; interdependent with community; family tasks are accomplished
- Family roles are flexible and appropriate for developmental stages
- Respect for family members is evident
- Family adapts to change
- Boundaries of family members are maintained
- Energy level of family supports activities of daily living
- Family resilience is evident
- Balance exists between autonomy and cohesiveness

### ▪▪▪▪▪ AUTHOR'S NOTE

The interventions found under Interrupted Family Processes focus on strengthening family functioning. Refer to Interrupted Family Processes and Readiness for Enhanced Parenting for interventions to promote family integrity, mutual support and positive functioning.

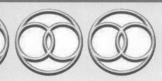

# READINESS FOR ENHANCED PARENTING

## DEFINITION

A pattern of providing an environment for children or other dependent client(s) that is sufficient to nurture growth and development and can be strengthened

## DEFINING CHARACTERISTICS

- Expresses willingness to enhance parenting
- Children or other dependent client(s) express satisfaction with home environment
- Emotional and tacit support of children or dependent client(s) is evident; bonding or attachment evident
- Physical and emotional needs of children/dependent client(s) are met
- Realistic expectations of children/dependent client(s) exhibited

### ▪▪▪▪▪ AUTHOR'S NOTE

Refer to Interrupted Family Processes for strategies to support effective family functioning and Readiness for Enhanced Resiliency for strategies to enhance parenting.

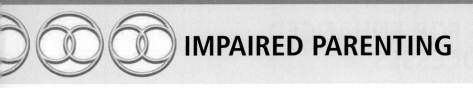

# IMPAIRED PARENTING

**Impaired Parenting**

Risk for Impaired Parent–Infant Attachment
Parental Role Conflict
Related to Effects of Illness and/or Hospitalization of a Child

## DEFINITION

State in which one or more caregivers demonstrate a real or potential inability to provide a constructive environment that nurtures the growth and development of his or her or their child (children)

## DEFINING CHARACTERISTICS

### Major (Must Be Present, One or More)

Inappropriate and/or non-nurturing parenting behaviors
Lack of parental attachment behavior

### Minor (May Be Present)

Frequent verbalization of dissatisfaction or disappointment with infant/child
Verbalization of frustration with role
Verbalization of perceived or actual inadequacy
Diminished or inappropriate visual, tactile, or auditory stimulation of infant
Evidence of abuse or neglect of child
Growth and development lag in infant/child

## RELATED FACTORS

Individuals or families who may be at risk for developing or experiencing parenting difficulties

### Parent(s)

| | | |
|---|---|---|
| Single | Addicted to drugs | Adolescent |
| Terminally ill | Abusive | Acutely disabled |
| Psychiatric disorder | Accident victim | Alcoholic |

### Child

| | | |
|---|---|---|
| Of unwanted pregnancy | With undesired | Terminally ill |
| With hyperactive | characteristics | Of undesired gender |
| characteristics | Mentally handicapped | Physically handicapped |

### Situational (Personal, Environmental)

*Related to interruption of bonding process secondary to:*
Illness (child, parent)      Relocation      Incarceration
*Related to separation from nuclear family*
*Related to lack of knowledge*
*Related to inconsistent caregivers or techniques*
*Related to relationship problems (specify):*
Marital discord      Stepparents      Divorce
Live-in partner      Separation      Relocation
*Related to little external support and/or socially isolated family*
*Related to lack of available role model*

*Related to ineffective adaptation to stressors associated with*

| | | |
|---|---|---|
| Illness | Economic problems | New baby |
| Substance abuse | Elder care | |

## Maturational

**Adolescent**
*Related to the conflict of meeting own needs over child's*
*Related to history of ineffective relationships with own parents*
*Related to parental history of abusive relationship with parents*
*Related to unrealistic expectations of child by parent*
*Related to unrealistic expectations of self by parent*
*Related to unrealistic expectations of parent by child*
*Related to unmet psychosocial needs of child by parent*

■■■■■■ **AUTHOR'S NOTE**

The family environment should provide the basic needs for a child's physical growth and development: stimulation of the child's emotional, social, and cognitive potential; consistent, stable reinforcement to learn impulse control; reality testing; freedom to share emotions; and moral stability (Pfeffer, 1981). This environment nurtures a child to develop, as Pfeffer (1981) states, "the ability to disengage from the family constellation as part of a process of lifelong individualization." It is the role of parents to provide such an environment. Most parenting difficulties stem from lack of knowledge or inability to manage stressors constructively. The ability to parent effectively is at high risk when the child or parent has a condition that increases stress on the family unit (e.g., illness, financial problems)." The phenomenon of parenting is relevant to many disciplines, including nursing" (Gage, Everett, & Bullock, 2006, p. 56).

   *Impaired Parenting* describes a parent experiencing difficulty creating or continuing a nurturing environment for a child. *Parental Role Conflict* describes a parent or parents whose previously effective functioning is challenged by external factors. In certain situations, such as illness, divorce, or remarriage, role confusion and conflict are expected. If parents do not receive assistance in adapting their role to external factors, *Parental Role Conflict* can lead to *Impaired Parenting*. "*The family is the primary social institution in which parenting takes place*" (Gage, Eververt, & Bullock, 2006, p. 57).

■■■■■ **ERRORS IN DIAGNOSTIC STATEMENTS**

### Impaired Parenting related to child abuse

Child abuse is a sign of family dysfunction. Usually, each situation involves an abusing adult and a knowing non-abusing adult; the treatment plan must include both. Thus, the diagnosis *Disabled Family Coping* would be more descriptive. *Impaired Parenting* is most appropriate when an external factor challenges the parents. External factors do not cause child abuse; rather, emotional disturbances and ineffective coping do.

**NOC**
Child Development
(Specify), Family
Coping, Family
Environment:
Internal, Family
Functioning, Parent-
Infant Attachment

## ➤ Goal

The parent/primary caregiver will acknowledge a problem with parenting skills.

### Indicators

- Provide a safe environment for child.
- Describe resource available for assistance with improvement of parenting skills.

**NIC**
Parenting
Promotion,
Developmental
Enhancement,
Anticipatory
Guidance, Parent
Education, Behavior
Management

## ➤ General Interventions

### Encourage Parents to Express Frustrations
### Regarding Role Responsibilities, Parenting, or Both.

Convey empathy.
Reserve judgment.
Convey/Offer educational information based on assessment

Help foster realistic expectations.

Encourage discussion of feelings regarding unmet expectations.

Discuss strategies that might increase the likelihood of expectations being met (e.g., discussing with partner, child; setting personal goals).

**R:** Parents who are encouraged to discuss their parenting expectations and who agree to support each other's decisions have less family tension (Hockenberry & Wilson, 2009).

## Educate Parents on Normal Growth and Development and Age-Related Expected Behaviors (Refer to Delayed Growth and Development).

**R:** Certain levels of stress interfere with the parent's ability to show patience and understanding (Hockenberry & Wilson, 2009). There is a real need for health care providers to assess parents and their parenting skills, "...the importance of addressing the needs of both the parents and children at the health visit as well as understanding the social and emotional dynamics of the parent-child relationship in effectively helping parents with child-rearing challenges" (Regalado, Sareen, Inkelas, Wissow, & Halfon, 2004, p. 1958).

## Explore with Parents the Child's Problem Behavior.

Frequency, duration

Context (when, where, triggers)

Consequences (parental attention, discipline, inconsistencies in response)

Behavior desired by parents

## Discuss Positive Parenting Techniques.

Convey to child that he or she is loved.

Catch child being good; use good eye contact.

Set aside "special time" when parent guarantees a time with child without interruptions.

Ignore minor transgressions by having no physical contact, eye contact, or discussion of the behavior.

Practice active listening. Describe what child is saying, reflect back the child's feelings, and do not judge.

Use "I" statements when disapproving of behavior. Focus on the act, not the child, as undesirable.

Positive reinforcement is an effective and recommended discipline technique for all ages (Banks, 2002). Redirecting is effective for infant to school age, whereas verbal instruction/explanation is most effective for school-age and adolescents (Banks, 2002).

**R:** Parents need confidence, as well as skill, to be comfortable in their new role. The nurse is in the enviable position of being able to assist families by providing information on parenting.

**R:** Observations of parent–child interactions should be guided by attention to the reciprocal aspect. Interactive "mismatch" may hamper parenting behaviors, evidenced when an infant is demanding and a parent lacks resilience or when the child's behavior is normal and the parents' expectations are unrealistic.

## Explain the Discipline Technique of "Time Out," Which Is a Method to Stop Misconduct, Convey Disapproval, and Provide Both Parent and Child Time to Regroup (Christophersen, 1992; Herman-Staab, 1994). Time Out Is Most Effective for the Toddler and School Age Child (Banks, 2002).

### Outline the Procedure.

Place or bring the child to a chair in a quiet place with few distractions (not the child's room or an isolated place).

Instruct child to stay in the chair. Set timer for 1 min of quiet time for each year of age.

Start the timer when the child is quiet.

If the child misbehaves, cries, or gets off the chair, reset the timer.

When the timer goes off, tell the child it is okay to get up.

**R:** The "time out" approach avoids many problems of other disciplinary approaches (e.g., arguing, physical punishment, loss of control; Hockenberry & Wilson, 2009).

### *Explain to the Child:*

This is not a game.

Practice it once when the child is behaving.

Explain rules and then ask the child questions to ensure understanding (if older than 3 years).

**R:** Discipline should be implemented at the time of an undesired behavior to increase effectiveness (Hockenberry & Wilson, 2009).

### *Remember:*

Do not warn child before sending for time out. If time out is appropriate, use it; do not threaten.

If child laughs during time out, ignore it.

Be sure no television is on or can be seen.

Do not look at or talk to or about child during time out.

Do not act angry; remain calm.

Keep yourself busy; let the child see you and what he or she is missing.

Do not give up or give in.

**R:** Behavioral modification techniques can be implemented effectively only when parents are consistent (Hockenberry & Wilson, 2009)." Parenting style was considered to be an important influence on children's social adjustment" (Gage, Everett, & Bullock, 2006, p.60).

**R:** Discipline should be implemented at the time of an undesired behavior to increase effectiveness (Hockenberry & Wilson, 2009).

## If Additional Sources of Conflict Arise, Refer to the Specific Nursing Diagnosis (e.g., Caregiver Role Strain, Fatigue).

## Take Opportunities to Role-Model Effective Parenting Skills; If Relevant, Share Some Frustrations You Have Experienced with Your Child to Help Normalize the Frustrations.

## Clarify the Strengths of the Parents or Family.

## Role-Play Asking for Help or Disciplining a Child.

## Provide General Parenting Guidelines.

Routine assessment of parent child interactions is an important aspect in providing anticipatory guidance about discipline (Regalado, Sareen, Inkelas, Wissow, & Halfon, 2004; Banks, 2002)

Practice open, honest dialogues. Never threaten (e.g., "If you are bad, I won't take you to the movies").

Do not lecture. Tell the child he or she was wrong and let it go. Spend time talking about pleasant experiences.

Compliment children on their achievements. Make each child feel important and special. Especially tell a child when he or she has been good; try not to focus on negative behavior.

Do not be afraid to hold and hug (boys as well as girls).

Set limits and keep them. Expect cooperation. Encourage the child to participate in activities that conform to your values. Do not be trapped by, "But everybody else can."

Let the child help you as much as possible." Nurses can encourage parents in their roles beyond childbearing, help them to solve problems, perform parenting tasks, and understand what is developmentally appropriate" (Gage, Everett, & Bullock, 2006, p. 57).

Discipline the child by restricting activity. Sit a younger child in a chair for 3 to 5 min. If the child gets up, reprimand once and put him or her back. Continue until the child sits for the prescribed time. For an older child, restrict bicycle riding or movie going (pick an activity that is important to him or her).

Make sure the discipline corresponds to the unacceptable behavior. Allow children opportunities to make mistakes and to express anger verbally.

Stay in control. Try not to discipline when you are irritated.

When long explanations are needed, give them after the discipline.

Remember to examine what you are doing when you are not disciplining your child (e.g., enjoying each other, loving each other).

Never reprimand a child in front of another person (child or adult). Take the child aside and talk.

Never decide you cannot control a child's destructive behavior. Examine your present response. Are you threatening? Do you follow through with the punishment or do you give in? Has the child learned you do not mean what you say?

Be a good model (the child learns from you whether you intend it or not). Never lie to a child even when you think it is better; the child must learn that you will not lie, no matter what.

Give each child a responsibility suited to his or her age, such as picking up toys, making beds, or drying dishes. Expect the child to complete the task.

Share your feelings with children (happiness, sadness, anger). Respect and be considerate of the child's feelings and of his or her right to be human.

**R:** Reasoning is not appropriate with young children, who cannot "see the other side" (Hockenberry & Wilson, 2009).

**R:** Children learn to be responsible adults by having responsibilities as children.

**R:** Ignoring problem behavior can minimize or eliminate it (Hockenberry & Wilson, 2009).

## Initiate Health Teaching and Referrals as Indicated.

Community resources—counseling, social service, parenting classes
Support groups—self-help, church

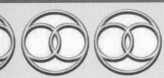

# RISK FOR IMPAIRED PARENT–INFANT ATTACHMENT

## DEFINITION

State in which there is a risk for a disruption of a nurturing, protective, interactive process between a parent/primary caregiver and infant

## RISK FACTORS

Refer to Related Factors.

## RELATED FACTORS

### Pathophysiologic

*Related to interruption of attachment process secondary to:*
Parental illness      Infant illness

### Treatment-Related

*Related to barriers to attachment secondary to:*
Lack of privacy      Intensive care monitoring    Structured "visitation"
Equipment  Restricted visitors

### Situational (Personal, Environmental)

*Related to unrealistic expectations (e.g., of child, of self)*
*Related to unplanned pregnancy*
*Related to disappointment with infant (e.g., gender, appearance)*
*Related to life event stressors associated with new baby and other responsibilities secondary to:*
Health issues          Substance abuse          Mental illness
Relationship difficulties      Economic difficulties
*Related to lack of knowledge and/or available role model for parental role*
*Related to physical disabilities of parent (e.g., blindness, paralysis, deafness)*
*Related to being emotionally unprepared due to premature delivery of infant*

## Maturational

### Adolescent
*Related to difficulty delaying own gratification for the gratification of the infant*

■■■■■■ **AUTHOR'S NOTE**

This new diagnosis describes a parent or caregiver at risk for attachment difficulties with his or her infant. Barriers to attachment can be the environment, knowledge, anxiety, and health of parent or infant. This diagnosis is appropriate as a risk or high-risk diagnosis. If the nurse diagnoses a problem in infant–parent attachment, the diagnosis *Risk for Impaired Parenting related to difficulties in parent–child attachment* would be more useful so that the nurse could focus on improving attachment and preventing destructive parenting patterns.

■■■■■■ **ERRORS IN DIAGNOSTIC STATEMENTS**

### Risk for Impaired Parent–Infant Attachment related to husband not being the biologic father

The related factor is certainly a risk factor associated with attachment problems; however, this information is confidential and requires caution to protect its disclosure. If a family shares this information during an assessment or interaction, the nurse should record it exactly in quotes in the progress notes. The nurse can write the nursing diagnosis as *Risk for Impaired Parent–Infant Attachment related to possible rejection of infant by father*.

**NOC**
Refer to *Impaired Parenting*

➤ **Goal**

The parent will demonstrate increased attachment behaviors, such as holding infant close, smiling and talking to infant, and seeking eye contact with infant.

### Indicators

- Be supported in his or her need to be involved in infant's care.
- Begin to verbalize positive feelings regarding infant.

**NIC**
Refer to *Impaired Parenting*

➤ **General Interventions**

## Assess Causative or Contributing Factors.

### Maternal

Unwanted pregnancy
Prolonged or difficult labor and delivery
Postpartum pain or fatigue
Lack of positive support system (mother, spouse, friends)
Lack of positive role model (mother, relative, neighbor)
Inability to prepare emotionally for an unexpected delivery

## Inadequate Coping Patterns (One or Both Parents)

Alcoholic
Drug addict
Marital difficulties (separation, divorce, violence)
Change in lifestyle related to new role
Adolescent parent
Career change (e.g., working woman to mother)
Illness in family

### Infant

Premature, defective, ill
Multiple birth

## Eliminate or Reduce Contributing Factors, If Possible.

### Illness, Pain, Fatigue

Establish with mother what infant care activities are feasible.
Provide mother with uninterrupted sleep periods of at least 2 h during the day and 4 h at night.
Provide relief for discomforts.

Episiotomy:

- Evaluate degree of pain.
- Assess for hematomas and abscesses.
- Provide with comfort measures (ice, warm compresses, analgesics*).

Hemorrhoids:

- Prevent and treat constipation.
- Provide comfort measures (compresses with witch hazel, suppositories,* analgesics*).

Breast engorgement of nursing mother:

- Encourage woman to nurse as frequently as possible.
- Apply warm compresses (shower) before nursing.
- Apply cold compresses after nursing.
- Try hand massage, hand expressing, or breast pump between nursing.
- Offer mild analgesics.
- See *Ineffective Breastfeeding.*

Breast engorgement of non-nursing mother:

- Offer analgesics as ordered.
- Apply ice packs.
- Encourage use of a good supporting brassiere that covers the entire breast.

### Lack of Experience or Positive Mothering Role Model

Explore with mother her feelings and attitudes concerning her own mother.
Assist her to identify someone who is a positive mother; encourage her to seek that client's aid.
Outline the teaching program available during hospitalization.
Determine who will assist her at home initially.
Identify community programs and reference material that can increase her learning about child care after discharge (see References/Bibliography).

### Lack of Positive Support System

Identify parent's support system; assess its strengths and weaknesses.
Assess the need for counseling.
Encourage parents to express feelings about the experience and about the future.
Be an active listener to the parents.
Observe the parents interacting with the infant.
Assess for resources (financial, emotional) already available to the family.
Be aware of resources available both within the hospital and in the community.
Counsel the parents on assessed needs.
Refer to hospital or community services.

### Barriers to Practicing Cultural Beliefs That May Affect the Family Unit During Hospitalization

Support mother–infant–family beliefs.
Integrate culture and traditions into routine care.
Identify community resources.

---

*May require a primary care professional's order.

### Elimination of Institutional Barriers That Inhibit Individualizing of Care

Sensitize staff to practicing family-centered care.
Use families to review practice and policies.
Encourage cultural sensitization of staff.

**R:** The use of birthing rooms enhances the bonding process because of the decrease in interruptions.

## Provide Opportunities for the Process of Mutual Interaction.

### Promote Bonding in the Immediate Postdelivery Phase.

Encourage mother to hold infant after birth (may need a short recovery period).
Provide skin-to-skin contact if desired; keep room warm (72° to 76° F) or use a heat panel over the infant.
Provide mother with an opportunity to breast-feed immediately after delivery, if desired.
Delay administration of silver nitrate to allow for eye contact.
Give family as much time as they need together with minimum interruption from staff (the "sensitive period" lasts from 30 to 90 min).
Encourage father to hold infant.

**R:** Research indicates that there is a "sensitive period" during the newborn's first minutes and hours of life during which the child is beautifully equipped to meet and interact with the parents. Close contact at this time and in the days to follow is most beneficial to the bonding process (Klaus & Kennell, 1976).

### Facilitate the Attachment Process During the Postpartum Phase.

Check mother regularly for signs of fatigue, especially if she had anesthesia.
Offer flexible rooming-in to the mother; establish with her the care she will assume initially and support her requests for assistance.
Discuss future involvement of the father in the infant's care (if desired, plan opportunities for father to participate in his child's care during visits).

**R:** The period from birth to 3 days is important for the father–child relationship.

### Provide Support to the Parents.

Listen to the mother's replay of her labor and delivery experience.
Allow for verbalization of feelings.
Indicate acceptance of feelings.
Point out the infant's strengths and individual characteristics to the parents.
Demonstrate the infant's responses to the parents.
Have a system of follow-up after discharge, especially for families considered at risk (e.g., telephone call or a home visit by the community health nurse).
Be aware of resources and support groups available within the hospital and community; refer the family as needed.

**R:** In a longitudinal study of the interaction between 49 premature infants and their mothers, Zahr (1991) found that maternal rating of the infant's temperament and availability of support system were the most significant variables that correlated with a positive mother–infant interaction at 4 and 8 months postpartum.

### Assess the Need to Support the Parents' Emerging Confidence in Child Care.

Observe the parents interacting with the infant.
Support each parent's strengths.
Assist each parent in those areas in which he or she is uncomfortable (role modeling).
Have handouts and audiovisual aids available for parents to view at odd hours.
Assess for level of knowledge in growth and development; provide information as needed.
Help parents understand infant's cues and temperament.
See References/Bibliography for recommended printed material on parenting and child care.

**R:** Seeing, touching, and caring for the infant promotes attachment (Klaus & Kennell, 1976).

### When Immediate Separation of the Child from the Parents is Necessary Because of Prematurity or Illness, Provide for Bonding/Attachment Experiences, as Possible.

Invite parents to see and touch infant as soon as possible.

Encourage parents to spend prolonged time with infant.

Support activities such as skin-to-skin holding, containment of infant with parental hands in the isolette, and basic caregiving activities.

If infant is transported to another facility and separated from mother:

- Have staff make frequent calls to mother.
- Encourage family to spend time in NICU; bring back verbal reports and pictures of infant.
- Explore family and community resources to provide means of rejoining mother and infant as soon as possible.

**R:** When caring for families of high-risk newborns, nurses can foster attachment and reduce anxiety by letting parents know through frequent communication that they are welcome partners in their child's care.

**R:** Parents are reluctant to form attachments to a sick infant because of their fear of loss. This reluctance creates tremendous guilt.

**R:** Parents must be given the opportunity for grief work in the case of an ill or impaired infant before attachment can begin.

## For Adoptive Parents:

Counsel adoptive parents that many emotions are normal on first interaction with their children.

Counsel adoptive parents about the possibility of postadoption depression.

Encourage adoptive parents to seek parenting classes before receiving their infant.

**R:** In a research study of 24 first-time adoptive mothers, Koepke, Anglin, Austin, and Delesalle (1991) found that adoptive mothers began developing affectional ties to their babies at much the same time and in as individual a way as birth mothers. Adoptive mothers may be as susceptible as birth mothers to periods of sadness and maternal depression.

## Initiate Referrals, as Needed.

Consult with community agencies for follow-up visits if indicated.

Refer parents to pertinent organizations (see References/Bibliography).

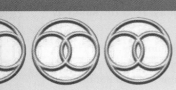

# PARENTAL ROLE CONFLICT

## DEFINITION

State in which a parent or primary caregiver experiences or perceives a change in role in response to external factors (e.g., illness, hospitalization, divorce, separation), pitch of child with special needs

## DEFINING CHARACTERISTICS

### Major (Must Be Present, One or More)

Parent(s) express(es) concerns about changes in parental role

Demonstrated disruption in care and/or caretaking routines

## Minor (May Be Present)

Parent(s) express(es) concerns/feelings of inadequacy to provide for child's physical and emotional needs during hospitalization or in the home

Parent(s) express(es) concerns about effect of child's illness on other children

Parent(s) express(es) concerns about care of siblings at home

Parent(s) express(es) concern about perceived loss of control over decisions relating to the child

# RELATED FACTORS

## Situational (Personal, Environmental)

***Related to separation from child secondary to:***

Birth of a child with a congenital defect and/or chronic illness

Hospitalization of a child with an acute or chronic illness

Change in acuity, prognosis, or environment of care (e.g., transfer to or from ICU)

***Related to fear of involvement secondary to invasive or restrictive treatment modalities (e.g., isolation, intubation)***

***Related to interruption of family life secondary to:***

Home care of a child with special needs (e.g., apnea monitoring, postural drainage, hyperalimentation)

Frequent visits to hospital

Addition of new family member (aging relative, newborn)

***Related to change in ability to parent secondary to:***

| | | |
|---|---|---|
| Illness of parent | Remarriage | Travel requirements |
| Dating | Work responsibilities | Death |
| Divorce | | |

> ■■■■■■ **AUTHOR'S NOTE**
>
> See *Impaired Parenting.*

**NOC**
Caregiver Adaptation to Child's Hospitalization, Caregiver Home Care Readiness, Coping, Family Environment: Internal Family Functioning, Parenting

## ➤ Goal

The parent and child will demonstrate control over decision making.

### Indicators

- Express feelings regarding the situation.
- Identify sources of support.

**NIC**
Caregiver Support, Role Enhancement, Anticipatory Guidance, Family Involvement Promotion, Counseling Referrals

## ➤ General Interventions

### Assess the Present Situation.

Parents' and children's perceptions of and responses to situation

Parental understanding of the effects of the situation on children and their typical responses

Changes in parenting practices and daily routines (employment or change in child care arrangements)

Other related stressors (financial, job-related)

Level of conflict between parents

Social support for both parents

> **R:** Adjustment to the condition may be accompanied by feelings of quilt, self-accusation, anger, and bitterness (Hockenberry & Wilson, 2009).

## Encourage the Involvement of Fathers in Care.

Foster his strengths.

Provide an appropriate place for grieving.

Encourage the sharing of grief.

Include the father in care.

**R:** Nursing strategies based on an empowerment model are the most effective in helping parents resolve role conflict and move through role transition.

## Help Parents with Limit Setting with the Child.

Explain the boundaries of acceptable behavior.

Expect the child to perform age-appropriate self-care activities when able.

Assign age-appropriate chores.

Expect the child to participate in his or her care.

**R:** These strategies can help parents acquire parenting behaviors that will be effective in caring for their ill child in the hospital or the home on a temporary or long-term basis.

## Encourage Parents to Address Siblings' Responses.

Help parents talk to siblings about the child's condition.

Encourage parents to spend special time with siblings, acknowledge that negative feelings are normal, and allow some participation in the child's care.

Allow siblings a life outside of caregiving.

**R:** Siblings need age-appropriate explanations of the situation. They need to be prepared for the physical changes and possible role changes (Hockenberry & Wilson, 2009).

## Assist Family to Increase Decision-Making Abilities (Dunst, Trivette, & Deal, 1988a; Smith, 1999).

Emphasize parental responsibility for meeting needs and solving problems.

Emphasize building on parental strengths.

Provide active and reflective listening.

Offer normative help that is congruent with parental appraisal of need.

Promote acquisition of competencies.

Use parent–professional collaboration as the mechanism for meeting needs.

Allow locus of control to reside with the parent.

Accept and support parental decisions.

**R:** Respecting parents as the experts in caring for their child promotes more confidence and collaboration with caregivers (Baker, 1994).

## Support Siblings (Hockenberry & Wilson, 2009).

Listen to the siblings' feelings. Accept reasonable anger. Praise when they have been patient or very helpful.

Explain their sibling's condition and limit their responsibilities of care taking.

**R:** Siblings experience loneliness, increased responsibilities, fear, jealousy, guilt and resentment (Hockenberry & Wilson, 2009).

## Encourage Expression of Feelings (Hockenberry & Wilson, 2009).

Describe behavior, e.g., "You seem angry most of the time."

Provide understanding, e.g., "Being angry is only natural."

Help focus on feelings: "Do you wonder why this has happened to your child (or siblings)?"

**R:** Siblings will experience being pushed to the background and a disruption in special events, e.g., holidays, vacations. Their parents may be emotionally and physically unavailable for them (Hockenberry & Wilson, 2009).

### Facilitate Parent–Nurse Partnerships.

Acknowledge the parents' overall competence and their unique expertise.

Explain everything related to care. Engage parents in team meetings.

Negotiate differences, be flexible, and offer respite.

**R:** Respecting parents as the experts in caring for their child promotes more confidence and collaboration with caregivers (Baker, 1994).

### Initiate Teaching and Referrals as Needed.

Ensure that the school nurse is aware of the situation.

Initiate referrals as needed, e.g., in home care, day care, respite care.

Identify local and national disease—oriented organizations, e.g., National Information Center for children and youth with disabilities (800-695-0285, www.Nichcy.org).

Refer to *Caregiver Role Strain* for additional interventions.

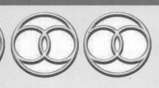

# PARENTAL ROLE CONFLICT

## ▶ Related to Effects of Illness and/or Hospitalization of a Child

**NOC**
See *Parental Role Conflict*

### ➤ Goals

The parent will demonstrate control over decision making concerning the child and collaborate with health professionals to make decisions about the care of the child.

#### Indicators

- Relate information about the child's health status and treatment plan.
- Participate in caring for the child in the home/hospital setting to the degree desired.
- Verbalize feelings about the child's illness and the hospitalization.
- Identify and use available support systems that allow parent time and energy to cope with ill child's needs.

**NIC**
See *Parental Role Conflict*

### ➤ General Interventions

#### Help Adapt Parenting Role During Illness (Newton, 2000).

Use role-supplementation strategies and role cues to help parents adapt parenting role to meet the child's needs.

Role model parenting behaviors appropriate to child's developmental stage and medical condition.

Instruct parents to continue limit-setting strategies and demonstrations of caring behaviors (e.g., touching, hugging despite hospitalization and equipment).

Provide information to empower parents to adapt parenting role to the situation of hospitalization and/or chronic illness.

Provide information about hospital routines and policies, such as visiting hours, mealtimes, division routines, medical and nursing routines, rooming-in, and so forth.

Introduce self and other health care workers involved in the child's care; explain the role of each team member.

Explain procedures and tests to parents; help them interpret these activities to the child; discuss child's age-appropriate range of responses.

Assess usual parenting role or interpretation of real or perceived parental role.

Assess parental knowledge about child's normal growth and development, safety issues, and so forth; offer supplemental information as appropriate (see *Delayed Growth and Development*).

Teach parents special skills needed to provide for the physical and health care needs of the child.

**R:** Parental stress may be mediated by

- Helping parents feel they are part of the team caring for their child and that they have all the information that is known about their child's condition
- Allowing parents to comfort their child
- Comforting the parent
- Treating the child as an individual, such as using the child's name, approaching the child in an age-appropriate manner, and talking to the child even if the child is comatose

## Facilitate Communication About Condition and Treatment Plan.

Foster open communication between self and parents, allowing time for questions, frequent repetition of information; provide direct and honest answers.

Facilitate open communication between parents and other members of the health care team.

Approach parents with new information; do not make them assume the responsibility for seeking the information.

When parents cannot be with their child, facilitate communication through telephone calls; allow parents to call primary nurse or nurse caring for child.

Facilitate interdisciplinary communication so all members of the health care team have congruent and consistent information to share with the family.

Minimize waiting time for parents whenever possible.

Assess parental understanding of the child's illness.

Explain and interpret medical terminology to parents to foster their understanding of the child's condition:

- What is the reason for the child's hospitalization?
- What is going to be done to the child during hospitalization?
- Will the child be awake for the procedures?
- Will the child feel pain or discomfort?
- Where will it hurt?
- What will be done for the discomfort?
- Will the procedure change the child in any way? Is the change temporary or permanent?
- Who may visit the child? When?
- What may be brought to the hospital from home?
- How long will the child be in the hospital?
- Will there be any restrictions for the child at home?

Role-model interpreting events to child; help parents interpret to child and other family members.

Respect confidentiality of information; share information about child with parents only; instruct other family members to obtain information from parents.

**R:** Parents may be hampered in their acquisition of new effective parenting behaviors by feelings of anxiety, guilt, powerlessness, and diminished competence, and by lack of information or unfamiliarity with hospital surroundings, personnel, and systems.

## Support Continued Decision Making.

Allow parents to help formulate plan of care for their child.

Use parents as a source of information about the child, his or her usual behaviors, reactions, and preferences.

Recognize parents as experts about their child.

Allow parents to be present during treatments and procedures if they desire.

Involve parents in decisions about the child's care, giving them choices whenever possible.

**R:** Based on the promotion of self-determination, decision-making capabilities, and self-efficacy, the family-centered empowerment model requires three beliefs: (1) parents are competent in or have the capacity to become competent in the care of their child; (2) parents must be given opportunities to display competencies in the care of their children; and (3) parents need the necessary information to make informed decisions and to obtain resources to meet needs, and thus acquire control over their child's care (Dunst, Trivette, Davis & Wheeldreyer, 1988).

**R:** Pass and Pass (1987) suggest providing parents with a list of questions they should be asking about their child's hospitalization.

## Allow Parents to Participate in Care of Their Child to the Degree They Desire.

Provide for 24-h rooming-in for at least one parent and extended visiting for other family members.

Collaborate and negotiate about parental tasks they wish to continue to do, tasks they wish others to assume, tasks they wish to share, and tasks they want to learn.

Assess parental ability to comfort the child; use comfort strategies that parents have indicated for the child.

Allow parents to have uninterrupted time with the child.

Provide consistent caregivers for the family through primary nursing; explain the primary nurse's role, responsibilities, and commitment to the parent and child.

Explore with parents their personal responsibilities (i.e., work schedule, sibling care, household responsibilities, responsibilities to extended family); assist them to establish a schedule that allows sufficient caregiving time for the child or visiting time with the hospitalized child without frustration in meeting other role responsibilities (e.g., if visiting is not possible until evening hours, delay child's bath time and allow parent to bathe child then).

**R:** Support and enhancement of role transition for parents of an ill child can best be achieved in a setting that is guided by principles of family-centered care and by a nursing process that also is guided by this family-focused philosophy.

## Support Parental Ability to Normalize the Hospital/Home Environment.

Orient parents and child to hospital setting before admission, if possible, through pre-hospitalization or pre-transfer tour.

Orient parents to the hospital environment: kitchen, playroom, tub room, treatment room, and parents' lounge.

Instruct parents how to obtain needed supplies for self and child.

Orient parents to other hospital areas: cafeteria, chapel, gift shop, library, Ronald McDonald House.

Encourage parents to bring clothing and toys from home.

Allow parents to prepare home-cooked food or bring food from home if desired.

Encourage families to eat meals together.

Provide for sibling visitation. Help parents prepare siblings for the visit.

Construct daily routine around home routine as indicated by parent(s).

Provide privacy for parent–child interactions (e.g., privacy for breast-feeding, family time for teens and parents).

Provide parents with comfortable visiting and sleeping accommodations at the bedside, if possible, for easy access to the child.

Attempt to minimize stressors of the unit/division (e.g., noise level, over access by hospital personnel, unplanned client care) that disrupt quiet/rest periods.

Provide age-appropriate developmental (school) and diversional activities for the child to provide for parenting opportunities.

Encourage parents to take the child on leaves from the hospital, including visits home, as possible.

Use an interdisciplinary approach to care planning to minimize the length of hospitalization.

**R:** Nursing interventions should be oriented to preparing the parent for potential stressors in an effort to decrease anxiety, thus enabling parents to spend more energy on normalizing the environment for their hospitalized children.

## Help Verbalize Feelings About the Child's Illness or Hospitalization.

Encourage parents to express feelings and concerns about the child's illness or hospitalization and about the perceived need for parental role change.

Provide opportunities for parents to be alone, not in the presence of the child, so they may feel free to express feelings, frustrations, and fears.

Indicate acceptance of parental feelings.

Identify staff members who have established a therapeutic relationship with the parents.

Provide opportunities for parents to talk about themselves, events related to hospitalization/illness, and real/perceived conflicts and changes in their role, whether temporary or permanent.

**R:** Knafl and Dixon (1984) found that 24% of the fathers in their study reported role expansion as a result of the hospitalization of their child. Expansion included the responsibility for monitoring the child's care.

**R:** Alexander and coworkers (1988) found a significant level of high anxiety in non–rooming-in fathers with greater numbers of children at home, suggesting a shift in home responsibilities.

## Provide for Physical and Emotional Needs of Parents.

Assess and facilitate parental ability to meet self-care needs (e.g., rest, nutrition, activity, privacy).

Allow parents to determine the caregiving schedule to correspond with a schedule to meet their own needs.

Assess support systems: parent to parent, family, friends, minister, and so forth.

Assess, acknowledge, and facilitate family strengths.

Facilitate and reinforce effective coping strategies used by parents.

Continue to listen to parental concerns regarding the child and parental role.

Continue to assess additional stressors in the family setting.

**R:** Alexander and coworkers (1988) found significantly higher anxiety levels in non–rooming-in parents of hospitalized children, especially as the duration of hospitalization increased.

## Initiate Referrals, If Indicated.

Chaplain, social service, community agencies (respite care), parent self-help groups

Provide information to parents for self-referral.

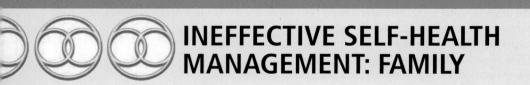

# INEFFECTIVE SELF-HEALTH MANAGEMENT: FAMILY

## DEFINITION

Pattern in which the family experiences or is at risk to experience difficulty integrating into daily living a program for treatment of illness and the sequealae of illness that meets specific health goals

## DEFINING CHARACTERISTICS

### Major (Must Be Present)

Inappropriate family activities for meeting the goals of a treatment or prevention program

### Minor

Acceleration (expected or unexpected) of illness symptoms of a family member

Lack of attention to illness and its sequealae

Verbalized desire to manage the treatment of illness and prevention of sequealae

Verbalized difficulty with regulation/integration of one or more prescribed regimens for treatment of illness and its effects or prevention of complications

Verbalized that family did not take action to reduce risk factors for progression of illness and sequealae

## RELATED FACTORS

Refer to *Ineffective Self-Health Management*.

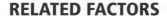 **AUTHOR'S NOTE**

Refer to *Ineffective Self-Health Management*.

**ERRORS IN DIAGNOSTIC STATEMENTS**

Refer to *Ineffective Self-Health Management*.

**KEY CONCEPTS**

Refer to *Ineffective Self-Health Management*.

## Focus Assessment Criteria

Refer to *Ineffective Self-Health Management*.

## General Interventions

Refer to *Ineffective Self-Health Management*.

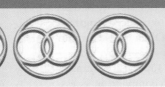 # IMPAIRED HOME MAINTENANCE

## DEFINITION

State in which a client or family experiences or is at risk to experience difficulty in maintaining a safe, hygienic, growth-producing home environment

## DEFINING CHARACTERISTICS

### Major (Must Be Present, One or More)

*Expressions or observations of*

| | | |
|---|---|---|
| Difficulty maintaining home hygiene | Difficulty maintaining a safe home | Inability to keep up home |
| | | Lack of sufficient finances |

### Minor (May Be Present)

| | | |
|---|---|---|
| Repeated infections | Infestations | Accumulated wastes |
| Unwashed utensils | Offensive odors | Overcrowding |

## RELATED FACTORS

### Pathophysiologic

*Related to compromised functional ability secondary to chronic debilitating disease*

| | | |
|---|---|---|
| Diabetes mellitus | Arthritis | Chronic obstructive |
| Multiple sclerosis | Congestive heart failure | pulmonary disease (COPD) |

Cerebrovascular accident          Parkinson's disease          Muscular dystrophy
Cancer

## Situational (Personal, Environmental)

*Related to change in functional ability of (specify family member) secondary to:*
Injury (fractured limb, spinal cord injury)
Surgery (amputation, ostomy)
Impaired mental status (memory lapses, depression, anxiety–severe panic)
Substance abuse (alcohol, drugs)
*Related to unavailable support system*
*Related to loss of family member*
*Related to lack of knowledge*
*Related to insufficient finances*

## Maturational

### Infant
*Related to multiple care requirements secondary to:*
High-risk newborn

### Older Adult
*Related to multiple care requirements secondary to:*
Family member with deficits (cognitive, motor, sensory)

## ■■■■■■ AUTHOR'S NOTE

With rising life expectancy and declining mortality rates, the numbers of older adults are steadily increasing, with many living alone at home. Eighty percent of people 65 years or older report one or more chronic diseases. Of adults 65 to 74 years of age, 20% report activity limitations, and 15% cannot perform at least one activity of daily living (ADL) independently (Miller, 2009). The shift from health care primarily in hospitals to reduced lengths of stay has resulted in the discharge of many functionally compromised people to their homes. Often a false assumption is that someone will assume the management of household responsibilities until the client has recovered.

*Impaired Home Maintenance* describes situations in which a client or family needs teaching, supervision, or assistance to manage the household. Usually, a community health nurse is the best professional to complete an assessment of the home and the client's functioning there. Nurses in acute settings can make referrals for home visits for assessment.

A nurse who diagnoses a need for teaching to prevent household problems may use *Risk for Impaired Home Maintenance related to insufficient knowledge of (specify)*.

## ■■■■■■ ERRORS IN DIAGNOSTIC STATEMENTS

### Impaired Home Maintenance related to caregiver burnout

Caregiver burnout is not a sign of or related factor for *Impaired Home Maintenance*. It is associated with *Caregiver Role Strain*. *Impaired Home Maintenance* also may be present if multiple responsibilities overwhelm the caregiver. In this situation, both diagnoses are needed because the interventions for them differ.

## Pediatric Considerations

- Children depend on family members to manage home care.
- Trends in the treatment of children with chronic illness or disability include home care, early discharge, focus on developmental age, and assessment of strengths and uniqueness. Interventions are geared toward the entire family rather than just the ill child (Hockenberry & Wilson, 2009).
- High-risk graduates of neonatal intensive care units (NICUs) require technically complex home care. Discharge is planned as early as possible to contain cost and to help reduce adverse effects of hospitalization on the family system.

## Geriatric Considerations

- Older people have greater incidences of chronic disease, impaired function, and diminished economic resources, and a smaller social network than do younger people (Miller, 2009).
- After 75 years of age, most people living in the community live alone. Of older people living alone, 60% own their home (Miller, 2009).
- Functional ability includes ADLs and also instrumental activities of daily living (IADLs)—those skills needed to live independently (e.g., procuring food, cooking, using the telephone, housekeeping, handling finances). IADLs are connected integrally to physical and cognitive abilities. The older adult who lives alone is at great risk of being institutionalized if he or she cannot perform IADLs. The possibility is great that no social network can meet these deficits (Miller, 2009).
- Approximately 9 of 10 older people have one or more chronic health problems with differing effects on function. Chronic conditions cause approximately 60% of people older than 75 years to limit their ADLs (Holzapfil, 1998).
- Along with diminished cognitive or physical ability, the older client frequently has diminished financial resources, sporadic kin, or few neighborhood social supports. He or she also may live in substandard housing or housing that does not allow simple adaptation to meet individual physical or cognitive deficits (Miller, 2009).
- In some cultures and family structures, older adults can seek assistance in some areas of home management and still retain a sense of independence. These people have determined that, by choosing selective resources to meet their needs, they will be able to maintain independent living for a longer time (Miller, 2009).

**NOC**
Family Functioning

## ➤ Goal

The client or caretaker will express satisfaction with home situation.

### Indicators

- Identify factors that restrict self-care and home management.
- Demonstrate ability to perform skills necessary for care of the home.

**NIC**
Home Maintenance Assistance, Environmental Management: Safety, Environmental Management

## ➤ General Interventions

The following interventions apply to many with impaired home maintenance, regardless of etiology.

## Assess for Causative or Contributing Factors.

Lack of knowledge
Insufficient funds
Lack of necessary equipment or aids
Inability (illness, sensory deficits, motor deficits) to perform household activities
Impaired cognitive functioning
Impaired emotional functioning

## Reduce or Eliminate Causative or Contributing Factors, If Possible.

### Lack of Knowledge

Determine with client and family the information they need to learn:

- Monitoring skills (pulse, circulation, urine)
- Medication administration (procedure, side effects, precautions)
- Treatment/procedures
- Equipment use/maintenance
- Safety issues (e.g., environmental)
- Community resources
- Follow-up care
- Anticipatory guidance (e.g., emotional and social needs, alternatives to home care)

Initiate teaching; give detailed written instruction.

### Insufficient Funds

Consult with social service department for assistance.

Consult with service organizations (e.g., American Heart Association, The Lung Association, American Cancer Society) for assistance.

### Lack of Necessary Equipment or Aids

Determine type of equipment needed, considering availability, cost, and durability.

Seek assistance from agencies that rent or loan supplies:
- Teach care and maintenance of supplies to increase length of use.
- Consider adapting equipment to reduce cost.

### Inability to Perform Household Activities

Determine type of assistance needed (e.g., meals, housework, transportation); assist client to obtain it.

#### Meals

Discuss with relatives the possibility of freezing complete meals that require only heating (e.g., small containers of soup, stews, casseroles).

Determine availability of meal services for ill people (e.g., Meals on Wheels, church groups).

Teach people about nutritious foods that are easily prepared (e.g., hard-boiled eggs, tuna fish, peanut butter).

#### Housework

Encourage client to contract with an adolescent for light housekeeping.

Refer client to community agency for assistance.

#### Transportation

Determine availability of transportation for shopping and health care.

Suggest client request rides with neighbors to places they drive routinely.

### Impaired Cognitive Functioning

Assess client's ability to maintain a safe household.

Refer to *Risk for Injury* related to lack of awareness of hazards.

Initiate appropriate referrals.

### Impaired Emotional Functioning

Assess severity of the dysfunction.

Refer to *Ineffective Coping* for additional assessment and interventions.

**R:** In determining a client's ability to perform self-care at home, the nurse must assess his or her ability to function and protect self. The nurse considers motor and sensory deficits and mental status (Miller, 2009).

### Initiate Health Teaching and Referrals, as Indicated.

Refer to community-nursing agency for a home visit.

**R:** A home visit is essential to assess and evaluate what services are needed. Third-party payers will usually reimburse for this type of assessment visit.

Refer to community agencies (e.g., visitors, meal programs, homemakers, adult day care).

Refer to support groups (e.g., local Alzheimer's Association, American Cancer Society).

**R:** Discharge planning begins at admission, with the nurse determining anticipated needs after discharge: client's self-care ability, availability of support, homemaker services, equipment needs, community nursing services, therapy (physical, speech, occupational; Green, 1998).

**R:** The home environment must be assessed for safety before discharge: location of bathroom, access to water, cooking facilities, and environmental barriers (stairs, narrow doorways).

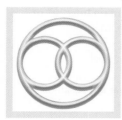

This section will focus on the use of nursing diagnoses in the community. This organization will allow for all nursing diagnoses with the client as the community to be grouped together for clarity.

This section will include all the NANDA-approved community diagnoses and other NANDA-approved diagnoses with community application. In Part One, there are many diagnoses that have an individual focus but would be useful in the community—for example, *Imbalanced Nutrition related to frequent intake of high-fat and salty foods as evidenced by reports of an average intake of fast foods of over 10 to 15 meals a week*. If a community is forced to relocate, the diagnosis *Anticipatory Grieving related to sale of apartment and forced relocation of tenants as manifested by anger, crying and fear* might apply.

Students can be introduced to community nursing with a focus on a small geographic population such as a neighborhood, assisted-living residents, or a group of women in a shelter. Students may also address some common-interest communities such as a senior citizen center, church community, or local chapter of Women against Rape.

## KEY CONCEPTS

1. "In community settings, there is a generally broader focus on both physical and mental health than on the disease per se and on the variables that affect health directly or indirectly, such as lifestyle, family interaction patterns and community resources (public transportation and adequate housing)" (Aroskar, 1979, p. 36).
2. Community health care differs from home health care:
   Community Health Care: Continuous
   • Targets populations
   • Focuses on groups that do not seek care
   • Emphasizes wellness and primary prevention
   Home Health Care: Episodic
   • Targets individuals, families
   • Focuses on individuals who seek care
   • Emphasizes restoring health after an acute episode
3. Community competence describes the healthy functioning of the total community unit. A competent community has four important characteristics (Cattrell, 1976; Allender & Spradley, 2006):
   • It collaborates effectively to identify community needs and problems.
   • It achieves a working consensus on goals and priorities.
   • It agrees on ways and means to implement the agreed-on goals.
   • It collaborates effectively in the required actions.
4. The essential conditions for community competence and health are (Cattrell, 1976; Allender & Spradley, 2006):
   • A high degree of awareness that "we are community"
   • Use of natural resources while taking steps to conserve them for future generations
   • Open recognition of subgroups and encouragement of their participation in community affairs
   • Readiness to meet crises
   • Problem solving: community identifies, analyzes, and organizes to meet its own needs

*(continued)*

■■■■■■ **KEY CONCEPTS** *Continued*

- Open channels of communication that allow information to flow among all subgroups of citizens in all directions
- Desire to make each resource available to all members of the community
- Legitimate and effective ways to settle disputes
- Encouragement of maximum citizen participation in decision making
- Promotion of high-level wellness among all its members

5. Community refers "to a collection of people who interact with one another and whose common interests or characteristics form a basis for a sense of unity or belonging" (Allender & Spradley, 2006, p. 6).

6. There are three types of communities (Allender & Spradley, 2006):
- Common-interest is a collection of people locally or widespread with a shared interest or goal.
- Geographic is defined as a group in a certain geographic boundary.
- Community of solution is a group of people who come together to address a problem that affects all of them.

7. Examples of each type of community:
Geographic Community
- City
- Town
- Neighborhood
- County, state
- Country, world
- Prison, jail

Common-Interest Community
- Church members
- Disabled individuals
- Pregnant teens
- Women Against Rape
- Mothers Against Drunk Driving (MADD)
- Nurse Practitioners

Community of Solutions
- County Water Department
- City Health Department
- Disaster team
- Environmental Protection Agency
- Ambulance service
- Health center

8. Communities have six common components (Clemen-Stone et al., 2002):
- *People:* People are the most important resource or core of the community. Functional, cohesive communities have shared values.
- *Goals/needs:* Goals and needs of individuals and groups in the community reflect the community goals and needs. As in Maslow's hierarchy, a community must have its needs of physiology, safety, and social affiliation fulfilled before meeting higher needs of esteem and self-actualization.
- *Community environment:* The environment (climate, natural resources, buildings, food, water supply, flora, animals, insects, economics, health and welfare services, leadership, social networks, recreation, and religion) has major effects on health.
- *Service systems:* These are a network of agencies and organizations in the community that help to meet the basic needs (social welfare, education, economic) and the health needs of the community.
- *Boundaries:* These define communities. Some boundaries are concrete, such as a geographic or political entity (e.g., cities, states) or a situation (e.g., home, school, work). Interests define conceptual boundaries (e.g., book clubs).

9. Healthy People 2010 focuses on nine leading health indicators that "reflect the major public heath concerns in the United States and were chosen based on their ability to motivate action, the availability of data to measure their progress, and their relevance as broad public health issues" (USDHHS PHS, 2000, p. 11). Refer to Box II.5 for a list of the nine Health Indicators.

*(continued)*

■ ■ ■ ■ ■ ■  **KEY CONCEPTS** *Continued*

10. Communities (local, state) can uses these ten health indicators to assess their current health status and to monitor it over time (Edelman & Mandell, 2006).

11. Rural communities have fewer than 2,500 residents. Rural people are more self-reliant and reluctant to seek assistance from others. Researchers have found that rural people "define health as the ability to work and to do what needs to be done" (Bushy, 1990, p. 89). They do not value comfort, cosmetic issues, and health promotion. They access health care services when they cannot work (Bushy, 1990).

12. Rural communities often resist outsiders' ideas and prefer health care providers who live in their community. Because people all know one another, however, they are reluctant to ask for help or share problems for fear their neighbors will find out (Bushy, 1990).

## Community Assessment (Allender & Spradley, 2006; Hunt & Rosenthal, 2000) _____

The community assessment can be utilized in its entirety or in segments if a focused assessment is desired. This assessment will direct the collection of data to determine the presence of effective functioning or ineffective functioning.

### Sources of Data

Individuals
Groups, sub-groups (e.g., adolescents, homeless, elders)
Maps
Chamber of Commerce
Public Library
Health planning boards
Farm labor boards
Social service programs
Health department (local, county health)
Local government
Educational programs
Web sites (www. followed by two-letter abbreviation for state, e.g., www.ca.gov)
World Health Organization (WHO)
National Institutes of Health (NIH)
U.S. Public Health Services
U.S. Bureau of Census

---

**BOX II.5  THE NINE LEADING HEALTH INDICATORS THAT REFLECT THE MAJOR PUBLIC HEALTH CONCERNS IN THE UNITED STATES**

Physical activity

Overweight and obesity

Tobacco use

Substance abuse

Responsible sexual behavior

Mental health

Injury and violence

Environmental quality

Immunizations

## Methods of Data Collection

- Windshield survey
- Community resident interviews
- Participant observations
- Descriptive epidemiologic studies
- Focus groups

### *Geographic*

1. Location
   - Neighborhood, city, county, state
2. Physical environment
   - Site of natural disaster (floods, earthquakes, volcano, hurricanes, tornadoes
3. Recreational opportunities
4. Climate
   - Heat or cold extremes
   - Rain or snow extremes
5. Flora and fauna
   - Poisonous plants, diseased animals, venomous animal, insects
6. Man-made environment
   - Housing, dams, water supply, chemical waste, air pollution
   - Industrial pollutants, air quality

### *Population Demographics*

1. Size
2. Density
   - High/low
3. Composition
   - Gender ratio
   - Age distribution
   - Ethnic origins
   - Race distributions
   - Other (e.g., married, single, gay)
4. Characteristics
   - Mobility
   - Socioeconomic status
   - Unemployment rates
   - Educational level
   - Types of employment
   - Migrants, transients (e.g., snow birds)

**DATA ANALYSIS QUESTIONS**
- What are the population size and age distributions?
- What is the distribution of gender, races, and marital status?
- What is the distribution of educational levels, occupations, and income?

# Functional Health Patterns (Edelman & Mandle, 2006; Allender & Spradley, 2006; Hunt & Rosenthal, 2000)

This section provides a comprehensive assessment of a community, using the Functional Health Patterns (Gordon, 1994). It is also designed to allow a focus assessment on only one functional health pattern, e.g., nutrition of a community. Data analysis questions follow each pattern for assistance in determining if there is effective functioning, a problem, or a risk for a problem.

## Health Perception–Health Maintenance Pattern

Mortality rates (age-related, maternal, and neonatal)
Ten leading causes of death

Morbidity rates of: Cancer, coronary hearth disease, alcoholism, substance abuse, communicable diseases
(TB, STDs, HIV)
Mental illness
Crime rates and types
Motor vehicle accidents, alcohol/drug related

## Environmental Hazards

Natural disasters, extreme climates, toxins, venomous insects, reptiles, animals, and poisonous plants

## Health Care Services

Hospital services, nursing homes, assisted living facilities, ambulatory services
Occupational school health, health department, community services, health centers, home services

## Protective Services

Police, fire, disaster response plan, ambulance services
Environmental protection services

## Support Available

Financial, food, housing, clothing, and counseling

**DATA
ANALYSIS
QUESTIONS**
- What are the major health problems?
- How has the community responded to the major health problems?
- Are they satisfied with the results?
- What health promotion programs are available? Affordable?
- What health services are believed to be needed?
- Is there a group (cultural, ethnic, poor, transients) whose health needs are not addressed?
- How do the unemployed and uninsured access health care?
- What is the incidence of alcohol/drug related crimes and accidents?
- What is the community's perception of safety?
- What are the climate hazards?
- How does the community reduce risks of injury in extreme weather?
- What are the flora and fauna hazards?
- How does the community reduce risks of injury?

## Nutritional–Metabolic Pattern

Access to food
Cost of food
Sources of food stores, markets, fast food, nutritional services (e.g., WIC, Meals on Wheels)
Incidence of malnourished, overweight or obesity
Water supply (source, testing results)

**DATA
ANALYSIS
QUESTIONS**
- How does the cost of food compare with other communities?
- How often is fast food consumed?
- Are there food programs for children, elderly, poor?
- What types of foods are in the school (cafeteria, vending machines)?

## Elimination Pattern

Sanitation (water supply, sewage disposal, trash and garbage disposal, rodent and vermin control)
Ecologic concerns (recycling, types of hazardous waste)

**DATA
ANALYSIS
QUESTIONS**
- Are hazardous wastes under control?
- Are dumps or disposables a risk to water contamination?
- Are the disaster plans current?
- What is the air pollution index?

## Activity–Exercise Pattern

Transportation (options, costs, access?)
Recreation facilities (types, costs, access?)
Frequency of walking, riding bikes, play areas (access, condition, safety)
Housing (availability, quality, cost)

**DATA
ANALYSIS
QUESTIONS**

- How adequate is the transportation system?
- Are recreation facilities used?
- Are there barriers to using these facilities (cost, access, handicap-friendly)?
- Are these safe play areas for children?
- Is housing adequate, safe, affordable?

## Cognitive–Perception Pattern

Educational levels
Process of community decisions
Decision-makers (community, business, faith-based)
Educational facilities (public, private, adult education, higher education, health education programs)—
quality, availability, cost
Communication (publications, radio and TV stations, informal network)

**DATA
ANALYSIS
QUESTIONS**

- How are the schools rated (county, state, national)?
- What is the dropout rate?
- What are the reasons for dropouts?
- Is adult education available?
- What educational programs are available for residents with English as a second language skills?
- Do health related agencies work together?

## Role–Relationship Pattern

Community sponsored events (faith-based, senior centers, parenting classes, children's activities)
Socioeconomic groups
Ethnic-racial groups
Communications methods (newspapers, flyers, bulletins, radio, TV)

**DATA
ANALYSIS
QUESTIONS**

- How is information communicated to the residents?
- Are there public meetings?
- Do residents interact with each other?
- Is there a friendly atmosphere?
- What are the roles of domestic violence, violence, child abuse, elder abuse?
- What is the divorce rate?

## Sleep–Rest Pattern

Noise sources (cars, airplanes, industrial)

**DATA
ANALYSIS
QUESTIONS**

- How is the noise level controlled?

## Coping–Stress Tolerance Pattern

Assistance Programs (local, faith-based, state, federal)
Crisis intervention programs (mental health services, crisis centers, telephone help lines)
History of unresolved conflict (racial, gangs)
Crimes (types, drug-related)

**DATA
ANALYSIS
QUESTIONS**

- Are assistance programs accessible for all residents?
- Is there a problem with prostitution or pornography?
- What are the crime statistics?

- Are residents satisfied with assistance programs?
- What is the community response to crisis? Anger? Indifference? Isolation? Helpless? Overwhelmed?
- What are the barriers to effective coping?

## Sexuality–Reproductive Pattern

Average size of family
Reproduction (birth rate, teen pregnancies, prenatal care, abortion facilities)
Birth control resources
Educational programs (sex education, childbirth education classes, parenting classes)

**DATA ANALYSIS QUESTIONS**
- Are family planning services available to all residents?
- Is there family counseling available and affordable?
- Is sex education supported in schools and community?

## Value–Belief Pattern

Community origins
Community traditions
Religions in community
Social programs

**DATA ANALYSIS QUESTIONS**
- What are the community's priorities?
- Do most residents feel they are valued in the community?
- Are all ethnic groups accepted?
- Are all religious groups accepted?

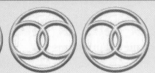

# READINESS FOR ENHANCED COMMUNITY COPING

## DEFINITION

A state in which a community's pattern for adaptation and problem solving is satisfactory for meeting the demands or needs of the community, but the community desires to improve management of current and future problems/stressors

## DEFINING CHARACTERISTIC

### Major (Must Be Present)

Successful coping with a previous crisis

### Minor (May Be Present)

Active planning by community for predicted stressors
Active problem solving by community when faced with issues
Agreement that community is responsible for stress management
Positive communication among community members
Positive communication between community/aggregates and large community
Programs available for recreation and relaxation
Resources sufficient for managing stressors

## RELATED FACTORS

Not applicable.

■■■■■■ **AUTHOR'S NOTE**

This diagnosis can be used to describe a community that wishes to improve an already effective pattern of coping. For a community to be able to be assisted to a higher level of functioning, its basic needs for food, shelter, safety, a clean environment, and a supportive network must first be addressed. When these needs are met, programs can focus on higher functioning, such as wellness and self-actualization. Community programs can be designed after a community assessment and because of community requests. They can focus on enhancing health promotion with topics related to optimal nutrition, weight control, regular exercise programs, constructive stress management, social support, role responsibilities, and preparing for and coping with life cycle events such as retirement, parenting, and pregnancy.

| **NOC** |
| :--- |
| Community Competence, Community Health Status, Community Risk Control |

## ➤ Goal

The community (specify type of community, e.g., the town of Mullica Hill, the southeast neighborhood of south Tucson) will provide programs to improve (specify type of focus, e.g., Nutrition).

### Indicators

- Identify health promotion needs as (specify: e.g., daily decrease in low-fat foods, increase in fruits and vegetables)
- Access resources needed (specify: e.g., local experts, nutritionist, college students)
- Develop programs (specify: health fair, school cafeteria, printed material) based on needs assessment

| **NIC** |
| :--- |
| Program Development, Risk Identification, Community Health Development, Environmental Risk Protection |

## ➤ Interventions

**Conduct Focus Groups to Discuss Programs to Assist Residents with Positive Coping with Developmental Tasks.**

Arrange focus groups according to age groups including diverse groups.

**R:** Focus groups assessments can increase community members' participation in community programs (Clark, Cary, & Diemert, 2003).

## Plan Programs Targeted for a Specific Population.

*Adolescents (13 to 18 years)*
Career planning          Stress management
*Young Adults (18 to 35 years)*
Career selection         Constructive relationships
Balancing one's life     Parenting issues
*Middle Age (35 to 65 years)*
Launching children       Reciprocal relationships
Aging parents            Quality leisure time
*Older Adults (65 years and older)*
Retirement issues        Balancing one's life       Anticipated losses
                         Facts and myths of aging

*All Ages*
Civic planning           Meeting needs of all community members
Crisis intervention      Grieving
                         Community involvement

**R:** Life cycle events are predictable developmental tasks of young adults, middle adults, and older adults. (Refer to Key Concepts for specifics.) Programs in the community can be planned to assist persons with adapting successfully to life cycle events (Clemen-Stone et al., 2002).

## Discuss Programs that Promote High-Level Wellness.

- Optimal nutrition
- Weight control

- Exercise programs
- Socialization programs
- Effective problem-solving
- Injury prevention
- Environmental quality

## Define the Target Health Promotion Needs.

Analyze assessment of community. Prioritize the needs:
Organize the focus of group responses
Probability of success
Cost-benefit ratio (e.g., resources available)

## Select a Health Promotion Program.

Identify target population (e.g., entire community, older adults, adolescents).
Delineate a timetable for the planning and implementation stages.

**R:** Focus groups can identify residents' assessment of health needs and promote their involvement in community programming (Clark, Cary, & Ciemart, 2003).

## Meet with Community Groups (Health Centers, Faith-Based Groups, Government Agencies) to Review Findings of Focus Groups and to Discuss Collaborative Programming.

**R:** Community building can develop new and existing leadership and strengthen community organizations and inter-organizational collaboration (McLeroy et al., 2003).

## Plan the Program.

- Develop detailed program objectives and the evaluation framework to be used.

| | |
|---|---|
| Content | Time needed |
| Ideal teaching method for targeting group | Teaching aids (e.g., large- print materials) |

- Establish resources needed and sources.

| | |
|---|---|
| Space | Transportation facilities |
| Optimal day of week | Optimal time of year |
| Supplies, audiovisual equipment | Financial (budgeted, donations) |

- Market the program.

| | |
|---|---|
| Media (e.g., newspaper, TV, radio) | Posters (food market, train station) |
| Flyers (distribute via school to home) | Word of mouth (religious organizations, community |
| Guest speaker (community clubs, schools) | clubs, schools) |

**R:** The community health nurse, as an advocate and community liaison, collaborates with other disciplines and agencies to match resources with community-identified needs for program success (Edelman & Mandle, 2006).

## Provide Program and Evaluate Whether Desired Results (Objectives) Were Achieved.

| | |
|---|---|
| Number of participants | Negative feedback |
| Objectives achieved | Actual expenditures vs. budgeted |
| Statistics (e.g., bicycle accidents) | Participant evaluations |
| Adequate planning | Revisions for future planning |
| | Shared responsibility |

**R:** Evaluation will determine if the program was completely effective, partly effective, or ineffective in achieving the program objectives (Edleman & Mandle, 2006).

Determine the strengths and limitations of the program and plan a new approach if indicated.

**R:** Community health-promotion programs must demonstrate effectiveness to earn continued community and economic support (Edelman & Mandle, 2006).

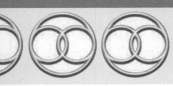

# INEFFECTIVE COMMUNITY COPING

## DEFINITION

The state in which a community's pattern of activities for adaptation and problem solving is unsatisfactory for meeting the demands or needs of the community

## DEFINING CHARACTERISTICS

### Major (Must Be Present)

Community does not meet its own expectations
Unresolved community conflicts
Expressed difficulty in meeting demands for change
Expressed vulnerability

### Minor (May Be Present)

| | | |
|---|---|---|
| Angry | Bitter | Indifferent |
| Apathetic | Helpless | Hopeless |
| Overwhelmed | | Violent Outbursts |

## RISK FACTORS

Presence of risk factors (see Related Factors)

## RELATED FACTORS

### Situational

*Related to lack of knowledge of resources*
*Related to inadequate communication patterns*
*Related to inadequate community cohesiveness*
*Related to inadequate problem solving*
*Related to inadequate community destruction secondary to:\**

| | |
|---|---|
| Flood | Hurricane |
| Earthquake | Epidemic |
| Avalanche | |

*Related to traumatic effects of:\**

| | |
|---|---|
| Airplane crash | Industrial disaster |
| Large fire | Environmental accident |

*Related to threat to community safety (e.g., murder, rape, kidnapping, robberies)\**
*Related to sudden rise in community unemployment*

### Maturational

*Related to inadequate resources for:*

| | |
|---|---|
| Children | Working parents |
| Adolescents | Older Adult |

---

\* These represent risk factors for *Risk for Ineffective Community Coping*. Refer to Author's Notes for additional clarification.

■■■■■■ **AUTHOR'S NOTE**

*Ineffective Community Coping* is a diagnosis of a community that does not have a constructive system in place to cope with events or changes that occur. The focus of interventions is to improve community dialogue, planning, and resource identification.

   When a community has experienced a natural disaster (e.g., hurricane, flood), a threat to safety (e.g., murder, violence, rape), or a man-made disaster (e.g., airplane crash, large fire), the focus should be on preventive strategies. The diagnosis *Risk for Ineffective Community Coping* is more appropriate when the community has been a victim of a disaster or a violent crime.

---

**NOC**
Community Competence, Community Health Status, Community Risk Control

➤ **Goal**

The community will engage in effective problem solving.

### Indicators

- Identify problem.
- Access information to improve coping.
- Use communication channels to access assistance.

---

**NIC**
Community Health Development, Environmental Risk Protection, Program Development, Risk Identification

➤ **General Interventions**

### Assess for Causative or Contributing Factors.

Refer to Related Factors.

### Provide Opportunities for Community Members (e.g., Schools, Churches, Synagogues, Town Hall) to Meet and Discuss the Situation.

Demonstrate acceptance of their anger, withdrawal, or denial.
Correct misinformation as needed.
Discourage blaming.

**R:** certain behaviors or beliefs (e.g., anxiety, fear, value conflicts) can interfere with problem solving. They should be explored in discussions (Clemen-Stone et al., 2002).

## Provide for Effective Communication (Allender & Spradley, 2006, p. 453).

Allow for and address questions.
Convey the facts.
Convey seriousness.
Be clear, simple and repetitive.
Present solutions and suggestions.
Address real and perceived needs.

**R:** In order for communication to effectively elicit action, it must be believable, current, clear, authoritative, and predictive of the probability of future events (Allender & Spradley, 2006).

## Promote Community Competence in Coping.

Focus on community goals, not individuals' goals.
Engage subgroups into group discussions and planning.
Ensure resource access for all members (e.g., flexible hours for working members).
Devise a method for formal disagreements.
Evaluate each decision's impact on all community members.

**R:** In order for a community to cope effectively, it must function collectively, not as individuals. (Allender & Spradley, 2006).

## Establish a Community Information Center at the Local Library to Access Information and Support, e.g., Telephone, On-line.

**R:** "The public library has the resources and expertise to address the need for prompt, reliable and relevant information in any conflict or crisis situation" (Will, 2001).

## Identify the Collaborative Resources that Can Be Accessed in the Health Department, Faith-Based Organization, Social Services, and Health Care Provider Agencies.

**R:** Inter-organizational collaboration draws upon each other's strengths and increases community participation (Zahner & Corrado, 2004).

## Use the Community Information Center (e.g., Local Library) to Inform Residents of Ongoing Activities and Progress.

**R:** Open channels of communication can reduce speculation, anger, and apathy (Allender & Spradley, 2006).

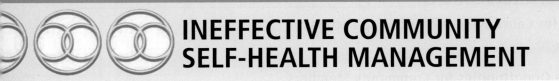

# INEFFECTIVE COMMUNITY SELF-HEALTH MANAGEMENT

## DEFINITION

Pattern in which the community experiences or is at risk to experience difficulty integrating a program for treatment of illness and the sequelae of illness and reduction of risk situations (e.g., safety, pollution)

## DEFINING CHARACTERISTICS

### Major (Must Be Present, One or More)

Verbalized difficulty in meeting health needs in communities
Acceleration (expected or unexpected) of illness(es)
Morbidity, mortality rates above norm

## RELATED FACTORS

### Situational (Environmental)

*Related to unavailability of community programs for (specify):*

| | | |
|---|---|---|
| Prevention of diseases | Screening for diseases | Immunizations |
| Dental care | Accident prevention | Fire safety |
| Smoking cessation | Substance abuse | Alcohol abuse |
| Child abuse | | |

*Related to problem accessing program secondary to:*

| | | |
|---|---|---|
| Inadequate communication | Limited hours | Lack of transportation |
| Insufficient funds | | |

*Related to complexity of population's needs*
*Related to lack of awareness of availability*
*Related to multiple needs of vulnerable groups (specify):*

| | | |
|---|---|---|
| Homeless | Pregnant teenagers | Below poverty level |
| Home-bound individuals | | |

*Related to unavailable or insufficient health care agencies*

■■■■■ **AUTHOR'S NOTE**

This diagnosis describes a community that is experiencing unsatisfactory management of its health problems. This diagnosis can also describe a community with evidence that a population is underserved because of lack of availability of, access to, or knowledge of health care resources. Community nurses, using the results of community assessments, can identify at-risk groups and overall community needs. In addition, they assess health systems, transportation, social services, and access.

**NOC**

Participation: Health Care Decisions, Risk Control, Risk Detection

➤ **Goals**

This community will:

- Identify needed community resources
- Promote the use of community resources for health problems

**NIC**

Decision-Making Support, Health System Guidance, Risk Identification, Community Health Development, Risk Identification

➤ **General Interventions**

## Using Health Department Data (Local, County, State, National), Identify Major Health Problems and Associated Risks, for Example:

- Obesity
- Heart disease
- Asthma
- Automobile accidents

**R:** These data will provide accurate statistics (Allender & Spradley, 2006).

## Organize Focus Groups to Assess Health Needs and Assets. Include Different Age Groups, Ethnic/Racial Groups, and Residents with Varied Lengths of Residence (Clarke et al., 2003).

Initiate discussion with (Clarke et al., 2003, p. 458):

- What is it like to live in this community?
- What could make life in this community better?
- What kinds of things could improve the health of people who live in this community?
- What could the health department do to improve the health of people who live in this community?
- What could you, or people you know, do to improve life in this community?

**R:** "Focus groups specifically targeted to all segments of the population proved to be an effective mechanism to elicit broad community input regarding health needs and assets" (Clark et al., 2003, p. 462).

## Meet with Community Groups (Health Centers, Faith-Based Groups, Government Agencies) to Review Findings of Focus Groups and to Discuss Collaborative Planning.

**R:** Community building can develop new and existing leadership and strengthen community organizations and inter-organizational collaboration (McLeroy et al., 2003).

## Organize Response Data.

Rank-order entire sample.

Group responses of selected groups (e.g., age, gender, income level, disabled).

**R:** The cost of health-related programs and limited resources makes priority identification imperative (Edelman & Mandle, 2006).

## Analyze the Findings.

### *What Overall Health Problems Are Reported?*

### *What Are the Health Concerns of:*

| | |
|---|---|
| Older population | Households with children up to 20 years of age |
| Single-parent households | Respondents younger than 45 years |
| People below poverty level | Uninsured |
| Adolescents | New immigrants |

**R:** Health care program planning provides an orderly structure for organizing large quantities of data to achieve community health goals successfully (Clemen-Stone et al., 2002).

## Evaluate Community Resources.

What resources are available for the health problems identified?
Are there utilization or access problems with the services?
How does the population learn about services?
Identify problems that do not have community services available.

**R:** Evaluation of resources available is needed to match activities planned and to determine if funding is needed for additional resources (Edelman & Mandle, 2006).

## If Services Are Unavailable, Pursue Program Development.

### *Examine and Evaluate Similar Programs in Other Communities.*

| | | |
|---|---|---|
| Basic information | Purpose, goals | Services available |
| Funding | Cost to participants | Accessibility of services |

## Meet with Appropriate People to Discuss Findings (Survey, On-Site Visits). Address the Following:

Presence of community support
Available expertise and technology in community
Financial support

## Identify Appropriate Community Sources of Assistance.

| | | |
|---|---|---|
| Hospital departments | Health departments | Faith-based organizations |
| Chamber of Commerce | Health care professionals | Industry |
| Private foundations | Public assistance agencies | Professional societies |

## Collaborate with University Faculty for Collaborative Grant Writing.

**R:** The financial support of health care programs can often come from private or public sources.

## Plan the Program (Refer to Readiness for Enhanced Community Coping for Interventions for Community Planning).

## If Services Are Available But Are Underutilized, Assess for (Bamberger et al., 2000):

### *System Barriers*

| | |
|---|---|
| Hours of operation (inconvenient) | Location of services (access, aesthetics, distance) |
| Efficiency and atmosphere | Cost |
| Complicated appointment system | Unfriendly |

### *Personal Barriers*

| | |
|---|---|
| Mistrust | Competing life priorities |
| Powerlessness | Illiteracy |

Lacking resources
(e.g., telephone, transportation, child care, finances)

Unpredictable work schedule
Non–English speaking

**R:** Unless the barriers to accessing health care services are identified and eliminated, these services will continue to be underused (Bamberger et al., 2000).

## Evaluate Vulnerable Population's Access to Health Care and Knowledge of Risk Factors.

Rural families, elderly
Homeless

Migrant workers
Those below poverty level

New immigrants

**R:** Access to care is a social justice issue (Allender & Spradley, 2006).

## Make a Priority of Ensuring that Basic Needs for Food, Shelter, Clothing, and Safety Are Met Before Attempting to Address Higher Health Needs.

**R:** Physiologic needs must be met before a person can focus on meeting higher needs for personal well-being and health-seeking behavior (Maslow, 1970).

## Provide Information Regarding Illness Prevention, Health Promotion, and Health Services to Vulnerable Populations (e.g., Federally-funded Community Health Centers).

Be sure reading material is appropriate for targeted group (e.g., reading level, language, pictures).
Use posters, flyers.
Select locations that the targeted populating uses regularly:

Grocery, convenience stores
Religious services
Meetings

Day care centers
Laundromat
Sporting events

School activities
Community fairs

**R:** Vulnerable populations (poor, uninsured, ethnic minorities) report no regular source of care, no ambulatory visits within the preceding 12 months, and fair or poor health status (USDHHS, 2000). They have higher premature death rates, high morbidities, low functional status, and low quality of life (Leight, 2003).

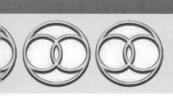

# CONTAMINATION: COMMUNITY

**Contamination: Community**

**Risk for Contamination: Community**

## DEFINITION

Exposure to environmental contaminants in doses sufficient to cause adverse health effects

## DEFINING CHARACTERISTICS

Clusters of patients seeking care for similar signs or symptoms
Signs and symptoms are dependent on the causative agent. Causative agents include pesticides, chemicals, biologics, waste, radiation, and pollution.
See *Contamination: Individual* for specific contaminant-related health effects.

Large numbers of patients with rapidly fatal illnesses

Sick, dying or dead animals or fish; absence of insects

Measurement of contaminants exceeding acceptable levels

# RELATED FACTORS

## Pathophysiologic

Presence of bacteria, viruses, toxins

## Treatment-Related

Insufficient or absent use of decontamination protocol

Inappropriate or no use of protective clothing

## Situational

Acts of bioterrorism; flooding, earthquakes, natural disasters

Sewer line leaks

Industrial plant emissions; intentional or accidental discharge of contaminants by industries or businesses

Physical factors: Climactic conditions such as temperature, wind; geographic area

Social factors: Crowding, sanitation, poverty, lack of access to health care

Biological factors: Presence of vectors (mosquitoes, ticks, rodents)

## Environmental Factors

Contamination of aquifers by septic tanks

Intentional/accidental contamination of food and water supply

Exposure to heavy metals or chemicals, atmospheric pollutants, radiation, bioterrorism, disaster; concomitant or previous exposures

## Maturational Factors

Community dynamics (participation, power and decision-making structure, collaborative efforts)

---

## ■■■■■■ KEY CONCEPTS

### Generic Considerations

- Bioterrorism is the intentional use of microorganisms or toxins derived from living organisms to cause death or disease in humans, animals, or plants on which we depend (Ashford et al., 2003).
- The time period between exposure and the onset of symptoms may vary from hours to weeks. Nurses need to be familiar with the most likely agents to be used and their consequences (Veenema, 2002).
- Children are often exposed to toxicants through the agricultural and home use of pesticides or the ingestion of pesticide residues on food or in water. Children are more vulnerable than adults to experiencing delayed effects. Some pesticides may interfere with the physiologic processes of the child, including the immune, respiratory, and neurologic systems (Children's Environmental Health Network, 2004).
- More than 70,000 individual industrial chemicals are registered with the Environmental Protection Agency (EPA) for commercial use, and an average of 2300 new chemicals are introduced each year. All humans are now exposed to synthetic pollutants in drinking water, air, and the food supply, as well as in consumer products and home pesticides.
- Indoor pesticide residues can persist for weeks after use leaving pregnant women at risk, especially in urban areas. In studies of pregnant women living in New York City, 70% to 80% tested positive for pesticide exposure during their pregnancy (Berkowitz et al., 2003).
- The Air Pollution and Respiratory Health Program tracks indoor and outdoor air quality and associated health effects. Of particular concern is the impact of wildfires, debris fires following natural disasters, carbon monoxide poisoning, and molds (www.cdc.gov/nceh/airpollution/about.htm).

*(continued)*

▪▪▪▪▪▪ **KEY CONCEPTS** *Continued*

- The World Health Organization (2005) ranks indoor air pollution as the eighth most important risk factor when considering the global burden of disease. In developing countries, it is the most lethal killer after malnutrition, unsafe sex, and lack of water and sanitation, and is responsible for 1.6 million deaths a year due to pneumonia, chronic respiratory disease, and lung cancer (www.who.int/mediacentre/factsheets/fs292/en/index/html).

- The amount and duration of radiation exposure affects the severity or type of health effect. Internal exposure occurs through ingestion of radioactive material (food/water contamination). External exposure occurs through direct contact with radioactive material. The primary health effect from chronic radiation exposure is cancer; however, additional effects include DNA mutations and teratogenic mutations. Acute health effects include burns and radiation poisoning. The symptoms of radiation poisoning vary with the level of exposure and include nausea, fatigue, changes in blood chemistries, hemorrhage, damage to the central nervous system, and eventual death. Children and fetuses are particularly susceptible to the effects of radiation exposure (EPA, 2004).

- Radon enters homes through soil and water. Radon gas decays into particles that are trapped in the lungs. The risk of radon-related lung cancer is particularly elevated for smokers. Although children have been reported to have greater risk than adults of certain types of cancer from radiation, there are currently no conclusive data on whether children are at greater risk than adults from radon exposure (EPA, 2004).

- Contamination of water and food occurs when microorganisms, bacteria, and viruses that live in soil and in the gastrointestinal tract of animals enter the water supply from the direct disposal of waste into streams or lakes or from run-off from wooded areas, pastures, septic tanks, and sewage plants into streams or groundwater. Contamination of drinking water source by sewage can occur from raw sewage overflow, septic tanks, leaking sewer lines, land application of sludge, and partially treated wastewater. Nitrates, metals, toxic materials, and salts may also contaminate water (http://extoxnet.orst.edu/faqs/safedrink.sewage.htm).

- Contamination events may occur as a result of accidents or intentional acts. Biological agents include bacteria, viruses, fungi, other microorganisms, and their associated toxins. They may adversely affect health in several ways ranging from mild, allergic reactions to serious medical conditions, even death. The organisms are widespread in the natural environment and are found in water, soil, plants, and animals (www.osha-slc.govSLTC/biological agents/index.html).

- Exposure to biological agents occurs through direct contact with a hazardous substance, liquid (droplets or aerosols), inhalation of vapors or aerosols, or ingestion. Routes of transmission of infectious agents are contact, droplet, airborne, common vehicle, and vector borne (U.S. Army Medical Research Institute of Infectious Diseases, 2004).

- The mode of transmission of the specific agents will determine the category of isolation precaution used (standard, airborne, droplet, and contact isolation) (Veenema, 2006).

- Isolation precautions are used to reduce and prevent the spread of contamination and to protect health care workers from being exposed (http://www.cdc.gov/ncidod/ dhap/gl_isolation_ptII.htm/).

- Hazardous waste is any waste (liquid, sludge, solid, or gas) that may pose a threat to human health or the environment due to its quantity or characteristics. Industrial and commercial plants and businesses (chemical, electroplating, auto manufacturers, lumber treating, dry cleaners, photo processing, petroleum refineries, and hospitals) generate hazardous waste. Households also produce hazardous waste (pesticides, cleaning agents, paint and solvents, fluorescent light bulbs) (http://dnr.mo./gov/env/hwp/index.html).

- Untreated sewage that ends up in recreational drinking water, in groundwater, and in basements after flooding adversely affects human health and the environment. Each year, swimming in water contaminated by sewage overflows causes 1.8 million to 3.5 million illnesses. Drinking contaminated water causes an additional 500,000 illnesses (www.nrdc.org.water/pollution/sewage.asp)

# Focus Assessment Criteria

## Subjective Data

### *Assess for Defining Characteristics.*

Clusters of community members reporting the following:

- Respiratory/cardiac: Difficulty breathing, cough, flu symptoms, irregular heart beat
- Gastrointestinal: stomach ache, diarrhea, cramping, nausea, vomiting
- Neurologic: muscle weaknesses, joint and muscle aches, visual changes
- Dermatologic: skin lesions, pustules, skin irritation, itching, blistering, burns
- Exposure to radiation
- Pregnancies resulting in birth defects
- Unusual liquids, sprays, or vapors at work or home
- Dead or dying animals in area
- Explosions or bombs
- Employment or home located near industrial, agricultural, or commercial businesses

## Objective Data

Clusters of community members with the following:

- Neurologic: Hallucinations, confusion, seizures, decreased level of consciousness, pupil changes, and blurred vision
- Pulmonary: Labored breathing, cyanosis
- Cardiac: Cardiac dysrhythmia, hypertension, hypotension,
- Integumentary: Skin lesions (rash, pustules, scabs), blisters, ulcerations, burns, erythema, dry or moist desquamation, jaundice
- Fever
- Cancers (thyroid, skin, leukemia)
- Birth defects
- Radiation sickness: Weakness, hair loss, changes in blood chemistries, hemorrhage, diminished organ function

### *Assess for Related Factors.*

Refer to Related Factors.

## Goal

Community utilizes health surveillance data system to monitor for contamination incidents.
Community will participate in mass casualty and disaster readiness drills.
Community will utilize disaster plan to evacuate and triage affected members.
Community exposure to contaminants will be minimized.
Community health effects associated with contamination will be minimized.

# General Interventions

## Monitor for Contamination Incidents Using Health Surveillance Data.

**R:** Early surveillance and detection are critical components of preparation for potential biological attacks (Veenema, 2006).

## Provide Accurate Information on Risks Involved, Preventive Measures, and Use of Antibiotics and Vaccines.

Encourage community members to talk to others about their fears.
Provide general supportive measures (food, water, shelter).

**R:** Interventions aimed at supporting coping help the community deal with feelings of fear, helplessness, and loss of control that are normal reactions in a crisis situation.

# Specific Interventions

## Prevention:

Identify community risk factors and develop programs to prevent disasters from occurring.

**Preparedness:**

Plan for communication, evacuation, rescue, and victim care.
Schedule mass casualty and disaster readiness drills.

**Response:**

Identify contaminants in the environment.
Educate community about the environmental contaminant.
Collaborate with other agencies (local health department, EMS, state and federal agencies).
Rescue, triage, stabilize, transport, and treat affected community members.

**Recovery:**

Act to repair, rebuild, or relocate; mental health services should assist in psychological recovery (adapted from Allender & Spradley, 2006).

**Decontamination Procedure:**

Primary decontamination of exposed personnel is agent specific.

- Remove contaminated clothing.
- Use copious amounts of water and soap or diluted (0.5%) sodium hypochlorite.

Secondary decontamination from clothing or equipment of those exposed—use proper physical protection.

**R:** Decontamination procedure prevents exposure of additional community members and health care workers.

Employ appropriate isolation precautions: universal, airborne, droplet, and contact isolation.

**R:** Precautions prevent cross-contamination by agent.

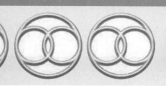

# RISK FOR CONTAMINATION: COMMUNITY

## DEFINITION

Community: Accentuated risk of exposure to environmental contaminants in doses sufficient to cause adverse health effects

## RISK FACTORS

See Related Factors under *Contamination: Community*

### ■■■■■■ KEY CONCEPTS

See Key Concepts under *Contamination: Community*

## Focus Assessment Criteria

### Assess for Related Factors.

Refer to Related Factors under *Contamination: Community*.

## Goal

Community utilizes health surveillance data system to monitor for contamination incidents.
Community will participate in mass casualty and disaster readiness drills.
Community will remain free of contamination-related health effects.

## General Interventions

### Monitor for Contamination Incidents Using Health Surveillance Data.

**R:** Early detection of environmental contamination will decrease the risk of actual contamination occurring.

### Provide Accurate Information on Risks Involved and Preventive Measures.

Encourage community members to talk to others about their fears.

**R:** Interventions aimed at supporting coping help the community deal with feelings of fear, helplessness, and loss of control that are normal reactions in a crisis situation.

## Specific Interventions

### Identify Community Risk Factors and Develop Programs to Prevent Disasters from Occurring.

Notify agencies authorized to protect the environment of contaminants in the area.
Modify the environment to minimize risk.

**R:** Modification of the environment will decrease the risk of actual contamination occurring.

## Part Four
# HEALTH PROMOTION/WELLNESS NURSING DIAGNOSES

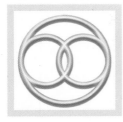

This section organizes all the Health Promotion/Wellness Diagnoses for individuals. All these diagnoses are organized under *Health-Seeking Behaviors*. *Health–Seeking Behaviors* is a broad nursing diagnosis that can be useful if a specific wellness diagnosis does not address the targeted health topic. Some of the diagnoses included in this section represent unhealthy lifestyles. They have been included with a health promotion focus e.g., Stress Overload, Sedentary Lifestyle.

Wellness nursing diagnoses are "a clinical judgment about an individual, group or community in transition from a specific level of wellness to a higher level of wellness" (NANDA, 2007, p. 10). A valid wellness nursing diagnosis has two requirements: (1) the person has a desire for increased wellness in a particular area and (2) the person is currently functioning effectively in a particular area.

Wellness nursing diagnoses are one-part statements with no related factors. The goals established by the person or group will direct their actions to enhance their health.

There is still confusion about the clinical usefulness of this type of diagnosis. This author takes the position that some of these diagnoses can be strengthened and are clinically useful, such as *Readiness for Enhanced Parenting* or *Readiness for Enhanced Community Coping*. The clinical usefulness of others, for example, *Readiness for Enhanced Power*, *Readiness for Enhanced Urinary Elimination*, and other similar diagnoses, is questionable. Under each diagnosis, Author's Notes will elaborate on the clinical usefulness of the diagnosis.

Clinically, data that represent strengths can be important for nurses to know. These strengths can assist the nurse in selecting interventions to reduce or prevent a problem in another health pattern. If nurses want to designate strength, it should be documented as strength on the assessment form or care plan. If the client desires assistance in promoting a higher level of function, *Readiness for Enhanced (specify)* would be useful in certain settings, e.g. schools, community centers, older-assisted living facilities. Interested clinicians can utilize these health-promotion/wellness diagnoses and are invited to share their work with NANDA and this author.

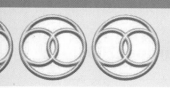

# HEALTH-SEEKING BEHAVIORS

## DEFINITION

Health-Seeking Behaviors: State in which a person in stable health actively seeks ways to alter personal health habits and/or the environment to move toward a higher level of wellness*

## DEFINING CHARACTERISTICS

### Major (Must Be Present)

Expressed or observed desire to seek information for health promotion.

### Minor (May Be Present)

Expressed of observed desire for increased control of health.
Expression of concern about current environmental conditions on health status.
Stated or observed unfamiliarity with wellness community resources.
Demonstrated or observed lack of knowledge of health-promotion behaviors.

### ▪▪▪▪▪ AUTHOR'S NOTE

This diagnosis can be used to focus on a personal or lifestyle change in a specific area that is effective and can be enhanced. If the specific wellness diagnoses do not target the specific area of wellness, this diagnosis can be used—for example, *Health-Seeking Behaviors: Cross-Training Exercise Program*.

### ▪▪▪▪▪ KEY CONCEPTS

- Healthy People 2010 has two major goals (2000):
- Increase quality and years of healthy life
- Eliminate health disparities

*(continued)*

---

*Stable health status is defined as the following: age-appropriate illness prevention measures are achieved; client reports good or excellent health; and signs and symptoms of disease, if present, are controlled.

■■■■■■ **KEY CONCEPTS** *Continued*

- Health promotion addresses strategies to assist people to live at the highest level of well-being as possible (Edelman & Mandle, 2006).
- All persons can be assisted to a healthier lifestyle if motivated and informed. If the person has deficits in his or her lifestyle, other nursing diagnoses apply, such as *Risk Prone Health Behavior* or *Imbalanced Nutrition*.
- Some individuals regularly engage in healthy choices. These individuals may desire to increase the strength of these choices to be even healthier in one or more areas, such as decision-making or nutrition.
- The nurse is an advocate for healthier lifestyles and personal behavior. This person does not need to be motivated; instead, the nurse will direct him or her to sources of information and strategies to increase wellness in the desired area.
- The nurse must be careful not to judge the overall health practices of the individual as barriers to increase wellness in a specific area. For example, a woman may smoke and also consume a very balanced low-fat, low-CHO diet; if she desires, she could improve her already nutritious diet. Her smoking habit can be addressed under *Risk Prone Health Behavior*.

## Health Promotion/Wellness Assessment (Carpenito-Moyet, 2007; Gordon, 2003; Edelman & Mande, 2006)

### Subjective Data

#### Health Perception–Health Management Pattern

Ask the person to place a check in front of a category that they observe regularly; place two checks if they are perfect in the category (Breslow, 2004):

- Three meals a day at regular times and no snacking
- Breakfast every day
- Moderate exercise two or three times a week
- 7 to 8 hours of sleep, not more or less
- No smoking
- Moderate weight
- No alcohol or in moderation

#### What Is the Person/Family's Perception of Their Overall Health?

- What personal practices maintain their health?
- What sources does the person or family access to maintain or improve their healthy lifestyle?

#### Nutrition–Metabolic Pattern

- What is the person's body mass index (BMI)?
- Typical daily fluid intake
- Supplements (vitamins, types of snacks)
- Daily intake of whole grain or enriched breads, cereals, rice or pasta.
- Two pieces of fruit daily
- Unlimited raw, non-starch vegetables daily
- Skim or low-fat dairy products
- Meats and poultry trimmed of fat and skin
- No fried foods/snacks
- Do you see a relationship among stress and tension, emotional upsets, and your diet or eating habits?

#### Elimination Pattern

- Bowel elimination pattern? (Describe)
  - Frequency, character
- Urinary elimination? (Describe)
  - Character (amber, yellow, straw-colored)

## Activity–Exercise Pattern

- Exercise pattern? Type, frequency
- Leisure activities? Frequency
- Energy level? (High, moderate, adequate, low)
- Are there barriers to exercising?
- What are five things that you do to play?
- What things do you do that make you feel good?

## Sleep–Rest Pattern

- Satisfied and rested?
  - Average hours of sleep per night
  - Relaxation periods? How often, how long.

## Cognitive–Perceptual Pattern

Satisfied with:

- Decision-making?
- Memory?
- Ability to learn?

Describe briefly your educational background.

## Self-Perception–Self-Concept Pattern

Describe how you feel about:

- Yourself
- Your body? Changes?

Do you have trouble expressing anger, sadness, happiness, love, and/or sexuality?
What are your major strengths or personal qualities?
What are your weaknesses or negative aspects?
In your life right now, what is your most meaningful activity?
How many more years do you expect to live, and how do you think you will die?
How do you imagine your future?
What would you like to accomplish in your future? Are there changes you need to make to accomplish this?

# List the Most Important Events, Crises, Transitions, and/ or Changes (Positive or Negative) in Your Life.

Take time to reflect on how they affected you. Place an asterisk in front of one or two that were especially important.

## Roles–Relationships Pattern

- Satisfied with job? Need a change?
- Satisfied with role responsibilities?
- Describe your relationship with your family/partner.
- Describe your friendships (close, casual).
- List the most important people in your life right now and why they are important.

## Sexuality–Reproductive Pattern

- Is sex an important aspect of your life?
- Are you currently in a sexual relationship?
- What would you want to change about your current sexual relationship?

## Coping–Stress Tolerance Pattern

- List the most regular sources of stress in your life. How could you make them less stressful?
- How do you usually respond to stressful situations? (get angry, withdraw, take it out on others, get sick, drink, eat?)

- What situations make you feel calm or relaxed?
- What situations make you feel anxious or upset? What can you do to make yourself feel better?

### Values–Beliefs Pattern

- Write ten things you most value in life.
- Would you describe yourself as a religious or spiritual person?
- How do your beliefs help you?

| NOC |
|---|
| Adherence Behavior, Health Beliefs, Health Promoting Behaviors, Well-Being |

## ➤ Generic Goals

The person will express a desire to move from wellness to a higher level of wellness in (specify), for example, nutrition, decision-making.

### Indicators

Identify two new strategies (specify) to enhance well-being.

| NIC |
|---|
| Health Education, Risk Identification, Values Classification, Behavior Modification, Coping Enhancement, Knowledge: Health Resources |

## ➤ Generic Interventions

The following interventions are appropriate for any health promotion/wellness nursing diagnosis that focuses on lifestyle changes and choices, for example, *Readiness for Enhanced Nutrition*, *Parenting*, *Sleep*, *Breastfeeding*, *Family Coping* and *Family Processes*. These areas of wellness and health promotion can be found readily in the self-help literature and on the Internet. Some of the interventions for the wellness diagnoses, such as *Readiness for Enhanced Grieving*, *Readiness for Enhanced Coping* or *Readiness for Enhanced Decision-Making* can be found in Section Two, Part One under the individual nursing diagnoses. For example, in *Decisional Conflict* there are interventions that can promote better decision-making even for someone already making good decisions.

### Complete Assessment of One or More or All Functional Health Patterns as the Individual Desires.

**R:** This structured assessment provides the individual with an opportunity to focus on segments of their health behavior and/or lifestyle to judge their satisfaction or desire for enhancement.

### Renew Data with Person or Group.

- Does the person/group report good or excellent health?
- Does the person desire to learn a behavior to maximize health in a specific pattern?

**R:** Every day clients decide what they're going to eat, whether they will exercise, and other lifestyle choices (Bodenheimer, MacGregor, & Sharifi, 2005).

### Encourage the Person/Group to Select Only One Wellness Focus at a Time

**R:** Addressing multiple behavioral changes at one time is time consuming, which may discourage the change (Bodenheimer, MacGregor, & Sharifi, 2005).

### Refer to Educational Resources on a Particular Focus (Printed, Web Sites). Examples of Generic Data-bases/Web Sites Include:

- www.seekwellness.com/wellness/
- www.cdc.gov/—Centers for Disease Central and Prevention
- www.agingblueprint.org—focuses on aging well
- www.nhlbi.nih.gov—US Department of Health and Human Services
- www.ahrq.gov—US Preventive Services Task Force
- www.health.gov—various health topics
- www.nih.gov—National Institutes of Health
- www.fda.gov—Food and Drug Administration
- www.mbmi.org—Mind-Body Medical Institute
- www.ahha.org—American Holistic Health Association

**R:** Self-management tools for autonomous or highly motivated individuals are assistive technologies such as smart treadmills, online education and support groups, and self-help books that are utilized independently (Barrett, 2005).

## Advise the Person to Contact the Nurse to Discuss the Outcome of Resource Review via Telephone or e-Mail.

**R:** Motivated, autonomous clients can be supported via the telephone or e-mail, which is efficient and cost-effective for them (Piette, 2005).

## Discuss the Strategies or Targeted Behavior Changes. Have the Person Record Realistic Goals and Time Frames that Are Highly Specific:

- For example, Goal—I will reduce my daily intake of CHO.
- Indicators—Reduce cookie intake from five to two each day.
- Change pasta to multigrain pasta.
- Reduce potato intake by 50% and replace the 50% with root vegetables.

**R:** In order to increase self-efficacy, the person must be successful. Success is more predictable if goals and indicators are concrete and achievable (Bodenheimer, MacGregor, & Sharifi, 2005).

## Ask the Person If You Can Contact Him or Her at Designated Intervals (Every Month, at 4 to 6 Months, at 1 Year); Call or E-Mail Person to Discuss Progress.

**R:** All types of clients, motivated or not, can benefit from support from their health care professional.

## Advise the Person that This Process Can Be Repeated as They Desire in Other Functional Health Patterns.

**R:** Enhanced wellness can be a continuous, lifelong journey with the client as navigator and the health care professional as the travel agent.

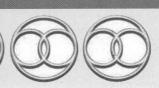

# INEFFECTIVE HEALTH MAINTENANCE

Ineffective Health Maintenance

Related to Insufficient Knowledge of Effects of Tobacco Use and Self-Help Resources Available
Related to Increased Food Consumption in Response to Stressors and Insufficient Energy
 Expenditure for Intake

## DEFINITION

State in which a person or group experiences or is at risk of experiencing a disruption in health because of an unhealthy lifestyle or lack of knowledge to manage a condition

## DEFINING CHARACTERISTICS (IN THE ABSENCE OF DISEASE)

### Major (Must Be Present, One or More)

**Reports or demonstrates an unhealthy practice or lifestyle, such as:**

| | | |
|---|---|---|
| Reckless driving | Excessive sun exposure | Inadequate dental care |
| High-fat diet | Substance abuse | Inadequate hygiene |
| Overeating | Sedentary lifestyle | Inadequate oral hygiene |

## Minor (May Be Present)

**Reports or demonstrates:**

*Skin and nails*

| | |
|---|---|
| Malodorous | Skin lesions (pustules, rashes, dry or scaly skin) |
| Unexplained scars | Unusual color, pallor |
| Sunburn | |

*Respiratory system*

| | | |
|---|---|---|
| Frequent infections | Dyspnea with exertion | Chronic cough |

*Oral cavity*

Frequent sores (on tongue, buccal mucosa)
Loss of teeth at early age
Lesions associated with lack of oral care or substance abuse (leukoplakia, fistulas)

*Gastrointestinal system and nutrition*

| | | |
|---|---|---|
| Obesity | Chronic bowel irregularity | Chronic anemia |
| Chronic dyspepsia | Anorexia | Cachexia |

*Musculoskeletal system*

Frequent muscle strain, backaches, neck pain
Diminished flexibility and muscle strength

*Genitourinary system*

Frequent sexually transmitted infections
Frequent use of potentially unhealthful over-the-counter products (e.g., chemical douches, perfumed vaginal products, nasal sprays)

*Constitutional*

| | | |
|---|---|---|
| Chronic fatigue | Headaches | Apathy |

*Psychoemotional*

Emotional fragility
Frequent feelings of being overwhelmed

# RELATED FACTORS

Various factors can produce *Ineffective Health Maintenance*. Common causes are listed next.

## Situational (Personal, Environmental)

**Related to:**

| | |
|---|---|
| Information misinterpretation | Lack of access to adequate health care services |
| Lack of motivation | Inadequate health teaching |
| Lack of education or readiness | Impaired ability to understand secondary to: (specify) |

## Maturational

Table II.20 lists age-related conditions.
**Related to lack of education of age-related risk factors. Examples include the following:**

### Child

| | | |
|---|---|---|
| Sexuality and sexual development | Inactivity | Poor nutrition |
| | Substance abuse | Safety hazards |

### Adolescent

| | | |
|---|---|---|
| Same as children practices | Substance abuse | Vehicle safety |

### Adult

| | | |
|---|---|---|
| Parenthood | Safety practices | Sexual function |

### Older Adult

| | |
|---|---|
| Effects of aging | Sensory deficits |

## TABLE II.20  PRIMARY AND SECONDARY PREVENTION FOR AGE-RELATED CONDITIONS

| Developmental Level | Primary Prevention | Secondary Prevention |
|---|---|---|
| Infancy (0–1 year) | Parent education<br>  Infant safety<br>  Nutrition<br>  Breast feeding<br>Sensory stimulation<br>  Infant massage and touch<br>  Visual stimulation<br>    Activity<br>    Colors<br>  Auditory stimulation<br>    Verbal<br>    Music<br>Immunizations<br>  DPT or DTaP<br>  IPV, Hib<br>  Hepatitis B<br>Rotavirus<br>  Pneumococcal<br>Meningococcal<br>  Influenza<br>Oral hygiene<br>  Teething biscuits<br>  Fluoride (if needed > 6 months)<br>  Avoid sugared food and drink | Complete physical examination every<br>2–3 months<br>Screening at birth<br>  Congenital hip dysplasia<br>  PKU<br>  G-6-PD deficiency in blacks, Mediterranean, and Far<br>  Eastern origin children<br>  Sickle cell<br>  Hemoglobin or hematocrit (for anemia)<br>  Cystic fibrosis<br>  Vision (startle reflex)<br>  Hearing (response to and localization of sounds)<br>TB test at 12 months<br>Developmental assessments<br>Screen and intervene for high risk<br>  Low birth weight<br>  Maternal substance abuse during pregnancy<br>    Alcohol: fetal alcohol syndrome<br>    Cigarettes: SIDS<br>    Drugs: addicted neonate, AIDS<br>  Maternal infections during pregnancy |
| Preschool (1–5 years) | Parent education<br>  Teething<br>  Discipline<br>  Nutrition<br>  Accident prevention<br>  Normal growth and development<br>Child education<br>  Dental self-care<br>  Dressing<br>  Bathing with assistance<br>  Feeding self-care<br>Immunizations<br>  DTaP<br>  IPV<br>  MMR<br>  HIB<br>  *H. influenzae*<br>  Varicella<br>  Hepatitis A (high risk)<br>  Pneumococcal<br>  Hepatitis B<br>Dental/oral hygiene<br>  Fluoride treatments<br>  Fluoridated water | Complete physical examination between 2 and 3 years and<br>  preschool (UA, CBC)<br>TB test at 3 years<br>Development assessments (annual)<br>  Speech development<br>  Hearing<br>  Vision<br>Screen and intervene<br>  Lead poisoning<br>  Developmental lag<br>  Neglect or abuse<br>  Strong family history of arteriosclerotic diseases (e.g., MI, CVA,<br>  peripheral vascular disease), diabetes, hypertension, gout, or<br>  hyperlipidemia—fasting serum cholesterol at age 2 years, then<br>  every 3–5 years if normal<br>  Strabismus<br>  Hearing deficit<br>  Vision deficit |
| School age (6–11 years) | Health education of child<br>  "Basic 4" nutrition<br>  Accident prevention<br>  Outdoor safety<br>  Substance abuse counsel<br>  Anticipatory guidance for physical changes at<br>  puberty<br>Immunizations<br>  Tetanus age 11–12<br>  MMR<br>  DtaP  boosters between<br>  TOPV  4 and 6 years<br>  Pneumococcal (high risk) | Complete physical examination<br>TB test every 3 years (at ages 6 and 9)<br>Developmental assessments<br>  Language<br>  Vision: Snellen charts at school<br>    6–8 years, use "E" chart<br>    Over 8 years, use alphabet chart<br>  Hearing: audiogram<br>Cholesterol profile, if high risk, every 3–5 years<br>Serum cholesterol one time (not high risk) |

*(continued)*

**TABLE II.20 PRIMARY AND SECONDARY PREVENTION FOR AGE-RELATED CONDITIONS (Continued)**

| Developmental Level | Primary Prevention | Secondary Prevention |
|---|---|---|
| | Varicella (at age 11–12 if no history of infection)<br>Gardisil (HPV) series of three for girls, may begin at 9 years old<br>Dental hygiene every 6–12 months<br>   Continue fluoridation<br>Complete physical examination | |
| Adolescence (12–19 years) | Health education<br>  Proper nutrition and healthful diets<br>  Sex education<br>    Choices<br>    Risks<br>    Precautions<br>    Sexually transmitted diseases<br>  Safe driving skills<br>  Adult challenges<br>    Seeking employment and career choices<br>    Dating and marriage<br>    Confrontation with substance abuse<br>  Safety in athletics, water<br>  Skin care<br>Dental hygiene every 6–12 months<br>Immunizations<br>  Hepatitis B, Hepatitis A series if needed<br>  TOPV booster at 12–14 years<br>  Gardisil (HPV) (series of three for girls ages 11–26) | Complete physical exam yearly<br>  Blood pressure<br>  Cholesterol profile<br>  PPD test at 12 years and yearly if high risk<br>  RPR, CBC, U/A<br>  Female: breast self-exam (BSE)<br>  Male: testicular self-exam (TSE)<br>  Female, Pap and pelvic exam yearly after 3 years of onset of sexual activity or at age 21<br>urine gonorrhea and chlamydia tests with yearly PE's<br>screening and interventions if high risk<br>  Depression<br>  Suicide<br>  Substance abuse<br>  Pregnancy<br>Family history of alcoholism or domestic violence<br>Sexually Transmitted Infections |
| Young adult (20–39 years) | Health education<br>  Weight management with good nutrition as BMR changes<br>  Low-cholesterol diet<br>Lifestyle counseling<br>  Stress management skills<br>  Safe driving<br>  Family planning<br>  Divorce<br>  Sexual practices<br>  Parenting skills<br>  Regular exercise<br>  Environmental health choices<br>  Alcohol, drug use<br>  Use of hearing protection devices<br>Dental hygiene every 6–12 months<br>Immunizations<br>  Tetanus (Td or Tdap. at 20 years and every 10 years<br>  Female: rubella, if serum negative for antibodies<br>  Hepatitis B for high-risk people | Complete physical exam at about 20 years, then every 5–6 years<br>Female: BSE monthly, Pap 1–2 years unless high risk<br>Male: TSE monthly<br>Parents-to-be: high-risk screening for Down syndrome, Tay-Sachs<br>Female pregnant: RPR, rubella titer, Rh factor, amniocentesis for women 35 years or older (if desired)<br>All females: baseline mammography between ages 35 and 40<br>If high risk, Female with previous breast cancer: annual mammography at 35 years and yearly after, a female with mother or sister who has had breast cancer, same as above<br>Family history colorectal cancer or high risk: annual stool guaiac, digital rectal, and colonoscopy at intervals determined after baseline colonoscopy.<br>PPD if high risk<br>Glaucoma screening at 35 years and along with routine physical exams<br>Cholesterol profile every 5 years, if normal<br>Cholesterol profile every 1 year if borderline |
| Middle-aged adult (40–59 years) | Health education: continue with young adult<br>Midlife changes, male and female counseling (see also Young adult)<br>  "Empty nest syndrome"<br>  Anticipatory guidance for retirement<br>  Grandparenting<br>Dental hygiene every 6–12 months<br>Immunizations<br>  Tetanus (Td, Tdap) every 10 years<br>  Influenza—annual if high risk (i.e., major chronic disease [COPD, CAD])<br>  Pneumococcal—every 5–6 years | Complete physical exam every 5–6 years with complete laboratory evaluation (serum/urine tests, x-ray, ECG)<br>Dexascan (screening for high risk men and women for osteoporosis) once then as needed<br>Female: BSE monthly<br>Male: TSE monthly<br>PSA yearly after age 40 for Blacks and Hispanics and after age 50 for others<br>All females: mammogram every 1–2 years (40–49 years) then annual mammography 50 years and over<br>Schiotz's tonometry (glaucoma) every 3–5 years<br>Colonoscopy at 50 and 51, then at intervals determined after baseline colonoscopy.<br>Stool guaiac annually at 50 and yearly after |

*(continued)*

## TABLE II.20  PRIMARY AND SECONDARY PREVENTION FOR AGE-RELATED CONDITIONS (Continued)

| Developmental Level | Primary Prevention | Secondary Prevention |
|---|---|---|
| Older adult (60–74 years) | Health education: continue with previous counseling<br>  Home safety<br>  Retirement<br>  Loss of spouse, relatives, friends<br>  Special health needs<br>    Nutritional changes<br>    Changes in hearing or vision<br>  Dental/oral hygiene every 6–12 months<br>Immunizations<br>  Tetanus every 10 years<br>  Influenza—annual<br>  Pneumococcal—every 5–6 years<br>Zoster | Complete physical exam every 2 years with laboratory assessments<br>Blood pressure annually<br>Female: BSE monthly, Pap every 1–3 years annual mammogram<br>Male: TSE monthly, PSA yearly<br>Annual stool guaiac<br>Colonoscopy (interval determined by baseline results)<br>Complete eye exam yearly<br>Dexascan once and as needed<br>Screen for high risk<br>  Depression<br>  Suicide<br>  Alcohol/drug abuse<br>  "Elder abuse" |
| Old-age adult (75 years and over) | Health education: continue counseling<br>Anticipatory guidance<br>  Dying and death<br>  Loss of spouse, relatives, friends<br>  Increasing dependency on others<br>Dental/oral hygiene every 6–12 months<br>Immunizations<br>  Tetanus every 10 years<br>  Influenza—annual<br>  Pneumococcal—if not already received | Complete physical exam annually<br>Female: annual mammogram, colonoscopy (interval determined by baseline results)<br>Schiotz's tonometry every 3–5 years |

## AUTHOR'S NOTE

The nursing diagnosis *Ineffective Health Maintenance* applies to both well and ill populations. Health is a dynamic, ever-changing state defined by the individual based on his or her perception of highest level of functioning (e.g., a marathon runner's definition of health will differ from a paraplegic person's). Because clients are responsible for their own health, *Ineffective Health Maintenance* represents a diagnosis that the person is motivated to treat. An important associated nursing responsibility involves raising client consciousness that better health is possible.

This diagnosis is appropriate for a person expressing a desire to change an unhealthy lifestyle. Examples are excessive dissatisfaction with occupation; lack of exercise; failure to be refreshed after rest; diet high in fat, salt, simple carbohydrates; tobacco use; obesity; excessive alcohol use; and insufficient social support.

The nursing diagnosis *Risk for Ineffective Health Maintenance* is useful to describe a person who needs teaching or referrals before discharge from an acute care center to prevent problems with health maintenance after discharge or in community settings.

*Health-Seeking Behaviors* is used to describe a person or group desiring health teaching related to the promotion and maintenance of high-level wellness (e.g., preventive behavior, age-related screening, optimal nutrition) or, according to NANDA, "seeking ways to alter personal health habits in order to move to a higher level of health." In most cases, this diagnosis describes an asymptomatic person. It also can be used in cases of chronic disease to help that person attain higher wellness in a particular area. Different from good health, high-level wellness is defined as an integrated method of functioning oriented toward maximizing potential). For example, a woman with multiple sclerosis and many physical problems could learn breast self-examination or relaxation exercises using *Health-Seeking Behaviors: Breast self-examination*.

*Health-Seeking Behaviors* is best written as a one-part diagnostic statement with the sought-after health practice specified (e.g., *Health-Seeking Behaviors: Breast self-examination*). Using "related to" is unnecessary; it is understood that all people with Health-Seeking Behaviors are motivated to achieve a higher level of health. Related factors could not represent causative or contributing factors, unless the nurse wants to repeat the same factors for each client (e.g., *Health-Seeking Behaviors: Breast self-examination related to desire to maximize health*).

As focus shifts from an illness/treatment-oriented to a health-oriented health care system, *Ineffective Health Maintenance* and *Health-Seeking Behaviors* are becoming increasingly significant. The increasingly high acuity and shortened lengths of stay in hospitals require nurses to be creative in addressing health promotion (e.g., by using printed materials, television instruction, and community-based programs).

# ■■■■■ ERRORS IN DIAGNOSTIC STATEMENTS

1. *Ineffective Health Maintenance related to refusal to quit smoking*

   Refusal to quit smoking represents significant data that require further clarification. Is the person making an informed decision? Does the person know the effects of smoking on respiratory and cardiovascular functioning? Does the person know where to acquire assistance to stop smoking? If the answers are "yes," then *Ineffective Health Maintenance* is incorrect. On the other hand, if the person is not fully aware of the deleterious effects of smoking or the availability of self-help resources, *Ineffective Health Maintenance related to insufficient knowledge of effects of tobacco use and self-help resources available* may be appropriate.

   *Note:* The nurse should be cautioned about timing attempts to encourage a person to quit smoking or control eating after an acute episode, such as myocardial infarction. In such a situation, denying the person his or her usual coping mechanism, no matter how unhealthy, may be more problematic to overall health. The nurse should emphasize teaching so the person can make informed choices, not merely prohibit certain choices.

2. *Health-Seeking Behaviors related to increased alcohol and tobacco use in response to marital break-up and heavy family demands*

   This diagnosis is inappropriate for this person, who wants to alter personal habits but is not in good or excellent health. A more appropriate focus would be to promote constructive stress management without tobacco or alcohol through the nursing diagnosis *Ineffective Coping related to inability to constructively manage the stressors associated with marital break-up and family demands*.

# ■■■■■ KEY CONCEPTS

## Generic Considerations

- Many people view health as the absence of disease. Rather, health can be viewed as a return (or recovery) to a previous state or to a heightened awareness of full potential and life meaning.
- Control of major health problems in the United States depends directly on modification of individual behavior and habits of living.
  - The U.S. poverty line is $18,850 for a family of four (US Bureau of Census, 2004). The overall poverty rate is 13 %, about 40 million people with 38% being children under 5. (Ibid)
  - In addition to addressing lifestyles to promote wellness, total health depends on (Edelman & Mandle, 2006):
  - Eradication of poverty and ignorance
  - Availability of jobs
  - Adequate housing, transportation, and recreation
  - Public safety
  - Aesthetically pleasing and beneficial environment
- The goals of prevention are as follows:
  - Avoidance of disease through healthy lifestyles
  - Decreased mortality from disease through early detection and intervention
  - Improved quality of life
- The three levels of prevention are primary, secondary, and tertiary.
- *Primary prevention* involves actions that prevent disease and accidents and promote well-being. Key concepts are as follows:

| Concept | Examples |
|---|---|
| Wellness | Diet low in salt, sugar, and fat |
| A lifestyle that incorporates the principles of health promotion and is directed by self- | Regular exercise and stress management; elimination of smoking; minimal alcohol intake responsibility |
| Self-help | |
| Mutual sharing with others who have similar needs | La Leche League; childbirth education; assertiveness training; specific written resources (books, pamphlets, magazines); public media |
| Safety | Adherence to speed limits; use of seat belts and car seats; proper storage of household poisons |
| Immunizations | *Children:* Hepatitis B series |
| | *Nonpregnant women of childbearing age:* rubella if antibody titer is negative |
| | *Elderly:* influenza, pneumonia |

*(continued)*

■■■■■■ **KEY CONCEPTS** *Continued*

- *Secondary prevention* concerns actions that promote early detection of disease and subsequent intervention: regular examination by a health professional and self-examination.
- Tasks of screening are to
  - Identify major disabling conditions.
  - Investigate personal and social benefits of early detection and intervention for asymptomatic people with the condition (e.g., facilitate family coping, minimize disability and cost, prevent premature death, improve productivity, decrease overall morbidity and mortality).
  - Identify those at high risk for specific conditions through *personal health history* (e.g., concurrent disease such as diabetes mellitus means higher risk for hypertension), *family health history* (e.g., breast cancer, diabetes, hypertension), and *social history* (e.g., substance abuse—cancer, heart disease; sexual patterns—venereal disease; domestic violence—person abuse).
  - Identify tests and procedures that accurately detect the condition (Who will do them? How often are they done? Who bears the cost?).
  - Plan a strategy for disseminating screening information to health care professionals and the public.
  - Plan evaluation of screening effectiveness.
- Types of screening include the following:
  - Physical findings (periodic examinations by health care professionals and self-examinations of breasts, testicles, and skin)
  - Survey of risk factors (smoking, alcohol abuse)
  - Laboratory tests (serum—e.g., sickle cell in African-Americans, phenylketonuria in newborns; urine—e.g., renal disease in older adults; x-ray—e.g., dental caries, chest tuberculosis)
- *Tertiary prevention* involves actions that restore and rehabilitate and prevent complications in cases of illness. Examples for a person with coronary artery disease would be:
  - Restorative (surgery, such as coronary artery bypass, angioplasty, and medications)
  - Rehabilitative (stress management, exercise program, stop smoking)
- Potential barriers to prevention are found both in the health care system and in clients. The system may be
  - Disease oriented rather than health oriented
  - Composed of health care professionals who have learned to focus on fragmented systems of the human body rather than on a holistic approach
  - Functioning in a financial system that rewards treatment, not prevention, of illness
  - Difficult to reach or previously shown to be unsatisfactory
- Clients may:
  - Believe that outside forces (fate, luck) determine health/illness (external locus of control)
  - Perceive the needed behavior as unacceptable or uncomfortable
  - Practice unhealthy sociocultural behaviors (e.g., obesity considered desirable, salt prevalent in diet)
  - Experience psychological impediments to practicing healthy behaviors
  - Lack financial resources

## Health Promotion Behaviors

- A person is motivated to pursue health promotion behaviors if (Pender, Murdaugh, & Parsons, 2006):
  - The change is desired and has value
  - The change will produce positive results
  - It is likely that they will be successful
- Several factors influence motivation (Pender et al., 2006):
  - Previous experiences.
  - Past is a predictor for future behavior.
  - Perceived benefits of action
  - Perceived barriers e.g. discomfort, expense, time, dexterity,
  - Perceived health status
  - Cognitive impairments
  - Problems with mobility, dexterity, strength, agility

- "Self-management support is the assistance caregivers give clients with chronic diseases in order to encourage daily decision that improve health related behaviors and clinical outcomes" (Bodenheimer, MacGregor, & Sharifi, 2005, p. 4).
- Clients are helped to choose health behaviors in a collaborative partnership with the caregivers (Bodenheimer et al., 2005).
- Refer to Ineffective Self-Health Management for key concepts on health education, self-efficacy, and barriers to learning.
- Motivational interviewing is a readiness to change model in which readiness = importance × confidence. Techniques are used to assess readiness to change (importance and confidence) and to encourage clients to increase their readiness (Rollnik, Mason, & Butler, 2000).

## Literacy

Health literacy is "the degree to which individuals have that capacity to obtain, process and understand basic health information and services needed to make appropriate health decisions" (Cutilli, 2005).

- Those with the highest incidence of low literacy:
- Are poor
- Live in the South and West
- Do not have a high school diploma
- Are members of an ethnic/cultural minority over 65
- Have physical/mental disabilities
- Are homeless or inmates

## Stress

Refer to Anxiety and Ineffective Coping for specific information on anxiety and ineffective coping.

- Stress is always present in all persons. Stress is the physical, psychological, social, or spiritual effect of life's pressures and events (Edelman & Mandle, 2006).
- Stress is an interactive process in response to the loss or threat of loss of homeostasis or well-being (Cahill, 2002).
- Stress is a psychological, emotional state experienced by an individual in response to a specific stressor or demand that results in harm, either temporary or permanent, to the person (Ridner, 2004, p. 539).
- Excessive stress requires recognition, perception and adaptation (Cadhill, 2001).
- A chronic state of stress or repeated episodes of psychological stress (depression, anger, hostility, anxiety) can lead to cardiovascular disease, arteriosclerosis, headaches, and gastrointestinal disorders (Edelman & Mandle, 2006).
- In response to stress, individuals initiate or increase unhealthy behaviors such as overeating, sedentary lifestyle, excessive use of drugs or alcohol, smoking, and social isolation (USDHHS, 2000).

## Nutrition

See Key Concepts for *Imbalanced Nutrition*.

## Exercise

- Regular exercise can increase
- Cardiovascular–respiratory endurance          Delivery of nutrients to tissue
- Muscle strength          Tolerance for psychological stress
- Muscle endurance          Ability to reduce body fat content
- Flexibility
- Vigorous exercise sessions should include a warm-up phase (10 min at a slow pace), endurance exercises, and a cool-down phase (5 to 10 min of a slow pace and stretching).
- Current beliefs regarding optimal exercise are as follows:
  - Emphasize physical activity over "exercise."
  - Moderate physical activity is very beneficial.
  - Intermittent physical activity that accumulates to 30 or more min is beneficial.
- To enhance long-term exercise, the person should (Moore & Charvat, 2002):
  - Respond to relapses with a plan to prevent recurrences.

- Set realistic goals.
- Keep an exercise log.
- Exercise with a friend.

## Weight Reduction

- Overeating is a complex problem with physical, social, and psychological components.
- Eighty percent of children of two obese parents will become obese, as opposed to 40% with one obese parent and 7% with no obese parent (Buiten & Metzger, 2000).
- Body mass index (BMI) is a ratio of weight and height that estimates total body fat (Dudek, 2006). According to the third National Health and Nutrition Examination Survey (NHANES III), 54.9 million Americans 20 years and older are overweight (BMI 25 to 29.9) or obese (BMI >30; Dudek, 2006).
- An excess of 50 to 100 calories each day will cause a 5- to 10-lb gain in 1 year (Dudek, 2006).
- Fluctuations in body weight are common, especially in women. Daily weights can be misleading and disheartening. Body measurements are a better gauge of losses.
- Regular exercise causes lean muscle mass to increase. Because muscle weighs more than fat, the scale may reflect a weight gain.
- Restrictive diets usually do not last and fail to establish healthy eating patterns. A better approach is modifying existing eating habits (Wiereng & Oldham, 2002).

## Tobacco Use

- "Tobacco use is the leading preventable cause of disease and premature death in the US" (MMWR 11/2008, p. 1). It has been proven that tobacco use causes the following cancers: lung, bronchial, larygeal, oral cavity, pharyngeal, esophageal, stomach, pancreatic, kidney, urinary bladder, cervical and acute myelogenous leukemia. (Ibid)
- Cigarette smoke causes more than 4000 chemicals, 250 of which are toxic, to be absorbed in the blood and swallowed into the gastrointestinal (GI) tract to act directly in the oral cavity and respiratory system (Andrews, 1998; Mayo Clinic, 2009).
- In the US, 22.3% of men and 17.4% of women smoke. In America Indian / Alaska Natives, the rate for smokers is 36.4% (CDC, 2008).

The effects of smoking or second-hand smoke on women are:

- Women smoking during reproductive age are at risk for difficulty conceiving, infertility, spontaneous abortion, premature rupture of membranes, low birth weight, neonatal mortality, stillbirth Preterm delivery and sudden infant death syndrome (SIDS) (MMWR 8/2008).
- Women who smoke are at risk for early menopause, decreased bone density, and osteoporosis (Miller, 2009).
- Smoking has immediate and long-term effects on the cardiovascular system. *Immediate effects* are vasoconstriction and decreased oxygenation of the blood, elevated blood pressure, increased heart rate and possible dysrhythmias, and increased work of the heart. *Long-term effects* are an increased risk for coronary artery disease, stroke, hyperlipidemia, and myocardial infarction. Smoking also contributes to hypertension, peripheral vascular disease (e.g., leg ulcers), and chronically abnormal arterial blood gases (low oxygen, or $Po_2$, and high carbon dioxide, or $Pco_2$).
- Use of smokeless tobacco (snuff, chewing tobacco) is associated with yellow teeth, gum recession, cavities, oral leukoplakia (premalignant lesions), oral cancer, pancreatic cancer, stroke and cardiovascular disease, higher cholesterol levels, gastric ulcers, heart disease and nicotine addiction. At least 12 million Americans are at risk, mostly male teens and male adults (National Cancer Institute, 2009).
- Nicotine is the primary addicting substance in tobacco smoke and juice. Clients with tobacco addiction need special assistance with short-term withdrawal and long-term maintenance of a tobacco-free life.
- *Passive smoking or secondhand smoke* is the inhalation of tobacco smoke by nonsmokers. Secondhand smoke contains formaldehyde, arsenic, cadmium, benzene, ammonia, carbon monoxide, methanol, hydrogen cyanide and polonium. Secondhand smoke has been shown to have negative health effects (Andrews, 1998; Pletsch, 2002; Mayo Clinic, 2009):
  - People with angina experience more discomfort in a smoke-filled room.
  - Bronchospasm increases when a person with asthma is exposed to tobacco smoke.
  - Children living with smoking parents have more upper respiratory, ear infections and dental caries than those living with nonsmokers.

- Passive smoking causes lung cancer, asthma, and bronchitis in nonsmokers.
- Pregnant women exposed to secondhand smoke have lower birth weight infants
- Sudden infant death syndrome is two to four times more common in infants whose mothers smoked during pregnancy.

## Osteoporosis

- Osteoporosis is classified as primary (associated with age- and menopause-related changes) or secondary (caused by medications or diseases; Miller, 2009).
- Age-related changes beginning around age 40 years decrease cortical bone by 3% per decade in men and women. Lifetime bone loss is 35% (women) and 23% (men) of cortical bone and 50% (women) and 33% (men) of trabecular bone (Miller, 2009).
- Osteoporosis is classified as primary (associated with age- and menopause-related changes) or secondary (caused by medications or diseases; Miller, 2009).
- Contributing factors to osteoporosis include loss of female hormones after menopause; hypogonadism; low calcium or vitamin D intake; insufficient exercise; small stature; fair skin; family history; cigarette smoking; excessive consumption of alcohol, caffeine, or protein; excessive use of aluminum-type antacids; long-term use of corticosteroids; therapy for chronic illness (bowel, kidney, liver); excessive thyroid replacement; excessive thyroid function (Hansen & Vondracek, 2004).

## Pediatric Considerations

- Anticipatory health promotion, or *anticipatory guidance*, is essential to comprehensive health care. It varies in content with a child's age and involves teaching families what is likely in upcoming weeks or months.
- Health maintenance begins with the prenatal visit and continues with comprehensive health supervision during the child's development
- The child depends on a parent/adult caregiver to provide a safe environment and promote health (e.g., immunizations, well check-ups, chronic disease management;
- Risk of ineffective health maintenance varies with a child's age and health status. For example, the toddler is at risk for accidental poisoning, whereas the adolescent is more likely to engage in high-risk behavior
- Malnutrition, lack of immunizations, or an unsafe environment may be related to deficient parental knowledge, impaired parenting, or barriers to health care (Hockenberry & Wilson, 2009).
- Many factors can influence a child's nutritional needs, including periods of rapid growth, stress, illness, metabolic errors, medications, and socioeconomic factors (e.g., inadequate income, poor housing, lack of food).
- By conservative estimates, more than one million youths run away from home each year. Alienated youth are frequently outside the health care system and tend to remain there unless efforts are made to identify and develop acceptable health services for them. The adoption of destructive lifestyles by many of these youths contributes heavily to physical and psychological morbidity and to alarmingly high mortality.
- Obesity and overweight rates in children have increased from 1988-1994 to 2003-2004 as follows (National Center for Health Statisitics, 2006):
  - Ages 2-5 years old from 7.2 to 13.9%.
  - Ages 6-11 years old from 11 to 19%
  - Ages 12-19 years old from 11to 17%
- Good weight management for children and adolescents focuses on weight maintenance or a slow weight loss, nutrient and energy needs, hunger prevention, preservation of lean body mass, and increased physical activity and growth.
- In a study of children who were clearly obese (> 90th percentile for weight and height), Myers and Vargas (2000) found that 35% of Hispanic parents did not perceive their child as obese. Eighteen percent of staff at the health center did not perceive the children as obese.
- About 3000 people younger than 18 years start smoking each day. About 75% of adolescents who smoke want to quit (DuRant & Smith, 1999).
- Nearly all long-term smokers begin before age 19 (CDC, 2004).
- More than 33% of high school students (more than 3 million) smoke cigarettes; almost 10% (more than 1 million) use smokeless tobacco (DuRant & Smith, 1999).

## Maternal Considerations

- Women smoking during reproductive age are at risk for difficulty conceiving, infertility, spontaneous abortion, premature rupture of membranes, low birth weight, neonatal mortality, stillbirth, preterm delivery and SIDS (CDC, 2008).

## Geriatric Considerations

- According to Miller (2009), health is the ability of older adults to function at their highest capacity, despite age-related changes and risk factors. Of all age-related changes, osteoporosis is most likely to have serious negative functional consequences, even without additional risk factors.
- About 70% of people older than 65 years rate their health as excellent (Miller, 2009).
- Differentiating between age-related changes and risk factors that affect the functioning of older people is important. Such risk factors as inadequate nutrition, fluid intake, exercise, and socialization can have more influence on functioning than can most age-related changes.
- Older adults have decreased sweating, shivering, peripheral circulation, subcutaneous tissue and inefficient vasconstriction. These age-related changes diminished ability to adapt to adverse temperatures and increase their risk of hypothermia and hyperthermia. This can also affect thermoregulation during and tolerance of physical activity (Miller, 2009).
- Regular exercise has been shown to correlate positively with increased self-esteem. Adult learning principles support encouraging exercise or regular activity that has meaning to the older person if compliance is expected. e.g. stretching exercises, walking.

## Transcultural Considerations

- Health and illness are culturally prescribed. One culture may view an obese person as strong and healthy, whereas another culture views that same person as weak and unhealthy. Nurses must remember that treatment strategies consistent with a person's cultural beliefs may have a better chance of success (Andrews & Boyle, 2008).
- A future orientation to illness, disease, and health care is necessary for prevention. The dominant US culture is oriented to the future, whereas other cultures have a present-oriented perception (e.g., African American, Hispanic, Southern Appalachian, traditional Chinese). Some members of these cultures, however, are future oriented.
- Some cultures believe that fate depends on God or other supernatural forces. Humans are at the mercy of these forces despite their behavior (Andrews & Boyle, 2008).
- Some Asian cultures believe in balance and harmony for health. They emphasize moderation and avoid excesses. In the *yin/yang theory*, the yin force in the universe represents female aspects of nature: cold and darkness. The yang force represents male aspects of nature: fullness, light, and warmth. An imbalance of yin and yang creates illness.
- In Hispanic and black cultures, health is maintained by the *hot/cold humoral theory*. This ancient Greek concept describes four body humors: yellow bile, black bile, phlegm, and blood. When these humors are balanced, health is present. Treatment of illness consists of restoring humoral balance by adding or deleting substances (e.g., foods, beverages, herbs, drugs) that are either hot or cold. For example, an earache is classified as cold and thus needs hot substances for treatment (Andrews & Boyle, 2008).
- Because the family is usually the client's most important social unit, the nurse can promote their help to support lifestyle changes (Andrews & Boyle, 2008).
- Blacks, Hispanics, and Asians in the United States smoke more than whites and have higher death rates from cancer. More emphasis on creating culturally based cessation programs and materials is needed (Koepke, Flay, & Johnson, 1990; CDC, 2006).
- Among Puerto Rican women, weight gain after marriage is considered positive, signifying that the husband is a good provider and that the wife is a good cook (Keller & Stevens, 1996).

# Focus Assessment Criteria

## Subjective Data

### *Assess for Defining Characteristics.*

**Health Status**
*Client's Description of Health*
*Immediate Health Concerns*
*Frequency of*

| | | |
|---|---|---|
| Bowel irregularity | Respiratory infections | Influenza |
| Urinary tract infections | Headaches | Fatigue |
| Mouth lesions | Skin rashes | Feeling overwhelmed |

### *Assess for Related Factors.*

**Influencing Factors: Health Management and Adherence Behavior**
What factors make it difficult to follow health advice?
What daily health management activities are practiced?
How much control does the person believe he or she has?

**Risk Factors**
*Family incidence of*

| | | |
|---|---|---|
| Cardiovascular disease | Abuse or violence | Hypertension |
| Drug or alcohol abuse | Cancer | Overweight/Obesity |
| Diabetes mellitus | Depression | Other (specify) |

*Health Habits*
Smoking (how much)
Alcohol
Drug use (prescribed, over-the-counter)
Dietary consumption of fat/salt/sugar, carbohydrates, protein; frequency and amount of portions
Exercise program

**Environmental Risk Factors**
Do you use seat belts or child restraints?
Is home child-proofed? (If appropriate, determine measures taken.)
Could any factors in the home or at work cause falls or accidents?
Could any other factors potentially threaten your health or cause injury?

**Preventive Health Screening Activities**
Self-examinations (breasts, testicles, blood pressure): indicate frequency and perceived problems
Last professional examination (dental, pelvic, rectal, vision, hearing, complete physical)
Last laboratory or other diagnostic testing (electrocardiogram, complete blood count, cholesterol, occult blood, Pap, chest x-ray, prostate-specific antigen [PSA])

## Objective Data

### *Assess for Defining Characteristics.*

General appearance   Weight   Height

For more information on Focus Assessment Criteria, visit http://thepoint.lww.com.

## ➤ Goal

The person or caregiver will verbalize intent to engage in health maintenance behaviors.

### *Indicators*

Identify barriers to health maintenance.

## ➤ General Interventions

### Assess for Barriers to Health Maintenance.

Refer to Related Factors.

### Explain Primary and Secondary Prevention Measures for Age (see Table II.21).

**R:** Many injuries, physical or mental disorders, or health-threatening situations can be prevented or decreased by immunizations, health education, safety programs, and healthy lifestyles or detected early with screening and treated promptly. (Murray, Zentner, & Yakimo,2009).

### Identify Strategies to Improve Access for the Vulnerable Populations (e.g., Uninsured, Displaced, Homeless, Poor).

- Community Centers, School-Based Clinics, Planned parenthood, faith-based clinics
- Pharmaceutical Companies Assistance Programs, generic alternative medications

**R:** Low-income families usually focus on meeting basic needs (food, shelter, and safety) and seeking help with curing illness, not preventing it. The cost of medications and office visits, hours of operations, and transportation are barriers for the poor.

### Assist Client and Family to Identify Behaviors that are Detrimental to Their Health.

- Tobacco use (Refer to Ineffective Health Maintenance)
- High fat, high carbohydrate, high calorie diets (Refer to Imbalance Nutrition)
- Sedentary life styles (Refer to Sedentary Lifestyle)
- Inadequate immunizations(refer to Ineffective Health Maintenance)
- Excessive Stress (Refer to Stress Overload)

**R:** Providing information and resources can help foster a sense that change is possible.

## ▶ Related to Insufficient Knowledge of Effects of Tobacco Use and Self-Help Resources Available*

- Identify benefits of abstinence from tobacco use.
- Verbalize commitment to personal health and desire to eliminate tobacco use.†
- Devise strategies to assist in smoking/chewing cessation.†

**NIC**
See *Ineffective Health Maintenance*

## ➤ Interventions

### Define Tobacco Use Behavior.

#### *Type and Quantity*

*Cigarettes*
Filter/nonfilter
Regular/reduced tar and nicotine
Pack-years

*Cigars*
Inhaled/not inhaled
Number/day, number of years

*Pipe*
Inhaled/not inhaled
Number of bowls/day

*Smokeless tobacco (chewing)*
Number of minutes/day
Number of years

#### *Associated Activities, Motivation, Previous Quitting Attempts (Leon, 2002)*

- When do you smoke first cigarette of the day?
- What triggers you to want a cigarette?
- What happens if you can't smoke for a few hours?
- When you are sick, do you still smoke?
- When did you last try to stop smoking, and what motivated you?
- Have you had any successes, and for how long?
- What were your three toughest obstacles to quitting, and what could we do about them?
- What made you start again?
- What is your present motivation for quitting?
- What method(s) do you think would be best for you to try now?
- Who or what has helped you when you tried to stop in the past?

**R:** Information that increases confidence in success may precipitate a decision to cease smoking (Andrews, 1998).

### Promote Understanding of Personal Tobacco Use Behavior.

#### *Identify Negative Aspects of Tobacco Use with Client.*

*Physical:* exercise intolerance, cough, sputum, frequent respiratory infections, dental disease, increased risk of diseases, premature facial wrinkling, bad breath

*Environmental:* burned clothing/furniture, discolored interiors of home/workplace, malodorous clothing/furniture, dirty ashtrays, house and occupational fires

---

*This nursing diagnosis can be used in two different situations – for the person who does not know the hazards of tobacco use and for the person who desires to quit.

†These outcome criteria are established only *if* the client desires to quit tobacco use. For the client who does not wish to change tobacco use behaviors, provide information regarding health risks and benefits so he or she makes an *informed* choice. Avoid being judgmental. Always "keep the door open" should the client later change his or her mind.

*Social:* inability to smoke in public places; offensive nature of tobacco use behaviors to family members, friends, coworkers

*Financial:* calculate monetary cost of client's habit with client

*Psychological:* unpleasant withdrawal symptoms when tobacco is not available (e.g., midnight "nicotine fits"), decreased self-esteem from dependency

## Identify Positive Aspects of Tobacco Use with Client (Use Client's Own Words). Have Person List All Reasons Why He or She Wants to Quit.

**R:** To assist a person to initiate a health behavior change, the nurse provides information to increase perceptions of the seriousness of the behavior and susceptibility to disease if behavior continues (Andrews, 1998; Murray, Zewntner, & Yakimo, 2009).

## Provide Information on Health Risks.

### Address Health Risks of Tobacco Use to Self. Refer to Key Concepts.

### Address Health Risks of Tobacco Use to Others. Refer to Key Concepts.

### Discuss the Benefits of Quitting.

| | | |
|---|---|---|
| Decreased pulse and blood pressure | Improved taste/smell | Lower risk of cancer, stroke, COPD, myocardial infarction |
| Decreased sputum production | | |
| Pulmonary mucosa regenerates | Improved dental hygiene | Increased social acceptance |
| | Improved circulation | Fewer respiratory infections |

**R:** To assist a person to initiate a health behavior change, the nurse provides information to increase perceptions of the seriousness of the behavior and susceptibility to disease if behavior continues (Andrews, 1998; Murray, Zewntner, & Yakimo, 2009).

## Explore Strategies Available to Quit.

Individual methods: self-help books and tapes, "cold turkey"

Group methods: contact local chapters of American Cancer Society, American Lung Association, and state-funded hotlines

Hypnosis, Acupuncture

Over-the-counter products: filters, tablet regimens, nontobacco cigarettes, nicotine-containing chewing gum

Prescription medications varenicline (Chantix), bupropian (Wellbutrin, Zyban), antidepressants

Transdermal nicotine patch: stress the hazards of smoking with patch

**R:** The best quit-smoking programs are those that combine multiple strategies (Stead & Perea, 2006).

## Discuss Strategies to Minimize Weight Gain and to Increase Exercise. Refer to Sedentary Lifestyle.

## Discuss Symptoms of Nicotine Withdrawal; Assist Client to Prepare for Them (Stead & Perea, 2008).

| | | |
|---|---|---|
| Craving for tobacco | Irritability | Tension |
| Difficulty concentrating | Restlessness | Headaches |
| Drowsiness | Increased Appetitie | Trouble Sleeping |

Advise:

To choose a time to quit of relatively low stress.

The severity of symptoms are related to duration of smoking and how many cigarettes smoked.

These symptoms occur whether the persons stops suddenly or cuts back.

Nicotine withdrawal usually takes 2-4 weeks.

**R:** Review of options available can enhance autonomy and decision-making.

## Plan with Client Strategies for Quitting.

### *Prepare to Stop.*

List all reasons for wanting to quit.

### *Determine When Smoking Is Most Desirable (e.g., Upon Awaking, After a Meal). Continue to Smoke but Delay Smoking for ½ to One Hour.*

Choose a quit date after 4 weeks of changing smoking patterns.
Enlist someone for support.
Reduce caffeine intake.
Throw away all tobacco, lighters, and ashtrays.
Clean car, clothes, and house of smell of smoke.
Have teeth cleaned.
Avoid tempting situations (e.g., alcohol use).
Put money saved from not smoking in a fund for your use only. Treat yourself with it.

### *Avoid Urges to Smoke.*

Spend more time with nonsmokers.
Engage in activities that cannot include smoking (e.g., exercising).
Keep low-calorie oral substitutes handy (e.g., gum, fruit).
Use a relaxation technique such as deep breathing.

### *Engage in the Following If Relapse Occurs.*

Stop smoking immediately.
Get rid of cigarettes.
Realize that relapse is common before successful quitting.
Learn from mistakes.
Set a new date.

**R:** Assessment of previous attempts to quit provides insight; which can increase motivation and success. Specific strategies can increase motivation

Pediatric Interventions

**Assess If Adolescent Knows Someone Who Smokes (Peers, Relatives).**
Use an open-ended, nonjudgmental approach (e.g., "What do you think about smoking?").

**Relate Short-Term Rather Than Long-Term Consequences of Smoking (e.g., Early Wrinkling of Skin, Yellow Stains on Teeth and Fingers, Tobacco Odor on Breath and Clothing, Gum Disease, Tooth Staining).**

**Emphasize Ostracization of Smokers (e.g., Standing Outside Buildings in the Cold to Smoke).**
**R:** Teenagers are very preoccupied with appearance and peer acceptance. The incidence of use of smokeless tobacco has increased in school-aged children, many of whom see it as less of a health hazard than smoking cigarettes

**Discuss Hazards of Smokeless Tobacco (Cancer of Mouth and Tongue, Tooth Erosion and Loss, Foul Breath, Gum Disease, Tooth Staining, Heart Disease).**

**Advise that Smokeless Tobacco in Your Mouth for 30 Minutes Is the Same as Smoking Three Cigarettes.**
**R:** Smokeless tobacco is not harmless and can cause serious health problems (National Cancer Institute (2006).

**Assist Adolescent Not to Start Smoking (DuRant & Smith, 1999).**
Counteract advertising images.
Practice assertive behavior.
Discuss smoking myths.

*(continued)*

**Pediatric
Interventions**
*Continued*

Address health consequences of tobacco use.

Most smokers would like to quit. Advise them to ask smokers if they would like to quit

**R:** Helping teens to appreciate that most smokers would like to quit may deter them from starting
(Hockenberry and Wilson, 2009).

**Maternal
Interventions**

### Explain the Adverse Effects of Smoking (Mitchell et al., 1999; CDC, 2006).
### During Pregnancy

- Crosses the placenta
- Reduces oxygen to the fetus
- Reduces transport of nutrients, calcium, glucose, hormones
- Causes low birth weight
- Causes stillbirths, congenital deformities

### In Infants and Children

- Contributes to allergies, otitis media, bronchitis, asthma, and sudden infant death syndrome

### If Desired, Establish a Plan to Decrease Number of Cigarettes Smoked per Day and, if Possible, Set a Date for Total Cessation.

### Approach Relapses as Temporary Setbacks.

### Identify Situations that Lead to Smoking.

**R:** Adverse effects are proportional to daily cigarettes smoked; thus, any decrease is beneficial.

## ▶ Related to Increased Food Consumption in Response to Stressors and Insufficient Energy Expenditure for Intake

**NOC**

Refer to *Ineffective Health Maintenance*

### ➤ Goal

The person will commit to a weight-loss program.

### *Indicators*

- Identify patterns of eating associated with consumption/energy expenditure imbalance.
- Identify stressors and effective response patterns.
- Describe the relationship among metabolism, intake, and exercise.
- Commit to exercise program (specify type, amount).
- Commit to reduced caloric intake program (adults only).
- Commit to eating a balanced diet.

**NIC**

Refer also to *Ineffective Health Maintenance,* Weight Reduction Assistance, Counseling, Mutual Goal Setting, Referral, Support Group

### ➤ Interventions

### Assess for Causative and Contributing Factors.

Lack of knowledge about
    Balanced nutritional intake
    Exercise requirements
Inappropriate response to external stressors
Lack of initiative, motivation
Imbalanced composition of foods (e.g., excess fat or simple carbohydrate intake)
Cultural, familial, genetic factors

Poor eating habits (e.g., eating out, eating on the run, skipping meals)
Sedentary lifestyle or occupation
Recent smoking cessation
Sabotage by family or significant others
Too much intake for energy expended

**R:** Identification of contributing factors can help plan specific strategies

## Increase Awareness of Components of Intake/Activity Balance.

Multiply female weight by 11 and male weight by 12 to determine calorie intake/day needed to maintain current weight. One pound of fat is roughly equivalent to 3500 cal. To lose 2 lb/week, a person must cut 7000 cal from weekly intake or increase exercise caloric expenditure.
Use exercise caloric expenditure charts to determine amount of calories burned per duration of activity.
Teach client that he or she may achieve weight-loss goals by combining reduction of caloric intake with energy expenditure (exercise).
Remind client that successful weight reduction/maintenance depends on a balance of reduced caloric intake and caloric expenditure through exercise.

**R:** Intake must be reduced to 500 cal/day less than requirement to obtain a 1 lb/week weight loss. To maintain ideal body weight, food consumed must equal physical activity daily (Roberts, 2000). Dieting without exercise decreases resting metabolic rate. Exercise, even without dieting, produces the best long-term effects (Roberts, 2000).

## Advise Client to Keep a Food Intake and Exercise Diary for 1 week.

| | | |
|---|---|---|
| Food intake/exercise | Location/time of meals | Emotions around meal time |
| People with whom client eats | Skipped meals | Snacks |

**R:** Overweight individuals often report that their intake is less than it actually is.

## Familiarize Client with Cues that Often Trigger Eating.

| | | |
|---|---|---|
| Another activity (e.g., watching TV) | Everyone else eating Standing up | Boredom or stress |

**R:** Often, inappropriate response to external cues, including stressors, facilitates or aggravates obesity. This response initiates an ineffective pattern in which the person eats in response to stress cues rather than physiologic hunger.

## Teach Basics of Balanced Nutritional Intake.

Choose a plan that encourages high intake of complex carbohydrates and limited intake of fat.
Know what you are eating. The "basic four" label is misleading (e.g., a chicken-fried steak is a protein converted to high fat content through its preparation [frying]).
Obtain more calories from fruits and vegetables than from meat and dairy products. Also, eat more chicken and fish, which contain less fat and fewer total calories than beef, removing the fat and skin.
Avoid salad dressings (216 to 308 calories per 2-oz serving).
Avoid fast food. (It has high fat and total caloric content.)
Dine in or make special requests in restaurants for food selection/preparation (e.g., salad dressing on side, no sauce on entree).
Plan meals in advance. If attending a party or restaurant, decide what to eat ahead of time and stick to it.
Adhere to grocery list.
Involve family in meal planning for better nutrition.
Buy the highest-quality beef (ground round = 10% fat; hamburger = 25% fat).
Choose a variety of foods.
Avoid serving family-style.
Drink eight to ten 8-oz glasses of water daily. Avoid sugary drinks (e.g.; juice, soda fruit drinks)
Measure foods and count calories; keep records.
Read labels on foods, noting amount and calories per serving.

Eat slowly.

Experiment with spices, substitutes, and low-calorie recipes.

Do not skip meals

**R:** Strategies to reduce the intake of food and high-calorie foods will enhance weight loss.

## Discuss Benefits of Exercise.

| | | |
|---|---|---|
| Reduces caloric absorption | Suppresses appetite | Improves self-esteem |
| Preserves lean muscle mass | Increases oxygen uptake | Increases restful sleep |
| Reduces depression, anxiety, stress | Increases caloric expenditure | Increases resistance to age-related degeneration |
| Improves body posture | Maintains weight loss | |
| Provides fun, recreation, diversion | Increases metabolic rate | |

**R:** Any increase in activity also increases energy output and caloric deficits. Weight loss without exercise decreases resting basal metabolism (Roberts, 2000).

## Assist Client to Identify Realistic Exercise Program.

Before beginning an exercise program, the person must consider
- Physical limitations (consult nurse or physician)
- Personal preferences
- Lifestyle, finances available
- Community resources
- Needed clothing and shoes
- Clients must learn to monitor pulse before, during, and after exercise to assist them to achieve target heart rate and not to exceed maximum advisable heart rate for age.

| Age | Maximum Heart Rate | Target Heart Rate |
|---|---|---|
| 30 | 190 | 133 to 162 |
| 40 | 180 | 126 to 153 |
| 50 | 170 | 119 to 145 |
| 60 | 160 | 112 to 136 |

**R:** Evaluating these factors can reduce barriers and increase success.

## Discuss Aspects of Starting the Exercise Program.

Advise that a regular exercise program should

- Be enjoyable
- Use a minimum of 400 calories in each session
- Sustain a heart rate of approximately 120 to 150 bpm
- Involve rhythmic, alternating contracting and relaxing of muscles
- Be integrated into the person's lifestyle 4 to 5 days/week for at least 30 to 60 min

Start slow and easy. Obtain clearance from physician.

Plan a daily walking program.

Start at 5 to 10 blocks for 0.5 to 1 mile/day; increase 1 block or 0.1 mile/week.

Gradually increase rate and length of walk; remember to progress slowly.

Avoid straining or pushing too hard and becoming overly fatigued.

Stop immediately if any of the following occur:

| | |
|---|---|
| Lightness or pain in chest | Dizziness |
| Severe breathlessness | Loss of muscle control |
| Lightheadedness | Nausea |

If pulse is 120 beats/minute (bpm) at 5 min or 100 bpm at 10 min after stopping exercise, or if shortness of breath occurs 10 min after exercise, slow down either the rate or the distance of walking.

If client cannot walk 5 blocks or 0.5 mile without signs of overexertion, decrease length of walking for 1 week to point before signs appear and then start to add 1 block/0.1 mile each week.

Walk at same rate; time with stopwatch or second hand on watch; after reaching 10 blocks (1 mile), try to increase speed.

Remember, increase only the rate or the distance of walking at one time.

Establish a regular time for exercise, with the goal of three to five times/week for 15 to 45 min and a heart rate of 80% of stress test or gross calculation (170 bpm for 20 to 29 years of age; decrease 10 bpm for each additional decade [e.g., 160 bpm for 30 to 39 years of age, 150 bpm for 40 to 49 years of age]).

Encourage significant others also to engage in walking program.

Add supplemental activity (e.g., parking far from destination, gardening, using stairs, spending weekends at activities that require walking).

Work up to 1 h of exercise per day at least 4 days per week.

Avoid lapses of more than 2 days between exercise sessions.

**R:** The most common reasons a person stops an exercise program is overexertion with resulting muscle and joint pain. The safest activities for the unconditioned obese person are walking, water aerobics, swimming, and cycling.

## Teach About the Risks of Obesity.

| | | |
|---|---|---|
| Vascular insufficiency | Arteriosclerosis | Heart disease |
| Hypertension | Left ventricular hypertrophy | Diabetes mellitus |
| Gallbladder disease | Complications of surgery | Respiratory disease |
| Joint degeneration (knees, hips, ankles) | Cancer (e.g., breast) | |
| High risk for falls | Poor healing ability | |
| Increased LDL cholesterol | Decreased HDL cholesterol | Lymphedema of legs |

**R:** The effects of excess weight are insidious and often not felt by the person until they threaten health or cause pain. Excess weight contributes to hypertension, type 2 diabetes, heart disease, sleep apnea, osteoarthritis, gallstones, stress incontinence, and high LDL and low HDL levels (Dudek, 2006). Weight loss of even 5% to 10% can lower blood pressure and improve glucose lipid profiles (Dennis, 2004).

## Assist Client to Increase Interest and Motivation.

Build a support system of people who value growth and you as an individual.

Be aware of rationalization (e.g., a lack of time may be a lack of prioritization).

Keep a list of positive outcomes and health benefits, e.g., sleep better, lower blood pressure,

**R:** Weight loss is a life changing event if it is to be sustained. Motivation must be maintained. Weight loss of even 5% to 10% can lower blood pressure and improve glucose lipid profiles (Dennis, 2004).

## Reduce Inappropriate Responses to Stressors.

Distinguish between urge and hunger.

Use distraction, relaxation, and imagery.

Use alternative response training:

- Make a list of external cues/situations that lead to off-target behavior.
- List constructive behaviors (e.g., take a walk) to replace off-target behaviors.
- Post the list of alternate constructive behaviors on the refrigerator.
- Reevaluate every 1 to 2 weeks whether plan is realistic and effective.

**R:** Overeating is often associated with boredom and stress.

## Initiate Health Teaching and Referrals, as Indicated.

Refer client to support groups (e.g., Weight Watchers, Overeaters Anonymous, TOPS).

**R:** Weight loss strategies are life long and may require assistance from programs and support groups.

**Pediatric
Interventions**

**Assist Child and Family to Realize the Shared Responsibility of Weight Control.**

Discuss with family the hazards of overweight children.

- Childhood obesity leads to adult obesity.
- Excess weight elevates blood pressure, heart rate, and cardiac output in children (see Key Concepts, Pediatric Considerations for other health dangers).
- As weight increases, activity decreases.

**R:** Refer to key concepts.

Use creative methods with small children to teach good nutrition

- Create a felt board with each day of the week. Using pictures of food groups, vegetables, grains, milk, meat, cheese, yogurt, fruits, have child stick them to the board for that day
- Read books that emphasize good food with more energy, strong muscles and bones etc.

**R:** Children respond favorable to activities that are a bridge between concrete experiences and abstract ideas (Murray, Zentner, & Yakimo.2009).

Collaborate with family on a dietary plan (Murray. Zentner, & Yakimo, 2009).

- Discuss the importance of balancing intake with activity. Explain that weight gain occurs with overeating, inadequate activity, or both. Limit TV, computer time. Stop eating in front of TV or while reading.
- Eat meals at table and engage in pleasant discussions.
- Avoid using food as a punishment or reward.
- Elicit the child's favorite foods; try to include reasonable amounts in the plan.
- Encourage child to try new foods (e.g., yogurt).
- Teach child how to self-monitor intake, eating only when hungry.
- Encourage child to eat healthy snacks (e.g., raw vegetables, no-fat popcorn).
- Help child avoid prepared and sugared foods.
- Advise parents to limit the high-calorie/high-fat foods in the house.
- Advise parents to replace whole milk with skim milk after child is 2 years of age.
- Advise parents not to force child to finish every bottle or meal.
- Advise parents not to use sweets as reward for finishing meal.
- Help child to avoid skipping meals.
- Set realistic goals and rewards of 1 to 4 lb/month; collaborate with parents for reward for adherence.
- Encourage them to decrease television watching, recreational computer use (1 h/day); elicit favorite shows.
- Plan family activity regularly (adult walking, child riding or skating).

**R:** Healthy eating and lifestyles should be a family oriented with all members involved for success. Overweight parents have overweight children who grow up to be overweight adults

Initiate referrals as indicated.
   If desired, enlist the help of the school nurse (e.g., weigh-ins, support).
   Consider summer camps for overweight teens.
   Make use of community resources (e.g., adolescent support groups).

**R:** Community resources may be needed to assist parents with lifestyle change.

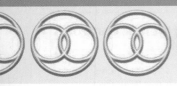

# RISK-PRONE HEALTH BEHAVIOR

## DEFINITION

State in which a person has an inability to modify lifestyle/behavior in a manner consistent with a change in health status

## DEFINING CHARACTERISTICS

### Major (must be present, one or more)

Minimizes health status change.
Failure to take action that prevents health problems.

## RELATED FACTORS

### Situational (personal, environmental)

*Related to:*
Low self-efficacy
Negative attitude toward health care
Multiple stressors
Inadequate social support
Inadequate resources
Inadequate finances
Multiple responsibilities
*Related to impaired ability to understand secondary to:*
Low literacy
Language barriers

### ■■■■■■ AUTHOR'S NOTE

This new nursing diagnosis replaces the NANDA diagnosis *Impaired Adjustment. Risk-Prone Health Behavior* has some commonalities with *Ineffective Health Maintenance* and *Noncompliance*. This author recommends that *Ineffective Health Maintenance* be used to describe a person with an unhealthy lifestyle that puts him or her at risk for a chronic health problem or disease. *Noncompliance* applies to a person who wants to comply, but factors are present that deter adherence.

*Risk-Prone Health Behavior* describes a person with a health problem who is not participating in management of the health problem because of lack of motivation, comprehension, or personal barriers.

### ■■■■■ ERRORS IN DIAGNOSTIC STATEMENTS

#### Risk-Prone Health Behavior related to high-fat diet and sedentary lifestyle

This diagnosis represents an unhealthy lifestyle. The related factors are actually signs and symptoms, not related factors; thus, the diagnosis would be *Ineffective Health Maintenance related to unknown etiology as evidenced by high-fat diet and sedentary lifestyle*. It is necessary for the nurse to assess what factors fall under "related to," such as lack of knowledge, inadequate time, or access barriers.

*Noncompliance related to unknown etiology as evidenced by reports it is not necessary to monitor blood glucose levels daily*
Since the person with diabetes does not desire to monitor blood glucose levels, the focus is on helping him or her understand the importance through motivation, attitude, and behavior changes. *Risk-Prone Health Behavior related to unknown etiology as evidenced by reports it is not necessary to monitor blood glucose levels daily* would be more appropriate because it would focus on behavior changes. *Noncompliance* should focus on barriers that do not relate to motivation.

■■■■■■ **KEY CONCEPTS**

### Generic Considerations

- "Self-management support is the assistance caregivers give clients with chronic diseases in order to encourage daily decision that improve health related behaviors and clinical outcomes" (Bodenheimer, MacGregor, & Sharifi, 2005, p. 4).
- Clients are helped to choose health behaviors in a collaborative partnership with the caregivers (Bodenheimer et al., 2005).
- Refer to *Ineffective Therapeutic Regimen Management* for key concepts on health education, self-efficacy, and barriers to learning.
- Motivational interviewing is a readiness to change model in which readiness = importance × confidence. Techniques are used to assess readiness to change (importance and confidence) and to encourage clients to increase their readiness (Rollnik, Mason, & Butler, 2000).

### *Literacy*

- Health literacy is "the degree to which individuals have that capacity to obtain, process and understand basic health information and services needed to make appropriate health decisions" (Cutilli, 2005).
- Those with the highest incidence of low literacy:
- Are poor
- Live in the South and West
- Have less than a high school diploma
- Are members of an ethnic/cultural minority over 65
- Have physical/mental disabilities
- Are homeless or inmates

## Focus Assessment Criteria

Literacy level (Murphy et al., 1993)

### *Have Person Read the Following Words:*

| | |
|---|---|
| Fat | Fatigue |
| Flu | Directed |
| Pill | Colitis |
| Allergic | Constipation |
| Jaundice | Osteoporosis |
| Anemia | |

Note: fat, flu, and pill are not scored. A score of 6 or fewer correct can indicate a person at risk for poor literacy.

- Assess knowledge of condition:
- Examples:
- Do you know what diabetes is?
- What would you like to know about hypertension?
- Do you know what to do to prevent complications of diabetes?
- Assess for barriers:
- What do you think is causing your BP (blood sugar or weight) to remain high?
- What could you do to decrease your BP (weight, blood sugar)?
- Would you like to stop smoking (or drinking alcohol)?
- What is preventing you?

**NOC**

Adherence Behavior, Symptom Control, Health Beliefs Treatment Behavior Illness/Injury

## ➤ Goals

The person will verbalize intent to modify one behavior to manage health problem indicators:

- Describe the health problem.
- Describe the relationship of present practices/behavior to decreased health.
- Engage in goal setting.

**NIC**
Health Education,
Mutual Goal Setting,
Self-responsibility,
Teaching: Disease
Process, Decision-
Making Process

## ➤ General Interventions _____

### If Low Literacy Is Suspected, Start with What the Person Is Most Stressed About.

- Speak simply.
- Repeat and ask person to repeat.
- Use pictures.
- Use appropriate examples.
- Demonstrate and ask for a return demonstration.
- Use videotapes and audiotapes.

**R:** Persons who are identified as having reading problems will have difficulty with most verbal instructions and patient education material (Kalichman et al., 2005).

### Engage in Collaborative Decision Making (Bodenheimer, MacGregor, & Shariffi, 2005).

- List some choices for improving the person's health.

For example: for diabetes
exercise                    healthy eating
medication                  blood glucose monitoring
client–defined choice

### Ask If There Is One Activity on the List They Would Like to Focus on.

**R:** Caregivers provide expertise and tools for care giving out health-related decisions made.

### Clients Are Responsible for Day-to-Day Decisions (Bodenheimer et al., 2005).

Provide information as directed by the client:

- Ask: What do you want to know about _____?
- Provide information the person wants to know.
- Ask the person if he/she understood.
- Ask if there are other questions.

**R:** Clients often receive too much or too little information. Learning chosen by the learner does improve health-related outcomes (Bodenheimer et al., 2005).

### Ask the Person to Repeat the Goal, Behavior or Activity.

**R:** Assessing understanding can improve comprehension and outcomes positively.

### Assess Readiness to Change.

- Determine how important the person thinks the behavior change is.

For example:
How important is it to you to increase your activity? Rate from 0–10.
0—not important      10—important

**R:** If the person does not think the behavior change is important to improved health, he or she is unlikely to initiate the change (Bodenheimer et al., 2005).

### Determine How Confident the Person Is to Make the Change.

For example:
How confident are you that you can get more exercise? Rate from 0–10.

- Determine if the person is ready for change.

- If the importance level is 7 or above, assess confidence level. If the importance level is low, provide more information regarding risks of not changing behavior.
- If the level of confidence is 4 or less, ask the person why it is not a 1.
- Ask person what is needed to change the low score to an 8.

**R:** If the importance and/or the confidence is low, an action plan with specific behavior changes would not reflect true collaboration.

## Collaboratively Set a Goal and an Action Plan that Are Realistic.

For example:
How often each week could you walk around the block two times?

**R:** The person's level of confidence will increase with success. Advice that is not easily achievable sets the person up for failure (Bodenheimer et al., 2005).

Ask the Person If You Can Call Him or Her in 2 Weeks to See How He or She Is Doing. Gradually Extend the Time to Monthly Calls.

**R:** Telephone support has been found to benefit persons with limited health literacy, those with multiple chronic health problems, and those with gaps in care (Piette, 2005).

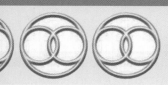

# EFFECTIVE BREASTFEEDING

## DEFINITION

Effective Breastfeeding: The state in which a mother–infant dyad exhibits adequate proficiency and satisfaction with the breastfeeding process

## DEFINING CHARACTERISTICS

### Major (Must Be Present)

Mother's ability to position infant at breast to promote a successful latch-on response
Infant content after feeding
Regular and sustained suckling/swallowing at the breast
Infant weight patterns appropriate for age
Effective mother–infant communication patterns (infant cues, maternal interpretation and response)

### Minor (May Be Present)

Signs or symptoms of oxytocin release (let-down or milk ejection reflex)
Adequate infant elimination patterns for age
Eagerness of infant to nurse
Maternal verbalization of satisfaction with breastfeeding

### ■■■■■■ AUTHOR'S NOTE

This diagnosis reportedly represents a newly proposed NANDA wellness diagnosis, defined as "a clinical judgment about an individual, family, or community in transition from a specific level of wellness to a higher level of wellness." The definition does not describe a mother–infant dyad seeking higher-level breastfeeding, but "adequate proficiency and satisfaction with the breastfeeding process." *This diagnosis Effective Breastfeeding should be changed to Readiness for Enhanced Breastfeeding for terminology which is consistent for wellness diagnoses.*

*(continued)*

■■■■■■ **AUTHOR'S NOTE** *Continued*

In the management of breastfeeding, nurses will encounter three situations covered by the following nursing diagnoses:

*Ineffective Breastfeeding*
*Risk for Ineffective Breastfeeding*
*Readiness for Enhanced Breastfeeding*

The nurse would use *Ineffective Breastfeeding* to describe an evaluation judgment of a mother's and infant's breastfeeding session for both ineffective and potentially ineffective breastfeeding. This evaluation results from the nurse observing or the mother reporting those signs and symptoms listed as defining characteristics. These signs and symptoms do not describe higher-level breastfeeding.

If the nurse cares for a mother reporting proficiency and satisfaction with breastfeeding and desiring additional teaching to achieve even greater proficiency and satisfaction, *Readiness for Enhanced Breastfeeding* would be appropriate. The focus of this teaching and continued support would not be on preventing ineffective breastfeeding or maintaining adequate proficiency and satisfaction, but on promoting higher-quality breastfeeding.

This diagnosis is not useful in its present form; instead, the nurse should use *Ineffective Breastfeeding* or *Risk for Ineffective Breastfeeding*. Nurses desiring to use a wellness nursing diagnosis could use *Readiness for Enhanced Breastfeeding*. Because this diagnosis is not on the NANDA list, nurses using it should send their experiences to NANDA.

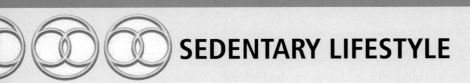

# SEDENTARY LIFESTYLE

## DEFINITION

The state in which an individual or group reports a habit of life that is characterized by a low physical activity level

## DEFINING CHARACTERISTICS

### Major (Must Be Present, One or More)

Chooses a daily routine lacking physical exercise
Demonstrates physical deconditioning
Verbalized preference for activities low in physical activity

## RELATED FACTORS

Pathophysiologic-related decreased endurance secondary to obesity.

### Situational (Personal, Environment)

*Related to inadequate knowledge of health benefits of physical activity*
*Related to inadequate knowledge of exercise routines*
*Related to insufficient resources (money, facilities)*
*Related to perceived lack of time*
*Related to lack of motivation*
*Related to lack of interest*
*Related to lack of injury*

■■■■■ **AUTHOR'S NOTE**

This is the first nursing diagnosis submitted by a nurse from another country and accepted by NANDA. Congratulations to J. Adolf Guirao-Goris of Valencia, Spain.

■■■■■ **KEY CONCEPTS**

### Generic Considerations

- Regular exercise can increase

| | |
|---|---|
| Cardiovascular-respiratory endurance | Delivery of nutrients to tissue |
| Muscle strength | Tolerance for psychological stress |
| Muscle endurance | Ability to reduce body fat content |
| Flexibility | |

- Vigorous exercise sessions should include a warm-up phase (10 minutes at a slow pace), endurance exercise, and a cool-down phase (5 to 10 minutes of a slow pace and stretching).
- Current beliefs regarding optimal exercise are as follows (Allison & Keller, 1997):
  Emphasize physical activity over "exercise."
  Moderate physical activity that accumulates to 30 or more minutes is beneficial.
  To enhance long-term exercise, the person should (Moore & Charvat, 2002):
  Respond to relapse with a plan to prevent recurrences.
  Set realistic goals.
  Keep an exercise log.
  Exercise with a friend.
- A regular pattern of moderate intensity physical activity of 30 minutes or more, which can be accumulated throughout the day, 4 to 5 times a week, can be beneficial. Previously, vigorous exercise was recommended for a continuous 30 minutes or more.
- Forty percent of adults are completely sedentary in their leisure time (Nies & Chruscial, 2002).
- At least 1 hour of walking per week can lower the risk of coronary heart disease in women (Lee et al., 2001).

 **Geriatric Considerations**

- Physical activity, healthful eating, social connections, meaningful involvement and access to health care can increase healthy aging (Young & Cochrane, 2004).
- Physical activity contributes to well-being, flexibility, strength, function, and chronic disease management (Taggart, 2002).
- Only 24% of older women exercise (Rogers et al., 2002).
- Tai Chi improved balance, functional mobility and fear of falling among older women (Taggart, 2002).
- Falls in older women are a major health concerns (Young & Cochrane, 2004).

## Focus Assessment Criteria

### Subjective Data

*Assess for Defining Characteristic.*

Regular exercise pattern (none, daily weekly).
Reports fatigue, shortness of breath with increased activity.

**NOC**
Knowledge: Health Behaviors, Physical Fitness

➤ ### Goal

The person will verbalize intent to or engage in increased physical activity.

*Indicators*

- Set a goal for weekly exercise.
- Identify a desired activity or exercise.

**NIC**
Exercise Promotion,
Exercise Therapy

## ➤ General Interventions

### Discuss Benefits of Exercise

| | | |
|---|---|---|
| Reduces caloric absorption | Improves body posture | Increases metabolic rate |
| Preserves lean muscle mass | Suppresses appetite | Improves self-esteem |
| Reduces depression, | Increases oxygen uptake | Increases restful sleep |
| anxiety stress | Increases caloric expenditure | Increases resistance to |
| Provides fun, recreation, diversion | Maintains weight loss | age-related degeneration |

**R:** The process of seeking and attaining positive lifestyle change is known as "empowering potential." It occurs in three stages: appraising readiness, changing, and integrating change. As a person strives to improve health, he or she moves through a process of introspection; planning new, healthier activities; coping with barriers and setbacks; and ultimately absorbing these new behaviors into everyday life.

**R:** The client is responsible for choosing a healthy pattern of living. The nurse is responsible for explaining the choices.

## Assist Client to Identify Realistic Exercise Program. Consider:

Physical limitations (consult nurse or physician)
Personal preferences
Lifestyle
Community resources
Needed clothing and shoes
Clients must learn to monitor pulse before, during, and after exercise to assist them to achieve target heart rate and not to exceed maximum advisable heart rate for age.

| Age | Maximum Heart Rate | Target Heart Rate |
|---|---|---|
| 30 | 190 | 133 to 162 |
| 40 | 180 | 126 to 153 |
| 50 | 170 | 119 to 145 |
| 60 | 160 | 112 to 136 |

**R:** A regular exercise program should be:

- Enjoyable
- Use a minimum of 400 calories in each session
- Sustain a heat rate of approximately 120 to 150 bpm
- Involve rhythmic, alternating contracting and relaxing of muscles
- Be integrated into the person's lifestyle of 4 to 5 days/week for at least 30 to 60 minutes.

## Discuss Aspects of Starting the Exercise Program.

Start slow and easy; obtain clearance from physician.
Read, consult experts, and talk with friends/coworkers who exercise.
Plan a daily walking program:

- Start at 5 to 10 blocks for 0.5 to 1 mile/day; increase 1 block or 0.1 mile/week.
- Gradually increase rate and length of walk; remember to progress slowly.
- Avoid straining or pushing too hard and becoming overly fatigued.
- Stop immediately if any of the following occur:

| | |
|---|---|
| Lightness or pain chest | Dizziness |
| Severe breathlessness | Loss of muscle control |
| Lightheadedness | Nausea |

If pulse is 120 beats/minute (bpm) at 4 minutes or 100 bpm at 10 minutes after stopping exercise, or if shortness of breath occurs 10 minutes after exercise, slow down either the rate or the distance of walking for 1 week to point before signs appear and then start to add 1 block/0.1 mile each week.
Walk at same rate; time with stopwatch or second hand on watch; after reaching 10 blocks (1 mile), try to increase speed.
Remember, increase only the rate or the distance of walking at one time.

Establish a regular time for exercise, with the goal of three to five times/week for 15 to 45 minutes and a heart rate of 80% of stress test or gross calculation (170 bpm for 20 to 29 years of age.) Decrease 10 bpm for each additional decade (e.g., 160 bpm for 30 to 39 years of age, 150 bpm for 40 to 49 years of age).

Encourage significant others also to engage in walking program.

Add supplemental activity (e.g., parking far from destination, gardening, using stairs, spending weekends at activities that require walking).

Work up to 1 hour of exercise per day at least 4 days per week.

Avoid lapses of more than 2 days between exercise sessions.

**R:** The safest activities for the unconditioned obese person are walking, water aerobics, and swimming.
**R:** Any increase in activity also increases energy output and caloric deficits.

## Assist Client to Increase Interest and Motivation.

Develop a contract listing realistic short- and long-term goals.

Keep intake/activity records.

Increase knowledge by reading and talking with health-conscious friends and coworkers.

Make new friends who are health conscious.

Get a friend to also follow the program or be a source of support.

Be aware of rationalization (e.g., a lack of time may be a lack of prioritization).

Keep a list of positive outcomes.

**R:** Friends have the most positive influence to keep on an exercise program (Resnick et al., 2002).

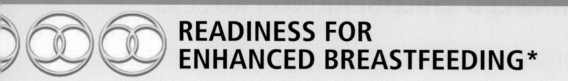

# READINESS FOR ENHANCED BREASTFEEDING*

## DEFINITION

Readiness for Enhanced Breastfeeding: The state in which a mother-infant dyad exhibits adequate proficiency and satisfaction with the breastfeeding process

## DEFINING CHARACTERISTICS

### Major (Must Be Present)

Mother's ability to position infant at breast to promote a successful latch-on response

Infant content after feeding

Regular and sustained suckling/swallowing at the breast

Infant weight patterns appropriate for age

Effective mother-infant communication patterns (infant cues, maternal interpretation and response)

### Minor (May Be Present)

Signs or symptoms of oxytocin release (let-down or milk ejection reflex)

Adequate infant elimination patterns for age

Eagerness of infant to nurse

Maternal verbalization of satisfaction with breastfeeding

---

*This diagnosis is not on the NANDA-I list but has been added for usefulness and clarity.

■■■■■■ **KEY CONCEPTS**

Refer to *Ineffective Breastfeeding*.

## Focus Assessment

Refer to *Ineffective Breastfeeding*.

| NOC |
| --- |
| Knowledge: breastfeeding. |

➤ **Goals**

The mother will report an increase in confidence and satisfaction with breastfeeding.

*Indicators*

Identify two new strategies (specify) to enhance breastfeeding.

| NIC |
| --- |
| Refer to Health-Seeking Behaviors |

➤ **Interventions**

Refer to the Internet for sites for resources and information on breastfeeding.
Refer to *Ineffective Breastfeeding for interventions to enhanced breastfeeding.*

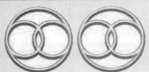

# READINESS FOR ENHANCED CHILDBEARING PROCESS

## DEFINITION (NANDA)

A pattern of preparing for, maintaining and strengthening a healthy pregnancy and child birth process and care of newborn.

## DEFINING CHARACTERISTICS (NANDA)

### During Pregnancy

Reports appropriate prenatal lifestyle (e.g. diet, elimination, sleep, bodily movement, exercise, personal hygiene
Reports appropriate physical preparations
Reports managing unpleasant symptoms in pregnancy
Demonstrates respect for unborn baby
Rep[orts a realistic birth plan
Prepares necessary new born care items
Seeks necessary newborn care items
Seeks necessary knowledge (e.g. of labor and delivery, newborn care
Reports available f support systems
Has regular prenatal health visits

### During Labor and Delivery

Reports lifestyle (e.g., diet, elimination, sleep bodily movement, personal hygiene) that is appropriate for the stage if labor
Responds appropriately to the onset of labor
Is proactive in labor and delivery
Uses relaxation techniques appropriate for the stage of labor

Demonstrates attachment behavior to the newborn baby

Utilizes support systems appropriately

## After Birth

Demonstrates appropriate baby feeding techniques

Demonstrates appropriate breast care

Demonstrates attachment behavior to the baby

Demonstrates basic baby care techniques

Provides safe environment for the baby

Reports appropriate postpartum lifestyle(e.g. diet, elimination, sleep, bodily movement, exercise, personal hygiene)

Utilizes support system appropriately

### AUTHOR'S NOTE

This new NANDA-I nursing diagnosis represents the comprehensive care that is needed to promote the following: healthy pregnancy, childbirth and the postpartum process, enhanced relationships (mother, father, infant, and siblings) and optimal care of the newborn. This care is beyond the scope possible in this text. Refer to a text on Maternal-Child Health for the specific interventions for this diagnosis.

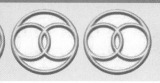

# READINESS FOR ENHANCED COMFORT

## DEFINITION (NANDA)

A pattern of ease, relief, and transcendence in physical, psychospiritual, environmental, and/or social dimensions that can be strengthened

## DEFINING CHARACTERISTICS (NANDA)

Expresses desire to enhance comfort

Expresses desire to enhance feeling of contentment

Expresses desire to enhance relaxation

Expresses desire to enhance resolution of complaints

### AUTHOR'S NOTE

This diagnosis is very general and therefore does not direct specific interventions. It encompasses physical, psychological, spiritual, environmental, and social dimensions. It would be more clinically useful to focus on a particular dimension, such as *Readiness for Enhanced Spiritual-Well Being*.

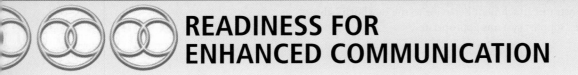

# READINESS FOR ENHANCED COMMUNICATION

## DEFINITION (NANDA)

A pattern of exchanging information and ideas with others that is sufficient for meeting one's needs and life's goals, and can be enhanced

## DEFINING CHARACTERISTICS (NANDA)

Able to speak a language
Able to write a language
Expresses feelings
Expresses satisfaction with ability to share ideas with others
Expresses satisfaction with ability to share information with others
Expresses willingness to enhance communication
Forms phases
Forms sentences
Forms words
Interprets nonverbal cures appropriately
Uses nonverbal cues appropriately

### ■■■■■■ AUTHOR'S NOTE

This diagnosis represents a person with good communications skills. Interventions to enhance communication skills can be found in Section 2 Part 1 in Impaired Communication and Impaired Verbal Communication.

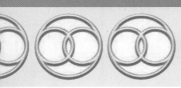

# READINESS FOR ENHANCED COPING

## DEFINITION

A pattern of cognitive and behavioral efforts to manage demands that is sufficient for well-being and can be strengthened

## DEFINING CHARACTERISTICS

Acknowledges power
Aware of possible environmental changes
Defines stressors as manageable
Seeks knowledge of new strategies
Seeks social support
Uses a broad range of emotion-oriented strategies
Uses a broad range of problem-oriented strategies
Uses spiritual resources

▨▨▨■■■ **KEY CONCEPTS**
Refer to Stress Overload for principles of effective coping.

## Focus Assessment

Refer to Health Promotion/Wellness Assessment under Self–Perception- Self-Concept Pattern.

## Goals

The individual/group will report increased satisfaction with coping with stressors.

### Indicators

Identify two new strategies (specify) to enhance coping with stressors

## Interventions

### If Anxiety Diminishes One's Effective Coping, Teach:

- Abdominal relaxation breathing
- Abdominal breathing with imagining a peaceful scene e.g. ocean, woods, mountains
Imagine the feel of the warm sand on your feet, sun on your face, the sound of water.

**R:** Relaxation techniques provide an opportunity to regroup prior to reacting.

### Explain Reframing (Varcarolis, 2006, p. 153)

Reassess the situation, ask yourself:
- What positive thing can out of the situation?
- What did I learn?
- What would I do differently next time?
- What might be going on with your (boss, partner, sister friend) that would cause him or her to say or do that?
- Is she or he stressed out or having problems?

**R:** Reframing provides one with the opportunity to analyze and consider reasons for behavior and alternative options.

### Acknowledge Stress Reducing Tips for Living (Varcarolis, 2008, p. 154):

- Exercise regularly, at least 3 times weekly
- Reduce caffeine intake
- Engage in meaningful, satisfying work
- Do not let work dominate your life
- Guard your personal freedom
- Choose your friends. Associate with gentle people
- Live with and love who you choose
- Structure your time as you see fit
- Set your own life goals

**R:** The stressors of life are heightened when others decide how you should live your life.

Refer to the Internet for sites for resources and information on stress reduction techniques.

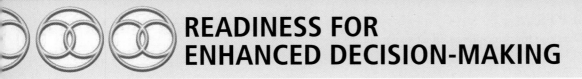

# READINESS FOR ENHANCED DECISION-MAKING

## DEFINITION

A pattern of choosing courses of action that is sufficient for meeting short- and long-term health-related goals and can be strengthened

## DEFINING CHARACTERISTICS

Expresses desire to enhance decision-making
Expresses desire to enhance congruency of decisions with personal and/or sociocultural values and goals
Expresses desire to enhance risk-benefit analysis of decisions
Expresses desire to enhance understanding of choices and the meaning of the choices
Expresses desire to enhance use of reliable evidence for decisions

### ▬▬▬▬▬ KEY CONCEPTS

Refer to *Decisional Conflict* for principles of effective decision-making.

## Focus Assessment

Refer to Health Promotion/Wellness Assessment under Cognitive–Perceptual Pattern.

**NOC**
Decision-Making,
Information
Processing

> ## Goals

The individual/group will report increased satisfaction with decision-making.

### Indicators

Identify two new strategies (specify) to enhance decision-making.

**NIC**
Decision-Making
Support, Mutual
Goal Setting

> ## Interventions

Refer to the Internet for sites for resources and information on decision-making.
Refer to Interventions for *Health-Seeking Behaviors* and *Decisional Conflict*.

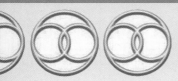

# READINESS FOR ENHANCED FLUID BALANCE

## DEFINITION

A pattern of equilibrium between fluid volume and chemical composition of body fluids that is sufficient for meeting physical needs and can be strengthened

## DEFINING CHARACTERISTICS

- Expresses willingness to enhance fluid balance
- Stable weight

- Moist mucous membranes
- Food and fluid intake adequate for daily needs
- Straw-colored urine with specific gravity within normal limits
- Good tissue turgor
- No excessive thirst
- Urine output appropriate for intake
- No evidence of edema of dehydration

## ▪▪▪▪▪▪ AUTHOR'S NOTE

If a person has a pattern of equilibrium between fluid volume and the chemical composition of body fluids that is sufficient for meeting physical needs, how can this be strengthened? Would it be more useful to focus on education under the diagnosis *Risk for Deficient Fluid Volume*?

## ▪▪▪▪▪▪ KEY CONCEPTS

Refer to *Imbalanced Nutrition* and *Deficient Fluid Volume* for Key Concepts on balanced nutrition and fluid volume.

| **NOC**
Fluid Balance, Hydration, Electrolyte Balance | ➤ | ## Goals |

The individual will report increased satisfaction with fluid balance.

### Indicators

Identify two new strategies (specify) to enhance fluid balance.

| **NIC**
Fluid/Electrolyte Management; See also Health-Seeking Behaviors | ➤ | ## Interventions |

Refer to the Internet for sites for resources and information on nutrition.
Refer to Interventions for *Health-Seeking Behavior* and *Deficient Fluid Balance*.

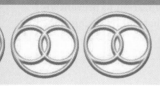

# READINESS FOR ENHANCED HOPE

## DEFINITION (NANDA)

A pattern of expectations and desires that is sufficient for mobilizing energy on one's own behalf and can be strengthened

## DEFINING CHARACTERISTICS (NANDA)

- Expresses expectations congruent with desires
- Sets achievable goals
- Conducts problem-solving to meet goals
- Expresses belief in possibilities
- Expresses a sense of spirituality and meaning to life
- Interconnected with others
- Expresses desire or agrees to enhanced hope

**KEY CONCEPTS**

Refer to *Hopelessness* for principles of hope.

## Focus Assessment

Refer to Health Promotion/Wellness Assessment under Self-Perception–Self-Concept Pattern.

**NOC**
See Hopelessness

**NIC**
Refer to Internet sites for Resources and Information on Hope, Refer to Hopelessness for Interventions to Promote Hope, Refer to Health-Seeking Behaviors for Generic Interventions.

➤ ## Goals

The individual/group will report increased hope.

### Indicators

Identify two new strategies (specify) to enhance hope.

## Interventions

Refer to *Hopelessness* for Interventions to Promote Hope.

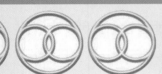

# READINESS FOR ENHANCED IMMUNIZATION STATUS

## DEFINITION (NANDA)

A pattern of conforming to local, national, and/or international standards of immunization to prevent infectious disease(s) that is sufficient to protect a person, family, or community and that can be strengthened

## DEFINING CHARACTERISTICS (NANDA)

- Obtains immunizations appropriate for age and health status
- Expresses knowledge of immunization standards
- Exhibits behavior to prevent infectious diseases
- Keeps records of immunizations
- Values immunizations as a health priority; describes possible problems associated with immunizations

■■■■■ **AUTHOR'S NOTE**

This diagnosis would apply to an individual or group that needs an immunization according to a national/international standard. All individuals qualify for immunization depending on their age or risk factors. An individual either is a candidate for immunizations or is not. The diagnosis *Risk for Altered Health Maintenance* would be more useful to describe an individual who needs immunizations and/or age-related screening such as mammograms. Thus, *Readiness for Enhanced Immunization* is not clinically useful.

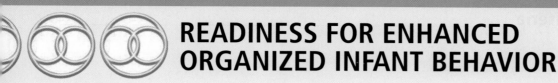

# READINESS FOR ENHANCED ORGANIZED INFANT BEHAVIOR

## DEFINITION

A pattern of modulation of the physiologic and behavioral systems of functioning of an infant (i.e., autonomic, motor, state, organizational, self-regulatory, and attention-interactional) that is satisfactory but that can be improved, resulting in higher levels of integration in response to environmental stimuli

## DEFINING CHARACTERISTICS (BLACKBURN & VANDENBERG, 1993)

### Autonomic System

- Regulated color and respiration
- Reduced visceral signals (e.g., smooth)
- Reduces tremors, twitches
- Digestive functioning, feeding tolerance

### Motor System

Smooth, well-modulated posture and tone
Synchronous smooth movements with:

- Hand/foot clasping
- Suck/suck searching
- Grasping
- Hand holding
- Hand-to-mouth activity
- Tucking

### State System

Well-differentiated range of states
Clear, robust sleep states
Focused, shiny-eyed alertness with intent or animated facial expressions
Active self-quieting/consoling "Ooh" face
Attentional smiling
Cooing

### ■■■■■ AUTHOR'S NOTE

This diagnosis describes an infant who is responding to the environment with stable and predictable autonomic, motor, and state cues. The focus of interventions is to promote continued stable development and to reduce excess environmental stimuli that may stress the infant. Because this is a wellness diagnosis, the use of related factors is not needed. The nurse can write the diagnostic statement as *Readiness for Enhanced Organized Infant Behavior as evidenced by ability to regulate autonomic, motor, and state systems to environmental stimuli*.

### ■■■■■ KEY CONCEPTS

#### Generic Considerations
See *Disorganized Infant Behavior*.

# Focus Assessment Criteria

## Objective Data

Refer to Defining Characteristics.

### *Reciprocal Interactions*

Eye contact                    Exploratory behavior
Mutual gazing                  Easy consolation
Reaching toward                Attending to social stimuli

---

**NOC**
Child Development:
Specify Age, Sleep,
Comfort Level

## ➤ Goals

The infant will continue age-appropriate growth and development and not experience excessive environmental stimuli. The parent(s) will demonstrate handling that promotes stability.

### *Indicators*

- Describe developmental needs of infant.
- Describe early signs of stress of exhaustion.
- Demonstrate:
  - Gentle, soothing touch
  - Melodic tone of voice, coos
  - Mutual gazing
  - Rhythmic movements
  - Acknowledgment of all baby's vocalizations
  - Recognition of soothing qualities of actions

---

**NIC**
Developmental
Care, Infant Care,
Sleep Enhancement,
Environmental
Management:
Comfort Parent
Education: Infant
Attachment
Promotion,
Caregiver Support,
Calming Technique

## ➤ General Interventions

### Explain to Parents the Effects of Excess Environmental Stress on the Infant

### Provide a List of Signs of Stress for Their Infant. Refer to **Disorganized Infant Behavior** for a List of Signs

### Teach Them to Terminate Stimulation If Infant Shows Signs of Stress

**R:** Premature infants must adapt to the extrauterine environment with underdeveloped body systems (Vandenberg, 1990). These infants can tolerate only one activity at a time (Blackburn, 1993).

## Role-Model Developmental Interventions

- Offer only when the infant is alert (if possible, show parents examples of alert and not alert).
- Begin with one stimulus at a time (touch, voice).
- Provide intervention for a short time.
- Increase interventions according to infant's cues.
- Provide frequent, short interventions instead of infrequent, long-term ones.
- Stimulation (visual, auditory, vestibular, tactile, olfactory, gustatory)
- Periods of alertness
- Sleep requirements

**R:** Parents need to understand that they must pace the type, amount, intensity, and timing of stimulation. Behavioral cues from the infant should guide these decisions (Becker, 1997).

## Explain, Role-Model, and Observe Parents Engaging in Developmental Interventions

### Visual

Eye-to-eye contact

Face-to-face experiences

High-contrast colors, geometric shapes (e.g., black and white shapes on paper mobile); up to 4 weeks, simple mobiles of four dessert-size paper plates with stripes, four-square checkerboards, a black dot, and a simple bull's eye, hung 10 to 13 inches from baby's eyes.

### Auditory

Use high-pitched vocalizations.

Play classical music softly.

Use a variety of voice inflections.

Avoid loud talking.

Call infant by name.

Avoid monotone speech patterns.

### Vestibular (Movement)

Rock baby in chair.

Place infant in sling and rock.

Close infant's fist around a soft toy.

Slowly change position during handling.

Provide head support.

### Tactile

Use firm, gentle touch as initial approach.

Use skin-to-skin contact in a warm room.

Provide alternative textures (e.g., sheepskin, velvet, satin).

Avoid stroking if responses are disorganized.

### Olfactory

Wear a light perfume.

### Gustatory

Allow non-nutritive sucking (e.g., pacifier, hand in mouth).

**R:** Individualized developmental care can improve developmental outcomes, weight gain, sleep, motor function, pain tolerance, and feeding. Parents are helped to understand the infant's needs, which will improve attachment and reduce fears (Als, Gilkerson, Duffy et al., 2003).

## Promote Adjustment and Stability in Caregiving Activities (Blackburn & Vandenberg, 1991; Merenstein & Gardner, 1998)

### Waking

Enter room slowly.

Turn on light and open curtains slowly.

Avoid walking baby if he or she is asleep.

### Changing

Keep room warm.

Gently change position; contain limbs during movement.

Stop changing if infant is irritable.

*Feeding*

Time feedings with alert states.
Hold infant close and, if needed, swaddle in a blanket.

*Bathing*

Ventral openness may be stressful. Cover body parts not being bathed.
Proceed slowly; allow for rest.
Offer a pacifier or hand to suck.
Eliminate unnecessary noise.
Use a soft, soothing voice.

**R:** Patterns for routine care should be adhered to in order to minimize stress and conserve energy (Blackburn & Vanderberg, 1991).

## Explain the Need to Reduce Environmental Stimuli When Taking the Infant Outside

Shelter the eyes from light.
Swaddle the infant so his or her hands can reach the mouth.
Protect from loud noises.

**R:** See above rationale.

## Praise Parent(s) on Interaction Patterns; Point Out Infant's Engaging Responses

**R:** Parental confidence can be increased and thus enhance bonding and nurturing behavior at home (Lawhon, 2002).

## Initiate Health Teaching and Referrals If Needed

Explain that developmental interventions will change with maturity. Refer to *Delayed Growth and Development* for specific age-related developmental needs.
Provide parent (s) with resources for assistance at home (e.g., community resources).
Refer to the Internet for sites for resources and information on preterm newborns.

**R:** Families of preterm infants need continued support and anticipatory guidance to improve the transition from the NICU to home (Vandenberg, 1999; Mouradian, Als, & Coster, 2000).

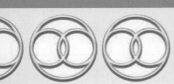

# READINESS FOR ENHANCED KNOWLEDGE (SPECIFY)

## DEFINITION (NANDA)

The presence of acquisition of cognitive information related to a specific topic is sufficient for meeting health-related goals and can be strengthened

## DEFINING CHARACTERISTICS (NANDA)

- Expresses an interest in learning
- Explains knowledge of the topic
- Behaviors congruent with expressed knowledge
- Describes previous experiences pertaining to the topic

■■■■■■ **AUTHOR'S NOTE**

*Readiness for Enhanced Knowledge* is very broad. All nursing diagnoses—actual, risk, and wellness—seek to enhance knowledge. Once the specific area of enhanced knowledge is identified, refer to that specific diagnosis, for example, *Readiness for Enhanced Nutrition, Grieving, Risk for Ineffective Parenting, Deficient Health Behavior,* or *Ineffective Therapeutic Regimen Management. Readiness for Enhanced Knowledge* is not needed because it lacks the reason for the desired or needed knowledge.

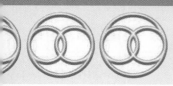

# READINESS FOR ENHANCED NUTRITION

## DEFINITION (NANDA)

A pattern of nutrient intake that is sufficient for meeting metabolic needs and can be strengthened

## DEFINING CHARACTERISTICS (NANDA)

- Expresses willingness to enhance nutrition
- Eats regularly
- Consumes adequate food and fluid
- Expresses knowledge of healthy food and fluid choices
- Follows an appropriate standard for intake (e.g., the food pyramid or American Diabetic Association guidelines)
- Safe preparation and storage for food and fluids
- Attitude toward eating and drinking is congruent with health goals

■■■■■■ **KEY CONCEPTS**

Refer to *Imbalanced Nutrition* for principles of balanced nutrition.

## Focus Assessment

Refer to Health Promotion/Wellness Assessment under Nutrition–Metabolic Pattern.

**NOC**
Nutritional Status, Teaching Nutrition

## ➤ Goals

The individual/group will report an increase in balanced nutrition.

### Indicators

Identify two new strategies (specify) to enhance nutrition

**NIC**
Nutrition Management, Nutrition Monitoring

## ➤ Generic Interventions

Refer to Internet sites for resources and information on nutrition:

- www.mypyramid.gov
- www.health.gov/dietaryguidelines
- www.lifestyleadvantage.org

Refer to *Health-Seeking Behaviors* for generic interventions.

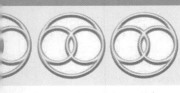

# READINESS FOR ENHANCED POWER

## DEFINITION (NANDA)

A pattern of participating knowingly in change that is sufficient for well-being and can be strengthened

## DEFINING CHARACTERISTICS (NANDA)

Expresses readiness to enhance awareness of possible changes to be made
Expresses readiness to enhance freedom to perform actions for change
Expresses readiness to enhance identification of choices that can be made for change
Expresses readiness to enhance involvement in creating change
Expresses readiness to enhance knowledge for participation in change
Expresses readiness to enhance participation in choices for daily living and health
Expresses readiness to enhance power

### ▪▪▪▪▪▪ KEY CONCEPTS

Refer to *Powerlessness* for principles of power and locus of control.

## Focus Assessments

Refer to *Powerlessness*.

**NOC**
Health Beliefs: Perceived Control, Participation: Health Care Decisions

## ➤ Goals

The individual/group will report increased power.

### *Indicators*

Identify two new strategies (specify) to enhance power.

**NIC**
Decision-making support, Self-responsibility Facilitation, Teaching: Individual

## ➤ Interventions

Refer to *Powerlessness* for strategies to increase power and to *Health-Seeking Behaviors* for generic interventions.

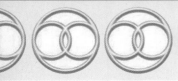

# READINESS FOR ENHANCED RELATIONSHIP

## DEFINITION (NANDA)

A pattern of mutual partnership that is sufficient to provide each other's needs and can be strengthened.

## DEFINING CHARACTERISTICS (NANDA)

Express desire to enhance communication between partners
Express satisfaction with sharing of information and ideas between partners

Express satisfaction with fulfilling physical and emotional needs by one's partner

Demonstrates mutual respect between partners

Meets developmental goals appropriate for family life-cycle stage

Demonstrates well-balanced autonomy and collaboration between partners

Demonstrates mutual support in daily activities between partners

identifies each other as a key person

Demonstrates understanding of partner's insufficient (physical, social)

Express satisfaction with complementary relation between partners

# Goals

The individual will report increased satisfaction with partnership.

## Indicators

Identify two new strategies (specify) to enhance partnership

# Interventions

## Teach to: (Murray, Zentner, & Yakimo, 2009, p. 563)

- Talk daily about feelings
- Elicit feelings of partner
- Explore " what if… conversations.

**R:** Regular sharing of feelings provide opportunities to solve small problems before they escalate.

## Vary Family Responsibilities, Schedule, Chores and Roles.

**R:** This can prepare the family to adapt during times of crisis.

## Engage Partner to Discuss Individual Problems, Validate Solutions or Ask for Partner's Opinion on the Problem.

**R:** This sharing promotes mutual respect.

## Establish a Support System that Can Help When Needed. Provide Such Support to Other Families or Individuals in Need.

**R:** Outside support is needed during crisises.

## During Times of High Stress or Crises, Share Feelings of Guilt, Anger, or Helplessness.

**R:** Discussion of feelings about the situation clarifies that the stress is situation related not about the partner.

## Engage in Activities Together as Partners, Family.

**R:** Isolating behaviors can increase fears and anger.

## Refer to the Internet for Sites for Resources for Coping with Difficult Family Situations (e.g., Death of Member, Ill Family Member).

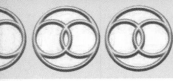

# READINESS FOR ENHANCED RELIGIOSITY

## DEFINITION (NANDA)

Ability to increase reliance on religious beliefs and/or participate in rituals of a particular faith tradition

## DEFINING CHARACTERISTICS (NANDA)

Expresses a desire to strengthen religious belief patterns:
- Comfort or religion in the past
- Questions belief patterns that are harmful
- Rejects belief patterns that are harmful
- Requests assistance expanding religious options
- Requests assistance to increase participation in prescribed religious beliefs
- Requests forgiveness
- Requests reconciliation
- Requests meeting with religious leaders/facilitators
- Requests religious materials and/or experiences

### ▪▪▪▪▪▪ AUTHOR'S NOTE

This diagnosis represents a variety of foci. Request for forgiveness may be related to an actual nursing diagnosis such as *Grieving, Ineffective Individual Coping,* or *Compromised Family Coping.* Further assessment is needed for interventions. Refer to *Impaired Religiosity* in Section II, Part One for additional information.

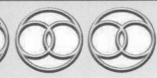

# READINESS FOR ENHANCED RESILIENCE

## DEFINITION (NANDA)

A pattern of positive responses to an adverse situation or crisis that can be strengthened to optimize human potential

## DEFINING CHARACTERISTICS (NANDA)

Access to resources
Effective use of conflict management strategies
Expressed desire to enhance resilience
Identifies support systems
Involvement in activities
Presence of a crisis
Sets goals
Use of effective communication skills
Verbalizes self control

Demonstrates positive outlook
Enhances personal coping skills
Identifies available resources
Increases positive relationships with others
Makes progress toward goals
Safe environment is maintained
Takes responsibilities for actions
Verbalizes an enhanced sense of control

# RELATED FACTORS

Demographics that increase chance
  of maladjustment
Inconsistent parenting
Low maternal education
Minority status
Poor impulse control
Psychological disorders
Condition
Violence

Drug used
Gender
Low intelligence
Large family size
Parental mental illness
Poverty
Vulnerability factors which encompass indices that
  exacerbate the negative reflects of the risk

## AUTHOR'S NOTE

This new NANDA- I diagnosis focuses on the concept of resilience. Resilience is a strength that one has, to allow one to persevere and overcome difficulties. When faced with a crisis or problem, resilient people respond constructively with solutions or effective adaption. Resilience is not a nursing diagnosis. It is an important and vital characteristic that can be nurtured and taught to children to assist them to cope with problematic life events.

The defining characteristics listed, describe enhanced or effective coping. In contrast, the related factors are contributing factors for ineffective coping.

This author recommends:

• Using Risk for Infective Coping related to the related factors listed above to assist someone to prevent ineffective coping
• Using Ineffective Coping related to the above related factors if Defining characteristics of Ineffective Coping exist. (Refer to Section 2 under Ineffective Coping for specific defining characteristics)
• Referring to the interventions for promoting resiliency in children and adults (Refer to index under resiliency for specific pages)

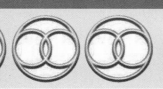

# READINESS FOR ENHANCED SELF-CARE

## DEFINITION (NANDA)

A pattern of performing activities for oneself that helps to meet health-related goals and can be strengthened

## DEFINING CHARACTERISTICS (NANDA)

Expresses a desire to enhance independence in maintaining life
Expresses desire to enhance independence in maintaining health
Expresses desire to enhance knowledge of strategies of self-care
Expresses a desire to enhance responsibility for self-care
Expresses desire to enhance self-care

## AUTHOR'S NOTE

This diagnosis focuses more on improving self-care activities. Refer to *Self-Care Deficits* for interventions to improve self-care.

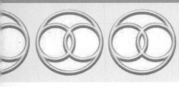

# READINESS FOR ENHANCED SELF-CONCEPT

## DEFINITION (NANDA)

A pattern of perceptions or ideas about the self that is sufficient for well-being and can be strengthened

## DEFINING CHARACTERISTICS (NANDA)

- Expresses willingness to enhance self-concept.
- Expresses satisfaction with thoughts about self, sense of worthiness, role performance, body image, and personal identity.
- Actions are congruent with expressed feelings and thoughts.
- Expresses confidence in abilities.
- Accepts strengths and limitations.

### ▰▰▰▰▰▰ KEY CONCEPTS

Refer to *Disturbed Self-Concept* for principles related to self-concept.

## Focus Assessment

Refer to Health Promotion/Wellness Assessment under Self-Perception–Self-Concept Pattern.

**NOC**
Quality of Life, Self-Esteem, Coping

### ➤ Goals

The individual will report increased self-concept in (specify situation).

### *Indicators*

Identify two new strategies (specify) to enhance self-concept.

**NIC**
Hope Instillation, Values Clarification, Coping Enhancement

### ➤ Interventions

Refer to *Disturbed Self-Concept* for interventions to improve self-concept.
Refer to *Health-Seeking Behaviors* for generic interventions.

# EFFECTIVE SELF-HEALTH MANAGEMENT: INDIVIDUAL

## DEFINITION (NANDA)

Individual: Pattern in which a person integrates into daily living a program for treatment of illness and its sequelae that is satisfactory for meeting health goals

## DEFINING CHARACTERISTICS (NANDA)

Appropriate choices of daily activities to meet the goals of a treatment or prevention program
Illness symptoms within a normal range of expectation

Verbalized desire to manage the treatment of illness and prevention of sequelae
Verbalized intent to reduce risk factors for progression of illness and sequelae

## RELATED FACTORS

Refer to Author's Note for an explanation.

### ■■■■■■ AUTHOR'S NOTE

*Effective Therapeutic Regimen Management* is the same as Readiness for Enhanced Self Health Management. Refer to Readiness for Enhanced Self-Health Management.

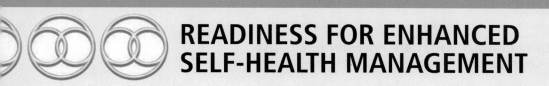

# READINESS FOR ENHANCED SELF-HEALTH MANAGEMENT

\* This diagnostic label was changed from Readiness for Enhanced Therapeutic Regimen Management by NANDA-I in 2008.

## DEFINING CHARACTERISTICS (NANDA)

- Expresses desire to manage the treatment of illness and prevention of sequelae.
- Choices of daily living are appropriate for meeting the goals of treatment or prevention.
- Expresses little to no difficulty with regulation/integration of one or more prescribed regimens for treatment of illness or prevention of complications.
- Describes reduction of risk factors for progression of illness and sequelae.
- No unexpected acceleration of illness symptoms.

### ■■■■■■ ERRORS IN DIAGNOSTIC STATEMENTS

**Readiness for Enhanced Self-Health Management related to internal locus of control**
This diagnosis does not need related factors, which would serve only to repeat characteristics of people who manage their conditions well (e.g., motivated, knowledgeable).

### ■■■■■■ KEY CONCEPTS

See *Ineffective Therapeutic Regimen Management*.

## Focus Assessment Criteria

### Subjective and Objective Data

#### Assess for Defining Characteristics

Is knowledgeable about:

- Illness/condition (severity, susceptibility to complications, prognosis, ability to cure it or control its progression)
- Treatment/diagnostic studies
- Preventive measures

Has a pattern of adherence to recommended health behaviors or regimen

Expresses a desire to increase ability to manage condition (progression, sequelae)

Reports that symptoms of condition are stable or diminished

For more information on Focus Assessment Criteria, visit http://thepoint.lww.com.

**NOC**
Compliance Behaviors, Knowledge: Treatment Regimen, Participation: Health Care Decisions, Risk Control

➤ ## Goal

The person will describe strategies to address progression or complications of condition should they arise.

### Indicators

• Discuss situations that can challenge continued successful management.
• Describe or demonstrate self-care techniques needed.

**NIC**
Behavior Modification, Mutual Goal Setting, Teaching: Individual, Decision-Making Support, Health System Guidance, Anticipatory Guidance

➤ ## General Interventions

### Discuss Possible Changes in Client's Condition that May Affect Illness and Usual Management

Exacerbation      Complications      Side effects of medication

### Advise Early Contact with Care Provider to Discuss Possible Changes in Management Regimen

**R:** The dynamic nature of chronic conditions necessitates knowledge of how to balance one's life to keep symptoms under control as much as possible (Lubin, 1995).

## Discuss How Increased Stress Can Negatively Affect Previous Successful Management and Possibly Decrease Resistance to Colds or Influenza

### Explore With Client His or Her Usual Level of Stress

Usual level of stress   Signs of overload

### Emphasize That Stress Accompanies Favorable and Unfavorable Life Events (e.g., Marriage, Divorce, Birth, Death, Vacations, Work)

Refer to *Stress Overload* for additional interventions.

**R:** Assisting the person to evaluate the effects of stress realistically can promote stress-reduction activities (Edelman & Mandle, 2005).

Refer to the Internet for resources and information on specific topics (e.g., amputation, diabetes mellitus).

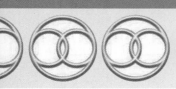

# READINESS FOR ENHANCED SLEEP

## DEFINITION

A pattern of natural, periodic suspension of consciousness that provides adequate rest, sustains a desired lifestyle and can be enhanced

## DEFINING CHARACTERISTICS

Amount of sleep is congruent with developmental needs

Expresses a feeling of being rested after sleep

Expresses willingness to enhance sleep

Follows sleep routines that promote sleep habits
Occasional use of medications to induce sleep

## ■■■■■■ KEY CONCEPTS

Refer to Health Promotion/Wellness Assessment under Elimination Pattern.

## Focus Assessment

Refer to Disturbed Sleep Pattern.

## Goals

The individual will report satisfactory sleep pattern.

### Indicators

Identify two new strategies (specify) to enhance sleep.

## Interventions

Refer to Disturbed Sleep patterns for strategies to promote sleep.

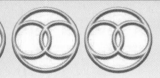

# READINESS FOR ENHANCED SPIRITUAL WELL-BEING

## DEFINITION

A person who experiences affirmation of life in a relationship with a higher power (as defined by the person), self, community, and environment that nurtures and celebrates wholeness

## DEFINING CHARACTERISTICS (CARSON, 1999)

- Inner strength that nurtures:
  - Sense of awareness
  - Inner peace
  - Sacred source
  - Unifying force
  - Trust relationships
- Intangible motivation and commitment directed toward ultimate values of love, meaning, hope, beauty, and truth.
- Trusts relations with or in the transcendent that provide bases for meaning and hope in life's experiences and love in one's relationships.
- Has meaning and purpose to existence.

## ■■■■■■ KEY CONCEPTS

- Growth in spirituality is a dynamic process in which an individual becomes increasingly aware of the meaning, purpose and values in life (Carson, 1999). Spiritual growth is a two-directional process: horizontal and vertical. The horizontal process increases the person's awareness of the transcendent values inherent in all relationships and activities of life (Carson, 1999). The vertical process moves the person into a closer relationship with

*(continued)*

■■■■■■■ **KEY CONCEPTS** *Continued*

a higher being, as conceived by the person. Carson illustrates that it is possible to develop spirituality through the horizontal process and not the vertical. For example, a person can define his or her spirituality in terms of relationships, art, or music without a relationship with a higher being, just as an individual can focus his or her spirituality on a higher being and may not express spirituality through other avenues.

- Faith is necessary for spiritual growth, particularly for a relationship to a higher being. Hope is also critical for spiritual development and integral to the horizontal and vertical processes (Carson, 1999).
- Research suggests that HIV-positive individuals who are spiritually well and who find meaning and purpose in life are also hardier (Carson & Green, 1992).
- Regardless of a person's religion or lack of belief in any, the process of spiritual growth is similar. The religious foundations that guide the growth are very different. When people are together on the level of spirituality, they meet on the level of the heart. On this level, all people are one. There is only one God, and it would seem logical that people's experiences of the transcendent would be similar. When the experiences are reframed into religious dogma, that is when disagreements begin (Carson, 1999).

Spirituality has been found especially important to caregivers of victims of chronic illness. Nurses can work to enhance spiritual well-being for them.

## Focus Assessment Criteria

Refer to Health Promotion/Wellness Assessment under Values–Beliefs Pattern.

**NOC**
Hope, Spiritual
Well-Being

➤ ## Goals

The person will express enhanced spiritual harmony and wholeness.

### *Indicators*

- Maintain previous relationship with higher being.
- Continue spiritual practices not detrimental to health.

**NIC**
Spiritual Growth
Facilitation, Spiritual
Support, Hope

➤ ## Interventions

Refer to the Internet for resources and information on spiritual health.
Refer to *Health-Seeking Behaviors* for additional generic interventions.

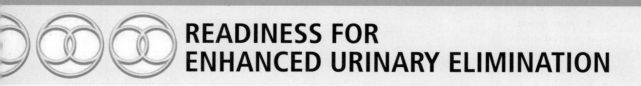

# READINESS FOR ENHANCED URINARY ELIMINATION

## DEFINITION (NANDA)

A pattern of urinary function that is sufficient for meeting eliminatory needs and can be strengthened

## DEFINING CHARACTERISTICS (NANDA)

- Expresses willingness to enhance urinary elimination.
- Urine is straw colored with no odor.
- Specific gravity is within normal limits.
- Amount of output is within normal limits for age and other factors.
- Positions self for emptying of bladder.
- Fluid intake is adequate for daily needs.

■■■■■■ **KEY CONCEPTS**

Refer to Health Promotion/Wellness Assessment under Elimination Pattern.

## Focus Assessment

Refer to *Impaired Urinary Elimination*.

**NOC**
Fluid Balance, Hydration, Electrolyte Balance

➤ ## Goals

The individual will report an increased balance in urinary elimination.

### *Indicators*

Identify two new strategies (specify) to enhance urinary elimination.

**NIC**
Education: Fluid/ Electrolyte

➤ ## Interventions

Refer to the Internet for resources and information on fluid balance:
- www.health.gov/dietaryguidelines
- www.seekwellness.com/wellness

See also *Health-Seeking Behaviors* for generic interventions.

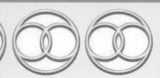

# STRESS OVERLOAD

## DEFINITION

State in which an individual or group experience overwhelming, excessive amounts and types of demands that require action

## DEFINING CHARACTERISTICS

### Physiologic

Headaches
Indigestion
Sleep difficulties
Restlessness
Fatigue

### Emotional

| | |
|---|---|
| Crying | Anger |
| Edginess | Impatience |
| Nervousness | Easily upset |
| Overwhelmed | Feeling sick |

### Cognitive

| | |
|---|---|
| Memory loss | Constant worry |
| Forgetfulness | Loss of humor |
| Difficulty making decisions | Trouble thinking clearly |

## Behavioral

| | |
|---|---|
| Isolation | Intolerance |
| Lack of intimacy | Compulsive eating |
| Excessive smoking | Resentment |

## RELATED FACTORS

The related factors for *Stress Overload* for one person can be multiple coexisting stressors that can be pathophysiologic, maturational, treatment related, situational, environmental, and/or personal.

### Pathophysiologic

Related to coping with:

- Acute illness (myocardial infarction, fractured hip)
- Chronic illness (arthritis, depression, COPD)
- Terminal illness
- New diagnosis (cancer, genital herpes, HIV, multiple sclerosis, diabetes mellitus)
- Disfiguring condition

### Situational (Personal, Environmental)

Related to actual or anticipated loss of a significant other secondary to:

| | |
|---|---|
| Death, dying | Moving |
| Divorce | Military duty |

Related to coping with:

| | |
|---|---|
| Dying | War |
| Assault | |

Related to actual or perceived change in socioeconomic status secondary to:

| | |
|---|---|
| Unemployment | New job |
| Promotion | Illness |
| Destruction of personal property | |

Related to coping with:

| | |
|---|---|
| Family violence | New family member |
| Substance abuse | Relationship problems |

### Maturation

Related to coping with:

| | |
|---|---|
| Retirement | Financial changes |
| Loss of residence | Functional losses |

■■■■■■ **AUTHOR'S NOTE**

This diagnosis represents a person in an overwhelming situation influenced by multiple varied stressors. If stress overload is not reduced, the person will deteriorate and is in danger of injury and illness.

■■■■■■ **KEY CONCEPTS**

Refer to *Anxiety* and *Ineffective Coping* for specific information on anxiety and ineffective coping.

- Stress is always present in all persons. Stress is the physical, psychological, social, or spiritual effect of life's pressures and events (Edelman & Mandle, 2006).
- Stress is an interactive process in response to the loss or threat of loss of homeostasis or well-being (Cahill, 2002).
- Stress is a psychological, emotional state experienced by an individual in response to a specific stressor or demand that results in harm, either temporary or permanent, to the person (Ridner, 2004, p. 539).

*(continued)*

■■■■■■ **KEY CONCEPTS** *Continued*

- Excessive stress requires recognition, perception and adaptation (Cadhill, 2001).
- A chronic state of stress or repeated episodes of psychological stress (depression, anger, hostility, anxiety) can lead to cardiovascular disease, arteriosclerosis, headaches, and gastrointestinal disorders (Edelman & Mandle, 2006).
- In response to stress, individuals initiate or increase unhealthy behaviors such as overeating, sedentary lifestyle, excessive use of drugs or alcohol, smoking, and social isolation (USDHHS, 2000).

## Focus Assessment

### Subjective/Objective

#### Ask Person to Rate His or Her Usual Level of Stress.

0 = little     10 = overwhelming

#### Ask Person to Describe How His or Her Stress Is Affecting the Ability to Function.

Work
Sleep
Relationships

#### Assess for Feelings of:

| | |
|---|---|
| Anger | Unhappiness |
| Impatience | Edginess |
| Despair | Boredom |
| Apathy | Easily upset |
| Lack of intimacy | Intolerance |

#### Assess for Cognitive Symptoms.

| | |
|---|---|
| Forgetfulness | Constant worry |
| Memory loss | Thoughts of abandonment |
| Difficulty making decisions | Loss of sense of humor |

#### Assess for Overuse of

| | |
|---|---|
| Sleep | Tobacco |
| Alcohol | Food |
| Drugs (prescription, street) | |

**NOC**
Well–Being: Health Beliefs; Anxiety Reduction; Coping; Knowledge: Health Promotion; Knowledge: Health Resources

## Goal

The person will verbalize intent to change two behaviors to decrease or manage stressors.

### Indicators

- Identify stressors that can be controlled and those that can not.
- Identify one successful behavior change to increase stress management.
- Identify one behavior to reduce or eliminate, to increase successful stress management.

**NIC**
Assist the Person to Appraise Their Present Stressors and Categorize Them as: Extrinsic (No Control); Intrinsic (Some Control)

## Interventions

**R:** Faced with overwhelming multiple stressors, the person can be assisted to differentiate which stressors can be modified or eliminated (Edelman & Mandel, 2006).

### Assist Them to Recognize Their Thoughts, Feelings, Actions, and Physiologic Responses.

**R:** Self-awareness can help the person reframe and reinterpret their experiences (Edelman & Mandle, 2006).

### Teach the Person How to Break the Cycle of Their Stress in a Traffic Jam and That There Are Increases in Heart Rate, Respirations, and Strong Feelings of Anger (Edelman & Mandle, 2006).

> Purposefully distract yourself by thinking of something pleasant.
> Engage in a diversional activity.
> Initiate relaxation breaking: inhale through nose, taking 4 seconds.
> Refer to resources to learn relaxation techniques such as audiotapes, printed material, yoga.

### Ask the Person to List One or Two Changes He or She Would Like to Make in the Next Week.

> Diet (eat one vegetable a day)
> Exercise (walk one to two blocks each day)
> **R:** In a person who is already overwhelmed, small changes in lifestyle may have a higher chance for success and will increase confidence (Bodenheimer, MacGregor, & Shariffi, 2005).

### If Sleep Disturbances Are Present, Refer to Insomnia.

> Ask what activity brings them feelings of peace, joy, and happiness. Ask them to incorporate one of these activities each week.
> **R:** Persons overwhelmed usually deny themselves such activities. Leisure can break the stress cycle (Wells-Federman, 2000).

### If Spiritual Needs Are Identified as Deficient, Refer to Spiritual Distress.

> Ask what is important, and if change is needed to include in life.
> **R:** Values clarification assists the overwhelmed person to identify what is meaningful and valued and if it is present in his or her actual living habits (Edelman & Mandle, 2006).

### Assist the Person to Set Realistic Goals to Achieve a More Balanced Health-Promoting Lifestyle (Wells-Federman, 2000).

> What is most important?
> What aspects of your life would you like to change most?
> What is the first step?
> When?
> **R:** Setting realistic goals with increase confidence and success (Bodenheimer, MacGregor, & Shariffi, 2005).

### Initiate Health Teaching and Referrals as Necessary.

> If person is engaged in substance or alcohol abuse, refer for drug and alcohol abuse.
> If person has severe depression or anxiety, refer for professional counseling.
> If family functioning is disabled, refer for family counseling.

# Manual of Collaborative Problems

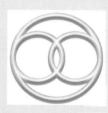

## Introduction

This Manual of Collaborative Problems presents 52 specific collaborative problems grouped under nine generic collaborative problem categories. Previously, collaborative problems have been labeled as *Potential Complication: (specify)* or *PC (specify)*. The terminology for collaborative problems has been revised in this edition to *Risk for Complications of (specify)* or *RC of (specify)*. These problems have been selected because of their high incidence or morbidity. Information on each generic collaborative problem is presented under the following subheads:

- Definition
- Author's Note: Discussion of the problem to clarify its clinical use
- Significant Laboratory/Diagnostic Assessment Criteria: Laboratory findings useful in monitoring

Discussions of the 52 specific collaborative problems cover the following information:

- Definition
- High-Risk Populations
- Nursing Goals: A statement specifying the nursing accountability for the collaborative problem. Indicators have been added to evaluate specific physiological status.
- General Interventions and Rationales: These specifically direct the nurse to:
  - Monitor for onset or early changes in status.
  - Initiate physician- or advanced practice nurse–prescribed interventions as indicated.
  - Initiate nurse-prescribed interventions as indicated.
  - Evaluate the effectiveness of these interventions.

A rationale statement in parentheses and italics explains why a sign or symptom is present or gives the scientific explanation for why an intervention produces the desired response. Keep in mind that for many of the collaborative problems in Section III, associated nursing diagnoses also can be predicted to be present. For example, a client with diabetes mellitus would receive care under the collaborative problem *RC of Hypo/Hyperglycemia* along with the nursing diagnosis *Risk for Ineffective Health Maintenance related to insufficient knowledge of (specify)*; a client with renal calculi would be under the collaborative problem *RC of Renal Calculi* and also the nursing diagnosis *Risk for Ineffective Self-Health Management related to insufficient knowledge of prevention of recurrence, dietary restrictions, and fluid requirements*.

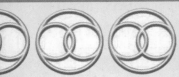

# RISK FOR COMPLICATIONS OF CARDIAC/VASCULAR DYSFUNCTION

Risk for Complications of Cardiac/Vascular Dysfunction

RC of Bleeding
RC of Decreased Cardiac Output
RC of Dysrhythmias
RC of Pulmonary Edema
RC of Deep Vein Thrombosis
RC of Hypovolemia
RC of Compartment Syndrome
RC of Pulmonary Embolism

## DEFINITION

Describes a person experiencing or at high risk to experience various cardiac and/or vascular dysfunctions

### ■■■■■ AUTHOR'S NOTE

The nurse can use this generic collaborative problem to describe a person at risk for several types of cardiovascular problems. For example, for a client in a critical care unit vulnerable to cardiovascular dysfunction, using *RC of Cardiac/Vascular Dysfunction* would direct nurses to monitor cardiovascular status for various problems, based on focus assessment findings. Nursing interventions for this client would focus on detecting and diagnosing abnormal functioning.

For a client with a specific cardiovascular complication, the nurse would add the applicable collaborative problem to the client's problem list, along with specific nursing interventions for that problem. For example, a Standard of Care for a client after myocardial infarction could contain the collaborative problem *RC of Cardiac/Vascular Dysfunction*, directing nurses to monitor cardiovascular status. If this client later experienced a dysrhythmia, the nurse would add *RC of Dysrhythmia* to the problem list, along with specific nursing management information (e.g., *RC of Dysrhythmia related to myocardial infarction*). When the risk factors or etiology is not directly related to the primary medical diagnosis, the nurse still should add them, if known (e.g., *RC of Hypo/Hyperglycemia related to diabetes mellitus* in a client who has sustained myocardial infarction).

For information on Focus Assessment Criteria, visit http://thepoint.lww.com.

## SIGNIFICANT LABORATORY/DIAGNOSTIC ASSESSMENT CRITERIA

Cardiac enzymes and proteins (Currently, the gross total values of CK, LDH, SGOT and or SGPT in the evaluation of cardiac injury are relatively low. Iso-enzymes or bands as well as troponins are the only ones usually used. Elevated with cardiac tissue damage [e.g., in myocardial infarction].)
Creatinine kinase (CK)
Creatinine phosphokinase, isoenzymes (e.g., CK-MB, CK-BB, CK-MM)
Creatinine kinase isoforms (CK-MB, CK-MM subforms)
Lactic dehydrogenase (LDH), isoenzymes
Myoglobin (troponin)
Brain–type natriuretic peptide (BNP) (hormones released as a peripheral response to cardiac impairment, e.g., heart failure)
C-reactive protein, P-selectin (markers of inflammation and necrosis)
Serum potassium (fluctuates with diuretic therapy, parenteral fluid replacement)
Serum calcium, magnesium, phosphate
White blood cell count (elevated with inflammation)
Erythrocyte sedimentation rate (elevated with inflammation, tissue injury)

Arterial blood gas (ABG) values (lowered $SaO_2$ indicates hypoxemia; elevated pH, alkalosis; lowered pH, acidosis)

Coagulation studies (elevated with anticoagulant and/or thrombolytic therapy or coagulopathies)

Hemoglobin and hematocrit (elevated with polycythemia, lowered with anemia)

Electrocardiograph with or without stress test

Doppler ultrasonic flow meter

Cardiac catheterization

Intravascular ultrasonography (IVU)

Electrophysiology studies

Computed tomography (CT), ultrafast computed tomography

Magnetic resonance imaging

Signal-averaged electrocardiography

Echocardiography with or without stress test

Phonocardiography

Exercise electrocardiography (ECG)

Perfusion imaging

Infarct imaging

Angiocardiography

Holter monitoring

Inflatable loop monitor

# ▶ Risk for Complications of Bleeding

## DEFINITION

Describes a person experiencing or at high risk to experience a decrease in blood volume

## HIGH-RISK POPULATIONS

- Intraoperative status
- Postoperative status

Post-procedural cannulation of any arterial vessel but particularly those at risk for retro-peritoneal bleed due to cannulation of femoral vessel

- Anaphylactic shock
- Trauma
- A history of bleeding disease or dysfunction
- Anticoagulant use, including over-the-counter use of aspirin or NSAIDs (nonsteroidal anti-inflammatory drugs)
- Chronic steroid use
- Acetaminophen use with associated liver dysfunction
- Anemia
- Liver disease
- Disseminated intravascular coagulation (DIC)
- Rupture of esophageal varices
- Dissecting aneurysms
- Trauma in pregnancy
- Pregnancy-related complications (Placenta previa, molar pregnancy, abruption placenta)

## Nursing Goals

The nurse will manage and minimize bleeding episodes.

*Indicators*

Refer to *Decreased Cardiac Output* for indicators

## General Interventions and Rationales

- Monitor fluid status; evaluate
  - Intake (parenteral and oral)
  - Output and other losses (urine, drainage, and vomiting), nasogastric tube *(Early detection of fluid deficit enables interventions to prevent shock.)*
- Monitor the surgical site for bleeding, dehiscence, and evisceration. *(Careful monitoring allows early detection of complications.)*
- Teach client to splint the surgical wound with a pillow when coughing, sneezing, or vomiting. *(Splinting reduces stress on suture line by equalizing pressure across the wound.)*
- Monitor for bleeding from esophageal varices

Hematemesis (vomiting blood)
Melena (black, sticky stools)
(Varices are delated tortuous veins in the lower esophagus. Portal hypertension caused by obstruction of the portal venous system from cirrhosis results in increased pressure on the vessels in the esophagus, making them fragile and at risk to bleed [Porth, 2007]).

- Test stools daily for occult blood if indicated. *(Signs of gastrointestinal bleeding may be detected early.)*
- If anticoagulant therapy, monitor for:

Bruises, nosebleeds
Bleeding gums
Hematuria
Severe headaches
Red or black stools (The prolonged clotting time of anticoagulants by anticoagulant therapy can cause spontaneous bleeding anywhere in the body. Hematuria is a common early sign.)

- Monitor for signs of bleeding with venous access devices e.g., IVs, long term venous access devices

Hematoma at site
Bleeding at site (Bleeding can occur several hours after insertion after blood pressure returns to normal and puts increased pressure on newly formed clot at the insertion site. It can also develop later, secondary to vascular erosion due infection)

- Monitor for bleeding during pregnancy and postpartum (refer to specific collaborative problems as *Risk for Complications of Placenta Previa*)
- Monitor for signs and symptoms of shock:
  - Increased pulse rate with normal or slightly decreased blood pressure, narrowing pulse pressure, decrease in mean or mean arterial pressure (MAP)
  - Urine output <5 mL/kg/h
  - Restlessness, agitation, decreased mentation
  - Increased respiratory rate, thirst
  - Diminished peripheral pulses
  - Cool, pale, moist, or cyanotic skin
  - Decreased oxygenation saturation ($SaO_2$, $SvO_2$), pulmonary artery pressures
  - Decreased hemoglobin/hematocrit, decreased cardiac output/index
  - Decreased central venous pressure
  - Decreased right atrial pressure
  - Decreased wedge pressure
  *(The compensatory response to decreased circulatory volume aims to increase oxygen delivery through increased heart and respiratory rates and decreased peripheral circulation [manifested by diminished peripheral pulses and cool skin]. Decreased oxygen to the brain alters mentation. Decreased circulation to the kidneys leads to decreased urine output. Hemoglobin and hematocrit values decline if bleeding is significant.)*
- If shock occurs, place client in the supine position unless contraindicated (e.g., head injury). *(This position increases blood return [preload] to the heart.)*

- Insert an IV line; use a large-bore catheter if blood replacement is anticipated. Initiate appropriate protocols for shock (e.g., vasopressor therapy). Refer also to *RC of Acidosis* or *RC of Alkalosis*, if indicated, for more information. *(Protocols aim to increase peripheral resistance and elevate blood pressure.)*
- Contact physician or advanced practice nurse with assessment data that may indicate bleeding. and to replace fluid losses at a rate sufficient to maintain urine output >0.5 mL/kg/h (e.g., saline or Ringer's lactate). *(This measure promotes optimal renal tissue perfusion.)*
- Restrict client's movement and activity. *(This helps decrease tissue demands for oxygen.)*
- Provide reassurance, simple explanations, and emotional support to help reduce anxiety. *(High anxiety increases metabolic demands for oxygen.)*
- Administer oxygen as ordered. (Diminished blood volume causes decreased circulating oxygen levels.)

# ▶ Risk for Complications of Decreased Cardiac Output

## DEFINITION

Describes a person experiencing or at high risk to experience inadequate blood supply for tissue & organ needs because of insufficient blood pumping by the heart

## HIGH-RISK POPULATIONS

Coronary artery disease (CAD) and its antecedents, including angina or the more preferred term acute coronary syndrome (ACS)

- Acute myocardial infarction
- Aortic or mitral valve disease with a murmur and/or history of rheumatic fever
- Cardiomyopathy
- Cardiac tamponade
- Hypothermia
- Septic shock
- Coarctation of the aorta
- Chronic obstructive pulmonary disease (COPD)
- Congenital heart disease
- Hypovolemia (e.g., due to severe bleeding or burns)
- Bradycardia
- Tachycardia
- Congestive heart failure
- Cardiogenic shock
- Hypertension

## Nursing Goals

The nurse will monitor and manage episodes of decreased cardiac output.

### Indicators:

Calm, alert, oriented
Oxygen saturation >95%
Normal sinus rhythm
No chest pain
No life-threatening dysrhythmias
Skin warm and dry
Usual skin color (appropriate for race)
Pulse: regular rhythm, rate 60–100 beats/min.
Respirations 16–20 breaths/min

Blood pressure >90/60, <140/90 mm Hg, MAP >70, or CVP >11
Urine output >5 mL/kg/h
Serum ph.7.35–7.45
Serum RCO$_2$ 35–45 mm Hg
SPO2 goals >95% for those without history of lung disease
Breath sounds without evidence of new, abnormal sounds (rales)
No presence of distended neck veins (JVD)

## General Interventions and Rationales

- Monitor for signs and symptoms of decreased cardiac output/index:
  - Increased, decreased, and/or irregular pulse rate
  - Increased respiratory rate
  - Decreased blood pressure, increased blood pressure
  - Abnormal heart sounds
  - Abnormal lung sounds (crackles, rales)
  - Decreased urine output (<5 mL/kg/hr)
  - Changes in mentation
  - Cool, moist, cyanotic, mottled skin
  - Delayed capillary refill time
  - Neck vein distention
  - Weak peripheral pulses
  - Abnormal pulmonary artery pressures
  - Abnormal renal artery pressures
  - Decreased mixed venous oxygen saturation
  - Electrocardiogram (ECG) changes
  - Dysrhythmias
  - Decreased SaO$_2$
  - Decreased (ScvO$_2$)

  *(Decreased cardiac output/index leads to insufficient oxygenated blood to meet the metabolic needs of tissues. Decreased circulating volume can result in hypoperfusion of the kidneys and decreased tissue perfusion with a compensatory response of decreased circulation to extremities and increased pulse and respiratory rates. Changes in mentation may result from cerebral hypoperfusion. Vasoconstriction and venous congestion in dependent areas [e.g., limbs] produce changes in skin and pulses.)*

- Initiate appropriate protocols or standing orders, depending on the underlying etiology of the problem affecting ventricular function. *(Nursing management differs based on etiology [e.g., measures to help increase preload for hypovolemia and to decrease preload for impaired ventricular contractility].)*
- Position the client with the legs elevated, unless ventricular function is impaired. *(This position can help increase preload and enhance cardiac output.)*
- During acute episodes, maintain absolute bed rest and minimize all controllable stressors. Administer IV morphine PRN according to protocol. (Morphine is the preferred agent in most cases.) Use with caution if client is hypotensive. *(These measures decrease metabolic demands.)*
- Assist client with measures to conserve strength, such as resting before and after activities (e.g., meals, baths). *(Adequate rest reduces oxygen consumption and decreases the risk of hypoxia.)*
- Monitor intake and output and weight. *(Changes can indicate fluid retention.)*
- In a client with impaired ventricular function, cautiously administer IV fluids. Consult with physician or advanced practice nurse if ordered rate exceeds 125 mL/h. Be sure to include any additional IV fluids (e.g., antibiotics) when calculating hourly allocation. *(A client with poorly functioning ventricles may not tolerate increased blood volumes.)*
- If decreased cardiac output results from hypovolemia, septic shock, or dysrhythmia, refer to the specific collaborative problem in this section.
- Administer inotropic and vasoactive agents (e.g., digoxin, dopamine, dobutamine) as prescribed to improve contractility.
- Assist with insertion and/or maintenance of mechanical cardiac assist devices as indicated (e.g., intraaortic balloon pumps, hemapump, ventricular assist devices).

## ▶ Risk for Complications of Dysrhythmias

## DEFINITION

Describes a person experiencing or at high risk to experience a disorder of the heart's conduction system that results in an abnormal heart rate, abnormal rhythm, or a combination of both

## HIGH-RISK POPULATIONS

A-type coronary artery disease (CAD):

- Angina
- Myocardial infarction (acute coronary syndrome [ACS])
- Congestive heart failure
- Hypoendocrine or hyperendocrine states
  Sepsis or severe sepsis/septic shock
- Increased intracranial pressure
- Electrolyte imbalance (calcium, potassium, magnesium, phosphorus)
- Atherosclerotic heart disease
- Medication side effects (e.g., aminophylline, dopamine, stimulants, digoxin, beta blockers, dobutamine, lidocaine, procainamide, quinidine, diuretics)
- COPD
- Cardiomyopathy, valvular heart disease
- Anemia
- Postoperative cardiac surgery
- Postoperative after any major anesthesia
- Trauma
- Sleep apnea

## Nursing Goals

The nurse will manage and minimize dysrhythmic episodes.

### Indicators

Refer to *Decreased Cardiac Output* indicators

## General Interventions and Rationales

- Monitor for signs and symptoms of dysrhythmias:
  - Abnormal rate, rhythm
  - Palpitations, chest pain, syncope, fatigue
  - Decreased $SaO_2$
  - ECG changes
  - Hypotension
  - Change in level of consciousness
  *(Ischemic tissue is electrically unstable, causing dysrhythmias. Certain congenital cardiac conditions, electrolyte imbalances, and medications also can cause disturbances in cardiac conduction.)*
- Initiate appropriate protocols depending on the type of dysrhythmia; this may include:
  - Supraventricular tachycardia: vagal stimulation (direct or indirect), IV calcium channel blockers, digoxin (IV), adenosine, diltiazem, adenocard, synchronized cardioversion, overdrive pacing
  - Atrial fibrillation: digitalization, electrical cardioversion, anticoagulant therapy
  - Premature ventricular contractions, ventricular tachycardia: IV lidocaine, IV procainamide, oxygen
  - Ventricular tachycardia: oxygen, lidocaine, procainamide, amiodarone, synchronized or unsynchronized cardioversion (dependent on presence of pulse)
  - Bradycardia or heart blocks: atropine, pacing, dopamine infusion, epinephrine infusion

- Ventricular fibrillation: cardiopulmonary resuscitation (CPR), defibrillation, epinephrine, lidocaine, bretylium
- Pulseless electrical activity: CPR, atropine (if rate bradycardic), epinephrine (diagnose and treat the cause)
- Asystole: CPR, epinephrine, atropine
- Administer supplemental oxygen *(It increases circulating oxygen levels and decreases cardiac workload.)*
- Monitor oxygen saturation ($SaO_2$) with pulse oximetry and ABGs as necessary.
- Monitor serum electrolyte levels (e.g., sodium, potassium, calcium, magnesium). *(High or low electrolyte levels may exacerbate a dysrhythmia.)*
- Monitor pacemaker and automatic implantable cardioverter (cardiac) defibrillator (AICD) therapy.

# ▶ Risk for Complications of Pulmonary Edema

## DEFINITION

Describes a person experiencing or at high risk to experience insufficient gas exchange because of accumulation of fluid related to left-sided heart failure or fluid overload

## HIGH-RISK POPULATIONS

- Hypertension
- Dysrhythmias
- Myocardial infarction
  - Acute cardiac syndrome (ACS)
  - Angina
- Congestive heart failure
- Cardiomyopathy
- Failed pacemaker, lead wires and/or generator
- Coronary artery disease
- Aortic or mitral cardiac valve disease
- Diabetes mellitus
- Inhalation of toxins
- Drug overdose
- Smoking
- Congenital heart defects
- Neurologic trauma

## Nursing Goals

The nurse will manage and minimize episodes of pulmonary edema.

### *Indicators*

Alert, calm, oriented
Symmetrical easy, rhythmic respirations
Warm, dry skin
Full breath sounds all lobes
No crackles and wheezing
Usual color (for race)
Refer to *RC of Decreased Cardiac Output* for additional indicators

## General Interventions and Rationales

- Monitor for signs and symptoms of pulmonary edema:
  - Dyspnea, cyanosis

- Tachypnea labored breathing
- Adventitious breath sounds, crackles
- Persistent cough or productive cough with frothy, pink-tinged sputum
- Abnormal ABGs
- Decreased $O_2$ saturation by pulse oximetry
- Decreased cardiac output/cardiac index
- Elevated pulmonary artery pressure
- Tachycardia
- Abnormal heart sounds ($S_3$)

Jugular vein distention (JVD)

*(Impaired pumping of left ventricle accompanied by decreased cardiac output and increased pulmonary venous pressure and pulmonary artery pressure produce pulmonary edema. Hypoxia produces increased capillary, causing fluid to enter pulmonary tissue and triggering signs and symptoms.)*

- If indicated, administer oxygen as prescribed.
- Initiate appropriate treatments according to protocol, which may include
  - Diuretics *(to decrease preload)*
  - Vasodilators *(to decrease preload & afterload)*
  - Positive inotropics (e.g., digitalis; *to enhance ventricular contractions)*
  - Morphine *(to decrease anxiety, preload and afterload, and metabolic demands)*
- Monitor urine parameters: specific gravity, intake/output, weight, and serum osmolality values. *(These values can help evaluate hydration.)*
- Take steps to maintain adequate hydration while avoiding overhydration. *(Adequate hydration helps liquefy pulmonary secretions; overhydration can increase preload and worsen pulmonary edema.)*
- Change client's position every 2 h with chest physical therapy. Determine which position provides optimum oxygenation by analyzing $PaO_2$ from pulse oximetry and/or ABG values with the client in various positions. *(Limiting time the client spends in positions that compromise oxygenation improves $PaO_2$.)*
- Place the client in high Fowler's position with legs dependent if dyspnea is severe. Encourage client to be out of bed and in a chair for meals. *(This positioning helps decrease venous return, increase venous pooling, and decrease preload.)*
- Encourage use of incentive spirometer, cough, and deep breathing every 2 h.
- Minimize controllable stressors (e.g., noise, long tests and procedures, strenuous activity); explain all procedures and treatments. *(These measures may reduce anxiety, which can help decrease metabolic demands.)*
- Continue monitoring cardiovascular status—vital signs & hemodynamic values, ABG values, cardiac output, fluid balance, weight, pulse oximeter, and urine output hourly. *(This monitoring helps evaluate response to treatment.)*

# ▶ Risk for Complications of Deep Vein Thrombosis

## DEFINITION

Describes a person experiencing venous clot formation because of blood stasis, vessel wall injury, or altered coagulation

## HIGH-RISK POPULATIONS (FETTERMAN & LEMBURG, 2004)

- Immobility >72 h
- Fractures (especially hip, pelvis & leg)
- Chemical irritation of vein
- Blood dyscrasias
- All major surgeries that involve general anesthesia and immobility in the operative course (pre-op, peri-op, and post-op combined), especially surgeries involving abdomen, pelvis & lower extremities.
- Orthopedic, urologic, or gynecologic surgery

- History of venous insufficiency
- Obesity
- Estrogen use (high dose)
- Cancer
- Heart failure
- Varicose veins
- Inflammatory bowel disease
- Pregnancy
- Severe COPD
- History of deep vein thrombosis (DVT) or pulmonary embolism
- Surgery greater than 30 min
- Over 40 years of age
- CVA
- MI
- Critical illness
- Indwelling central venous catheters
- Nephrotic syndrome

## Nursing Goals

The nurse will manage and minimize complications of DVT.

### Indicators

No leg pain
No leg edema
No pain with dorsiflexion of feet (Homans' sign)
No change in skin temperature or color

## General Interventions and Rationales

- Monitor the status of venous thrombosis, noting
  - Diminished or absent peripheral pulses (*Insufficient circulation causes pain and diminished peripheral pulses.*)
  - Unusual warmth and redness or coolness and cyanosis, increased leg swelling (*Unusual warmth and redness point to inflammation; coolness and cyanosis indicate vascular obstruction.*)
  - Increasing leg pain (*Leg pain results from tissue hypoxia.*)
  - Sudden, severe chest pain, increased dyspnea, tachypnea (*These findings may indicate mobilization of thrombi to the lungs.*)
  - Positive Homans' sign (*In a positive Homans' sign, dorsiflexion of the foot causes pain because of insufficient circulation.*)
  - Consult physician for use of below-knee antiembolic stockings or sequential pressure devices, low-dose dextran, or anticoagulant therapy for high-risk clients. (*These assist to reduce venous stasis.*)
- Refer to High-Risk Populations.
- Evaluate hydration status based on urine specific gravity, intake/output, weights, and serum osmolality. Take steps to ensure adequate hydration. (*Increased blood viscosity and coagulability and decreased cardiac output may contribute to thrombus formation.*)
- Encourage client to perform isotonic leg exercises. (*They promote venous return.*)
- Ambulate as soon as possible with at least 5 min of walking each waking hour. Avoid prolonged chair sitting with legs dependent. (*Walking contracts leg muscles, stimulates the venous pump, and reduces stasis.*)
- Elevate the affected extremity above the level of the heart. (*This positioning can help reduce interstitial swelling by promoting venous return.*)
- Discourage smoking. (*Nicotine can cause vasospasms.*)
- Administer anticoagulant therapy as the physician or advanced practice nurse prescribes, and monitor blood coagulation results daily. (*Anticoagulant therapy prevents extension of a thrombosis by delaying the clotting time of blood.*)
- For a client receiving anticoagulant therapy, monitor for early signs of abnormal bleeding (e.g., hematuria, bleeding gums, ecchymoses, petechiae, epistaxis). (*Prolonged clotting time can increase the risk of bleeding.*)

- Administer analgesics for leg pain as prescribed.
- Explain the importance of external compression devices (graded compression below-knee elastic stockings, sequential compression/decompression stockings [SCDs], intermittent external pneumatic compression [IERC] impulse boots). *(Venous return is increased; pooling is decreased. IRC and impulse boots increase the rate and velocity of venous flow and decrease hypercoagulability [Morton et al., 2005].)*

# ▶ Risk for Complications of Hypovolemia

## DEFINITION

Describes a person experiencing or at high risk to experience inadequate cellular oxygenation and inability to excrete waste products of metabolism secondary to decreased fluid volume (e.g., from bleeding, plasma loss, prolonged vomiting, or diarrhea)

## HIGH-RISK POPULATIONS

- Intraoperative status
- Postoperative status

Post-procedural cannulation of any arterial vessel but particularly those at risk for retro-peritoneal bleed due to cannulation of femoral vessel

- Anaphylactic shock
- Trauma
- Bleeding

A history of bleeding disease or dysfunction
Anticoagulant use, including over-the-counter use of aspirin or NSAIDs (nonsteroidal anti-inflammatory drugs)
Chronic steroid use
Acetaminophen with associated liver dysfunction
Anemia
Liver disease

- Diabetic ketoacidosis (DKA) or Hyperosmolar Hyperglycemic State (HHS) (Kitabchi, Haerian, & Rose, 2008)
- Prolonged vomiting or diarrhea
- Infants, children, elderly
- Acute pancreatitis
- Major burns
- Disseminated intravascular coagulation (DIC)
- Rupture of esophageal varices
- Dissecting aneurysms
- Prolonged pregnancy
- Trauma in pregnancy
- Diabetes insipidus
- Ascites
- Peritonitis
- Intestinal obstruction
- Sepsis (Bridges & Dukes, 2005)

## Nursing Goals

The nurse will manage and minimize hypovolemic episodes.

*Indicators*

Refer to *RC of Decreased Cardiac Output* for indicators

## General Interventions and Rationales

- Monitor fluid status; evaluate
- Intake (parenteral and oral)
- Output and other losses (urine, drainage, and vomiting), nasogastric tube *(Early detection of fluid deficit enables interventions to prevent shock.)*
- Monitor the surgical site for bleeding, dehiscence, and evisceration. *(Careful monitoring allows early detection of complications.)*
- Teach client to splint the surgical wound with a pillow when coughing, sneezing, or vomiting. *(Splinting reduces stress on suture line by equalizing pressure across the wound.)*
- Monitor for signs and symptoms of shock:
  - Increased pulse rate with normal or slightly decreased blood pressure, narrowing pulse pressure, decrease in mean or mean arterial pressure (MAP)
  - Urine output <5 mL/kg/h
  - Restlessness, agitation, decreased mentation
  - Increased respiratory rate, thirst
  - Diminished peripheral pulses
  - Cool, pale, moist, or cyanotic skin
  - Decreased oxygenation saturation ($SaO_2$, $SvO_2$), pulmonary artery pressures
  - Decreased hemoglobin/hematocrit, decreased cardiac output/index
  - Decreased central venous pressure
  - Decreased right atrial pressure
  - Decreased wedge pressure

  *(The compensatory response to decreased circulatory volume aims to increase oxygen delivery through increased heart and respiratory rates and decreased peripheral circulation [manifested by diminished peripheral pulses and cool skin]. Decreased oxygen to the brain alters mentation. Decreased circulation to the kidneys leads to decreased urine output. Hemoglobin and hematocrit values decline if bleeding is significant.)*
- If shock occurs, place client in the supine position unless contraindicated (e.g., head injury). *(This position increases blood return [preload] to the heart.)*
- Insert an IV line; use a large-bore catheter if blood replacement is anticipated. Initiate appropriate protocols for shock (e.g., vasopressor therapy). Refer also to *RC of Acidosis* or *RC of Alkalosis*, if indicated, for more information. *(Protocols aim to increase peripheral resistance and elevate blood pressure.)*
- Collaborate with physician or advanced practice nurse to replace fluid losses at a rate sufficient to maintain urine output >0.5 mL/kg/h (e.g., saline or Ringer's lactate). *(This measure promotes optimal renal tissue perfusion.)*
- Restrict client's movement and activity. *(This helps decrease tissue demands for oxygen.)*
- Provide reassurance, simple explanations, and emotional support to help reduce anxiety. *(High anxiety increases metabolic demands for oxygen.)*
- Administer oxygen as ordered.

# ▶ Risk for Complications of Compartment Syndrome

## DEFINITION

Describes a person experiencing increased pressure in a limited space, such as a fascial envelope, which compromises circulation and function, usually in the forearm or leg (Morton et al., 2005). Risk factors can either cause internal compression or external compression (Tumbarello, 2000).

## HIGH-RISK POPULATIONS

### Internal Factors

- Fractures
- Musculoskeletal surgery
- Injuries (crush, electrical, vascular)
- Allergic response (snake, insect bites)
- Excessive edema
- Thermal injuries
- Vascular obstruction
- Intramuscular bleeding

### External Factors

Extravasation of IV fluids
Procedural cannulation of vessel for diagnostic or interventional reasons

- Casts
- Prolonged use of tourniquet
- Tight dressings
- Tight closure of fascial detects
- Positioning during surgery
- Lying on limb for extended periods

## Nursing Goals

The nurse will manage and minimize compartment syndrome.

### Indicators

Pedal pulses 2+, equal
Capillary refill <3 sec
Warm extremities
No complaints of paresthesia (numbness), tingling
Minimal swelling
Ability to move toes or fingers

## General Interventions and Rationales

- Refer to nursing diagnosis *Risk for Peripheral Neurovascular Dysfunction* for specific extremity assessment techniques and prevention of compartment syndrome.
- Monitor for signs of compartment syndrome:

*Early Signs*
- Unrelieved or increasing pain
- Pain with passive stretch movement or flexion of toes or fingers
- Mottled or cyanotic skin
- Excessive swelling
- Delay in capillary refill
- Paresthesia
- Inability to move toes or fingers

*(Pain and paresthesia indicate compression of nerves and increasing pressure within muscle compartment. Passive stretching of muscles decreases muscle compartment, thus increasing pain. Delayed capillary refill or mottled or cyanotic skin indicates obstructed capillary blood flow.)*

*Late Signs*
- Pallor
- Diminished or absent pulse
- Cold skin

*(Arterial occlusion produces these late signs.)*

- Assess neurovascular function at least every hour for first 24 h. *(Peripheral neurovascular compromise may be the first sign [Tumbarello, 2000].)*
- Instruct client to report unusual, new, or different sensations (e.g., tingling, numbness, and/or decreased ability to move toes or fingers). *(Early detection of compromise can prevent serious impairment [Pellino et al., 1998; Morton et al., 2006].)*
- If signs of compartment syndrome occur, notify physician or advanced practice nurse and
  - Discontinue elevation and ice applications.
  - Loosen circumferential dressings, splints, casts per protocol. *(Elevation will impede perfusion.)*
- If invasive compartment monitoring system is used, follow procedure for use.
- Monitor and document compartment pressures according to protocol. Report elevated pressures promptly.
- Carefully maintain hydration. *(Hypovolemia can result from fluid volume shift.)*
- Evaluate cardiovascular and renal status; pulse, respiration, blood pressure and urine output. *(Eight liters of fluid can extravasate into a limb, causing hypovolemia, decreased renal function, and shock [Pellino et al., 1998].)*
- Notify the physician or advanced practice nurse of any early signs and symptoms of neurovascular compromise. *(The physician or advanced practice nurse will evaluate the cause and determine the necessary treatment, such as cast-splitting, removal of medical antishock trousers [MAST], removal of intraaortic balloon pump, surgery [e.g., fasciotomy].)*

# ▶ Risk for Complications of Pulmonary Embolism

## DEFINITION

Describes a person experiencing or at high risk to experience obstruction of one or more pulmonary arteries from a blood clot or air or fat embolus

## HIGH-RISK POPULATIONS

- Infection
- Prolonged immobilization
- Prolonged sitting/traveling
- Varicose veins
- Vascular injury
- Tumor
- Increased platelet count (e.g., from polycythemia, splenectomy)
- Thrombophlebitis
- Vascular disease
- Presence of foreign bodies (e.g., IV or central venous catheters)
- Heart disease (especially congestive heart failure)
- Surgery or trauma (especially of hip, pelvis, spine, lower extremities)
- Postoperative state
- Pregnancy
- Postpartum state
- Diabetes
- COPD
- History of previous pulmonary embolism or thrombophlebitis
- Smoking
- Obesity
- Oral contraceptive use, estrogen therapy
- Leg, pelvic fractures, injuries

- Increased coagulability (e.g., cancer)
- Sickle cell disease
- Thermal injuries
- Polycythemia
- Acute spinal cord injury
- Thrombus formation in heart from cardioversion, bacterial endocarditis, atrial fibrillation, or myocardial infarction
- Greater than 40 years old (Shaughnessy, 2007)
- Presence of venous thromboembolism (VTE) (Shaughnessy, 2007)
- For air embolism
  - Central line insertion or removal, sheaths
  - Central line tubing changes, manipulation, or disconnection

## Nursing Goals

The nurse will manage and minimize complications of pulmonary embolism.

### Indicators

No change in mentation or anxiety (Shaughnessy, 2007)
No chest pain
No dyspnea
Heart rate & respiratory rate within range for individual (Shaughnessy, 2007)
Normal sinus rhythm
Temperature, 98–99.5° F
No hemoptysis (Shaughnessy, 2007)

## General Interventions and Rationales

Screen for prevention and institute prophylaxis per protocol

- Consult with physician or advanced practice nurse for low-dose heparin therapy for a high-risk client until ambulatory (see Anticoagulant Therapy in RC of Medication Therapy Adverse Effects). *(Heparin therapy decreases platelet adhesiveness, reducing the risk of embolism.)*
- Refer to the nursing diagnosis *Risk for Ineffective Peripheral Tissue Perfusion* in Section II for information on preventing DVT.
- Monitor for signs and symptoms of pulmonary embolism:
  - Acute, sharp chest pain
  - Dyspnea, restlessness, cyanosis, decreased mental status or anxiety
  - Decreased oxygen saturation ($SaO_2$, $SvO_2$)
  - Tachycardia
  - Tachypnea (Shaughnessy, 2007)
  - Neck vein distention
  - Hypotension
  - Acute right ventricular dilation without parenchymal disease (on chest x-ray)
  - Confusion
  - Cardiac dysrhythmias (can be lethal)
  - Low-grade fever
  - Productive cough with blood-tinged sputum
  - Pleural friction rub or new murmur (Shaughnessy, 2007)
  - Crackles
  *(Occlusion of pulmonary arteries impedes blood flow to the distal lung, producing a hypoxic state.)*
- If these manifestations occur, promptly initiate protocols for shock.
  - Establish an IV line (for medication and fluid administration).
  - Administer fluid replacement therapy according to protocol.
  - Insert indwelling urinary (Foley) catheter (to monitor circulatory volume through urine output).
  - Initiate ECG monitoring and invasive hemodynamic monitoring (to detect dysrhythmias and guide therapy).

- Administer vasopressors to increase peripheral resistance and raise blood pressure.
- Administer digitalis glycosides and IV diuretics and antiarrhythmic agents, as indicated.
- Administer small IV doses of morphine (to reduce anxiety and decrease metabolic demands).
- Refer to *RC of Hypovolemic Shock* for additional interventions.
- Prepare for angiography and/or perfusion lung scans (to confirm diagnosis and detect the extent of atelectasis).

*(Because death from massive pulmonary embolism commonly occurs in the first 2 h after onset, prompt intervention is crucial.)*

- Initiate oxygen therapy; monitor oxygen saturation. *(This measure rapidly increases circulating oxygen levels.)*
- Monitor serum electrolyte levels, ABG values, blood urea nitrogen, and complete blood count results. *(These laboratory tests help determine perfusion and volume status.)*
  *Monitor D-Dimer & chest x-ray (aids in diagnosis) (Shaughnessy, 2007)*
- Initiate thrombolytic therapy (e.g., urokinase, streptokinase) per orders. *(Thrombolytics can cause lysis of emboli and increase pulmonary capillary perfusion.)*
- When prescribed after thrombolytic infusion, initiate heparin therapy (continuous IV infusion or intermittent). Monitor clotting times during heparin therapy. *(Heparin can slow or halt the underlying thrombotic process, helping prevent clot extension or recurrence.)*
- For a client receiving thrombolytics and/or anticoagulant therapy, monitor for signs of abnormal bleeding (e.g., hematuria, bleeding gums, ecchymosis, petechiae, epistaxis).

## For Air Embolism

- Before central line catheter insertion and tubing changes, place client in Trendelenburg's position and instruct him or her to perform Valsalva maneuver during the procedure. *(These measures increase intrathoracic pressure and help prevent air from entering the catheter.)*
- Follow instruction policies for central lines.
- Before central venous catheter, pulmonary artery catheter or transvenous pacing wire removal, place client in Trendelenburg's position and instruct to perform Valsalva maneuver or at least hold breath during the procedure. If spontaneously breathing, remove catheter during breath holding or expiration; if mechanically ventilated, remove during inspiratory phase of respiratory cycle (Lynn-McHale Wiegand & Carlson, 2005). After removal, immediately apply direct pressure to the catheterization site, and then apply a sterile nonpermeable dressing. Leave dressing in place for 24 to 48 h. *(These measures help prevent air entry.)*
- Monitor for signs and symptoms of air embolism during dressing and IV tubing changes and after any accidental separation of IV connections:
  - Sucking sound on insertion
  - Dyspnea
  - Tachypnea
  - Wheezing
  - Substernal chest pain
  - Anxiety

*(Air embolism can occur with IV tubing changes, with accidental tubing separation, and during catheter insertion, removal and disconnection. [For example, a client can aspirate as much as 200 mL of air from a deep breath during subclavian line disconnection.] Entry of air into the pulmonary arterial system can obstruct blood flow, causing bronchoconstriction of the affected lung area.)*

- If air embolism is suspected
  - Place client in steep Trendelenburg's position on left side. *(This position displaces air away from pulmonary valve and prevents more air from entering.)*
  - Administer oxygen through face mask according to protocol. *(This promotes diffusion of nitrogen, which compresses an air embolism in about 80% of cases.)*
  - Initiate protocols for respiratory or cardiac arrest if indicated.

## For RC of Fat Embolism

- Monitor for sign and symptoms of fat embolism:
  - Tachypnea more than 30/min

- Sudden onset of chest pain or dyspnea
- Restlessness, apprehension
- Confusion
- Elevated temperature above 103° F
- Increased pulse rate more than 140/min
- Petechial skin rash (12 to 96 h postoperative)

*(These changes are the result of hypoxemia. Fatty acids attack red blood cells and platelets to form microaggregates, which impair circulation to vital organs, such as the brain. Fatty globules passing through the pulmonary vasculature cause a chemical reaction that decreases lung compliance and ventilation/perfusion ratio and raises body temperature. Rash results from capillary fragility. Common sites are conjunctiva, axilla, chest, and neck [Pellino et al., 1998].)*

- Minimize movement of a fractured extremity for the first 3 days after the injury. *(Immobilization minimizes further tissue trauma and reduces the risk of embolism dislodgement [Pellino et al., 1998].)*
- Ensure adequate hydration. *(Optimal hydration dilutes the irritating fatty acids through the system [Pellino et al., 1998].)*
- Monitor intake/output, urine color, and specific gravity. *(These data reflect hydration status.)*

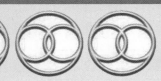

# RISK FOR COMPLICATIONS OF RESPIRATORY DYSFUNCTION

**Risk for Complications of Respiratory Dysfunction**

RC of Hypoxemia
RC of Atelectasis, Pneumonia
RC of Tracheobronchial Constriction
RC of Pneumothorax

## DEFINITION

Respiratory Dysfunction:
Describes a person experiencing or at high risk to experience various respiratory problems

### ■■■■■ AUTHOR'S NOTE

The nurse uses the generic collaborative problem *RC of Respiratory Dysfunction* to describe a person at risk for several types of respiratory problems and to identify the nursing focus—monitoring respiratory status for detection and diagnosis of abnormal functioning. Nursing management of a specific respiratory complication is then described under the appropriate collaborative problem for that complication. For example, a nurse using *RC of Respiratory Dysfunction* for a client in whom hypoxemia later develops would then add *RC of Hypoxemia* to the client's problem list. If the risk factors or etiology were not related directly to the primary medical diagnosis, the nurse would add this information to the diagnostic statement (e.g. *RC of Hypoxemia related to COPD* in a client with chronic obstructive pulmonary disease [COPD] who experiences respiratory problems after gastric surgery).

For a person vulnerable to respiratory problems because of immobility or excessive tenacious secretions, the nurse should apply the nursing diagnosis *Risk for Ineffective Respiratory Function related to immobility* rather than *RC of Respiratory Dysfunction*.

For information on Focus Assessment Criteria, visit http://thepoint.lww.com.

## SIGNIFICANT LABORATORY/DIAGNOSTIC ASSESSMENT CRITERIA

Blood pH (elevated in alkalosis, lowered in acidosis)

Arterial blood gas (ABG) values:

- pH (elevated in alkalemia, lowered in acidemia) (more commonly referred to as alkalosis and or acidosis)
- $PCO_2$ (elevated in pulmonary disease, lowered in hyperventilation)
- $PO_2$ (lowered in pulmonary disease)
- $CO_2$ content (elevated in COPD, lowered in hyperventilation)

Sputum stain and culture
Chest x-ray
Pulmonary angiography
Bronchoscopy
Thoracentesis
Pulmonary function tests
Ventilation/perfusion scanning
Pulse oximetry
End-tidal carbon monitoring ($ETCO_2$)

# ▶ Risk for Complications of Hypoxemia

## DEFINITION

Describes a person experiencing or at high risk to experience insufficient plasma oxygen saturation ($PO_2$ less than normal for age) because of alveolar hypoventilation, pulmonary shunting, or ventilation–perfusion inequality

## HIGH-RISK POPULATIONS

- COPD
- Pneumonia
- Atelectasis
- Pulmonary edema
- Adult respiratory distress syndrome
- Central nervous system depression
- Medulla or spinal cord disorders
- Guillain-Barré syndrome
- Myasthenia gravis
- Muscular dystrophy
- Obesity
- Compromised chest wall movement (e.g., trauma)
- Drug overdose
- Head injury
- Near-drowning
- Multiple trauma
- Anemia and/or hypovolemia
- Pulmonary embolism

## Nursing Goals

The nurse will manage and minimize complications of hypoxemia.

### Indicators

Serum pH 7.35–7.45
$PaCO_2$ 35-45

$PaO_2$ 80-100
Pulse: regular rhythm, rate 60–100 beats/min
Respirations 16–20 breaths/min.
Blood pressure<140/90, >90/60 mmHg (MAP [mean arterial pressure] >70) (CVP >11)
Urine output >30 mL/h (use of a standardized volume that is weight based, i.e., >5 mL/kg/h)

# General Interventions and Rationales

- Monitor for signs of acid–base imbalance:
  - ABG analysis: pH < 7.35, $PaCO_2$ > 48 mm Hg *(ABG analysis helps evaluate gas exchange in the lungs. In mild to moderate COPD, the client may have a normal $PaCO_2$ level as chemoreceptors in the medulla respond to increased PaCO2 by increasing ventilation. In severe COPD, however, the client cannot sustain this increased ventilation, and the PaCO2 value gradually increases.)*
  - Increased and irregular pulse, and increased respiratory rate initially, followed by decreased rate. *(Respiratory acidosis develops as a result of excessive $CO_2$ retention. A client with respiratory acidosis from chronic disease at first experiences increased heart rate and respirations in an attempt to compensate for decreased oxygenation. After a while, the client breathes more slowly and with prolonged expiration. Eventually, the respiratory center may stop responding to the higher $CO_2$ levels, and breathing may stop abruptly.)*
  - Changes in mentation (somnolence, confusion, irritability, anxiety). *(Changes in mentation result from cerebral tissue hypoxia.)*
  - Decreased urine output (<5 mL/kg/h); cool, pale, or cyanotic skin. *(The compensatory response to decreased circulatory oxygen aims to increase blood oxygen by increasing heart and respiratory rates and to decrease circulation to the kidneys and extremities [marked by decreased pulses and skin changes].)*
- Administer low-flow (2 L/min) oxygen as needed through nasal cannula, if indicated. *(Oxygen therapy increases circulating oxygen levels. High flow rates increase $CO_2$ retention in people with COPD. Using a cannula rather than a mask may help reduce the client's fears of suffocation.)*
- Evaluate the effects of positioning on oxygenation, using ABG values as a guide. Change client's position every 2 h, avoiding positions that compromise oxygenation. *(This measure promotes optimal ventilation.)*
- Ensure adequate hydration. Teach client to avoid dehydrating beverages (e.g., caffeinated drinks, grapefruit juice). *(Optimal hydration helps liquefy secretions. Avoid milk-based products.)*
- Teach client effective coughing technique. *(Effective coughing moves mucus from the lower airways to the trachea for expectoration.)*
- If client cannot expectorate secretions, use coughing, chest physiotherapy, or both to move secretions up from the trachea for suctioning. *(Suctioning is effective only at the tracheal level.)*
- Administer supplemental oxygen before and after suctioning. *(This measure helps prevent decreased $PO_2$ as a result of suctioning.)*
- Obtain a sputum sample for culture and sensitivity and Gram stain testing. *(Sputum culture and sensitivity determine whether an infection is contributing to symptoms.)*
- Eliminate smoke and strong odors from the client's room. *(Irritation of the respiratory tract can exacerbate symptoms.)*
- Monitor the electrocardiogram for dysrhythmias secondary to altered oxygenation. *(Hypoxemia may precipitate cardiac dysrhythmias.)*
- Monitor for signs of right-sided congestive heart failure:
  - Elevated diastolic pressure
  - Distended neck veins
  - Edema
  - Elevated central venous pressure
  *(The combination of arterial hypoxemia and respiratory acidosis acts locally as a strong vasoconstrictor of pulmonary vessels. This leads to pulmonary arterial hypertension, increased right ventricular systolic pressure, and, eventually, right ventricular hypertrophy and failure.)*
- Refer to the nursing diagnosis *Activity Intolerance* in Section II for specific adaptive techniques to teach a client with chronic pulmonary insufficiency.

# ▶ Risk for Complications of **Atelectasis, Pneumonia**

## DEFINITION

Describes a person experiencing impaired respiratory functioning because of alveolar collapse, which can result in pneumonia*

## HIGH-RISK POPULATIONS

- Pulmonary edema
- Postoperative status (especially abdominal or thoracic surgery)
- Immobilization
- Decreased level of consciousness
- Nasogastric feedings
- Chronic lung disease (COPD, bronchiectasis, cystic fibrosis)
- Debilitation
- Decreased surfactant production
- Compression of lung tissue (e.g., from cancer, abdominal distention, obesity, pneumothorax)
- Airway obstruction

## Nursing Goals

The nurse will manage and minimize complications of atelectasis or pneumonia.

### Indicators

Alert, calm, oriented
Respiratory rate 16–20 breaths/min
Respirations easy, rhythmic
No change in usual skin color
(Inclusion of pulse oximetry values for those with and without a history of lung disease as well as ETCO$_2$)

## General Interventions and Rationales

- Monitor respiratory status and assess for signs and symptoms of inflammation:
  - Increased respiratory rate (tachypnea)
  - Fever and chills (sudden or insidious)
  - Productive cough
  - Diminished or absent breath sounds, rales or crackles (Ellstrom, 2006)
  - Pleuritic chest pain
  - Tachycardia
  - Marked dyspnea
  - Cyanosis
  - Lethargy

  *(Tracheobronchial inflammation, impaired alveolar capillary membrane function, edema, fever, and increased sputum production disrupt respiratory function and compromise the blood's oxygen-carrying capacity. Reduced chest wall compliance in older adults affects the quality of respiratory effort. In older adults, tachypnea [>26 respirations/min] is an early sign of pneumonia, often occurring 3 to 4 days before a confirmed diagnosis. Delirium or mental status changes are often seen early in pneumonia in older adults [Porth, 2007; Morton et al., 2006].)*

- Monitor for signs and symptoms of infection:
  - Fever of 101° F (39.4° C) or higher

---

*The nurse should use the nursing diagnosis *Risk for Ineffective Respiratory Function* for people at high risk for atelectasis and pneumonia, to focus on prevention. The collaborative problem *RC of Atelectasis, Pneumonia* is applicable only if the condition occurs.

- Chills
- Tachycardia
- *Manifestations of shock: restlessness or lethargy, confusion, decreased systolic blood pressure*

(*Endogenous pyrogens are released and reset the hypothalamic set point to febrile levels. The body temperature is sensed as "too cool"; shivering and vasoconstriction result to generate and consume heat. Core temperature rises to the new level of the set point, resulting in fever. White blood cells are released to destroy some pathogens. The impaired respiratory system cannot compensate; tissue hypoxia results [Porth, 2007; Morton et al., 2006].*)

- If fever occurs, provide cooling measures (e.g., reduced clothing and bed linen, tepid baths, increased fluids, hypothermia blanket). (*Reducing body temperature is necessary to lower metabolic rate and reduce oxygen consumption.*)
- Monitor for signs and symptoms of septic shock:
  - Altered body temperature (>38° C or <36° C)
  - Hypotension (/90, >90/60 mm Hg (MAP [mean arterial pressure] >70) (CVP >11)
  - Decreased level of consciousness
  - Weak, rapid pulse
  - Rapid, shallow respirations or $CO_2 < 32$

(Diminishing oxygen saturation as seen by pulse oximetry)

  - Cold, clammy skin
  - Oliguria (urine output < 5 mL/kg/h)

(*Septic shock is a systemic inflammatory response syndrome [SIRS] associated with infection because of microorganisms resulting in hypotension and perfusion abnormalities despite fluid resuscitation or vasopressors.*)

- Evaluate the effectiveness of cough suppressants and expectorants. (*A dry, hacking cough interferes with sleep and affects energy. Cough suppressants should be used judiciously, however, because complete depression of the cough reflex can lead to atelectasis by hindering movement of tracheobronchial secretions.*)
- Maintain oxygen therapy, as prescribed, and monitor its effectiveness. (*Oxygen therapy may help prevent dyspnea and also reduce the risk of pulmonary edema.*)
- Provide respiratory physiotherapy (e.g., chest percussion, postural drainage) to move thick, tenacious secretions along the tracheobronchial tree. (*Exudate in the alveoli and bronchospasms linked to increased bronchopulmonary secretions can decrease ventilatory effort and impair gas exchange.*)
- Teach client how to do diaphragmatic breathing. (*This technique increases tidal volume by maximizing diaphragmatic descent.*)
- Refer to *RC of Hypoxemia* for additional interventions.

(If intubated, use of the ventilator acquired pneumonia [VAP] bundle interventions for prevention of VAP) Elevation of the head of the bed 30 degrees at all times, mouth care every 2 h, DVT and PUD prophylaxis, percussion, vibration and lateral rotation.

# ▶ Risk for Complications of Tracheobronchial Constriction

## DEFINITION

Describes a person experiencing or at high risk to experience air flow limitations through the tracheobronchial tree because of asthma, bronchitis, emphysema, and/or allergic reaction

## HIGH-RISK POPULATIONS

- COPD
- Allergies
- Asthma
- Chronic bronchitis
- Viral infections (<6 months of age)
- Cystic fibrosis

## Nursing Goals

The nurse will manage and minimize episodes of tracheobronchial constriction.

### Indicators

Refer to RC of Hypoxemia for indicators

## General Interventions and Rationales

- Monitor respiratory status continuously during acute exacerbation; evaluate:
  - Use of accessory muscles
  - Respiratory rate, pulse rate, blood pressure
  - Breath sounds (e.g., wheezing) (stridor)
  - ABG values
  - Peripheral perfusion (skin color, pulses)
  - Level of consciousness

  *(A client's respiratory status can change rapidly, with specific changes depending on response to treatments, level of fatigue, and severity of the episode.)*
- Administer oxygen through nasal cannula at 2 to 3 L/min. *(Oxygen therapy reduces hypoxemic effects; cannula rather than mask may help minimize feelings of suffocation.)*
- Ensure adequate hydration either orally or intravenously. *(Good hydration status helps prevent tenacious, impacted mucus.)*
- During acute episodes, stay with client and have him or her breathe using pursed-lip or diaphragmatic breathing. *(A panicky, dyspneic client needs a nurse's constant presence to help gain control over his or her breathing.)*
- Maintain client in upright position. *(It promotes optimal lung expansion.)*
- Initiate interventions as prescribed by physician or advanced practice nurse, which may include anti-inflammatory agents, $\beta_2$-agonists, theophylline preparations, or corticosteroids (systemic or inhaled).
- Consult with physician or advanced practice nurse for possible intubation if work of breathing becomes increasingly difficult for the client. *(Exhaustion brought on by excessive respiratory effort can lead to pulmonary arrest.)*
- When indicated, initiate health teaching, using the nursing diagnosis *Risk for Ineffective Health Maintenance related to insufficient knowledge of (specify).*

### Pediatric Interventions and Rationales

- Refer also to General Interventions.
- Monitor respiratory status:
  - Pulse rate, respiratory rate
  - Use of accessory respiratory muscles, retractions, nasal flaring
  - Diaphoresis, cyanosis
  - Wheezing, cough

  *(Increased pulse and respiratory rate indicate hypoxia. Asthma often manifests as a cough rather than wheezing.)*
- Assess for signs of dehydration. *(Children with dyspnea may refuse fluids.)*
- Ensure adequate hydration. *(Good hydration helps prevent tenacious, impacted mucus.)*
- Evaluate child's and parents' understanding of condition, triggers, monitoring, and treatment.
- Ask child and/or parent to demonstrate use of inhaler, spacer, or nebulizer. *(Many drug failures result from improper use of equipment.)*
- Teach how to monitor peak expiratory flow rates (PEFR) twice daily, before and after treatments, in a diary.
  - Determine the child's personal-best values.
  - Instruct to increase medications if PEFR falls below 50% to 80% of personal best.
  - Instruct to use bronchodilator immediately if rate is below 50%, and seek emergency treatment if not improved immediately.

  *(PEFR monitoring is critical to effective prevention of acute exacerbations in children with moderate or severe asthma.)*

## ▶ Risk for Complications of Pneumothorax

## DEFINITION

Describes a person experiencing or at high risk to experience accumulation of air in the pleural space because of lung injury. (Spontaneous pneumothorax should always be considered in clients with or without history of lung disease when the onset is sudden and acute, accompanied with or without significant trauma)

## HIGH-RISK POPULATIONS

- Severe blunt or penetrating chest injury
- Postoperative status (cardiac or thoracic surgery)
- Mechanically ventilated with positive end-expiratory pressure
- Interstitial lung disease
- Insertion of central venous catheter
- Transbronchial biopsy
- Thoracentesis
- Post-procedural central line placement with subclavian approach

## Nursing Goals

The nurse will manage and minimize complications of pneumothorax

### Indicators

Refer to Hypoxemia for Indicators

## General Interventions and Rationales

- Monitor for signs and symptoms of pneumothorax:
  - Acute pleuritic chest pain
  - Dyspnea, tachypnea, tachycardia
  - Hyperresonant percussion sounds with loss of breath sounds over the affected side
  - Shifting of trachea

  *(Early detection and prompt intervention are necessary to prevent serious complications.)*
- Administer oxygen, if indicated. If chronic $CO_2$ retention occurs, limit the flow rate to no more than 2 L/min. *(Higher flow rates can depress ventilatory drive.)*
- Prepare for stat chest x-ray, ABGs, possible chest tube placement.
- Evaluate the need for analgesics to manage thoracic pain. *(Pain interferes with lung expansion on inspiration, compromising oxygenation.)*
- Reposition client every 2 h, keeping the unaffected lung in the dependent position. *(This position limits pain and improves oxygenation by better equalizing ventilation and perfusion.)*
- Explain and supervise deep breathing with sustained maximum inspiration. *(Deep breathing expands lungs and evacuates air from pleural space into chest drainage system [if present].)*
- Instruct person to avoid coughing except when necessary to clear secretions. *(Coughing increases pain.)*
- Minimize environmental stimuli, provide emotional support, and offer simple explanations for all procedures. *(These measures may help reduce anxiety, increasing respiratory rate.)*
- If use of a chest drainage system is indicated, follow institutional protocols for set-up, assessment, and maintenance.

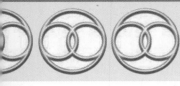

# RISK FOR COMPLICATIONS OF METABOLIC/ IMMUNE/HEMATOPOIETIC DYSFUNCTION

**Risk for Complications of Metabolic/Immune/Hematopoietic Dysfunction**

RC of Hypo/Hyperglycemia
RC of Negative Nitrogen Balance
RC of Electrolyte Imbalances
RC of Sepsis
RC of Acidosis (Metabolic, Respiratory)
RC of Alkalosis (Metabolic, Respiratory)
RC of Allergic Reaction
RC of Thrombocytopenia
RC of Opportunistic Infections
RC of Sickling Crisis

## DEFINITION

Describes a person experiencing or at high risk to experience various endocrine, immune, or metabolic dysfunctions

## ■■■■■■ AUTHOR'S NOTE

The nurse can use this generic collaborative problem to describe a person at risk for several types of metabolic and immune system problems. For example, for a client with pituitary dysfunction who is at risk for various metabolic problems, using *RC of Metabolic Dysfunction* directs nurses to monitor endocrine system function for specific problems, based on focus assessment findings. Under this collaborative problem, nursing interventions would focus on monitoring metabolic status to detect and diagnose abnormal functioning. If the client developed a specific complication, the nurse would add the appropriate specific collaborative problem, along with nursing management information, to the client's problem list. For a client with diabetes mellitus, the nurse would add the diagnostic statement *RC of Hypo/Hyperglycemia*. For a client receiving chemotherapy, the nurse would use *RC of Immunodeficiency*, a collaborative problem that encompasses leukopenia, thrombocytopenia, and erythrocytopenia. If thrombocytopenia were an isolated problem, it would warrant a separate diagnostic statement (i.e., *RC of Thrombocytopenia*).

For a client with a condition or undergoing a treatment that produces immunosuppression (e.g., acquired immunodeficiency syndrome [AIDS], graft-versus-host disease, immunosuppressant therapy), the collaborative problem *RC of Immunosuppression* would be appropriate. When conditions have or possibly could have affected coagulation (e.g., chronic renal failure, alcohol abuse, anticoagulant therapy), a collaborative problem such as *RC of Hemolysis* or *RC of Erythrocytopenia* would be indicated. If the risk factors or etiology were not directly related to the primary medical diagnosis, they could be added (e.g., *RC of Immunosuppression related to chronic corticosteroid therapy* in a client who has sustained a myocardial infarction).

For information on Focus Assessment Criteria, visit http://thepoint.lww.com.

## SIGNIFICANT LABORATORY/DIAGNOSTIC ASSESSMENT CRITERIA

Serum amylase (elevated in acute pancreatitis, lowered in chronic pancreatitis)
Serum albumin (lowered in malnutrition)
Lymphocyte count (lowered in malnutrition)
Serum calcium (elevated in hyperparathyroidism, certain cancers, and acute pancreatitis, lowered in hypoparathyroidism)
Blood pH (elevated in alkalosis, lowered in acidosis)
Serum glucose (elevated in diabetes mellitus and pancreatic insufficiency, lowered in pancreatic islet cell tumors)

Serum antidiuretic hormone (ADH) (elevated levels indicate syndrome of inappropriate antidiuretic hormone excretion [SIADH]), reduced levels indicate central diabetes insipidus)

Urine specific gravity (reflects the kidneys ability to concentrate and dilute urine)

Serum osmolarity (represents concentration of particles in blood)

Urine osmolarity (measures urine concentration—increased in Addison's disease, SIADH, dehydration renal disease; decreased in diabetes insipidus, psychogenic water drinking)

Serum glycosylated hemoglobin (Hgb A1c) (reflects mean glucose levels for preceding 2 to 3 months)

Urine acetone, urine glucose (present in diabetes mellitus)

Urine ketone bodies (present in uncontrolled diabetes)

Platelets (elevated in polycythemia and chronic granulocytic leukemia, lowered in anemia and acute leukemia)

Immunoglobulins (elevated in autoimmune disease)

Coagulation tests (elevated in thrombocytopenia, purpura, and hemophilia)

Prothrombin time (elevated in anticoagulant therapy, cirrhosis, and hepatitis)

Red blood cell (RBC) count (lowered in anemia, leukemia, and renal failure)

CT, MRI of targeted organ

Bone marrow aspirate with diagnostic pathology

Spinal tap with appropriate analysis, culture and sensitivity

# ▶ Risk for Complications of Hypo/Hyperglycemia

## DEFINITION

Describes a person experiencing or at high risk to experience a blood glucose level that is too low or too high for metabolic function*

### ■■■■■■ AUTHOR'S NOTE

In 2006, NANDA approved the nursing diagnosis, *Risk for Unstable Blood Sugar*. This author defines this condition as a collaborative problem. The nurse can choose which terminology is preferred. The student should consult with the instructor for direction.

## HIGH-RISK POPULATIONS

- Diabetes mellitus
- Parenteral nutrition
- Sepsis
- Enteral feedings
- Corticosteroid therapy
- Neonate of diabetic mother
- Small-for-gestational-age neonate
- Neonate of narcotic-addicted mother
- Thermal injuries (severe)
- Pancreatitis (hyperglycemia), cancer of pancreas
- Addison's disease (hypoglycemia)
- Adrenal gland hyperfunction
- Liver disease (hypoglycemia)

---

*If the person is not at risk for both, the diagnosis should specify the problem (e.g., *RC of Hyperglycemia related to corticosteroid therapy*).

## Nursing Goals

The nurse will manage and minimize episodes of hypoglycemia or hyperglycemia.

### Indicators

Alert, calm oriented
No complaints of dizziness
Warm, dry skin
No complaints of fatigue, nausea, abdominal pain, diaphoresis
Pulse: no significant increase
Respirations: no significant increase

## General Interventions and Rationales

Many labs and institutions require a repeat of or a second method of validation for treatment of "Critical Lab Values." The organizations define them and require them even for Point of Care (POC) testing for blood glucose values.

### For Hypoglycemia

- Monitor serum glucose level at the bedside before administering hypoglycemic agents and/or before meals and hour of sleep. *(Serum glucose is a more accurate parameter than urine glucose, which is affected by renal threshold and renal function.)*
- Monitor for signs and symptoms of hypoglycemia:
  - Blood glucose level below institutional guide, commonly 50–60 mg/dL
  - Pale, moist, cool skin
  - Tachycardia, diaphoresis
  - Jitteriness, irritability, nervousness (National Institutes of Health [NIH], 2003)
  - Hypoglycemia unawareness
  - Incoordination, difficulty speaking (NIH, 2003)
  - Drowsiness, confusion, lightheadedness (NIH, 2003)
  - Hunger (NIH, 2003)
  - Weakness (NIH, 2003)

  *(Hypoglycemia [insufficient glucose levels] can result from excessive insulin, insufficient food intake, excessive physical activity, excessive alcohol intake, medications, diseases, hormone or enzyme deficiencies, or tumors [NIH, 2003].) A rapid drop in blood glucose level stimulates the sympathetic system to produce adrenaline, which causes diaphoresis, cool skin, tachycardia, and jitteriness.*
- Check standard for hypoglycemia oral treatment. If client can swallow, give him or her ½ cup of fruit juice or non-diet soda; 1 cup of milk; 5-6 pieces of hard candy; 2-3 glucose tablets; or 1-2 teaspoons of sugar or honey, every 15 min until blood glucose level exceeds 69 mg/dL. Check glucose level prior to administering more glucose. *(Simple carbohydrates are metabolized quickly [NIH, 2003].)*
- If client cannot swallow, administer glucagon hydrochloride subcutaneously or 50 mL of 50% glucose in water intravenously (IV), according to protocol. *(Glucagon causes glycogenolysis in the liver when glycogen stores are adequate. In a client in critical condition who has been in a coma for some time, glycogen stores likely have already been used up, and IV glucose is the only effective treatment.)*
- Recheck blood glucose level 1 h after an initial blood glucose reading of greater than 69 mg/dL. *(Regular monitoring detects early signs of high or low levels.)*
- If indicated, consult with a dietitian to provide a complex carbohydrate snack at bedtime. *(This measure can help prevent hypoglycemia during the night.)*

### For Hyperglycemia

- Monitor for signs and symptoms of diabetic ketoacidosis:
  - Anion gap
  - Blood glucose level >300 mg/dL
  - Positive plasma ketone, acetone breath
  - Headache
  - Kussmaul's respirations

- Anorexia, nausea, vomiting
- Tachycardia
- Decreased blood pressure
- Polyuria, polydipsia
- Decreased serum sodium, potassium, and phosphate levels

*(When insulin is unavailable, blood glucose levels rise and the body metabolizes fat for energy-producing ketone bodies. Excessive ketone bodies cause headaches, nausea, vomiting, and abdominal pain. Respiratory rate and depth increase to help increase $CO_2$ excretion and reduce acidosis. Glucose inhibits water reabsorption in the renal glomerulus, leading to osmotic diuresis with severe loss of water, sodium, potassium, and phosphates. Diabetic ketoacidosis occurs in type I diabetes.)*

- If ketoacidosis occurs, initiate appropriate protocols to reverse dehydration, restore the insulin–glucagon ratio, and treat circulatory collapse, ketoacidosis, and electrolyte imbalance.
- Continue to monitor hydration status every 30 min; assess skin moisture and turgor, urine output and specific gravity, and fluid intake. *(Accurate assessments are needed during the acute stage [first 10–12 h] to prevent overhydration or underhydration.)*
- Continue to monitor blood glucose levels according to protocol. *(Careful monitoring enables early detection of medication-induced hypoglycemia or continued hyperglycemia.)*
- Monitor serum potassium, sodium, and phosphate levels. *(Acidosis causes hyperkalemia and hyponatremia. Insulin therapy promotes potassium and phosphate return to the cells, causing serum hypokalemia and hypophosphatemia.)*
- Monitor neurologic status every hour. *(Fluctuating glucose levels, acidosis, and fluid shifts can affect neurologic functioning.)*
- Carefully protect client's skin from microorganism invasion, injury, and shearing force; reposition every 1 to 2 h. *(Dehydration and tissue hypoxia increase the skin's vulnerability to injury.)*
- Do not allow a recovering client to drink large quantities of water. Give a conscious client ice chips to quench thirst. *(Excessive fluid intake can cause abdominal distention and vomiting.)*
- Monitor for signs and symptoms of hyperosmolar hyperglycemic nonketotic (HHNK) coma:
  - Blood glucose 600–2000 mg/dL
  - Serum sodium, potassium normal or elevated
  - Elevated hematocrit, blood urea nitrogen (BUN)
  - Nausea, vomiting
  - Hypotension, tachycardia
  - Dehydration, weight loss, poor skin turgor
  - Lethargy, stupor, coma
  - Elevated urine glucose (>2+)
  - Urine ketones negative or <2+
  - Polyuria

*(HHNK results from relative insulin deficiency. Hyperglycemia and hyperosmolality are present, but there is an absence of significant ketones. HHNK coma can be a response to acute stress [e.g., from myocardial infarction, burns, severe infection, dialysis, or hyperalimentation]. People with type II insulin-resistant diabetes who experience marked dehydration are especially at risk. Glucose inhibits water reabsorption in the renal glomerulus, leading to osmotic diuresis with loss of water, sodium, potassium, and phosphates. Cerebral impairment results from intracellular dehydration in the brain [Porth, 2007; Morton et al., 2006].)*

- Monitor cardiac function and circulatory status; evaluate:
  - Rate, rhythm (cardiac, respiratory)
  - Skin color
  - Capillary refill time, central venous pressure
  - Peripheral pulses
  - Serum potassium

*(Severe dehydration can cause reduced cardiac output and compensatory vasoconstriction. Cardiac dysrhythmias can result from potassium imbalances.)*

- Follow protocols for ketoacidosis, as indicated.
- Investigate for causes of ketoacidosis or hypoglycemia, and teach prevention and early management, using the nursing diagnosis *Risk for Ineffective Self-Health Management related to insufficient knowledge of (specify)* (see Section II).

**Pediatric Interventions and Rationales**

Refer also to General Interventions.

Consult with dietitian for nutritional management. *(The goal is a consistent, well-balanced diet to ensure normal growth and development.)*

If a child, evaluate child's growth and development. *(Poor control of glucose levels affects growth.)*

Teach about condition, insulin therapy, self-monitoring of glucose, nutrition, exercise, and prevention of complications. Consult with school nurse for management at school. *(Effective management is a team effort.)*

# ▶ Risk for Complications of Negative Nitrogen Balance

## DEFINITION

Describes a person experiencing or at risk to experience catabolism, when more nitrogen is excreted from tissue breakdown than is replaced by intake

## HIGH-RISK POPULATIONS

- Severe malnutrition
- Prolonged NPO state
- Elderly with chronic disease
- Uncontrolled diabetes
- Digestive disorders
- Prolonged use of glucose or saline IV therapy
- Inadequate enteral replacement
- Excessive catabolism (e.g., due to cancer, infection, burns, surgery, excess stress)
- Anorexia nervosa, bulimia
- Critical illness
- Chemotherapy
- Sepsis

## Nursing Goals

The nurse will manage and minimize negative nitrogen balance.

### Indicators

Temperature 98–99.5° F.
White blood count 4,300–10,800 mm$_3$
No extremity edema
Serum prealbumin 20–50 g/dL
Serum albumin 3.5–5 g/dL

## General Interventions and Rationales

- Establish the client's optimum weight for height. *(This establishes baseline goals.)*
- Weigh client daily at same time, wearing same amount of clothes, same scale, and same bedding. *(Monitoring weight helps detect excessive catabolism.)*
- Monitor for signs of negative nitrogen balance:
  - Weight loss
  - 24-h urine nitrogen balance below zero

  *(Cachexia results from increased metabolic demands, insufficient replacement, and anorexia. Impaired carbohydrate metabolism causes increased metabolism of fats and protein, which—especially with metabolic acidosis—can lead to negative nitrogen balance and weight loss.)*

- Monitor for signs and symptoms of hypoalbuminemia, which can have a rapid or insidious onset:
  - Emotional depression, fatigue *(These effects result from decreased energy supplies.)*
  - Muscle wasting *(This results from insufficient protein available for tissue repair.)*
  - Poorly healing wounds *(This results from insufficient protein available for tissue repair.)*
  - Edema *(Edema results from a plasma-to-interstitial fluid shift because of insufficient vascular osmotic pressure.)*
- Monitor laboratory values:
  - Serum prealbumin and transferring *(These values evaluate visceral protein. Prealbumin is a precursor to albumin and a much more sensitive measure of visceral protein.)*
  - BUN *(This value measures kidney clearance ability.)*
  - 24-h urine nitrogen *(Because the glomerulus reabsorbs 99% of what is filtered, measurement of urea nitrogen, a waste product of protein metabolism, gives data to calculate the nitrogen balance.)*
  - Electrolytes, osmolality *(These values help assess kidney function.)*
  - Total lymphocyte count *(Lymphocyte production requires protein.)*
- Continually reevaluate the client's energy/protein requirements. Consult with a registered dietitian for evaluation (e.g., indirect calorimetry test, anthropometric measures). *(The person's calorie/protein requirements will change depending on metabolic demands [e.g., from stress, fever, or infection].)*
- Administer total parenteral solutions, intralipid fat emulsions, and/or enteral formulas as prescribed by the physician or advanced practice nurse and in accordance with appropriate procedures and protocols. *(This client's increased caloric requirements for tissue repair cannot be met with routine IV therapy.)*
- For specific nursing interventions to increase oral nutrient intake, refer to the nursing diagnosis *Imbalanced Nutrition: Less Than Body Requirements* (see Section II).

## ▶ Risk for Complications of Electrolyte Imbalances*

- Risk for Complications of Hypokalemia
- Risk for Complications of Hyperkalemia
- Risk for Complications of Hyponatremia
- Risk for Complications of Hypernatremia
- Risk for Complications of Hypocalcemia
- Risk for Complications of Hypercalcemia
- Risk for Complications of Hypophosphatemia
- Risk for Complications of Hyperphosphatemia
- Risk for Complications of Hypomagnesemia
- Risk for Complications of Hypermagnesemia
- Risk for Complications of Hypochloremia
- Risk for Complications of Hyperchloremia

## DEFINITION

Describes a person experiencing or at risk to experience a deficit or excess of one or more electrolytes

## HIGH-RISK POPULATIONS

### For Hypokalemia

- Crash dieting
- Diabetic Ketoacidosis
- Metabolic or respiratory alkalosis
- Excessive intake of licorice

---

*For a person experiencing or at high risk to experience a deficit or excess in a single electrolyte, the diagnostic statement should specify the problem (e.g., *RC of Hypokalemia related to diuretic therapy*).

- Diuretic therapy
- Loss of gastrointestinal (GI) fluids (through excessive nasogastric suctioning, nausea, vomiting, or diarrhea)
- Steroid use
- Estrogen use
- Hyperaldosteronism
- Severe burns
- Decreased potassium intake
- Liver disease with ascites
- Renal tubular acidosis
- Malabsorption
- Severe catabolism
- Salt depletion
- Hemolysis
- Hypoaldosteronism
- Rhabdomyolysis
- Laxative abuse
- Villous adenoma
- Hyperglycemia
- Severe magnesium depletion

## For Hyperkalemia

- Renal failure
- Excessive potassium intake (oral or IV)
- Cell damage (e.g., from burns, trauma, surgery)
- Crushing injuries
- Potassium-sparing diuretic use
- Adrenal insufficiency
- Lupus
- Sickle cell disease
- Post-transplant
- Chemotherapy
- Metabolic acidosis
- Transfusion of old blood
- Internal hemorrhage
- Hypoaldosteronism
- Acidosis
- Rhabdomyolysis

## For Hyponatremia

- Water intoxication (oral or IV)
- Renal failure
- Gastric suctioning
- Vomiting, diarrhea
- Burns
- Potent diuretic use
- Excessive diaphoresis
- Excessive wound drainage
- Congestive heart failure
- Hyperglycemia
- Malabsorption syndrome
- Cystic fibrosis
- Addison's disease
- Psychogenic polydipsia

- Oxytocin administration
- Syndrome of inappropriate antidiuretic hormone (SIADH) (resulting from central nervous system [CNS] disorders, major trauma, malignancies, or endocrine disorders)
- Adrenal gland insufficiency
- Chronic illness (e.g., cirrhosis)
- Hypothyroidism (moderate, severe)

## For Hypernatremia

- Elderly, infants
- Inadequate fluid intake
- Heat stroke
- Diarrhea
- Severe insensible fluid loss (e.g., through hyperventilation or sweating)
- Diabetes insipidus
- Excessive sodium intake (oral, IV, medications)
- Hypertonic tube feeding
- Coma
- High protein feeding with inadequate $H_2O$ intake

## For Hypocalcemia

- Renal failure (increased phosphorus)
- Protein malnutrition (e.g., due to malabsorption)
- Inadequate calcium intake
- Diarrhea
- Burns
- Malignancy
- Hypoparathyroidism
- Vitamin D deficiency
- Osteoblastic tumors

## For Hypercalcemia

- Chronic renal failure
- Sarcoidosis and granulomatous disease
- Excessive vitamin D intake
- Hyperparathyroidism
- Decreased hypophosphatemia
- Bone tumors
- Cancers (Hodgkin's disease, myeloma, leukemia, neoplastic bone disease)
- Prolonged use of thiazide diuretics
- Paget's disease
- Parathyroid hormone-secreting tumors (e.g., lung, kidney)
- Hemodialysis
- Multiple fractures
- Prolonged immobilization
- Excessive calcium-containing antacids

## For Hypophosphatemia

- Diabetic ketoacidosis
- Prolonged use of IV dextrose solutions
- Malabsorption disorders
- Renal wasting of phosphorus
- Low-phosphate diet (oral, total parenteral nutrition)
- Rickets

- Excessive use of phosphate binders
- Osteomalacia
- Alcoholism

## For Hyperphosphatemia

- Excessive vitamin D intake
- Renal failure
- Healing fractures
- Bone tumors
- Hypoparathyroidism
- Hypocalcemia
- Phosphate laxatives
- Excessive IV or PO phosphate
- Chemotherapy
- Catabolism
- Lactic acidosis

## For Hypomagnesemia

- Malnutrition
- Prolonged diuretic use
- Chronic alcoholism
- Excessive lactation
- Severe diarrhea, nasogastric suctioning
- Cirrhosis
- Severe dehydration
- Ulcerative colitis
- Toxemia
- Burns
- Cisplatinum use
- Hyperthyroidism/Cushing's disease
- Prolonged IV therapy without magnesium

## For Hypermagnesemia

- Addison's disease
- Renal failure
- Severe dehydration with oliguria
- Excessive intake of magnesium-containing antacids, laxatives
- Thiazide use

## For Hypochloremia

- Loss of GI fluids (e.g., through vomiting, diarrhea, suctioning)
- Metabolic alkalosis
- Diabetic acidosis
- Prolonged use of IV dextrose
- Excessive diaphoresis
- Excessive diuretic use
- Ulcerative colitis
- Fever
- Acute infections
- Severe burns

## For Hyperchloremia

- Metabolic acidosis
- Severe diarrhea

- Excessive parenteral isotonic saline solution infusion
- Urinary diversion
- Renal failure
- Cushing's syndrome
- Hyperventilation
- Eclampsia
- Anemia
- Cardiac decompensation

## Nursing Goals

The nurse will manage and minimize episodes of electrolyte imbalance(s) using laboratory values and norms from organization.

### Indicators

Serum magnesium 1.3–2.4 mEq/L
Serum sodium 135–145 mEq/L
Serum potassium 3.8–5 mEq/L
Serum calcium 8.5–10.5 mg/dL
Serum phosphates 125–300 mg/dL
Serum chloride 98–108 mEq/L

## General Interventions

Identify the electrolyte imbalance(s) for which the client is vulnerable, and intervene as follows. (Refer to High-Risk Populations under the specific imbalance.)

### Risk for Complications of Hypo/Hyperkalemia

- Monitor for signs and symptoms of hyperkalemia:
  - Weakness to flaccid paralysis
  - Muscle irritability
  - Paresthesias
  - Nausea, abdominal cramping, or diarrhea
  - Oliguria
  - Electrocardiogram (ECG) changes: tall, tented T waves, ST segment depression, prolonged PR interval (>0.2 s), first-degree heart block, bradycardia, broadening of the QRS complex, eventual ventricular fibrillation, and cardiac standstill (Porth, 2007)

  *(Hyperkalemia can result from the kidney's decreased ability to excrete potassium or from excessive potassium intake. Acidosis increases the release of potassium from cells. Fluctuations in potassium level affect neuromuscular transmission, producing cardiac dysrhythmias, and reducing action of GI smooth muscle. There is an increase in cardiac irritability and cardiac monitoring may show early changes as premature ventricular beats.)*
- For a client with hyperkalemia
- Restrict potassium-rich foods, fluids, and IV solutions with potassium. *(High potassium levels necessitate a reduction in potassium intake.)*
- Provide range-of-motion (ROM) exercises to extremities. *(ROM improves muscle tone and reduces cramps.)*
- Per orders or protocols, give medications to reduce serum potassium levels, such as:
  - IV calcium *(To block effects on the heart muscle temporarily)*
  - Sodium bicarbonate, glucose, insulin *(To force potassium back into cells)*
  - Cation-exchange resins (e.g., Kayexalate, hemodialysis; *to force excretion of potassium*)
- Monitor for signs and symptoms of hypokalemia:
  - Weakness or flaccid paralysis
  - Decreased or absent deep tendon reflexes
  - Hypoventilation, change in consciousness
  - Polyuria
  - Hypotension
  - Paralytic ileus
  - ECG changes: U wave, low-voltage or inverted T wave, dysrhythmias, and prolonged QT interval

- Nausea, vomiting, anorexia

  *(Hypokalemia results from losses associated with vomiting, diarrhea, or diuretic therapy, or from insufficient potassium intake. Hypokalemia impairs neuromuscular transmission and reduces the efficiency of respiratory muscles. Kidneys are less sensitive to antidiuretic hormone and thus excrete large quantities of dilute urine. GI smooth muscle action also is reduced. Abnormally low potassium levels also impair electrical conduction of the heart [Porth, 2007].)*

- For a client with hypokalemia:
  - Encourage increased intake of potassium-rich foods. *(An increase in dietary potassium intake helps ensure potassium replacement.)*
  - If parenteral potassium replacement (always diluted) is instituted, do not exceed 10 mEq/h in adults. Monitor serum potassium levels during replacement. *(Excessive levels can cause cardiac dysrhythmias.)*
  - Observe the IV site for infiltration. *(Potassium is very caustic to tissues.)*
  - Monitor for discomfort at peripheral infusion site, consider lidocaine additive to reduce/prevent discomfort

## Risk for Complications of Hypo/Hypernatremia

- Monitor for signs and symptoms of hyponatremia:
  - CNS effects ranging from lethargy to coma, headache
  - Weakness
  - Abdominal pain
  - Muscle twitching or convulsions
  - Nausea, vomiting, diarrhea
  - Apprehension

  (Hyponatremia results from sodium loss through vomiting, diarrhea, or diuretic therapy; excessive fluid intake; or insufficient dietary sodium intake. Cellular edema, caused by osmosis, produces cerebral edema, weakness, and muscle cramps.)

- For a client with hyponatremia, initiate IV sodium chloride solutions and discontinue diuretic therapy, as ordered. *(These interventions prevent further sodium losses.)*
- Monitor for signs and symptoms of hypernatremia with fluid overload:
  - Thirst, decreased urine output
  - CNS effects ranging from agitation to convulsions
  - Elevated serum osmolality
  - Weight gain, edema
  - Elevated blood pressure
  - Tachycardia

  *(Hypernatremia results from excessive sodium intake or increased aldosterone output. Water is pulled from the cells, causing cellular dehydration and producing CNS symptoms. Thirst is a compensatory response to dilute sodium.)*

- For a client with hypernatremia:
  - Initiate fluid replacement in response to serum osmolality levels, as ordered. *(Rapid reduction in serum osmolality can cause cerebral edema and seizures.)*
  - Monitor for seizures. *(Sodium excess causes cerebral edema.)*
  - Monitor intake and output, weight. *(This evaluates fluid balance.)*

## Risk for Complications of Hypo/Hypercalcemia

- Monitor for signs and symptoms of hypocalcemia:
  - Altered mental status
  - Numbness or tingling in fingers and toes
  - Muscle cramps
  - Seizures
  - ECG changes: prolonged QT interval, prolonged ST segment, and dysrhythmias
  - Chvostek's or Trousseau's sign
  - Tetany

  *(Hypocalcemia can result from the kidney's inability to metabolize vitamin D [needed for calcium absorption]. Retention of phosphorus causes a reciprocal drop in serum calcium level. A low serum calcium level produces*

*increased neural excitability, resulting in muscle spasms [cardiac, facial, extremities] and CNS irritability [seizures]. It also causes cardiac muscle hyperactivity, as evidenced by ECG changes.)*

- For a client with hypocalcemia:
  - Per orders for acute hypocalcemia, administer calcium by way of IV bolus infusion.
  - Consult with the dietitian for a high-calcium, low-phosphorus diet. *(Lower serum calcium level necessitates dietary replacement.)*
  - Assess for hyperphosphatemia or hypomagnesemia. *(Hyperphosphatemia inhibits calcium absorption; in hypomagnesemia, the kidneys excrete calcium to retain magnesium.)*
  - Monitor for ECG changes: prolonged QT interval, irritable dysrhythmias, and atrioventricular conduction defects. *(Calcium imbalances can cause cardiac muscle hyperactivity.)*
- Monitor for signs and symptoms of hypercalcemia:
  - Altered mental status
  - Anorexia, nausea, vomiting, constipation
  - Numbness or tingling in fingers and toes
  - Muscle cramps, hypotoxicity
  - Deep bone pain
  - AV blocks (ECG)

  *(Insufficient calcium level reduces neuromuscular excitability, resulting in decreased muscle tone, numbness, anorexia, and mental lethargy.)*
- For a client with hypercalcemia:
  - Initiate normal saline IV therapy and loop diuretics, as ordered; avoid thiazide diuretics. *(IV fluids dilute serum calcium. Loop diuretics enhance calcium excretion; thiazide diuretics inhibit calcium excretion.)*
  - Per order, administer phosphorus preparations and mithramycin (contraindicated in clients with renal failure). *(These increase bone deposition of calcium.)*
  - Monitor for renal calculi (see *RC of Renal Calculi*).

## Risk for Complications of Hypo/Hyperphosphatemia

- Monitor for signs and symptoms of hypophosphatemia:
  - Muscle weakness, pain
  - Bleeding
  - Depressed white cell function
  - Confusion
  - Anorexia

  *(Phosphorus deficiency impairs cellular energy resources and oxygen delivery to tissues and also causes decreased platelet aggregation.)*
- For a client with hypophosphatemia, per order, replace phosphorus stores slowly by oral supplements, and discontinue phosphate binders. *(This helps prevent precipitation with calcium.)*
- Monitor for signs and symptoms of hyperphosphatemia:
  - Tetany
  - Numbness or tingling in fingers and toes
  - Soft tissue calcification
  - Chvostek's and Trousseau's signs
  - Coarse, dry skin

  *(Hyperphosphatemia can result from the kidneys' decreased ability to excrete phosphorus. Elevated phosphorus does not cause symptoms in itself, but contributes to tetany and other neuromuscular symptoms in the short term and to soft tissue calcification in the long term.)*
- For a client with hyperphosphatemia, administer phosphorus-binding antacids, calcium supplements, or vitamin D, and restrict phosphorus-rich foods. *(Supplements are needed to overcome vitamin D deficiency and to compensate for a calcium-poor diet. High phosphate decreases calcium, which increases parathyroid hormone [PTH]. PTH is ineffective in removing phosphates due to renal failure, but causes calcium reabsorption from bone and decreases tubular reabsorption of phosphate.)*

## Risk for Complications of Hypo/Hypermagnesemia

- Monitor for hypomagnesemia:
  - Dysphagia, nausea, anorexia

- Muscle weakness
- Facial tics
- Athetoid movements (slow, involuntary twisting movements)
- Cardiac dysrhythmias, flat or inverted T waves, prolonged QT intervals, tachycardia, depressed ST segment. Torsades, a specific type of ventricular dysrythmia, is associated with hypomagnesemia
- Confusion

*(Magnesium deficit causes neuromuscular changes and hyperexcitability.)*

- For a client with hypomagnesemia, initiate magnesium sulfate replacement (dietary for mild deficiency, parenteral for severe deficiency), as ordered.
- Initiate seizure precautions. *(This protects from injury.)*
- Monitor for hypermagnesemia:
  - Decreased blood pressure, bradycardia, decreased respirations
  - Flushing
  - Lethargy, muscle weakness
  - Peaked T waves

*(Magnesium excess causes depression of central and peripheral neuromuscular function, producing vasodilation.)*

- If respiratory depression occurs, consult with the physician for possible hemodialysis. *(Magnesium-free dialysate causes excretion.)*

## Risk for Complications of Hypo/Hyperchloremia

- Monitor for hypochloremia:
  - Hyperirritability
  - Slow respirations
  - Decreased blood pressure

*(Hypochloremia occurs with metabolic alkalosis, resulting in loss of calcium and potassium, which produces the symptoms.)*

- For a client with hypochloremia, see *RC of Alkalosis* for interventions.
- Monitor for hyperchloremia:
  - Weakness
  - Lethargy
  - Deep, rapid breathing

*(Metabolic acidosis causes loss of chloride ions.)*

- For a client with hyperchloremia, see *RC of Acidosis* for interventions.

# ▶ Risk for Complications of Sepsis

## DEFINITION

Describes a person experiencing or at high risk to experience a systemic response to the presence of pathogenic bacteria, viruses, fungi, or their toxins. The microorganisms may or may not be present in the bloodstream.

## HIGH-RISK POPULATIONS

- Extreme age (<1 year and >65 years)
- Drug dependency, alcoholism
- Burns, multiple trauma
- Infection (urinary, respiratory, wound)
- Immunosuppression
- Invasive lines (urinary, arterial, endotracheal, or central venous catheter)
- AIDS

- Disseminated intravascular coagulation
- Pressure ulcers
- Extensive slow-healing wounds
- Surgical procedures (GI, thoracic, cardiac)
- Diabetes mellitus
- Malnutrition
- Cancer
- Cirrhosis, pancreatitis
- Transplants
- Hypothermia
- Aspiration
- Chronic illness; diabetes, renal or hepatic failure

## Infants/Children

- Viral upper respiratory infection
- Bacterial enteritis
- Burns
- Urinary tract infections
- Bite wounds (e.g., dog, human)
- Craniofacial surgery
- Compromised host defenses

## Nursing Goals

The nurse will identify early signs of sepsis; and manage and monitor the complications of sepsis.

### Indicators

Temperature 98–99.5° F
Pulse 60–100 beats/min
Arterial oxygen saturation (pulse ox) >95%
Arterial carbon dioxide 35–45 mmHg
Urine output >5 kg/mL/h
Urine specific gravity 1.005–1.030

## General Interventions and Rationales

- Monitor for signs and symptoms of sepsis (Morton et al., 2006):
  - Temperature >38° C or <36° C
  - Heart rate >90 beats/min
  - Respiratory rate >20 breaths/min or $PaCO_2$ <32 torr (<4.3 kPa)
  - White blood cell (WBC) count >12,000 cells/$mm_3$, <4000 cells/$mm_3$, or >10% immature (band) forms

  Pan and or site specific cultures
  Serum lactic acid level
  APACHE 2 score
- Assess fluid status: monitor CVP and administer fluid boluses (500 ml every 20-30 minutes). Early Goal Directed Therapy (EGDT) with fluid replacement improves cardiac output, tissue perfusion, and oxygen delivery, improving mortality & morbidity. (*Sepsis causes vasodilation and capillary leak resulting in hypovolemia.*)
- Monitor blood pressure. Administer replacement fluids and vasopressors (especially norepinephrine) to maintain MAP >65. (*In EGDT, maintaining MAP >65 improves outcomes [Picard et al., 2006].*)
- Assess for evidence of adequate tissue perfusion: heart rate, respirations, urine output, mentation, $ScvO_2$/$SVO_2$. Maintain $ScvO_2$/$SVO_2$ >70%, urine output > 20 ml/hr. *EGDT directed by $ScvO_2$/$SVO_2$ (Monitoring reduces mortality [Picard et al., 2006].)*
- Early treatment with broad spectrum antibiotics. (*Beginning therapy within one hour of entering protocol improves mortality [Picard et al., 2006].*)

- Monitor serum cortisol levels. *(Treatment with low-dose steroids significantly reduces mortality in patients with septic shock and adrenal insufficiency [Picard et al., 2006].)*
- Monitor serum glucose levels. Use insulin (IV) to maintain tight glycemic control. *(Tight glycemic control improves patient outcomes [Picard et al., 2006].)*
- As ordered, administer activated protein C in eligible patients. Assess for signs and symptoms of bleeding or coagulopathy. *(Endogenous protein C interferes with clotting factors, preventing the formation of thrombin and gaurds against excess fibrinolysis. It also has anti-inflammatory properties [Dettenmeier, Swindell, Stroud, Arkins, & Howard, 2003; Picard et al., 2006].)*
- Monitor older adults for changes in mentation; weakness, malaise; normothermia or hypothermia; and anorexia. *(These clients do not exhibit the typical signs of infection. Usual presenting findings—fever, chills, tachypnea, tachycardia, and leukocytosis—frequently are absent in older adults with significant infection.)*
- If indicated, refer to *RC of Hypovolemic Shock* for more information.

**Pediatric Interventions and Rationales**

- Monitor temperature (temperature >41° C [105.8° F] implies bacteremia). Very young infants can be hypothermic.
- Monitor for behavior changes:
  - Quality of cry
  - Response to parental stimulation
  - State variation
  - Response to social stimulation
  *(These changes reflect compromised cerebral circulation.)*
- Monitor respiratory pattern. *(Tachypnea and acrocyanosis may reflect poor peripheral perfusion.)*
- Monitor blood pressure, peripheral pulses, and capillary refill times. *(Circulatory inadequacy can be present even with normal blood pressures. Maintaining MAP >65 mm Hg improves patient outcomes) [Dettenmeier et al., 2003; Picard et al., 2006].)*
- Monitor for cutaneous changes. *(Petechiae, ecchymoses of distal extremities, and diffuse erythroderma can manifest with sepsis due to coagulopathy/DIC.)*
- Monitor oxygen saturation. *(Pulse oximetry measures oxygen levels.)*

# ▶ Risk for Complications of Metabolic or Respiratory Acidosis

## DEFINITION

Describes a person experiencing or at high risk for experiencing an acid–base imbalance due to increased production of acids or excessive loss of base

## HIGH-RISK POPULATIONS

### For Respiratory Acidosis

- Hypoventilation
- Acute pulmonary edema
- Airway obstruction
- Pneumothorax
- Sedative overdose
- Severe pneumonia
- Chronic obstructive pulmonary disease
- Asthma
- CNS lesions
- Disorders of respiratory system, muscle and chest wall (myasthenia gravis, amyotrophic lateral sclerosis, Guillain-Barré syndrome)

## For Metabolic Acidosis

- Diabetes mellitus
- Lactic acidosis
- Late-phase salicylate poisoning
- Uremia
- Methanol or ethylene glycol ingestion
- Diarrhea
- Intestinal fistulas, malabsorption
- Intake of large quantities of isotonic saline or ammonium chloride
- Renal failure (acute or chronic)
- Massive rhabdomyolysis
- Poisoning
- Drug toxicity

## Nursing Goals

The nurse will manage and minimize complications of acidosis.

### Indicators

Refer to Electrolyte Imbalances for Indicators
Blood urea nitrogen 10–20 mg/dL
Creatinine 0.2–0.8 mg/dL
Alkaline phosphate 30–150 IU/mL
Serum prealbumin 1–3 g/dL
No muscle cramps

## General Interventions and Rationales

### For Metabolic Acidosis

- Monitor for signs and symptoms of metabolic acidosis:
  - Rapid, shallow respirations
  - Headache, lethargy, coma
  - Nausea and vomiting
  - Low plasma bicarbonate and pH of arterial blood
  - Behavior changes, drowsiness
  - Increased serum potassium
  - Increased serum chloride
  - $PCO_2$ <35 to 40 mm Hg
  - Decreased $HCO_3$

  *(Metabolic acidosis results from the kidney's inability to excrete hydrogen ions, phosphates, sulfates, and ketone bodies. Bicarbonate loss results when the kidney reduces its resorption. Hyperkalemia, hyperphosphatemia, and decreased bicarbonate levels aggravate metabolic acidosis. Excessive ketone bodies cause headaches, nausea, vomiting, and abdominal pain. Respiratory rate and depth increase to increase $CO_2$ excretion and reduce acidosis. Acidosis affects the CNS and can increase neuromuscular irritability because of the cellular exchange of hydrogen and potassium.)*
- For a client with metabolic acidosis:
  - Initiate IV fluid replacement as ordered, depending on the underlying etiology. *(Dehydration may result from gastric and urinary fluid losses.)*
  - If the etiology is diabetes mellitus, refer to *RC of Hypo/Hyperglycemia* for interventions.
  - Assess for signs and symptoms of hypocalcemia, hypokalemia, and alkalosis as acidosis is corrected. *(Rapid correction of acidosis may cause rapid excretion of calcium and potassium and rebound alkalosis.)*
  - Correct, per orders, any electrolyte imbalances. Refer to *RC of Electrolyte Imbalances* for specific interventions for each type of electrolyte imbalance.
  - Monitor arterial blood gas (ABG) values, urine pH. *(These values help evaluate the effectiveness of therapy.)*

## For Respiratory Acidosis

- Monitor for signs and symptoms of respiratory acidosis:
  - Tachycardia, dysrhythmias, bounding pulses
  - Blurred vision, papilledema
  - Diaphoresis
  - Nausea and/or vomiting
  - Restlessness, headaches
  - Dyspnea, hypoventilation
  - Increased respiratory effort
  - Decreased respiratory rate
  - Increased $PCO_2$
  - Normal or decreased $PO_2$
  - Increased serum calcium
  - Decreased sodium chloride
  - Decreased reflexes
  - Decreased level of consciousness

  *(Respiratory acidosis can occur when an impaired respiratory system cannot remove $CO_2$, or when compensatory mechanisms that stimulate increased cardiac and respiratory efforts to remove excess $CO_2$ are overtaxed. Elevated $PaCO_2$ is the chief criterion. Elevated $PaCO_2$ increases cerebral blood flow, which decreases perfusion to heart, kidneys, and GI tract.)*
- For a client with respiratory acidosis:
  - Improve ventilation by
    - Positioning with head of bed up *(To promote diaphragmatic descent)*
    - Coaching in deep-breathing with prolonged expiration *(To increase exhalation of $CO_2$)*
    - Aiding expectoration of mucus followed by suctioning, if needed *(To improve ventilation–perfusion)*
- Consult with physician or advanced practice nurse for possible use of mechanical ventilation if improvement does not occur after the preceding interventions.
- Administer oxygen after the client is breathing better. *(Use of oxygen is of no value if the client is not breathing effectively and can result in further deterioration and death.)*
- Promote optimal hydration. *(This helps liquefy secretions and prevent mucous plugs.)*
- Limit use of sedatives and tranquilizers. *(Both can cause respiratory depression.)*
- Initiate the first five interventions for respiratory acidosis to correct metabolic acidosis.

# ▶ Risk for Complications of Metabolic or Respiratory Alkalosis

## DEFINITION

Describes a person experiencing or at high risk for experiencing an acid–base imbalance due to excessive bicarbonate or loss of hydrogen ions

## HIGH-RISK POPULATIONS

### For Respiratory Alkalosis

- Pulmonary disease
- CNS disorders/lesions
- Hyperventilation
- Severe infection, fever
- Asthma

---

\*When indicated, the nurse should specify the diagnosis as either *RC of Metabolic Acidosis* or *RC of Respiratory Acidosis*.

- Overly vigorous mechanical ventilation
- Restricted diaphragmatic movement (e.g., due to obesity, pregnancy)
- Inadequate oxygen in inspired air
- Congestive heart failure
- Alcohol intoxication
- Cirrhosis
- Thyrotoxicosis
- Paraldehyde, epinephrine, early salicylate overdose
- Overrapid correction of metabolic acidosis

## For Metabolic Alkalosis

- Prolonged vomiting, gastric suctioning, diarrhea
- Use of potent diuretics (e.g., thiazides), with resultant hydrogen and potassium loss
- Corticosteroid therapy
- IV replacement with potassium-free IV solutions
- Primary and secondary hyperaldosteronism
- Adrenocortical hormone disease
- Prolonged hypercalcemia or hypokalemia
- Excessive correction of metabolic acidosis

# Nursing Goals

The nurse will manage and minimize complications of alkalosis.

### Indicators

See RC of Metabolic or Respiratory Acidosis for indicators.

# General Interventions and Rationales

## For Metabolic Alkalosis

- Monitor for early signs and symptoms of metabolic alkalosis:
  - Tingling of fingers, dizziness
  - Hypertonic muscles (tremors)
  - Hypoventilation (to conserve carbonic acid)
  - Increased $HCO_3$
  - Slightly increased $PCO_2$
  - Decreased serum chloride, serum potassium, serum calcium
  - Hypoventilation
  - Polydipsia
  
  (*A decrease in ionized calcium produces most symptoms.*)
- For a client with metabolic alkalosis:
  - Initiate order for parenteral fluids. (*To correct sodium, water, chloride deficits*)
  - Monitor carefully the administration of ammonium chloride if ordered. (*Ammonium chloride increases circulating hydrogen ions, which results in decreased pH. Treatment can cause too-rapid decrease in pH and hemolysis of RBCs.*)
  - Evaluate renal and hepatic function before administration of ammonium chloride. (*Impaired renal or hepatic function cannot accommodate increased hemolysis.*)
  - Administer sedatives and tranquilizers cautiously, if ordered. (*Both depress respiratory function.*)
  - Monitor ABG values, urine pH, serum electrolyte levels, and BUN. (*These values help evaluate response to treatment and detect rebound metabolic acidosis resulting from too-rapid correction.*)

## For Respiratory Alkalosis

- Monitor for respiratory alkalosis:
  - Lightheadedness

- Numbness, tingling
- Carpopedal spasm
- Muscle weakness
- Normal or decreased $HCO_3$
- Decreased $PCO_2$
- Decreased serum potassium
- Increased serum chloride
- Decreased serum calcium

*(Decrease in plasma carbonic acid content causes vasoconstriction, decreased cerebral blood flow, and decreased ionized calcium.)*

- For a client with respiratory alkalosis:
  - Determine the cause of hyperventilation. *(Different etiologies warrant different interventions [e.g., anxiety versus incorrect mechanical ventilation].)*
  - Calm the anxious person by maintaining eye contact and remaining with him or her. *(Anxiety increases respiratory rate and $CO_2$ retention.)*
  - Instruct the person to breathe slowly with you. *(This increases $CO_2$ retention.)*
  - Alternatively, have the anxious person breathe into a paper bag and rebreathe from the bag. *(This increases $PaCO_2$ as the person rebreathes his or her own exhaled $CO_2$.)*
  - If anxiety is causative, refer to the nursing diagnoses *Anxiety* and *Ineffective Breathing Patterns* in Section II for additional interventions.
  - Consult with physician or advanced practice nurse for use of sedation as necessary. *(Sedation can help reduce respiratory rate and anxiety.)*
  - Monitor ABG values and electrolyte levels (e.g., potassium, calcium). *(Monitoring these values helps evaluate the client's response to treatment.)*
  - As necessary, refer to *RC of Electrolyte Imbalances* for specific management of electrolyte imbalance.

# ▶ Risk for Complications of Allergic Reaction

## DEFINITION

Describes a person experiencing or at high risk to experience hypersensitivity and release of mediators to specific substances (antigens)

## HIGH-RISK POPULATIONS

- History of allergies
- Asthma
- Immunotherapy
- Individuals exposed to high-risk antigens:
  - Insect stings (e.g., bee, wasp, hornet, ant)
  - Animal bites/stings (e.g., stingray, snake, jellyfish)
  - Radiologic iodinated contrast media (e.g., used in arteriography, intravenous pyelography)
  - Transfusion of blood and blood products
- High-risk individuals exposed to:
  - High-risk medications (e.g., aspirin, antibiotics, opiates, local anesthetics, animal insulin, chymopapain)
  - High-risk foods (e.g., peanuts, chocolate, eggs, seafood, shellfish, strawberries, milk)
  - Chemicals (e.g., floor waxes, paint, soaps, perfume, new carpets)

## Nursing Goals

The nurse will manage and minimize complications of allergic reactions.

## Indicators

Calm, alert, oriented
No complaints of urticaria or pruritus
No complaints of tightness in throat
No complaints of shortness of breath or wheezing

## General Interventions and Rationales

- Carefully assess for history of allergic responses (e.g., rashes, difficulty breathing). *(Identifying a high-risk client allows precautions to prevent anaphylaxis.)*
- If the client has a history of allergic response, consult with physician or advanced practice nurse regarding skin tests, if indicated. *(Skin testing can confirm hypersensitivity.)*
- Monitor for signs and symptoms of localized allergic reaction:
  - Wheals, flares (due to histamine release)
  - Itching
  - Nontraumatic edema (perioral, periorbital)
  *(These early manifestations can indicate the beginning of a continuum of localized reaction to systemic reaction to anaphylactic shock.)*
- At the first sign of hypersensitivity, consult with physician or advanced practice nurse for pharmacologic intervention, such as antihistamines. *(Antihistamines are commonly used to treat mild localized reactions by inhibiting histamine release.)*
- Monitor for signs and symptoms of systemic allergic reaction and anaphylaxis:
  - Lightheadedness, skin flushing, and slight hypotension (resulting from histamine-induced vasodilation)
  - Throat or palate tightness, wheezing, hoarseness, dyspnea, and chest tightness (from smooth muscle contraction from prostaglandin release)
  - Irregular, increased pulse and decreased blood pressure (from leukotriene release, which constricts airways and coronary vessels)
  - Decreased level of consciousness, respiratory distress, and shock (resulting from severe hypotension, respiratory insufficiency, and tissue hypoxia)
  *(Within minutes, such reactions can progress to severe hypotension, decreased level of consciousness, and respiratory distress, and can prove rapidly fatal.)*
- Promptly initiate emergency protocol for anaphylaxis and/or stat page physician or advanced practice nurse.
  - Start an IV line. *(For rapid medication administration)*
  - Administer epinephrine IV or endotracheally. *(To produce peripheral vasoconstriction, which raises blood pressure and acts as a β agonist to promote bronchial smooth muscle relaxation, and to enhance inotropic and chronotropic cardiac activity)*
  - Administer oxygen; establish a patent airway if indicated. Have suction available. Oropharyngeal intubation may be required. *(Laryngeal edema interferes with breathing.)*
- Administer other medications, as ordered, which may include:
  - Corticosteroids *(To inhibit enzyme and WBC response to reduce bronchoconstriction)*
  - Aminophylline *(To produce bronchodilation)*
  - Vasopressors *(To counter profound hypotension)*
  - Diphenhydramine *(To prevent further antigen–antibody reaction)*
- Frequently evaluate response to therapy; assess:
  - Vital signs
  - Level of consciousness
  - Lung sounds, peak flows
  - Cardiac function
  - Intake and output
  - ABG values
  *(Careful monitoring is necessary to detect complications of shock and identify the need for additional interventions.)*
- After recovery, discuss with the client and family preventive measures for anaphylaxis and the need to carry an anaphylaxis kit, which contains injectable epinephrine and oral antihistamines for use in self-treating allergic reaction.

# ▶ Risk for Complications of Thrombocytopenia

## DEFINITION

Describes a person experiencing or at high risk to experience insufficient circulating platelets (less than 150,000). This decrease can be caused by a reduction in platelet production, a change in platelet distribution, platelet destruction, or vascular dilution

## HIGH-RISK POPULATIONS

### Decreased Platelet Production from

- Treatment for certain chronic diseases such as Crohn's and RA (Enbrel group)
- Chemotherapy
- Radiation therapy
- Bone marrow invasion by tumor
- Leukemia
- Heparin therapy
- Toxins
- Severe infection (sepsis)
- Alcoholism
- Aplastic anemia
- Human immunodeficiency virus (HIV)

### Increased Platelet Destruction from

- Antibodies
- Aspirin
- Alcohol
- Quinine, quinidine
- Digoxin
- Sulfonamides
- Entrapment in large spleen
- Infections (bacteremia, postviral infections)
- Renal disease
- Post-transfusion status
- Hypertension
- Hypothermia
- Viral infection (e.g., Epstein-Barr)
- HIV

### Increased Platelet Utilization from

- Disseminated intravascular coagulation
- Thrombotic thrombocytopenic purpura
- Liver disease
- Administration of several units of non–platelet-containing fluids

## Nursing Goals

The nurse will manage and minimize complications of decreased platelets.

### Indicators

Platelet count > 150,000/mm₃

# General Interventions and Rationales

- Monitor complete blood count (CBC), hemoglobin, coagulation tests, and platelet counts. *(These values help evaluate response to treatment and risk for bleeding. Platelet count <20,000/mm$_3$ indicates a high risk for intracranial bleeding.)*
- Assess for other factors that may lower platelet count in addition to the primary cause:
  - Abnormal hepatic function
  - Abnormal renal function
  - Infection, fever
  - Anticoagulant use
  - Alcohol use
  - Aspirin use
  - Administration of several units of non–platelet-containing fluids (e.g., packed RBCs)
  *(Assessment may identify factors that could be controllable.)*
- Monitor for signs and symptoms of spontaneous or excessive bleeding:
  - Spontaneous petechiae, ecchymoses, hematomas
  - Bleeding from nose or gums
  - Prolonged bleeding from invasive procedures such as venipunctures or bone marrow aspiration
  - Hematemesis or coffee-ground emesis
  - Hemoptysis
  - Hematuria
  - Vaginal bleeding
  - Rectal bleeding
  - Gross blood in stools
  - Black, tarry stools
  - Change in vital signs
  - Change in neurologic status (blurred vision, headache, disorientation)
  - Urine, feces, and emesis positive for occult blood
  - High pad/tampon count for menstruating women
  *(Constant monitoring is needed to ensure early detection of bleeding.)*
- Assess for systemic signs of bleeding and hypovolemia:
  - Increased pulse, increased respirations, decreased blood pressure
  - Changes in neurologic status (e.g., subtle mental status changes, blurred vision, headache, disorientation; *Changes in circulatory oxygen levels produce changes in cardiac, vascular, and neurologic functioning.*)
- If hemorrhage is suspected, refer to *RC of Hypovolemic Shock* for specific interventions.
- Anticipate platelet transfusion.
- Apply direct pressure for 5 to 10 min, then a pressure dressing, to all venipuncture sites. Monitor carefully for 24 h. *(These measures promote clotting and reduce blood loss.)*
- Treat nausea aggressively to prevent vomiting. *(Severe vomiting can cause GI bleeding.)*
- Minimize rectal probing. *(This avoids injury to rectal tissue and bleeding.)*
- Using the nursing diagnosis *Risk for Injury related to bleeding tendency* (see Section II), implement nursing interventions and teaching to reduce the risk of trauma.

# ▶ Risk for Complications of Opportunistic Infections

# DEFINITION

Describes a person experiencing or at high risk to experience an infection by an organism capable of causing disease only when immune system dysfunction is present

## HIGH-RISK POPULATIONS

- Immunosuppressive therapy (chemotherapy, antibiotics)
- Malignancy
- Sepsis
- AIDS
- Nutritional deficits
- Burns
- Trauma
- Extensive pressure ulcers
- Radiation therapy (long bones, skull, sternum)
- Elderly with chronic illness
- Drug/alcohol addiction

## Nursing Goals

The nurse will manage and minimize complications of immunodeficiency.

### Indicators

Temperature 98–99.5° F
Respirations 16–20 breaths/min
No cough
Alert, oriented
No seizures, no headache
Regular, formed stools
No herpetic or zoster lesions
No swallowing complaints
No change in vision
No weight loss
No new lesions, e.g., mouth
No lymphadenopathy

## General Interventions and Rationales

- Monitor CBC, WBC differential (neutrophils, lymphocytes), and absolute neutrophil count (WBC × neutrophil). *(These values help evaluate response to treatment.)*
- Monitor for signs and symptoms of primary or secondary infection:
  - Slightly increased temperature
  - Chills
  - Dysphagia
  - Adventitious breath sounds
  - Cloudy or foul-smelling urine
  - Complaints of urinary frequency, urgency, or dysuria
  - WBCs and bacteria in urine
  - Redness, change in skin temperature, swelling or unusual drainage in any area of disrupted skin integrity, including previous and current puncture sites
  - Irritation or ulceration of oral mucous membrane
  - Complaints of perineal or rectal pain and any unusual vaginal or rectal discharge
  - Increased hemorrhoidal pain, redness, or bleeding
  - Painful, pruritic skin lesions (herpes zoster), particularly in cervical or thoracic area
  - Change in WBC count, especially increased immature neutrophils
  *(In a client with severe neutropenia, usual inflammatory responses may be decreased or absent.)*
- Obtain culture specimens (e.g., urine, vaginal, rectal, mouth, sputum, stool, blood, skin lesions, indwelling lines) as ordered. *(Testing determines the type of causative organism and guides treatment.)*
- Monitor for signs and symptoms of sepsis. *(Gram-positive and gram-negative organisms can invade open wounds, causing septicemia. A debilitated client is at increased risk. Sepsis produces massive vasodilation, resulting in hypovolemia and subsequent tissue hypoxia. Hypoxia leads to decreased renal function and cardiac output,*

*triggering a compensatory response of increased respirations and heart rate in an attempt to correct hypoxia and acidosis. Bacteria in urine or blood indicates infection [Morton et al., 2005].)*

- Monitor for therapeutic and nontherapeutic effects of antibiotics.
- Monitor for signs and symptoms of opportunistic protozoal infections:
  - *Pneumocystis carinii* pneumonia: dry, nonproductive cough, low-grade fever, gradual to severe dyspnea
  - *Toxoplasma gondii* encephalitis: headache, lethargy, seizures
  - *Cryptosporidium* enteritis: watery diarrhea, nausea, abdominal cramps, malaise

  *(Clients with immunodeficiency are at risk for secondary diseases of opportunistic infections; protozoal infections are the most common and serious.)*
- Monitor for signs and symptoms of opportunistic viral infections:
  - Herpes simplex oral or perirectal abscesses: severe pain, bleeding, rectal discharge
  - Cytomegalovirus retinitis, colitis, pneumonitis, encephalitis, or other organ disease
  - Progressive multifocal leukoencephalopathy: headache, decreased mentation
  - Varicella zoster, disseminated (shingles)
- Monitor for signs and symptoms of opportunistic fungal infections:
  - *Candida albicans* stomatitis and esophagitis: exudate, complaints of unusual taste in mouth
  - *Cryptococcus neoformans* meningitis: fever, headaches, blurred vision, stiff neck, confusion
- Monitor for signs and symptoms of opportunistic bacterial infections, which commonly affect the pulmonary system:
  - *Mycobacterium avium* (intracellular disseminated)
  - *Mycobacterium tuberculosis* (extrapulmonary and pulmonary)
- Emphasize the need to report symptoms promptly. *(Early treatment of adverse manifestations often can prevent serious complications [e.g., septicemia] and also increases the likelihood of a favorable response to treatment.)*
- Explain the need to balance activity and rest and to consume a nutritious diet. *(Rest and a nutritious diet give energy for healing and enhancement of the body's defense system.)*
- Avoid or minimize invasive procedures (e.g., urinary catheterization, arterial or venous punctures, injections, rectal tubes, suppositories). *(This precaution helps prevent introduction of microorganisms.)*
- Explain the importance of adhering to medication regimen (prophylaxis and antiviral).
- Refer to the nursing diagnosis *Risk for Infection* in Section II for interventions to prevent introduction of microorganisms and to increase resistance.

# ▶ Risk for Complications of Sickling Crisis

## DEFINITION

Describes a person with sickle cell disease experiencing vascular occlusion by the sickled cells, which damages cells and tissue and causes hemolytic anemia, massive splenomegaly, and hypovolemic shock, acute chest syndrome, cerebrovascular accidents

## HIGH-RISK POPULATIONS

### People with Sickle Cell Disease with Precipitating Factors, such as:

- High altitude (>7000 ft above sea level)
- Unpressurized aircraft
- Dehydration (e.g., diaphoresis, diarrhea, vomiting)
- Strenuous physical activity
- Cold temperatures (e.g., iced liquids)
- Infection (e.g., respiratory, urinary, vaginal) parvovirus
- Ingestion of alcohol
- Cigarette smoking

## Nursing Goals

The nurse will manage and minimize the sickling crisis.

### Indicators

Pain control to a pre-established acceptable level
Oxygen saturation >95%
No or minimal bone pain
No or minimal abdominal pain
No or minimal chest pain
No or minimal fatigue
No or minimal headache
Urine output >5 mL/kg/h

## General Interventions and Rationales

- Monitor for signs and symptoms of anemia:
  - Lethargy
  - Weakness
  - Fatigue
  - Increased pallor
  - Dyspnea on exertion

  *(Because anemia is common with most of these clients and low hemoglobins are relatively tolerated, changes should be described in reference to person's baseline or acute symptoms [Rausch & Pollard, 1998].)*
- Monitor laboratory values, including CBC with reticulocyte count. *(Reticulocyte [normal level about 1%] elevation represents active erythropoiesis. Lack of elevation with anemia may represent a problem [Newcombe, 2002].)*
- Monitor for signs and symptoms of acute chest syndrome:
  - Fever
  - Acute chest pain

  *(Acute chest syndrome is the term used to represent the group of symptoms—acute pleuritic chest pain, fever, leukocytosis, and infiltrates on chest x-ray—seen in sickle cell disease [Rausch & Pollard, 1998]. This medical emergency may be caused by "sickling" leading to pulmonary infarction.)*
- Monitor for signs and symptoms of infection:
  - Fever
  - Pain
  - Chills
  - Increased WBCs

  *(Bacterial infection is a major cause of morbidity and mortality. Decreased spleen function [asplenia] results from sickle cell anemia. The loss of the spleen's ability to filter and destroy various infectious organisms increases the risk of infection [Porth, 2007].)*
- Monitor for changes in neurologic function:
  - Speech disturbances
  - Sudden headache
  - Numbness, tingling

  *(Cerebral infarction and intracranial hemorrhage are complications of sickle cell disease. Occlusion of nutrient arteries to major cerebral arteries causes progressive wall damage and eventual occlusion of the major vessel. Intracerebral hemorrhage may be secondary to hypoxic necrosis of vessel walls [Rausch & Pollard, 1998].)*
- Monitor for splenic dysfunction. *(The spleen is responsible for filtering blood to remove old bacteria. Sluggish circulation and increased viscosity of sickled cells causes splenic blockage. The normal acidotic and anoxic environment of the spleen stimulates sickling, which increases blood flow obstruction [Porth, 2007].)*
- Monitor for splenic sequestration crisis:
  - Sudden onset of lassitude
  - Very pale, listless
  - Rapid pulse
  - Shallow respirations
  - Low blood pressure

*(Increased obstruction of blood from the spleen together with rapid sickling can cause sudden pooling of blood into the spleen. This causes intravascular hypovolemia and hypoxia, progressing to shock [Rausch & Pollard, 1998].)*

- Instruct client to report the following:
  - Any acute illness
  - Severe joint or bone pain
  - Chest pain
  - Abdominal pain
  - Headaches, dizziness
  - Gastric distress
  - Priapism
  - Recurrent vomiting

  *(These symptoms may indicate vaso-occlusion in varied sites as a result of sickling. Some illnesses may predispose the client to dehydration [Rausch & Pollard, 1998].)*
- Initiate therapy per physician or nurse practitioner prescription (e.g., antisickling agents, analgesics, transfusions).
- Provide:
  - Bed rest
  - Fluids and foods high in folic acid
  - Warm compresses to areas of pain
  - Refer to the nursing diagnosis *Acute Pain* (see Section II, Part One) for interventions to manage the pain associated with a sickling crisis.

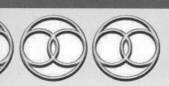

# RISK FOR COMPLICATIONS OF RENAL/URINARY DYSFUNCTION

**RC of Complications Renal/Urinary Dysfunction**

RC of Acute Urinary Retention
RC of Renal Insufficiency
RC of Renal Calculi

## DEFINITION

Describes a person experiencing or at high risk to experience various renal or urinary tract dysfunctions

### ■■■■■■ AUTHOR'S NOTE

The nurse can use this generic collaborative problem to describe a person at risk for several types of renal or urinary problems. For such a client (e.g., a client in a critical care unit, who is vulnerable to various renal/urinary problems), using *RC of Renal/Urinary Dysfunction* directs nurses to monitor renal and urinary status, based on the focus assessment, to detect and diagnose abnormal functioning. Nursing management of a specific renal or urinary complication would be addressed under the collaborative problem applying to the specific complication. For example, a standard of care for a client recovering from coronary bypass surgery could contain the collaborative problem *RC of Renal/Urinary Dysfunction*, directing the nurse to monitor renal and urinary status. If urinary retention developed in this client, the nurse would add *RC of Urinary Retention* to the problem list, along with specific nursing interventions to manage this problem. If the risk factors or etiology were not directly related to the primary medical diagnosis, the nurse still would specify them in the diagnostic statement (e.g., *RC of Renal Insufficiency related to chronic renal failure* in a client who has sustained a myocardial infarction).

Keep in mind that the nurse must differentiate those problems in bladder function that nurses can treat primarily as nursing diagnoses (e.g., incontinence, chronic urinary retention) from those that nurses manage using both nurse-prescribed and physician-prescribed interventions (e.g., acute urinary retention).

## SIGNIFICANT LABORATORY/DIAGNOSTIC ASSESSMENT CRITERIA_____

Hemoglobin (lowered in chronic renal disorders)
Prealbumin, albumin (lowered in renal disease)
Amylase (elevated with renal insufficiency)
pH, base excess, bicarbonate (lowered in metabolic acidosis, elevated in metabolic alkalosis)
Calcium (lowered in uremic acidosis)
Chloride (elevated with renal tubular acidosis)
Creatinine (elevated with kidney disease)
Magnesium (lowered in chronic nephritis)
Phosphorus (elevated with chronic glomerular disease, lowered with renal tubular acidosis)
Potassium (elevated in renal failure, lowered with chronic diuretic therapy, renal tubular acidosis)
Proteins (total, albumin, globulin) (lowered in nephritic syndrome)
Sodium (elevated with nephritis, lowered with chronic renal insufficiency)
Blood urea nitrogen (BUN) (elevated in acute or chronic renal failure)
Uric acid (elevated with chronic renal failure)
White blood cell (WBC) count (elevated with acute and lowered in chronic infections)
Urine (clean catch)
Blood (present with hemorrhagic cystitis, renal calculi, renal, bladder tumors)
Creatinine (elevated in acute/chronic glomerulonephritis, nephritis, lowered in advanced degeneration of kidneys)
pH (elevated with metabolic acidosis, lowered with metabolic alkalosis)
Specific gravity (elevated with dehydration, lowered with overhydration, renal tubular disease)
Myoglobin
Urine sodium and osmolarity
Culture and sensitivity
24-hour urine creatinine clearance
Renal ultrasound, magnetic resonance imaging
Kidneys, ureters, bladder x-ray
Renal biopsy
Renal angiography

## ▶ Risk for Complications of Acute Urinary Retention

## DEFINITION _____

Describes a person experiencing or at high risk to experience an acute abnormal accumulation of urine in the bladder and the inability to void due to a temporary situation (e.g., postoperative status) or to a condition reversible with surgery (e.g., prostatectomy) or medications

## HIGH-RISK POPULATIONS _____

- Postoperative status (e.g., surgery of the perineal area, lower abdomen)
- Postpartum status
- Anxiety
- Prostate enlargement, prostatitis
- Medication side effects (e.g., atropine, antidepressants, antihistamines)
- Postarteriography status
- Bladder outlet obstruction (infection, tumor)
- Impaired detrusor contractility

# Nursing Goals

The nurse will manage and minimize acute urinary retention episodes.

## Indicators

Urinary output >5mL/kg/h
Can verbalize bladder fullness
No complaints of lower abdominal pressure

# General Interventions and Rationales

- Monitor a postoperative client for urinary retention. *(Trauma to the detrusor muscle and injury to the pelvic nerves during surgery can inhibit bladder function. Anxiety and pain can cause spasms of the reflex sphincters. Bladder neck edema also can cause retention. Sedatives and narcotics can affect the CNS and effectiveness of smooth muscles [Porth, 2007].)*
- Monitor for urinary retention by palpating and percussing the suprapubic area for signs of bladder distention (overdistention, etc.). Instruct client to report bladder discomfort or inability to void. *(These problems may be early signs of urinary retention.)*
- Monitor for urinary retention in postpartum women. *(Labor and delivery can slacken the tone of the bladder wall temporarily, causing urinary retention.)*
- Encourage client to void within 6 to 8 hours after delivery. *(Desire to void may be diminished because of increased bladder capacity related to reduced intra-abdominal pressure after delivery.)*
- In a postpartum client, differentiate between bladder distention and uterine enlargement:
  - A distended bladder protrudes above the symphysis pubis.
  - When the nurse massages the uterus to return it to its midline position, the bladder protrudes further.
  - Percussion and palpation can distinguish between a rebounding bladder (from fluid) and a firm uterus.
  *(A distended bladder can push the uterus up and to the side and cause uterine relaxation.)*
- If client does not void within 8 to 10 h after surgery or complains of bladder discomfort, take the following steps:
  - Warm the bedpan.
  - Encourage client to get out of bed to use the bathroom, if possible.
  - Instruct a man to stand when urinating, if possible. If unable to stand, even sitting at the side of the bed helps.
  - Run water in the sink as client attempts to void.
  - Pour warm water over client's perineum.
  *(These measures help promote relaxation of the urinary sphincter and facilitate voiding.)*
- After the first voiding postdelivery or postsurgery, continue to monitor and to encourage client to void again in 1 hour or so. *(The first voiding usually does not empty the bladder completely.)*
- If the client still cannot void after 10 h, follow protocols for straight catheterization, as ordered by physician/advanced practice nurse. Consider bladder scanning to determine if the amount of urine in the bladder necessitates catheterization. *(Straight catheterization is preferable to indwelling catheterization because it carries less risk of urinary tract infection from ascending pathogens. Bladder scanning is not a risk for infection.)*
- For a client with chronic urinary retention, refer to the nursing diagnosis *Urinary Retention* in Section II.
- If person is voiding small amounts, use straight catheterization; if postvoid residual is >200 mL, leave catheter indwelling. Notify physician or advanced practice nurse.

# ▶ Risk for Complications of Renal Insufficiency

## DEFINITION

Describes a person experiencing or at high risk to experience a decrease in glomerular filtration rate that results in oliguria or anuria

## HIGH-RISK POPULATIONS

- Renal tubular necrosis from ischemic causes
  - Excessive diuretic use
  - Pulmonary embolism
  - Burns
  - Intrarenal thrombosis
  - Rhabdomyolysis
  - Renal infections
  - Renal artery stenosis/thrombosis
  - Peritonitis
  - Sepsis
  - Hypovolemia
  - Hypotension
  - Congestive heart failure
  - Myocardial infarction
  - Aneurysm
  - Aneurysm repair
- Renal tubular necrosis from toxicity
- Nonsteroidal anti-inflammatory drugs
  - Gout (hyperuricemia)
  - Hypercalcemia
  - Certain street drugs (e.g., PCP)
  - Gram-negative infection
  - Radiocontrast media
  - Aminoglycoside antibiotics
  - Antineoplastic agents
  - Methanol, carbon tetrachloride
  - Snake venom, poison mushroom
  - Phenacetin-type analgesics
  - Heavy metals
  - Insecticides, fungicides
  - Aminoglycosides
  - Diabetes mellitus
  - Primary hypertensive disease
  - Hemolysis (e.g., from transfusion reaction)

## Nursing Goals

The nurse will manage and minimize complications of renal insufficiency.

### Indicators

Urine specific gravity 1.005–1030
Urine output >5 mL/kg/h
Urine sodium 130–200 mEq/24 h
Blood urea nitrogen 10–20 mg/dL
Serum potassium 3.8–5 mEq/L

Serum sodium 135–145 mEq/L

Phosphorus 2.5–4.5 mg/dL

Creatinine clearance 100–150 mL of blood cleared/mm

## General Interventions and Rationales

- Monitor for early signs and symptoms of renal insufficiency:
  - Sustained elevated urine specific gravity, elevated urine sodium levels
  - Sustained insufficient urine output (<5 mL/kg/h), elevated blood pressure
  - Elevated BUN, serum creatinine, potassium, phosphorus, and ammonia; decreased creatinine clearance
  - Dependent edema (periorbital, pedal, pretibial, sacral)
  - Nocturia
  - Lethargy
  - Itching
  - Nausea/vomiting

  *(Hypovolemia and hypotension activate the renin–angiotensin system, increasing renal vasculature resistance, which decreases renal plasma flow and glomerular filtration rate. Decreased glomerular filtration rate eventually causes insufficient urine output and stimulates renin production, elevating the blood pressure in an attempt to increase blood flow to the kidney. Decreased excretion of urea and creatinine in the urine elevates BUN and creatinine levels. Dependent edema results from increased plasma hydrostatic pressure, salt and water retention, and/or decreased colloid osmotic pressure from plasma protein losses [Porth, 2007].)*

- Weigh the client daily at a minimum; more often, if indicated. Ensure accurate findings by weighing at the same time each day, on the same scale, and with the client wearing the same amount of clothing. *(Daily weights and intake and output records help evaluate fluid balance and guide fluid intake recommendations.)*

- Maintain strict intake and output records; determine the net fluid balance and compare with daily weight loss or gain for correlation. *(A 1-kg [2.2-lb] weight gain correlates with excess intake of 1 L.)*

- Explain prescribed fluid management goals. *(Client and family understanding may enhance cooperation.)*

- Adjust client's daily fluid intake so it approximates fluid loss plus 300–500 mL/day. *(Careful replacement therapy is necessary to prevent fluid overload.)*

- Distribute fluid intake fairly evenly throughout the entire day and night. It may be necessary to match fluid intake with loss every 8 h or even every hour if the client is critically imbalanced. *(Maintaining a constant fluid balance, without major fluctuations, is essential. Allowing toxins to accumulate because of poor hydration can cause complications such as nausea and sensorium changes.)*

- Encourage client to express feelings and frustrations; give positive feedback. *(Fluid and diet restrictions can be extremely frustrating. Emotional support can help reduce anxiety and may improve compliance with the treatment regimen.)*

- Consult with a dietitian regarding the fluid and diet plan. *(Important considerations in fluid management, requiring a specialist's attention, include the fluid content of nonliquid food, appropriate amount and type of liquids, liquid preferences, and sodium content.)*

- Administer oral medications with meals whenever possible. If medications must be administered between meals, give with the smallest amount of fluid necessary. *(This measure avoids using parts of the fluid allowance unnecessarily.)*

- Avoid continuous IV fluid infusion whenever possible. Dilute all necessary IV drugs in the smallest amount of fluid that is safe for IV administration. Use small IV bags and an IV controller or pump, if possible, to prevent accidental infusion of a large volume of fluid. *(Extremely accurate fluid infusion is necessary to prevent fluid overload.)*

- Monitor for signs and symptoms of metabolic acidosis:
  - Rapid, shallow respirations
  - Headaches
  - Nausea and vomiting
  - Low plasma pH
  - Behavioral changes, drowsiness, lethargy

  *(Acidosis results from the kidney's inability to excrete hydrogen ions, phosphates, sulfates, and ketone bodies. Bicarbonate loss results from decreased renal resorption. Hyperkalemia, hyperphosphatemia, and decreased*

*bicarbonate levels aggravate metabolic acidosis. Excessive ketone bodies cause headaches, nausea, vomiting, and abdominal pain. Respiratory rate and depth increase in an attempt to increase $CO_2$ excretion and thus reduce acidosis. Acidosis affects the CNS and can increase neuromuscular irritability because of the cellular exchange of hydrogen and potassium [Porth, 2007].)*

- For a client with metabolic acidosis, ensure adequate caloric intake while limiting fat and protein intake. Consult with a dietitian for an appropriate diet. *(Restricting fats and protein helps prevent accumulation of acidic end products.)*
- Assess for signs and symptoms of hypocalcemia, hypokalemia, and alkalosis as acidosis is corrected. *(Rapid correction of acidosis may cause rapid excretion of calcium and potassium and result in rebound alkalosis.)*
- Consult with the primary provider to initiate bicarbonate/acetate dialysis if the preceding measures do not correct metabolic acidosis:
  - Bicarbonate dialysis for severe acidosis: dialysate – $NaHCO_3$ = 100 mEq/L
  - Bicarbonate dialysis for moderate acidosis: dialysate – $NaHCO_3$ = 60 mEq/L

  *(The acetate anion, which the liver converts to bicarbonate, is used in dialysate to combat metabolic acidosis. Bicarbonate dialysis is indicated for clients with liver impairment, lactic acidosis, or severe acid–base imbalance.)*
- Monitor for signs and symptoms of hypernatremia with fluid overload:
  - Extreme thirst
  - CNS effects ranging from agitation to convulsion

  *(Hypernatremia results from excessive sodium intake or increased aldosterone output. Water is pulled from the cells, causing cellular dehydration and producing CNS symptoms. Thirst is a compensatory response aimed at diluting sodium.)*
- Maintain prescribed sodium restrictions. *(Hypernatremia must be corrected slowly to minimize CNS deterioration.)*
- Monitor for electrolyte imbalances:
  - Potassium
  - Calcium
  - Phosphorus
  - Sodium
  - Magnesium

  *(Refer to RC of Electrolyte Imbalances for specific signs and symptoms and interventions. Renal dysfunction can cause hyperkalemia, hypernatremia, hypocalcemia, hypermagnesemia, or hyperphosphatemia. Diuretic therapy can cause hypokalemia or hyponatremia.)*
- Monitor for gastrointestinal (GI) bleeding. *(Refer to RC of GI Bleeding for more information and specific interventions. The poor platelet aggregation and capillary fragility associated with high serum levels of nitrogenous wastes may aggravate bleeding. Heparinization required during dialysis in cases of gastric ulcer disease also may precipitate GI bleeding.)*
  - Monitor for manifestations of anemia:
  - Dyspnea
  - Fatigue
  - Tachycardia, palpitations
  - Pallor of nail beds and mucous membranes
  - Low hemoglobin and hematocrit levels
  - Easy bruising

  *(Chronic renal failure results in decreased red blood cell production and survival time because of elevated uremic toxins.)*
- Avoid unnecessary collection of blood specimens. *(Some blood loss occurs with every blood collection.)*
- Instruct client to use a soft toothbrush and to avoid vigorous nose blowing, constipation, and contact sports. *(Trauma prevention reduces the risk of bleeding and infection.)*
- Demonstrate the pressure method to control bleeding should it occur. *(Applying direct, constant pressure on a bleeding site can help prevent excessive blood loss.)*
- Monitor for manifestations of hypoalbuminemia:
  - Serum albumin level <3.5 g/dL; proteinuria (<100–150 mg protein/24 h)
  - Edema formation: pedal, facial, sacral
  - Hypovolemia
  - Increased hematocrit and hemoglobin levels

(Refer to *RC of Negative Nitrogen Balance* for more information and interventions. When albumin leaks into the urine because of changes in the glomerular electrostatic barrier or because of peritoneal dialysis, the liver responds by increasing production of plasma proteins. When the loss is great, the liver cannot compensate, and hypoalbuminemia results.)

- Monitor for hypervolemia. Evaluate daily:
  - Weight
  - Fluid intake and output records
  - Circumference of the edematous parts
  - Laboratory data: hematocrit, serum sodium, and plasma protein in specific serum albumin

  *(As glomerular filtration rate decreases and the functioning nephron mass continues to diminish, the kidneys lose the ability to concentrate urine and to excrete sodium and water, resulting in hypervolemia.)*

- Monitor for signs and symptoms of congestive heart failure and decreased cardiac output:
  - Gradual increase in heart rate
  - Increasing dyspnea
  - Diminished breath sounds, rales
  - Decreased systolic blood pressure
  - Presence of or increase in $S_3$ and/or $S_4$ heart sounds
  - Gallop rhythm
  - Peripheral edema
  - Distended neck veins

  *(Congestive heart failure can result from increased cardiac output, hypervolemia, dysrhythmias, and hypertension, reducing the ability of the left ventricle to eject blood, with subsequent decreased cardiac output and increased pulmonary vascular congestion.)*

- Encourage adherence to strict fluid restrictions: 800–1000 mL/24 h, or 24-h urine output plus 500 mL. *(Fluid restrictions are based on urine output. In an anuric client, restriction usually is 800 mL/day, which accounts for insensible losses from metabolism, the GI tract, perspiration, and respiration.)*

- Collaborate with physician, advanced practice nurse, or dietitian to plan an appropriate diet. Encourage adherence to a low-sodium diet (2–4 g/day). *(Sodium restrictions should be adjusted based on urine sodium excretion.)*

- If hemodialysis or peritoneal dialysis is initiated, follow institutional protocols.

### Pediatric Interventions and Rationales

- Assess for signs and symptoms unique to children with renal failure:
  - Growth failure
  - Bone deformities
  - Abnormal tooth development
  - Unexplained dehydration
  - Salt craving

  *(Children with renal insufficiency present differently from adults.)*

- Explore with parents child's response to exercise. *(Lethargy and reduced exercise tolerance are two early signs of renal insufficiency [Hockenberry & Wilson, 2009].)*

- Per orders, initiate treatment for anemia, hypertension, acidosis, and renal osteodystrophy. *(These represent the key nondialytic therapy goals.)*

- Consult with dietitian. *(Children with renal dysfunction present a challenge for obtaining adequate protein for growth and development and to prevent worsening of renal function [Hockenberry & Wilson, 2009].)*

## ▶ Risk for Complications of Renal Calculi

## DEFINITION

Describes a person with or at high risk for development of a solid concentration of mineral salts in the urinary tract.

## HIGH-RISK POPULATIONS

- History of renal calculi
- Urinary infection
- Urinary stasis, obstruction
- Immobility
- Hypercalcemia (dietary)
- Conditions that cause hypercalcemia
  - Hyperparathyroidism
  - Renal tubular acidosis
  - Myeloproliferative disease (leukemia, polycythemia vera, multiple myeloma)
  - Excessive excretion of uric acid
  - Inflammatory bowel disease
  - Gout
  - Dehydration

## Nursing Goals

The nurse will manage and minimize complications of renal calculi.

### Indicators

Temperature 98–99.5° F
Urine output >5 mL/kg/h
Urine specific gravity 1.005–1.030
Blood urea nitrogen 5–25 mg/dL
Clear urine
No flank pain

## General Interventions and Rationales

- Monitor for signs and symptoms of calculi:
  - Increased or decreased urine output
  - Sediment in urine
  - Flank or loin pain
  - Hematuria
  - Abdominal pain, distention, nausea, diarrhea
  *(Stones in the urinary tract can cause obstruction, infection, and edema, manifested by loin/flank pain, hematuria, and dysuria. Stones in the renal pelvis may raise urine production. Calculi-stimulating renointestinal reflexes can cause GI symptoms.)*
- Send urine for culture and sensitivity; send 24-hour urine for calcium oxalate, phosphorus, and uric acid. *(Tests are needed to determine type of stone and infection.)*
- Strain urine to obtain a stone sample; send samples to the laboratory for analysis. *(Acquiring a stone sample confirms stone formation and enables analysis of stone constituents.)*
- If the client complains of pain, consult with the physician or advanced practice nurse for aggressive therapy (e.g., narcotics, antispasmodics). *(Calculi can produce severe pain from spasms and proximity of the nerve plexus.)*
- Track the pain by documenting location, any radiation, duration, and intensity (using a rating scale of 0–10). *(This measure helps evaluate movement of calculi.)*

- Instruct the client to increase fluid intake, if not contraindicated. *(Increased fluid intake promotes increased urination, which can help facilitate stone passage and flush bacteria and blood from the urinary tract.)*
- Prepare person for KUB x-ray, excretory urography, and/or renal ultrasound.
- Monitor for signs and symptoms of pyelonephritis:
  - Fever, chills
  - Costovertebral angle pain (a dull, constant backache below the 12th rib)
  - Leukocytosis
  - Bacteria, blood, and pus in urine
  - Dysuria, frequency

  *(Urinary stasis or irritation of tissue by calculi can cause urinary tract infections. Signs and symptoms reflect various mechanisms. Bacteria can act as pyrogens by raising the hypothalamic thermostat through the production of endogenous pyrogen, which may be mediated through prostaglandins. Chills can occur when the temperature set-point of the hypothalamus changes rapidly. Costovertebral angle pain results from distention of the renal capsule. Leukocytosis reflects increased leukocytes to fight infection through phagocytosis. Bacteria and pus in urine indicate a urinary tract infection. Bacteria can irritate bladder tissue, causing spasms and frequency [Porth, 2007].)*
- Monitor for early signs and symptoms of renal insufficiency. (Refer to *RC of Renal Insufficiency*.)

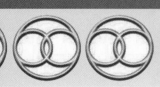

# RISK FOR COMPLICATIONS OF NEUROLOGIC/SENSORY DYSFUNCTION

**Risk for Complications of Neurologic/Sensory Dysfunction**

RC of Increased Intracranial Pressure
RC of Seizures
RC of Increased Intraocular Pressure
RC of Neuroleptic Malignant Syndrome (NMS)
RC of Alcohol Withdrawal

## DEFINITION

Describes a person experiencing or at high risk to experience various neurologic or sensory dysfunctions

## AUTHOR'S NOTE

The nurse can use this generic collaborative problem to describe a person at risk for several types of neurologic or sensory problems (e.g., a client recovering from cranial surgery or who has sustained multiple traumas). For such a person, using *RC of Neurologic/Sensory Dysfunction* directs nurses to monitor neurologic and sensory function based on focus assessment findings. Should a complication occur, the nurse would add the applicable specific collaborative problem (e.g., *RC of Increased Intracranial Pressure*) to the client's problem list to describe nursing management of the complication. If the risk factors or etiology were not related directly to the primary medical diagnosis or treatment, the nurse could add this information to the diagnostic statement. For example, for a client with a seizure disorder admitted for abdominal surgery, the nurse would add *RC of Seizures related to epilepsy* to the problem list.

In addition to the collaborative problem, the nurse should assess for other actual or potential responses that can compromise functioning. Some of these responses may represent nursing diagnoses (e.g., *Risk for Injury related to poor awareness of environmental hazards secondary to decreased sensorium*).

For information on Focus Assessment Criteria, visit http://thepoint.lww.com.

# SIGNIFICANT LABORATORY/DIAGNOSTIC ASSESSMENT CRITERIA_____

## Cerebrospinal Fluid
## Cloudy presentation (indicative of an infection)

Protein (increased in meningitis)
White blood cell (WBC) count (increased in meningitis)
Albumin (elevated with brain tumors)
Glucose (decreased with bacterial meningitis)

## Blood

WBC count (elevated with bacterial infection, decreased in viral infection)
Alcohol level
Glucose calcium
Mercury, lead levels if indicated

## Radiologic/Imaging

Skull, spine x-rays
Computed tomography (CT)
Magnetic resonance imaging (MRI)
Cerebral angiography
Position emission tomography (PET) (measures physiologic and biochemical process in the nervous system; can detect tumors, vascular diseases, and behavioral disturbances such as dementia or schizophrenia)
Myelography

## Other

Doppler
Lumbar puncture
Electroencephalography (EEG)
Continuous bedside cerebral blood flow monitoring

# ▶ Risk for Complications of Increased Intracranial Pressure

## DEFINITION _____

Describes a person experiencing or at high risk to experience increased pressure (>15 mm Hg) exerted by cerebrospinal fluid within the brain's ventricles or the subarachnoid space

## HIGH-RISK POPULATIONS _____

- Intracerebral mass (lesions, hematomas, tumors, abscesses)
- Blood clots
- Blockage of venous outflow
- Head injuries
- Reye's syndrome
- Meningitis
- Premature birth
- Cranial surgery

## Nursing Goals

The nurse will manage and minimize episodes of increased intracranial pressure (ICP).

### Indicators

Alert, oriented, calm or no change in usual cognitive status
No seizures
Appropriate speech
Pupils equal; reactive to light and accommodation
Intact extraocular movements
Pulse 60–100 beats/min
Respirations 16–20 breaths/min
BP >90/60, <140/90 mm Hg
Stable pulse pressure (difference between diastolic and systolic readings)
No nausea/vomiting
Mild to no headache
ICP monitoring to maintain the range indicated.

## General Interventions and Rationales

- Monitor for signs and symptoms of increased ICP.
  - Assess the following (Glascow Coma Scale [GCS]) (Hickey, 2006)
    - Best eye opening response: spontaneously, to auditory stimuli, to painful stimuli, or no response
    - Best motor response: obeys verbal commands, localizes pain, flexion–withdrawal, flexion–decorticate, extension–decerebrate, or no response
    - Best verbal response: oriented to person, place, and time; confused conversation; inappropriate speech; incomprehensible sounds; or no response

  *(Deficiencies of cerebral blood supply resulting from hemorrhage, hematoma, cerebral edema, thrombus, or emboli compromise cerebral tissue. These responses evaluate the client's ability to integrate commands with conscious and involuntary movement. The nurse can assess cortical function by evaluating eye opening and motor response. No response may indicate damage to the midbrain.)*
- Assess for changes in vital signs:
  - Pulse changes: slowing rate to 60 beats/min or lower or increasing rate to 100 beats/min or higher *(Bradycardia is a late sign of brain stem ischemia. Tachycardia may indicate hypothalamic ischemia and sympathetic discharge.)*
  - Respiratory irregularities: slowing rate with lengthening apneic periods *(Respiratory patterns vary depending on the site of impairment. Cheyne-Stokes breathing [a gradual increase followed by a gradual decrease, then a period of apnea] points to damage in both cerebral hemispheres, midbrain, and upper pons. Central neurogenic hyperventilation occurs with midbrain and upper pontine lesions. Ataxic breathing [irregular with random sequence of deep and shallow breaths] indicates pontine dysfunction. Hypoventilation and apnea occur with medullary lesions.)*
  - Rising blood pressure and/or widening pulse pressure
  - Bradycardia, increased systolic blood pressure, and increased pulse pressure *(These are late signs [known as Cushing Response] [Hickey, 2006] of brain stem ischemia leading to cerebral herniation.)*
- Assess pupillary responses. *(Changes indicate pressure on oculomotor or optic nerves.)*
  - Inspect the pupils with a bright pinpoint light to evaluate size, configuration, and reaction to light. Compare both eyes for similarities and differences. *(The oculomotor nerve [cranial nerve III] in the brain stem regulates pupil reactions.)*
  - Evaluate gaze to determine whether it is conjugate (paired, working together) or if eye movements are abnormal. *(Conjugate eye movements are regulated from parts of the cortex and brain stem.)*
  - Evaluate the ability of the eyes to adduct and abduct. *(Cranial nerve VI, or the abducens nerve, regulates abduction and adduction of the eyes. Cranial nerve IV, or the trochlear nerve, also regulates eye movement.)*
- Note any other signs and symptoms:
  - Vomiting *(Vomiting results from pressure on the medulla, which stimulates the brain's vomiting center.)*
  - Headache: constant, increasing in intensity, or aggravated by movement
  - Straining *(Compression of neural tissue increases ICP and causes pain.)*
  - Subtle changes (e.g., lethargy, restlessness, forced breathing, purposeless movements, changes in mentation; *These signs may be the earliest indicators of cranial pressure changes.)*

- Elevate the head of the bed 30 to 45 degrees unless contraindicated. *(Slight head elevation can aid venous drainage to reduce cerebrovascular congestion, thereby decreasing ICP. Positioning is very dependent upon the type of surgery done and the approach used and should always be clarified before repositioning.)*
- Avoid the following situations or maneuvers, which can increase ICP (Porth, 2002):
  - Carotid massage *(This slows the heart rate and reduces systemic circulation, which is followed by a sudden increase in circulation.)*
  - Neck flexion or extreme rotation; if intubated, do not use securing device with circumferential wrapping (Bhardwaj, Mirski, & Ulatowski, 2004). *(This inhibits jugular venous drainage, which increases cerebrovascular congestion and ICP.)*
  - Digital anal stimulation, breath-holding, straining *(These can initiate the Valsalva maneuver, which impairs venous return by constricting the jugular veins, thus increasing ICP.)*
  - Extreme flexion of the hips and knees *(Flexion increases intrathoracic pressure, which inhibits jugular venous drainage, increasing cerebrovascular congestion and, thus, ICP.)*
  - Rapid position changes
  - Seizures (Bhardwaj et al., 2004)
- Teach client to exhale during position changes. *(This helps prevent the Valsalva maneuver.)*
- Consult with the physician or nurse practitioner for stool softeners, if needed. *(Stool softeners prevent constipation and straining during defecation, which can trigger the Valsalva maneuver.)*
- Maintain a quiet, calm, softly lit environment. Schedule several lengthy periods of uninterrupted rest daily. Cluster necessary procedures and activities to minimize interruptions. *(These measures promote rest and decrease stimulation, both of which can help decrease ICP.)*
- Avoid sequential performance of activities that increase ICP (e.g., coughing, suctioning, repositioning, bathing). *(Research has validated that such sequential activities can cause a cumulative increase in ICP [Porth, 2007].)*
- Monitor temperature. As indicated, initiate external hypothermia or hyperthermia measures per orders and institutional protocol. *(Impaired hypothalamic function can interfere with temperature regulation, necessitating intervention. Hypothermia may reduce ICP, whereas hyperthermia may increase it. Prevent shivering which can increase ICP [Bhardwaj et al., 2004].)*
- Limit suctioning time to 10 s at a time; hyperoxygenate client both before and after suctioning. *(These measures help prevent hypercapnia, which can increase cerebral vasodilation and raise ICP, and prevent hypoxia, which may increase cerebral ischemia.)*
- Consult with physician or advanced practice nurse about administering prophylactic lidocaine before suctioning. *(This measure may help prevent acute intracranial hypertension [Morton et al., 2006].)*
- Maintain optimal ventilation through proper positioning and suctioning as needed. *(These measures help prevent hypoxemia and hypercapnia, suctioning when not needed causes agitation and increases ICP [Bhardwaj et al., 2004].)*
- Monitor arterial blood gas (ABG) values. *(ABG values help evaluate gas exchange in the lungs and determine circulating oxygen level and arterial $CO_2$. It is recommended that arterial $O_2$ be between 90 and 100 torr, and that arterial $CO_2$ be between 25 and 30 mm Hg, to prevent cerebral ischemia and cerebrovascular congestion, which increase ICP.)*
- If indicated, initiate protocols or collaborate with physician or advanced practice nurse for drug therapy, which may include the following (Morton et al., 2006):
  - Sedation, barbiturates *(These drugs reduce cerebral metabolic rate, contributing to decreased ICP.)*
  - Anticonvulsants *(These agents help prevent seizures, which increase cerebral metabolic rate.)*
  - Osmotic diuretics *(These agents draw water from brain tissue to the plasma to reduce cerebral edema.)*
  - Nonosmotic diuretics *(These agents draw sodium and water from edematous areas to reduce cerebral edema.)*
  - Steroids *(These drugs can reduce capillary permeability, limiting cerebral edema.)*
  - Paralytics *(These drugs reduce cerebral metabolic rate promoting decreased ICP [Bhardwaj et al., 2004].)*
- Carefully monitor hydration status; evaluate fluid intake and output, serum osmolality, and urine specific gravity and osmolality. *(Dehydration from diuretic therapy can cause hypotension and decreased cardiac output.)*
- If intravenous (IV) fluid therapy is prescribed, carefully administer IV fluids with an infusion pump. *(Careful IV fluid administration is necessary to prevent overhydration, which increases ICP.)*
- If using an ICP monitoring device, refer to the procedure manual for guidelines (e.g., ventriculostomy, subarachnoid bolt, epidural monitor).

## ▶ Risk for Complications of Seizures

## DEFINITION

Describes a person experiencing or at high risk to experience paroxysmal episodes of involuntary muscular contraction (tonus) and relaxation (clonus)

## HIGH-RISK POPULATIONS

- Perinatal injuries
- Family history of seizure disorder
- Cerebral cortex lesions
- Head injury
- Infectious disorder (e.g., meningitis)
- Cerebral circulatory disturbance (e.g., cerebral palsy, stroke)
- Brain tumor
- Alcohol overdose or withdrawal
- Drug overdose or withdrawal (e.g., theophylline)
- Electrolyte imbalances (e.g., hypocalcemia, pyridoxine deficiency)
- Hypoglycemia
- High fever
- Eclampsia
- Metabolic abnormalities (renal, hepatic, electrolyte)
- Poisoning (mercury, lead, carbon monoxide)

## Nursing Goals

The nurse will manage and minimize seizure episode.

### Indicators

No seizures or uncomplicated seizures

## General Interventions and Rationales

- Determine whether the client senses an aura before onset of seizure activity. If so, reinforce safety measures to take during an aura (e.g., lie down, pull car over to roadside and shut off ignition).
- If seizure activity occurs, observe and document the following (Hickey, 2006):
  - Where seizure began
  - Type of movements, parts of body involved
  - Changes in pupil size or position
  - Urinary or bowel incontinence
  - Duration
  - Unconsciousness (duration)
  - Behavior after seizure
  - Weakness, paralysis after seizure
  - Sleep after seizure (postictal period)
  *(Progression of seizure activity may assist in identifying its anatomic focus.)*
- Provide privacy during and after seizure activity. *(To protect the client from embarrassment)*
- During seizure activity, take measures to ensure adequate ventilation (e.g., loosen clothing). *Do not* try to force an airway or tongue blade through clenched teeth. *(Strong clonic/tonic movements can cause airway occlusion. Forced airway insertion can cause injury.)*
- During seizure activity, gently guide movements to prevent injury. Do not attempt to restrict movements. *(Physical restraint could result in musculoskeletal injury.)*
- If the client is sitting when seizure activity occurs, ease him or her to the floor and place something soft under his or her head. *(These measures help prevent injury.)*

- After seizure activity subsides, position client on the side. *(This position helps prevent aspiration of secretions.)*
- Allow person to sleep after seizure activity; reorient on awakening. *(The person may experience amnesia; reorientation can help him or her regain a sense of control and can help reduce anxiety.)*
- If person continues to have generalized convulsions, notify physician or advanced practice nurse and initiate protocol:
  - Establish airway.
  - Suction PRN.
  - Administer oxygen through nasal catheter.
  - Initiate an IV line.
  *(Status epilepticus is a medical emergency with a 10% mortality rate. Impaired respiration can cause systemic and cerebral hypoxia. IV administration of a rapid-acting anticonvulsant [e.g., diazepam] is indicated [Hickey, 2006].)*
- Keep the bed in a low position with the siderails up, and pad the siderails with blankets. *(These precautions help prevent injury from fall or trauma.)*
- If the client's condition is chronic, evaluate the need for teaching self-management techniques. Use the nursing diagnosis *Risk for Ineffective Self-Health Management related to insufficient knowledge of condition, medication regimen, safety measures, and community resources* (see Section II).

# ▶ Risk for Complications of Increased Intraocular Pressure

## DEFINITION

Describes a person experiencing or at high risk to experience increased aqueous humor production or resistance to outflow, which can cause compression of nerve fibers and blood vessels in the optic disc

## HIGH-RISK POPULATION

- Glaucoma
- Corneal transplant
- Radiation therapy
- Eye trauma
- Ophthalmic surgery

## Nursing Goals

The nurse will manage and minimize increased intraocular pressure.

### Indicators

No complaints of eyebrow pain
No complaints of nausea
No complaints of halos around lights

## General Interventions and Rationales

- Reinforce prescribed postoperative activity restrictions, which may include avoiding the following:
  - Bending at the waist
  - Making sudden head movements
  - Valsalva maneuver (e.g., straining during bowel movements)
  *(These activities can increase intraocular pressure.)*
- Reinforce the need to wear eye protection (patch and shield). *(These protect the eye from trauma.)*
- Monitor for bleeding, dehiscence, and evisceration. *(Ocular tissue is vulnerable to these problems because of its high vascularity and fragile vessels.)*

- Monitor for signs and symptoms of increased intraocular pressure:
  - Eyebrow pain
  - Nausea
  - Halos around lights

  *(Intraocular pressure may increase in response to surgery or owing to medications, such as steroid eye drops.)*
- Administer an antiemetic if nausea develops. *(Vomiting increases intraocular pressure and must be avoided.)*
- Monitor visual acuity and note any changes (e.g., halos around lights). *(Factors that can alter vision include blood in the vitreous or from the incision, infection, dislocation of the lens implant, redetachment of the retina, and increased intraocular pressure.)*
- Position client on the back with the head elevated; turn on the unaffected side. *(This positioning can help reduce pressure in the affected eye.)*
- Maintain a quiet environment; limit external stimuli and activities. *(These measures can help reduce stress and may promote a decrease in intraocular pressure.)*

Ensure that the client understands the importance of following the positional limitations if they are indicated. *(Postoperative positioning may be very specific for surgical procedures where gas has been injected into the eye.)*

Use appropriate care and caution in application of eye drops, avoiding contamination of the eye dropper and the eye. *(Postoperative eye infections can result in failed surgery and loss of vision.)*

# ▶ Risk for Complications of Neuroleptic Malignant Syndrome (NMS)

## DEFINITION

Describes a person experiencing or at high risk to experience an acute, life-threatening reaction to neuroleptic medication. The pathophysiology of NMS is poorly understood, but like other forms of extrapyramidal symptoms, there appear to be neuroleptic-induced dopaminergic blockade and dopamine depletion in the CNS, particularly in the basal ganglia and hypothalamus, which causes the various symptoms. It is most often characterized by the rapid onset of severe muscular rigidity [peripheral musculoskeletal muscle is susceptible to dopamine blockade (Bhardwaj et al., 2004)], autonomic instability, hyperthermia, and deteriorating mental state. It occurs in 1% of clients receiving neuroleptic agents.

## HIGH-RISK POPULATIONS

- Use of neuroleptics, especially the higher-potency drugs haloperidol, fluphenazine, and chlorpromazine
- Use of long-acting depot neuroleptics
- Use of neuroleptic medications in combination with:
  - Concurrent lithium therapy
  - Physiologic stress
  - Nutritional deficiencies
  - Concurrent organic brain syndrome
  - Physical exhaustion
  - Dehydration
  - Acquired immunodeficiency syndrome (AIDS)
  - Restraints
  - Anticholinergic drugs
  - Agitation
  - Mood disorders
  - High temperature and humidity
  - Alcoholism (Bhardwaj et al., 2004)
  - Agitation (Bhardwaj et al., 2004)
- High doses of neuroleptics
- Concurrent use of two or more neuroleptics

- Previous history of NMS
- Male gender, younger than 40 years of age (80% of cases)
- Undergoing "rapid neuroleptization," especially if administered by injections
- Initial 2 weeks of therapy, although it can occur at any point in neuroleptic therapy (e.g., 16% within 24 h of administration)
- Discontinuation of antiparkinsonian drugs

## Nursing Goals

The nurse will manage and minimize NMS episodes.

### Indicators

No complaints of muscle aches, cramp, rigidity
Usual skin color
No complaints of dyspnea
No urinary incontinence
BP >90/60, <140/90 mm Hg
Heart rate 60–100 beats/min
No evidence of diaphoresis
Normal deep tendon response
Urine color pale to amber

## General Interventions and Rationales

- Hold doses of all neuroleptic drugs and drugs with anticholinergic properties, and notify physician.
- Maintain airway. Provide a calm environment. *(Any client with altered level of consciousness is at risk for airway compromise and hypoventilation. Chest wall muscle rigidity also contributes.)*
- Recognize and treat promptly cardiac dysrhythmias and blood pressure instabilities as necessary.
- Monitor for signs and symptoms.
  - Severe extrapyramidal symptoms:
    - Muscular rigidity
    - Dysarthria
    - Dysphagia (difficulty swallowing)
    - Excess salivation
    - Myoglobinuria (urine turning red)
    - Akinesis
    - Cogwheel rigidity
    - Muteness
    - Waxy flexibility
    - Exaggerated deep tendon reflexes
  - Autonomic dysfunction:
    - Tachycardia
    - Diaphoresis
    - Urinary incontinence
    - Labile or sustained hypertension
    - Hypotension (abnormal blood pressure)
    - Dyspnea
    - Tachypnea
    - Pallor
    - Cardiac dysrhythmias
  - Fever above 100° F
  - Behavioral changes or fluctuations (e.g., confusion, delirium, agitation, coma, catatonic-like posturing, combativeness)
  - Dehydration
  - Malnutrition

  *(The underlying pathophysiology is not well understood but appears to be related to the blockage or depletion of the CNS neurotransmitter dopamine. Signs and symptoms of NMS appear to be related to the degree and sites of*

*involvement of dopamine blockade. For example, dopamine blockade in the nigrostriatal pathway appears to cause muscular rigidity; dopamine impairment in the preoptic anterior hypothalamus, which regulates temperature, appears to cause fever; dopamine disturbance in the spinal cord may cause autonomic dysfunction.)*

- Monitor for abnormal laboratory findings:
  - Elevated creatine phosphokinase
  - Elevated WBC count
  - Elevated liver functions
  - ABG
  - Electrolytes

*(As the body reacts to dopamine depletion, WBC count rises, creatine phosphokinase is elevated because of micronecrosis of the skeletal muscles, and hepatic enzymes are elevated. Blood gas determinations measure the degree of autonomic instability. Electrolytes measure the effect of autonomic instability and micronecrosis on the body systems.)*

- Assess vital signs frequently (blood pressure; temperature, pulse, respiration; and electrocardiogram) for signs of respiratory and cardiovascular decompensation.
- Monitor degree of rigidity through deep tendon reflexes. If rigidity is worsening, further measures must be taken because it can affect the muscles of the vital organs. *(Deep tendon reflexes indicate objectively whether the rigidity is worsening or improving.)*
- Institute seizure precautions.
- Monitor fluid intake and output and for signs of renal decompensation. *(Excessive muscle breakdown [micronecrosis] can cause myoglobinuria and renal failure.)*
- Auscultate and evaluate lungs for pulmonary stasis and embolus. *(Dysphagia can lead to aspiration pneumonia. Immobility places a person at risk for pulmonary stasis or embolus.)*
- If dantrolene is ordered to help decrease muscle rigidity, remain alert for:
  - Liver toxicity
  - Phlebitis and tissue damage (if administered IV)

*(Dantrolene, a skeletal muscle relaxant, acts at the level of the sarcoplasmic reticulum, complementing the effects of a dopaminergic agent.)*

- Apply cooling blankets, antipyretic medications, and cool sponge baths (to control fever).
- If dysphagia is present:
  - Monitor food intake closely.
  - Provide soft or liquid diet.
  - Tube feedings or total parenteral nutrition if nutritional status continues to decline
  - Refer also to *Impaired Swallowing.*
- Refer to *Risk for Impaired Skin Integrity* to prevent pressure ulcers. *(Profuse diaphoresis, dehydration, urinary incontinence, and contracted limbs set the stage for skin breakdown.)*
- Provide mouth care and suctioning as needed. *(Dysphagia can cause increased salivation.)*
- Apply eye lubricants & tape eyelids closed as needed. *(These prevent exposure keratitis secondary to inadequate blinking.)*
- After recovery:
  - Teach client and significant others the importance of maintaining proper nutrition, sleep, and exercise. *(Physiologic depletion predisposes the person to NMS.)*
  - Review manifestations of NMS and teach client and significant others to seek immediate medical help if stiffness, fever, excess sweating, and racing pulse occur. *(Early detection can prevent serious complications; NMS has an 11.6% mortality rate.)*
- Institute seizure precautions.

## ▶ Risk for Complications of Alcohol Withdrawal

## DEFINITION

Describes a person experiencing or at high risk to experience the complications of alcohol withdrawal (e.g., delirium tremens, autonomic hyperactivity, seizures, alcohol hallucinosis, and hypertension)

## HIGH-RISK POPULATIONS

Alcoholics

## Nursing Goals

The nurse will manage and minimize alcohol withdrawal complications.

### Indicators

No seizure activity
Calm, oriented
Temperature 98–99.5° F
Pulse 60–100 beats/min
BP >90/60, <140/90 mm Hg
No reports of hallucinations
No tremors

## General Interventions and Rationales

- Carefully attempt to determine if the client abuses alcohol. Consult with the family regarding their perception of alcohol consumption. Explain why accurate information is necessary. *(It is critical to identify high-risk people so potentially fatal withdrawal symptoms can be prevented.)*
- Obtain history of previous withdrawals.
  - Delirium tremens:
    - Time of onset
    - Manifestation
  - Seizures:
    - Time of onset
    - Type

*(Withdrawal occurs 6 to 96 h after drinking ends. Withdrawal can occur in people who are considered "social drinkers" [6 oz of alcohol daily for a period of 3 to 4 weeks]. Withdrawal patterns may resemble those of previous episodes. Seizure patterns unlike previous episodes may indicate another underlying pathology.)*

- Obtain a complete history of prescription and nonprescription drugs taken. *(Benzodiazepine or barbiturate withdrawal may mimic alcohol withdrawal and complicate the picture.)*
- Consult with the primary provider regarding the risk of the client and initiation of benzodiazepine therapy, with dosage determined by assessment findings. *(Benzodiazepine requirements in alcohol withdrawal are highly variable and client specific. Fixed schedules may over sedate or under sedate.)*
- Observe for the desired effects of benzodiazepine therapy:
  - Relief from withdrawal symptoms
  - Peaceful sleep but rousable

*(Benzodiazepines are the drugs of choice in controlling withdrawal symptoms. Neuroleptics cause hypotension and lower seizure threshold. Barbiturates may effectively control symptoms of withdrawal but have no advantages over benzodiazepines.)*

- Monitor for indicators of a drop in blood alcohol level and determine the time of onset:
  - Anxiety
  - Insomnia
  - Mild tachycardia
  - Tremors

- Sensory hyperacuity
- Low-grade fever
- Disorientation
- Dehydration

*(Once a level drops 100 mg/dL below the person's normal, withdrawal typically occurs. These symptoms can last up to 5 days. Withdrawal results in a hypermetabolic state from adrenergic excess and possible alteration of prostaglandin E₁ levels.)*

- Monitor for withdrawal seizures.
  - Determine time of onset.
  - Refer also to *RC of Seizures.*

  *(Withdrawal seizures can occur 6 to 96 h after drinking ends. They are usually nonfocal and grand mal, last minutes or less, and occur singly or in clusters of two to six.)*
- Monitor for and intervene promptly in cases of status epilepticus. Follow institution's emergency protocol. *(Status epilepticus is life-threatening if not controlled immediately with IV diazepam.)*
- Monitor for delirium tremens.
  - Delirium component (vivid hallucinations, confusion, extreme disorientation, and fluctuating levels of awareness)
  - Extreme hyperadrenergic stimulation (tachycardia, hypertension or hypotension, extreme tremor, agitation, diaphoresis, and fever)

  *(Delirium tremens appears on days 3-5 after cessation of drinking and resolve within 5 days) [Bhardwaj et al., 2004].)*
- Monitor and determine onset of alcohol hallucinosis, which involves visual, auditory, and tactile hallucinations (however, the person senses that the hallucinations are not real and is aware of surroundings). *(Alcohol hallucinosis occurs 6 to 96 h after abstinence and can last up to 3 days.)*
- Monitor vital signs at least every 2 h:
  - Temperature, pulse, and respiration
  - Blood pressure

  *(Clients in withdrawal have elevated heart rate, respirations, and fever. Clients experiencing delirium tremens can be expected to have a low-grade fever. Rectal temperature greater than 37.7° C [99.9° F] is a clue to possible infection.)*
- Maintain the client's IV running continuously. *(This is necessary for fluid replacement and dextrose, thiamine bolus, benzodiazepine, and magnesium sulfate administration. Chlordiazepoxide and diazepam should not be given IM because of unpredictable absorption.)*
- Refer to the nursing diagnosis *Ineffective Denial* for interventions for substance abuse.

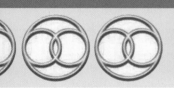

# RISK FOR COMPLICATIONS OF GASTRO-INTESTINAL/HEPATIC/BILIARY DYSFUNCTION

**Risk for Complications of Gastrointestinal/Hepatic/Biliary Dysfunction**

RC of Paralytic Ileus
RC of GI Bleeding
RC of Hepatic Dysfunction
RC of Hyperbilirubinemia

## DEFINITION

Describes a person experiencing or at high risk to experience compromised function in the gastrointestinal (GI), hepatic, or biliary systems. (*Note:* These three systems are grouped together for classification purposes. In a clinical situation, the nurse would use either *RC of Gastrointestinal Dysfunctional*, *RC of Hepatic Dysfunction*, *RC of Bleeding* or *RC of Biliary Dysfunction* to specify the applicable system.)

▨▩▦▧■■ **AUTHOR'S NOTE**

The nurse can use these generic collaborative problems to describe a person at risk for various problems affecting the GI, hepatic, or biliary systems. Doing so focuses nursing interventions on monitoring GI, hepatic, or biliary status to detect and diagnose abnormal functioning. Should a complication develop, the nurse would add the applicable specific collaborative problem (e.g., *RC of GI Bleeding, RC of Hepatic Dysfunction*) to the problem list, specifying appropriate nursing management.

In most cases, along with these collaborative problems, the nurse treats other associated responses, using nursing diagnoses (e.g., *Impaired Comfort related to accumulation of bilirubin pigment and bile salts*).

For information on Focus Assessment Criteria, visit http://thepoint.lww.com.

## SIGNIFICANT LABORATORY/DIAGNOSTIC ASSESSMENT CRITERIA_____

Urinalysis (to detect low amylase levels, which indicate pancreatic insufficiency)
Serum *Helicobacter pylori* (*H. pylori*) (positive as a risk factor for peptic ulcer disease)
Serum albumin (lowered in chronic liver disease)
Serum amylase (elevated in biliary tract disease)
Serum lipase (elevated in pancreatitis)
Serum calcium (high total calcium levels in cancer of liver, pancreas, and other organs)
Stool specimen (can be analyzed for blood, parasites, fat)
Bilirubin (elevated in hepatic disease, newborn hyperbilirubinemia)
Potassium (lowered in liver disease with ascites, vomiting, diarrhea)
Blood urea nitrogen (BUN; increased in hepatic failure)
Prothrombin time (elevated in cirrhosis, hepatitis)
Hemoglobin, hematocrit (decreased with bleeding)
Sodium (decreased with dehydration)
Platelets (decreased with liver disease or bleeding)
Serum ammonia level elevated in liver dysfunction
Hepatitis panel for primary differential diagnosis of diseases of the liver
Abdominal x-ray
Ultrasound (to detect masses, obstruction, gallstones)
CT scan, MRI (to evaluate sot tissue for abscesses, tumors, sources of bleeding)
Colonoscopy, barium enema
Endoscopy, upper GI series
Endoscopic retrograde cholangiopancreatography (ERCP)

## ▶ Risk for Complications of Paralytic Ileus

## DEFINITION _____

Describes a person experiencing or at high risk to experience neurogenic or functional bowel obstruction

## HIGH-RISK POPULATIONS _____

- Thrombosis or embolus to mesenteric vessels
- Any major surgery with use of general anesthesia and subsequent limitation of mobility, as well as minor surgery of the abdomen
- Postoperative status (bowel, retroperitoneal, or spinal cord surgery)
- Electrolyte imbalances (e.g., hypokalemia)
- Hypokalemia
- Postshock status

- Hypovolemia
- Post-trauma (e.g., spinal cord injury)
- Strangulated hernias
- Congenital bowel deformities
- Uremia
- Spinal cord lesion

## Nursing Goals

The nurse will manage and minimize complications of paralytic ileus.

### Indicators

Bowel sounds present
No nausea and vomiting
No abdominal distention

## General Interventions and Rationales

- In a postoperative client, monitor bowel function, looking for:
  - Bowel sounds in all quadrants returning within 24 to 48 h of surgery
  - Flatus and defecation resuming by the second or third postoperative day
  *(Surgery and anesthesia decrease innervation of the bowel, reducing peristalsis and possibly leading to transient paralytic ileus [Porth, 2007].)*
- Do not allow client any fluids until bowel sounds are present. When indicated, begin with small amounts of clear liquids only. Monitor client's response to resumption of fluid and food intake, and note the nature and amount of any emesis or stools. *(The client will not tolerate fluids until bowel sounds resume.)*
- Monitor for signs of paralytic ileus—primarily pain, typically localized, sharp, and intermittent; hiccups; nausea/vomiting; constipation; distended abdomen; rebound tenderness. *(Intraoperative manipulation of abdominal organs and the depressive effects of narcotics and anesthetics on peristalsis can cause paralytic ileus, typically developing between the third and fifth postoperative day.)*
- If paralytic ileus is related to hypovolemia, refer to *RC of Hypovolemia* for more information and specific interventions.

# ▶ Risk for Complications of GI Bleeding

## DEFINITION

Describes a person experiencing or at high risk to experience GI bleeding

## HIGH-RISK POPULATIONS

- Prolonged mechanical ventilation
- Disorders of GI, hepatic, and biliary systems
- Transfusion of 5 U (or more) of blood
- Recent stress (e.g., trauma, sepsis), prolonged mechanical ventilation
- Esophageal varices
- Peptic ulcer
- Colon cancer
- Platelet deficiency
- Coagulopathy
- Shock, hypotension
- Major surgery (>3 h)

- Head injury
- Severe vascular disease
- Burns (>35% of body)
- Daily use of aspirin or nonsteroidal anti-inflammatory drugs (NSAIDs)

## Infants/Children (Hockenberry & Wilson, 2009)

- Neonate (*swallowed maternal blood, *hemorrhagic disease, anal fissure, stress ulcers, enterocolitis, vascular malformations)
- 6 months (same as above except [*], intussusception, lymphonodular hyperplasia)
- 6 months to 5 years (same as above, epistaxis, esophagitis, varices, gastritis, Meckel's diverticulum, Henoch-Schönlein purpura, polyps)
- 5 to 18 years (same as above, Mallory-Weiss tear, peptic ulcer, chronic ulcerative colitis, Crohn's disease, hemorrhoids)

# Nursing Goals

The nurse will manage and minimize complications of GI bleeding.

## Indicators

Negatives stool occult blood
Calm, oriented
Refer to *RC of Hypovolemia* for indicators

# General Interventions and Rationales

- Initiate prophylaxis protocol for persons on mechanical ventilation. *(These individuals are high risk for GI bleeding.)*
- Monitor for signs and symptoms of GI bleeding:
  - Nausea
  - Hematemesis
  - Blood in stool
  - Decreased hematocrit or hemoglobin
  - Hypotension, tachycardia
  - Diarrhea or constipation
  - Anorexia

  *(Clinical manifestations depend on the amount and duration of GI bleeding. Early detection enables prompt intervention to minimize complications.)*
- Monitor for occult blood in gastric aspirates and bowel movements.
- Monitor gastric pH every 2 to 4 h. *(Maintenance of gastric pH <5 has decreased bleeding complications by 89%.)*
- Use pH paper that has a range from 0 to 7.5. Use good light to interpret the color on the pH paper.
  - Position client on the left side lying down. *(The left side down position allows the tip of the nasogastric [NG] or gastrostomy tube to move into the greater curvature of the stomach and usually below the level of gastric fluid.)*
  - Use two syringes (>30 mL) to obtain the aspirate. Aspirate a gastric sample and discard. Use aspirate in the second syringe for testing. *(The first aspirate clears the tube of antacids and other substances that can alter the pH of the sample.)*
- Evaluate for other factors that affect the pH reading:
  - Medications (e.g., cimetidine)
  - Tube feeding
  - Irrigations

  *(False-positive and false-negative findings can result when aspirate contains certain substances. Most investigators recommend a range of 3.5 to 5.0.)*
- Monitor vital signs often, particularly blood pressure and pulse. *(Careful monitoring can detect early changes in blood volume.)*

- Consult with physician/advanced practice nurse for the specific prescription for titration ranges of pH and antacid administration.
- If NG intubation is prescribed, use a large-bore (18-gauge) tube and follow protocols for insertion and client care. *(An NG tube can remove irritating gastric secretions, blood, and clots and can reduce abdominal distention.)*
- Follow the protocol for gastric lavage, if ordered. *(Lavage provides local vasoconstriction and may help control GI bleeding.)*
- Monitor hemoglobin, hematocrit, red blood cell count, platelets, prothrombin time, partial thromboplastin time, type blood and cross match, and blood urea nitrogen (BUN) values. *(These values reflect the effectiveness of therapy.)*
- If hypovolemia occurs, refer to *RC of Hypovolemia* for more information and specific interventions.
- Prepare for transfusion per physician/advanced practice nurse order. *(Doing so can reestablish volume status. Use of warmed blood products is better tolerated and safer.)*

Provide client education and obtain consent for transfusion of blood products in advance.
(This helps to alleviate anxiety and facilitate the transfusion if it becomes necessary. Consent obtained in advance should always be re-affirmed before proceeding.)

# ▶ Risk for Complications of Hepatic Dysfunction

## DEFINITION

Describes a person experiencing or at high risk to experience progressive liver dysfunction

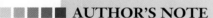 **AUTHOR'S NOTE**

In 2006, NANDA accepted the nursing diagnosis, *Risk for Impaired Liver Function*. This author maintains that this is a collaborative problem. Nurses can choose to use either terminology. Students should consult with their faculty for direction.

## HIGH-RISK POPULATIONS

### Infections

- Hepatitis A, B, C, D, E, non-A, non-B, non-C
- Herpes simplex virus (types 1 and 2)
- Epstein-Barr virus
- Varicella zoster
- Dengue fever virus
- Rift Valley fever virus

### Drugs/Toxins

- Industrial substances (chlorinated hydrocarbons, phosphorus)
- *Amanita phalloides* (mushrooms)
- Aflatoxin (herb)
- Medications (isoniazid, rifampin, halothane, methyldopa, tetracycline, valproic acid, monoamine oxidase inhibitors, phenytoin, nicotinic acid, tricyclic antidepressants, isoflurane, ketoconazole, cotrimethoprim, sulfasalazine, pyrimethamine, octreotide, antivirals)
- Acetaminophen toxicity
- Cocaine
- Alcohol

## Hypoperfusion (Shock Liver)

- Venous obstructions
- Budd-Chiari syndrome
- Veno-occlusive disease
- Ischemia

## Metabolic Disorders

- Hyperbilirubinemia
- Wilson's disease
- Tyrosinemia
- Heat stroke
- Galactosemia
- Nutritional deficiencies

## Surgery

(Traumatized liver)
- Jejunoileal bypass
- Partial hepatectomy
- Liver transplant failure

## Other

- Reye's syndrome
- Acute fatty liver of pregnancy
- Massive malignant infiltration
- Autoimmune hepatitis
- Rh incompatibility
- Ingestion of raw contaminated fish
- Thalassemia

# Nursing Goals

The nurse will manage and minimize the complications of hepatic dysfunction.

## Indicators

Prothrombin time (PT) 11–12.5 sec
Partial prothrombin time (PTT) 60–70 sec
Aspartate aminotransferase (AST) male 7–21 u/L, female 6–18 u/L
Alanine aminotransferase (ALT) 5–35 u/L
Alkaline phosphatase 30–150 u/L
Serum electrolytes within normal range

# General Interventions and Rationales

- Monitor for signs and symptoms of hepatic dysfunction:
  - Anorexia, indigestion *(GI effects result from circulating toxins.)*
  - Jaundice *(Yellowed skin and sclera result from excessive bilirubin production.)*
  - Petechiae, ecchymoses *(These skin changes reflect impaired synthesis of clotting factors.)*
  - Clay-colored stools *(This can result from decreased bile in stools.)*
  - Elevated liver function tests (e.g., serum bilirubin, serum transaminase) *(Elevated values indicate extensive liver damage.)*
  - Prolonged prothrombin time *(This reflects reduced production of clotting factors.)*
- With hepatic dysfunction, monitor for hemorrhage. *(The liver has a central role in hemostasis. Decreased platelet count results from impaired production of new platelets from the bone marrow. Decreased clearance of old platelets by the reticuloendothelial system also results. In addition, synthesis of coagulation factors [II, V, VII, IX, and X] is impaired, resulting in bleeding. The most frequent site is the upper GI tract. Other sites include the nasopharynx, lungs, retroperitoneum, kidneys, and intracranial and skin puncture sites [Porth, 2007].)*

- Teach client to report any unusual bleeding (e.g., in the mouth after brushing teeth). (*Mucous membranes are prone to injury because of their high surface vascularity.*)
- Monitor for portal systemic encephalopathy by assessing:
  - General appearance and behavior
  - Orientation
  - Speech patterns
  - Laboratory values: blood pH and ammonia level
  (*Profound liver failure results in accumulation of ammonia and other toxic metabolites in the blood. The blood–brain barrier permeability increases, and both toxins and plasma proteins leak from capillaries to the extracellular space, causing cerebral edema.*)
- Monitor for signs and symptoms of (refer to the index under each electrolyte for specific signs and symptoms):
  - Hypoglycemia (*Hypoglycemia is caused by loss of glycogen stores in the liver from damaged cells and decreased serum concentrations of glucose, insulin, and growth hormones.*)
  - Hypokalemia (*Potassium losses occur from vomiting, NG suctioning, diuretics, or excessive renal losses.*)
  - Hypophosphatemia (*The loss of potassium ions causes the proportional loss of magnesium ions. Increased phosphate loss, transcellular shifts, and decreased phosphate intake contribute to hypophosphatemia.*)
- Monitor for acid–base disturbances. Hepatocellular necrosis can result in accumulation of organic anions, resulting in metabolic acidosis. (*People with ascites often have metabolic alkalosis from increased bicarbonate levels resulting from increased sodium/hydrogen exchange in the distal tubule.*)
- Assess for side effects of medications. Avoid administering narcotics, sedatives, and tranquilizers and exposing the client to ammonia products. (*Liver dysfunction results in decreased metabolism of certain medications [e.g., opiates, sedatives, tranquilizers], increasing the risk of toxicity from high drug blood levels. Ammonia products should be avoided because of the client's already high serum ammonia level.*)
- Monitor for signs and symptoms of renal failure. (Refer to *RC of Renal Failure* for more information.) (*Obstructed hepatic blood flow results in decreased blood to the kidneys, impairing glomerular filtration and leading to fluid retention and decreased urinary output.*)
- Monitor for hypertension. (*Fluid retention and overload can cause hypertension.*)
- Teach client and family to report signs and symptoms of complications, such as:
  - Increased abdominal girth (*It may indicate worsening portal hypertension.*)
  - Rapid weight loss or gain (*Weight loss points to negative nitrogen balance; weight gain points to fluid retention.*)
  - Bleeding (*Unusual bleeding indicates decreased prothrombin time and clotting factors.*)
  - Tremors (*They can result from impaired neurotransmission because of failure of the liver to detoxify enzymes that act as false neurotransmitters.*)
  - Confusion (*This can result from cerebral hypoxia caused by high serum ammonia levels resulting from the liver's impaired ability to convert ammonia to urea.*)

# ❯ Risk for Complications of Hyperbilirubinemia

## DEFINITION

Describes a neonate with or at high risk for development of excessive serum bilirubin levels (>0.15 mg/dL)

## HIGH-RISK POPULATIONS (SIMPSON & CREEHAN, 2007)

### Newborn

- Birthweight <1500 g
- Preterm delivery
- Male sex
- Hypothermia
- Asphyxia

- Hypoalbuminemia
- Sepsis
- Meningitis
- Polycythemia (Hct > 65%)
- Drugs that affect albumin binding
- Congenital hypothyroidism
- Bruising
- Poor feeding
- Inborn errors of metabolism

## Maternal

- Oxytocin
- Forceps or vacuum delivery
- Blood incompatibilities
- Diabetes
- East Asian heritage
- Gestational hypertension
- Family history of jaundice, liver disease, anemia, or splenectomy

## Nursing Goals

The nurse will manage and minimize complications of hyperbilirubinemia.

### Indicators

Bilirubin level < 0.15 mg/dL

## General Interventions and Rationales

- Prevent cold stress. (*Metabolism of brown adipose tissue releases nonesterified free fatty acids, which compete with bilirubin for albumin-binding sites.*)
- Ensure adequate hydration and intake. (*Optimal fluid and feedings facilitate bilirubin excretion.*)
- Differentiate physiologic jaundice from pathologic jaundice. Physiologic jaundice requires no treatment, whereas pathologic jaundice does.
  - Physiologic jaundice:
    - Benign
    - Onset 3 to 6 days (breast-feeding jaundice)
    - Onset 5 to 15 days (breast milk jaundice)
  - Pathologic jaundice:
    - Rapidly rises
    - Onset first 24 h of life
- Screen for high-risk infants.
  - Evaluate for presence of jaundice.
    - Face (early sign of bilirubin level >5 mg/dL)
    - Trunk/sternum (seen with levels >10 mg/dL)
    - Lower body (seen with levels >15 mg/dL)
- Assess for ecchymoses, abrasions, or petechiae. (*Extravasated hemoglobin in the tissue will add to normal hemoglobin breakdown and increase bilirubin production.*)
- Monitor for bilirubin-induced neurologic dysfunction. (*Bilirubin deposits in the basal ganglia and at nerve terminals cause encephalopathy in 25% of preterm infants and 2% of healthy term infants.*)
  - Behavior change: lethargy, somnolence progressing to convulsions and coma
  - Muscle tone abnormalities
  - Shrill, high-pitched cry
  - Poor sucking
- Initiate phototherapy according to protocol, if indicated. (*Phototherapy breaks down bilirubin into water-soluble products that can be excreted.*)
- If phototherapy is performed, ensure optimal hydration. Weigh infant daily to assess fluid status. (*Phototherapy increases fluid loss through diaphoresis.*)

- Protect infant's eyes during phototherapy treatment. Use Plexiglas shields; ensure that lids are closed before applying shields. Provide periods out of light with eye shields removed. *(These precautions help ensure safe treatment.)*
- Monitor for eye discharge, excessive pressure on lids, and corneal irritation. *(These complications may result from use of eye shields.)*
- Turn infant frequently during phototherapy. *(Any areas not exposed to light will remain jaundiced.)*
- Monitor temperature, checking it at least every 4 h. *(A nude infant is vulnerable to hypothermia; use of radiant warmers increases the risk of hyperthermia.)*
- Prepare parents for home phototherapy. *(Term infants older than 48 h with bilirubin levels >14 mg/dL but <18 mg/mL are candidates.)*
- Explain procedure.
  - Teach warning signs of neurotoxicity.
  - Provide written instructions.
  - Arrange for daily home health nurse visits.

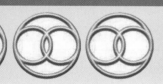

# RISK FOR COMPLICATIONS OF MUSCULAR/SKELETAL DYSFUNCTION

**Risk for Complications of Muscular/Skeletal Dysfunction**

RC of Pathologic Fractures
RC of Joint Dislocation

## DEFINITION

Describes a person experiencing or at high risk to experience various musculoskeletal problems

## ■■■■■■ AUTHOR'S NOTE

The nurse can use this generic collaborative problem to describe people at risk for several types of musculoskeletal problems (e.g., all clients who have sustained multiple trauma). This collaborative problem focuses nursing management on assessing musculoskeletal status to detect and to diagnose abnormalities.

For a client exhibiting a specific musculoskeletal problem, the nurse would add the applicable collaborative problem (e.g., *RC of Pathologic Fractures*) to the problem list. If the risk factors or etiology were not related directly to the primary medical diagnoses, the nurse would add this information to the diagnostic statement (e.g., *RC of Pathologic Fractures related to osteoporosis*).

Because musculoskeletal problems typically affect daily functioning, the nurse must assess the client's functional patterns for evidence of impairment. Findings may have significant implications—for instance, a casted leg that prevents a woman from assuming her favorite sleeping position and impairs her ability to perform housework. After identifying any such problems, the nurse should use nursing diagnoses to address specific responses of actual or potential altered functioning.

For information on Focus Assessment Criteria, visit http://thepoint.lww.com.

## SIGNIFICANT LABORATORY/DIAGNOSTIC ASSESSMENT CRITERIA

### Laboratory

Serum calcium (decreased in osteoporosis)
Serum phosphorus (decreased in osteoporosis)
Sedimentation rate (increased in inflammatory disorders)

## Diagnostic

Bone density test (DXA)
X-ray
Computed tomography (CT) scan
Magnetic resonance imaging (MRI)
Bone scan
Aspiration

# ❱ Risk for Complications of Pathologic Fractures

## DEFINITION

Describes a person experiencing or at high risk to experience a fracture unrelated to trauma because of defects in bone structure

## HIGH-RISK POPULATIONS

- Osteopenia
- Osteoporosis
- Cushing's syndrome
- Malnutrition
- Long-term corticosteroid therapy
- Osteogenesis imperfecta
- Bone tumors (primary or metastatic)
- Paget's disease
- Prolonged immobility
- Irradiation fraction
- Rickets
- Osteomalacia
- Hyperparathyroidism
- Multiple myeloma
- Lymphatic leukemia
- Cystic bone disease
- Infection

## Nursing Goals

The nurse will manage and minimize complications of pathologic fractures.
No new onset of pain.
No changes in height.

## General Interventions and Rationales

- Monitor for signs and symptoms of pathologic fractures:
  - Localized pain that is continuous and unrelenting (back, neck, or extremities)
  - Visible bone deformity
  - Crepitation on movement
  - Loss of movement or use
  - Localized soft tissue edema
  - Skin discoloration

*(Detection of pathologic fractures enables prompt intervention to prevent or minimize further complications.)*

- In a client with osteoporosis, monitor for signs and symptoms of vertebral, hip, and wrist fractures, such as:
  - Pain in the lower back, neck, or wrist
  - Localized tenderness
  - Pain radiating to abdomen and flank
  - Spasm of paravertebral muscles

  *(Progressive osteoporosis more readily affects bones with high amounts of trabecular tissue [e.g., hip, vertebrae, wrist].)*
- Promote weight-bearing activities as soon as possible. *(Weight bearing prevents bone demineralization.)*
- Teach measures to help prevent injury and promote weight bearing, such as:
  - Using smooth movements to avoid pulling or pushing on limbs
  - Supporting the extremities when turning in bed
  - Lifting the buttocks up slightly when sitting to provide weight bearing to the legs and arms
- Monitor x-ray results and serum calcium levels. *(These diagnostic findings help evaluate the client's risk for fractures.)*
- If a fracture is suspected, maintain proper alignment and immobilize the site using pillows or a splint; notify the physician or advanced practice nurse promptly. *(Timely, appropriate intervention can prevent or minimize soft tissue damage.)*
  - Teach client and family measures to prevent or delay bone demineralization, using the nursing diagnosis *Health-Seeking Behaviors: Management of osteoporosis.*
  - Provide calcium supplementation, as ordered
  - Provide vitamin D supplementation, as ordered

# ▶ Risk for Complications of Joint Dislocation

## DEFINITION

Describes a person experiencing or at high risk to experience displacement of a bone from its position in a joint

## HIGH-RISK POPULATIONS

- Total hip replacement
- Total knee replacement
- Fractured hip, knee, shoulder

## FOR INFANTS/CHILDREN

- Birth trauma (e.g., breech, firstborn)
- Sports
- Cerebral palsy (hip)

## Nursing Goals

The nurse will manage and minimize complications of joint dislocation.

### Indicators

Hip in abduction or neutral position
Aligned affected extremity

## General Interventions and Rationales

- Maintain correct positioning.
  - Hip: Maintain the hip in abduction, neutral rotation, or slight external rotation.

- Hip: Avoid hip flexion over 60 degrees.
- Knee: Slightly elevated from hip; avoid using bed knee gatch or placing pillows under the knee (to prevent flexion contractures). Place pillows under the calf.
  *(Specific positions are used to prevent prosthesis dislocation.)*
- Assess for signs of joint (hip, knee) dislocation:
  - *Hip*
    - Acute groin pain in operative hip
    - Shortening of leg with external rotation
  - *Hip, Knee, Shoulder*
    - "Popping" sound heard by client
    - Bulge at surgical site
    - Inability to move
    - Pain with mobility
  *(Until the surrounding muscles and joint capsule heal, joint dislocation may occur if positioning exceeds the limits of the prosthesis, as in flexing or hyperextending the knee or abducting the hip >45 degrees.)*
- The client may be turned toward either side unless contraindicated. Always maintain an abduction pillow when turning; limit the use of Fowler's position. *(If proper positioning is maintained, including the abduction pillow, clients may safely be turned toward the operative and nonoperative side. This promotes circulation and decreases the potential for pressure ulcer formation as a result of immobility. A prolonged Fowler's position can dislocate the prosthesis.)*
- Monitor for shoulder joint dislocation/subluxation. *(Total shoulder arthroplasty has a higher risk of joint dislocation/subluxation because the shoulder is capable of movement in three planes [flexion/extension, abduction/adduction, internal/external rotation].)*

**Pediatric Interventions and Rationales**

- Evaluate newborn for developmental dysplasia of the hip
- "Clunk" sound of subluxation or dislocation (Barlow test)
- Abducting and lifting hip back in place (Ortolani test)
  *(These maneuvers test for instability.)*
- For infants older than 6 months, assess for
- Asymmetry
  - Abduction and full extension limitations
  - Shortened flexed thigh length on dysplasic side
  *(After 6 months, the Barlow and Ortolani tests are often falsely negative because of diminished laxity.)*

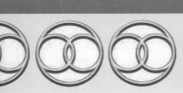

# RISKS FOR COMPLICATIONS OF REPRODUCTIVE DYSFUNCTION

**Risks for Complications of Reproductive Dysfunction**

RC of Prenatal Bleeding
RC of Preterm Labor
RC of Pregnancy-Associated Hypertension
RC of Nonreassuring Fetal Status
RC of Postpartum Hemorrhage

## DEFINITION

Describes a person experiencing or at high risk to experience a problem in reproductive system functioning

■■■■■ **AUTHOR'S NOTE**

This generic collaborative problem provides a category under which to classify more specific collaborative problems affecting the reproductive system. Unlike the other generic collaborative problems (e.g., *RC of Respiratory Dysfunction*, *RC of Cardiac Dysfunction*), it is of little clinical use by itself. So, instead of adding this generic collaborative problem to a client's problem list, the nurse should use the appropriate specific collaborative problem, such as *RC of Non-reassuring Fetal Status* or *RC of Postpartum Hemorrhage*.

For information on Focus Assessment Criteria, visit http://thepoint.lww.com.

## SIGNIFICANT LABORATORY/DIAGNOSTIC ASSESSMENT CRITERIA_____

Complete blood count (CBC) with differential
Hemoglobin and hematocrit (H/H)
Platelets (Plt)
PT, PTT, fibrinogen, fibrinogen degradation products (if patient is actively bleeding)
Blood type and Rh
Culture for gonorrhea and Chlamydia
Human papillomavirus (HPV), positive strains in cervical cancer
Gram's stain for diplococci
Group B streptococcus culture (if positive, it increases risk for UTI, pyelonephritis, chorioamnionitis, preterm labor, premature rupture of membranes, postpartum infection, neonatal infections)
Rapid plasma reagin test (RPR; positive in syphilis)
Cervical, urethral smears (positive in infections)
Pap smear (positive in dysplasia, carcinoma)
Fetal pH (lowered in hypoxia)
Western blot test (positive for human immunodeficiency virus [HIV])
Radiologic/imaging
Ultrasound imaging
Doppler
Electronic fetal monitoring

## ▶ Risk for Complications of Prenatal Bleeding

## DEFINITION _____

Describes a woman experiencing or at high risk to experience bleeding during pregnancy

## HIGH-RISK POPULATIONS _____

- Incompetent cervix
- Spontaneous therapeutic abortion
- Ectopic pregnancy
- Gestational trophoblastic disease (hydatidiform mole)
- Cervical carcinoma
- Cervicitis
- Genital tract trauma
- Disseminated intravascular coagulation

### For Placenta Previa (Late Pregnancy) (Simpson & Creehan, 2007)

- Previous placenta previa

- Previous cesarean section
- Induced or spontaneous abortions involving suction curettage
- Multiparity
- Uterine abnormalities
- Advanced maternal age (>35 years)
- Cigarette smoking
- Multiple gestation
- Fetal hydrops
- Large placenta
- Uterine anomalies
- Fibroid tumors
- Endometritis
- African-American or Asian ethnicity

## For Abruptio Placentae (Late Pregnancy) (Simpson & Creehan, 2007)

- Hypertension
- Very short umbilical cord
- Trauma
- Precipitous labor
- Uterine abnormalities
- Poor nutrition, especially folic acid deficiency
- Partial abruption of current pregnancy
- History of abruption
- Preterm premature rupture of membranes <34 weeks' gestation
- Prior cesarean delivery
- High parity
- Oxytocin induction resulting in uterine hyperstimulation
- Cocaine/amphetamine use
- Cigarette smoking
- Rapid decompression of the uterus such as in the birth of the first of multiple fetuses or with polyhydramnios
- Uterine fibroids at the placental implantation site
- Use of intrauterine pressure catheters during labor

# Nursing Goals

The nurse will manage and minimize complications of prenatal bleeding.

## Indicators

Refer to Hypovolemia.

# General Interventions and Rationales

- Teach the client to report unusual bleeding immediately.
- If bleeding occurs, notify physician or midwife and monitor:
  - Amount, character, color
  - Cramps, contractions, pain, or tenderness
  - Vital signs, hematocrit
  - Urine output
- Start and maintain two large bore (16-g or 18-g) intravenous (IV) if actively bleeding or hypovolemic, according to protocol.
- Monitor fetal heart tones (refer to *RC of Nonreassuring Fetal Status* for specific guidelines).
- Do not perform vaginal or rectal examinations until placenta previa has been ruled out. *(These procedures can tear the placenta, causing life-threatening hemorrhage.)*
- Maintain client in a lateral recumbent position. *(This position displaces the uterus which reduces compression on the vena cava. This improves maternal cardiac output and increases perfusion to the fetus.)*
- Administer oxygen by face mask at a rate of 8 L/min, as indicated. *(Supplemental oxygen therapy increases maternal circulating oxygen to the fetus.)*

- If signs of shock occur, refer to *RC of Hypovolemic shock* for more information on nursing management.
- Refer to the nursing diagnosis *Grieving* for interventions to provide support.

# ▶ Risk for Complications of Preterm Labor

## DEFINITION

Describes a woman experiencing or at high risk to experience expulsion of a viable fetus after the 20th and before completing the 36th week of gestation.

## HIGH-RISK POPULATIONS (SIMPSON & CREEHAN, 2007; GILBERT, 2007)

- Previous preterm birth
- Premature membrane rupture
- Multifetal gestation
- Age (younger than 17 years or older than 35 years)
- Hydramnios
- Uterine anomalies
- Cervical dilation >2 cm by 32 weeks' gestation
- Diethylstilbestrol exposure in utero
- Cervical incompetence
- Cervical shortening <1 cm at 32 weeks' gestation
- Cocaine/amphetamine abuse
- Preterm bleeding
- Uterine irritability
- Reproductive tract infection
- Low socioeconomic status
- Maternal medical conditions (e.g., infection, renal disease, hypertension, anemia, heart disease)
- Previous second-trimester abortions
- Closely spaced pregnancies
- Low-weight, small-stature mother
- Physical abuse/trauma
- Heavy work outside home/prolonged standing
- Poor weight gain
- Tobacco use
- Bacterial vaginosis
- Non-white race

## Nursing Goals

The nurse will manage and minimize complications of preterm labor.

### Indicators

No c/o of cramping, pain
No c/o of backache
No c/o of pelvic pressure
No change in vaginal secretions
No vaginal bleeding or spotting
Urinalysis within normal limits

## General Interventions and Rationales

- Teach client to watch for and report (Mattson & Smith, 2004):
  - Uterine contractions, menstrual-like cramps, abdominal tightening

- Low backache
- Pelvic pressure or fullness
- Change in amount or character of vaginal secretions
- Nausea, vomiting and diarrhea
- Vaginal spotting or bleeding
- Urinary tract infection
- General sense of discomfort or unease

*(Early detection of impending premature labor enables interventions to ensure successful delivery and decrease the risk of complications.)*

- Once labor begins, stay with the client and provide emotional support. *(Reassurance and support can help the client prepare for and cope with premature birth.)*
- Assess for client's level of anxiety and presence of economic or family stressors.
- Maintain constant bed rest. *(Bed rest is thought to reduce pressure of the fetal presenting part on the cervix, thus improving uterine blood flow.)*
- Assess for domestic violence and provide appropriate intervention and referrals as needed.
- Ensure optimal hydration (oral and/or IV). *(Hydration inhibits the release of antidiuretic hormone and oxytocin from the posterior pituitary gland and increases uterine blood flow, thereby stabilizing decidual lysosomes [Gilbert, 2007].)*
- Monitor fetal heart rate.
- Have patient empty bladder every 2 hours while awake. *(This will prevent bladder pressure.)*
- If IV tocolytic therapy (e.g., magnesium sulfate, ritodrine, nifedipine, indomethacin) is prescribed, refer to protocol for preparation (e.g., baseline laboratory tests, electrocardiogram [ECG]) and administration.
- During IV tocolytic therapy (Mandeville & Troiano, 2002; Gilbert, 2007):
  - Establish a baseline and then assess pulse, respirations, blood pressure, and breath sounds every 15 min during loading doses, with dosage increases, or with unstable vital signs and every hour during maintenance. *(Cardiopulmonary complications of tocolytic therapy can be fatal; close monitoring is essential.)*
  - With magnesium sulfate, assess deep tendon reflexes and level of consciousness every hour and ensure antidote calcium gluconate is available at bedside. *(Hypermagnesemia can cause central nervous system [CNS] depression.)*
  - Monitor and record fetal heat rate and uterine activity continuously. *(This information is necessary to evaluate the effectiveness of the therapy and its effects on the fetus.)*
  - Obtain laboratory studies including a complete blood cell count with differential, blood glucose, urea nitrogen and serum electrolytes to monitor maternal response to drug therapy.
  - *With ritodrine, assess urine for ketones hourly or with every void; auscultate breath sounds and assess for cough, chest pain, or shortness of breath every 2 h.*
  - Maintain total fluid intake <2500 mL/24 h to avoid fluid overload.
  - Measure and record hourly intake and output and a daily weight during infusion.
  - Maintain bed rest in lateral recumbent position. *(This position increases uterine perfusion.)*
- Notify physician or midwife if the following occur (Mandeville & Troiano, 2002):
  - Respiratory rate <12/min or >24/min
  - Abnormal breath sounds, signs and symptoms of dyspnea, or mild coughing
  - Pulse rate >120 beats/min, systolic pressure <90 mm Hg or diastolic pressure <50 mm Hg or >90 mm Hg
  - Decreasing deep tendon reflexes or level of consciousness
  - Fetal heart rate above 160 beats/min or nonreassuring fetal heart rate tracing
  - Six or more uterine contractions per minute
  - ECG changes
  - Urinary output <30 mL/h
  - Suspected magnesium sulfate toxicity
  - Symptoms of placental abruption
  - $SaO_2$ <95%

# ▶ Risk for Complications of Pregnancy-Associated Hypertension

## DEFINITION

Describes a woman experiencing or at high risk to experience a multisystem disease characterized by vasoconstriction, endothelial cell damage, hypertension (systolic pressure 140 mm Hg or higher or diastolic pressure 90 mm Hg or higher), proteinuria, and edema during pregnancy (Simpson & Creehan, 2007; Gilbert, 2007; Mattson & Smith, 2004; ACOG, 2002)

## HIGH-RISK POPULATIONS

- Primigravida
- Younger than 19 years of age
- Older than 35 years of age
- History of pregnancy-associated hypertension
- Chronic hypertensive disease
- Pre-existing renal disease
- Diabetes mellitus
- Vascular disease
- Multifetal pregnancy
- Fetal hydrops
- Hydatidiform mole
- Family history of preeclampsia or eclampsia
- Obesity

## Nursing Goals

The nurse will manage and minimize complications of hypertension.

### Indicators

BP >90/60, <140/90
Tendon response 2+
No complaints of headaches
Urine output 30 mL/h
No complaints of nausea and vomiting
No complaints of visual disturbances
No complaints of dyspnea
No complaints of epigastric pain
No change in level of consciousness

## General Interventions and Rationales

- Monitor blood pressure and compare readings to those taken earlier in the pregnancy. *(Midway through pregnancy, blood pressure commonly is lower than the woman's usual reading; thus, any elevation—even if readings still are within normal limits—may be significant.)*
- Monitor daily weights. *(Sudden weight gain of 2 lb or more can indicate tissue or occult edema.)*
- Monitor for edema, particularly in the ankles, fingers, and face. *(Edema results from sodium retention related to decreased glomerular filtration.)*
- Monitor laboratory results for proteinuria and increased plasma uric acid levels. *(Peripheral arterial vasoconstriction leads to decreased glomerular filtration.)*
- Monitor fetal well-being by means of serial ultrasounds to estimate fetal growth, amniotic fluid index (AFI) studies, biophysical profile (BPP) with nonstress test, and daily fetal movement counts to assess uteroplacental perfusion (Gilbert, 2007).
- Assess for and teach client to report (Mandeville & Troiano, 2002):
  - Visual disturbances, such as blurred vision or scotomata

- Headaches
- Rapid onset of edema
- Dyspnea
- Decreased urine output
- Nausea and vomiting
- Change in level of consciousness
- Epigastric or right upper quadrant pain

*(These are indicators of cerebral edema, pulmonary edema, and gastrointestinal [GI], renal, or hepatic impairments.)*

- Teach a client exhibiting mild hypertension with minimal or no edema or proteinuria to:
  - Restrict activities and rest in bed most of the day.
  - Increase dietary protein intake to compensate for losses in urine.
  - Measure and record intake, output, and weight daily.
- For a client with progressive or severe hypertension and/or proteinuria, hospitalization may be indicated with:
  - Complete bed rest in left lateral position
  - Daily weight, intake and output monitoring
  - Daily urinalysis for protein and casts
  - Liver function tests, uric acid test, BUN, serum creatinine, platelet count, hematocrit
  - Magnesium sulfate therapy, sedation
- Ensure that the client gets as much undisturbed rest as possible. *(Adequate rest promotes relaxation and may help reduce hypertension and decrease the risk of seizure activity.)*
- Assess deep tendon reflexes of biceps and quadriceps and compare responses on each side (Reeder et al., 1997). *(CNS irritability increases the reflex response.)*
- Assess for signs and symptoms of impending convulsion:
  - Epigastric or right upper quadrant pain
  - Headache and blurred vision
  - Increasing hyperreflexia
  - Development or worsening of clonus (alternating contraction and relaxation [e.g., twitching])
  *(Convulsions are a sign of cerebral hemorrhage.)*
- Assess fetal heart tones for incidence of late decelerations, absent long-term variability, or bradycardia. *(Decreased placental perfusion causes late deceleration; hypoxia causes bradycardia [Mandeville & Troiano, 2001].)*
- Consult with physician or advanced practice nurse regarding low-dose aspirin therapy or calcium supplements for high-risk women during pregnancy. *(Studies have shown these therapies to reduce pregnancy-associated hypertension in high-risk women.)*
- If seizures occur, refer to *RC of Seizures* for nursing interventions.
- Refer to *RC of Preterm Labor* for nursing interventions with magnesium sulfate therapy.

# ▶ Risk for Complications of Nonreassuring Fetal Status

## DEFINITION

Describes a fetus experiencing or at high risk to experience a disruption of the physiologic exchange of nutrients, oxygen, and metabolites (ACOG, 2005; Simpson & Creehan, 2007; Feinstein, Torgerson, & Atterbury, 2003; Gilbert, 2007)

## HIGH-RISK POPULATIONS

### Fetal Factors

- Prematurity
- Intrauterine growth retardation

- Atresia of umbilical cord
- Cord compression
- Placental insufficiency
- Infection
- Multiple gestation
- Congenital anomalies
- Dysmaturity
- Acute hemolytic crisis
- Rh disease

## Maternal Factors

- Chronic hypertension, pregnancy-associated hypertension
- Diabetes mellitus
- Third-trimester bleeding
- Maternal hypoxia (e.g., respiratory insufficiency)
- Maternal infection
- Hypotension
- Seizures
- Uterine hyperstimulation
- Prolonged uterine contractions
- Abruptio placentae
- Cardiovascular disease
- Substance abuse
- Malnutrition

## Nursing Goals

The nurse will manage and minimize episodes of nonreassuring fetal status.

### Indicators

Refer to assessment criteria under Interventions.

## General Interventions and Rationales

- Determine baseline fetal heart tones and evaluate as reassuring if:
  - Rate of 110–160 bpm
  - Regular rhythm
  - Presence of moderate variability (normal fetal rate has a fine irregularity of 6–25 bpm)
  - Presence of accelerations
  - Absence of decrease from baseline
  - Early decelerations (transient slowing of fetal heart rate with compression of the contraction causing parasympathetic stimulation)
- Monitor for nonreassuring fetal heart rate or rhythm, including:
  - Minimal baseline variability (<5 bpm)
  - Tachycardia (>160 bpm)
  - Bradycardia (<110 bpm)
  - Late decelerations (visually apparent gradual decrease of fetal heart rate below baseline; the onset, nadir and recovery of the deceleration occur after the onset, peak and recovery of the contraction)
  - Variable decelerations, caused by compression of the umbilical cord
  - Sinusoidal pattern (smooth, repetitive undulation of baseline)
  *(Fetal hypoxia, maternal drugs, maternal anemia, or dysrhythmias can cause changes in fetal heart rate [Merenstein & Gardner, 1998].)*
- If tachycardia occurs, assess:
  - Maternal temperature *(Fetal tachycardia occurs when maternal core temperature rises. It may increase before the mother's temperature can be measured orally or rectally.)*
  - Maternal intake, output, and urine specific gravity *(Maternal dehydration can cause fetal tachycardia.)*
  - Maternal anxiety level *(Severe anxiety can increase fetal heart rate.)*

- Maternal medication use *(Certain medications used by the mother can cause increased fetal heart rate [e.g., atropine, terbutaline, ritodrine hydrochloride, scopolamine].)*
  - Increase maternal hydration *(Maternal dehydration can cause fetal tachycardia.)*
- Notify the physician or advanced practice nurse of the situation and your assessment findings.
- Position the mother on her left side. *(This position decreases occlusion of the inferior vena cava by displacing the uterus, promoting venous return to the heart.)*
- If decreased variability occurs, evaluate possible causes, which can include:
  - Sleeping fetus
  - Effects of narcotics or sedatives
  - Fetal hypoxia
  - Maternal position
- If nonreassuring fetal heart patterns continue, notify the physician or advanced practice nurse and take the following steps (Feinstein, Torgerson, & Atterbury, 2003):
  - Change maternal position from side to side.
  - Administer oxygen by face mask at a flow rate of 8–10 L/min, according to protocol. *(This increases oxygen delivery to the fetus.)*
  - Hydrate with a bolus of IV fluid
  - Consider amnioinfusion according to protocol.
  - Consider tocolysis according to protocol.
  - Consider fetal scalp blood sample according to protocol. *(To evaluate fetal pH and metabolic status)*
  - If fetal scalp monitoring is not immediately available, perform fetal scalp stimulation with a gloved finger. *(A well-oxygenated fetus will respond with an acceleration of 15 bpm in amplitude or more for a duration of 15 sec or more, which usually reflects a pH of 7.0 or greater [Feinstein, Torgerson, & Atterbury 2003].)*
  - Discontinue oxytocin infusion, if indicated, according to protocol.
- Initiate continuous electronic fetal monitoring according to protocol, if indicated.
- Remain with the mother and partner, provide information, and give them opportunities to share concerns and fears. *(This ensures constant monitoring and also may help reduce the mother's anxiety.)*
- Coach mother on breathing techniques to reduce anxiety and decrease hyperventilation.
- If the mother's condition worsens or if fetal pH is 7.2 or below, anticipate a cesarean section and assist as indicated.
- If mild variable decelerations occur, change the mother's position from supine to lateral or from one side to the other. *(Position shifts may relieve cord compression.)*
- If severe variable decelerations occur, take the following steps:
  - Notify the physician or advanced practice nurse.
  - Discontinue oxytocin infusion per protocol.
  - Perform a vaginal examination to assess for cord prolapse.
  - Shift the mother's position to left side lying and evaluate fetal heart rate; if not improved, turn the mother on her right side.
  - If these position changes do not improve fetal heart rate, or if cord is prolapsed, help the mother assume a knee–chest position. *(This reduces pressure on the cord and increases perfusion to the fetus.)*
  - Administer oxygen by face mask at a rate of 8 to 10 L/min, according to protocol. *(This increases oxygen delivery to the fetus.)*
  - Assess for improvement in fetal heart rate within 1 min.
- Anticipate an emergency vaginal delivery or cesarean section if the mother's condition worsens, if cord prolapse occurs, and/or if fetal pH is 7.2 or lower.

# ▶ Risk for Complications of Postpartum Hemorrhage

## DEFINITION

Describes a woman who is experiencing or is at high risk to experience acute blood loss greater than 500 mL after vaginal birth or greater than 1000 mL after cesarean birth within the first 24 h postpartum (primary hemorrhage) or occurring after 24 h and before the 6th week postpartum (secondary hemorrhage).

## HIGH-RISK POPULATIONS (SIMPSON & CREEHAN, 2001; ACOG, 2006) _____

- Problematic third stage of labor
- Overdistended uterus (e.g., due to hydramnios, large fetus, multiple gestation)
- Prolonged labor
- Precipitous labor/birth
- Oxytocin induction/augmentation
- Multiparity
- Maternal exhaustion
- Instrument delivery
- History of uterine atony
- Uterine fibroids
- History of postpartum hemorrhage
- Excessive analgesic or anesthesia use
- Preeclampsia
- Retained placental fragments
- Trauma to genital tract
- Maternal systemic disease (leukemia, thrombocytopenia, blood dyscrasia)
- Chorioamnionitis
- Asian or Hispanic ethnicity

## Nursing Goals _____

The nurse will manage and minimize postpartum bleeding.

### Indicators

Refer to Hypovolemia
Firm uterus

## General Interventions and Rationales _____

- Assess the uterine fundus every 5 min for the first hour postpartum and PRN thereafter for the first 24 h; evaluate:
  - Height (normally should be at the level of the umbilicus after delivery)
  - Size (when contracted, should be about the size of a large grapefruit)
  - Consistency (should feel firm)
  
  *(A boggy or relaxed uterus will not control bleeding by compression of the uterine muscle fibers.)*
- If the uterus is relaxed or relaxing, massage it with firm but gentle circular strokes until it contracts. *(Massage stimulates the uterine muscle to contract.)*
- Avoid routine massage or over massaging the uterus. *(Unnecessary massage can cause pain and muscle fatigue, with subsequent uterine relaxation.)*
- Monitor blood pressure and pulse every 15 min for 1 h, then every 30 min for the next hour, and then once every hour until the mother's condition stabilizes. *(Careful vital sign monitoring provides accurate evaluation of hemodynamic status.)*
- Monitor perineal blood loss. Keep a record of the number of pads used and the amount of saturation. *(Continuous seepage of blood with a firm uterus can indicate cervical or vaginal lacerations. Bleeding after the first 24 hours can indicate retained placental fragments or subinvolution.)*
- Obtain hemoglobin and hematocrit levels. Report a decrease to the physician or midwife. *(A decrease in the hemoglobin value of 1.0–1.5 g/dL and a four-point drop in hematocrit indicate a blood loss of 450–500 mL.)*
- Monitor bladder size and urine output with the same frequency as for vital signs. *(A distended bladder can displace the uterus and increase uterine atony.)*
- If bleeding becomes excessive, if the uterus fails to contract, or if vital sign changes occur, notify the physician or advanced practice nurse.
- If the woman exhibits signs of shock, refer to RC of Hypovolemic Shock for nursing interventions.

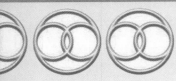

# RISK FOR COMPLICATIONS OF MEDICATION THERAPY ADVERSE EFFECTS*

**Risk for Complications of Medication Therapy Adverse Effects**

RC of Anticoagulant Therapy Adverse Effects
RC of Antianxiety Therapy Adverse Effects
RC of Adrenocorticosteroid Therapy Adverse Effects
RC of Antineoplastic Therapy Adverse Effects
RC of Anticonvulsant Therapy Adverse Effects
RC of Antidepressant Therapy Adverse Effects
RC of Antiarrhythmic Therapy Adverse Effects
RC of Antipsychotic Therapy Adverse Effects
RC of Antihypertensive Therapy Adverse Effects
RC of β-Adrenergic Blocker Therapy Adverse Effects
RC of Calcium Channel Blocker Therapy Adverse Effects
RC of Angiotensin-Converting Enzyme Inhibitor Therapy and Angiotension Receptor Blocker
    Therapy Adverse Effects
RC of Diuretic Therapy Adverse Effects

## DEFINITION

Describes a client experiencing or at high risk to experience potentially serious effects or reactions related to medication therapy

## AUTHOR'S NOTE

The nurse can use these collaborative problems to describe a client who has experienced or who is at risk for adverse effects of medication therapy. In contrast to side effects, which are troublesome and annoying but rarely serious, adverse effects are unusual, unexpected, and potentially serious reactions. Adverse drug reactions are drug-induced toxic reactions. Examples of adverse effects include dysrhythmias, gastric ulcers, blood dyscrasias, and anaphylactic reactions; examples of side effects include drowsiness, dry mouth, nausea, and weakness. Side effects usually can be managed by changing the dose, form, route of administration, or diet, or by using preventive measures with continuation of the medication. Adverse effects may require discontinuation of the medication. A care plan will not contain a collaborative problem for every medication that the client is taking. Nurses routinely teach clients about side effects of medications and monitor for side effects as part of the standard of care for every client. These collaborative problems are indicated for clients who are at high risk for adverse effects or reactions because of the duration of the therapy, high predictability of their occurrence, the potential seriousness if they occur, and previous history of an adverse response. Students may add these collaborative problems to care plans. Practicing nurses could have access to standardized plans for *Medication Therapy Adverse Effects* for major medications.

## HIGH-RISK POPULATIONS

- Prolonged medication therapy
- History of hypersensitivity
- History of adverse reactions
- High single or daily doses

---

*This section is intended as an overview of the nursing accountability for adverse effects of medication therapy. It is not intended to provide the reader with complete information on individual drugs, which can be found in pharmacology texts or manuals.

Changes in daily doses

- Multiple medication therapy
- Mental instability
- Hepatic insufficiency
- Renal insufficiency
- Disease or condition that increases the risk of a specific adverse response (e.g., history of gastric ulcer)

# ▶ Risk for Complications of Anticoagulant Therapy Adverse Effects

## HIGH-RISK POPULATIONS FOR ADVERSE EFFECTS

- Diabetes mellitus
- Hypothyroidism
- Gastrointestinal (GI) bleeding
- Bleeding tendency
- Hyperlipidemia
- Elderly women
- Vitamin K deficiency
- Debilitation
- Congestive heart failure
- Children
- Mild hepatic or renal dysfunction
- Tuberculosis
- Pregnancy
- Immediately postpartum

## Nursing Goals

The nurse will monitor for or assist the client and family to identify and minimize adverse effects.

### Indicators

Identify signs and symptoms that need immediate reporting.

## General Interventions and Rationales

- Refer also to a pharmacology text for specific information on the individual drug.
- Assess for contraindications to anticoagulant therapy:
  - History of hypersensitivity
  - Wounds
  - Presence of active bleeding
  - Blood dyscrasias
  - Anticipated or recent surgery
  - GI ulcers
  - Subacute bacterial endocarditis
  - Pericarditis
  - Severe hypertension
  - Impaired renal function
  - Impaired hepatic function
  - Hemorrhagic cerebrovascular accident
  - Use of drugs that affect platelet formation (e.g., salicylates, dipyridamole, NSAIDs)
  - Presence of drainage tubes
  - Eclampsia

- Hemorrhagic tendencies
- Threatened abortion
- Ascorbic acid deficiency
- Spinal puncture
- Regional anesthesia
- Pregnancy (coumadin)
- Inadequate lab facilities
- Compliance risk
- Spinal puncture
- Explain possible adverse effects:
  - *Systemic*
    - Hypersensitivity (fever, chills, runny nose, headache, nausea, vomiting, rash, itching, tearing)
    - Bleeding, hemorrhage
      fatigue/malaise/lethargy
      alopecia
      rash
      fever
      cold intolerance
      anemia
  - *Gastrointestinal*
  - Vomiting
  - Diarrhea
      abdominal cramps
      hepatitis
      flatulence/bloating
  - *Cardiovascular*
  - Hypertension
  - Chest pain
      edema
      vasculitis
  - *Renal*
  - Impaired renal function
  - *Neurological*
  - Dizziness
      paresthesias
- Monitor for and reduce the severity of adverse effects.
- Monitor laboratory results of activated partial thromboplastin time (APTT) for heparin therapy and prothrombin time (PT) and international normalized ratio (INR) for oral therapy. Report values over target for therapeutic range. *(The therapeutic range for PT is 1.3–1.5 × control or INR of 2.0–3.0.)*
- Monitor for signs of bleeding (e.g., bleeding gums, skin bruises, dark stools, hematuria, epistaxis).
- For a client receiving heparin therapy, have protamine sulfate available during administration. For warfarin, the antidote is vitamin K. *(Protamine sulfate is the antidote to reverse the effects of heparin.)*
- Carefully monitor older adult clients. *(They are more sensitive to the effects of anticoagulants.)*
- Consult with the pharmacist about medications that can potentiate (e.g., antibiotics, cimetidine, salicylates, phenytoin, acetaminophen, antifungals, NSAIDs, bismuth) or inhibit (e.g., barbiturates, dicloxacillin, carbamazepine, nafcillin, bile acid binding agents, griseofulvins) anticoagulant action.
- Monitor for signs and symptoms of heparin-induced thrombocytopenia (fever, weakness, difficulty speaking, seizures, yellowing of skin/eyes, dark or bloody urine, petechiae). *(Antibodies directed against platelet membrane are produced in the presence of heparin, causing increased platelet consumption.)*
- Reduce hematomas and bleeding at injection sites.
- Use small-gauge needles.
- Do not massage sites.
- Rotate sites.
- Use subcutaneous route.
- Apply steady pressure for 1–2 min.

*(These techniques reduce the trauma to tissues and avoid highly vascular areas [e.g., muscles].)*

- Instruct client to avoid use of razors or to use electric razors.
- Instruct client to avoid pregnancy while on therapy. *(Warfarin is toxic to fetuses.)*
- Teach client and family how to prevent or reduce the severity of adverse effects.
  - Instruct them to monitor for and report signs of bleeding.
  - Tell them to inform physicians, dentists, and other health care providers of anticoagulant therapy before invasive procedures. *(Precautions may be needed to prevent bleeding.)*
  - Instruct them to contact physician or advanced practice nurse immediately after the onset of a fever or rash. *(These can indicate an infection or allergic response.)*
  - Tell them that it takes 2–10 days for PT levels to return to normal after warfarin (Coumadin) is stopped.
  - Explain that certain medications can inhibit or potentiate anticoagulant effect, and advise them to consult with a pharmacist before taking any prescribed or over-the-counter drug (e.g., aspirin, antibiotics, ibuprofen, diuretics). Teach them to avoid foods high in vitamin K; such foods include turnip greens, asparagus, broccoli, watercress, cabbage, beef liver, lettuce, and green tea. *(Vitamin K decreases anticoagulant action.)*
  - Teach client to avoid alcohol, which potentates the effects of the anticoagulant if hepatic disease is also present.
  - Instruct client to wear Medic-Alert identification.
  - Stress the importance of regular follow-up care and regular monitoring of blood levels
  - Instruct the client and family to report the following:

| | |
|---|---|
| Bleeding | Dark stools |
| Fever | Chills |
| Sore throat, difficulty speaking | Itching |
| Dark urine | Yellowing of skin or eyes |
| Mouth sores | severe headache |
| New rash | Major illness |
| Persistent abdominal pain | Episode of fainting |

## ▶ Risk for Complications of Antianxiety Therapy Adverse Effects

## HIGH-RISK POPULATIONS FOR ADVERSE EFFECTS

- Children
- Older adults
- Impaired liver or kidney function
- Psychosis
- Depression
- Pregnancy or breast-feeding
- Severe muscle weakness
- Limited pulmonary reserves

## Nursing Goals

The nurse will monitor for or assist the client and family to identify and minimize adverse effects.

### Indicators

Will report signs and symptoms that need immediate reporting.

# General Interventions and Rationales

- Refer also to a pharmacology text for specific information on the individual drug.
- Assess for contraindications to antianxiety therapy:
- Hypersensitivity
- Impaired consciousness
- Compromised respiratory function
- Shock
- Porphyria
- History of drug or alcohol (for benzodiazepines) abuse
- Undiagnosed neurologic disorders
- Glaucoma, paralytic ileus, prostatic hypertrophy (for benzodiazepines)
- Pregnancy or breast-feeding
- Alcohol use
- Severe, uncontrolled pain
- Narrow-angle glaucoma
- CNS depression
- Explain possible adverse effects:
  - *Systemic*
  - Hypersensitivity (pruritus, rash, hypotension)
  - Hair loss
  - Drug dependency
  - Sleep disturbances
      drowsiness
      dry mouth
      blurred vision
      altered libido
      appetite change
      weight change
  - *Cardiovascular*
  - Decreased heart rate, blood pressure
  - Transient tachycardia, bradycardia
  - Edema
  - *Central Nervous System*
  - Impaired judgment
  - Paradoxical excitement
  - Excessive drowsiness
  - Tremors
  - Dizziness
  - Slurred speech
  - Confusion
  - Dysphagia
  - Headache
      ataxia
      amnesia
  - *Respiratory*
  - Respiratory depression
  - *Hematologic*
  - Leukopenia
  - *Ophthalmic*
  - Blurred vision
  - *Genitourinary*
  - Urine retention
  - *Hepatic*
  - Jaundice
  - Monitor for and reduce the severity of adverse effects.

- Monitor for history of drug dependency
- Evaluate the client's mental status before drug administration. Consult the physician or advanced practice nurse if the client exhibits confusion or excessive drowsiness.
- Evaluate the client's risk for injury; see *Risk for Injury* for more information.
- Monitor for signs of overdose (e.g., slurred speech, continued somnolence, respiratory depression, confusion).
- Monitor for signs of tolerance (e.g., increased anxiety, wakefulness).
  - Teach client and family how to prevent or reduce the severity of adverse effects.
  - Instruct client never to discontinue taking the medication abruptly after long-term use. (*Abrupt cessation can cause vomiting, tremors, and convulsions.*)
  - Teach family or significant others the signs of overdose (e.g., slurred speech, continued somnolence, respiratory depression, confusion).
  - Remind client and family that alcohol and other sedatives potentiate the action of the medication.
  - Instruct client to avoid driving and other hazardous activities when drowsy.
  - Discuss the possibility of drug tolerance and dependence with long-term use.
  - Instruct the client and family to report the following signs or symptoms:

| | |
|---|---|
| Slurred speech | Vivid dreams |
| Continued somnolence | Euphoria |
| Confusion | Hallucinations |
| Respiratory insufficiency | Sore throat |
| Hostility, rage | Fever |
| Muscle spasms | Mouth ulcers |

# ▶ Risk for Complications of Adrenocorticosteroid Therapy Adverse Effects

## HIGH-RISK POPULATIONS FOR ADVERSE EFFECTS

- Acquired immunodeficiency syndrome (AIDS)
- Thrombophlebitis
- Congestive heart failure
- Diabetes mellitus
- Hypothyroidism
- Glaucoma
- Osteoporosis
- Myasthenia gravis
- Bleeding ulcers
- Seizure disorders or mental illness
- Older adults
- Pregnancy or breast-feeding
- Severe stress, trauma, or illness
    systemic fungal infection

## Nursing Goals

The nurse will monitor for or assist the client and family to identify and minimize adverse effects.

*Indicators*

Will identify signs and symptoms that need immediate reporting

## General Interventions and Rationales

- Refer also to a pharmacology text for specific information on the individual drug.
- Assess for contraindications to steroid therapy:

| | |
|---|---|
| History of hypersensitivity | Hypertension |
| | Active peptic ulcer disease |
| Active tuberculosis | Active fungus infection |
| Herpes | Cardiac disease |

- Explain possible adverse effects:
  - *Systemic*
    Hypersensitivity (rash, hives, hypotension, respiratory distress, anaphylaxis)
    Increased susceptibility to infection
    Acute adrenal insufficiency (response to abrupt cessation after 2 weeks of therapy)
    Hypokalemia
    Delayed wound healing
    Hypertriglyceridemia
    Acne
    Insomnia
    Ecchymosis
    Hyperglycemia
    Appetite change
  - *Central Nervous System*

    | | |
    |---|---|
    | Hallucinations | Psychosis |
    | Headaches | Papilledema |
    | Mood swings | anxiety |
    | Depression | |

  - *Ophthalmic*

    | | |
    |---|---|
    | Glaucoma | Cataracts |

  - *Cardiovascular*

    | | |
    |---|---|
    | Thrombophlebitis | Hypertension |
    | Embolism | Edema |
    | Dysrhythmias | |

  - *Gastrointestinal*

    | | |
    |---|---|
    | Bleeding | Pancreatitis (especially children) |
    | Ulcers | Nausea/vomiting |
    | Dyspepsia | |

  - *Musculoskeletal*

    | | |
    |---|---|
    | Osteoporosis | Growth retardation in children |
    | Muscle wasting | Buffalo hump |

    Monitor for adverse effects.
  - Establish baseline assessment data.

    | | |
    |---|---|
    | Weight | Serum potassium |
    | Complete blood count (CBC) | Blood glucose |
    | | Serum sodium |
    | Blood pressure | |

  - Monitor:

    | | |
    |---|---|
    | Weight | Blood glucose |
    | CBC | Serum sodium |
    | Blood pressure | Stool for guaiac |
    | Serum potassium | |

  - Report changes in monitored data.
- Teach the client and family how to prevent or reduce the severity of adverse effects.
  - Instruct to take the medication with food or milk. *(This reduces gastric distress.)*
  - Advise to weigh self daily at the same time and wearing the same clothes each time. *(Weight gain may indicate fluid retention.)*
  - Instruct to avoid people with infections. *(The client's compromised immune system increases his or her vulnerability to infection.)*
  - Advise to consult with a physician, advanced practice nurse, or pharmacist before taking any over-the-counter drugs. *(Serious drug interactions can occur.)*

- Instruct to inform physicians, advanced practice nurse, dentists, and other health care providers of therapy before any invasive procedure. *(Precautions should be taken to prevent bleeding.)*
- Instruct to contact the physician or advanced practice nurse if signs of infection occur.
- Teach to take medication in the morning. *(This can help reduce adrenal suppression and decrease insomnia.)*
- Instruct to wear Medic-Alert identification. *(He or she may need more medication in an emergency.)*
- Warn never to discontinue the medication without consulting the physician or advanced practice nurse about side effects. *(The medication needs to be weaned because adrenal function needs a gradual return time.)*
- Limit sodium intake to 6 g/day. *(Excess sodium will increase fluid retention.)*
- Discuss the possible problems of weight gain and sodium retention (refer to *Imbalanced Nutrition: More Than Body Requirements* and *Excess Fluid Volume* for more information).
- Explain possible drug-induced appearance changes (e.g., moon face, hirsutism, abnormal fat distribution).
- Encourage client to establish a system to prevent dosage omission or double dosage (e.g., check sheet, prefilled daily dose containers, or place with toothbrush).
- Explain the risk for hyperglycemia. *(Steroids interfere with glucose metabolism.)*
- Instruct the client and family to report the following signs and symptoms:
  - Gastric pain
  - Darkened stool color
  - Unusual weight gain
  - Vomiting
  - Sore throat, fever
  - Adrenal insufficiency (fatigue, anorexia, palpitations, nausea, vomiting, diarrhea, weight loss, mood swings)
  - Menstrual irregularities
  - Change in vision, eye pain
  - Persistent, severe headache
  - Leg pain, cramps
  - Excessive thirst, hunger, urination
  - Diarrhea
  - Change in mental status
  - Dizziness
  - Palpitations
  - Fatigue, weakness

# ▶ Risk for Complications of Antineoplastic Therapy Adverse Effects

## HIGH-RISK POPULATIONS FOR ADVERSE EFFECTS

- Debilitation
- Bone marrow depression
- Malignant infiltration of kidney
- Malignant infiltration of bone marrow
- Liver dysfunction
- Renal insufficiency
- Older adult
- Children

## Nursing Goals

The nurse will monitor for or assist the client and family to identify and minimize adverse events.

*Indicators*

Will identify signs and symptoms that need immediate reporting.

## General Interventions and Rationales

- Refer also to a pharmacology text for specific information on the individual drug.
- Assess for contraindications to antineoplastic therapy:
  - Hypersensitivity to the drug
  - Radiation therapy within the previous 4 weeks
  - Severe bone marrow depression
  - Breast-feeding
  - First trimester of pregnancy
- Explain possible adverse effects:
  - *Systemic*
    Hypersensitivity (pruritus, rash, chills, fever, difficulty breathing, anaphylaxis)
    Immunosuppression
    Alopecia
    Fever
    Rash
    Infection
    Thrombocytopenia
    SIADH
  - *Cardiovascular*
    Congestive heart failure
    Dysrhythmias
  - *Respiratory*
    Pulmonary fibrosis
  - *Central Nervous System*

    | | |
    |---|---|
    | Confusion | Depression |
    | Headaches | Dizziness |
    | Weakness | Neurotoxicity |

  - *Hematologic*

    | | |
    |---|---|
    | Leukopenia | Anemia |
    | Bleeding | Hyperuricemia |
    | Thrombocytopenia | Electrolyte imbalances |
    | Agranulocytosis | |

  - *Gastrointestinal*

    | | |
    |---|---|
    | Diarrhea | Enteritis |
    | Anorexia | Intestinal ulcers |
    | Vomiting | Paralytic ulcer |
    | Mucositis | |

  - *Hepatic*
    Hepatotoxicity
  - *Genitourinary/Reproductive*

    | | |
    |---|---|
    | Renal failure | Decreased sperm count |
    | Amenorrhea | Hemorrhagic cystitis |
    | Sterility | Renal calculi |

- Take steps to reduce extravasation of vesicant medications (agents that cause severe necrosis if they leak from blood vessels into tissue). Examples of vesicant medications are amsacrine, bisantrene, dactinomycin, dacarbazine, daunorubicin, estramustine, nitrogen mustard, plicamycin, vinblastine, vincristine, and vindesine.
- Preventive measures are as follows:
  - Avoid infusing vesicants over joints, bony prominences, tendons, neurovascular bundles, or the antecubital fossa.
  - Avoid multiple punctures of the same vein within 24 h.
  - Administer the drug through a long-term venous catheter.

- Do not administer the drug if edema is present or blood return is absent.
  - If peripheral IV site is used, evaluate its status and whether it is less than 24 h old.
  - Observe the infusion continuously if it is peripheral.
  - Provide infusion through a central line and check every 1–2 h.
  - Infuse vesicant before any other medications, even antiemetics.
- Monitor during drug infusion.
  - Assess patency of IV infusion line.
  - Observe tissue at the IV site every 30 min for the following:
    - Swelling (most common)
    - Leakage
    - Burning/pain (not always present)
    - Inflammation
    - Erythema (not seen initially)
    - Hyperpigmentation
- If extravasation occurs, take the following steps:
  - Stop administration of drug.
  - Leave needle in place.
  - Gently aspirate residual drug and blood in tubing or needle.
  - Avoid applying direct pressure on site.
  - Give antidote as ordered by physician or institutional policy.
  - If plant alkaloid extravasation, apply warm compresses 15 to 20 min q.i.d. for 24 h.
  - If anthracycline extravasation, apply ice for 15–20 min every 3–4 h for 24–48 h.
  - Instruct on local care:
    - Elevate limb for 48 h.
    - After 48 h, encourage to use limb normally.
- Monitor for and reduce the severity of adverse effects.
  - Document a baseline assessment of vital signs, cardiac rhythm, and weight. Monitor daily. *(This facilitates subsequent assessments for adverse reactions.)*
  - Ensure that baseline electrolyte, blood chemistry, bone marrow, and renal and hepatic function studies are done before administering the first dose. *(This enables monitoring for adverse reactions.)*
  - Ensure adequate hydration, at least 2 L/day. *(Good hydration can help prevent kidney damage from rapid destruction of cells.)*
  - Monitor for early signs of infection. *(Bone marrow suppression increases the risk of infection.)*
  - Monitor for sodium, potassium, magnesium, phosphate, and calcium imbalances. *(Electrolyte imbalances are commonly precipitated by renal injury, vomiting, and diarrhea.)*
  - Monitor for renal insufficiency: insufficient urine output, elevated specific gravity, elevated urine sodium levels. *(Certain antineoplastics have toxic effects on renal glomeruli and tubules.)*
  - Monitor for renal calculi: flank pain, nausea, vomiting, abdominal pain; refer to *RC of Renal Calculi* if it occurs. *(Rapid lysis of tumor cells can produce hyperuricemia.)*
  - Monitor for neurotoxicity: paresthesias, gait disturbance, disorientation, confusion, foot drop or wrist drop, fine motor activity disturbances. *(Some antineoplastics impair neural conduction.)*
- Teach the client and family how to prevent or reduce the severity of adverse effects.
  - Stress the importance of follow-up assessments and laboratory tests. *(This can help detect adverse effects early.)*
  - Instruct to avoid crowds and people with infectious diseases. *(A client receiving antineoplastic therapy is very susceptible to infectious diseases.)*
  - Teach to monitor weight and intake and output daily. *(Regular monitoring can detect adverse effects early.)*
  - Instruct to consult with primary health care provider before taking any over-the-counter drugs. *(Serious drug interactions can occur.)*
  - Advise to avoid live vaccines. *(A compromised immune system increases the risk for onset of disease.)*
  - Refer to appropriate nursing diagnoses for selected responses (e.g., *Imbalanced Nutrition, Impaired Oral Mucous Membranes*).
- Instruct the client and family to report the following signs and symptoms:
  - Fever (>100° F)
  - Chills, sweating

- Diarrhea
- Severe cough
- Sore throat
- Unusual bleeding
- Burning on urination
- Muscle cramps
- Flulike symptoms
- Pain, swelling at IV site
- Abdominal pain
- Confusion, dizziness
- Decreased urine output

# ▶ Risk for Complications of Anticonvulsant Therapy Adverse Effects

## HIGH-RISK POPULATIONS FOR ADVERSE EFFECTS

- Hepatic insufficiency
- Renal insufficiency
- Coagulation problems
- Hyperthyroidism
- Diabetes mellitus
- Older adults
- Debilitation
- Cardiac dysfunction
- Glaucoma
- Myocardial insufficiency
  MAOI use within 14 days

## Nursing Goals

The nurse will monitor for or assist the client and family to identify and minimize adverse effects.

## General Interventions and Rationales

- Refer also to a pharmacology text for specific information on the individual drug.
- Assess for contraindications to anticonvulsant therapy (Arcangelo & Peterson, 2005):
  - Hypersensitivity
  - Bone marrow depression
  - Heart block, sinus bradycardia (Dilantin)
  - Pregnancy
  - Hepatic insufficiency (Depakote)
  - Blood dyscrasias
  - Respiratory obstruction
- Explain possible adverse effects:
  - *Systemic*
    | | |
    |---|---|
    | Hypersensitivity (excessive side effects, rashes) | Lupus-like reactions |
    | | Folate deficiency |
    | SIADH | hyponatremia |
    | Fatigue/weakness | suicidality |
  - *Central Nervous System*
    | | |
    |---|---|
    | Depression | Personality changes |
    | Irritability | Tremors |
    | Ataxia | Cognitive impairment |

  Blurred vision             nystagmus
  Dizziness                  withdrawal seizures
- *Cardiovascular*
  A-V block
- *Hematologic*
  Leukopenia                 Anemias
  Bone marrow suppression    Thrombocytopenia
  agranulocytosis
- *Gastrointestinal*
  Gingival hyperplasia (with hydantoin)
  Pancreatitis
- *Hepatic*
  Hepatitis
  Elevated liver enzymes
- *Genitourinary*
  Albuminuria                Impotence
  Urine retention            Renal calculi
  Monitor for and reduce the severity of adverse effects.
- Document baseline information on seizures: type, frequency, usual time, presence of aura, precipitating factors.
- Administer medication at regular intervals. *(Regular administration helps prevent fluctuating serum drug levels.)*
- Keep a flow record of serum drug levels; report levels outside the therapeutic range. *(Seizures can occur with lower levels; higher levels can cause toxicity.)*
- Monitor hepatic and blood count studies. *(These studies can detect blood dyscrasias and hepatic dysfunction.)*
- Monitor for sore throat, persistent fatigue, fever, and infections. *(These signs and symptoms can indicate blood dyscrasias.)*
- Take vital signs before and after parenteral drug administration. *(Vital signs demonstrate the drug's effect on cardiac function.)*
- When administering the drug IV, monitor vital signs closely and give the drug slowly. *(Close monitoring can enable early detection of bradycardia, hypotension, and respiratory depression.)*
- Teach the client and family how to prevent or reduce the severity of adverse effects.
  - Stress not to alter the dosage or abruptly discontinue the medication. *(Changing the regimen can precipitate severe seizures.)*
  - Emphasize the importance of taking the medication on time, around-the-clock if needed. *(Regular administration helps maintain therapeutic drug levels.)*
  - Instruct to consult with a pharmacist before taking any medications (e.g., aspirin, oral contraceptives, folic acid). *(Certain medications reduce the effects of anticonvulsants.)*
  - Stress the importance of maintaining a proper diet; encourage to consult with a physician or advanced practice nurse to determine the need for supplements. *(Some anticonvulsants interfere with vitamin and mineral absorption.)*

Avoid azoles, MAO inhibitors, protease inhibitors, acteominophen, ginkgo biloba, and macrolide antibiotics while on medication.

Medications that can decrease the effect of the medications include cimetidine, warfarin and tramadol. Grapefruit can interfere with absorption of the medication.

# ◗ Risk for Complications of Antidepressant Therapy Adverse Effects

## HIGH-RISK POPULATIONS FOR ADVERSE EFFECTS

- Increased ocular pressure
- Impaired renal function
- Impaired hepatic function
- Urine retention
- Diabetes mellitus
- Seizure disorder
- Hyperthyroidism
- Parkinson's disease
- Pregnancy or breast-feeding
- Electroconvulsive therapy
- Cardiovascular disease
- Schizophrenia, psychosis
- Older adults
    patients under 25
    diuretic users

## Nursing Goals

The nurse will monitor for or assist the client and family to identify and minimize adverse effects.

## General Interventions and Rationales

- Refer also to a pharmacology text for specific information on the individual drug.
- Assess for contraindications to antidepressant therapy:
  - Hypersensitivity
  - Narrow-angle glaucoma
  - Acute recovery phase after myocardial infarction
  - Severe renal impairment
  - Severe hepatic impairment
  - Prostatic hypertrophy
  - Cerebrovascular disease
  - Cardiovascular disease
  - Schizophrenia (for monoamine oxidase [MAO] inhibitors)
  - Anesthesia administration within the past 1–2 weeks (for MAO inhibitors)
  - Hypertension (for MAO inhibitors)
  - Concomitant use of MAO inhibitors and tricyclics
  - Seizure disorder (for tricyclics)
  - Ingestion of foods containing tyramine (for MAO inhibitors)
  - Concomitant use of MAO inhibitors, sympathomimetics, narcotics, sedatives, hypnotics, barbiturates, phenothiazines, alcohol, street drugs, and antihypertensives
- Explain possible adverse effects:
  - *Systemic*
      Hypersensitivity (rash, petechiae, urticaria, photosensitivity)
      Diaphoresis
      Hyponatremia
      SuicidalityDry mouth
      Sweating
      Anorexia
      Weight gain

- *Central Nervous System*

| | |
|---|---|
| Nightmares | Tremors |
| Ataxia | Delusions |
| Seizures | Agitation |
| Paresthesias | Hypomania |
| Extrapyramidal symptoms | Confusion |
| Mania | Hallucinations |

- *Cardiovascular*

| | |
|---|---|
| Orthostatic hypotension (MAO inhibitors) | Tachycardia |
| Hypertension crisis (MAO inhibitors) | Dysrhythmias (MAO inhibitors) |

- *Hematologic*
  - Blood dyscrasias
  - Bone marrow suppression
- *Gastrointestinal*
  - Paralytic ileus
  - Vomiting
  - Diarrhea/ constipation
- *Hepatic*
  - Hepatotoxicity
- *Genitourinary*

| | |
|---|---|
| Urine retention | Impotence |
| Prostatic hypertrophy | Nocturia |
| Acute renal failure | Priapism (MAO inhibitors) |
| Ejaculatory dysfunction | |

- *Endocrine*
  - Altered blood glucose levels
  - SIADH
- Monitor for and reduce the severity of adverse effects.
- Consult with a pharmacist regarding potential interactions with the client's other medications. *(MAO inhibitors cause many adverse interactions.)*
- Document baseline pulse, cardiac rhythm, and blood pressure. *(Antidepressants can seriously affect cardiac function; baseline assessment enables accurate monitoring during drug therapy.)*
- Ensure that baseline blood, renal, and hepatic function studies are done. *(Baseline values allow monitoring for changes.)*
- Record signs and symptoms of depression before initiating therapy. *(This information facilitates evaluation of the client's response to therapy.)*
- Monitor weight and intake and output, and assess for edema. *(Some antidepressants can cause fluid retention and anorexia.)*
- Teach the client and family how to prevent or reduce the severity of adverse effects.
- Stress that alcohol potentiates medication effects.
- Instruct the client to consult a pharmacist before taking any over-the-counter drugs. *(Many medications interact with antidepressants.)*
- Warn the client not to adjust dosage or discontinue medication without consulting a physician or nurse.
- For a client taking an MAO inhibitor, stress the importance of avoiding certain foods containing tyramine, such as avocados, bananas, fava beans, raisins, figs, aged cheeses, sour cream, red wines, sherry, beer, yeast, yogurt, pickled herring, chicken liver, aged meats, fermented sausages, chocolate, caffeine, soy sauce, licorice. *(These foods have a pressor effect, which may cause a hypertensive reaction.)*
- Instruct the client to continue to avoid hazardous foods and medications for several weeks after the medication is discontinued. *(MAO enzyme regeneration takes several weeks.)*
- Advise family members to watch for and report signs of hypomania or exaggerated symptoms in the client.
- Explain that MAO inhibitors must be discontinued 1 week before anesthesia administration. *(MAO inhibitors can have serious interactions with anesthetics and narcotics.)*
- For diaphoresis-related electrolyte depletion associated with selective serotonin reuptake inhibitors, instruct to:
  - Avoid caffeine.

- Avoid activity in hot weather.
- Drink 8 oz of fluids with electrolytes every 30 min.
- Instruct the client to report the following signs and symptoms:
  - Hypertensive reaction (headache, neck stiffness, palpitations, sweating, nausea, photophobia)
  - Visual disturbances
  - Yellowed skin or eyes
  - Rash
  - Abdominal pain
  - Pruritus
  - Urinary problems
  - Seizures
  - Changes in mental status

# ▶ Risk for Complications of Antiarrhythmic Therapy Adverse Effects

## HIGH-RISK POPULATIONS FOR ADVERSE EFFECTS

- Hypertension
- Diabetes mellitus
- Children
- Older adults
- Impaired hepatic function
- Impaired renal function
- Cardiomegaly
- Pulmonary pathology
- Thyrotoxicosis
- Peripheral vascular disease
- Atrioventricular conduction abnormalities
- Congestive heart failure
- Hypotension
- Digitalis intoxication
- Potassium imbalance

## Nursing Goals

The nurse will monitor for or assist the client and family to identify and minimize adverse effects.

## General Interventions and Rationales

- Refer also to a pharmacology text for specific information on the individual drug.
- Assess for contraindications to antiarrhythmic therapy (Arcangelo & Peterson, 2005):

| | |
|---|---|
| Hypersensitivity | Myasthenia gravis |
| Ventricular fibrillation (digoxin) | Cardiac, renal, or hepatic failure |
| Thrombocytopenia purpura | Heart block (diltiazem, metoprolol, propranolol) |
| | Ventricular tachycardia (digoxin) |

- Explain possible adverse effects:
  - *Systemic*
    - Hypersensitivity (rash, difficulty breathing, heightened side effects)
    - Lupus like reaction
  - *Cardiovascular*
    - Worsening or new dysrhythmia
    - Hypotension
    - Cardiotoxicity (widened QRS complex >25%, ventricular extrasystoles, absent P waves)

- *Central Nervous System*
  Dizziness
  Apprehension
- *Hematologic*
  Agranulocytosis
- Monitor for and reduce the severity of adverse effects.
  - Establish a baseline assessment of blood pressure, heart rate, respiratory rate, peripheral pulses, lung sounds, and intake and output. (*Baseline assessment facilitates evaluation for adverse reactions to drug therapy.*)
  - Report any electrolyte imbalance, acid–base imbalance, or oxygenation problems. (*Dysrhythmias are aggravated by these conditions.*)
  - Withhold the dose and consult the physician or advanced practice nurse if the client experiences a significant drop in blood pressure, bradycardia, worsening dysrhythmia, or a new dysrhythmia after receiving the medication. (*These signs may indicate an adverse reaction.*)
  - During parenteral administration, have emergency drugs (e.g., vasopressors, cardiac glycosides, diuretics) available and resuscitation equipment on hand; use microdrip infusion equipment to ensure close regulation of IV flow rate.
- Teach the client and family how to prevent or reduce the severity of adverse effects.
  - Stress the importance of ongoing follow-up with the primary health care providerand/or cardiologist
  - Emphasize the need to take the medication on time and to avoid "doubling up" on doses. (*A regular schedule prevents toxic blood levels.*)
  - Instruct to take the medication with food. (*This can help minimize GI distress.*)
  - Teach to monitor pulse and blood pressure daily. (*Careful monitoring can detect early signs of adverse effects.*)
  - Advise to consult a pharmacist before taking any over-the-counter drugs. (*Possible drug interactions may alter cardiac stability.*)
- Instruct the client and family to report the following signs and symptoms:
  - Dizziness, faintness
  - Palpitations
  - Visual disturbances
  - Hallucinations
  - Confusion
  - Headache
  - 1- to 2-lb weight gain
  - Coldness and numbness in extremities

# ▶ Risk for Complications of Antipsychotic Therapy Adverse Effects

## HIGH-RISK POPULATIONS FOR ADVERSE EFFECTS _____

- Glaucoma
- Prostatic hypertrophy
  elderly
  demented
- Epilepsy
- Diabetes mellitus
- Severe hypertension
- Ulcers
- Cardiovascular disease
- Chronic respiratory disorders
- Hepatic insufficiency
- Pregnancy or breast-feeding
- Exposure to extreme heat, phosphorus insecticides, or pesticides

## Nursing Goals

The nurse will monitor for or assist the client and family to identify and minimize adverse effects.

## General Interventions and Rationales

- Refer also to a pharmacology text for specific information on the individual drug.
- Assess for contraindications to antipsychotic therapy:
  - Bone marrow suppression
  - Blood dyscrasias
  - Parkinson's disease
  - Hepatic insufficiency
  - Renal insufficiency
  - Cerebral arteriosclerosis
  - Coronary artery disease
  - Circulatory collapse
  - Mitral insufficiency
  - Severe hypotension
  - Alcoholism, drug abuse
  - Subcortical brain damage
  - Comatose states
  - Explain possible adverse effects:
- *Systemic*
  - Hypersensitivity (rash, abdominal pain, jaundice, blood dyscrasias)
  - Photosensitivity
  - Fever
  - Weight change
- *Cardiovascular*

| | |
|---|---|
| Hypertension | Orthostatic hypotension |
| Palpitations | QT prolongation |

- *Central Nervous System*
  - Extrapyramidal (acute dystonia, akathisia, pseudoparkinsonism)

| | |
|---|---|
| Hyperreflexia | Tardive dyskinesia |
| Cerebral edema | Neuroleptic malignant syndrome |
| Sleep disturbances | Bizarre dreams |
| Anxiety | Drowsiness |

- *Gastrointestinal*
  - Constipation
  - Paralytic ileus
  - Fecal impaction
- *Hematologic*

| | |
|---|---|
| Agranulocytosis | Thrombocytopenia |
| Leukopenia | Purpura |
| Leukocytosis | Pancytopenia |
| Anemias | |

- *Ophthalmic*

| | |
|---|---|
| Ptosis | Lens opacities |
| Pigmentary retinopathy | |

- *Respiratory*

| | |
|---|---|
| Laryngospasm | Dyspnea |
| Bronchospasm | |

- *Genitourinary*

| | |
|---|---|
| Urine retention | Incontinence |
| Enuresis | Impotence |

- *Endocrine*

| | |
|---|---|
| Gynecomastia | Glycosuria |
| Altered libido | Hyperglycemia |
| Amenorrhea | Galactorrhea |

- Monitor for and reduce the severity of adverse effects.
  Document a baseline assessment of blood pressure (sitting, standing, and lying), pulse, and temperature. *(Baseline assessment facilitates monitoring for adverse reactions.)*
  Ensure that baseline bone marrow, renal, and hepatic function studies are done before administering the first dose. *(Results of these studies enable monitoring for changes.)*
  After parenteral administration, keep the client flat and monitor blood pressure. *(These measures help reduce hypotensive effects.)*
  Monitor blood pressure during initial treatment. *(Blood pressure monitoring detects early hypotensive effects.)*
  Assess bowel and bladder functioning. *(Anticholinergic and antiadrenergic effects decrease sensory stimulation to the bowel and bladder.)*
  Observe for fine, wormlike movements of the tongue. *(Early detection of tardive dyskinesia enables prompt intervention and possible reversal of its course.)*
  Monitor for acute dystonic reactions, neck spasms, eye rolling, dysphagia, convulsions. *(Early detection of these signs may indicate the need for dose reduction.)*
  Ensure optimal hydration; evaluate urine specific gravity regularly. *(Dehydration increases susceptibility to dystonic reactions.)*
  Monitor for signs and symptoms of blood dyscrasias: decreased white cells, platelets, and red cells; sore throat; fever; malaise. *(Antipsychotic medication can cause bone marrow suppression.)*
  Monitor weight. *(Antipsychotic medication can cause hypothyroidism, commonly marked by weight gain.)*
  Monitor for neuroleptic malignant syndrome; refer to *RC of Neuroleptic Malignant Syndrome* for interventions. *(Neuroleptic malignant syndrome is a potentially dangerous adverse effect of antipsychotic drug therapy.)*
- Teach the client and family how to prevent or reduce the severity of adverse effects.
  - Instruct to consult a pharmacist before taking any over-the-counter drugs. *(Serious drug interactions can occur with various over-the-counter medications.)*
  - Stress the need to continue the medication regimen as prescribed and never abruptly stop taking it. *(Abrupt cessation can cause vomiting, tremors, and psychotic behavior.)*
  - Caution the client to protect himself from sun exposure with clothing, hat, sunglasses, and sunscreen. *(Photosensitivity is a common side effect of antipsychotic therapy.)*
  - Warn against using alcohol, barbiturates, or sedatives. *(Their effects are potentiated in combination with antipsychotic medication.)*
- Instruct the client and family to report the following signs and symptoms:

| | |
|---|---|
| Urine retention | Fine, wormlike tongue movements |
| Visual disturbances | Neck spasms |
| Fever | Dysphagia |
| Sore throat | Eye rolling |
| Signs of infection | Involuntary chewing, puckering |
| Tremors | Puffing movements |
| Abdominal pain | |

# ▶ Risk for Complications of Antihypertensive Therapy Adverse Effects

- β-Adrenergic Blocker Therapy Adverse Effects
- Calcium Channel Blocker Therapy Adverse Effects
- Angiotensin-Converting Enzyme Inhibitor and Angiotensin Receptor Blocker Therapy Adverse Effects
- Diuretic Therapy Adverse Effects

■■■■■ ■ **AUTHOR'S NOTE**

Antihypertensive medications are classified into nine groups: central adrenergic agents, ganglionic blockers, peripherally acting catecholamine depleters, α-adrenergic blockers, calcium channel blockers, β-adrenergic blockers, vascular smooth muscle relaxants, angiotensin-converting enzymes, and diuretics. Because their sites of action differ greatly, it is not useful to present a generic collaborative problem of *RC of Antihypertensive Therapy Adverse Effects*. Instead, three classifications are addressed: β-adrenergic blockers, calcium channel blockers, and angiotensin-converting enzymes. For information on other classifications, consult a pharmacology text.

# ▶ Risk for Complications of β-Adrenergic Blocker Therapy Adverse Effects

## HIGH-RISK POPULATIONS FOR ADVERSE EFFECTS

- Diabetes mellitus
- Severe liver disease
- Pregnancy or breast-feeding
- Chronic bronchitis, emphysema

asthma/bronchospasm

bradycardia

2ND or 3RD degree heart failure

pheochromocytoma

- Peripheral vascular insufficiency
- Allergic rhinitis
- Renal insufficiency
- Hepatic insufficiency
- Myasthenia gravis

## Nursing Goals

The nurse will monitor for or assist the client and family to identify and minimize adverse effects.

## General Interventions and Rationales

- Refer also to a pharmacology text for specific information on the individual drug.
- Assess for contraindications to β-adrenergic blockers (Arcangelo & Peterson, 2005):
  - Hypersensitivity
  - Sinus bradycardia
  - Second- or third-degree heart block
  - PR interval greater than 0.24 s on electrocardiogram (ECG)
  - Heart (except carvedilol, metoprolol)
  - Cardiogenic shock
  - MAO inhibitor or tricyclic antidepressant therapy
  - Asthma (for nonselective β-adrenergic blockers)
  - Diabetes
  - Hyperlipidemia
  - Peripheral
  - Arterial insufficiency
  - Pregnancy—first trimester
- Explain possible adverse effects:
  - *Systemic*
    Hypersensitivity (rash, pruritus)
    Increased triglycerides

Decreased high-density lipoproteins (HDL)
Feeling of cold
Lethargy
Leg pain
- *Central Nervous System*

| | |
|---|---|
| Depression | Memory loss |
| Paresthesias | Bizarre dreams |
| Insomnia | Hallucinations |
| Behavior changes | Catatonia |
| Vertigo | |

- *Cardiovascular*

| | |
|---|---|
| Bradycardia | Cerebrovascular accident |
| Edema | Tachycardia |
| Hypotension | Peripheral arterial insufficiency |
| Arrthymia | Raymauds phenomenon |

Congestive heart failure
- *Hematologic*
  Agranulocytosis
  Thrombocytopenia
  Eosinophilia
- *Gastrointestinal*

| | |
|---|---|
| Diarrhea | Vomiting |
| Ischemic colitis | Gastric pain |

- *Hepatic*
  Hepatomegaly
- *Respiratory*

| | |
|---|---|
| Bronchospasm | Dyspnea |
| Rales | |

- *Endocrine*
  Hypoglycemia or hyperglycemia
- *Genitourinary*
  Difficulty urinating
  Elevated blood urea nitrogen and serum transaminase
- *Ophthalmic*
  Blurred vision
- Monitor for and reduce the severity of adverse effects.
  - Establish a baseline assessment of pulse, blood pressure (lying, sitting, standing), lung fields, and peripheral pulses. *(Baseline assessment facilitates monitoring for adverse reactions.)*
  - Ensure that baseline renal, hepatic, glucose, and blood studies are done before drug therapy begins. *(Results of these studies enable monitoring for changes.)*
  - Establish with the physician or advanced practice nurse the parameters (blood pressure, pulse) that call for withholding the medication. *(Hypotension and bradycardia can reduce cardiac output.)*
  - Monitor intake, output, and weight and assess for edema. *(Reduced cardiac output can cause fluid accumulation.)*
  - Monitor for congestive heart failure. *(β-Adrenergic blockers can compromise cardiac function.)*
  - Monitor for hypoglycemia in a client with diabetes. *(β-Adrenergic blockers interfere with the conversion of glycogen to glucose by occupying β-adrenergic receptor sites.)*
- Teach the client how to prevent or reduce the severity of adverse effects.
  - Stress the importance of continuing the medication regimen as prescribed, and warn client never to discontinue the drug abruptly. *(Abrupt cessation may precipitate dysrhythmias or angina.)*
  - Emphasize the need to monitor pulse and blood pressure daily. Explain the pulse and blood pressure values that indicate the need to withhold the medication.
  - Instruct to weigh self daily, at the same time each day and wearing the same clothes every time; tell client to report any weight gain of 1 lb or more. *(Weight gain may indicate fluid retention resulting from decreased cardiac output.)*

Instruct to taper slowly. Abrupt withdrawal insomeone with CAD can cause exacerbation of angina, MI or arrthymia

- Explain the need to protect hands and feet from prolonged exposure to cold. (β-*Adrenergic blockers decrease circulation in the skin and extremities.*)
- Instruct to consult with primary health care provider before exercising. (*The medication impedes the body's adaptive response to stress.*)
- Stress the importance of follow-up laboratory tests. (*Significant abnormalities in liver or renal function studies and blood count may be seen.*)
- Instruct the client and family to report the following signs and symptoms:
  - 1- to 2-lb weight gain
  - Edema
  - Difficulty breathing
  - Pulse or blood pressure above or below pre-established parameters
  - Dark urine
  - Difficult urination
  - Visual disturbances
  - Sore throat
  - Fever
  - Sleep disturbances
  - Memory loss
  - Mental changes
  - Behavioral changes

# ▶ Risk for Complications of Calcium Channel Blocker Therapy Adverse Effects

## HIGH-RISK POPULATIONS FOR ADVERSE EFFECTS

- Renal insufficiency
- Hepatic insufficiency
- Hypotension
- Decreased left ventricular function
- Pregnancy or breast-feeding
- Digitalis therapy
- β-Adrenergic blocker therapy
  - Congestive Heart failure
  - Impaired liver/renal function

## Nursing Goals

The nurse will monitor for or assist the client and family to identify and minimize adverse effects.

## General Interventions and Rationales

- Refer also to a pharmacology text for specific information on the individual drug.
- Assess for contraindications to calcium channel blocker therapy:
  - Severe left ventricular dysfunction
  - Sick sinus syndrome
  - Second- or third-degree heart block
  - Cardiogenic shock
  - Acute myocardial infarction (with diltiazem)
  - IV use of verapamil and β-adrenergic blockers
  - Symptomatic hypotension
  - Advanced congestive heart failure

- Explain possible adverse effects:
  - *Systemic*
    Hypersensitivity (rash, pruritus, extreme hypotension)
    Hair loss
    Sweating, chills
  - *Central Nervous System*

    | Tremors | Insomnia |
    | --- | --- |
    | Confusion | Headache |
    | Mood changes | |

  - *Cardiovascular*

    | Palpitations | Heart failure |
    | --- | --- |
    | Myocardial infarction | Bradycardia |
    | Hypotension | Third-degree heart block (with verapamil) |
    | Arrthymias | peripheral edema |

  - *Gastrointestinal*

    | Diarrhea | Cramping |
    | --- | --- |
    | Constipation | dyspepsia |

  - *Hepatic*
    Elevated liver enzymes
  - *Respiratory*

    | Dyspnea | Pulmonary edema |
    | --- | --- |
    | Wheezing | |

  - *Musculoskeletal*

    | Muscle cramping | Inflammation |
    | --- | --- |
    | Joint stiffness | |

  - *Genitourinary*

    | Impotence | Menstrual irregularities |
    | --- | --- |

- Monitor for and reduce the severity of adverse effects.
  - Establish a baseline assessment of pulse, blood pressure, cardiac rhythm, and lung fields. *(Baseline data facilitate detection of adverse reactions.)*
  - Ensure that baseline hepatic function studies are performed before starting drug therapy. *(Calcium channel blockers can cause liver enzyme elevation.)*
  - Carefully monitor blood pressure and heart rate during initial stages of therapy. *(Bradycardia and hypotension may occur.)*
  - Monitor for congestive heart failure. *(Decreased cardiac output can compromise heart function.)*
  - Establish with the physician or advanced practice nurse the parameters (blood pressure, pulse) for withholding the medication. *(Hypotension and bradycardia can reduce cardiac output.)*
  - Monitor intake and output and weight, and assess for edema. *(Reduced cardiac output can cause fluid accumulation.)*
  - Teach the client and family how to prevent or reduce the severity of adverse effects. Refer to *RC of β-Adrenergic Blocker Therapy Adverse Effects* for specific interventions.
  - Instruct the client and family to report the following signs and symptoms:
    - 1- to 2-lb weight gain
    - Edema
    - Difficulty breathing
    - Pulse or blood pressure above or below pre-established parameters
    - Sleep disturbances
    - Mental changes
  - Instruct not to stop or miss medication doses. *(Withdrawal hypertension can occur.)*
  - Instruct not to chew, divide, or crush. *(Medication will be absorbed too quickly.)*

# ▶ Risk for Complications of Angiotensin-Converting Enzyme Inhibitor and Angiotension Receptor Blocker Therapy Adverse Effects

## HIGH-RISK POPULATIONS FOR ADVERSE EFFECTS

- Severe renal dysfunction
- Systemic lupuslike syndrome
- Reduced white blood cell count
- Valvular stenosis
- Diabetes mellitus
- Pregnancy or breast-feeding
    Congestive heart failure
    Volume depletion
    Hyponatremia
    hyperkalemia
- Autoimmune disease (for captopril)
- Coronary disease (for captopril)
- Cerebrovascular disease (for captopril)
- Medication therapy that causes leukopenia or agranulocytosis
- Collagen vascular disease (for enalapril)

## Nursing Goals

The nurse will monitor for or assist the client and family to identify and minimize adverse effects.

## General Interventions and Rationales

- Refer also to a pharmacology text for specific information on the individual drug.
- Assess for contraindications to angiotensin-converting enzyme inhibitor therapy:
  - History of adverse effects
  - Renal stenosis (bilateral, unilateral)
  - Previous hypersensitivity
  - Pregnancy
  - Explain possible adverse effects:
  - *Systemic*
      Hypersensitivity (urticaria; rash; angioedema of face, throat, and extremities; difficulty breathing; stridor)
      Photosensitivity
      Alopecia
  - *Central Nervous System*
      | | |
      |---|---|
      | Vertigo | Insomnia |
      | Fainting | Headache |
  - *Cardiovascular*
      | | |
      |---|---|
      | Tachycardia | Angina pectoris |
      | Congestive heart failure | Chest pain |
      | Hypotension | Palpitations |
      | Pericarditis | Flushing |
      | | Raynaud's disease |
  - *Gastrointestinal*
      | | |
      |---|---|
      | Loss of taste | Diarrhea |
      | Vomiting | Peptic ulcer |
      | Anorexia | |
  - *Hematologic*
      | | |
      |---|---|
      | Neutropenia | Eosinophilia |

        Agranulocytosis        Hyperkalemia

        Hemolytic anemia

- *Musculoskeletal*

        Joint pain

- *Genitourinary*

        Proteinuria        Urinary frequency

        Polyuria        Renal insufficiency

        Oliguria        Elevated BUN/creatinine

- *Respiratory*

        Cough        URI symptoms

- Monitor for and reduce the severity of adverse effects.
  - Establish a baseline assessment of pulse, blood pressure (lying, sitting, and standing), cardiac rhythm, and lung fields. *(Baseline assessment data are vital to evaluating response to therapy and identifying adverse reactions.)*
  - Ensure that baseline electrolyte, blood, and renal and hepatic function studies are performed. *(The medication can cause liver enzyme elevation and hypokalemia.)*

Repeat BUN/creatinine and electrolytes in 4-6 weeks then periodically
  - Carefully monitor blood pressure and heart rate during initial stages of therapy. *(Bradycardia and hypotension may occur.)*
  - Monitor for congestive heart failure. *(Decreased cardiac output can compromise heart function.)*
  - Establish with the physician or advanced practice nurse the parameters (blood pressure, pulse) for withholding the medication. *(Hypotension and bradycardia can reduce cardiac output.)*
  - Monitor intake and output and weight, and assess for edema. *(Reduced cardiac output can cause fluid accumulation.)*
- Teach the client and family how to prevent or reduce the severity of adverse effects.
  - Refer to *PRC of β-Adrenergic Blocker Therapy Adverse Effects.*
  - Stress the importance of follow-up laboratory tests. *(Significant abnormalities in urinary protein and blood counts can occur.)*
- Instruct the client and family to report the following signs and symptoms:
  - 1- to 2-lb weight gain
  - Edema
  - Difficulty breathing
  - Pulse or blood pressure above or below pre-established parameters
  - Dark urine
  - Difficult urination
  - Visual disturbances
  - Sore throat
  - Fever
  - Sleep disturbances
  - Memory loss
  - Mental changes
  - Behavioral changes

## ▶ Risk for Complications of Diuretic Therapy Adverse Effects

## HIGH RISK POPULATIONS FOR ADVERSE EFFECTS

- Diabetes mellitus
- Acute MI
- Arrthymias
- Impaired liver function
- History of gout

- History of pancreatitis
- Elderly
- SLE

## Nursing Goals

The nurse will monitor for and assist the client and family to identify and minimize adverse effects.

## General Interventions and Rationales

- Refer to a pharmacology text for specific information on the individual drug
- Assess for contraindications to diuretic therapy
  - History of adverse effects
  - Sulfa allergy
  - Anuria
  - Electrolyte imbalance
  - Hepatic coma
- Explain possible side effects
  - *Systemic*
    Hypokalemia
    Electrolyte imbalance
    Metabolic alkalosis
    Dehydration
    Ototoxicity/ tinnitus
      Blurred vision
    Hyperuricemia
    Hypocalcemia
    Hyperglycemia
    hypomagnesemia
      leukopenia
      muscle cramps
    anorexia
    rash
    pruritus
    tinnitus
  - *Central Nervous System*
    Paresthesias
    Photosensitivity
  - *Cardiovascular*
    Hypovalemia
    Anemia
    Vasculitis
    Orthostatic hypotension
  - *Gastrointestinal*
    Abdominal cramps
    Diarrhea
    Nausea/vomiting
    Cholestatic jaundice
    pancreatitis
  - *Hematologic*
    Thrombosis
    Thromobcytopenia
    Leukopenia
  - *Genitourinary*
    Interstitial nephritis
    Urinary frequency
- Monitor for and reduce the severity of adverse effects

- Identify a base line of pulse and blood presue (lying, sitting and standing)
- Monitor lab results, especially electrolytes.
- Establish with the provider the parameters (blood pressure) for withholding the medication
- Monitor intake and output and weight daiily
- Teach the aptient and family how to prevent the severity of adverse events
- Stress the importance of follow-up laboratory tests
- Instruct the patient to change position slowly
- Instruct the patient and family to report the following signs and symptoms:
  - 1 to 2 lb weight gain
  - edema
  - shortness of breath
  - visual and hearing disturbances
  - blood pressure below established parameters
  - dark urine
  - muscle cramps
  - increased lethargy
  - abdominal pain

# Updated NANDA Diagnoses

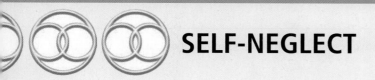

## SELF-NEGLECT

### DEFINITION (NANDA)

A constellation of culturally framed behaviors involving one or more self-care activities in which there is a failure to maintain a socially accepted standard of health and well-being (Gibbons, Lauder, and Ludwick, 2006).

### DEFINING CHARACTERISTICS (NANDA)

- Inadequate personal hygiene
- Inadequate environmental hygiene
- Non-adherence to health activities

### RELATED FACTORS (NANDA)

- Capgras syndrome
- Cognitive impairment (e.g., dementia)
- Depression
- Learning disability
- Fear of institutionalization
- Frontal lobe dysfunction and executive processing ability
- Functional impairment
- Lifestyle/Choice
- Maintaining control
- Malingering
- Obsessive-compulsive disorder
- Schizotypal personal disorders
- Substance abuse
- Major life stressor

### ■■■■■■ AUTHOR'S NOTES

This diagnosis focuses on three problems: self-care problems, home hygiene, and non-compliance. Presently, three nursing diagnoses would more specifically describe the focus as *Self-Care Deficit*, *Altered Home Management*, and *Ineffective Self-Health Management*. Refer to these diagnoses in the index.

# IMPAIRED INDIVIDUAL RESILIENCE

## DEFINITION (NANDA)

Decreased ability to sustain a pattern of positive responses to an adverse situation or crisis

## DEFINING CHARACTERISTICS (NANDA)

- Decreased interest in academic activities
- Decreased interest in vocational activities
- Depression, guilt, shame
- Isolation
- Low self-esteem
- Lower perceived health status
- Renewed elevation of distress
- Social isolation
- Using maladaptive coping skills (i.e., drug use, violence, etc.)

## RELATED FACTORS (NANDA)

- Demographics that increase chance of maladjustment
- Drug use
- Inconsistent parenting
- Low intelligence
- Low maternal education
- Large family size
- Minority status
- Parental mental illness
- Poor impulse control
- Poverty, violence
- Psychological disorders
- Vulnerability factors which encompass indices that exacerbate the negative effects of the risk condition

■■■■■■ **AUTHOR'S NOTES**

This new NANDA-I diagnosis does not represent a nursing diagnosis. The defining characteristics are not defining resilience but in fact a variety of coping problems or mental disorders. Most of the related factors are prejudicial, pejorative, and cannot be changed by interventions. One related factor listed—poor impulse control—is a sign/symptom of hyperactivity disorders and some mental disorders. Resilience is a strength that can be taught and nurtured in children. Resilient individuals and families can cope in adverse situations and crises. They problem solve and adapt their functioning to the situation. For example, when a mother of a family of five had to undergo chemotherapy, the family formulated a plan together to divide the responsibilities previously managed by the mother. When an individual or family has inadequate resilience, they are a t risk for ineffective coping. Refer to Ineffective Coping, Compromised or Disabled Family Coping for Key Concepts, Goals and Interventions/ Rationale.

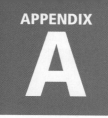

# Nursing Diagnoses Grouped Under Functional Health Patterns*

## 1. Health Perception–Health Management

Falls, Risk for
Growth and Development, Delayed
    Adult Failure to Thrive
    Growth, Risk for Altered
    Development, Risk for Altered
†Health Behavior, Risk-Prone
Health Maintenance, Impaired
    †Surgical Recovery, Delayed
Health-Seeking Behaviors
†Immunization Status, Readiness for Enhanced
Lifestyle, Sedentary
Noncompliance
Risk for Injury
    Risk for Suffocation
    Risk for Poisoning
    Risk for Trauma
Injury, Risk for
    Perioperative Positioning
    †Wandering
†Sudden Infant Death Syndrome, Risk for

## 2. Nutritional–Metabolic

Body Temperature, Risk for Imbalanced
    Hypothermia
    Hyperthermia
    Thermoregulation, Ineffective
Deficient Fluid Volume
Excess Fluid Volume
Deficient Fluid Volume, Risk for
Electrolyte Imbalances, Risk for
Fluid Balance, Readiness for Enhanced
Infection, Risk for
‡Infection Transmission, Risk for
Jaundice, Neonatal
Latex Allergy
Latex Allergy, Risk for
Nutrition, Imbalanced: Less Than Body Requirements
    Breastfeeding, Effective
    Breastfeeding, Ineffective
    †Breastfeeding, Readiness for Enhanced
    Breastfeeding, Interrupted
    Dentition, Impaired
    Feeding Pattern, Ineffective Infant
    Swallowing, Impaired
Nutrition, Imbalanced: More Than Body Requirements
Nutrition, Imbalanced: Risk for More Than Body Requirements
Nutrition, Readiness for Enhanced
Protection, Ineffective
    Tissue Integrity, Impaired
        Oral Mucous Membrane, Altered
        Skin Integrity, Impaired

## 3. Elimination

Constipation
Constipation, Risk for

Perceived Constipation
Diarrhea
Bowel Incontinence
Urinary Elimination, Impaired
Urinary Elimination, Readiness for Enhanced
Overflow Urinary Incontinence
Total Urinary Incontinence
Functional Urinary Incontinence
Reflex Urinary Incontinence
Renal Perfusion, Risk for impaired
Urge Urinary Incontinence
Urge Urinary Incontinence, Risk for
Stress Urinary Incontinence
‡Maturational Enuresis

## 4. Activity–Exercise

Activity Intolerance
Activity Planning, Ineffective
Adaptive Capacity, Intracranial Decreased
Bleeding, Risk for
Cardiac Output, Decreased
Disuse Syndrome
Deficient Diversional Activity
Home Maintenance, Impaired
Infant Behavior, Disorganized
Infant Behavior, Risk for Disorganized
Infant Behavior, Readiness for Enhanced Organized
Mobility, Impaired Physical
    Bed Mobility, Impaired
    Walking, Impaired
    Wheelchair Mobility, Impaired
    Wheelchair Transfer Ability, Impaired
Peripheral Neurovascular Dysfunction, Risk for
‡Respiratory Function, Risk for Impaired
    Dysfunctional Ventilatory Weaning Response
    Ineffective Airway Clearance
    Ineffective Breathing Patterns
    Impaired Gas Exchange
    Ventilation, Inability to Sustain Spontaneous
‡Self-Care Deficit Syndrome (Specify):
(‡Instrumental, Feeding, Bathing/Hygiene, Dressing/Grooming, Toileting)
    †Self-Care, Readiness for Enhanced
Self-Health Management, Ineffective
Self-Health Management Readiness for Enhanced
Self-Health Management: Family, Ineffective
Shock, Risk for
Tissue Perfusion, Ineffective (Specify Type)
Cardiac Perfusion, Risk for Decreased
Cerebral Tissue Perfusion, Risk for
Gastrointestinal Motility, Dysfunction
Gastrointestinal Motility, Risk for Dysfunctional
Gastrointestinal Tissue perfusion, Risk for Ineffective
Peripheral Tissue Perfusion, Ineffective
Renal Perfusion, Risk for Impaired
Vascular Trauma, Risk for

*The Functional Health Patterns were identified in Gordon, M. (1982). *Nursing diagnosis: Process and application.* New York: McGraw-Hill, with minor changes by the author.
†These diagnoses were accepted by the North American Nursing Diagnosis Association (NANDA) in 2008.
‡These diagnoses are not currently on the NANDA list but have been included for clarity and usefulness.

## 5. Sleep–Rest

Disturbed Sleep Pattern
   Insomnia
   Sleep Deprivation
†Sleep, Readiness for Enhanced

## 6. Cognitive–Perceptual

Comfort, Impaired
   Acute Pain
   Chronic Pain
   Nausea
   Comfort, Readiness for Enhanced
Confusion
   Acute Confusion
   Chronic Confusion
Decisional Conflict
Decision-Making, Readiness for Enhanced
Dysreflexia
Dysreflexia, Risk for Autonomic
Environmental Interpretation Syndrome, Impaired
Deficient Knowledge (specify)
†Knowledge, Readiness for Enhanced
Risk for Aspiration
Disturbed Sensory Perception: (Specify):
(Visual, Auditory, Kinesthetic, Gustatory, Tactile, Olfactory)
Memory, Impaired
Unilateral Neglect

## 7. Self-Perception

Anxiety
   Death Anxiety
Fatigue
Fear
†Hope, Readiness for Enhanced
Hopelessness
†Power, Readiness for Enhanced
Powerlessness
Powerlessness, Risk for
‡Disturbed Self-Concept
   Disturbed Body Image
   Disturbed Personal Identity
      Disturbed Self-Esteem
         Chronic Low Self-Esteem
         Situational Low Self-Esteem
         Situational Low Self-Esteem, Risk for
Self-Concept, Readiness for Enhanced
Self-Neglect
Stress Overload

## 8. Role–Relationship

‡Communication, Impaired
   Communication, Impaired Verbal
Communication, Readiness for Enhanced
Family Processes, Interrupted
   Family Processes, Dysfunctional: Alcoholism
Family Processes, Readiness for Enhanced
†Grieving
   Grieving, Anticipatory
   †Grieving, Complicated
   Grieving, Readiness for Enhanced
†Chronic Sorrow

Loneliness, Risk for
Parent–Infant Attachment, Risk for Impaired
Parenting, Impaired
Parenting, Readiness for Enhanced
Parental Role Conflict
Readiness for Enhanced Relationship
Role Performance, Ineffective
Social Interaction, Impaired
Social Isolation

## 9. Sexuality–Reproductive

Childbearing Process, Readiness for Enhanced
Maternal/Fetal Dyad, Risk for Disturbed
Sexual Dysfunction
Sexuality Patterns, Altered

## 10. Coping–Stress Tolerance

Caregiver Role Strain
Coping, Ineffective
   Defensive Coping
   Ineffective Denial
Coping: Compromised, Family
Coping: Readiness for Enhanced Family
Coping: Ineffective Community
Coping, Readiness for Enhanced
Coping, Readiness for Enhanced Community
Disabled Family Coping
Disturbed Energy Field
Post-trauma Response
   Rape Trauma Syndrome
Post-trauma Syndrome, Risk for
Relocation Stress Syndrome
Relocation Stress Syndrome, Risk for
Resilience, Risk for Compromised
Resilience, Impaired Individual
Resilience, Readiness for Enhanced
‡Self-Harm, Risk for
   Self-Abuse, Risk for
   Self-Mutilation
   Self-Mutilation, Risk for
Suicide, Risk for
Violence  Risk for Self-Directed
Violence, Risk for Other Directed

## 11. Value–Belief

†Moral Distress
Spiritual Distress
Spiritual Distress, Risk for
Spiritual Well-Being, Readiness for
   Enhanced
   Religiosity, Impaired
   †Religiosity, Readiness for Enhanced
   Religiosity, Risk for Impaired

---

†These diagnoses were accepted by the North American Nursing Diagnosis Association (NANDA) in 2006.
‡These diagnoses are not currently on the NANDA list but have been included for clarity and usefulness.

# Nursing Admission Data Base

**NURSING ADMISSION DATA BASE**

Date _____ Arrival Time _____ Contact Person _____ Phone _____

ADMITTED FROM:   ___ Home alone   ___ Home with relative   ___ Long-term care
                   ___ Homeless     ___ Home with ‾‾‾‾‾          facility
                   ___ ER           ___ (Specify)     ___ Other _____

MODE OF ARRIVAL:  ___ Wheelchair   ___ Ambulance   ___ Stretcher

REASON FOR HOSPITALIZATION: _____
_____
_____

LAST HOSPITAL ADMISSION: Date _____ Reason _____

PAST MEDICAL HISTORY: _____
_____

| MEDICATION<br>(Prescription/Over-the-Counter) | DOSAGE | LAST DOSE | FREQUENCY |
|---|---|---|---|
| | | | |
| | | | |
| | | | |
| | | | |
| | | | |

**HEALTH MAINTENANCE–PERCEPTION PATTERN**

USE OF:

Tobacco:   ___ None ___ Quit (date) ___ Pipe ___ Cigar ___<1 pk/day
              ___ 1–2 pks/day ___ >2 pks/day Pks/year history _____

Alcohol:  ___ Date of last drink ___ Amount/type
          ___ No. of days in a month when alcohol is consumed

Other Drugs: ___ No ___ Yes  Type _____ Use _____

Allergies (drugs, food, tape, dyes): _____ Reaction _____
_____

**ACTIVITY–EXERCISE PATTERN**

SELF-CARE ABILITY:

   0 = Independent    1 = Assistive device    2 = Assistance from others
   3 = Assistance from person and equipment    4 = Dependent/Unable

| | 0 | 1 | 2 | 3 | 4 |
|---|---|---|---|---|---|
| Eating/Drinking | | | | | |
| Bathing | | | | | |
| Dressing/Grooming | | | | | |
| Toileting | | | | | |
| Bed Mobility | | | | | |
| Transferring | | | | | |
| Ambulating | | | | | |
| Stair Climbing | | | | | |
| Shopping | | | | | |
| Cooking | | | | | |
| Home Maintenance | | | | | |

ASSISTIVE DEVICES: ___ None ___ Crutches ___ Bedside commode ___ Walker
                  ___ Cane ___ Splint/Brace ___ Wheelchair ___ Other

CODE: (1) Not applicable (2) Unable to acquire
      (3) Not a priority at this time  (4) Other (specify in notes)

Side One

**NUTRITION–METABOLIC PATTERN**

Special Diet/Supplements _____

Previous Dietary Instruction: ___ Yes ___ No

Appetite: ___ Normal ___ Increased ___ Decreased ___ Decreased taste sensation
___ Nausea ___ Vomiting

Weight Fluctuations Last 6 Months: ___ None _____ lbs. Gained/Lost

Swallowing difficulty: ___ None ___ Solids ___ Liquids

Dentures: ___ Upper (_ Partial _ Full) ___ Lower (_ Partial _ Full)
With Person ___ Yes ___ No

History of Skin/Healing Problems: ___ None ___ Abnormal Healing ___ Rash
___ Dryness ___ Excess Perspiration


**ELIMINATION PATTERN**

Bowel Habits: ___ # BMs/day ___ Date of last BM ___ Within normal limits
___ Constipation ___ Diarrhea ___ Incontinence
___ Ostomy: Type: ___ Appliance ___ Self-care ___ Yes ___ No

Bladder Habits: ___ WNL ___ Frequency ___ Dysuria ___ Nocturia ___ Urgency
___ Hematuria ___ Retention

Incontinency: ___ No ___ Yes ___ Total ___ Daytime ___ Nighttime
___ Occasional ___ Difficulty delaying voiding
___ Difficulty reaching toilet

Assistive Devices: ___ Intermittent catheterization
___ Indwelling catheter ___ External catheter
___ Incontinent briefs


**SLEEP–REST PATTERN**

Habits: ___ hrs/night ___ AM nap ___ PM nap
Feel rested after sleep ___ Yes ___ No

Problems: ___ None ___ Early waking ___ Insomnia ___ Nightmares


**COGNITIVE–PERCEPTUAL PATTERN**

Mental Status: ___ Alert ___ Receptive aphasia ___ Poor historian
___ Oriented ___ Confused ___ Combative ___ Unresponsive

Speech: ___ Normal ___ Slurred ___ Garbled ___ Expressive aphasia
Spoken language _____ Interpreter _____

Language Spoken: ___ English ___ Spanish ___ Other _____

Ability to Read English: ___ Yes ___ No _____

Ability to Communicate: ___ Yes ___ No _____

Ability to Comprehend: ___ Yes ___ No _____

Level of Anxiety: ___ Mild ___ Moderate ___ Severe ___ Panic

Interactive Skills: ___ Appropriate ___ Other _____

Hearing: ___ WNL ___ Impaired (_ Right _ Left) ___ Deaf (_ Right _ Left)
___ Hearing Aid

Vision: ___ WNL ___ Eyeglasses ___ Contact lens
___ Impaired ___ Right ___ Left
___ Blind ___ Right ___ Left
___ Prosthesis ___ Right ___ Left

Vertigo: ___ Yes ___ No    memory intact ___ Yes ___ No

Discomfort/Pain: ___ None ___ Acute ___ Chronic ___ Description _____
_____

Pain Management: _____


**COPING–STRESS TOLERANCE/SELF-PERCEPTION/SELF-CONCEPT PATTERN**

Major concerns regarding hospitalization or illness (financial, self-care): _____
_____

Major loss/change in past year: ___ No ___ Yes _____

Fear of Violence ___ Yes ___ No  Who _____

Outlook on Future _____ (rate 1–poor–to 10–very optimistic)

CODE:  (1) Not applicable (2) Unable to acquire
(3) Not a priority at this time (4) Other (specify in notes)

Side Two

**SEXUALITY–REPRODUCTIVE PATTERN**
LMP: _____ Gravida _____ Para _____ Birth Control _____
Menstrual/Hormonal Problems: ___ Yes ___ No _____
Last Pap Smear: _____ Hx of Abnormal PAP _____
Monthly Self-Breast/Testicular Exam: ___ Yes ___ No  Last Mammogram: _____
Sexual Concerns: _____
_____

**ROLE–RELATIONSHIP PATTERN**
Marital status: _____ Lives with _____
Occupation: _____
Employment Status: ___ Employed ___ Short-term disability
_____ Long-term disability ___ Unemployed
Support System: ___ Spouse ___ Neighbors/Friends ___ None
_____ Family in same residence ___ Family in separate residence
_____ Other _____
Family concerns regarding hospitalization: _____
_____

**VALUE–BELIEF PATTERN**
Religion: _____
Religious Restrictions: ___ No ___ Yes (Specify) _____
Request Chaplain Visitation at This Time: ___ Yes ___ No

**PHYSICAL ASSESSMENT (Objective)**

**1. CLINICAL DATA**
Age _____ Height _____ Weight _____ (Actual/Approximate) BMI _____
Temperature _____
Pulse: ___ Strong ___ Weak ___ Regular ___ Irregular
Blood Pressure: Right Arm ___ Left Arm ___ Sitting ___ Lying ___

**2. RESPIRATORY/CIRCULATORY**
Rate _____
Quality: ___ WNL ___ Shallow ___ Rapid ___ Labored ___ Other _____
Cough: ___ No ___ Yes/Describe _____
Auscultation:
Upper rt lobes ___ WNL ___ Decreased ___ Absent ___ Abnormal sounds ___
Upper lt lobes ___ WNL ___ Decreased ___ Absent ___ Abnormal sounds ___
Lower rt lobes ___ WNL ___ Decreased ___ Absent ___ Abnormal sounds ___
Lower lt lobes ___ WNL ___ Decreased ___ Absent ___ Abnormal sounds ___
Right Pedal Pulse: ___ Strong ___ Weak ___ Absent
Left Pedal Pulse: ___ Strong ___ Weak ___ Absent

**3. METABOLIC–INTEGUMENTARY**
SKIN:
Color: ___ WNL ___ Pale ___ Cyanotic ___ Ashen ___ Jaundice ___ Other ___
Temperature: ___ WNL ___ Warm ___ Cool
Edema: ___ No ___ Yes/Description/location _____
Lesions: ___ None ___ Yes/Description/location _____
Bruises: ___ None ___ Yes/Description/location _____
Reddened: ___ No ___ Yes/Description/location _____
Pruritus: ___ No ___ Yes/Description/location _____
Tubes: Specify _____
Changes _____ None, If Yes/Description/location _____
MOUTH:
Gums: ___ WNL ___ White plaque ___ Lesions ___ Other _____
Teeth: ___ WNL ___ Other _____
ABDOMEN:
Bowel Sounds: ___ Present ___ Absent

Side Three

**4. NEURO/SENSORY**

Pupils: \_\_\_\_ Equal \_\_\_\_ Unequal

  Left:  • • • • • • •

  Right: • • • • • • •

Reactive to light:

  Left: \_\_\_\_ Yes \_\_\_\_ No/Specify _____

  Right: \_\_\_\_ Yes \_\_\_\_ No/Specify _____

Eyes: \_\_\_\_ Clear \_\_\_\_ Draining \_\_\_\_ Reddened \_\_\_\_ Other _____

**5. MUSCULAR–SKELETAL**

Range of Motion: \_\_\_\_ Full \_\_\_\_ Other _____

Balance and Gait: \_\_\_\_ Steady \_\_\_\_ Unsteady

Hand Grasps: \_\_\_\_ Equal \_\_\_\_ Strong \_\_\_\_ Weakness/Paralysis (\_ Right \_ Left)

Leg Muscles: \_\_\_\_ Equal \_\_\_\_ Strong \_\_\_\_ Weakness/Paralysis (\_ Right \_ Left)

**DISCHARGE PLANNING**

Lives: Alone \_\_\_\_ With _____ No known residence _____

Intended Destination Post Discharge: \_\_\_\_ Home \_\_\_\_ Undetermined \_\_\_\_ Other \_\_\_\_

Previous Utilization of Community Resources:

  \_\_\_\_ Home care/Hospice \_\_\_\_ Adult day care \_\_\_\_ Church groups \_\_\_\_ Other _____

  \_\_\_\_ Meals on Wheels \_\_\_\_ Homemaker/Home health aide \_\_\_\_ Community support group

Post-discharge Transportation:

  \_\_\_\_ Car \_\_\_\_ Ambulance \_\_\_\_ Bus/Taxi

  \_\_\_\_ Unable to determine at this time

Anticipated Financial Assistance Post-discharge?: \_\_\_\_ No \_\_\_\_ Yes _____

Anticipated Problems with Self-care Post-discharge?: \_\_\_\_ No \_\_\_\_ Yes _____

Assistive Devices Needed Post-discharge?: \_\_\_\_ No \_\_\_\_ Yes _____

Referrals: (record date)

  Discharge Coordinator _____ Home Health _____

  Social Service _____

Other Comments: _____

_____

SIGNATURE/TITLE _____ Date _____

Side Four

# Bibliography

*Citations listed under the general category are used throughout the book*

## General References

Abdellah, F. G., & Levine, E. (1965). *Better patient care through nursing research.* New York: Macmillan.

Alfaro-LeFevre, R. (1998). *Applying nursing process: A step-by-step guide* (6th ed.). Philadelphia: Lippincott Williams & Wilkins.

Allender, J., & Spradley, B. (2006). *Community health nursing* (4th ed.). Philadelphia: Lippincott Williams & Wilkins.

American Nurses Association. (1980). *ANA social policy statement.* Washington, DC: Author.

American Psychiatric Association. (2004). *DSM IV-TR: Diagnostic and statistical manual of mental disorders* (4th ed., text revision). Washington, DC: Author.

Andrews, M., & Boyle, J. (2008). *Transcultural concepts in nursing* (5th ed.). Philadelphia: Lippincott Williams & Wilkins.

Archangelo, V. P., & Peterson, A. (2006) *Pharmacotherapeutics for advanced practice* (2nd ed.). Philadelphia: Lippincott Williams & Wilkins.

Aspinall, M. J., & Tanner, C. (1981). *Decision-making in patient care.* New York: Appleton-Century-Crofts.

Bickley, B. (2003). *A guide to physical examination and history taking* (8th ed.). Philadelphia: Lippincott Williams & Wilkins.

Block, G. J., & Nolan, J. W. (1986). *Health assessment for professional nursing: A developmental approach* (2nd ed.). New York: Appleton-Century-Crofts.

Boyd, M. A. (2005). *Psychiatric nursing: Contemporary practice* (3rd ed.). Philadelphia: Lippincott Williams & Wilkins.

Bulechek, G. M., Butcher, G. M., & Dochterman, J. M. (Eds.). (2008). *Nursing interventions: Treatments for nursing diagnoses* (5th ed.). Philadelphia: W. B. Saunders.

Bulechek, G., & McCloskey, J. (1985). Nursing interventions: Treatments for potential nursing diagnoses. In R. M. Carroll-Johnson (Ed.), *Classification of nursing diagnoses: Proceedings of the eighth national conference.* Philadelphia: J. B. Lippincott.

Carpenito-Moyet, L. J. (2009). *Nursing care plans and documentation: Nursing diagnoses and collaborative problems* (5th ed.). Philadelphia: Lippincott Williams & Wilkins.

Carpenito-Moyet, L. J. (2007). *Understanding the nursing process: Concept mappping and care planning for students.* Philadelphia: Lippincott Williams & Wilkins.

Carpenito, L. J. (1995). *Nurse practitioner and physician discipline specific expertise in primary care.* Unpublished manuscript.

Clemen-Stone, E., Eigasti, D. G., & McGuire, S. L. (2001). *Comprehensive family and community health nursing* (6th ed.). St. Louis: Mosby–Year Book.

Curtin, L., & Flaherty, M. J. (1982). *Nursing ethics.* Bowie, MD: Brady Communications.

Dudek, S. (2006). *Nutrition handbook for nursing practice* (5th ed.). Philadelphia: Lippincott Williams & Wilkins.

Edelman, C. H., & Mandle, C. (2006). *Health promotion throughout the life span* (6th ed.). St. Louis: Mosby–Year Book.

Giger, J., & Davidhizar, R. (2009). *Transcultural nursing: Assessment and intervention* (6th ed.). St. Louis: Mosby–Year Book.

Gordon, M. (1994). *Nursing diagnosis: Process and application.* St. Louis: Mosby–Year Book.

Gordon, M. (1982). Historical perspective: The National Group for Classification of Nursing Diagnoses. In M. J. Kim & D. A. Moritz (Eds.), *Classification of nursing diagnoses: Proceedings of the fourth national conference.* New York: McGraw-Hill.

Grondin, L., Lussier, R., Phaneuf, M., & Riopelle, L. (2005). *Planification des soins infirmiers.* Montreal: Les Editions de la Cheneliere.

Henderson, U., & Nite, G. (1960). *Principles and practice of nursing* (5th ed.). New York: Macmillan.

Hickey, J. (2006). *The clinical practice of neurological and neurosurgical nursing* (5th ed.). Philadelphia: Lippincott Williams & Wilkins.

Hockenberry, M. J., Wilson, D., & Winkelstein, M.L. (2008) *Wong's nursing care of infants and children* (7th ed.). Elsevier.

Hockenberry, M. J., & Wilson, D. (2009). *Essentials of pediatric nursing.* Elsevier.

Luis, M. T. (2008). *Diagnostico de enfermeria* (2nd ed.). Barcelona: Doyma.

Matteson, M. A., & McConnell, E. S. (1988). *Gerontological nursing: Concepts and practices.* Philadelphia: W. B. Saunders.

May, K. A., & Mahlmeister, L. R. (1994). *Maternal and neonatal nursing: Family-centered care* (3rd ed.). Philadelphia: J. B. Lippincott.

McCourt, A. (1991). Syndromes in nursing. In R. M. Carroll-Johnson (Ed.), *Classification of nursing diagnoses: Proceedings of the ninth NANDA national conference.* Philadelphia: J. B. Lippincott.

Miller, C. (2009). *Nursing for wellness in older adults* (5th ed.). Philadelphia. Lippincott Williams & Wilkins.

Mitchell, G. J. (1991). Nursing Diagnosis: An Ethical Analysis. *Image: The Journal of Nursing Scholarship.* 23, 99-103.

Mohr, W. K. (2007). *Psychiatric–mental health nursing: Adaptation and growth* (6th ed.). Philadelphia: Lippincott Williams & Wilkins.

Moorhead, S., Johnson, M., Maas, M., & Swanson, E. (2008). Nursing outcomes classification (NOC). St. Louis: Mosby.

Morton, P., Fontaine, D., Hudak, C., & Gallo, B. (2005). *Critical care nursing* (8th ed.). Philadelphia: Lippincott Williams & Wilkins.

Murray, R. B., Zentner, J. P., & Yakimo, R. (2009). *Health promotion strategies through the life span* (8th ed.). Upper Saddle River, NJ: Pearson Prentice Hall.

Norris, J., & Kunes-Connell, M. (1987). Self-esteem disturbance: A clinical validation study. In A. McLane (Ed.), *Classification of nursing diagnoses: Proceedings of the seventh NANDA national conference.* St. Louis: C. V. Mosby.

North American Nursing Diagnosis Association. (2002). *Nursing diagnosis: Definitions and classification 2001–2002.* Philadelphia: Author.

North American Nursing Diagnosis Association. (1992). *Taxonomy of nursing diagnoses.* Philadelphia: Author.

North American Nursing Diagnosis Association. (2009). Nursing diagnoses: Definitions and Classifications 2009-2010. Ames, IA: Wiley–Blackwell.

Pillitteri, A. (2009). *Maternal and child health nursing* (5th ed.). Philadelphia: Lippincott Williams & Wilkins.

Popkess-Vawter, S. (1984). Strength-oriented nursing diagnoses. In M. J. Kim, G. McFarland, & A. McLane (Eds.), *Classification of nursing diagnoses.* St. Louis: C. V. Mosby.

Porth, C. (2007). *Pathophysiology* (7th ed.). Philadelphia: Lippincott Williams & Wilkins.

Smeltzer, S., Bare, B., Hinkle, J., & Cheever, K. (2008). *Brunner & Suddarth's textbook of medical-surgical nursing* (11th ed.). Philadelphia: Lippincott Williams & Wilkins.

Stuart, G. W., & Sundeen, S. (2002). *Principles and practice of psychiatric nursing* (6th ed.). St. Louis: Mosby–Year Book.

Varcarolis, E., Carson, V. B., & Shoemaker, N. C. (2006). *Foundations of psychiatric mental health nursing* (4th ed.). Philadelphia: W. B. Saunders.

Varcarolis, E. M. (2007) *Manual of psychiatric nursing care plans* (3rd ed.). St. Louis: Saunders.

Weber, J., & Kelley, J. (2003). *Health assessment in nursing.* Philadelphia: Lippincott Williams & Wilkins.

Wong, D. (2003). *Nursing care of infants and children* (7th ed.). St. Louis: Mosby-Year Book.

# Section One

Fry, V. S. (1953). The creative approach to nursing. *American Journal of Nursing, 53*, 301–302.

Gordon, M. (1990). Towards theory-based diagnostic categories. *Nursing Diagnoses, 1*(1), 5–11.

Henderson, U., & Nite, G. (1960). *Principles and practice of nursing* (5th ed.). New York: Macmillan.

Levin, R. F., Krainovitch, B. C., Bahrenburg, E., & Mitchell, C. A. (1989). Diagnostic content validity of nursing diagnoses. *Image: The Journal of Nursing Scholarship, 21*(1), 40–44.

North American Nursing Diagnosis Association. (2008). *Classification of nursing diagnosis.* Philadelphia: NANDA.

Pearson, L. (2009). Annual update of how each state stands on legislative issues affecting advanced practice. *Nurse Practitioner, 26*(1), 26, 47–57.

Seahill, L. (1991). Nursing diagnosis vs. goal oriented treatment planning in inpatient child psychiatry. *Image: The Journal of Nursing Scholarship, 23*, 95–97.

Wallace, D., & Ivey, J. (1989). The bifocal clinical nursing model: Descriptions and application to patients receiving thrombolytic or anticoagulant therapy. *Journal of Cardiovascular Nursing, 4*(1), 33–45.

# Part One: Individual Nursing Diagnoses

## Activity Intolerance

Balfour, I. C. (1991). Pediatric cardiac rehabilitation. *American Journal of Diseases of Children, 145*, 627–630, Day 1984.

Cohen, J., Gorenberg, B., & Schroeder, B. (2000). A study of functional status among elders at two academic nursing centers. *Home Care Provider, 5*(3), 108–112.

Corcoran, P. J. (1991). Use it or lose it—the hazards of bed rest and inactivity. *Western Journal of Medicine, 154*, 536–538.

Fleg, J. L. (1986). Alterations in cardiovascular structure and function with advancing age. *American Journal of Cardiology, 5*(7), 33C–44C.

Magnan, M. A. (1987). *Activity intolerance: Toward a nursing theory of activity.* Paper presented at the Fifth Annual Symposium of the Michigan Nursing Diagnosis Association, Detroit, MI.

Punzal, P. A., Ries, A. L., Kaplan, R. M., & Prewitt, L. M. (1991). Maximum intensity exercise training in patients with chronic obstructive pulmonary disease. *Chest, 100*, 618-623.

Rees, K., Taylor, R. S., Singh, S., et al. (2004). Exercise based rehabilitation for heart failure. *Cochrane Database Systems Review* (3), CD003331.

Sarna, L., & Bialous, S. A. (2004). Why tobacco is a women's health issue. *Nursing Clinics of North America, 39*(1), 165–180.

## Pulmonary

Bauldoff, G., Hoffman, L., Sciurba, F., & Zullo, T. (1996). Home based upper arm exercises training for patients with chronic obstructive pulmonary disease. *Heart and Lung, 25*(4), 288–294.

Breslin, E. H. (1992). Dyspnea-limited response in chronic obstructive pulmonary disease: Reduced unsupported arm activities. *Rehabilitation Nursing, 17*, 12–20.

Klesges, R. C., Eck, L. H., Mellon, M. W., Fulliton, W., Somes, G. W., & Hanson, C. L. (1989). The accuracy of self-reports of physical activity. *Medicine and Science in Sports and Exercise, 22*, 690–697.

## Anxiety

Alexeeva, I., Thomas, B. C., & Pelletier, G. (2008). Psychosocial characteristics of cancer patients who choose to attend an educational session on cancer-related fatigue. *Cancer Nursing, 31*(5), 408–414.

Blanchard, C. M., Courneya, K. S., & Larng, D. (2001). Effects of acute exercise on state anxiety in breast cancer survivors. *Oncology Nursing Forum, 28*(10), 1617–21.

Brant, J. M. (1998). The art of palliative care: Living with hope, dying with dignity. *Oncology Nursing Forum, 25*(6), 995–1004.

Courts, N. F., Barba, B. E., & Tesh, A. (2001). Family caregivers attitudes towards aging, caregiving, and nursing home placement. *Journal of Gerontological Nursing, 27*(8), 44–52.

Grainger, R. (1990). Anxiety interrupters. *American Journal of Nursing, 90*(2), 14–15.

Grealish, L., Lomasney, A., & Whiteman, B. (2000). Foot massage. A nursing intervention to modify the distressing symptoms of pain and nausea in patients hospitalized with cancer. *Cancer Nursing, 23*, 237–243.

Hunt, B., & Rosenthal, D. (2000). Rehabilitation counselors' experiences with client death and death anxiety. *Journal of Rehabilitation, 66*(4), 44–50.

Jones, P. E., & Jakob, D. F. (1984). Anxiety revisited from a practice perspective. In M. J. Kim, G. K. McFarland, & A. M. McLane (Eds.), *Classification of nursing diagnoses: Proceedings of the fifth national conference.* St. Louis: C. V. Mosby.

Leske, J. (1993). Anxiety of elective surgical patients, family members. *AORN Journal, 57*, 1091–1103.

Lugina, H. I., Christenson, K., et al. (2001). Change in maternal concerns during midwifery 6 weeks postpartum period. *Journal of Midwifery and Women's Health, 46*(4), 248–257.

Lyons, B. A. (2002). Cognitive self-care skills: A model for managing stressful lifestyles. *Nursing Clinics of North America, 37*(2), 285–294.

May, R. (1977). *The meaning of anxiety.* New York: W. W. Norton.

Maynard, C. K. (2004). Assess and manage somatization. *Holistic Nursing Practice, 18*(2), 54–60.

Nelson, K. A., Walsh, D., Behrens, C., Zhukovsky, D. S., Lipnickey, V., & Brady, D. (2000). The dying cancer patient. *Seminars in Oncology, 27*(1), 84–89.

Stephenson, N. L., Weinrich, S. P., & Tavakoli, A. S. (2000). The effects of foot reflexology on anxiety and pain in patients with breast and lung cancer. *Oncology Nursing Forum, 27*, 67–72.

Tarsitano, B. P. (1992). Structured preoperative teaching. In G. Bulechek & J. McCloskey (Eds.), *Nursing interventions: Essential nursing interventions.* Philadelphia: W. B. Saunders.

Taylor-Loughran, A., O'Brien, M., LaChapelle, R., & Rangel, S. (1989). Defining characteristics of the nursing diagnoses fear and anxiety: A validation study. *Applied Nursing Research, 2*, 178–186.

Tusaie, K., & Dyer, J. (2004). Resilience: A historical review of construct. *Holistic Nursing Practice, 18*(1), 3–8.

Whitley, G. (1994). Concept analysis in nursing diagnosis research. In R. Carroll-Johnson & M. Paquette, *Classification of nursing diagnosis: Proceedings of the tenth conference.* Philadelphia: J. B. Lippincott.

Wong, H. L. C., Lopez-Nahas, V., & Molassiotis, A. (2001). Effects of music therapy on anxiety in ventilator dependent patients. *Heart Lung Journal of Acute Critical Care, 30*(5), 376–87.

Yokom, C. J. (1984). The differentiation of fear and anxiety. In M. J. Kim, G. K. McFarland, & A. M. McLane (Eds.), *Classification of nursing diagnoses: Proceedings of the fifth national conference.* St. Louis: C. V. Mosby.

## Death Anxiety

Silveira, M. J., DiPiero, A., Garrity, M. S., et al. (2000). Patients' knowledge of options at the end of life. Ignorance in the face of death. *JAMA, 284*(19), 2483–2488.

## Risk for Imbalanced Body Temperature

Ball, J. & Bindler, R. (2008). *Pediatric nursing: Caring for children* (4th ed.). Upper Saddle River, NJ: Pearson Prentice Hall.

DeFabio, D. C. (2000). Fluid and nutrient maintenance before, during and after exercise. *Journal of Sports Chiropractic and Rehabilitation, 14*(2), 21–24, 42–43.

Edwards, S. L. (1999). Hypothermia. *Professional Nurse, 14*(4), 253.

Fallis, W. M. (2000). Oral measurement of temperature in orally intubated critical care patients: State-of-the-science review. *American Journal of Critical Care, 9*(5): 334-43.

Giuliano, K. K., Giuliano, A. J., Scott, S. S., et al. (2000). Temperature measurement in critically ill adults: A comparison of tympanic and oral methods. *American Journal of Critical Care, 9*(4), 254–261.

Puterbough, C. (1991). Hypothermia related to exposure and surgical inteventions. *Today's OR Nurse, 13*(7): 32-33.

Smith, L. S. (2004). Temperature measurement in critical care adults: A comparison of thermometry and measurement routes. *Biological Research for Nursing, 6*(2), 117.

Wilkinson, J., & Van Leuven, K. (2007). *Fundamentals of nursing: Theory, concepts & applications.* Philadelphia: F. A. Davis Company.

## Ineffective Thermoregulation

Peterec, S. (2007). The premature newborn. In F. Oski (Ed.). *Principles and practices of pediatrics* (5th ed.). Philadelphia: Lippincott Williams & Wilkins.

Puterbough, C. (1991). Hypothermia related to exposure and surgical interventions. *Today's OR Nurse, 13*(7), 32-33.

Varda, K. E., & Behnke, R. S. (2000). The effect of timing of initial bath on newborn temperature. *JOGNN 29*(1), 27-32.

## Bowel Incontinence

Fauci, A. S., Braunwald, E., Kasper, D. L., Hauser, S. L., Longo, D. L., Jameson, J. L., Loscalzo, J. (2008). Caregiver role strain. In *Harrison's principles of internal medicine* (17th ed.). New York: McGraw-Hill.

Weeks, S. K., Hubbartt, E., & Michaels, T. K. (2000). Keys to bowel success. *Rehabilitation Nursing, 25*(2), 66-69.

## Effective and Ineffective Breastfeeding

Ertem, I. O., Votto, N., & Leventhal, J. M. (2001). The timing and predictors of the early termination of breastfeeding. *Pediatrics, 107*(3), 543-548.

Ortiz, J., McGilligan, K. & Kelly, P. (2004). Duration of breast milk expression among working mother's enrolled in an employer-sponsored location program. *Pediatric Nursing, 30*(2), 111-119.

## Caregiver Role Strain

Clipp, E., & George, L. (1990). Caregiver needs and patterns of social support. *Journal of Gerontology, 45*(3; Suppl), 102-111.

Dilworth-Anderson, P., Williams, I. C., & Gibson, B. E. (2002). Issues of race, rthnicity, and culture in caregiving research: A 20-year review (1980-2000). *The Gerontologist, 42*(2), 237-272.

Gaynor, S. (1990). The effects of home care on caregivers. *Image: The Journal of Nursing Scholarship, 22*, 208-212.

Hagen, B. (2001). Nursing home placement. *Journal of Gerontological Nursing, 27*(2), 44-53.

Lazarus, R. S., & Folkman, S. (1984). *Stress, appraisal and coping*. New York: Springer.

Lindgren, C. (1990). Burnout and social support in family caregivers. *Western Journal of Nursing Research*, 12,469-481.

Pearlin, L., Mullan, J., Semple, S., & Skaff, M. (1990). Caregiving and the stress process: An overview of concepts and their measures. *The Gerontologist, 30*, 583-594.

Shields, C. (1992). Family interaction and caregivers of Alzheimer's disease patients: Correlates of depression. *Family Process, 31*(3), 19-32.

Smith, G., Smith, M., & Toseland, R. (1991). Problems identified by family caregivers in counseling. *The Gerontologist, 31*(1), 15-22.

Tusaie, K. & Dyer, J. (2004). Resilience: A historical review of construct. *Holistic Nursing Practice, 18*(1), 3-8.

Winslow, B., & Carter, P. (1999). Patterns of Burden in wives who care for husbands with dementia. *Nursing Clinics of North America, 34*(2), 275-287.

Wong, D. L. (1991). Transition from hospital to home for children with complex medical care. *Journal of Pediatric Oncology, 8*(1), 3-9.

Young, M. G. (2001). Providing care for the caregiver. *Patient Care for the Nurse Practitioner, 2*, 36-47.

## Resources for the Consumer

Alzheimer's Disease and Related Disorders, Inc., National Headquarters, 70 East Lake Street, Chicago, IL 60601-5997.

American Association of Retired Persons, 1909 K Street NW, Washington, DC 20049.

Children of Aging Parents, 2761 Trenton Road, Levittown, PA 19056.

National Association for Home Care, 519 C Street, NE, Stanton Park, Washington, DC 20002.

National Association of Area Agencies on Aging, 600 Maryland Avenue, SW, Suite 208, Washington, DC 20024 www.patientcarenp.com (information on caregiving).

## Impaired Comfort

Agency for Health Care Policy and Research. (1992). *Acute pain management: Operative or medical procedures and trauma*. Rockville, MD: Author.

Agency for Health Care Policy and Research. (1994). *Management of cancer pain*. Rockville, MD: Author.

American Pain Society. (2003). Opioid analgesics. In *Principles of analgesic use in the treatment of acute pain and cancer pain* (5th ed., pp. 13-41). Glenview, IL: American Pain Society.

Carr, D. B. (Ed.). (2005). Genetics, pain, and analgesia. *Pain Clinical Updates (International Association for the Study of Pain), 13*(3).

Davis, D. C. (1996). The discomforts of pregnancy. *JOGNN, 25*(1), 73-81.

Dunwoody, C., Krenziscbek, D., Pasero, C., Rathmell, J., & Polomano, R. (2008). Assessment, physiological monitoring, and consequences of inadequately treated pain. *Pain Management Nursing, 9*(1), S11-21.

Eckert, R. M. (2001). Understanding anticipatory nausea. *Continuing Education, 28*(10), 1553-1560.

Elia, N., Lysakowski, C., & Tramer, M. (2005). Does multimodal analgesia with acetaminophen, nonsteroidal antinflammatory drugs, or selective cyclooxygenase-2 inhibitors and patient-controlled analgesia morphine offer advantages over morphine alone? *Anesthesiology, 103*(6), 1296-1304.

Ezzone, S., Baker, C., Rosselet, R., & Terepka, E. (1998). Music as an adjunct to antiemetic therapy. *Oncology Nursing Forum, 25*(9), 1551-1556.

Ferrell, B. R. (1995). The impact of pain on quality of life. *Nursing Clinics of North America, 30*, 609-624.

Field, T., Peck, M., Hernandez Reif, M., et al. (2000). Postburn itching, pain and psychological symptoms are reduced with massage therapy. *Journal of Burn Care Rehabilitation, 21*(3), 189-193.

Foltz, A. T., Gaines, G., & Gullatte, M. (1996). Recalled side effects and self-care actions of patients receiving inpatient chemotherapy. *Oncology Nursing Forum, 23*(4), 679-683.

Herr, K., et al. (2006). Pain assessment in the nonverbal patient: Position statement with clinical practice recommendations. *Pain Management Nursing*, (2), 44-52.

Hester, N. (1979). The preoperational child's reaction to immunization. *Nursing Research, 28*, 250-255.

Jarzyna, D. (2005). Opioid tolerance: A perioperative nursing challenge, *MEDSURG Nursing, 14*(6), 371-378.

Lowe, N. K. (1996). The pain and discomfort of labor and birth. *JOGNN, 25*(1), 82-92.

Lovering, S. (2006). Cultural attitudes and beliefs about pain. *Journal of Transcultural Nursing, 17*(4), 389-395.

Ludwig-Beymer, P. (1989). Transcultural aspects of pain. In J. Boyle & M. Andrews (Eds.), *Transcultural concepts in nursing*. Glenview, IL: Scott, Foresman.

Lussier, D., Huskey, A., & Portenoy, R. (2004). Adjuvant analgesics in cancer pain management. *Oncologist, 9*, 571-591.

McCaffrey, M., & Portenoy, R. (1999). Acetaminophen and nonsteroidal anti-inflammatory drugs (NSAIDs). In M. McCaffrey & Pasero, C. (Eds.), *Pain: Clinical manual* (2nd ed., pp. 129-160). New York: Mosby.

McGuire, D., Sheidler, V., & Polomano, R. C. (2000). Pain. In S. Groenwald, M. Frogge, M. Goodman, & C. Yarbo (Eds.). *Cancer nursing: Principles and practice* (5th ed.). Boston: Jones and Bartlett.

Mitra, S., & Sinatra, R. (2004). Perioperative management of acute pain in the opioid-dependent patient. *Anesthesiology, 101*(1), 212-227.

Pasero, C., & McCaffery, M. (2004). Pain control: Comfort-function goals. *AJN, 104*(9), 77.

Pasero, C., Paice, J., & McCaffery, M. (2004). Basic mechanisms underlying the causes and effects of pain. In M. McCaffery & C. Pasero, (Eds.), *Clinical pain manual* (pp. 15-34). New York: Mosby.

Perkins, F., & Kehlet, H. (2000). Chronic pain as an outcome of surgery: A review of predictive factors. *Anesthesiology, 92*(4), 123-133.

Savage, S., et al. (2001). *Definitions related to the use of opioids for the treatment of pain: A consensus document from the American Academy of Pain Medicine, the American Pain Society, and the American Society of Addiction Medicine*. Glenview, IL: Author.

Sloman, R. (1995). Relaxation and relief of cancer pain. *Nursing Clinics of North America, 30*, 697-709.

Thorns, A., & Edmonds, P. (2000). The management of pruritus in palliative care patients. *European Journal of Palliative Care, 7*(1), 9-12.

Voda, A., & Randall, M. (1982). Nausea and vomiting of pregnancy. In C. Norris (Ed.), *Concept clarification in nursing*. Rockville, MD: Aspen Systems.

Weber, S. E. (1996). Cultural aspects of pain in childbearing women. *JOGNN, 25*(1), 67-72.

Zborowski, M. (1952). Cultural components in response to pain. *Journal of Social Issues, 8*, 16-30.

## Impaired Communication

Iezzoni, L. F., O'Day, B., Keleen, M. A., & Harker, H. (2004). Improving patient care: Communicating about health care: Observations from persons who are deaf or hard of hearing. *Annals of Internal Medicine, 140*(5), 356–362.

Koester, L. S., Karkowski, A. M., & Traci, M. A. (1998). How do deaf and hearing-impaired mothers regain eye contact when their infants look away? *American Annals of the Deaf, 143*(1), 5–13.

Lindeblade, P. O., & McDonald, M. (1995). Removing communication barriers for the hearing-impaired elderly. *Med-Surg Nursing, 4*(5), 379–385.

Underwood, C. (2004). How can we best deliver an inclusive health service? *Primary Health Care, 14*(9), 20–21.

## Confusion

Anderson, C. (1999). Delirium and confusion are not interchangeable terms [letter to editor]. *Oncology Nursing Forum, 26*(3), 497–498.

Bishop, B. (2006). Worsening confusion in a geriatric patient. *Journal for Nurse Practitioners, 2*(1), 61–2.

Cacchione, P.Z., Culp, K., Laing, J., Tripp-Reimer, T. (2005). Clinical profile of acute confusion in the long-term care setting. *Clinical Nursing Research, 12*(2), 145-58.

Dellasega, C. (1998). Assessment of cognition in the elderly. *Nursing Clinics of North America, 33*(3), 395–406.

Dennis, H. (1984). Remotivation therapy groups. In I. M. Burnside (Ed.), *Working with the elderly group: Process and techniques* (2nd ed.). Monterey, CA: Jones & Bartlett.

Foreman, M. D., Mion, L. C. Tyrostad, L., & Flitcher, K. (1999). Standard of practice protocol: Acute confusion/delirium. *Geriatric Nursing, 20*(3), 147–152.

Gerdner, L. (1999). Individualized music intervention protocol. *Journal of Gerontological Nursing, 25*(10), 10–16.

Hall, G. R. (1991). Altered thought processes: Dementia. In M. Maas, K. Buckwalter, & M. Hardy (Eds.), *Nursing diagnoses and interventions for the elderly*. Menlo Park, CA: Addison-Wesley.

Hall, G. R. (1994). Caring for people with Alzheimer's disease using the conceptual model of progressively lowered stress threshold in the clinical setting. *Nursing Clinics of North America, 29*, 129–141.

Hall, G. R., & Buckwalter, K. C. (1987). Progressively lowered stress threshold: A conceptual model for care of adults with Alzheimer's disease. *Archives of Psychiatric Nursing, 1*, 399–406.

Janssens, J. P., Krause, K. H., (2004). Pneumonia in the very old. *The Lancet Infectious Diseases, 4*(2), 112-24.

Rasin, J. (1990). Confusion. *Nursing Clinics of North America, 25*, 909–918.

Rateau, M. R. (2000). Confusion and aggression in restrained elderly persons undergoing hip repair surgery. *Applied Nursing Research, 13*(1), 50–54.

Roberts, B. L. (2001). Managing delirium in adult intensive care patients. *Critical Care Nurse, 21*(1), 48–55.

Young, M. G. (2001). Providing care for the caregiver. *Patient Care for the Nurse Practitioner*, 36–48.

## Constipation

DiPiro, J., Talbert, R., Hayes, P., Yee, G., Matzke, G., & Posey, L. M. (2001). *Pharmacotherapy* (4th ed.). Norwalk, CT: Appleton & Lange.

Hadley, S. K., & Gaarder, S. M. (2005). Treatment of irritable bowel syndrome. *American Family Physician, 71*(12), 2501–6.

Schaefer, D., & Cheskin, L. (1998). Constipation in the elderly. *American Family Physician, 58*(4), 907–914.

Shua-Haim, J. Sabo, M., & Ross, J. (1999). Constipation in the elderly: A practical approach. *Clinical Geriatrics, 7*(12), 91–99.

Weeks, S. K., Hubbartt, E., & Michaels, T. K. (2000). Keys to bowel success. *Rehabilitation Nursing, 25*(2), 66–80.

## Ineffective Coping

Bartek, J. K., Lindeman, M., & Hawks, J. H. (1999). Clinical validation of characteristics of the alcoholic family. *Nursing Diagnosis, 10*(4), 158–68.

Bodenheimer, T., MacGregor, K., & Shariffi, C. (2005). Helping patients manage their chronic conditions. Retrieved February 21, 2009 from www.chef.org/publications.

Calarco, M., & Krone, K. (1991). An integrated nursing model of depressive behavior in adults. *Nursing Clinics of North America, 26*, 573–583.

Comfort, M., Sockloff, A., Loverro, J., & Kaltenbach, K. (2003). Multiple predictors of substance abuse, women's treatments and outcomes: A prospective longitudal study. *Addiction Behavior, 28*(2), 199–224.

Depression Guideline Panel. (1993). *Depression in primary care: Detection, diagnosis and treatment quick reference guide for clinicians, no. 5*. AHCPR Pub. No. 93-0552. Rockville, MD: U.S. Department of Health Care Policy and Research.

Finkelman, A. W. (2000). Self-management for psychiatric patient at home. *Home Care Provider, 5*(6), 95–101.

Flaskerud, J. H. (1984). A comparison of perceptions of problematic behavior by six minority groups and mental health professionals. *Nursing Research, 33*, 190–197.

Hamburg, D. A., & Adams, J. E. (1953). A perspective on coping behavior. *Archives of General Psychiatry, 17*, 1–20.

Lazarus, R. (1985). The costs and benefits of denial. In A. Monat, & R. Lazarus (Eds.), *Stress and coping: An anthology* (2nd ed.). New York: Columbia.

Lazarus, R., & Folkman, S. (1984). *Stress, appraisal and coping*. New York: Springer.

Lyon, B. L. (2002). Cognitive self-care skills: A model for managing stressful lifestyles. *Nursing Clinics of North America, 37*(2), 285–294.

Miller, P. (1983). Family health and psychosocial response to cardiovascular diseases. *Health Values, 7*(6), 10–15.

Prochasaska, J., DiClemente, C. C., & Norcross, J. C. (1982). In search of how people change. *American Psychology, 47*(8), 1102–1104.

Selye, H. (1974). *Stress without distress*. Philadelphia: J. B. Lippincott.

Simons, R. L., & West, G. E. (1984). Life changes, coping resources and health among the elderly. *International Journal of Aging and Human Development, 20*, 173–189.

Willis, L., Thomas, P., Garry, P. J., & Goodwin, J. (1987). A prospective study of response to stressful life events in initially healthy elders. *Journal of Gerontology, 42*, 627–630.

## Substance Abuse

Bodenheimer, T., MacGregor, K., & Shariffi, C. (2005). Helping patients manage their chronic conditions. Retrieved February 21, 2009 from www.chef.org/publications.

Ewing, J. A. (1984). Detecting alcoholism: The CAGE questionnaire. *Journal of the American Medical Association, 252*, 1905–1907.

Kappas-Larson, P., & Lathrop, L. (1993). Early detection and intervention for hazardous ethanol use. *Nurse Practitioner, 18*(7), 50–55.

Metzger, L. (1988). *From denial to recovery: Counseling problem drinkers, alcoholics, and their families*. San Francisco: Jossey-Bass.

Smith-DiJulio, K. (2006). People who depend on alcohol. In E. M. Varcarolis (Ed.), *Foundations of psychiatric mental health nursing* (6th ed.). Philadelphia: W. B. Saunders.

## Disabled Family Coping

Aiken, M. M. (1990). Documenting sexual abuses in prepubertal girls. *American Journal of Maternal–Child Nursing, 15*, 176–177.

Blair, K. (1986). The battered woman: Is she a silent partner? *Nurse Practitioner, 11*(6), 38.

Browne, K. (1989). The health visitor's role in screening for child abuse. *Health Visitor, 62*(3), 275–277.

Bullock, L. F., & McFarlane, J. (1989). Higher prevalence of low birth-weight infants born to battered women. *American Journal of Nursing, 89*, 1153–1155.

Bullock, L. F., McFarlane, J., Bateman, L., & Miller, V. (1989). Characteristics of battered women in a primary care setting. *Nursing Practitioner, 14*, 47–55.

Centers for Disease Control and Prevention. (2003). *Male batterers*. www.edc.gov/ncipc/factsheets/malebat.htm.

Carlson-Catalano, J. (1998). Nursing diagnoses and interventions for post–acute phase battered women. *Nursing Diagnosis, 9*(3), 101–109.

Chescheir, N. (1996) Violence against women: response from clinicians. *Journal of Emergency Medicine, 27*, 766–768.

Cowen, P. S. (1999). Child neglect: Injuries of omission. *Pediatric Nursing, 25*(4), 401–418.

Else, L., et al. (1993). Personality characteristics of men who physically abuse women. *Hospital and Community Psychiatry, 44*(10), 54–62.

Patterson, M. M. (1998). Child abuse: Assessment and interventions. *Orthopedic Nursing, 17*(1), 49–56.

Sammons, L. (1981). Battered and pregnant. *Maternal-Child Nursing Journal, 6,* 246–250.

Smith-DiJulio, K., & Holzapfel, S. K. (2006). Families in crises: Family violence. In E. M. Varcarolis, V. M. Carson, & N. C. Shoemaker (Eds.), *Foundations of psychiatric mental health nursing* (5th ed.). Philadelphia: W. B. Saunders.

Willis, D., & Porche, D. (2004). Male battering of intimate partners: Theoretical underpinnings, approaches and interventions. *Nursing Clinics of North America, 39*(1), 271–282.

## Child Abuse

Besharov, D. J. (1990). Gaining control over child abuse reports: Public agencies must address both under reporting and over reporting. *Public Welfare,* Spring, 34–40.

USDHHS (2006). Child maltreatment. Retrieved February 10, 2009 from www.acf.hhs.gov/programs/cb/stats_research/index.htm#can.

Kauffman, C. K., Neill, M. K., & Thomas, J. N. (1986). The abusive parent. In S. H. Johnson (Ed.), *High-risk parenting: Assessment and nursing strategies for families at risk.* Philadelphia: J. B. Lippincott.

Wissow, L. (1994). Child maltreatment. In M. Crocetti & M. A. Barone (Eds.), *Oski's principles and practice of pediatrics* (2nd ed.). Philadelphia: J. B. Lippincott.

## Elder Abuse/Neglect

Anetzberger, G. J. (1987). *The etiology of elder abuse by adult offspring.* Springfield, IL: Charles C. Thomas.

Anetzberger, G. J. (2001). Elder abuse identification and referral: The importance of screening tools and referral protocols. *Journal of Elder Abuse & Neglect, 13*(2), 3–22.

Fulmer, T., & Paveza, G. (1998). Neglect in the elderly. *Nursing Clinics of North America, 33*(3), 457–466.

Steinmetz, S. K. (1988). *Duty bound: Elder abuse and family care.* Newberry Park, CA: Sage.

Winslow, B. W. (1998). Family caregiving and the use of formal community support services: A qualitative case study. *Issues in Mental Health Nursing, 19*(1), 11–27.

## Resources

National Center on Elder Abuse. (2003). elder abuse/mistreatment defined. Available at www.elderabusecenter.org/default.cfm?p=mistreatment.cfm.

## Ineffective Community Coping

Allender, J., & Spradley, B. (2006). *Community health nursing* (4th ed.). Philadelphia: Lippincott Williams & Wilkins.

Aroskar, M. (1979). Ethical issues in community health nursing. *Nursing Clinics of North America, 14,* 35–44.

## Readiness for Enhanced Community Coping

Archer, S. E. (1983). Marketing public health nursing services. *Nursing Outlook, 31,* 49–53.

Bushy, A. (1990). Rural determinants in family health: Considerations for community nurse. *Family and Community Health, 12*(4), 89–94.

## Decisional Conflict

Blackhall, L. J., Murphy, S. T. Frank, G., Michel, V., & Azen, S. (1995). Ethnicity and attitudes toward patient autonomy. *JAMA, 74*(3), 1820–1825.

Cicirelli, V., & MacLean, A. P. (2000). Hastening death: A comparison of two end-of-life decisions. *Death Studies, 24*(3), 401–419.

Davis, A. J. (1989). Clinical nurses' ethical decision making in situations of informed consent. *Advanced Nursing Science, 11*(3), 63–69.

Geary, C. M. B. (1987). Nursing grand rounds: The patient with viral cardiomyopathy. *Journal of Cardiovascular Nursing, 2*(1), 48–52.

Jerewski, M. A. (1993). Consenting to DNR: Critical care nurses' interactions with patients and family members. *American Journal of Critical Care, 23*(6), 458–465.

Sims, S. L., Boland, D. L., & O'Neill, C. A. (1992). Decision making in home health care. *Western Journal of Nursing Research, 14,* 186–200.

Soholt, D. (1990). *A life experience: Making a health care treatment decision.* Unpublished master's thesis. Brookings, SD: South Dakota State University.

## Diarrhea

Bennett, R. (2000). Acute gastroenteritis and associated conditions. In L. R. Barker, J. Burton, & P. Zieve (Eds.), *Principles of ambulatory medicine.* Baltimore: Williams & Wilkins.

Brown, K. C. (1991). Dietary management of acute childhood diarrhea: Optimal timing of feeding and appropriate use of milk and mixed diets. *Journal of Pediatrics, 118,* S92–S98.

Fuhrman, M. P. (1999). Diarrhea and tube feeding. *Nutritional Clinical Practice, 14*(2), 83–84.

Goldman, L., & Ausiello, D. (2004). *Cecil Textbook of Medicine, Volume 1*(22nd ed.). Philadelphia: W. B. Saunders.

Jabbar, A., & Wright, R. A. (2003). Gastroenteritis and antibiotic-associated diarrhea. *Primary Care, 30*(1), 63-80.

Larson, C. E. (2000). Evidence-based practice. Safety and efficacy of oral rehydration therapy for treatment of diarrhea and gastroenteritis in pediatrics. *Pediatric Nursing, 26*(2), 177–179.

## Risk for Compromised Human Dignity

Haddock, J. (1994). Towards further clarification of the concept "dignity." *Journal of Advanced Nursing, 24*(5), 924–931.

Mairis, E. (1994). Concept clarification of professional practice—dignity. *Journal of Advanced Nursing, 19*(5), 947–953.

Reed, P., Smith, P., Fletcher, M., & Bradding, A. (2003). Promoting the dignity of the child in hospital. *Nursing Ethics, 10*(1), 67–78.

Shotton, L. & Seedhouse, D. (1998). Practical dignity in caring. *Nursing Ethics, 5*(3), 246–255.

Walsh, K. & Kowanko, I. *(2002).* Nurses' and patients' perceptions of dignity. *International Journal of Nursing Practice, 8*(3), 143–151.

## Disuse Syndrome

Christian, B. J. (1982). Immobilization: Psychosocial aspects. In C. Norris (Ed.), *Concept clarification in nursing.* Rockville, MD: Aspen Publications.

Goldman, L., & Ausiello, D. (2004). *Cecil Textbook of Medicine, Vol. 1* (22nd ed.). Philadelphia: W. B. Saunders.

Goodgame, R. (2006). A Bayesian approach to infectious diarrhea in adults. *Gastroenterology Clinics of North America, 35*(2): 249-73.

Jabbar, A., & Wright, R. A. (2003). Gastroenteritis and antibiotic-associated diarrhea. *Primary Care, 30*(1), 63–80.

Maher, A. Salmond, S., & Pellino, T. (1998). *Orthopedic nursing* (2nd ed.). Philadelphia: W. B. Saunders.

McKinley, W. O., Jackson, A. B., Cardenas, D. D., & Devivo, M. J. (1999). Long-term medical complications after traumatic spinal cord injury. *Archives of Physical Medical Rehabilitation, 80*(11), 1402–1410.

Wright, S. (1989). Nursing strategies: Altered musculoskeletal function. In R. L. Foster, M. M. Hunsberger, & J. J. T. Anderson (Eds.), *Family-centered nursing care of children.* Philadelphia: W. B. Saunders.

## Deficient Diversional Activity

Barba, B. E., Tesh, A. S., & Courts, N. F. (2002). Promoting thriving in nursing homes. *The Eden Alternative Journal of Gerontological Nursing, 28*(3), 7.

Rantz, M. (1991). Diversional activity deficit. In M. Maas, K. Buckwalter, & M. Hardy (Eds.), *Nursing diagnoses and interventions for the elderly.* Redwood City, CA: Addison-Wesley Nursing.

Rode, D., Capitulo, K.L., Fishman, M., & Holden, G. (1998). The Therapeutic Use of Technology. *The American Journal of Nursing, 98*(12): 32-35.

## Dysreflexia

Bennett, C. (2003). Urgent urological management of the paraplegic/quadriplegic patient. *Urologic Nursing, 23*(6), 436–437.

Black, K., & DeSantis, N. (1999). Medical complications common to spinal-cord injury and brain injured patients. *Topics in Spinal Cord Injury Rehabilitation, 5*(2), 47–75.

Kavchak-Keyes, M. A. (2000). Autonomic hyperreflexia. *Rehabilitation Nursing, 25*(1), 31–35.

McClain, W., Shields, C., & Sixsmith, D. (1999). Autonomic dysreflexia presenting as a severe headache. *American Journal of Emergency Medicine, 17*(3), 238–240.

Silver, J. R. (2000). Early autonomic dysreflexia. *Spinal Cord, 38,* 229–233.

Teasell, R., Arnold, J., & Delaney, G. (1996). Sympathetic nervous system dysfunction in high level spinal cord injuries. *Physical Medicine and Rehabilitation, 10*(1), 37–55.

Travers, P. (1999). Autonomic dysreflexia: A clinical rehabilitation problem. *Rehabilitation Nursing, 24*(1), 9–23.

## Energy Field Disturbance

Bradley, D. B. (1987). Energy fields: Implications for nurses. *Journal of Holistic Nursing, 5*(1), 32–35.

Denison, B. (2004). Touch the pain away. *Holistic Nursing Practice, 18*(3), 142–151.

Krieger, D. (1987). *Living the therapeutic touch: Healing as a lifestyle.* New York: Dodd, Mead.

Macrae, J. (1988). *Therapeutic touch: A practical guide.* New York: Knopf.

Meehan, T. C. (1991). Therapeutic touch. In G. Bulechek & J. McCloskey (Eds.), *Nursing interventions: Essential nursing treatments.* Philadelphia: W. B. Saunders.

Meehan, T. C. (1998). Therapeutic touch as nursing intervention. *Journal of Advanced Nursing, 28*(1), 117–125.

Quinn, J. F. (1989). Therapeutic touch as energy exchange: Replication and extension. *Nursing Science Quarterly, 2*(2), 79–87.

Quinn, J., & Strelkauskas, A. (1993). Psychoimmunologic effects of therapeutic touch on practitioners and recently bereaved recipients: A pilot study. *Advances in Nursing Science, 15*(4), 13–26.

Straneva, J. A. (2000). Therapeutic touch coming of age. *Holistic Nursing Practice, 14*(3), 1–13.

Umbreit, A. W. (2000). Healing touch: Applications in the acute care setting. *ACCN Clinical Issues of Advanced Practice in Acute Critical Care, 11*(1), 105–119.

## Interrupted Family Processes

Carson, V. M, & Smith-DiJulio, K. (2006). Family violence. In E. M. Varcarolis, V. M. Carson, & N. C. Shoemaker (Eds.), *Foundations of psychiatric mental health nursing* (5th ed.). Philadelphia: W. B. Saunders.

Clark, J., & Gwin, R. (2001). Psychological responses of the family. In S. Groenwald, M. Frogge, M. Goodman, & C. Yarbo (Eds.), *Cancer nursing: Principles and practice* (3rd ed.). Boston: Jones and Bartlett.

Duvall, E. M. (1977). *Marriage and family development* (5th ed.). Philadelphia: J. B. Lippincott.

Fife, B. L. (1985). A model for predicting the adaptation of families to medical crisis: An analysis of role integration. *Image: Journal of Nursing Scholarship, 18*(4), 108–112.

Hashizume, S., & Takano, J. (1983). Nursing care of Japanese American patients. In M. S. Orque, B. Bloch, & L. S. A. Monroy (Eds.), *Ethnic nursing care: A multicultural approach.* St. Louis: C. V. Mosby.

Kurnat, E., & Moore, C. (1999). The impact of a chronic condition on the families of children with asthma. *Pediatric Nursing, 25*(3), 288–292.

Nugent, K., Hughes, R., Ball, B., & Davis, K., (1992). A practice model for pediatric support groups. *Pediatric Nursing, 18*(1), 11–16.

## Alcoholism

Captain, C. (1989). Family recovery from alcoholism. *Nursing Clinics of North America, 24,* 55–67.

Collins, R. L., Leonard, K., & Searles, J. (1990). *Alcohol and the family: Research and clinical perspectives.* New York: Guilford Press.

Grisham, K., & Estes, N. (1982). Dynamics of alcoholic families. In N. Estes & M. E. Heinemann (Eds.), *Alcoholism: Development, consequences and interventions.* St. Louis: Mosby–Year Book.

Kellett, S. K. (2000). Do women carry more emotional baggage? Gender difference in contact length to a community alcohol treatment alcohol treatment service. *Journal of Substance Use, 5*(3), 211–217.

Smith-DiJulio, K. (2006). Care of the chemically impaired. In E. M. Varcarolis, V.M. Carson, & N. C. Shoemaker (Eds.), *Foundations of psychiatric mental health nursing* (5th ed.). Philadelphia: W. B. Saunders.

Starling, B. P., & Martin, A. C. (1990). Adult survivors of parental alcoholism: Implications for primary care. *Nursing Practice, 15*(7), 16–24.

Vanicelli, M. (1987). Treatment of alcoholic couples in outpatient group therapy. *Group 11, 4,* 247–257.

Wegscheider, S. (1981). *Another chance.* Palo Alto, CA: Science and Behavior Books.

Wing, D. M. (1991). Goal setting and recovery from alcoholism. *Archives of Psychiatry in Nursing, 5,* 178–184.

Wing, D. M. (1994). Understanding alcoholism relapse. *Nurse Practitioner, 19*(4), 67–69.

## Fatigue

Barsevick, A.M., Dudley, W., Beek, S., Sweeney, C., Whitmer, K., & Nail, L. (2004). A randomized clinical trial of energy conservation for patients with cancer-related fatigue. *Cancer,* 100: 1302-1310.

Dzurec, L. C. (2000). Fatigue and relatedness experiences of inordinately tired women: Fourth quarter. *Journal of Nursing Scholarship, 32*(4), 339–345.

Gardner, D. L. (1992). Fatigue in postpartum women. *Applied Nursing Research, 4*(5), 57–62.

Gardner, D. L., & Campbell, B. (1991). Assessing postpartum fatigue. *Maternal–Child Nursing Journal, 16,* 264–266.

Greenberg, D., Sawicka, J., Eisenthal, S., & Ross, D. (1992). Fatigue syndrome due to localized radiation. *Journal of Pain and Symptom Management, 7*(1), 38–45.

Hargreaves, M. (1977). The fatigue syndrome. *Practitioner, 218,* 841–843.

Jiricka, M. K. (2002). Alterations in activity tolerance. In C. M. Porth (Ed.), *Pathophysiology: Concepts of altered health states* (6th ed.). Philadelphia: Lippincott Williams & Wilkins.

Longino, C. F., & Kart, C. S. (1982). Explicating activity theory: A formal replication. *Journal of Gerontology, 37,* 713–722.

Nail, L., & Winningham, M. (1997). Fatigue. In S. Groenwald, M. Frogge, M. Goodman, & C. Yarbo (Eds.), *Cancer nursing: Principles and practice* (4th ed.). Boston: Jones and Bartlett.

Rhoten, D. (1982). Fatigue and the postsurgical patient. In C. Norris (Ed.), *Concept clarification in nursing.* Rockville, MD: Aspen Systems.

Tilden, V. P., & Weinert, C. (1987). Social support and the chronically ill individual. *Nursing Clinics of North America, 22,* 613–620.

## Fear

Bennett, S.J. Cordes, D., Westmoreland, G., Castro, R., & Donnelly, E. (2000). Self-care strategies for symptom management in patients with chronic heart failure. *Nursing Research,* 49(3): 139-145.

Broome, M. E., Bates, T. A., Lillis, P. P., & McGahee, T. W. (1990). Children's medical fears, coping behaviors, and pain perceptions during a lumbar puncture. *Oncology Nursing Forum, 17,* 361–367.

Cesarone, D. (1991). Fear. In M. Maas, K. Buckwalter, & M. Hardy (Eds.), *Nursing diagnoses and interventions for the elderly.* Redwood City, CA: Addison-Wesley Nursing.

Crossley, M.L. (2003). 'Let me explain': narrative emplotment and one patient's experience of oral cancer. *Social Science & Medicine,* 56(3): 439-48.

Nicastro, E., & Whetsell, M. V. (1999). Children's fears. *Journal of Pediatric Nursing, 14*(6), 392–402.

## Deficient and Excess Fluid Volume

Maughan, R., Leiper, J., & Shirreffs, S. (1997). Factors influencing the restoration of fluid and electrolyte balance after exercise in the heat. *British Journal of Sports Medicine, 31*(3), 175–182.

Sansevero, A. (1997). Dehydration in the elderly: Strategies for prevention and management. *Nurse Practitioner: American Journal of Primary Health Care, 22*(4), 41–42, 51–52, 54–57.

Terry, M., O'Brien, S., & Derstein, M. (1998). Lower-extremity edema: Evaluation and diagnosis. *Wounds: A Compendium of Clinical Research and Practice, 10*(4), 118–124.

Zembruski, C. (1997). GN management. A three-dimensional approach to hydration of elders: Administration, clinical staff, and in-service education. *Geriatric Nursing: American Journal of Care for the Aging, 18*(1), 20–26.

## Grieving

Bateman, A. L. (1999). Understanding the process of grieving and loss: A critical social thinking perspective. *Journal of American Psychiatric Nurses Association, 5*(5), 139–149.

Caserta, M. S., Lund, D. A., & Dimond, M. F. (1985). Assessing interviewer effects in a longitudinal study of bereaved elderly adults. *Journal of Gerontology, 40,* 637–640.

Cutcliffe, J. R. (2004). The inspiration of hope in bereavement counseling. *Issues in Mental Health Nursing, 25*(2), 165–190.

Mallinson, R. K. (1999). The lived experience of AIDS-related multiple losses by HIV-negative gay men. *Journal of the Association of Nurses in AIDS Care, 10*(5), 22–31.

Mina, C. (1985). A program for helping grieving parents. *Maternal–Child Nursing Journal, 10*, 118–121.

Pallikkathayil, L., & Flood, M. (1991). Adolescent suicide. *Nursing Clinics of North America, 26*(3), 623–630.

Rando, T. A. (1984). *Grief, dying, and death: Clinical interventions for caregivers.* Champaign, IL: Research Press.

Vanezis, M., & McGee, A. (1999). Mediating factors in the grieving process of the suddenly bereaved. *British Journal of Nursing, 8*(14), 932–937.

Vickers, J. L., & Carlisle, C. (2000). Choices and control: Parental experiences in pediatric terminal home care. *Journal of Pediatric Oncology Nursing, 17*(1), 12–21.

Worden, W. (2002). *Grief counseling and grief therapy* (3rd ed.). New York: Springer.

## Adult Failure to Thrive

Bergland, A. (2001). Thriving—a useful theoretical perspective to capture the experience of well-being among frail elderly in nursing homes? *Journal of Advanced Nursing 36*(3), 426–432.

Gosline, M. B. (2003). Client participation to enhance socialization for frail elders. *Geriatric Nursing, 24*(5), 286–289.

Haight, B. K. (2002). Thriving: A life span theory. *Journal of Gerontological Nursing, 28*(3), 14–22.

Kimball, M. J., & Williams-Burgess, C. (1995). Failure to thrive: The silent epidemic of the elderly. *Archives of Psychiatric Nursing, 9*(2), 99–105.

Kono, A., Kai, I., Sakato, C., et al. (2004). Frequency of going outdoors: A predictor of functional and psychosocial change among ambulatory frail elders living at home. *Journals of Gerontology Series A: Biological Sciences and Medical Sciences, 59*(3), 275–280.

Loeher, K.E., Bank, A.L., & MacNeill, S.E. (2004). Nursing home transition and depressive symptoms in older medical rehabilitation patients. *Clinical Gerontology, 27*(1/2), 59–70.

Loughlin, A. (2004). Depression and social support: Effective treatments for homebound elderly adults. *Journal of Gerontological Nursing, 30*(5), 11–15.

Newbern, V. B., & Krowchuk, H. V. (1994). Failure to thrive in elderly people: A conceptual analysis. *Journal of Advanced Nursing,* 840–849.

Tusaie, K. & Dyer, J. (2004). Resilience: A historical review of construct. *Holistic Nursing Practice, 18*(1), 3–8.

Wagnil, G. & Young H. M. (1990). Resilience among older women. *Image: Journal of Nursing Scholarship, 22*, 252–255.

## Ineffective Health Maintenance

Moore, S. M., & Charvat, J. M. (2002). Using the CHANGE intervention to enhance long-term exercise. *Nursing Clinics of North America, 37*(2), 273–281.

U.S. Department of Health and Human Services. (2001). Public Health Service. *Healthy people 2010.* Washington, DC: U.S. Government Printing Office.

U.S. Department of Health and Human Services. (1998). *Clinician's handbook of preventive services* (2nd ed.). Washington, DC: U.S. Government Printing Office.

## Tobacco Use

Andrews, J. (1998). Optimizing smoking cessation strategies. *Nurse Practitioner, 23*(8), 47–48, 51–52, 57, 61, 64, 67.

Centers for Disease Control and Prevention. (2000). Selected cigarette smoking initiation and quitting behaviors among high school students–US. *MMWR, 47,* 386.

Centers for Disease Control and Prevention. (2004). www.cdc.gov/health/tobacco.htm.

DuRant, R., & Smith, J. (1999). Adolescent tobacco use and cessation. *Primary Care, 26*(3), 553–576.

Mitchell, B., Sobel, H. L., & Alexander, M. H. (1999). The adverse health effects of tobacco and tobacco-related products. *Primary Care, 26*(3), 463–498.

National Cancer Institute. (2006). Surveillance for cancers associated with tobacco use—United States, 1999-2004. Retrieved February 9, 2009 from www.cdc.gov/mmwr/preview/mmwrhtml/ss5708a1.htm.

Pletsch, P. K. (2002). Reduction of primary and secondary smoke exposure for low-income black pregnant women. *Nursing Clinics of North America, 37*(2), 315–326.

Stead, L. T., & Perea, F. B. (2008). Nictotine replacement therapy for smoking cessation. *Cochrane Database.* September Review (1) CD1000/46.

Stead, L. T. & Perea, F. R. (2006). Telephone counseling for smoking cessation. *Cochrane Database.* System Review (3) CD002850.

U.S. Census Bureau. (2006). *Statistical Abstract of US.* Washington, DC: U.S. Government Printing Office.

## Obesity

Buiten, C., & Metzger, B. (2000). Childhood obesity and risk of cardiovascular disease: A review of the science. *Pediatric Nursing, 26*(1), 13–18.

Dennis, K. (2004). Weight management in women. *Nursing Clinics of North America, 39*(14), 231–241.

National Centers for Health Statistics. (2006). Prevalence of Overweight Among Children and Adolescents. Retrieved February 9, 2009 from www.cdc.gov/nchs/products/pubs/pubd/hestats/overweight/overwght_child_03.htm.

Wiereng, M. E., & Oldham, K. K. (2002). Weight control: A lifestyle-modification model for improving health. *Nursing Clinics of North America, 37*(2), 303–311.

## Osteoporosis

Eastell, R., Boyle, I., Compston, J., et al. (1998). Management of male osteoporosis: Report of UIC Consensus Group. *Quarterly Journal of Medicine, 91*(2), 71–92.

Hansen, L. B., & Vondracek, S. F. (2004). Prevention and treatment of nonpostmenopausal osteoporosis. *American Journal of Health System Pharmacy, 61*(24), 2637-2654.

Lindsay, R. (1989). Osteoporosis: An updated approach to prevention and management. *Geriatrics, 44*(1), 45–54.

Sommers, M. S., Johnson, S. A., & Berry, T. A. (2007). *Diseases and disorders: A nursing therapeutic manual* (3rd ed.). Philadelphia: F. A. Davis.

Woodhead, G., & Moss, M. (1998). Osteoporosis: Diagnosis and prevention. *Nursing Practitioner, 23*(11), 18, 23–24, 26–27, 31–32, 34–35.

### Internet Resources

Centers for Disease Control and Prevention. www.cdc.gov/tobacco.

Professional Assisted Cessation Therapy (PACT). www.endsmoking.org.

Campaign for Tobacco-Free Kids. www.tobaccofreekids.org.

Tobacco.org. www.tobacco.org.

www.cdc.gov/aging.htm.

Mayo Clinic. www.mayo.edu.

American Society of Aging. The Live Well, Live Long: Health Promotion and Disease Prevention for Older Adults. www.cdc.gov/agency.htm.

## Health-Seeking Behaviors

Leon, L. (2002). Smoking cessation—developing a workable program. *Nursing Spectrum, FL9*(18), 12–13.

Nyamathi, A. (1989). Comprehensive health seeking and coping paradigm. *Journal of Advanced Nursing, 14*, 281–290.

Tusaie, K., & Dyer, J. (2004). Resilience: A historical review of construct. *Holistic Nursing Practice, 18*(1), 3–8.

Woodhead, G. (1996). The management of cholesterol in coronary heart disease. *Nurse Practitioner, 21*(9), 45, 48, 51, 53.

## Impaired Home Maintenance

Green, K. (1998). *Home care survival guide.* Philadelphia: Lippincott.

Holzapfil, S. (1998). The elderly. In E. Varcarolis (Ed.). *Foundations of psychiatric mental health nursing* (3rd ed.). Philadelphia: W. B. Saunders.

## Hopelessness

Bayat, M., Erdem, E., & Kuzucu, E. G. (2008). Depression, anxiety, hopelessness, and social support levels of parents of children with cancer. *Journal of Pediatric Oncology Nursing,* July 22 PMD: 18648089.

Benzein, E. G., & Berg, A. C. (2005). The level of a relation between hope, hopelessness and fatigue in patients and family members in palliative care. *Palliative Medicine, 19*(3), 234–40.

Breussard, L., Myers, R., & Meaux, J. (2008). The impact of hurricanes Katrina and Rita on Louisiana school nurses. *Journal of School Nursing*, 24(2), 78-82 (PMD: 18363442).

Cashin, A., Potter, E., & Butler, T. (2008). The relationship between exercise and hopelessness in prison. *Journal of Psychiatric Mental Health Nursing*, 15(1), 66-71 (PMD 18186831).

Chen, M.L. (2003). Pain and hope in patients with cancer: A role for cognition. *Cancer Nursing*, 26(1), 61–7.

Christman, N. J. (1990). Uncertainty and adjustment during radiotherapy. *Nursing Research*, 39(1), 17–20, 47.

Clarke, D. M., Cook, K., Smith, G. C., & Piterman, L. (2008). What do general practitioners think depression is? A taxonomy of distress and depression for general practice. *Australian Medical Journal*, June 16, 188 (PMD: 18558909).

Davies, H. N. (1993). Hope as a coping strategy for the spinal cord injured individual. *Axone*, 15(2), 40–45.

Engel, G. (1989). A life setting conducive to illness: The giving up–given up complex. *Annals of Internal Medicine*, 69, 293–300.

Fiedorowicz, J. G., Leon, A. C., Keller, M. B., Solomon, D. A., Rice, J. P., & Corvall, W. H. (2008). Do risk factors for suicidal behavior differ by affective disorder polarity? *Psychology Medicine*, July 30:1–9 PMD: 18667100.

Giarratano, G., Orlando, S., Savage, J. (2008). Perinatal nursing in uncertain times: the Katrina effect. *American Journal of Maternal Child Nursing* 34(4): 249-57. PMD: 18664907.

Goldston, D. B., Reboussin, B. A., & Daniel, S. S. (2006). Predictors of suicide attempts: State and trait components. *Journal of Abnormal Psychology*, 115(4), 842–849.

Hammell, K. W., Miller, W. C., Forwell, S. J., Forman, B. E., & Jacobsen, B. A. (2008). Fatigue and spinal cord injury: A qualitative analysis. *Spinal Cord*, June 10 PMD 18542089.

Herth, K. (1993). Hope in the family caregiver of terminally ill people. *Journal of Advanced Nursing*, 18, 538-547.

Hinds, P., Martin, J., & Vogel, R. (1987). Nursing strategies to influence adolescent hopefulness during oncologic illness. *Journal of the Association of Pediatric Oncology Nurses*, 4(1/2), 14–23.

Jackson, B. S. (1993). Hope and wound healing. *Journal of Enterostomal Therapy in Nursing*, 20(2), 73–77.

Jennings, P. (1997). The aging spirit. Faith and hope—therapeutic tools for case managers. *Aging Today*, 18(2), 17.

Korner, I. N. (1970). Hope as a method of coping. *Journal of Consultation and Clinical Psychology*, 34, 134–139.

Kübler-Ross, E. (1975). *Death: The final stage of growth*. Englewood Cliffs, NJ: Prentice-Hall.

Kylma, J. (2005). Dynamics of hope in adults living with HIV/AIDS: A substantive theory. *Journal of Advanced Nursing*, 52(6), 620–30.

Kylma, J. (2005). Despair and hopelessness in the context of HIV—a meta-synthesis on qualitative research findings. *Journal of Clinical Nursing*, 14(7), 813–821.

Kylma, J., Vehvilainen-Julkunen, K., & Lahdevita, J. (2001). Hope, despair, and hopelessness in living with HIV/AIDS: A grounded theory study. *Journal of Advanced Nursing*, 33(6), 764–775.

Kylma, J., Vehvilainen-Julkunen, K., & Lahdevita, J. (2001). Voluntary caregivers' observations on the dynamics of hope across continuum of HIV/AIDS: A focus group study. *Journal of the Association of Nurses AIDS Care*, 12(2), 88–100.

LeGresley, A. (1991). Validation of hopelessness: Perceptions of the critically ill. In R. M. Carroll-Johnson (Ed.), *Classification of nursing diagnoses: Proceedings of the ninth conference*. Philadelphia: J. B. Lippincott.

Leininger, M. (1978). *Transcultural nursing: Concepts, theories, and practices*. New York: John Wiley & Sons.

Lin, H.R., and Bauer-Wu, S.M. (2003). Psycho-spiritual well-being in patients with advanced cancer: An integrative review of the literature. *Journal of Advanced Nursing*, 44(1), 69–80.

Lohne, V., & Severinsson, E. (2006). The power of hope: Patients' experiences of hope a year later after acute spinal cord injury. *Journal of Critical Nursing*, 15(3), 315–23.

Mallinson, R. K. (1999). The lived experience of AIDS-related multiple losses by HIV-negative gay men. *Journal of the Association of Nurses in AIDS Care*, 10(5), 22–31.

McMillan, D., Gilbody, S., Baresford, E., & Neilly, L. (2007). Can we predict suicide and non-fatal self-harm with the Beck Hopelessness Scale? A meta-analysis. *Psychology Medicine*, 1–10, PMID: 17202001.

Miller, J. F. (1989). Hope inspiring strategies of the critically ill. *Applied Nursing Research*, 2(1), 23–29.

Mok, E., Cahn, F., Chan, V., & Yeung, E. (2003). Family experience caring for terminally ill patients with cancer in Hong Kong. *Cancer Nursing*, 26(4), 267–75.

Notewotney, M. L. (1989). Assessment of hope in patients with cancer: Development of an instrument. *Oncology Nursing Forum*, 16, 57–61.

Okkonen, E., & Vanhanen, H. (2006). Family support, and subjective health of a patient in connection with coronary artery bypass surgery. *Heart Lung*, 35(4), 234–44.

Owen, D. C. (1989). Nurses' perspectives on the meaning of hope in patients with cancer: A qualitative study. *Oncology Nursing Forum*, 16, 75–79.

Parse, R. R. (1990). Parse's research methodology within an illustration of the lived experience of hope. *Nursing Science Quarterly*, 3(3), 9–17.

Plummer, E. M. (1988). Measurement of hope in the elderly hospitalized institutionalized person. *New York State Nurses' Association*, 19(3), 8–11.

Popovish, J.M., Fox, P.G., & Burns, K.R. (2003). "Hope" in the recovery from stroke in the U.S. *International Journal of Psychiatric Nursing Research*, 8(2), 905–920.

Reed, P. G. (1986). Developmental resources and depression in the elderly. *Nursing Research*, 35, 368–373.

Stotland, E. (1969). *The psychology of hope*. San Francisco: Jossey-Bass.

Tollett, J. H., & Thomas, S. P. (1995). A theory-based nursing intervention to instill hope in homeless veterans. *Advanced Nursing Science*, 18(2), 76–90.

Wagner, J. L., Smith, G., Ferguson, P. L., Horton, S., & Wilson, E. (2008). A hopelessness model of depressive symptoms in youth with epilepsy. *Journal of Pediatric Psychiatry*, June 6 PMD: 18539619.

Watson, J. (1979). *Nursing: The philosophy and science of caring*. Boston: Little, Brown.

Ye, S. C., & Yeh, H. F. (2007). Using complementary therapy with a hemo-dialysis patient with colon cancer and a sense of hopelessness. *Hu Li Za Zhi (Chinese)*, 54(5): 93-8.

Yu D. S., Lee, D. T., Kwong, A. N., Thompson, D. R., & Woo, J. (2008). Living with chronic heart failure: A review of qualitative studies of older people. *Journal of Advanced Nursing*, 61(5), 474–83. PMD: 18261056.

## Disorganized Infant Behavior

Acute Pain Management Guideline Panel. (1992a). *Acute pain management in infants, children, and adolescents: Operative and medical procedures*. Quick Reference Guide for Clinicians, AHCPR Pub. No. 92-0020. Rockville, MD: Agency for Health Care Policy and Research, Public Health Service, U.S. Department of Health and Human Services.

Acute Pain Management Guideline Panel. (1992b). *Acute pain management: Operative or medical procedures and trauma*. Clinical Practice Guideline, AHCPR Pub. No. 92-0032. Rockville, MD: Agency for Health Care Policy and Research, Public Health Service, U.S. Department of Health and Human Services.

Aita, M. & Snider, L. (2003). The art of developmental care in NICU: A concept analysis. *Journal of Advanced Nursing*, 41(3), 223.

Als, H., Gilkerson, L., Duffy, F. H., et al. (2003). A three-center, randomized, controlled trial of individualized developmental care for very low birth weight preterm infants: Medical, neurodevelopmental, parenting and caregiving effects. *Journal of Developmental and Behavioral Pediatrics*, 24(6), 399.

Als, H. (1986). A synactive model of neonatal behavioral organization: Framework for the assessment of neurobehavioral development in the premature infant and for the support of infants and parents in the neonatal intensive care environment. *Physical and Occupational Therapy in Pediatrics*, 6, 3–53.

Blackburn, S. (1993). Assessment and management of neurologic dysfunction. In C. Kenner, A. Brueggemeyer, & L. Gunderson (Eds.), *Comprehensive neonatal nursing*. Philadelphia: W. B. Saunders.

Blackburn, S., & Vandenberg, K. (1993). Assessment and management of neonatal neurobehavioral development. In C. Kenner, A. Brueggemeyer, & L. Gunderson (Eds.), *Comprehensive neonatal nursing*. Philadelphia: W. B. Saunders.

Bozzette, M. (1993). Observations of pain behavior in the NICU: An exploratory study. *Journal of Perinatal and Neonatal Nursing*, 7(1), 76–87.

Harrison, L., et al. (1996). Effects of gentle human touch on preterm infants: Pilot study results. *Neonatal Network*, 15(2), 35–41.

Merenstein, G. B., & Gardner, S. L. (1998). *Handbook of neonatal intensive care* (4th ed.). St. Louis: Mosby–Year Book.

Thomas, K. A. (1989). How the NICU environment sounds to a preterm infant. *MCN: American Journal of Maternal–Child Nursing, 14,* 249–251.

Vandenberg, K. (1990). The management of oral nippling in the sick neonate, the disorganized feeder. *Neonatal Network, 9*(1), 9–16.

Williamson, P. S., & Williamson, M. L. (1983). Physiologic stress reduction by local anesthetic during newborn circumcision. *Pediatrics, 7,* 36–40.

Yecco, G. J. (1993). Neurobehavioral development and developmental support of premature infants. *Journal of Perinatal and Neonatal Nursing, 7*(1), 56–65.

## Risk for Infection/Infection Transmission

Bertin, M. L. (1999). Communicable diseases: Infection prevention for nurses at work and at home. *Nursing Clinics of North America, 34*(2), 509–526.

Centers for Disease Control and Prevention. (2000). Guidelines for prevention of transmission of human immunodeficiency virus and hepatitis B virus to health-care and public safety workers. *MMWR, 49,* 5–15.

Centers for Disease Control and Prevention. (2002). Guidelines for hand hygiene in health care settings. Retrieved February 14, 2009 from www.cdc.gov/handhygiene.

Centers for Disease Control and Prevention. (2005). Antiretroviral postexposure prophylaxis after sexual, injection-druguse, or other nonoccupational exposure to HIV in the United States. Retrieved February 19, 2009 from www.cdc.gov/mmwr/preview/mmwrhtml/rr5402al.htm.

Centers for Disease Control and Prevention. (2007). HIV, pregnancy and childbirth. Retrieved October 2008 from www.cdc.gov/hiv/topics/prenatal/resources.

Centers for Disease Control and Prevention. (2001). *U.S. HIV and AIDS cases reported through December 2001.* Atlanta, GA: Department of Health and Human Services.

Centers for Disease Control and Prevention. (2008). HIV Transmission Rates in US. Retrieved February 25, 2009 from www.cdc.gov/hiv/topics/surveillance/resources/factsheets/transmission.htm.

Hall, H., Song, R., Rhodes, P., Prejeanm, J., Qian, A., Lee, L., et al. (2008). Estimates of HIV incidence in US. *JAMA, 300*(5), 520–529.

Kovach, T. (1990). Nip it in the bud: Controlling wound infection with preoperative shaving. *Today's O.R. Nurse, 9,* 23–26.

Owen, M., & Grier, M. (1987). *Infection risk assessment guide.* Orange, CA: Unpublished.

Sharbaugh, R. J. (1999). The risk of occupational exposure and infection with infectious disease. *Nursing Clinics of North America, 34*(2), 493–508.

### Internet Resources

Association for Professionals in Infection Control. www.apic.org.
Centers for Disease Control and Prevention. www.cdc.gov.
National Center for Infectious Disease. www.cdc.gov/ncidod/nicid.htm.

## Risk for Injury

Baumann, S. L. (1999). Defying gravity and fears: The prevention of falls in community-dwelling older adults. *Clinical Excellence for Nurse Practitioners, 3*(5), 254–261.

Lipsitz, L. A., & Fullerton, K. J. (1986). Postprandial blood pressure reduction in health elderly. *Journal of the American Geriatrics Society, 34,* 267–270.

National Safety Council. (2007). Retrieved February 12, 2009 from www.nsc.org/weekly_articles.

Schoenfelder, D. P. (2000). A fall prevention program for elderly individuals. *Journal of Gerontological Nursing, 26*(3), 43–45.

### Child Safety

American Medical Association Board of Trustees. (1991). Use of infant walkers. *American Journal of Diseases of Children, 145,* 933–934.

### Perioperative

AORN. (2009). *Perioperative Standards and recommended practices.* Denver: Association of Perioperative Registered Nurses.

Martin, J. T. (2000). Positioning aged patients. *Geriatric Anesthesia, 18,* 1.

Rothrock, J. C. (2003). *Alexander's care of the patient in surgery* (12th ed.). St. Louis: Mosby.

Smith, K. (1990). Positioning principles. *AORN Journal, 52,* 1196–1198, 1200–1202.

Spry, C. (2008). *Essentials of perioperative nursing.* Boston: Jones and Bartlett.

## Latex Allergy Response

Kleinbeck, S., English, L., Sherley, M. A., & Howes, J. (1998). A criterion-referenced measure of latex allergy knowledge. *AORN, 68*(3), 384–392.

Reddy, S. (1998). Latex allergy. *American Family Physician, 57*(1), 93–100.

## Risk for Loneliness

Bidwell, R. J., & Deisher, R. W. (1991). Adolescent sexuality: Current issues. *Pediatric Annals, 20,* 293–302.

Elsen, J., & Blegen, M. (1991). Social isolation. In M. Maas, K. Buckwalter, & M. Hardy (Eds.), *Nursing diagnoses and interventions for the elderly.* Redwood City, CA: Addison-Wesley Nursing.

Hillestad, E. A. (1984). Toward understanding of loneliness. In *Proceedings of Conference on Spirituality.* Milwaukee, WI: Marquette University.

Longino, C. F., & Karl, C. S. (1982). Explicating activity theory: A formal replication. *Journal of Gerontology, 37,* 713–722.

Mallinson, R. K. (1999). The lived experience of AIDS-related multiple losses by HIV-negative gay men. *Journal of Association of Nurses in AIDS Care, 10*(5), 22–31.

Maslow, A. H. (1968). *Towards a psychology of being* (2nd ed.). New York: Van Nostrand.

Santrock, J. (2004). *Life-Span Development* (9th ed.). Boston: McGraw-Hill.

## Risk Prone Health Management

Bandura, A. (1982). Self-efficacy mechanism in human agency. *American Psychology, 37*(3), 122–147.

Bodenheimer, T., Lorig, K., Holman, H., et al. (2002). Patient self-management of chronic disease in primary care. *JAMA, 288*(19), 2469.

Bodenheimer, T., MacGregor, K., & Sharifi, C. (2005). *Helping patients manage their chronic conditions.* Retrieved January 10, 2007 from www.chef.org/publications.

Butler, C., Rollnick, S., Cohen, D., et al. (1999). Motivational consulting versus brief advice for smokers in general practice: A randomized trial. *British Journal of General Practice, 49,* 611–616.

Cutilli, C. C. (2005). Health literacy? What you need to know. *Orthopaedic Nursing, 24*(3), 227–231.

Gallant, M. H., Beaulieu, M. C., & Carnevale, F. A. (2002). Partnership: An analysis of the concept within the nurse-client relationship. *Journal of Advanced Nursing, 40*(2), 149.

Kalichman, S. C., Cain, D., Fuhel, A., et al. (2005). Assessing medication adherence self-efficacy among low-literacy patients: Development of a pictographic visual analogue scale. *Health Education Research, 20*(1), 24–35.

Murphy, S. A. (1993). Coping strategies of abstainers from alcohol up to three years post-treatment. *Image: Journal of Nursing Scholarship, 25*(2), 87.

Piette, J. D. (2005). Using telephone support to manage chronic disease. California Healthcare Foundation. Retrieved January 6, 2007 from www.chef.org/topics/chronicdisease/index.cfm.

Prochasaska, J., DiClemente, C. C., & Norcross, J. C. (1992). In search of how people change. *American Psychology, 47*(8), 1102–1104.

Rakel, B. (1991). Knowledge deficit. In M. Maas, K. Buckwalter, & M. Hardy (Eds.), *Nursing diagnoses and interventions for the elderly.* Redwood City, CA: Addison-Wesley Nursing.

Rakel, B. A. (1992). Interventions related to teaching. In G. Bulechek & J. McCloskey (Eds.), *Nursing interventions* (2nd ed.). Philadelphia: W. B. Saunders.

Redman, B., & Thomas, S. (1996). Patient teaching. In G. Bulechek & J. McCloskey (Eds.), *Nursing interventions* (3rd ed.). Philadelphia: W. B. Saunders.

Rollnick, S., Mason, P., & Butler, C. (2000). *Health behavior change: A guide for practitioners.* Edinburgh: Churchill Livingstone.

Zerwich, J. (1992). Laying the groundwork for family self-help: Locating families, building trust and building strength. *Public Health Nursing, 9*(1), 15–21.

Zimmerman, G., Olsen, C. & Bosworth, M. (2000). A "Stages of Change" approach to helping patients change behavior. *American Family Physicians, 61*(5), 1409–1416.

## Impaired Physical Mobility

Addams, S. & Clough, J. A. (1998). Modalities for mobilization. In A. B. Mahler, S. Salmond, & T. Pellino (Eds.), *Orthopedic nursing*. Philadelphia: W. B. Saunders.

Berg, K., Hines, M., & Allen, S. (2002). Wheelchair users at home: Few modifications and many injurious falls. *American Journal of Public Health, 92*(1), 48.

Defloor, T., & Grypdonck, M. H. (1999). Sitting posture and prevention of pressure ulcers. *Applied Nursing Research, 12*(3), 136.

Hoeman, S.P. (2002). Movement, functional mobility, and activities of daily living. In Hoeman, S. P. (Ed.), *Rehabilitation nursing: Process, application, and outcomes* (3rd ed.). St. Louis: Mosby.

Kasper, C. E. (1993). Alterations in skeletal muscle related to impaired physical mobility: An empirical model. *Research and Nursing Health, 16*, 265–273.

Minkel, J. L. (2000). Seating and mobility considerations for people with spinal cord injury. *Physical Therapy, 80*(7), 701.

Pellino, T., Polacek, L. P., Preston, A., Bell, N., & Evans, R. (1998). Complications of orthopedic disorders and orthopedic surgery. In A. Maher, S. Salomond, & T. Pellino (Eds.), *Orthopaedic nursing* (2nd ed.). Philadelphia: W. B. Saunders.

Wound, Ostomy, and Continence Nurses Society. (2003). *Guideline for prevention of management of pressure ulcers* (WOCN clinical practice guideline, no. 2). Glenview, IL: Author.

## Moral Distress

Angus, D. C., Barnato, A. E., & Linde-Zwirbe, W. T., et al. (2004). Use of intensive care at end of life in US: An epidemiological study. *Critical Care Medicine, 32*, 638–48.

Caswell, D., & Cryer, H. G. (1995). Case study: When the nurse and physician don't agree. *Journal of Cardiovascular Nursing, 9*, 30–42.

Corley, M., Elswick, R., Gorman, M., & Clor, T. (2001). Development and evaluation of a moral distress scale. *Journal of Advanced Nursing, 33*(2), 250–256.

Corley, M., Minick, P., Elswick, R., & Jacobs, M. (2005). Nurse moral distress and ethical work environments. *Nursing Ethics, 12*(4), 381–389.

Elpern, E., Covert, B., & Kleinpell, R. (2005). Moral distress of staff nurses in a medical intensive care unit. *American Journal of Critical Care, 14*(6), 523–530.

Gutierrez, K.M. (2005). Critical care nurses' perceptions of and responses to moral distress. *Dimensions of Critical Care Nursing, 24*(5): 229–41.

Hanna, D. (2004). Moral distress: The state of the science. *Research and Theory for Nursing Practice: An International Journal, 18*(1), 73–93.

Kramer, F. A. (1974). Public accountability and organizational humanism. *Public Personnel Management, 3*(5)385.

Teno, J. M., Claridge, B. R., Casey, V., Welch, L. C., Wettle, T., Shield, R., et al. (2004). Family perspectives on end-of-life care at the last place of care. *Journal of the American Medical Association, 291*, 88-93.

Tiedje, L. B. (2000). Moral distress in perinatal nursing. *Journal of Perinatal & Neonatal Nursing, 14*(2), 36-43.

Wilkinson, J. M. (1988). Moral distress in nursing practice: Experience and effect. *Kansas Nurse, 63*(11), 8.

## Noncompliance

Cassells, J. M., & Redman, B. K. (1989). Preparing students to be moral agents in clinical nursing practice. *Nursing Clinics of North America, 24*, 463–473.

Hussey, L., & Gilliland, K. (1989). Compliance, low literacy and locus of control. *Nursing Clinics of North America, 24*, 605–611.

Lubin, I. M., & Larsen, P. D. (2006). Chronic Illness/Impact and Interventions. Boston: Jones & Bartlett.

Whatley, J. H. (1991). Effects of health locus of control and social network on adolescent risk taking. *Pediatric Nursing, 17*(2), 239–240.

Wysocki, T., & Wayne, W. (1992). Childhood diabetes and the family. *Practical Diabetology, 11*(20), 29–32.

## Imbalanced Nutrition: Less Than Body Requirements

Evans-Stoner, N. (1997). Nutrition assessment. *Nursing Clinic of North America, 32*(4) 637–650.

Foltz, A. (1997). Nutritional disturbances. In S. Groenwald, M. Frogge, M. Goodman, & C. Yarbo (Eds.), *Cancer nursing: Principles and practices* (4th ed.). Boston: Jones and Bartlett.

Jeng, C., Yang, H., & Tsai, J. (2000). Comparison of exercise self-efficacy and exercise test results between mild-moderate and severe lung function impairment patients with chronic obstructive pulmonary disease. *Nursing Research, 8*(1): 13-25.

Mahan, L. K., & Arlin, M. T. (1996). *Food, nutrition and diet therapy* (9th ed.). Philadelphia: W. B. Saunders.

Overfield, T. (1985). *Biologic variation in health and illness: Race, age, and sex differences.* Menlo Park, CA: Addison-Wesley.

Smeltzer, S., Bare, B., Hinkle, J., & Cheever, K. (2008). *Brunner & Suddarth's textbook of medical-surgical nursing* (11th ed.). Philadelphia: Lippincott, Williams & Wilkins.

White, R., & Ashworth, A. (2000). How drug therapy can affect, threaten and compromise nutritional status. *Journal Human Nutrition and Dieting, 13*, 119–129.

## Impaired Swallowing

Emick-Herring, B., & Wood, P. (1990). A team approach to neurologically based swallowing disorders. *Rehabilitation Nursing, 15*, 126–132.

Grober, M. (Ed.). (1984). *Dysphagia.* Oxford, UK: Butterworth-Heinemann.

## Impaired Parenting

Ahmann, E. (2002). Promoting positive parenting: An annotated bibliography. *Pediatric Nursing, 28*(4), 382.

Banks, J. B. (2002). Childhood discipline: Challenges for clinicians and parents. *American Family Physician, 66*(8), 1447-1452.

Christopherson, E. R. (1992). Discipline. *Pediatric Clinics of North America, 39*, 395–411.

Coffey, J. S. (2006, January- February). Parenting a child with chronic illness: A metasynthesis. *Pediatric Nursing, 32*(1), 51-59.

Family Pediatrics Report of the Task Force on the Family. (2003, June 2). *Pediatrics,* Retrieved September 6, 2008 from MasterFILE Premier database.

Friedman, M. M., Bowden, V. R., & Jones, E. G. (2003). Family nursing: Research, theory, and practice (5th ed.). Upper Saddle River, NJ: Prentice Hall.

Gage, J., Everett, K., & Bullock, L. (2006). Integrative review of parenting in nursing research. *Journal of Nursing Scholarship, 38*(1), 56-62. Retrieved September 6, 2008 from CINAHL Plus with Full Text database.

Hallstrom, B. M., Runeson, I., & Elander, G. (2002). Observed parental needs during their child's hospitalization. *Journal of Pediatric Nursing, 17*(2),140-148.

Herman-Staab, B. (1994). Screening, management and appropriate referral for pediatric behavior problems. *Nurse Practitioner, 19*(7), 40–49.

Klaus, M., & Kennell, J. (1976). *Maternal-infant bonding.* St. Louis: C.V. Mosby.

Koepke, J., Anglin, S., Austin, J., & Delesalle, J. (1991). Becoming parents: Feelings of adoptive mothers. *Pediatric Nursing, 17*(4), 337–340.

Melynk, B. M., Feinstein, N. F., Alpert-Gills, L., Fairbank, E., Hugh, F. C., Sinkin, R. A., Stone, P. W., Small, L., Tu, X., & Gross, S.J. (2006). Reducing premature infant's length of stay and improving parents' mental health outcomes with the creating opportunities for parent empowerment (COPE) neonatal intensive care unit program: A randomized, controlled trial. *Pediatrics, 118*(5), e1414-e1427.

Melynk, B.M., Feinstein, N., & Fairbanks, E. (2006). Two decades of evidence to support implementation of the COPE program as standard practice with parents of young unexpectedly hospitalized/critically ill children and premature infants. *Pediatric Nursing, 32*(5), 475-480.

Merenstein, G., & Gardner, S. (1998). *Handbook of neonatal intensive care* (4th ed.). St. Louis: Mosby-Year Book.

Pfeffer, C. R. (1981). Development issues among children of separation and divorce. In I. R. Stuart & L. E. Abt (Eds.), *Children of separation and divorce: Management and treatment.* New York: Van Nostrand Reinhold.

Rivera-Adino, J., & Lopez, L. (2000). When culture complicates care. *RN, 63*(7), 47.

## Parent-Infant Attachment

Brown, W., Pearl, L., & Carrasco, R. (1991). Evolving models of family-centered services in neonatal intensive care. *Children's Health Care, 20,* 50–52.

Goulet, C., Bell, L., & Tribble, D. (1998). A concept analysis of parent–infant attachment. *Journal of Advanced Nursing, 28*(5), 1071–1081.

Lawhon, G. (2002). Integrated Nursing Care: Vital issues important in the humane care of the newborn. *Seminars in Neonatology, 7,* 441.

Mercer, R., & Ferketich S. (1990). Predictors of parental attachment during early parenthood. *Journal of Advanced Nursing, 15*(3), 268–280.

Regalado, M., Harvinder, S., Inkelas, M., Wissow, L., & Halfon, N. (2004). Parents' discipline of young children: Results from the National Survey of Early Childhood Health. *Pediatrics, 113*(6), 1952-1958.

Wittkowski, A., Wieck, A., & Mann, S. (2007). An evaluation of two bonding questionnaires: A comparison of the Mother-to Infant Bonding Scale with the Postpartum Bonding Questionnaire in a sample of primiparous mothers. *Archives of Women's Mental Health, 10*(4), 171-175. Retrieved October, 10, 2008 from CINAHL with Full Text database.

## Parental Role Conflict

Baker, N. A. (1994). Avoid collisions with challenging families. *Maternal–Child Nursing Journal, 19,* 97–101.

Clements, D., Copeland, L., & Loftus, M. (1990). Critical times for families with a chronically ill child. *Pediatric Nursing, 16*(2), 157–161.

Dunst, C. J., Trivette, C. M., Davis, M., & Wheeldreyer, J. C. (1988). Enabling and empowering families of children with health impairments. *Children's Health Care, 17,* 71–81.

Gallo, A. (1991). Family adaptation in childhood chronic illness. *Journal of Pediatric Health Care, 5,* 78–85.

Melnyk, B., Feinstein, N., Moldenhouer, Z., & Small, L. (2001). Coping in parents of children who are chronically ill. *Pediatrics, 27*(6), 548–558.

Schepp, K. (1991). Factors influencing the coping effort of mothers of hospitalized children. *Nursing Research, 40,* 42–45.

Smith, L. (1999). Family-centered decision-making: A model for parent participation. *Journal of Neonatal Nursing, 5*(6), 31–33.

Thurman, K. (1991). Parameters for establishing family-centered neonatal intensive care services. *Children's Health Care, 20*(1), 34–40.

## Risk for Peripheral Neurovascular Dysfunction

Altizer, L. (2004). Compartment Syndrome. *Orthopedic Nursing, 23*(6), 391–396.

Bourne, R. B., & Rorabeck, C. H. (1989). Compartmental syndrome of the lower leg. *Clinical Orthopaedics and Related Research, 240,* 97–104.

Fahey, V., & Milzarek, A. (1999). Extra-anatomic bypass surgery. *Journal of Vascular Nursing, 17*(3), 71–75.

Harris, I., Kadir, A., & Donald, G. (2006). Continuous compartment pressure monitoring for tibia fractures: Does it influence outcome? *The Journal of TRAUMA Injury, Infection, and Critical Care, 60*(6), 1330-1335.

Kakar, S., Firoozabadi, R., McKean, J., & Tornetta, P. (2007). Diastolic blood pressure in patients with tibia fractures under anesthesia: Implications for the diagnosis of compartment syndrome. *Journal of Orthopedic Trauma, 21,* 99-103.

Kracun, M. D., & Wooten, C. L. (1998). Crush injuries: A case of entrapment. *Critical Care Nursing Quarterly, 21*(2), 81–86.

Miller, N. C., & Askew, A. E. (2007). Tibia fractures: An overview of evaluation and treatment. *Orthopaedic Nursing, 26*(4), 216-223.

Peck, S. (1991). Crush syndrome. *Orthopaedic Nursing, 9*(3), 33–40.

Pellino, T., Polacek, L. P., Preston, A., Bell, N., & Evans, R. (1998). Complications of orthopedic disorders and orthopedic surgery. In A. Maher, S. Salomond, & T. Pellino (Eds.), *Orthopaedic nursing* (2nd ed.). Philadelphia: W. B. Saunders.

Redemann, S. (2002). Modalities for immobilization. In A. B. Maher, S. W. Salmond & T. A. Pellino (Eds.), *Orthopedic Nursing* (3rd ed, p. 303). Philadelphia: W. B. Saunders.

Ross, D. (1991). Acute compartmental syndrome. *Orthopaedic Nursing, 10*(2), 33–38.

## Post-Trauma / Rape Trauma Syndrome

Adams, C., & Fay, J. (1989). *Free of the shadows.* Oakland, CA: New Harbinger.

American Bar Association (2004). Commission on domestic violence. American Bar Association, 14(3).

Burgess, A. W. (1995). Rape trauma syndrome: A nursing diagnosis. *Occupational Health Nursing, 33*(8), 405–410.

Burgess, A. W., Dowdell, R. N., & Prentley, R. (2000). Sexual abuse of nursing home residents. *Journal of Psychosocial Nursing, 38*(6), 10–18.

Carson V. M., & Smith-DiJulio, K. (2006). Sexual assault. In E. Varcarolis, V. M. Carson, & N. C. Shoemaker (Eds.), *Foundations of psychiatric–mental health nursing* (5th ed.). Philadelphia: W. B. Saunders.

Charron, H. S. (1998). Anxiety disorders. In E. M. Varcarolis (Ed.), *Foundations of psychiatric mental health nursing* (3rd ed.). Philadelphia: W. B. Saunders.

Ellis, G. M. (1994). Acquaintance rape. *Perspectives in Psychiatric Care, 30,* 11–16.

Fielo, S. (1987). How does crime affect the elderly? *Geriatric Nursing, 8*(2), 80–83.

Foley, T., & Darvies, M. (1987). *Rape: Nursing care of victims.* St. Louis: C. V. Mosby.

Foubert, J. D. (2000). The longitudinal effects of a rape-prevention program on fraternity men's attitudes, behavioral intent and behavior. *Journal of American College Health, 48*(1), 158–163.

Francis, S. (1993). Rape and sexual assault. In B. S. Johnson (Ed.), *Psychiatric–mental health nursing: Adaptation and growth.* Philadelphia: J. B. Lippincott.

French, K., Beynon, C., & Delaforce, J. (2007). Alcohol: Is the true (Rape Drug). *Nursing Standard, 21*(29), 26–27.

Goldstein, M.Z. (2005). *Comprehensive textbook of psychiatry, Vol. 2* (8th ed., pp. 3828–3834). Philadelphia: Lippincott Williams & Wilkins.

Heinrich, L. (1987). Care of the female rape victim. *Nursing Practitioner, 12*(11), 9.

Horowitz, M. J. (1986). Stress response syndromes: A review of post-traumatic and adjustment disorders. *Hospital and Community Psychiatry, 37,* 241–248.

Kagawa-Singer, M. (2005). The cultural context of death rituals and mourning practices. *Oncology Nursing Forum, 25*(10), 1752–1756.

Ledrayt, L. E. (1998). SANE development and operation guide. *Journal of Emergency Nursing, 24*(2), 197–98.

Ledray, L. E. (2001). Evidence collection and care of the sexually assault survivor: SANE-SART response. Retrieved February 21, 2009 from www.vaw.umn.edu/documents/commissioned/2forensicvidence.htlm.

Petter, L. M., & Whitehill, D. L. (1998). Management of female sexual assault. *American Family Physician, 58*(4), 920–926.

Pfefferbaum, B., Gurwich, R. H., McDonald, N. B., et al. (2000). Post-traumatic stress among young children after the death of a friend or acquaintance in a terrorist bombing. *Psychiatric Services, 51*(3), 386–388.

Rape Abuse and Incest National Network. (2002). Retrieved February 10, 2007 from www.rainn.org/news/ncvs2002.

Rotter, J. C. (2000). Family grief and mourning. *Family Journal, 8*(3), 275–279.

Smith-DiJulio, K. (1998). Evidence of maladaptive responses to crisis: Rape. In E. Varcarolis (Ed.), *Foundations of psychiatric–mental health nursing* (3rd ed.). Philadelphia: W. B. Saunders.

Symes, L. (2000). Arriving at readiness to recover emotionally after sexual assault. *Archives of Psychiatric Nursing, 14*(1), 30–38.

## Powerlessness

Aujoulat, I., d'Hoore, W., & Deccache, A. (2006). Patient empowerment in theory and practice: Polysemy or cacophony? *Patient Education and Counseling, 66*(1), 13–20.

Burkhart, P.V., & Rayens, M.K. (2005). Self-concept and health focus of control: Factors related to children's adherence to recommended asthma regimen. *Pediatric Nursing, 31*(5), 404–409.

Carroll, S. M. (2007). Silent, slow lifeworld: The communication experience of nonvocal ventilated patients. *Qualitative Health Research, 17*(9), 1165-77.

Chang, B. (1978). Generalized expectancy, situational perception and morale among the institutionalized aged. *Nursing Research, 27,* 316–324.

Corrradi, R. B., (2007). Turning passive into active: A building block of ego and fundamental mechanism of defense. *Journal of American Academy of Psychoanalysis and Dynamic Psychiatry, 35*(3), 393-416.

Eklund, M., & Backstrom, M. (2006). The role of perceived control for the perception of health by patients with persistent mental illness. *Scandinavian Journal of Occupational Therapy, 13*(4), 249–56.

Fuller, S. (1978). Inhibiting helplessness in elderly people. *Journal of Gerontological Nursing, 4,* 18–21.

Garrett, P. W., Dickson, H. G., Young, L., & Whelan, A. K. (2008). "The Happy Migrant Effect": Perceptions of negative experiences of healthcare by patients with little or no English: A qualitative study across seven language groups. *Quality and Safety in Health Care, 17*(2), 101–103.

Johansson, K., Salantera, S., & Katajisto, J. (2007). Empowering orthpaedic patients through preadmission education: Results from a clinical study. Patient Education Counseling. Accessed February 5, 2007 at www.ncbi.nlm.nih.gov/entrez/query.fcgi?CMD=search&DB=pubmed.

Klam, J., McLay, M., & Grabke, D. (2006). Personal empowerment program: Addressing health concerns in people with schizophrenia. *Journal of Psychosocial Nursing and Mental Health Services, 44*(8), 20–8.

Lambert, V. A., & Lambert, C. E. (1981). Role theory and the concept of powerlessness. *Journal of Psychosocial Nursing and Mental Health Services, 19*(9), 11–14.

Neufeld, A., Harrison, M. J., Stewart, M., & Hughes, K. (2008). *Qualitative Health Research, 18*(3), 301-10.

O'Heath, K. (1991). Powerlessness. In M. Maas, K. Buckwalter, & M. Hardy (Eds.), *Nursing diagnoses and interventions for the elderly.* Redwood City, CA: Addison-Wesley Nursing.

Oudshoorn, A., Ward-Griffin, C., & McWilliam, C. (2007). Client-nurse relationships in home-based palliative care: A critical analysis of power relations. *Journal of Clinical Nursing, 16*(8), 1435-43.

Sand, L., Strang, P., & Milberg, A. (2008). Dying cancer patients' experiences of powerlessness and helplessness. *Support Care Cancer, 16*(7), 853-62.

Seligman, M. (1975). *Helplessness: On depression, development, and death.* San Francisco: W. H. Freeman.

Simmons, R., & West, G. (1984–85). Life changes, coping resources and health among the elderly. *International Journal of Aging and Human Development, 20,* 173–189.

Stang, I., & Mittelmark, M. B. (2008). Learning as an empowerment process in breast cancer self-help groups. *Journal of Clinical Nursing,* August [epub ahead of print]

Weaver, T., & Narsavage, G. (1992). Physiological and psychological variables related to functional status in chronic obstructive pulmonary disease. *Nursing Research, 41,* 286–291.

Yu, D. S., Lee, D. T., Kwong, A. N., Thompson, D. R., & Woo, J. (2008). Living with chronic heart failure: a review of qualitative studies of older people. *Journal of Advanced Nursing, 61*(5), 474-83.

## Ineffective Protection

Agency for Health Care Policy and Research [AHCPR] Panel for the Prediction and Prevention of Pressure Ulcers in Adults. (1992, May). *Pressure ulcers in adults: Prediction and prevention.* Clinical Practice Guidelines Number 3, AHCPR, Bulletin No. 92-0047. Rockville, MD: Agency for Health Care Policy & Research, Public Health Services, U.S. Department of Health and Human Services.

Bates-Jensen, B. M. (1999). Chronic wound assessment. *Nursing Clinics of North America, 34*(4), 799–846.

Boynton, P. R., Jaworski, D., & Paustian, C. (1999). Meeting the challenges of healing chronic wounds in older adults. *Nursing Clinics of North America, 34*(4), 921–932.

Maklebust, J. (1998). Caring for homecare patients with pressure ulcers. *Home Healthcare Nurse, 17*(5), 307–315.

Maklebust, J., & Sieggreen, M. (2006). *Pressure ulcers: Guidelines for prevention and nursing management* (3rd ed.). Springhouse, PA: Springhouse.

Wysocki, A. (1999). Skin anatomy, physiology and pathophysiology. *Nursing Clinics of North America, 34*(4), 777–798.

## Impaired Oral Mucous Membrane

Beck, S. L. (2001). Mucositis. In S. L. Groenwald, M. Goodman, M. H. Frogge, & C. H. Yarbro (Eds.), *Cancer symptom management* (4th ed.). Boston: Jones & Bartlett Publishers.

Berry, A. M., Davidson, P. M., & Masters, J. (2007). Systemic literature review of oral hygiene practices for intensive care patients receiving mechanical ventilation. *American Journal of Critical Care, 16*(4), 552-562.

Clarkson, J. (2005). Palifermin improves oral mucositis after high-dose chemotherapy and radiation plus stem cell transplantation in people with hematological cancers. *Cancer Treatment Reviews, 31* (5); 413-416. Retrieved August 25, 2008 at www.sciencedirect.com/science.

Clarkson, J. E., Worthington, H. V., & Eden, O. B. (2007). Interventions for treating oral mucositis for patients with cancer receiving treatment. *Cochrane Database,* 1 Art. No. CD001973. Retrieved August 25, 2008 at www.cochrane.org.

Fournier, F., Dubois, D., Pronnier, P. (2005). Effects of gingival and dental plaque antiseptic decontamination on nosocomial infections acquired in the intensive care unit: A double-blind placebo-controlled multicenter study. *Critical Care Medicine, 33*(8): 1728-1735.

Kemp, J., & Brackett, H. (2001). Mucositis. In R. A. Gates, R. M. Fink (Eds.), *Oncology nursing secrets* (pp. 245–249). Philadelphia: Hanley & Belfus.

National Cancer Institute. (2008). *Oral complications of chemotherapy and head/neck radiation.* Retrieved September 2, 2008 at www.cancergov/cancertopics/pdq.

National Comprehensive Cancer Network. (2008). *Oral mucositis is often underrecognized and undertreated.* Retrieved September 2, 2008 at www.nccn.org/professionals/meetings/13thannual/highlights.

Oncology Nursing Society. (2007). Mucositis: What interventions are effective for managing oral mucositis in people receiving treatment for cancer, ONS PEP Cards.

## Relocation Stress

Adshead, H., Nelson, H., Gooderally, V., & Gollogly, P. (1991). Guidelines for successful relocation. *Nursing Standard, 5*(28), 32–35.

Anderzén, I., Arnetz, B. B., Söderström, T., & Söderman, E. (1997). Stress and sensitization in children: A controlled prospective psychophysiological study of children exposed to international relocation. *Journal of Psychosomatic Research, 43*(3), 259–269.

Armer, J. M. (1996). An exploration of factors influencing adjustment among relocating rural elders. *Image, 28*(1), 35–39.

Beirne, N. F., Patterson, M. N., Galie, M., & Goodman, P. (1995). Effects of a fast-track closing on a nursing facility population. *Health and Social Work, 20,* 117–123.

Davies, S., Nolan, M. (2004). Making the move: relatives' experiences of the transition to a new home. *Health Soc Care Community, 12*(6), 517–523.

Flanagan, V., Slattery, M. J., Chase, N. S., Meade, S. K., & Cronenwett, L. R. (1996). Mothers' perceptions of the quality of their infants' back transfer: Pilot study results. *Neonatal Network, 15*(2), 27–33.

Fried, T. R., Gillick, M. R., & Lipsitz, L. A. (1997). Short-term functional outcomes of long-term care residents with pneumonia treated with and without hospital transfer. *Journal of American Geriatrics Society, 45*(3), 302–306.

Gass, K. A., Gaustad, G., Oberst, M. T., & Hughes, S. (1992). Relocation appraisal, functional independence, morale, and health of nursing home residents. *Issues in Mental Health Nursing, 13,* 239–253.

Gibbins, S. A., & Chapman, J. S. (1996). Holding on: Perceptions of premature infants' transfers. *Journal of Obstetric, Gynecologic, and Neonatal Nursing, 25*(2), 147–153.

Haight, B. K. (1995). Suicide risk in frail elderly people relocated to nursing homes. *Geriatric Nursing, 16,* 104–107.

Harkulich, J., & Brugler, C. (1991). Relocation and the resident. *Activities, Adaptation and Aging, 15*(4), 51–60.

Harkulich, J. T., & Brugler, C. J. (1992). Relocation stress. In K. Gettrust & P. Brabec (Eds.), *Nursing diagnosis in clinical practice: Guides for care planning.* Louisville, KY: Delmar.

Houser. D. (1974). Safer care of MI patient. *Nursing 74, 4*(7), 42–47.

Hulewat, P. (1996). Resettlement: A cultural and psychological crisis. *Social Work, 41*(2), 129–135.

Johnson, R. A. (1996). The meaning of relocation among elderly religious sisters. *Western Journal of Nursing Research, 18*(2), 172–185.

Johnson, R. A., & Hlava, C. (1994). Translocation of elders: Maintaining the spirit. *Geriatric Nursing, 15,* 209–212.

Johnson, R. A., & Tripp-Reimer, T. (2001). Relocation among ethnic elders. *Journal of Gerontological Nursing, 27*(6), 22–27.

Kaisik, B. H., & Ceslowitz, S. B. (1996). Easing the fear of nursing home placements: The value of stress inoculation. *Geriatric Nursing, 17*(4), 182–186.

Kosasih, J. B., Borca, H. H., Wenninger, W. J., & Duthie, E. (1998). Nursing home rehabilitation after acute rehabilitation: Predictors and outcomes. *Archives of Physical Medical Rehabilitation, 79*(6), 670–673.

Lander, S. M., Brazill, A. L., & Landrigan, P. M. (1997). Intrainstitutional relocation. Effects on residents' behavior and psychosocial functioning. *Journal of Gerontological Nursing, 23*(4), 35–41.

Lethbridge, B., Somboom, O. P., & Shea, H. L. (1976). The transfer process. *Canadian Nurse, 72*, 39–40.

Loeher, K.E., Bank, A.L., McNeil, S.E., et al. (2004). Nursing home translation and depressive symptoms in older medical rehabilitation patients. *Clinical Gerontology, 27*(12), 59–70.

Longino, C. F., & Bradley, D. E. (2006). Internal and international migration. In R. H. Binstock & L. K. George (Eds.), *Handbook of aging and social services* (6th ed., pp. 76–93). San Diego: Academic Press.

Meacham, C. L., & Brandriet, L. M. (1997). The response of family and residents to long-term care placement. *Clinical Gerontologist, 18*(1), 63–66.

Miles, M. S. (1999). Parents who received transfer preparation had lower anxiety about their children's transfer from the pediatric intensive care unit to a general pediatric ward. *Applied Nursing Research, 12*(3), 114–120.

Miller, S. (1995). *After the boxes are unpacked.* Denver: Focus on the Family.

Minckley, B. B., Burrows, D., Ehrat, K., Harper, L., Jenkin, S. A., Minckley, W. F., Page, B., Schramm, D. E., & Wood, C. (1979). Myocardial infarct stress-of-transfer inventory: Development of a research tool. *Nursing Research, 28*, 4–9.

Mitchell, M. G. (1999). The effects of relocation of elderly. *Perspectives in Gerontological Nursing, 23*(1), 2–7.

Mitchell, M. L., Courtney, M., & Coyer, F. (2003). Understanding uncertainty and minimizing families' anxiety at the time of transfer from intensive care. *Nursing Health Science, 5*(3): 207–211.

Osborne, O. H., Murphy, H. Leichman, S. S., Griffin, M., Hagerott, R. J., Ekland, E. S., & Thomas, M. D. (1990). Forced relocation of hospitalized psychiatric patients. *Archives of Psychiatric Nursing, 4*, 221–227.

Puskar, K. R. (1986). The usefulness of Mahler's phases of the separation–individuation process in providing a theoretical framework for understanding relocation. *Maternal–Child Nursing Journal, 15*(1), 15–22.

Puskar, K. R. (1990). Relocation support groups for corporate wives. *American Association of Occupational Health Nurses Journal, 38*(1), 25–31.

Puskar, K. R., & Dvorsak, K. G. (1991). Relocation stress in adolescents: Helping teenagers cope with a moving dilemma. *Pediatric Nursing, 17*, 295–298.

Puskar, K. R., & Rohay, J. M. (1999). School relocation and stress in teens. *Journal of School Nursing, 15*(1), 16–22.

Reinardy, J. R. (1995). Relocation to a new environment: Decisional control and the move to a nursing home. *Health and Social Work, 20*(1), 31–38.

Smider, N. A., Essex, M. J., & Ryff, C. D. (1996). Adaptation to community relocation: The interactive influence of psychological resources and contextual factors. *Psychology of Aging, 11*(2), 362–372.

Tracey, J. P., & DeYoung, S. L. (2004). Moving to an assisted living facility: The transitional experience of elderly individuals. *Journal of Gerontology Nursing, 30*(10), 26–32.

Vernberg, E. M. (1990). Experiences with peers following relocation during early adolescence. *American Journal of Orthopsychiatry, 60*, 466–472.

Wilson, S. A. (1997). The transition to nursing home life: A comparison of planned and unplanned admissions. *Journal of Advanced Nursing, 26*(5), 864–871.

## Risk for Ineffective Respiratory Function

Chan, L. (1998). Effectiveness of a music therapy intervention on relaxation and anxiety for patients receiving ventilation assistance. *Heart and Lung, 27*(3), 169–176.

Change, V. (1995). Protocol for prevention of complications of endotracheal intubation. *Critical Care Nurse, 13*(4), 19–26.

Chulay, M. (2005). Suctioning: Endotracheal or tracheostomy tube. In D. J. Lynn-McHale Wiegand, & K. K. Carlson (Eds.), *AACN procedure manual for critical care* (5th ed., pp. 62-70). St.Louis: Elsevier Saunders.

Curley, M., & Fackler, J. (1998). Weaning from mechanical ventilation: Patterns in young children recovering from acute hypoxemic respiratory failure. *American Journal of Critical Care, 7*(5), 335–345.

Geisman, L. K. (1989). Advances in weaning from mechanical ventilation. *Critical Care Nursing Clinics of North America, 1*, 697–705.

Grif-Alspach, J. (2006). *Core curriculum for critical care nursing* (6th ed.). St. Louis: Elsevier.

Halm, M. A., & Krisko-Hagel, K. (2008). Instilling normal saline with suctioning: Beneficial technique or potentially harmful sacred cow? *American Journal of Critical Care, 17*(5), 469–472.

Henneman, E. A. (2001). Liberating patients from mechanical ventilation, a team approach, *Critical Care Nursing, 21*(3), 25.

Huckabay, L., & Daderian, A. (1989). Effect of choices on breathing exercises post open heart surgery. *Dimensions of Critical Care Nursing, 9*, 190–201.

Institute for Healthcare Improvement. (2008). Implement the ventilator bundle: Elevation of the head of the bed. Retrieved October 1, 2008 from www.ihi.org/IHI/Topics/CriticalCare/IntensiveCare/Changes/IndividualChanges/Elevationoftheheadofthebed.htm.

Jenny, J., & Logan, J. (1991). Analyzing expert nursing practice to develop a new nursing diagnosis: Dysfunctional ventilatory weaning response. In R. M. Carroll-Johnson (Ed.), *Classification of nursing diagnoses: Proceedings of the ninth conference.* Philadelphia: J. B. Lippincott.

Jenny, J., & Logan, J. (1994). Promoting ventilator independence. *Dimensions of Critical Care Nursing, 13*, 29–37.

Jenny, J., & Logan, J. (1998). Caring and comfort metaphors used by critical care patients. *Image, 30*(2), 197–208.

Logan, J., & Jenny, J. (1990). Deriving a new nursing diagnosis through qualitative research: Dysfunctional ventilatory weaning response. *Nursing Diagnosis, 1*(1), 37–43.

Logan, J., & Jenny, J. (1991). Interventions for the nursing diagnosis Dysfunctional Ventilatory Weaning Response: A qualitative study. In R. M. Carroll-Johnson (Ed.), *Classification of nursing diagnosis: Proceedings of the ninth conference.* Philadelphia: J. B. Lippincott.

Mannino, D. M., Homa, D. M., Pertowski, C. A., et al. (1999). Surveillance for asthma—United States, 1960–1995. *Morbidity and Mortality Weekly Report CDC Surveillance Summaries, 47*, 1–27.

Marini, J. J. (1991). Editorials. *New England Journal of Medicine, 324*, 1496–1498.

McCarley, C. (1999). A model of chronic dyspnea. *Image, 31*(3), 231–236.

Munro, C. L., & Grap, M. J. (2004). Oral health and care in the intensive care unit: State of the science. *American Journal of Critical Care, 13*(1), 25-34.

Owen, C. (1999). New directions in asthma management. *American Journal of Nursing, 99*(3), 26–34.

Schmierer, T. (2000). Prevention of allergies and asthma starts in pregnancy. Retrieved October 4, 2000 at www.advancefornurses.com/pastarticles/aug28_00cover.html.

Slutsky, A. S. (1993). ACCP consensus conference: Mechanical ventilation. *Chest, 104*, 1833–1859.

Tobin, M. J. (1994). Mechanical ventilation. *New England Journal of Medicine, 330*, 1056–1061.

Treloar, D. M., & Stechmiller, J. K. (1995). Use of a clinical assessment tool for orally intubated patients. *American Journal of Critical Care, 4*, 355–360.

Truesdell, C. (2000). Helping patients with COPD manage episodes of acute shortness of breath. *MedSurg Nursing, 9*(4), 178–182.

Venes, D. (2006). *Taber's cyclopedic medical dictionary* (20th ed.). Philadelphia: FA Davis Co.

### Internet Resources

Agency for Healthcare Research and Quality. www.ahrq.gov/.

Allergy and Asthma Web Page. www.cs.unc.edu/~kupstas/FAQ1.html.

Asthma and Allergy Foundation of America. www.aafa.org/.

Asthma Management Model. www.nbibisupport.com/asthma/research.html.

Global Initiative for Obstructive Lung Disease. www.coldcopd.com.

Joint Council of Allergy, Asthma, and Immunology. www.icaai.org/.

Quitting Smoking Guidelines. www.surgeongeneral.gov/tobacco/default.htm.

QuitNet. www.quitnet.org.

## Sedentary Lifestyle

Allison, M., & Keller, C. (1997). Physical activity in the elderly: Benefits and intervention strategies. *Nursing Practice, 22*(8), 53–54.

Lee, K. A. (2001). Sleep and fatigue. *Annual Review of Nursing Research, 19,* 249–273.

Nies, M. A., & Chruscial, H. L. (2002). Neighborhood and physical activity outcomes in women: Regional comparisons. *Nursing Clinics of North America, 37*(2), 295–301.

Resnick, B., Orwig, D., & Magaziner, J. (2002). The effect of social support on exercise behavior in older adults. *Clinical Nursing Research, 11*(1), 52.

Rogers, L. Q., Matevey, C., Hopkins-Price, P., et al. (2002). Exploring social cognitive theory constructs for promoting exercise among breast cancer patients. *Cancer Nursing, 27*(6), 462–473.

Taggart, H. M. (2002). Effects of Tai Chi exercise on balance, functional mobility, and fear of falling among older women. *Applied Nursing Research, 15*(4), 235–242.

Young, H. M., & Cochrane, B. B. (2004). Healthy aging for older women. *Nursing Clinics of North America, 39*(1), 131–143.

## Self-Care Deficit Syndrome

Maher, A. B., Salmond, S. W., & Pellino, T. (1998). *Orthopedic nursing* (2nd ed.). Philadelphia: W. B. Saunders.

Mosher, R. B., & Moore, J. B. (1998). The relationship of self-concept & self-care in children with cancer. *Nursing Science Quarterly, 11*(3), 116–122.

Tracey, C. (1992). Hygiene assistance. In G. Bulechek & J. McCloskey (Eds.), *Nursing interventions: Essential nursing treatments.* Philadelphia: W. B. Saunders.

## Disturbed Self-Concept

Bergamasco, E. C., Rossi, L., da Amancio C. G., & Carvalho, E. C. (2002). Body image of patients with burn sequellae. *Burns, 28,* 47–52.

Camp-Sorrell, D. (2007). Chemotherapy: Toxicity management. In C. Yarbro, M. H. Frogge, M. Goodman, & S. Groenwald, *Career nursing* (6th ed.). Boston: Jones and Bartlett.

Carscadden, J. S. *Above the cutting edge: A workbook for people who want to stop self-injury.* London, Ontario: London Psychiatric Hospital.

Friedman-Campbell, M., & Hart, C. A. (1984). Theoretical strategies and nursing interventions to promote psychological adaptation to spinal cord injuries and disability. *Journal of Neurosurgical Nursing, 16,* 335–342.

Hunter, K., Linn, M., & Harris, R. (1981–82). Characteristics of high and low self-esteem in the elderly. *International Journal of Aging and Human Development, 14,* 117–126.

Johnson, B.S. (1995) *Child, adolescent and family psychiatric nursing.* Philadelphia: J. B. Lippincott

Leuner, J., Coler, M., & Norris, J. (1994). Self-esteem. In M. Rantz & P. LeMone (Eds.), *Classification of nursing diagnosis: Proceedings of the eleventh conference.* Glendale, CA: CINAHL.

Meisenhelder, J. B. (1995). Self-esteem: A closer look at clinical interventions. *International Journal of Nursing studies, 22,* 125-127.

Morse, K. (1997). Responding to threats to integrity to self. *Science, 19*(4), 21–36.

Murray, M. F. (2000). Coping with change: Self-talk. *Hospital Practice, 31*(5), 118–120.

Norris, J., & Kunes-Connell, M. (1985). Self-esteem disturbance. *Nursing Clinics of North America, 20,* 745–761.

Norris, J., & Kunes-Connell, M. (1987). Self-esteem disturbance: A clinical validation study. In A. McLane (Ed.), *Classification of nursing diagnoses: Proceedings of the seventh conference.* St. Louis: C. V. Mosby.

Pierce, J., & Wardle, J. (1997), Cause and effect beliefs and self-esteem of overweight children. *Journal of Child Psychology and Psychiatry and Allied Disciplines, 38*(6), 645–650.

Price, B. (1990). A model for body-image care. *Journal of Advanced Nursing, 5,* 585–593.

Scipien, G. M., Chard, M. A., Howe, J., & Barnard, M. U. (1990). *Pediatric nursing care.* St. Louis: C. V. Mosby.

Specht, J. A., King, G. A., & Francis, P. V. (1998). A preliminary study of strategies for maintaining self-esteem in adolescents with physical disabilities. *Canadian Journal of Rehabilitation, 11*(3), 109–116.

Van-Dongen, C. J. (1998). Self-esteem among persons with severe mental illness. *Issues in Mental Health Nursing, 19*(1), 29–40.

Winkelstein, M. L. (1989). Fostering positive self-concept in the school-age child. *Pediatric Nursing, 15,* 229–233.

## Risk for Self-Harm

Carscadden, J. S. (1993a). *On the cutting edge: A guide for working with people who self injure.* London, Ontario: London Psychiatric Hospital.

Carscadden, J. S. (1993b). *Above the cutting edge: A workbook for people who want to stop self injury.* London, Ontario: London Psychiatric Hospital.

Carscadden, J. S. (1997). *Beyond the cutting edge: A survival kit for families of self-injurers.* London, Ontario: London Psychiatric Hospital.

Carscadden, J. S. (1998). *Premise for practice (relationship management team).* London, Ontario: London Psychiatric Hospital.

Dawson, D. F., & MacMillan, H. L. (1993). *Relationship management of the borderline patient: From understanding to treatment.* New York: Brunner/Mazel Publishers.

Egan, M. P., Rivera, S. G., Robillard, R. R., & Hanson, A. (1997). The no suicide contract: Helpful or harmful? *Journal of Psychosocial Nursing, 35*(3).

Hatton, C., & Valente, S. (1977). Assessment of suicidal risk. In C. Hatton (Ed.), *Suicide: Assessment and intervention.* New York: Appleton-Century-Crofts.

Luoma, J. B., Martin, C. E., & Pearson, J. L. (2002). Contact with mental health and primary care providers before suicide: A review of the evidence. *American Journal of Psychiatry, 159,* 909–916.

Mallinson, R. K. (1999). The lived experiences of AIDS-related multiple losses by HIV-negative gay men. *Journal of the Association of Nurses in AIDS Care, 10*(5), 22–31.

McIntosh, J. L. (1985). Suicide among the elderly: Levels and trends. *American Journal of Orthopsychiatry, 55*(4), 288–293.

Mellick, E., Buckwalter, K. C., & Stolley, J. M. (1992). Suicide among elderly white men: Development of a profile. *Journal of Psychosocial Nursing, 30*(2), 29–34.

Ortiz, M. (2006). Staying alive: A suicide prevention overview. *Journal of Psychosocial Nursing and Mental Health Services, 44*(12), 43–49.

Schultz, J.M., & Videbeck, S.L. (2002). *Lippincott's manual of psychiatric care plans.* Philadelphia: Lippincott Williams & Wilkins.

Seigel, K., & Meyer, I. (1999). Hope and resilience in suicide ideation and behavior of gay and bisexual men following notification of HIV infection. *AIDS Education & Prevention, 11*(1), 53–64.

## Disturbed Sensory Perception

Drury, J., & Akins, J. (1991). Sensory–perceptual alterations. In M. Maas, K. Buckwalter, & M. Hardy (Eds.), *Nursing diagnoses and interventions for the elderly.* Menlo Park, CA: Addison-Wesley Nursing.

Wilson, L. D. (1993). Sensory perceptual alteration: Diagnosis, prediction and intervention in the hospitalized adult. *Nursing Clinics of North America, 28,* 747–765.

## Ineffective Sexuality Patterns

Alteneder, R. & Hartzekk, D. (1999). Addressing couples' sexuality concerns during the childbearing period: Use of the PLISSIT model. *Journal of Obstetric, Gynecologic, and Neonatal Nursing, 26*(6), 651–658.

Annon, J. S. (1976). The PLISS + model: A proposed conceptual scheme for the behavioral treatment of sexual problems. *Journal of Sex Education and Therapy, 2,* 211–215.

Barclay, L., Donoron, J., & Genovese, A. (1996). Men's experiences during their partner's first pregnancy: A grounded theory analysis. *Australian Journal of Advanced Nursing, 13*(3), 12–24.

Donoran, J. (1995). The process of analysis during a grounded theory study of men during their partners' pregnancies. *Australian Journal of Advanced Nursing, 21*(4), 708–715.

Gilbert, E., & Harmon, J. (1998). *Manual of high risk pregnancy and delivery* (2nd ed.). St. Louis: Mosby-Year Book.

Gray, J. (1995). *Mars and Venus in the bedroom: A guide to lasting romance and passion.* New York: HarperCollins.

Horn, B. (1993). Cultural beliefs and teenage pregnancy. *Nurse Practitioner, 8*(8), 35, 39, 74.

Katzun, L. (1990). Chronic illness and sexuality. *American Journal of Nursing, 90,* 57–59.

Polomeno, V. (1999). Sex and babies: Pregnant couples' postnatal sexual concerns. *Journal of Prenatal Education, 8*(4), 9–18.

Smith, M. (1993). Pediatric sexuality: Promoting normal sexual development in children. *Nurse Practitioner, 18,* 37–44.

Waterhouse, J. (1993). Discussing sexual concerns with health care professionals. *Journal of Holistic Nursing, 11*, 125–134.

Waterhouse, J., & Metcalfe, M. (1991). Attitudes toward nurses discussing sexual concerns with patients. *Journal of Advanced Nursing, 16*, 1048–1054.

Wilmoth, M. C. (1993). Development and testing of the sexual behaviors questionnaire. *Dissertation Abstracts International, 54*, 6137B–6138B.

Wilmoth, M. C. (1994a). Strategies for becoming comfortable with sexual assessment. *Oncology Nursing News, 12*(2), 6–7.

Wilmoth, M. C. (1994b). Nurses' and patients' perspectives on sexuality: Bridging the gap. *Innovations in Oncology Nursing, 10*, 34–36.

## Disturbed Sleep Pattern

Blissit, P. (2001). Sleep, memory and learning. *Journal of Neurosurgical Nursing, 33*(4), 208–215.

Cureton-Lane, R. A., & Fontaine, D. K. (1997). Sleep in pediatric ICU. *American Journal of Critical Care, 6*(1), 56–63.

Dines-Kalinowski, C. M. (2000). Dream weaver. *Nursing Management, 33*(4), 48–49.

Hammer, B. (1991). Sleep pattern disturbance. In M. Maas, K. Buckwalter, & M. Hardy (Eds.), *Nursing diagnoses and interventions for the elderly*. Redwood City, CA: Addison-Wesley Nursing.

Hayashi, Y., & Endo, S. (1982). All-night sleep polygraphic recordings of healthy aged persons: REM and slow-wave sleep. *Sleep, 5*, 277–283.

Landis, C., & Moe, K. (2004). Sleep and menopause. *Nursing Clinics of North America, 39*(1), 97–115.

Larkin, V., & Butler, M. (2000). The implications of rest and sleep following childbirth. *British Journal of Midwifery, 8*(7), 438–442.

## Impaired Social Interaction

Johnson, B.S.(1995) *Child, adolescent and family psychiatric nursing*. Philadelphia: J. B. Lippincott

Maroni, J. (1989). Impaired social interactions. In G. McFarland, & E. McFarlane (Eds.), *Nursing diagnosis and interventions*. St. Louis: C. V. Mosby.

McFarland, G., Wasli, E., & Gerety, E. (1996). *Nursing diagnoses and process in psychiatric mental health nursing* (5th ed.). Philadelphia: J. B. Lippincott.

## Chronic Sorrow

Burke, M. L., Hainsworth, M. A., Eakes, G. G., & Lindgren, C. L. (1992). Current knowledge and research on chronic sorrow: A foundation for inquiry. *Death Studies, 16*(3), 231–245.

Eakes, G. G., Burke, M. L., & Hainsworth, M. A. (1998). Middle-range theory of chronic sorrow. *Image: Journal of Nursing Scholarship, 30*, 179.

Eakes, G. G. (1995). Chronic sorrow: The lived experience of parents of chronically mentally ill individuals. *Archives of Psychiatric Nursing, 9*(2), 77–84.

Gamino, L. A., Hogan, N. S., & Sewell, K. W. (2002). Feeling the absence: A content analysis from the Scott and White grief study. *Death Studies, 26*(10), 793.

Kearney, P. M., & Griffin, T. (2001). Between joy and sorrow: Being a parent of a child with developmental disability. *Journal of Advanced Nursing, 34*(5), 582–592.

Lindgren, C. L., Burke, M. L., Hainsworth, M. A., & Eakes, G. G. (1992). Chronic sorrow: A lifespan concept. *Scholarly Inquiry for Nursing Practice, 24*(6), 27–42.

Mallow, G. E., & Bechtel, G. (1999). Chronic sorrow: The experience of parents with children who are developmentally disabled. *Journal of Psychosocial Nursing, 37*(7), 31–35.

Melnyk, B., Feinstein, N., Moldenhouer, Z., & Small, L. (2001). Coping of parents of children who are chronically ill. *Pediatric Nursing, 27*(6), 548–558.

Monsen, R. B. (1999). Mothers' experiences of living worried when parenting children with spina bifida. *Journal of Pediatric Nursing, 14*(3), 157–163.

Northington, L. (2000). Chronic sorrow in caregivers of school age children with sickle cell disease: A grounded theory approach. *Issues in Comprehensive Pediatric Nursing, 23*(3), 141–154.

Teel, C. (1991). Chronic sorrow: Analysis of the concept. *Journal of Advanced Nursing, 16*(11), 1311–1319.

## Spiritual Distress

Bearon, L., & Koenig, H. (1990). Religious cognitions and use of prayer in health and illness. *The Gerontologist, 30*, 249–253.

Brennan, M.R. (1994). *Spirituality in the homebound elderly*. Doctoral dissertation, The Catholic University of America. Ann Arbor, MI: UMI.

Burkhart, L., & Solari-Twadell, A. (2001). Spirituality and religiousness: Differentiating the diagnoses through a review of the nursing diagnosis. *12*(2), 44–54.

Burkhart, M. A. (1994). Becoming and connecting: Elements of spirituality for women. *Holistic Nursing Practice, 8*, 12–21.

Cameron, M. E. (1998). Clinical sidebar. *Image, 30*(3), 275–280.

Carson, V. B. (1999). *Mental health nursing: The nurse-patient journey* (2nd ed.). Philadelphia: W. B. Saunders.

Carson, V. B., & Green, H. (1992). Spiritual well-being: A predictor of hardiness in patients with acquired immunodeficiency syndrome. *Journal of Professional Nursing, 8*, 209–220.

Corbett, K. (1998). Patterns of spirituality in persons with advanced HIV disease. *Research in Nursing and Health, 21*(2), 143–153.

Emblen, J. D., & Halstead, L. (1993). Spiritual needs and interventions: Comparing the views of patients, nurses and chaplains. *Clinical Nurse Specialist, 7*, 175–182.

Fowler, J. W. (1981). *Stages of faith development*. New York: HarperCollins.

Halstead, H. L. (1995). Spirituality in the elderly. In M. Stanley & P. G. Beare (Eds.), *Gerontological nursing* (pp. 415–425). Philadelphia: F. A. Davis.

Hinton, J. (1999). The progress of awareness and acceptance of dying assessed in cancer patients and their caring relatives. *Palliative Medicine, 13*(1), 19–35.

Kemp, C. (2001). Spiritual care interventions. In B. Ferrell & N. Coyle (Eds.), *Textbook of palliative nursing* (pp. 440–455). New York: Oxford.

Kendrick, K. D., & Robinson, S. (2000). Spirituality: Its relevance and purpose for clinical nursing in the new millennium. *Journal of Clinical Nursing, 9*(5), 701–705.

Millison, M. B. (1995). A review of the research on spiritual care and hospice. *The Hospice Journal, 10*, 3–17.

Mindel, C. H., & Vaughan, C. E. (1978). A multidimensional approach to religiosity and disengagement. *Journal of Gerontology, 33*, 103–108.

Moberg, D. O. (1984). Subjective measures of spiritual well-being. *Review of Religious Research, 25*, 351–364.

O'Brien, M.E. (2003). *Spirituality in nursing: Standing on holy ground* (2nd ed.). Boston: Jones and Bartlett.

Piles, C. L. (1990). Providing spiritual care. *Nurse Educator, 15*(1), 36–41.

Quintero, C. (1993). Blood administration in pediatric Jehovah's Witness. *Pediatric Nursing, 19*(1), 46–48.

Ryan, E. (1985). Selecting an instrument to measure spiritual distress. *Oncology Nursing Forum, 12*(2), 93–94, 99.

Ryan, M. C., & Patterson, J. (1987). Loneliness in the elderly. *Journal of Gerontological Nursing, 13*(5), 6–12.

Seymour, R. E. (1995). *Aging without apology: Living the senior years with integrity and faith*. Valley Forge, PA: Judson Press.

Sodestrom, K. E., & Martinson, I..M. (1987). Patients' spiritual coping strategies: A study of nurse and patient perspectives. *Oncology Nursing Forum, 14*(2), 41–46.

Stoll, R. I. (1984). Spiritual assessment: A nursing perspective. In R. Fehring (Ed.). *Proceedings of the conference on spirituality*. Milwaukee: Marquette University.

Taylor, E. Spiritual assessment. In B. Ferrell & N. Coyle (Eds.), *Textbook of palliative nursing* (pp. 397–406). New York: Oxford.

Wald, F. S., & Bailey, C. (1990). Nurturing the spiritual component in care for the terminally ill. *CARING Magazine, 9*(11), 64–68.

## Stress Overload

Bodenheimer, T., MacGregor, K., & Sharifi, C. (2005). Helping patients manage their chronic conditions. Retrieved January 10, 2007 from www.chef.org/publications.

Ridner, S.H. (2004). Psychological distress: Concept analysis. *Journal of Advanced Nursing, 45*(5): 536-45.

## Risk for Sudden Infant Death Syndrome

American Academy of Pediatrics. (2000). Task force on infant sleep position and Sudden Infant Death Syndrome: Changing concepts of

Sudden Infant Death Syndrome; Implications for infants' sleeping environment and sleep position. *Pediatrics, 105*(3), 650–656.

Anderson, J. E. (2000). Co-sleeping: Can we ever put the issue to rest? *Contemporary Pediatrics, 17*(6), 98–102, 109–110, 113–114.

Kliegman, R. M., Jensen, H. B., & Behrman, R. E. (2007). *Nelson textbook of pediatrics* (18th ed.). Philadelphia: W. B. Saunders.

Moon, R. Y. (2001). Are you talking to parents about SIDS? *Contemporary Pediatrics, 18*(3), 122–131.

Poyser, K. (2000). Cot death: Reducing the risk and reaching out to the public. *Community Practice, 73*(12), 878–880.

Sherratt, S. (1999). The pros & cons of movement monitors. *British Journal of Midwifery, 7*(9), 569–572.

### Disturbed Thought Processes

Baker, P. (1995). Accepting the inner voices. *Nursing Times, 91*(31), 59–61.

Maier-Lorentz, M. (2000). Effective nursing interventions for the management of Alzheimer's disease. *Journal of Neuroscience Nursing, 32*(3), 153–157.

### Ineffective Tissue Perfusion

Burch, K., Todd, K., Crosby, F., Ventura, M., Lohr, G., & Grace, M. L. (1991). PVD: Nurse patient interventions. *Journal of Vascular Nursing, 9*(4), 13–16.

Sieggreen, M. (1987). Healing of physical wounds. *Nursing Clinics of North America, 22,* 439–448.

Sieggreen, M. (1999). Assessment of clients with vascular disorders. In S. Black, P. Hawkes, & A. Keene (Eds.). *Medical surgical nursing* (6th ed.). Philadelphia: W. B. Saunders.

### Unilateral Neglect

Kalbach, L. R. (1991). Unilateral neglect: Mechanisms and nursing care. *Journal of Neuroscience Nursing, 23*(2), 125–129.

Lin, K. (1996). Right-hemispheric activation approaches to neglect rehabilitation post stroke. *American Journal of Occupational Therapy, 50*(7), 504–514.

Mitchell, P. H., Hodges, L. C., Muwaswes, M., & Walleck, C. A. (1992). *AANN's neuroscience nursing* (2nd ed.). Norwalk, CT: Appleton & Lange.

### Impaired Urinary Elimination

Ball, J., & Bindler, R. (2008). *Pediatric Nursing: Caring for Children* (4th ed.). Upper Saddle River, NJ: Pearson Prentice Hall.

Carpenter, R. O. (1999). Disorders of elimination. In J. McMillan, C. D. DeAngelis, R. Feigin, & J. B. Warshaw (Eds.), *Oski's pediatrics: Principles and practice* (3rd ed.). Philadelphia: Lippincott Williams & Wilkins.

Dougherty, M. (1998). Current status of research on pelvic muscles strengthening techniques. *Journal of Wound, Ostomy and Continence, 25*(3), 75–83.

Fanti, J. A., Newman, D. K., & Colling, J. (1996). *Urinary incontinence in adults: Acute and chronic management, Clinical practice guidelines No. 2.* Rockville, MD: U.S. Department of Health and Human Services.

Kelleher, R. (1997). Daytime and nighttime wetting in children: A review of management. *Journal of the Society of Pediatric Nurses, 2*(2), 73–82.

Longstaffe, S., Mofatt, M., & Whalen, J. C. (2000). Behavioral and self-concept changes after six months of enuresis treatment: A randomized controlled trial. *Pediatrics,* 105 Supplement, 935–940.

Macauley, M., Pettersen, L., Fader, M., Brooks, R., & Cottenden, A. (2004). A multicenter evaluation of absorbent products for children with incontinence and disabilities. *Journal of WOCH, 31*(4), 235–244.

Morison, M. (1998). Family attitudes to bed-wetting and their influence on treatment. *Professional Nurse, 13*(5), 321–325.

Perrin, L., Dauphinee, S. W., Corcos, S.W., Hanley, J. A., & Kuchel, G. A. (2005). Pelvic floor muscle training with biofeedback and bladder training in elderly women. *Journal of Wound, Ostomy and Continence Care, 32*(3), 186-199.

Resnik, N. M., & Yalla, S. V. (1985). Geriatiric incontinence and voiding dysfunction. In W. C. Walsh (Ed.), *Campbell's urology* (pp.1218-1223). Philadelphia: W. B. Saunders.

Sampselle, C., & DeLancey, J. (1998). Anatomy of female continence. *Journal of Wound, Ostomy and Continence Nursing, 25*(3), 63–74.

Scardillo, J., & Aronovitch, S. A. (1999). Successfully managing incontinence-related irritant dermatitis across the lifespan. *Ostomy Wound Management, 45*(4), 36–44.

Steeman, E., & Defever, M. (1998). Urinary Incontinence among elderly pesons who live at home. *Nursing Clinics of North America, 33*(4), 25-32.

Wilkinson, J., & Van Leuven, K. (2007). *Fundamentals of nursing: Theory, concepts & applications.* Philadelphia: F. A. Davis Company.

### Risk for Violence

Carson, V. B., & Alvarez, C. (2006). Anger and aggression. In E. M. Varcarolis, V. B. Carson, & N. C. Shoemaker (Eds.), *Foundations of psychiatric–mental health nursing* (5th ed.). Philadelphia: W. B. Saunders.

Davies, W. H., & Flannery, D. (1998). Post-traumatic stress disorder in children and adolescents exposed to violence. *Pediatric Clinics of North America, 45*(2), 341–353.

Dowd, M. D. (1998). Consequences of violence. *Pediatric Clinics of North America, 45*(2), 333–339.

Edari, R., & McManus, P. (1998). Risk and resiliency factors for violence. *Pediatric Clinics of North America, 45*(2), 293–303.

Farrell, S., Harmon, R., & Hastings, S. (1998). Nursing management of acute psychotic episodes. *Nursing Clinics of North America, 33*(1), 187–200.

Norris, M., & Kennedy, C. (1992). How patients perceive the seclusion process. *Journal of Psychosocial Nursing.* 23(6), 7-13

Veenema, G. (2001). Children's exposure to community violence. *Journal of Nursing Scholarship, 33*(2), 167–173.

Willis, E., & Strasburger, V. (1998). Media violence. *Pediatric Clinics of North America, 45*(2), 319–331.

### Wandering

Algase, D. L. (1999). Wandering in dementia. *Annual Review in Nursing Research, 17*(2), 185–217.

Altus, D. E., Mathews, R. M., Xaverius, P. K., Engelman, K. K., & Nolan B. D. (2000). Evaluation of an electronic monitoring system for people who wander. *American Journal of Alzheimer's Disease, 15*(2), 121–125.

Brown, J. B., Bedford, N. K., & White, S. J. (1999). *Gerontological protocols for nurse practitioners.* Philadelphia: Lippincott Williams & Wilkins.

Cohen-Mansfield, J. (1998). The effects of an enhanced environment on nursing home residents who pace. *Gerontologist, 38*(2), 199–208.

Logsdon, R. G., McCurry, T. L., Gibbons, L. E., Kukuli, W. A., & Larson, E. B. (1998). Wandering: A significant problem among community-residing individuals with Alzheimer's disease. *Journal of Gerontological Behavioral, Psychological and Social Science, 53B*(5), 294–299.

Maier-Lorentz, M. M. (2000). Effective nursing interventions for the management of Alzheimer's disease. *Journal of Neuroscience Nursing, 32*(2), 117–125.

Meiner, S. E. (2000). Wandering problems need ongoing nursing planning: A case study. *Geriatric Nursing.* 21(2), 101–106.

Pack, R. (2000). The "ins and outs" of wandering. *Nursing Homes, 49*(8), 55–59.

## Part Three: Community

### Contamination

Ashford, D. A., Kaiser, R. M., Bales, M. E., Shutt, K. Patrawalla, A., McShan, A., Tappero, J. W., Perkins, B. A., & Dannenberg, A. L. (2003). Planning against biological terrorism: Lessons from outbreak investigations. *Emerging Infectious Diseases,* [serial online] 2003 May. Retrieved August 1, 2008 from www.cdc.gov/ncidod/EID/vol9no5/02-0388.htm.

Berkowitz, G. S., Obel, J., Deych, E., Lapinski, R., Godbold, J., & Liu, Z. (2003). Exposure to indoor pesticides during pregnancy in a multiethnic, urban cohort. *Environmental Health Perspectives, 111*(1), 79-84.

Children's Environmental Health Network. (2004). Resource guide on children's environmental health. Retrieved August 1, 2008 from www.cehn.org.

Centers for Disease Control and Prevention. Air pollution and respiratory health. Retrieved August 1, 2008 from www.cdc.gov.nceh/airpollution/about.htm.

Centers for Disease Control and Prevention. Emergency preparedness & response. Retrieved August 1, 2008 from www.bt.cdc.gov.agent.

Environmental Protection Agency. (2008). A citizen's guide to radon: The guide to protecting yourself and your family from radon. Pub # EPA 402-K-02-006. Retrieved August 1, 2008 from www.epa.gov/iaq/radon/pubs/citguide.html.

Environmental Protection Agency. (2008). Hazardous waste. Retrieved August 12, 2008 from www.epa.gov/osw/hazwaste.htm.

Environmental Protection Agency. (2006). National Pesticide Program FY Annual Report 2006. Retrieved August 12, 2008 from www.epa.gov/oppfead1/annual/2006/06annual-rpt.pdf.

Environmental Protection Agency. (2004). Understanding radiation health effects. Retrieved August 12, 2008 from www.epa.gov/radiation/understand/health_effects.html.

ExtoxNet. (1997). Contamination of water and soil by sewage and water treatment sludge. Retrieved August 12, 2008 from www.extoxnet.orst.edu/faqs.

International Council of Nurses. Terrorism and bioterrorism: Nursing preparedness. Nursing Matters Fact Sheet. Retrieved August 1, 2008 from www.icn.ch/matters_bio.htm.

National Resources Defense Council. Sewage pollution threatens public health. Retrieved August 12, 2008 from www.nrdc.org/water/pollution/sewage.asp.

Siegel, J.D., Rhinehart, E., Jackson, M., Chiarello, L., & the Healthcare Infection Control Practices Advisory Committee. 2007 guideline for isolation precautions: Preventing transmission of infectious agents in healthcare settings, June 2007. Retrieved August 12, 2008 from www.cdc.gov/ncidod/dhqp/pdf/isolation2007.pdf.

U.S. Army Medical Research Institute of Infectious Diseases. (2004). *USAMRIID's medical management of biological casualties handbook* (6th ed.). Frederick, MD: Author.

U.S. Department of Labor. *Safety and health topics: Biological agents.* Retrieved August 12, 2008 from www.osha.gov/SLTC/biologicalagents/index.html.

Veenema, T., & Toke, J. (2006). Early detection and surveillance for biopreparedness and emerging infectious diseases. *Online Journal of Issues in Nursing, 11*(1). Retrieved August 1, 2008 from www.nursingworld.org/MainMenuCategories/ANAMarketplace/ANAPeriodicals/OJIN.aspx.

Veenema, T. G. (2002). Chemical and biological terrorism: Current updates for nurse educators. *Nursing Education Perspectives, 23*(2), 62-71.

Veenema, T. G. (2003). *Disaster nursing and emergency preparedness for chemical, biological and radiological terrorism and other hazards.* New York: Springer.

World Health Organization. (2005). Indoor air pollution and health. Fact sheet #292. Retrieved August 12, 2008 from www.who.int/mediacentre/factsheets/fs292/en/.

## Part Four: Health Promotion And Wellness

Bodenheimer, T., MacGregor, K., & Sharifi, C. (2005). Helping patients manage their chronic conditions. Retrieved January 10, 2007 from www.chef.org/publications.

Butler, C., Rollnick, S., Cohen, D., et al. (1999). Motivational consulting versus brief advice for smokers in general practice: A randomized trial. *British Journal of General Practice, 49,* 611–616.

Cutilli, C. C. (2005). Health literacy? What you need to know. *Orthopaedic Nursing, 24*(3), 227–231.

Kalichman, S. C., Cain, D., Fuhel, A., et al. (2005). Assessing medication adherence self-efficacy among low-literacy patients: Development of a pictographic visual analogue scale. *Health Education Research, 20*(1), 24–35.

Murphy, S. A. (1993). Coping strategies of abstainers from alcohol up to three years post-treatment. *Image: Journal of Nursing Scholarship, 25*(2), 87.

Piette, J. D. (2005). Using telephone support to manage chronic disease. California Healthcare Foundation. Retrieved January 6, 2007 from www.chef.org/topics/chronicdisease/index.cfm.

Rollnick, S., Mason, P., & Butler, C. (2000). *Health behavior change: A guide for practitioners.* Edinburgh: Churchill Livingstone.

## Section Three: Collaborative Problems

Altizer, L. (November 2004). Compartment syndrome. *Orthopaedic Nursing, 23*(6), 391-396.

American College of Obstetricians and Gynecologists. (2002). *Diagnosis and management of preeclampsia and eclampsia.* Practice Bulletin #33. Washington, DC: Author.

American College of Obstetricians and Gynecologists. (2003). *Management of preterm labor.* Practice Bulletin #43, July. Washington, DC: Author.

American College of Obstetricians and Gynecologists. (2005). *Intrapartum fetal heart rate monitoring.* Practice Bulletin #70, December. Washington, DC: Author.

American College of Obstetricians and Gynecologists (2006). *Postpartum hemorrhage.* Practice Bulletin #76, Washington, DC: Author.

Arcangelo, V., & Peters, J. (2001). *Pharmacology for nurse practitioners.* Philadelphia: Lippincott Williams & Wilkins.

Baird, M. S., Keen, J. H., & Swearingen, P. L. (2005). *Manual of critical care nursing: Nursing interventions and collaborative management* (5th ed.). St Louis, Missouri: Elsevier Mosby.

Bhardwaj, A., Mirski, M. A., & Ulatowski, J. A. (2004). *Handbook of neurocritical care.* Totowa, New Jersey: Humana Press.

Bridges, E. J., & Dukes, M. S. (2005). Cardiovascular aspects of septic shock: Pathophysiology, monitoring, and treatment. *Critical Care Nurse, 25*(2), 14-42.

Byrne, B. (2002). Deep vein thrombosis prophylaxis. *Journal of Vascular Nursing, 20*(2), 53–59.

Clarke-Pearson, D. L., Dodge, R. K., Synan, I., McClelland, R. C., & Maxwell, G. L. (2003). Venous thromboembolism prohylaxis: Patients at high risk to fail intermittent pneumatic compression. *Obstetrics & Gynecology, 101,* 157-163.

Cukierman, T., Gatt, M. E., Hiller, N., & Chajek-Shaul, T. (2005). A fracture diagnosis. *New England Journal of Medicine, 353,* 509-514.

de Feiter, P., van Hooft, M. A. A., Beets-Tan, R. G., & Brink, P. R. G. (2007). Fat embolism syndrome: Yes or no? *The Journal of TRAUMA Injury, Infection, and Critical Care, 63*(2), 429-431.

Deglin, J. H., & Vallerand, A. H. (2007). *Davis's drug guide for nurses* (10th ed.). Philadelphia: F. A. Davis Company.

Esche, C. A. (2005). Resiliency: a factor to consider when facilitating the transition from hospital to home in older adults. *Geriatric Nursing, 26* (4), 218-222.

Ellstrom, K. (2006). The pulmonary system. In J. Grif-Alspach (Ed.), *Core curriculum for critical care nursing* (6th ed., pp. 45-183). St. Louis: Saunders-Elsevier.

Feinstein, N., Torgerson, K.L., & Atterbury, J. (Eds.). (2003). *Fetal Heart Monitoring Principles & Practices* (3rd ed.). Dubuque, IA: Kendall-Hunt.

Fetterman, L. G., & Lemburg, L. (2004). A silent killer—Often preventable. *American Journal of Critical Care, 13*(5), 431-436.

Gilbert, E.S. (2007). *Manual of High Risk Pregnancy & Delivery* (4th ed.). St. Louis: Mosby.

Harris, I., Kadir, A., & Donald, G. (2006). Continuous compartment pressure monitoring for tibia fractures: Does it influence outcome? *The Journal of TRAUMA Injury, Infection, and Critical Care, 60*(6), 1330-1335.

Hickey, J. V. (2006). *The clinical practice of neurological and neurosurgical nursing* (5th ed.). Philadelphia: Lippincott Williams & Wilkins.

Kakar, S., Firoozabadi, R., McKean, J., & Tornetta, P. (2007). Diastolic blood pressure in patients with tibia fractures under anesthesia: Implications for the diagnosis of compartment syndrome. *Journal of Orthopedic Trauma, 21,* 99-103.

Kee, J. L. (2004). *Handbook of laboratory & diagnostic tests with nursing implications* (5th ed.). New Jersey: Pearson Education, Prentice Hall.

Kitabchi, A. E., Haerian, H., & Rose, B. D. (2008). *Treatment of diabetic ketoacidosis and hyperosmolar hyperglycemic state.* Retrieved November 14, 2008, from www.UpToDate.com.

Lehne, R. A. (2004). *Pharmacology for nursing care* (5th ed.). St Louis: W. B. Saunders.

Lewis, S. M., Heitkemper, M. M., Dirksen, S. R., O'Brien, P. G., Giddens, J. F., & Bucher, L. (2004). *Medical-Surgical Nursing: Assessment and management of clinical problems* (6th ed.). St Louis: Mosby.

Lynn-McHale Wiegand, D. J., & Carlson, K. K. (2005). *AACN procedure manual for critical care.* St. Louis, Missouri: Elsevier.

Mandeville, L. K., & Troiano, N. H. (2002). *High-risk & critical care intrapartum nursing* (2nd ed.). Philadelphia: Lippincott.

Mattson, S., & Smith, J. E. (2004). *Core curriculum for maternal-newborn nursing* (3rd ed.). St. Louis: Elsevier Saunders.

Meyer, N., Pennington, W. T., Dewitt, D., & Schmeling, G. (2007). Isolated cerebral fat emboli syndrome in multiply injured patients: A review of three cases and the literature. *The Journal of TRAUMA Injury, Infection, and Critical Care, 63*(6), 1395-1402.

Miller, N. C., & Askew, A. E. (2007). Tibia fractures: An overview of evaluation and treatment. *Orthopaedic Nursing, 26*(4), 216-223.

Newcombe, P. (2002). Pathophysiology of sickle cell disease crisis. *Emergency Nurse, 9*(9), 9–22.

Nucifora, G., Hysko, F., Vit, A., & Vasciaveo, A. (2007). Pulmonary fat embolism: Common and unusual computed tomography findings. *Journal of Computer Assisted Tomography, 31*(5), 806-807.

Rausch, M., & Pollard, D. (1998). Management of the patient with sickle cell disease. *Journal of Intravenous Nursing, 21*(1), 27–40.

Redemann, S. (2002). Modalities for immobilization. In A. B. Maher, S. W. Salmond, & T. A. Pellino (Eds.), *Orthopedic nursing* (3rd ed., p. 303). Philadelphia: W. B. Saunders.

Sahjian, M., & Frakes, M. (2007). Crush injuries: Pathophysiology and current treatment. *The Nurse Practitioner: The American Journal of Primary Health Care, 32*(9), 13-18.

Sanofi-Aventis. (2007). Lovenox. Retrieved December 20, 2007 from http://products.sanofi-aventis.us/lovenox/lovenox.html.

Schiff, R. L., Kahn, S. R., Shrier, I., Strulovitch, C., Hammouda, W., Cohen, E., et al. (2005). Identifying othapedic patients at high risk for venous thromboembolism despite thromboprophylaxis. *Chest, 128*, 3364-3371.

Shaughnessy, K. (2007). Massive pulmonary embolism. *Critical Care Nurse, 27(1), 39-51.*

Simpson, K. R., & Creehan, P. A. (2007). *AWHONN's perinatal nursing* (3rd ed.). Philadelphia: Lippincott Williams & Wilkins.

Tinetti, M. E. (2003). Preventing falls in the elderly person. *New England Journal of Medicine, 348*, 42-49.

Titler, M., Dochterman, J., Xie, X., Kanak, M., Fei, Q., Picone, D., et al. (2006). Nursing interventions and other factors associated with discharge disposition in elders patients after hip surgery. *Nursing Research,* 55 (4), 231-242.

Tumbarello, C. (2000). Acute extremity compartmental syndrome. *Journal of Trauma Nursing,* 7(2), 30–36.

Walker-Bone, K., Walter, G., & Cooper, C. (2002). Recent developments in the epidemiology of osteoporosis. *Current Opinion in Rheumatology, 14*(4), 411-415.

Wong, M., Tsui, H., Yung, S., Chan, K., & Cheng, J. (2004). Continuous pulse oximeter monitoring for inapparent hypoxemia after long bone fractures. *The Journal of TRAUMA Injury, Infection, and Critical Care, 56*(2), 356-362.

# Index

*Note:* Page numbers followed by *b*, *f* and *t* indicate boxes, figures and tables, respectively. Nursing diagnoses are indicated by initial capitals.

## A

AA (Alcoholics Anonymous), 216
AAP (American Academy of Pediatrics), 651
Abbreviated grief, 293
Abruptio placentae, 922
Absent grief, 293
Abstinence, in substance abuse, 217
Abuse. *See also* Other-Directed Violence, Risk for
  alcohol, 204, 213, *588t*, 719–720, 723
  child, 722, 730–733
  defined, 714
  domestic, 701, 715–718, 727–729, 733
  elder, 451, 718
  Ineffective Coping, 205
  self, 561, 571–573
  sexual, 549
  substance, 213, 215–217, 539
Accessory to sex, 450
Accidents. *See* Injury, Risk for
Ace bandages, 397
Acetate anion, 896
Acetone, 867
Acetylcholine, 169
Achieved decision, 45
Acid–base imbalance, 861
Acidosis
  overview, 895–896
  Risk for Complications of, 880–882
Acquaintance rape, 451
Acquired immunodeficiency
  syndrome (AIDS). *See* Human
  immunodeficiency virus
ACS (acute coronary syndrome), 847
Acting-out behavior, in Anxiety, 75
Action stage, Stages of Change Model, 581
Activated partial thromboplastin time (APTT), 932
Active assistive ROM, 392
Active listening, 748
Active resistive ROM, 392
Active ROM, 392
Activities of daily living (ADLs), 519
Activity
  Anxiety, 81
  assessing physiology response to, *63t*
  Constipation, 186

effects on peristalsis, 104
Falls, Risk for, 369
Grieving, 287–288
Hopelessness, 316–317
Hyperthermia, 95
Imbalanced Nutrition: More than Body
  Requirements, 442
Ineffective Health Maintenance,
  796–797
Ineffective Health Maintenance,
  Related to Increased Food
  Consumption in Response to
  Stressors and Insufficient Energy
  Expenditure for Intake, 805–809
Sedentary Lifestyle, 815–817
Activity Intolerance, 60–65
  defining characteristics of, 60
  definition of, 60
  focus assessment criteria, 63–64
  goals of interventions for, 64
  interventions for, 64–65
  related factors in, 60–62
  Related to Insufficient Knowledge
    of Adaptive Techniques Needed
    Secondary to COPD, 66–69
  Related to Insufficient Knowledge
    of Adaptive Techniques Needed
    Secondary to Impaired Cardiac
    Function, 69–71
Activity Planning, Ineffective, 71–72
Activity–exercise pattern
  community nursing diagnoses, 770
  functional health patterns, *32b*
  Health-Seeking Behaviors, 787
Activity/Rest domain, *11t*
Actual nursing diagnoses, 13–14, 41
Acupressure, 151
Acupuncture, 151
Acute chest syndrome, 890
Acute Confusion. *See* Confusion, Acute
Acute coronary syndrome (ACS), 847
Acute diarrhea. *See* Diarrhea
Acute Pain. *See* Pain, Acute
Acute tiredness, 254
Acute Urinary Retention, Risk for
  Complications of, 892–893
AD. *See* Autonomic Dysreflexia
ADA (Americans with Disabilities Act) of
  1990, 160
Adaptive coping mechanisms, 75
Addendum care plans, 49

Addiction
  defined, 133
  versus drug tolerance, 136
Addiction risk, 133
Adequate perfusion, 497
ADH (antidiuretic hormone), 867
ADLs (activities of daily living), 519
Adolescents
  age-related conditions, prevention of,
    *792t*
  daily nutritional requirements, *417t*
  Delayed Growth and Development, 300
  Disturbed Self-Esteem, 553
  Fatigue, 254
  Fear, 261–262
  Hopelessness, 310
  Impaired Comfort, 129
  Impaired Parenting, 747
  Impaired Social Interaction, 613
  Ineffective Coping, 200
  Ineffective Health Maintenance, 790
  Ineffective Sexuality Patterns, 587,
    592–593
  Infection, Risk for, 331
  Injury, Risk for, 361–362
  Other-Directed Violence, Risk for, 703
  Parent–Infant Attachment, Impaired,
    Risk for, 751
  Powerlessness, 457
  Rape Trauma Syndrome, 451–452
  Relocation Stress Syndrome, 486
  Self-Harm, Risk for, 561
Adrenocorticosteroid Therapy Adverse
  Effects, Risk for Complications of,
  935–937
Adults
  daily nutritional requirements, *417t*
  Disturbed Sleep Pattern, 603–605
  Fear, 261
  Hopelessness, 310
  Imbalanced Nutrition: More than Body
    Requirements, 440
  Impaired Social Interaction, 613
  Ineffective Health Maintenance, 790
  Ineffective Sexuality Patterns, 587
  Rape Trauma Syndrome, 451–452
Advanced practice, 5
Advent Christian Church (Seventh-Day
  Adventist), religious beliefs of,
  *632b–633b*
AFI (amniotic fluid index) studies, 925

**983**